Textbook of Oral and Maxillofacial Surgery

Third Edition

Edited by

Prof. Dr. Neelima Anil Malik BDS, MDS (Bom), FIAOS

Principal, Professor and Head
Department of Oral and Maxillofacial Surgery
Krishna Institute of Medical Sciences Deemed University's
School of Dental Sciences and Hospital
Karad, Dist. Satara, Maharashtra, India
Former Dean
Nair Hospital Dental College, Mumbai, Maharashtra, India
Former Professor and Head and Professor Emeritus
Department of Oral and Maxillofacial Surgery
Nair Hospital Dental College (NHDC)
Mumbai, Maharashtra, India
Former Recognized Undergraduate and Postgraduate Teacher of
University of Mumbai and
Maharashtra University of Health Sciences
Former Honorary Advisor and Consultant
Armed Forces Medical College (Dental Faculty)
Pune, Maharashtra, India
First Lady President of Association of
Oral and Maxillofacial Surgeons of India, 2003
Gold and Silver Medalist
Nair Hospital Dental College (NHDC), Bombay University
Recipient of Mumbai Mayor's Award, 2006
Recipient of Outstanding Teacher Award, 2011
Award given by Bitein—Premier Indian Dental Portal

Foreword

SG Damle

JAYPEE BROTHERS MEDICAL PUBLISHERS (P) LTD.

New Delhi • Panama City • London • Dhaka • Kathmandu

Jaypee Brothers Medical Publishers (P) Ltd.

Headquarters

Jaypee Brothers Medical Publishers (P) Ltd.
4838/24, Ansari Road, Daryaganj
New Delhi 110 002, India
Phone: +91-11-43574357
Fax: +91-11-43574314
Email: jaypee@jaypeebrothers.com

Overseas Offices

J.P. Medical Ltd.
83, Victoria Street, London
SW1H 0HW (UK)
Phone: +44-2031708910
Fax: +02-03-0086180
Email: info@jpmedpub.com

Jaypee-Highlights Medical Publishers Inc.
City of Knowledge, Bld. 237, Clayton
Panama City, Panama
Phone: + 507-301-0496
Fax: + 507- 301-0499
Email: cservice@jphmedical.com

Jaypee Brothers Medical Publishers (P) Ltd
17/1-B Babar Road, Block-B, Shaymali
Mohammadpur, Dhaka-1207
Bangladesh
Mobile: +08801912003485
Email: jaypeedhaka@gmail.com

Jaypee Brothers Medical Publishers (P) Ltd
Shorakhute, Kathmandu
Nepal
Phone: +00977-9841528578
Email: jaypee.nepal@gmail.com

Website: www.jaypeebrothers.com
Website: www.jaypeedigital.com

© 2012, Jaypee Brothers Medical Publishers

Inquiries for bulk sales may be solicited at: jaypee@jaypeebrothers.com

This book has been published in good faith that the contents provided by the contributors contained herein are original, and is intended for educational purposes only. While every effort is made to ensure accuracy of information, the publisher and the editor specifically disclaim any damage, liability, or loss incurred, directly or indirectly, from the use or application of any of the contents of this work. If not specifically stated, all figures and tables are courtesy of the editor. Where appropriate, the readers should consult with a specialist or contact the manufacturer of the drug or device.

Textbook of Oral and Maxillofacial Surgery

First Edition: 2002

Reprint: 2005

Second Edition: 2008

Reprint: 2010

Third Edition: **2012**

ISBN 978-93-5025-938-2

Printed at: Ajanta Offset & Packagings Ltd., New Delhi

Dedicated to

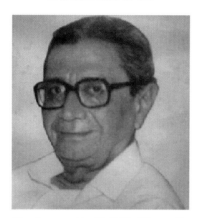

Professor Dr M.S.N. Ginwalla
Pioneer of Oral and Maxillofacial Surgery (India)
LDSc (Bom 1938), DDS (McGill Canada,1940), FICD, FIAOS, FAMS, JP
Postgraduate Course (MSc) in Maxillofacial and Plastic Surgery
University of Toronto,Canada,1942, under Dr F Risdon
Former Professor of Oral Surgery
Honorary Plastic Surgeon
Bai Yamunabai Laxman (BYL) Nair Charitable Hospital
Bombay, Maharashtra, India, 1945 to 1947
Honorary Plastic Surgeon
St George's and King Edward Memorial (KEM) Hospital
Bombay, Maharashtra, India, 1945 to 1955
Former Dean, Professor and Head and Professor Emeritus
Department of Maxillofacial, Plastic and Oral Surgery
Nair Hospital Dental College, Mumbai, Maharashtra, India
14-06-1963 to 13-06-1973 (Dean)
and
To all my esteemed teachers
with
Love and respect
and
To my husband Dr Anil Malik
and
To my daughter Dr Shambhvi Anil Malik

Contributors

Alka R Halbe MBBS, DA, MD (Anesthesiology) (Bom)
Former Professor
Department of Anesthesiology
Topiwala Nair Medical College and Hospital
Mumbai, Maharashtra, India
(Chapter 13)

Amit Date MDS (Bom)
Former Fellow
Head and Neck Services
Tata Memorial Hospital
Mumbai, Maharashtra, India
(Chapter 47)

Anil KD'Cruz MS, DNB
Chief
Head and Neck Services
Director
Tata Memorial Hospital
Mumbai, Maharashtra, India
(Chapter 47)

Anil S Malik BDS, MDS (Orthodontics) (Bom)
Former Professor and PG Teacher
Department of Orthodontics and
Dentofacial Orthopedics
Padmashree DY Patil Dental College and Hospital
Navi Mumbai, Maharashtra, India
(Chapters 24 and 25)

Beena M Kamdar MBBS, DA, MD (Anesthesiology) (Bom)
Former Professor and Head
Department of Anesthesiology
Topiwala Nair Medical College and Hospital
Mumbai, Maharashtra, India
(Chapters 11 and 19)

BH Sripathi Rao BDS, MDS (MAHE, Manipal)
Consultant Oral and Maxillofacial Surgeon
Mangalore, Karnataka, India
Principal, Professor and Head
Department of Oral and Maxillofacial Surgery
Yenepoya Dental College and Hospital
Mangalore, Karnataka, India
(Chapter 37)

Gauri Pantavaidya MS
Former Specialist Registrar
Head and Neck Services
Tata Memorial Hospital
Mumbai, Maharashtra, India
(Chapter 47)

Indula D Panchal MBBS, DA, MD (Anesthesiology) (Bom), DGO, MNAMS
Honorary Consultant, Anesthesiologist
Sir Hurkisondas Hospital and Research Center and
Jagjivan Ram Western Railways Hospital
Mumbai, Maharashtra, India
Former Professor and Head
Department of Anesthesiology
Topiwala Nair Medical College and Hospital
Mumbai, Maharashtra, India
(Chapter 12)

Manju N Gandhi MBBS, DA, MD (Anesthesiology) (Bom)
Former Professor
Department of Anesthesiology
Topiwala Nair Medical College and Hospital
Mumbai, Maharashtra, India
(Chapter 15)

Manju N Guhagarkar BDS, MDS (Bom)
Consultant Oral and Maxillofacial Surgeon
Mumbai, Maharashtra, India
Former Lecturer
Department of Oral and Maxillofacial Surgery
Nair Hospital Dental College
Mumbai, Maharashtra, India
(Chapters 1, 2, 4, 5 and 6)

Mushtaq I Parkar BDS, MDS (Bom)
Consultant Oral and Maxillofacial Surgeon
Professor
Department of Oral and Maxillofacial Surgery
Krishna Institute of Medical Sciences
Deemed University's
School of Dental Sciences and Hospital
Karad, Dist. Satara
Maharashtra, India
*(Chapters 7, 8, 9, 39, 40, 41, 54 and some updates in many
chapters, Appendices 1 and 2)*

Neelam A Andrade BDS, MDS (Bom)
Professor and Head
Department of Oral and Maxillofacial Surgery
Nair Hospital Dental College
Mumbai, Maharashtra, India
(Chapter 35)

Neelima Anil Malik BDS, MDS (Bom), FIAOS
Principal, Professor and Head
Department of Oral and Maxillofacial Surgery
Krishna Institute of Medical Sciences Deemed University's
School of Dental Sciences and Hospital
Karad, Dist. Satara, Maharashtra, India
(Chapters 3, 10, 21, 22, 23, 24, 25, 26, 27, 28, 29, 30, 31, 32, 33, 34, 36, 39, 40, 41, 42, 43, 44, 45, 46, 53, 54, 55)

Prashant A Punde BDS, MDS
Lecturer
Department of Oral and Maxillofacial Surgery
Krishna Institute of Medical Sciences
Deemed University's
School of Dental Sciences and Hospital
Karad, Dist. Satara, Maharashtra, India
(Chapter 54)

R Pradhan BSc, BDS, MDS, FICD, FDSRCPS (Glasgow)
Fellow
Indian Board of Association of Oral and Maxillofacial
Surgeon's of India
Former Head, Dean
Faculty of Dental Sciences
UP King George's University of Dental Sciences, Lucknow
Uttar Pradesh, India
Principal
UP Dental College and Research Centre
Lucknow, Uttar Pradesh, India
(Chapter 48)

Rupa K Sharma MBBS, DA, MD (Anesthesiology), DGO (Bom)
Former Professor
Department of Anesthesiology
Topiwala Nair Medical College and Hospital
Mumbai, Maharashtra, India
(Chapters 16 and 17)

Shambhvi Anil Malik BDS, MDS (Mumbai)
Diplomate, Certified Implantologist
DGI/Steinbeis University
Germany (Recognized in the European Union)
Consultant Prosthodontist
(Chapter 49)

Shubha N Mohite MBBS, DA, MD (Anesthesiology) (Bom)
Postgraduate Diploma in Educational Management
University of Mumbai
Mumbai, Maharashtra, India
Former Professor
Department of Anesthesiology
Topiwala Nair Medical College and Hospital
Mumbai, Maharashtra, India
(Chapter 18)

Sunali Khanna MDS, DNB, MNAMS
Lecturer
Department of Oral Medicine and Radiology
Nair Hospital Dental College
Mumbai, Maharashtra, India
(Chapter 51)

Swaran Arora MS, FRCS, LLM
Consultant Plastic Surgeon
Mumbai, Maharashtra, India
Former Professor and Head
Department of Plastic Surgery
Sir JJ Group of Hospitals and Grant Medical College
Mumbai, Maharashtra, India
(Chapter 38 and Clinical Photographs of Chapter 46)

Vandana S Trasi MBBS, DA, MD (Anesthesiology) (Bom)
Former Professor
Department of Anesthesiology
Topiwala Nair Medical College and Hospital
Mumbai, Maharashtra, India
(Chapter 20)

Vandana V Laheri MBBS, DA, MD (Anesthesiology) (Bom)
Former Professor
Department of Anesthesiology
Topiwala Nair Medical College and Hospital
Mumbai, Maharashtra, India
(Chapter 14 and All Illustrations for Chapters 12 to 20)

Vidya Rattan Chaudhary BDS, MDS (Bom)
Professor and Head
Unit of Oral and Maxillofacial Surgery
Oral Health Science Center
Postgraduate Institute of Medical
Education and Research
Chandigarh, India
(Chapters 50 and 52, Surgery Photographs of Chapter 55)

Dr SG Damle
Director
Medical Education and Public Health
Joint Municipal Commisioner (JMC)
Municipal Corporation of Greater Mumbai
Mumbai, Maharashtra, India

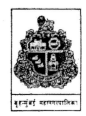

Foreword

It is my privilege to write a few words about the *Textbook of Oral and Maxillofacial Surgery*.

Textbook of Oral and Maxillofacial Surgery is well-orchestrated effort by the editor, Professor Dr (Mrs) Neelima Anil Malik, Head, Department of Oral and Maxillofacial Surgery, Nair Hospital Dental College (NHDC), Mumbai, Maharashtra, India. She is an academician par excellence. This, coupled with her skills and expertise in the field of oral and maxillofacial surgery, makes her an epitome for an ideal oral and maxillofacial surgeon and an eminent teacher.

The hallmark of the book is an extensive, pointwise coverage of the vast subject of oral and maxillofacial surgery in accordance with the syllabus of Dental Council of India and universities all over India. I am confident that the lucid well-illustrated book with easy language and concise tables will make an interesting and informative reading for undergraduate students.

The book has been authored by dedicated, outstanding, experienced clinicians and eminent teachers from India and will provide guidelines to safe and sound operative techniques suitable for the Indian subcontinent. The information provided in the book is the latest, taking into account the advances in science and technology in dentistry.

The editor deserves a hearty congratulation for all the efforts and hard work, she has undertaken. I am sure that the book will guide students into gaining an insight into the vast field of oral and maxillofacial surgery.

SG Damle
Dean, Nair Hospital Dental College (NHDC)
Mumbai, Maharashtra, India
Director, Medical Education and Public Health
Joint Municipal Commisioner (JMC)
Municipal Corporation of Greater Mumbai
Mumbai, Maharashtra, India

Preface to the Third Edition

My dear students and teachers,

It gives me an immense pleasure to connect with you all again, through this third edition of my *Textbook of Oral and Maxillofacial Surgery*.

This year, I have been voted as "Outstanding Teacher" (2011) by all my readers, well-wishers, all over the country, through The Premier Indian Dental Portal—Bitein. It always feels nice to be loved, appreciated and it encourages me more to contribute to the field of oral and maxillofacial surgery in my own humble way. Again 'a big thank to everybody'.

I am presenting this updated third edition of my book to you all and wish that you will always support me by reading this textbook.

The highlight of this new edition is the updated knowledge and inclusion of new chapters dedicated to the new technology—Recent Advances in Oral and Maxillofacial Surgery, Cone Beam Computerized Tomography (CBCT), Lasers, Piezosurgery. An additional chapter is also added to implantology section. This would not have been possible without the unconditional support from my contributors for this edition—Professor Vidya Rattan, Professor Mushtaq I Parkar, Dr Shambhvi Anil Malik, Dr Prashant A Punde, Dr Nilesh Patil, Dr Mounesh Kumar and Dr Jayant Landge.

The new technology gives the power of precision in clinician's hands, but we have to keep in mind that it keeps transforming at faster pace. As professionals, we need to change, learn, evolve, grow and more importantly, do it almost overnight. Using the latest technology to the best of our advantage, is no longer a bonus—it is a requirement. The volume of information is overwhelming. The solution is to adopt a timeless methodology for how to separate the 'wheat from the chaff'. We have tried to give comprehensive information of most of the updates in clinical practice. I hope its application in day-to-day clinical practice will benefit the patients.

I once again thank God almighty for his blessings in all my endeavors.

I also wish to convey my thanks to my earlier contributors, and of course, to M/s Jaypee Brothers Medical Publishers (P) Ltd, New Delhi, India, without their contribution, this third edition would not have been possible.

Recently, Shri Jitendar P Vij (Chairman and Managing Director), M/s Jaypee Brothers Medical Publishers (P) Ltd, New Delhi, India, has celebrated his successful 45 years of service in medical publishing.

During his journey, he has imparted knowledge to countless students, through his books, all over the world, and in turn, touched so many souls. My humble tribute to the passionate publisher Shri Jitendar P Vij. He has an amazing foresight in choosing his authors and he personally gives the much-needed support and encouragement.

My family members, my husband Dr Anil Malik, my daughter Dr Shambhvi Anil Malik, my friends and well-wishers have also contributed towards the success, by constant encouragement and support.

All the very best,
With warm regards,
Truly yours,
Love you all,
Neelima Anil Malik

Preface to the Third Edition

Preface to the First Edition

This textbook is the natural outcome of having worked at one of the prime dental teaching institutes in India, where there is abundance of variety of clinical materials and excellent infrastructure, with my teachers, colleagues and good friends over the past twenty-seven years in various capacities. This text also represents many years of combined clinical research and experience at our institute.

The field of Oral and Maxillofacial Surgery has witnessed significant changes over the last two decades. These changes have improved our knowledge and understanding of the diagnosis and management of oral and maxillofacial surgical problems. The basic aim of this textbook is to incorporate this updated information and provide concise description of various oral and maxillofacial surgical procedures and current concepts and contemporary information.

The unique feature of this book is that it incorporates all of those various subjects, which are usually found in separate textbooks. We have taken efforts to present every chapter with updated text and to provide clear illustrations, wherever required.

The information given and the chapters mentioned in this book are based on the curriculum prescribed for undergraduate program for all universities in India.

We felt the need to incorporate the extensive section on anesthesiology, as this aspect is not covered adequately in currently available standard textbooks in the subject. For the first time in the history, the anesthesiology chapters are supplemented with color illustrations.

It has been observed that the current trend of the undergraduate students is not to refer to many textbooks, may be because of either the time factor or the lack of availability of books, etc. We, therefore, desired to accommodate maximum information in one single textbook (Local anesthesia is not included, as many good books are available).

The purpose of this book is to present as lucid and simple text as possible in the point format, without sacrificing the biological concepts.

Pains taking efforts are also made to create illustrations and to provide maximum clinical pictures in most of the chapters, which is an essential feature of the book.

The earlier publications by our predecessors and prominent workers in the field served as a valuable source of reference material for this book.

The book is basically intended for dental undergraduates, but would certainly be useful for postgraduates, general practitioners and teachers in the field.

I humbly request the teachers throughout the country to give suggestions, contributions for future additions.

As we begin with the first century of the new millennium, we hope that this textbook will provide the data and reference source to assist the clinician and others to face the oral and maxillofacial problems.

"Never must the physician say the disease is incurable. By that admission he denies God, our creator, he doubts Nature with her profuseness of hidden powers and mysteries."

Paracelsus

I am very happy to present this textbook to the students all over the country, in the year, when I have been selected as "President Elect" of the Association of Oral and Maxillofacial Surgeons of India. I am grateful to all the members for giving me this opportunity to serve the fraternity.

Neelima Anil Malik

Acknowledgments

For the last many many years, I always dreamt of presenting a *Textbook of Oral and Maxillofacial Surgery* to the students all over the country.

First and foremost I have to thank "The Supreme Power—God" for giving me energy, inspiration and courage to complete this arduous task and to make my dream come true. Without "His" blessings nothing is possible.

I acknowledge my gratitude to Professor Dr SG Damle, Dean, Nair Hospital Dental College and Director, Medical Education and Public Health, Municipal Corporation of Greater Mumbai, Maharashtra, India. I am indebted to him for providing the facilities and opportunities, that made it possible to conduct the various clinical research and patient care, over the years, from which the clinical material for this text has been obtained. His constant encouragement and appreciation of the good work has always given us a boost.

My acknowledgments are also due to my all undergraduate teachers, who made the subject of oral and maxillofacial surgery so interesting, which inspired me to join the postgraduate studies in the subject.

I am indebted to my postgraduate teachers Professor Dr AP Chitre, Professor Dr KHC Kapadia and Professor Dr SK Dewan for their encouragement and guidance throughout my training program.

I would fail in my duty, if I do not mention late Dr Mrs Dhun Battiwala, who taught me my very first dental extraction. She and Dr AD'Costa supported me and helped me to continue my postgraduate studies along with the teaching job in the subject of oral and maxillofacial surgery, by exchanging their teaching posts with me. I am grateful to both of them.

A book of this magnitude was possible, only with cooperation of many individuals.

I would like to express my deep appreciation to all the contributors, whose untiring efforts have made this textbook possible.

My special thanks to the staff of the Anesthesiology Department of Topiwala Nair Medical College (TNMC) and Hospitals, Mumbai, Maharashtra, India, who have been always supportive for many many years and their contribution towards this book is also immense. Special credit goes to Professor Dr Mrs Divekar (Ex-Professor and Head of the Anesthesiology at TNMC) who developed the present 'state-of-the-art' anesthesiology department at our institute. And later on, more advances were carried forward by Professor Dr Mrs Panchal—Previous Professor and Head of the Department of Anesthesiology at TNMC and Current Professor and Head of the Department, Professor Dr Mrs Kamdar. Their excellent techniques and constant support has always made our life easy and given us the opportunity for excellent patient care.

Professor Dr JN Khanna also deserves special mention, as I have had opportunity to work with him and to enrich my knowledge and skill and share the responsibility of the department of oral and maxillofacial surgery at Nair Hospital Dental College (NHDC), Mumbai, Maharashtra, India.

I acknowledge the unconditional assistance given to me in my day-to-day work, by my Associate Professor, Dr M Deshpande and Senior Lecturer, Dr P Solanki, and I also thank all teaching and nonteaching staff members of the department.

My special thanks to all my present and past postgraduate students for the stimulation and encouragement, I derived from their enthusiasm and interest in the field of Oral and Maxillofacial Surgery.

I am grateful and indebted to the following for their knowledge and assistance in specific areas:

- Dr Mrs Vandana Laheri (Associate Professor of Anesthesiology at TNMC) and my ever-helping good friend, for complete color diagrams and illustrations provided for the anesthesiology chapters. She has also given me unconditional assistance for scanning, preparing other text diagrams, etc.
- Dr Ajit Pillai (Resident in Anesthesiology at TNMC) for line diagrams and some of the sketches illustrated in the book.

- Mr Pradeep Sahani (Commercial Artist) for some of the illustrations and photographs in the book.
- Mr A Sawant—For preparation of the initial computerized typescripts of the entire textbook.

Thank you all for your kind support and understanding.

I would like to thank Dr MI Parkar, our past student/resident and currently practicing Surgeon of oral and maxillofacial surgery, and teacher at Yerala Medical Trust's Dental College and Hospital at Navi Mumbai, Maharashtra, India, for his immense contribution towards the completion of this book.

Finally, my deep appreciation and love to my husband Dr Anil Malik for his personal sacrifice and constant support in permitting me to undertake and accomplish such a difficult endeavor and to my beloved daughter Dr Shambhvi Anil Malik for her motivation, inspiration and encouragement.

I am also grateful to Shri Jitendar P Vij (Chairman and Managing Director), Jaypee Brothers Medical Publishers (P) Ltd. New Delhi, India, who personally encouraged me to write the textbook.

On the occasion of releasing this third edition, I wish to thank profusely Shri Jitendar P Vij (Chairman and Managing Director), Mr Tarun Duneja (Director-Publishing) for publishing this book in excellent form. I thank the entire staff of Mumbai branch especially Mr CS Gawde (Branch Manager) and Mr Ramesh Krishnamachari (Commissioning Editor) for their cooperation and help.

I also wish to thank Mr KK Raman (Production Manager), Mr Sunil Kumar Dogra, Mr Manoj Pahuja, Mr Dinesh Joshi, Ms Samina Khan and Mr Gyanendra Kumar, for giving competent technical support which has helped me to bring out this edition with added color and excellence.

Last but not least, I would like to mention that I am indebted to individuals (including patients) too numerous to mention separately.

Contents

Section 5: Maxillofacial Trauma

Section 9: Orofacial Clefts

Section 10: Maxillary Sinus and its Implications

Section 11: Orofacial and Neck Infections

Section 14: Implantology in Oral and Maxillofacial Surgery

Section 15: Hemorrhage and Shock

Section 16: Miscellaneous

Section 17: Recent Advances in Oral and Maxillofacial Surgery

S E C T I O N

Principles of Oral and Maxillofacial Surgery

1

1 Introduction to Oral and Maxillofacial Surgery

Chapter Outline

- ❖ Scope
- ❖ Multidisciplinary Team Approach
- ❖ Newer Advances

DEFINITION

Oral and maxillofacial surgery is a branch of dentistry, that deals with the art of diagnosis and treatment of various diseases, injuries and defects involving the orofacial region.

Other specialties dealing with the cranio-oromaxillofacial region include the plastic surgery, neurosurgery, ENT surgery and ophthalmology, etc. Although, there is a considerable overlapping between these branches, in the past few years, a definite delineation has been made among each of these specialties. The oral and maxillofacial surgeon has carved a special niche in the multidisciplinary approach to craniofacial pathologies.

The field of oral and maxillofacial surgery has evolved through the ages. From extracting teeth by tying a thread around the tooth to refined techniques of today, the field has come a long way. Andre Fouchard is considered to be the father of dental surgery. Pioneers like Lister in the practice of asepsis, Wells in the introduction of anesthetic techniques, Bell in the field of orthognathic surgery, Gillie and Champy in the treatment of fractures have established a scientific basis to oral and maxillofacial surgical procedures. It is to them, we owe the modern day practice of oral and maxillofacial surgery.

SCOPE

The scope of oral and maxillofacial surgery depends on the qualifications and capabilities of the person. There is a definite distinction in the case selection for an undergraduate, trained in oral surgery, and a postgraduate, trained in oral and maxillofacial surgery and for cases that require multidisciplinary approach.

Oral and maxillofacial surgery essentially deals with the treatment of the following conditions:

1. Simple and complicated extractions of teeth and related management.
2. Treatment of cysts and tumors of both odontogenic and nonodontogenic origin, involving the jaw bones.
3. Management of disorders of maxillary sinuses.
4. Initial and definitive management of traumatic injuries of soft and hard tissues of orofacial region.
5. Temporomandibular joint disorders including internal derangement and ankylosis.
6. Salivary gland diseases and their management.
7. Diagnosis and management of dentofacial deformities, either acquired, developmental or congenital (including clefts of the lip and palate).
8. Management of orofacial infections involving the soft and hard tissues.
9. Preprosthetic surgical procedures including implantology.

10. Precancerous lesions such as, oral submucous fibrosis and leukoplakia.
11. Detection and management of oral cancer.
12. Management of orofacial pain.
13. Reconstruction of missing portion of jaw bones with bone graft/distraction osteogenesis.
14. Detection and management of facial neuropathy.

An undergraduate trained in oral surgery: It is expected to deal with simple exodontia, complications arising from routine extractions like, tooth/root fractures, tissue laceration, postextraction bleeding, minor post-extraction infections, immediate management of medical emergencies in the dental office and minor surgical procedures like apicoectomy and alveoloplasty.

A postgraduate student in Oral and Maxillofacial surgery: It deals with both the outpatient department cases as well as the patients admitted in the indoor ward. Beginning with complicated exodontia, the postgraduate program gradually trains the student to become a full fledged oral and maxillofacial surgeon, capable of handling the various pathologies of the face and the jaw bones.

MULTIDISCIPLINARY TEAM APPROACH

Cleft Lip and Palate

The oral and maxillofacial surgeon forms an important part of the cleft lip and palate management team, that comprises of the plastic surgeon, the pediatric surgeon, the orthodontist, the pedodontist, and the speech therapist. The oral and maxillofacial surgeon plays an important role in the primary as well as secondary closure of the palate, as well as in the correction of residual deformities of the maxilla and the mandible at a later stage.

Craniofacial Syndromes

The oral and maxillofacial surgeon also forms a part of the core group, consisting of neurosurgeon, plastic surgeon and ENT surgeon involved in treating craniofacial abnormalities, especially syndromal, like Crouzon's syndrome or Goldenhar syndrome, etc.

Trauma Unit

The oral and maxillofacial surgeon is also involved in the trauma unit along with orthopedic surgeon, general surgeon and plastic surgeon.

The oral surgeon, thus, forms an important link between the various specialties in the treatment of craniofacial pathologies.

NEWER ADVANCES

The field of oral and maxillofacial surgery is constantly evolving and adapting newer techniques, to refine the surgical procedures, and to achieve precision with minimally invasive techniques. One such technique that has revolutionized the treatment of facial deformities is distraction osteogenesis. The technique deals with the elongation of the bone by gradual callus distraction.

It is extremely difficult to outline the scope of a subject, where there is a constant adaptation with the introduction of research based technology and techniques. The students are advised to keep themselves updated with new literature on the subject.

2 Art of Diagnosis

The advent of the new century is marked by technological advances that have revolutionized science in every field as in medicine. Newer diagnostic aids and treatment modalities are being developed and introduced facilitating easier and quicker diagnosis and thereby improving patient care and treatment.

The first step towards treating any patient is making a correct diagnosis. The diagnostic sequence can be divided into five levels:

1. History taking
2. Clinical examination
3. Radiological analysis
4. Laboratory investigations
5. Interpretation and final diagnosis.

The first four steps help in obtaining a clinical database that can be then interpreted by the clinician to arrive at a final diagnosis.

The aims and objectives of this preoperative assessment are to decide:

1. The choice of anesthesia.
2. Whether the patient can withstand general anesthesia.
3. Whether the patient can withstand the trauma of surgery.
4. Any abnormalities in the patients general health, that need to be taken care of, prior to surgery.
5. Choice of premedication.
6. Treatment plan that will suit/benefit the patient the most.

▉ HISTORY TAKING

The aim of history taking is to obtain a correct account of the patient's problems, taking into consideration his/her symptoms, general condition, lifestyle, and socioeconomic background.

Art of History Taking

While talking to the patient, the clinician should establish a rapport with him/her, both by eye contact and positive body language. This goes a long way in eliciting information from the patient. The patient should be encouraged to narrate his problems in his own words, if possible in a chronological order. It can be compared to a story told in the patient's own words. The clinician can help the patient in unfolding his/her story by asking a few gentle questions like "Is there a change in the swelling during the course of the day?" or "Does the pain spread to any adjoining area?"

Steps in History Taking

Obtaining General Information

The first step in history taking is to obtain general information about the patient regarding the name, age, sex, marital status, address, race and occupation.

Chief Complaints

The chief complaint ascertains the principal reason as to why the patient is seeking medical attention. The following details are recorded:
1. All the symptoms, chronologically, in the patient's own words.
2. The onset, duration and progress of each of these symptoms.
3. Any treatment taken earlier for the condition, and the patient's response to the same.
4. A previous history of similar symptoms and treatment taken for the same, along with the outcome.
5. If the patient gives a history of trauma, additional history regarding unconsciousness, vomiting, bleeding from mouth, ear, nose or throat, retro/anterograde amnesia is obtained.

Past/Present Medical History

A detailed picture of the general medical status of the patient is obtained, which may or may not bear relevance to the chief complaint, the management of the patient and outcome of the treatment. The medical history questionnaire should include a detailed history of the following:
1. *Cardiovascular disorders* like myocardial infarction, ischemic heart disease, rheumatic heart disease, angina, valvular septal defect, hypertension and congestive cardiac failure. All the medications taken by the patient are listed including details about anticoagulants, antihypertensive drug therapy.
2. *Diseases of the respiratory system such* as chronic obstructive pulmonary disease, bronchial asthma, pneumonia, pleuritis, bronchitis, upper respiratory tract infections. These patients may be on bronchodilators, antihistaminics or steroid therapy. Any disease of the respiratory system significantly affects the anesthetic management of the patient. A history of sleep apnea may be obtained from the relatives. This condition is commonly seen in patients with severe mandibular retrusion secondary to bilateral temporomandibular joint ankylosis.
3. *Neurologic conditions* like, epilepsy, hemiparaplegia and past history of head injury and medications taken for the same. If the patient is an epileptic, then the last episode of seizure and the frequency of seizure episodes are recorded.
4. *Diseases of the endocrine system* including thyroid disorders, diabetes, adrenal pheochromocytoma, and multiple endocrine neoplasia and medications taken for the same. If the patient is a diabetic, care must be taken to mention his/her latest blood sugar values and the route of administration of the antidiabetic therapy, i.e. oral drugs or insulin injections.
5. *Hematological disorders* like anemias, leukemia, hemophilia, platelet count abnormalities, etc. and the last available blood reports pertaining to the condition.
6. *Infectious diseases* like tuberculosis, syphilis, viral hepatitis, herpes, and other sexually transmitted diseases.
7. *Reproductive system* like pregnancy, lactation, last menstrual cycle, number of children, abortions and use of oral contraceptives. Many common antibiotics are known to have interactions with oral contraceptives rendering them ineffective. The patient must then be advised to practice alternate methods of birth control for the period.
8. *Gastric disorders* like peptic ulcer, acidity problems, vomiting, and diarrhea.
9. *Renal pathologies* like glomerulonephritis, nephrotic syndrome, renal failure, and patients on dialysis.
10. *Disorders of the liver* like cirrhosis, alcoholic liver disease, hepatitis.
11. *Autoimmune disorders* like systemic lupus erythematosus, scleroderma, requiring long term corticosteroid therapy.
12. *Psychiatric ailments* and treatment taken for the same.
13. *Digestive system* loss of appetite, loss of weight, polydipsia, polyuria.
14. Allergy to any drug.
15. Childhood illness/birth trauma.
16. Details of previous hospitalization, blood transfusions and surgeries.

17. Past/present history of radiation therapy.
18. Current/past medications taken, e.g. NSAIDs for chronic inflammatory lesions, aspirin, anticoagulant therapy, anti-Koch's therapy, steroid therapy for autoimmune disorders.

Any of the above conditions can alter the patient's response to surgery and influence both the anesthetic and surgical management of the patient as well as postoperative recovery and wound healing.

Personal and Family History

This part of the history deals with both the personal habits as well as social history of the patient. It gives an overview of the patient's lifestyle. This gives a better perspective of the patient apart from contributing to the diagnosis of the disease as well as outcome of the treatment.

1. Habits like chewing tobacco, quicklime, areca nut, *pan masala*, *gutkha*, chronic alcoholism, chronic smoking, drug abuse and frequent exposure to commercial sex workers.
2. A detailed history of the immediate family of the patient, with their age, general health status, medical ailments, cause and age at the time of death of any deceased member is recorded. A family history of epilepsy, cardiac disorders, diabetes, bleeding disorders, and tuberculosis is of particular importance.

◼ CLINICAL EXAMINATION

The clinical examination of the patient begins as he/she enters the clinic. The patient's gait, composure, as well as speech reflect his/her general condition and psychological status. In this chapter, we will restrict ourselves to the orofacial region. For a detailed review of the other systems, one can refer to standard textbooks on surgery.

After the history taking, the patient's vital signs are first recorded, i.e. blood pressure, pulse, temperature and respiratory rate.

When examining the patient, the clinician should be well-versed with the four aspects of examination, i.e. inspection, palpation, percussion and auscultation. Of these percussion has least importance in the maxillofacial region.

We will now discuss the different aspects of examination and their clinical application to the orofacial region.

Extraoral Examination

Extraoral examination can be divided into frontal and profile examination. The following structures are examined:
1. Face
2. Skin and soft tissue
3. Skull
4. Bony skeleton of the face
5. Temporomandibular joints
6. Lymphatic systems
7. Salivary glands
8. Eyes.

Inspection

Face: At the onset of the examination, the face is first observed for any signs of asymmetry, swelling, etc. The proportion of the upper, middle and lower thirds of the face is noted along with their relation to each other. The facial morphology is identified (dolicocephalic, mesencephalic or brachycephalic).

Skin and soft tissue: The color and texture of the skin is indicative of many underlying systemic problems (Table 2.1).

Skull: While inspecting the orofacial region, the clinician should begin from the cranium and the frontal bone and proceed downwards. Any abnormality in the size and shape of the cranium is indicative of a probable congenital abnormality. Special care should be taken in trauma patients to detect head injuries. Edema, laceration, swelling and any depression in the contour of the skull vault are indicative of a head injury. Similarly any depression in the frontal bone is indicative of head injury.

Eyes: The eyes are examined for any soft tissue injury to the cornea or conjunctiva. Pallor is indicative of anemia, icterus is indicative of jaundice, and exophthalmous in absence of trauma is suggestive of thyroid disorders. Any injury to the orbital skeleton and contents presents as any one or a combination of following signs—subconjunctival hemorrhage, circumorbital ecchymosis/edema, enophthalmos, exophthalmos, change in the level of the orbital contents, or increased inter canthal distance.

Nose: When inspecting the nose, the following aspects are taken into consideration: (1) depression of the nasal bridge, deviation of the nasal septum; commonly seen in fractures of the nasal bones; and (2) obliteration of

Table 2.1: Colored texture of skin versus expected complications	
Colors	*Expected complications etiology*
Pallor	Temporary—shock, hemorrhage, intense emotion
	Persistent anemia
Abnormal redness	Overheating, extreme exertion, sunburn, febrile exanthematous and inflammatory skin diseases
Local redness	Telangiectasia, especially on the face
Cyanosis	Defective oxygenation of the blood, excessive decrease in the hemoglobin level
Subicteric, lemon yellow, daffodil tints	Pernicious anemia, acholuric jaundice
Yellow, orange or dark olive green color	Obstructive jaundice
Palms—orange yellow	Carotenemia (presence of excessive lipid soluble yellow pigments in the plasma, distinguished from jaundice as it does not stain the conjunctiva)
Absence of pigmentation	Generalized—albinism
	Localized—piebaldism
Patches of white and darkly pigmented skin	Vitiligo
Pale skin with diminished pigmentation	Hypopituitarism/hypogonadism
Brown to dark brown pigmentation of the affected parts of the skin	Addison's disease
Dry, scaly skin	Protein deficiency

the lateral wall of the nose and deviation of the nasal septum; as with tumors of the maxilla; maxillary sinus and the nose. In patients with cleft lip, special attention should be given to the alar base width, the columella and the deviation of the nose. Any evidence of nasal discharge, epistaxis or loss of smell (partial or complete) should be recorded.

Malar and paranasal regions: Two important things to be inspected in the paranasal region are any swelling present in the region, due to a cystic or tumorous lesion in the maxilla and hypoplasia of the paranasal area. Hypoplasia of the paranasal area can be a true hypoplasia or pseudohypoplasia secondary to mandibular prognathism. In trauma patients, the malar region has to be inspected for any "dimpling" along the contour of the zygomatic arch or depression of the zygomaticomalar complex. This is best appreciated from a bird's eye view (from above and behind the patient).

In addition, the clinician must evaluate any facial asymmetry, facial swelling, extraoral draining sinuses, scars, color and texture of the skin, and any signs of ecchymosis, hemorrhage, lacerations and abrasions. All patients with facial asymmetry/swelling have to be inspected from either below or from above and behind.

Areas best appreciated in the profile are the paranasal area, the frontal bone, the nasal projection,

the chin and the mandibular plane. Profile inspection is very important for patients who have to undergo orthognathic surgery.

Ears: Due to their close proximity to the temporomandibular joints, a close inspection of the ears is must, especially in trauma cases. Very often, there is frank bleeding from one or both the ears, indicative of a fracture of the condyle. Another condition where abnormality of the ear is seen is the Goldenhar syndrome, where the external ear may be missing with just ear tags present. The ear is examined for any evidence of frank infection or pus discharge. The patient's complaints of tinnitus or hearing impairment are recorded.

Lips: Few lesions involving the lips include clefts, ulcerative and nonulcerative growths, angular cheilitis, herpes infections, etc.

Palpation

Palpation must be done gently, without causing much distress to the patient. A quick and thorough palpation helps the clinician to establish his/her primary diagnosis. Palpation of the bony skeleton is begun from the frontal bone and proceeds downwards. Palpation of the facial skeleton is carried out simultaneously, bilaterally, starting from the supraorbital ridges, proceeding in the following order; the lateral orbital rim, the medial orbital rim, the infraorbital rim, the bridge of the nose and lateral nasal walls, the paranasal regions, the zygomatic bone and the arch contour, the temporomandibular joints, the posterior border of the ramus, the angle and the continuity of the inferior border of the mandible. The temporomandibular joints are usually palpated by placing the index fingers of both the hands just anteroinferior to the tragus of the ear. They can also be palpated intrameatally in a similar fashion. The joints are examined for any tenderness, clicking, crepitus on opening or closing of the mouth. The range of opening and left and right lateral excursions are checked and abnormalities are noted. The muscles of mastication are palpated for tenderness.

In a patient with a history of trauma, any step deformity, abnormal mobility of fragments, tenderness, reduced movements of the temporomandibular joints is indicative of a fracture in that area.

A facial swelling that is infective in nature will be soft, fluctuant, warm and tender on palpation. A facial swelling that is neoplastic or cystic in origin is usually firm to bony hard, with expansion of either or both the buccal and lingual cortical plates and may or may not be tender. If there is perforation of the cortical plate, the swelling will be soft on palpation in that region. Thinning of the buccal cortex is many a times indicated by a typical eggshell crackling sound on palpation. The inferior border is also examined for expansion. Expansion of the lingual cortex is very characteristic of ameloblastoma. An equal expansion in all directions is indicative of ossifying or cementifying fibroma. Lesions of bony origin are always bony hard to palpation, whereas vascular lesions produce a bruit or thrill.

For salivary gland disorders, the parotid and the submandibular glands are palpated extraorally. The parotid gland can be palpated in the preauricular, inferior auricular, and postauricular regions. The submandibular gland is checked by bimanual palpation by placing a finger of one hand in the submandibular region and another intraorally in the floor of the mouth.

When examining the eyes, the eyelids are gently separated to detect soft tissue injuries and hemorrhage, the extent of hemorrhage, if any, and if the patient is conscious, the vision is tested on each side in all the directions.

The preauricular, submandibular, submental, and cervical lymph nodes are palpated for enlargement, tenderness, mobility and consistency. The submandibular nodes are best palpated from behind by asking

Table 2.2: Palpating lymph nodes and probable associated conditions

Lymph nodes	Condition
Tender, mobile, enlarged	Acute infection
Nontender, mobile, enlarged	Chronic infection
Matted, nontender	Tuberculosis
Fixed, enlarged	Squamous cell Ca
Rubbery, enlarged	Lymphomas

the patient to flex his head forward and relax his neck muscles (Table 2.2).

Auscultation

Auscultation is mainly used in two conditions in the orofacial region:
1. Vascular lesions to hear bruits.
2. Temporomandibular joint pathological processes or to hear the joint movements.

Once the extraoral examination is complete, the oral opening should be measured prior to intraoral examination. Oral opening or maximal incisal opening is a distance measured between the incisal edges of the maxillary and mandibular central incisors.

Intraoral Examination

The structures to be examined during intraoral examination are as follows:
1. Buccal, labial and alveolar mucosa.
2. Hard and soft palate.
3. Floor of the mouth and tongue.
4. Retromolar region.
5. Posterior pharyngeal wall and faucial pillars.
6. Salivary glands and their orifices.
7. Dentition and occlusion.

Inspection

When the patient opens his mouth, the first thing the clinician sees is the oral hygiene. A fetid odor is indicative of a poor oral hygiene or an infective process in the oral cavity. The mucosa is inspected for color, texture, and presence of ulceration, growth or draining sinuses.

The size of the tongue, its mobility and surface are inspected. The tongue is then depressed to visualize the uvula, soft palate, and the lateral and posterior pharyngeal walls. Any deviation of the uvula, abnormal movement of the soft palate, mass at the base of the tongue, posterior pharyngeal walls and any swelling of the lateral and retropharyngeal space is identified.

The floor of the mouth is examined and a note of any inflammation, mass, hematoma is noted. The presence of a hematoma is usually indicative of a fracture in that region. A raised floor of the mouth in a patient having an abscess is suggestive of Ludwig's angina.

The salivary gland orifices are examined for any signs of inflammation or pus discharge.

The dentition is then examined, and a mention of missing, carious, mobile, restored and malposed teeth is made. The occlusion is checked and any deviation from the normal canine and molar relation, posterior gagging, anterior open bite, deep bite, reverse overjet, overjet is recorded. The arch form and the curve of Spee are also recorded.

The periodontal tissues are examined for the color and texture of the gingiva. Any sign of recession, hyperplasia, infection is noted.

Edentulous ridges are thoroughly examined for the form of the ridge, any soft tissue abnormality, bony abnormalities like tori, bony protuberances, etc. and the presence of any remnant root pieces.

Palpation

Intraoral palpation is similar to what is described extraorally. An extra- or intraosseous swelling is palpated to record the consistency and extent of the swelling. Further, palpation will reveal whether the swelling is sessile or pedunculated, and any breach in the buccal or lingual cortical plates.

Vascular lesions may produce a bruit or thrill, which can be appreciated on palpation.

In trauma patients, the palpation begins in the anterior maxillary region, and proceeds behind the zygomatic buttress to the tuberosity region. The anterior border of the ramus is then palpated, coming downward to the vestibule and to the anterior mandibular region. Any signs of tenderness or step are recorded. Holding the alveolar fragments between the fingers of the two hands and exerting pressure, checks the alveolar mobility. The maxillary mobility is checked at different levels by placing the fingers of one hand at the alar base, middle third of the nose and the nasal bridge, and exerting gentle pressure with the other hand on the maxillary anterior dentoalveolar segment. Any mobility of the teeth is checked.

The salivary glands are milked to check for normal salivary flow and quantity of the saliva.

Once the clinical examination is complete, the clinician has a general idea regarding the location, extent, and clinical nature of the lesion. A tentative diagnosis is established in the clinician's mind. This is put down as the provisional diagnosis. Radiological studies and other biochemical investigations, which will be discussed next, then support this provisional diagnosis.

■ CLINICAL DIAGNOSTIC AIDS

Radiological Examination

Radiological imaging is one of the most important diagnostic aids available to the clinician. Apart from the site and extent of the lesion, the radiological picture also to some extent reveals the nature of the lesion, since each lesion has its radiological presentation. For example, a multilocular lesion may be indicative of an ameloblastoma or a giant cell lesion or an odontogenic myxoma. Fibro-osseous lesions exhibit a mixed radio-paque-radiolucent lesion. Chronic osteomyelitis may have a moth-eaten appearance radiographically.

Apart from determining the site and extent of an obvious lesion, radiographs also enable the clinician to pick up silent lesions (incidental findings). With the advances in information technology, the field of radiology has been revolutionized. The acquirement and storage of data has been simplified to a minute volume of tissue, and with the help of a computer, an integration of these data images has been made possible. It is possible today for the clinician to have an accurate picture of the lesion before surgical intervention.

We divide this section into two parts:
1. Conventional radiography
2. Specialized imaging.

Conventional Radiography

Conventional radiography can be further divided into intraoral views and extraoral views.

Intraoral Radiographs

1. *Intraoral periapical view*—areas best appreciated are as follows:

- Teeth
- Periapical region
- Lamina dura and periodontal ligament space
- Supporting alveolar bone.

This view is useful in locating changes in the teeth and periapical tissues.

Indications in oral surgery

- Studying impacted third molars.
- Periapical lesion.
- Relation of the maxillary sinus to the teeth.
- Localizing fractured or remnant root pieces.
- Localizing foreign bodies, in interdental/periodontal regions.
- Differentiating between cystic and tumorous lesions.
- Locating the exact extent of the periapical lesion, especially in the maxilla.
- In trauma cases to identify dentoalveolar fractures and to rule out tooth fractures.

Advantages: Excellent view of the teeth and periapical region with minimal distortion.

Disadvantages: It cannot be used when the oral opening is reduced or for extensive lesions.

2. A. *Occlusal view of the mandible*—areas best appreciated are as follows:
   - Floor of the mouth.
   - Lingual aspect of the mandible.
   - Lower arch contour and continuity.
   B. *Occlusal view of the maxilla*—areas best appreciated:
   - Hard palate
   - Contour and continuity of the upper arch.

Indications in oral surgery

1. Locate impacted wisdom teeth.
2. Locate ectopic/supernumerary teeth.
3. Check for buccal/palatal cortical plate expansion.
4. Localization of salivary calculus in the submandibular salivary duct.
5. Study the hard palate and its lesions like palatine tori, palatal tumors.
6. Locate presence of foreign bodies in the soft tissues.
7. Study the tumors arising on the lingual aspect of the mandible, like mandibular osteomas.

Advantages

1. The only view that gives excellent visualization of the hard palate and the floor of the mouth.
2. When used in correlation with periapical views, they help to give an idea of the buccopalatal/lingual position of the object under consideration.

Extraoral Radiographs

1. *Orthopantomogram*—areas best appreciated are as follows:
   The temporomandibular joint, posterior and anterior border of the ramus, the ramus, the angle and the body of the mandible, the continuity of the inferior border of the mandible, the pterygomaxillary fissures, the maxillary tuberosity, the maxillary sinuses, and the teeth.

2. *Lateral oblique view of mandible*—areas best appreciated are as follows:
   - Two lateral oblique projections are required, each showing a different area of the mandible to its best advantage, i.e. the regions of the body and the ramus.
   - The mandibular body projection demonstrates the premolar-molar region and the inferior border of the mandible.
   - The ramus projection demonstrates the mandibular ramus from the angle to the condyle.
   - Third molar regions of both the maxilla and mandible are well-visualized.

3. *Posteroanterior view or Water's Position (occipitomental projection)* areas best appreciated are as follows:
   - Maxillary sinuses
   - Frontal and the ethmoid sinuses
   - Frontozygomatic suture
   - Supraorbital and infraorbital rims
   - Nasal cavity
   - Position of the coronoid process of the mandible between the maxilla and the zygomatic arch.

4. *Posteroanterior view of mandible*—areas best appreciated are as follows:
   - Body of the mandible
   - Inferior border, anterior border of the ramus.
   - Condylar neck
   - Nasal cavity.

The shadow of the vertebrae does not allow visualization of the mandibular symphysis region.

5. *Transorbital view*—area best appreciated mandibular condylar neck. Useful in the diagnosis of subcondylar fractures.

6. *Transcranial view*—areas best appreciated are as follows:
   • Glenoid fossa
   • Articular eminence
   • Condylar heads and their relation to one another.
   This view is taken in mouth open and closed positions for TM joint internal derangements, dislocation and subluxation.

7. *Lateral cephalogram view*—areas best appreciated are as follows:
   • Skull
   • Facial bones
   • Paranasal air sinuses
   • Hard palate
   • Nasopharyngeal tissues
   • Soft tissue outline of the face.
   Using the various cephalometric points, the relation between the maxilla, mandible and the skull, as well as their dental components can be established.

8. *Posteroanterior view of skull*—areas best appreciated are as follows:
   • Skull
   • Frontal and ethmoidal air sinuses
   • Nasal fossa and orbits.

9. *Lateral skull view*—areas best appreciated are skull and the bones of the middle third of the face.

10. *Submentovertex view (Jug Handle view)*—areas best appreciated are as follows:
    • Base of the skull
    • Position and orientation of the condyles
    • Sphenoidal air sinuses
    • Curvature of the inferior border of the mandible
    • Lateral wall of the maxillary sinus
    • Projection of the zygomatic arch
    • Medial and lateral pterygoid plates, and
    • Foramina at the base of the skull

11. *Chest X-ray (posteroanterior view)*—areas appreciated are as follows:
    • Bony skeleton, that is, ribs, sternum, and the vertebral column
    • Position of the trachea and the tracheal passage
    • Size, shape and position of the heart and aorta
    • Size and position of the diaphragm
    • Lung fields

Specialized Imaging

Tomogram

Tomography is the term used to refer to all types of body sectional radiographic techniques. The tomographic techniques used in maxillofacial surgery can be divided into two categories:
A. Conventional tomography.
B. Computed tomography.
A. *Conventional tomography:* During tomography the radiographic tube moves in one direction, the film moves in the opposite direction, and the fulcrum in the system remains stationary. The level of fulcrum is represented in the patient, as the layer of interest, where the anatomic structures are in sharp focus. All the points above and below this plane are blurred. Tomography is most often used for imaging of the temporomandibular joints, and occasionally to examine other facial structures, e.g. orbital cavity.
B. *Computed tomography (CT):* Computed tomography was first introduced in the mid 1970s. The CT scanners basically produce a digital data measuring the extent of X-ray transmission through an object. This numerical information is transformed into a density scale and used to reconstruct a visual image.

Advantages of a CT scan over conventional radiographs
1. Better visualization of structures in various minute levels and planes.
2. Greater geometric precision.
3. Three-dimensional view of the facial structures.
4. Sensitivity to discriminate between objects with small difference in density like blood and fat or blood and CSF.
5. Better visualization of the paranasal and orbital structures.
6. Exact localization of the lesions and their extent.

Ultrasonography

Ultrasonography uses the principle of echo, obtained from sound waves, as they pass through various structures. These echos are recorded and converted into a visual image. It has limited applications in the maxillofacial region and has low specificity. It is mainly used for imaging the salivary glands.

Magnetic Resonance Imaging

Magnetic resonance imaging (MRI) was introduced into clinical practice in the 1980s, and in a very short-time has gained immense importance in the field of diagnostic radiology. The MRI is unquestionably the best imaging modality available for lesions encountered in the central nervous system, the musculoskeletal system, and the cardiovascular system. It is a computer based tomographic technique that is developed to image tissues using positron emission from isotopes, or signals derived from the nuclear magnetic resonance properties of protons in the tissue water.

Applications in maxillofacial region: The MRI is an excellent imaging modality for soft tissues and has superseded CT scans in the evaluation of the imaging of the temporomandibular joint and the tumors of the nasopharynx, parapharyngeal area, salivary glands, tongue and oropharynx.

Radionuclide Imaging

Nuclear medicine utilizes radioactive compounds having affinity to particular tissues. These agents when injected into the patient, concentrate in large volumes in the target tissues and these tissues are studied under both dynamic and static conditions. The scans obtained are called scintigraphy or radionuclide scans. The most common radiopharmaceuticals used are, ^{99m}Technetium (^{99m}Tc), methylene diphosphonate, and ^{67}Gallium (^{67}Ga). The various structures best examined in the maxillofacial region are, the bony structures, the salivary glands, the thyroid, and the parathyroids. A "hot" area on the scintigram indicates increased tracer uptake and thereby increased vascular activity in the region, e.g. acute osteomyelitis, vascular uptake of a bone graft. A decreased uptake will be represented by a 'cold' area indicating reduced vascularity, e.g. a cyst or a necrotic area.

The technique of radionuclide imaging has high sensitivity and low specificity. It can detect early, silent lesions that are not visible radiographically. A single bone scan is sufficient to evaluate the entire bony skeleton of the body, preventing the necessity for repeated radiographs.

Applications of radionuclide imaging in the maxillofacial region

1. To detect salivary gland disorders.
2. To detect early silent lesions of the bony skeleton.
3. For early detection of metastasis from a primary malignant lesion.
4. For early detection of spread of infections like tuberculosis.

5. For evaluation of graft uptake postoperatively. A free graft will begin to show tracer uptake at the ends first, and gradually progresses to the center as the days progress. A cold area is indicative of graft rejection. A vascularized graft shows good tracer uptake throughout the graft immediate postoperatively.
6. To evaluate the progress of the treatment given to the patient, e.g. in patients with tuberculous lesions of the jaw bones, repeated scintigrams can be used to evaluate the pre and post extent and activity of the lesion.

Sialography

Sialography is a radiographic technique to detect and monitor salivary gland disease. The technique is used to examine all the ductal and acinar systems of the major salivary glands, especially the parotid and submandibular glands. The procedure reveals the integrity and location of the salivary glands.
1. Detection of sialoliths or foreign bodies.
2. Evaluation of the extent of ductal damage secondary to infection.
3. Evaluation of suspected neoplasms, as to the location, extent and size.
4. Evaluation of fistulae, diverticulae and strictures.
5. Diagnosis of autoimmune disorders like Sjögren's syndrome and Miculick's disease.

Arthrography

Arthrography is the introduction of an opaque contrast material in the joint space, so as to permit evaluation of structures that would otherwise be radiographically invisible. Arthrography has immense importance in temporomandibular joint imaging, to delineate the upper and lower joint compartments, the articular disc (the meniscus). It is contraindicated in acute infections and in patients with sensitivity to the contrast media.

Angiography

This is a method for studying the intracranial and extracranial vessels. A suitable radiopaque contrast medium is injected percutaneously into the carotid artery in the neck or into a vertebral artery, either by catheterization of a major blood vessel such as the femoral, axillary, brachial, or subclavian arteries. Radiographs are taken in various planes in the following few seconds. The arterial, capillary and venous circulation can be studied and abnormalities in the distribution, size, position and lumen of the vessels can be studied. In the maxillofacial region this technique is particularly useful in the study of the distribution pattern of the external carotid artery and the diagnosis of aneurysms, arteriovenous malformations and their feeder vessels, and vascular tumors. The procedure can also be coupled with identification and embolization of the feeder vessel in AV malformation prior to surgery.

Electrocardiogram

Electrocardiogram (ECG) records the changes in the electrical potential in association with the contraction of the heart.

It is useful to:
1. Determine the changes in the cardiac rate and rhythm.
2. Determine the changes in the impulse generation and conduction.
3. Detect areas of infarction.
4. Determine valvular dysfunction (stenosis and regurgitation).
5. Detect changes in the heart size.

Electrocardiogram (ECG) is advised in the following:
1. Patients above the age of 40 years.
2. In known cases of heart ailments.
3. In known cases of renal disorders.
4. In known cases of thyroid disorders.

◼ DIAGNOSTIC INVESTIGATIONS

Routine Hematological Investigations

Hemoglobin

Hemoglobin (Hb) indicates the oxygen carrying capacity of blood.

Normal value:

Females   : 12 to 16 gm%
Males   : 14 to 18 gm%

A decreased value is indicative of anemia (less than 12 gm% in adults). The most common cause of anemia is iron deficiency due to decreased intake of essential compounds, viz. vitamin B_1, B_6, B_{12}, iron, vitamin C. Other causes of anemia are decreased absorption of iron and vitamin B_6 as in sprue and pernicious anemia, respectively. Bone marrow depression, increased blood loss as in bleeding piles, gastric/duodenal ulcers, heavy

menstrual flow, hemoptysis and postpartum bleeding are also other causes.

Patients with low hemoglobin must be referred to the proper specialists for identification of the cause and necessary treatment prior to any surgical procedure.

Complete Blood Count

Complete blood count (CBC) includes the red blood cell count, white blood cell count, differential white blood cell count, an estimation of platelet number and a description of blood smear.
1. Helps to determine the nutritional status.
2. Helps to detect the presence of infection.
3. Helps to detect/rule out bleeding disorders.
4. Helps to decide whether the patient's immune response will be adequate to facilitate postoperative recovery.

Red blood cell count

Normal value:

Females : 4.5 to 5.5 million cells per cu mm
Males : 4.5 to 6.2 million cells per cu mm

A decrease in the red blood cell count is seen in anemia, pellagra, hemorrhage and liver disease. An increase is seen in polycythemia and extreme dehydration.

White blood cell count

Normal value:

Females : 5000 to 10000 cells per cu mm
Males : 5000 to 10000 cells per cu mm
Children below 7 years : 6000 to 15000 cells per cu mm

White cell count is increased (leukocytosis) in acute infections, uremia, leukemia and with steroid therapy. The count is decreased (leukopenia) in aplastic anemia, radiation therapy, infectious mononucleosis, malaria, AIDS, enteric fever and drug poisoning.

A physiological increase in the WBC count is seen in pregnancy, exposure to heat and cold, muscular exercise and emotional stress.

Differential white blood cell count

This count is the cell type distribution of the total white cell blood count.

Polymorphonuclear leukocytes (neutrophils): 50 to 70 percent.

Neutrophils are increased in infections, granulocytic leukemia, postsurgery, after severe exercise, severe hemorrhage and burns. The count is decreased in aplastic anemia, viral infections and in patients undergoing radiation or dialysis.

Lymphocytes: 25 to 40 percent.
Lymphocytes are increased in viral infections, tuberculosis, mononucleosis, syphilis, whooping cough, and lymphocytic leukemia. The count is decreased with stress, uremia and in steroid therapy.

Monocytes: 3 to 8 percent.
Monocytes are increased in monocytic leukemia, tuberculosis, chronic inflammation, collagen diseases (rheumatoid arthritis, systemic lupus erythematosus), subacute bacterial endocarditis, malaria, typhoid, kala-azar and protozoal infections.

Eosinophils: 1 to 8 percent.
Eosinophil count is increased in allergies, parasitic infection, collagen vascular diseases, Addison's disease and malignancy. Eosinophilia can be classified as:
1. Parasitic—helminthiasis, filariasis.
2. Allergic—asthma, urticaria, dermatitis.
3. Skin related—scabies, eczema, pemphigus.

The count is reduced in stress, steroid therapy, adrenocorticotropic hormone excess and in Cushing's syndrome.

Basophils: 0 to 1 percent.
Basophil count is increased in polycythemia, and chronic myeloid leukemia. The count is decreased in stress, steroid therapy, acute rheumatic fever and thyrotoxicosis.

Platelet count

Normal value: 1,50000 to 400000 cells per cu mm.
Platelet count is increased in malignancy, postsurgery or postsplenectomy, rheumatoid arthritis, iron deficiency anemia, trauma, and acute hemorrhage. The count is decreased in idiopathic thrombocytic purpura, marrow invasion or aplasia, hypersplenism, disseminated intravascular coagulation, cirrhosis of liver, massive transfusions, viral infections and infectious mononucleosis.

Erythrocyte sedimentation rate

Normal value:

Females : 0 to 20 mm/hour
Males : 0 to 10 mm/hour by Wintrobe's method.
Erythrocyte sedimentation rate (ESR) is a nonspecific test and values above normal are indicative of chronic infections, infarctions, trauma and inflammatory processes.

Coagulation Tests

Bleeding time: About 3 to 5 minutes by Duke's method (use of filter paper).
Bleeding time is the lag between the start of bleeding and the beginning of clot formation. It is increased in thrombocytopenia, capillary wall abnormalities (vitamin C deficiency), and platelet abnormalities which may be drug induced (use of aspirin, warfarin).

Clotting time: About 4 to 10 minutes by Lee-White method (use of capillary tube).
Clotting time indicates the time interval beginning from the formation of platelet plug to the completion of vasoconstriction and clot formation. Prolonged clotting time is seen in thrombocytopenia, hypersplenism, clotting factor deficiency and use of anticoagulants.

Prothrombin time: Usually 12 to 14 seconds. This value is always given with a control. Values within 2 seconds of the control are considered to be normal. It measures the extrinsic and the common pathways of the coagulation cascade. The prothrombin time is prolonged in factor I, II, V, VII, and X deficiency and in anticoagulant therapy, cirrhosis of liver, hepatitis, obstructive jaundice, colitis, celiac disease, sprue and salicylate therapy.

Partial thromboplastin time: Usually 25 to 45 seconds. This value is always given with a control. Values within 4 seconds of the control are considered to be normal. It is prolonged in factor I, II, V, VII, IX, X, XI and XII deficiencies and in patients undergoing heparin therapy.

Thromboplastin generation time: The normal range is 12 seconds or less. It is used to differentiate specific factor deficiencies, namely, V, VIII, IX, X, XI, and XII.

Biochemical Analysis

Renal Function Tests

Blood urea nitrogen

Normal value: 10 to 20 mg/100 ml
Decreased levels are associated with advanced liver disease and low protein diets.
Increased levels are seen in renal disorders and are associated with decreased glomerular filtration rate.

Serum creatinine

Normal value: 0.7 to 1.4 mg/100 ml
Increased values are associated with impaired renal functions and muscle diseases. Serum creatinine is a

more sensitive indicator of glomerular filtration rate than blood urea nitrogen.

Serum Electrolytes

Sodium

Normal value: 135 to 145 mEq/L

Hyponatremia is associated with cirrhosis of liver, congestive cardiac failure, adrenal insufficiency, nephritis, excessive use of diuretics, and water intoxication. Hypernatremia is associated with excessive water loss due to diarrhea, vomiting, and sweating and in diabetes mellitus.

Potassium

Normal value: 3.2 to 5.5 mEq/L

Hyperkalemia is associated with the release of cellular potassium secondary to surgery, crush injuries, hemolysis of red blood cells, renal failure and acidosis. Hypokalemia is seen in excessive fluid loss through the gastrointestinal tract or urinary tract.

Chloride

Normal value: 95 to 105 mEq/L

These levels fluctuate according to the serum sodium levels.

Liver Function Tests

Alkaline phosphatase

Normal value: 1.5 to 4.5 Bodansky Units.

Increase is associated with hepatic obstruction, and in any increase in the osteoblastic activity as in Paget's disease and Cherubism.

Serum albumin

Normal value: 3.5 to 5.0 gm/100 ml

Increase in serum albumin is associated with dehydration. Decrease in serum albumin levels is seen in kidney disorders such as nephritis, chronic glomerulonephritis, gastrointestinal diseases such as ulcerative colitis, and protein losing enteropathy, and liver diseases such as Laennec's cirrhosis and hepatocellular damage secondary to hepatitis.

Serum bilirubin

Normal value:

- Total bilirubin less than 0.8 mg/100 ml
- Direct bilirubin less than 0.5 mg/100 ml
- Indirect bilirubin less than 0.3 mg/100 ml

Bilirubin is an important measure of hepatic function. It is measured in two forms, direct (conjugated) and total (conjugated and unconjugated). The difference between the two represents the unconjugated form.

Serum glutamic oxaloacetic transaminase
Normal value: 10 to 50 mU/ml

Serum glutamic oxaloacetic transaminase (SGOT) levels are elevated in myocardial infarction, hepatitis, cirrhosis and liver neoplasms, hepatic necrosis.

The levels are reduced in beriberi, uncontrolled diabetes mellitus with acidosis.

Serum glutamic pyruvic transaminase

Normal value: 6 to 36 mU/ml

Serum glutamic pyruvic transaminase (SGPT) levels are elevated in myocardial infarction, and liver damage. The levels are more elevated in liver damage.

Serum calcium

Normal values: 8.5 and 10.5 mg/100 ml.

Increased values are associated with excessive osteolysis, as in hyperparathyroidism and malignancies with bone metastasis. Decreased values are associated with hypoparathyroidism, pseudohypoparathyroidism, tetany, hypoalbuminemia, acute pancreatitis, renal failure and starvation.

Serum phosphorus: The normal values for serum phosphorus is between 2.5 and 4.5 mg/100 ml. Increased levels are associated with hypoparathyroidism, pseudohypoparathyroidism, secondary hyperparathyroidism caused by chronic renal failure and metabolic acidosis. Decreased levels are associated with primary hyperparathyroidism, vitamin D deficiency, malabsorption diseases, and chronic antacid usage.

Blood glucose: The normal fasting glucose value is between 65 and 110 mg/100 ml of blood.

The normal postprandial glucose level is 120 to 160 mg/100 ml of blood.

Increased levels are seen in diabetes mellitus, Cushing's syndrome, pancreatitis, and pheochromocytoma. Decreased levels are indicative of hypoglycemia.

Blood gases: Blood gases are measured when there is an altered ventilatory status, hypoxemia, hypocapnia, hypercapnia, and pH disturbances. The parameters measured and their normal values are:

1. Partial pressure of oxygen (PO_2) 80 to 95 mm Hg
2. Oxygen saturation (SaO_2) 93 to 98 percent

3. Partial pressure of CO_2 (PCO_2) 36 to 43 mm Hg
4. Bicarbonate (HCO_3) content 20 to 30 mEq/L
5. Arterial pH 7.35 to 7.45.

Specific Investigations

ELISA for HIV 1 and 2 Antibodies

Enzyme linked immunosorbent assay (ELISA) is used as a screening test for HIV infected patients. Two positive tests by different methods are confirmatory for HIV infection.

Australia Antigen Test

This is a test to detect presence or absence of hepatitis B virus. It was first introduced by Blumberg and his colleagues in 1965. A positive result is indicative of a hepatitis B carrier.

Urine Analysis

Usually 100 ml of the first morning sample is collected in a sterile container.

Normal values

Color and appearance—straw yellow; clear.
Turbidity is indicative of presence of cells and casts.

Specific gravity—1.001 to 1.035
pH: 4.6 to 8.0

Chemical examination
- RBC count: Male — 0 to 3/high power field (HPF)
  Female — 0 to 5/HPF
- WBC count 0 to 4/HPF
- Epithelial cells—occasional
- Hyaline casts—occasional
- Bacteria—none (presence is indicative of urinary tract infection).
- Blood—negative (presence is indicative of trauma, infection, menses, renal stones, transfusion reaction).
- Bilirubin and bile pigments—negative (presence is indicative of hepatitis or obstructive jaundice).
- Glucose—negative (presence is indicative of diabetes mellitus, pancreatitis, shock, coronary thrombosis).
- Ketones—negative (presence is indicative of pregnancy, diabetic ketoacidosis, hyperthyroidism, fever, starvation).
- Proteins—Usually 35 mg of proteins are seen in a 24-hour urine sample. Albumin may normally be

present in the urine. The other proteins that may be excreted in the urine are globulin, Bence Jones protein, mucin and hemoglobin. Bence Jones protein is synthesized in the plasma cells and its presence is indicative of multiple myelomatosis. Presence of hemoglobin is indicative of hemolysis with urinary tract bleeding.

Proteinurea occurs in the following conditions:
- *Prerenal causes:* Postural, severe infections and fever and cerebral injury.
- *Renal:* Glomerulonephritis and diabetic glomerulosclerosis.
- *Postrenal:* Inflammation of the ureter and the urinary bladder.

Bacterial Culture and Antibiotic Sensitivity tests

Cultures can be obtained from the throat, sputum, draining pus, urine or stools. Cultures from the oral cavity can be obtained either by gathering exudative material or by aspiration with a needle and syringe or by use of a swab. A throat or pus culture is obtained by collecting the sample on an autoclaved swab stick. A transport medium must be used when the sample cannot be inoculated immediately onto a primary culture medium. ***For smear and culture in suspected cases of tuberculosis, the sample is sent in normal*** saline. The culture is then grown on any of the various culture media available, for example blood agar or chocolate agar. Antibiotic sensitivity testing evaluates the susceptibility of the isolated pathogenic organism to various antibiotics. The testing is carried out either by agar disc diffusion method, with small paper discs impregnated with the standard concentrations of the antibiotics or by serial dilution method, in tubes containing serial dilutions of various antibiotics.

Histopathological Evaluation

Histopathological evaluation is the final and confirmatory test for a lesion.

Exfoliative Cytology

First introduced by Papanicolaou and Traunt for the detection of uterine cancer. This technique is particularly used for diagnosing lesions of the epithelial surfaces. Scrapings from the surface of the lesion are collected with the help of a wooden spatula and a smear is prepared. The smear is then stained with a suitable stain, like Gram stain, and the cells are studied. This technique is of immense value in diagnosing malignant lesions of the oral cavity.

The study of the cells is reported as falling into one of the five categories:

- *Class 1:* Normal
- *Class 2:* Atypical (presence of minimal atypia but no evidence of malignancy)
- *Class 3:* Intermediate (Wider atypia, that may suggest cancer, but not clear cut)
- *Class 4:* Suggestive of cancer (Few cells with malignant characteristics, many cells with borderline characteristics)
- *Class 5:* Positive for cancer (cells obviously malignant).

Fine Needle Aspiration Cytology

Fine needle aspiration cytology (FNAC) uses a fine needle (23-26G) to aspirate the contents of the lesion. A smear is prepared, stained and studied. This test may not be significant at times.

■ BIOPSY

The term biopsy most often indicates the removal of tissue from a living subject for histological evaluation and analysis. It is important for the clinician to obtain a proper specimen from the lesion for evaluation.

Punch Biopsy

A small part of the lesion is obtained as specimen using a punch. This technique is of particular use in mucosal lesions from inaccessible regions that cannot be reached by conventional methods. The technique produces some amount of crushing or distortion of the tissues.

Incisional Biopsy

When there is a large diffuse lesion, a "representative" section of the lesion is incised with the help of a scalpel along with the normal tissue and sent for histopathological evaluation. The depth of the biopsy should be enough to obtain a representative area of the lesion. Usually an elliptical, wedge-shaped tissue is obtained with the "V" of the wedge converging into the deeper tissues.

Excisional Biopsy

Excisional biopsy is taken if the lesion is extremely small in size. In these cases, the entire lesion is excised in toto at the same sitting and sent for histopathological examination. It is a combination of diagnostic and ablative procedure and is suitable for lesions < 1 cm.

With all the investigations in hand, the clinician has a clear picture of the type, the location, extent and behavior of the lesion. A final diagnosis is then obtained and a suitable medical or surgical line of treatment is decided upon.

■ BIBLIOGRAPHY

1. Daniel M Laskin. Oral and Maxillofacial Surgery, 1st Indian edition, Vol. 1.
2. Goaz, White. Oral Radiology – Principles and Interpretation. 3rd edition.
3. Hutchinson's Clinical Methods. Michael Swash. 19th edition.
4. Killey HC, Seaward GR, Kay LW. An Outline of Oral Surgery. 4th revised reprint Vol. 1.
5. Paul H Kwon, Daniel M Laskin. Clinician's Manual of Oral and Maxillofacial Surgery. 2nd edition.
6. Peterson Ellis, Hupp Sweker. Contemporary Oral and Maxillofacial Surgery. 4th edition.

3 Diagnostic Imaging

Fast moving, fast changing 'Infotech industry' is dominating our lives today. With the new technologies, it is very difficult to keep pace with the latest. There is widespread impact of computers and information technology on health sciences too. A term 'medical informatics' is coined nearly 25 years back. Rapid technological advances in the imaging science and industry have had a significant impact on diagnostic imaging, with the promise of increased accuracy and sensitivity in clinical diagnosis. Imaging science has kept pace with the latest technological developments and has been at the cutting edge of advances in diagnostic science. Scene is changed from the older static imaging (anatomical data) to latest dynamic imaging (pathophysiological data).

W Roentgen's image of the bones of his hand in 1895, made it possible for the surgeons to learn about the internal structures of their patients, by means other than exploratory surgery. The chronicle of the subsequent development of diagnostic radiology is one of improved image technical quality, reduced patient radiation risk and increased differentiation of nonosseous tissues.

The CT scan is the current practical culmination in all three areas. The theoretical basis for computed tomography, i.e. CT was first described by Johann Radon in 1917. In 1969, Godfrey Hounsfield, by introducing first clinical CT scanner technology, revolutionized diagnostic imaging, for which he and Allen Cormack received a Nobel Prize in 1979. After this breakthrough, latest technologies have also further revolutionized diagnostic radiology in the field of maxillofacial surgery. Application of these technical advances has assisted us in (i) the definition of aberrant anatomy, (ii) planning of complex surgical procedures and (iii) evaluating operative results.

In spite of the high costs, there are so many newer diagnostic modalities like ultrasound, scintigraphy, computed tomography (CT), magnetic resonance imaging (MRI), etc. that are now widely used throughout the most affluent countries. The significance of any new information, however, always must be adjudicated in the light of clinical symptoms. From the plethora of these newly available diagnostic imaging modalities, clinicians must select the 'right choice'.

Diagnostic imaging in oral and maxillofacial surgery encompasses a broad range of knowledge, skills and technologies.

Diagnostic imaging procedure involves six distinct elements
1. Source
2. Subject

3. Acquisition
4. Storage/retrieval/transmission/communication
5. Viewing/analysis/display
6. Human element/clinician.

Although in practice all these elements may be implemented in a complex integrated approach, it is important to review them individually for proper selection of imaging modality for a particular patient.

1. *Source*—while choosing the source of imaging, it is very important to know the type of tissue (bony or soft) and the disease. Source also should be selected with the aim of causing minimum damage to human subject and environment.
   a. Tissue and disease—selective energy band.
   b. Minimizing damage to human subject and environment.
2. *Subject*
   a. Better understanding of how a given energy source interacts with normal or abnormal tissues, organs, etc.
   b. Early diagnosis without compromising the specificity/sensitivity.
3. *Acquisition*
   a. More accurate, sensitive and robust image receptors.
   b. Cost, long term market stability, compatibility and availability of the equipment is also an important factor.
4. *Storage/retrieval/transmission/communication*
   a. Reliability, security, cost
   b. Universal and system dependent exchange of information
5. *Viewing/analysis/display*
   a. Uniform quality across all outpatient devices.
   b. Advanced imaging, approaches for image enhancement, analysis, modeling and visualization.
6. *Human element—clinician*
   a. Keep pace with ever changing field.
   b. Selection of optimal tool for diagnostic task.
   c. Going beyond visual diagnosis.

A typical source of excitation/illumination for diagnostic imaging includes a selective band of electromagnetic waves, generated externally or internally with respect to human subject. The interaction of this energy source and human tissue is the most critical parameter in the selection of the appropriate modality for a given diagnostic task. Selection of an image acquisition system then becomes a function of the first two elements. Once the image has been acquired,

it can be stored for future retrieval and communication or immediately viewed and analyzed by the clinician. All the above-mentioned six elements have to address several technical and clinical challenges in a given clinical set-up.

Imaging has two roles
1. The identification of an abnormality in terms of presence, site, size and nature (if possible).
2. Provision of information necessary for decision, for planning of surgical or other treatment.
   The imaging objectives—depend on many factors
   A. 1. The amount/type of information required.
      2. The time period of the treatment rendered.
   B. Decision will depend upon integration of the above factors.
      1. When to image?
      2. Which imaging modality to use?
      3. Design a procedure specific to the patient's clinical needs.
   C. To define the precise extent of the lesion than to make specific diagnosis.

FUNDAMENTAL TENET OF IMAGING MODALITY

1. To yield maximum accurate diagnostic information.
2. To maximize benefit/risk ratio.

The imaging modality is chosen, not necessary, because it costs the least or produces the lowest radiation exposure or is available in the vicinity.

DIAGNOSTIC IMAGING—AS LOW AS REASONABLE ACHIEVABLE PRINCIPLE

As low as reasonably achievable (ALARA) for X-ray exposure.

SELECTION OF IMAGING MODALITY

- Improved technical image quality
- Reduced patient radiation risk
- Increased differentiation of nonosseous tissue

The Goal 'Gold standard' of imaging modalities:
- To develop a 'virtual operative environment'
- To preview patient's anatomy in both two and three-dimensional formats
- To analyze and measure the patient's deviation from normal

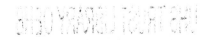

- To simulate an optimized and practical operative solution before surgery
- To have more accurate method of intraoperative navigation and measurements
- Efficient and accurate transfer of information
- Accurate documentation and quantification of the lesion.

We have to understand that 'the complex architecture of the facial skeleton and its contents have created a challenge to the surgeon to find a surgical access and to the radiologist to image'. *No other anatomic region in the body has got such a complexity. The complexity of the facial architecture is not only due to the multiplicity of its components, but also to the intricacy of their geometric relationships.*

The imaging modalities are broadly classified into two groups:

1. ***Invasive or interventional imaging:*** This is rapidly changing technology, mostly used for diagnostic, therapeutic and curative purposes.

   Examples—embolization, delivery of cytotoxic drugs, calculus destruction, angiography, angioplasty, etc.

2. ***Noninvasive imaging***
   - Plain conventional radiography
   - Magnetic resonance imaging (MRI)
   - Radionuclide studies—scintigraphy—bone scan
   - Ultrasonography (USG)
   - Computed tomography

We will be discussing noninvasive imaging modalities used in oral and maxillofacial surgical field (Tables 3.1 to 3.3).

Table 3.1: X-ray and nuclear medicine imaging both use ionizing radiation	
X-ray imaging	*Nuclear medicine imaging*
Produced by differential absorption of X-rays by the body tissue	Obtained by mapping the distribution of radioactivity of an injected body tissue radionuclide within the body.
Depicts anatomic architecture of bone	Reflects physiologic status to assess viability, vascularity and metabolic activity of bone.
Often insensitive until pathology is well-established.	Ability to detect early physiological changes. Metabolic alteration at 5–10% level can be detected within 48 hours.
At least 30–50% of mineral content change is required.	
Can be detected after 10 days–3 weeks	

Table 3.2: Advantages of MRI versus CT scan	
MRI	*CT scan*
Noninvasive—no ionizing radiation	Large radiation dose
Vessels shown without IV contrast	IV contrast necessary for soft tissue, blood vessels enhancement
Direct multiplanar easy imaging	Axial images reformatting requires large radiation
High soft tissue contrast reduction	
Safe procedure	
Can be repeated again following previous studies	

Table 3.3: Advantages of CT versus MRI	
CT scan	*MRI*
Widely available in most countries	A scarce resource in many countries
No claustrophobia	Long time—claustrophobia, discomfort
Few restrictions	Very expensive
Less expensive than MRI	Restrictions—metal implants, pace makers, intraocular foreign bodies, ferromagnetic clips, neurostimulator units
	Motion—image suffers

Plain Conventional Radiography

Plain conventional radiography is a versatile diagnostic tool.

Shortfalls

- Two-dimensional record of three-dimensional object
- Superimposition of various structures above and below, in the pathway of X-ray in the region of interest.
- Requires multiple projections
- Difficult to detect subtle pathology or trauma
- Limited value, poor understanding of the relationship of normal to abnormal structures.

That is why, traditional conventional radiography is being replaced by the newer modalities for their obvious advantages.

Magnetic Resonance Imaging (Figs 3.1 to 3.8)

- In 1946, Block and Purcell described the phenomenon of magnetic resonance and won the Nobel Prize in 1952
- In 1972, Lauterbur used it for the first-time for medical imaging
- Most innovative, noninvasive technique
- Magnetic resonance imaging (MRI) is considered as cornerstone of medical imaging
- It employs radiofrequency radiation in the presence of carefully controlled magnetic fields

- It produces high quality cross-sectional images of the body in any plane
- New MRI scanner designs bring about motion and fat suppression, which can achieve faster scan sequences
- Addition of surface coils improves resolution and decreases scan time
- MRI shows superior soft tissue contrast

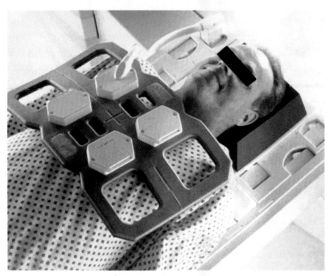

Fig. 3.2A: Surface coils

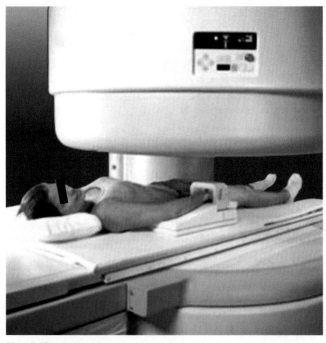

Fig. 3.2B: Open MRI machine. Most MRI machines have a long tunnel, which can lead to discomfort and a sense of claustrophobia. An 'Open MRI' is a 'C' shaped machine, which is open on three sides. This makes the entire procedure very comfortable without claustrophobia

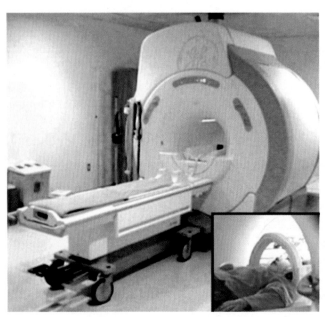

Fig. 3.1: An old MRI scanner machine

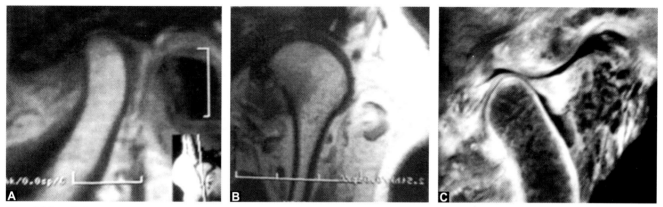

Figs 3.3A to C: (A) Normal temporomandibular joint (TMJ) MRI scan image in sagittal view, (B) Normal TMJ MRI scan image in coronal view, (C) Dissection of normal TMJ region (anatomy specimen)

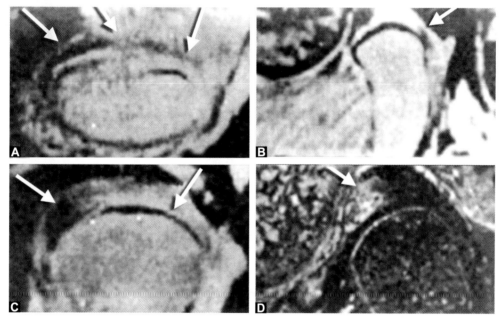

Figs 3.4A to D: Comparison of MRI of normal TMJ with cryosection of the same specimen. (A) Axial scan, (B) Sagittal scan, (C) Coronal scan of TMJ showing normal position of the disk in all planes, (D) Cryosection confirms the findings of the MRI scan

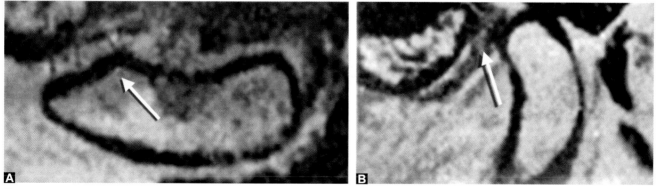

Figs 3.5A and B: MRI axial and sagittal view: (A) Axial view of (L) TMJ gives the information, that there is a flattening of anterior aspect of the condyle and presence of osteophyte (arrow), (B) Sagittal view of (L) TMJ shows slightly anteriorly placed disk (arrow). Osteophyte is not seen in this view

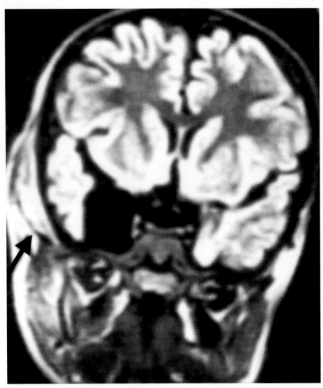

Fig. 3.6: MRI scan for 4-year-old male child shows the involvement of infratemporal space due to odontogenic infection (arrow)

- Easier multiplanar imaging
- Sensitivity and accuracy of 100 percent in detecting small tumors
- IV contrast increases sensitivity
- Modality of choice for nasopharynx, tongue, skull base pathology.
- Decreases the artifact scatter seen in CT due to dental fillings, metallic crowns, etc.

Limitations of MRI

- Inability to image bone due to lack of signal from cortical bone
- Knowledge of normal MR anatomy is necessary, for detection of pathology and interpretation
- Motion artifacts due to long-time procedures.

Though in India, MRI is not very popular in the field of maxillofacial surgery, mainly because of nonavailability and high cost factor, its best application is in the evaluation of the TMJ disk deformities (Figs 3.3A to C).

The standard plane of MRI used to study TMJ disk deformities is usually sagittal plane (Figs 3.4 and 3.5). It can be also used for evaluation of various spaces of head and neck region.

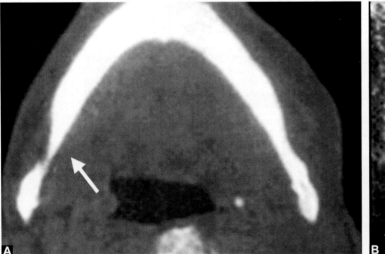
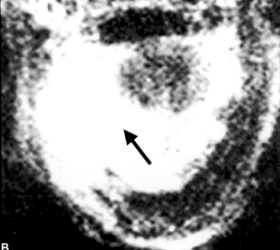

Figs 3.7A and B: MRI gives indication of the soft tissue growth which can be missed in CT scan: (A) CT scan for (R) mandibular retromolar area was declared as negative involvement, (B) MRI scan for the same patient gives positive imaging of the retromolar area with soft tissue growth seen (arrow). Biopsy report proved as squamous cell carcinoma

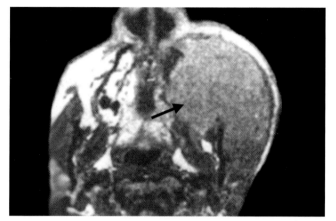

Fig. 3.8: MRI scan of the (L) maxillary sinus showing tumor

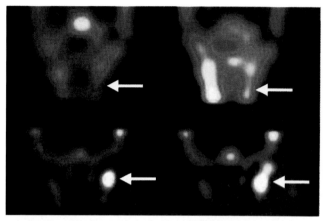

Fig. 3.10: Bone scan of the skull showing malignant tissue in the bone, not detected by other imaging modalities

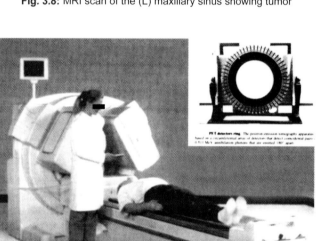

Fig. 3.9: Spect rotating camera system. A modern triple-headed gamma camera with a scanning couch. The heads are mounted on a rotating gantry and can be moved into a variety of geometrics

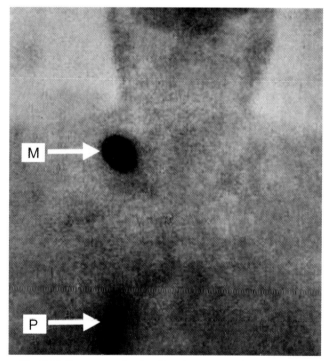

Fig. 3.11: Bone scan showing P—primary tumor, M—metastasis

Radionuclide Bone/Skeletal Scan or Scintigraphy (Figs 3.9 to 3.16)

- Radionuclide ^{99m}Technetium labeled phosphate (^{99m}Tc-P)
- First introduced by Subramanian and Macfee—1971
- IV injection in small, safe amounts of radioactive elements, such as ^{99m}Tc-P or ^{67}Gallium is used
- Highly sensitive to blood flow and metabolic activity of bone tissue
- Accumulation within the skeleton. Fifty percent deposition is seen in one hour
- Remainder of the radioactive element, disperses in the soft tissues
- It is excreted via the urinary tract

- After the injection, patient is encouraged to drink several glasses of water and encouraged to go for frequent micturation
- This type of hydration reduces the radiation and accelerates the soft tissue clearance and enhances image quality of skeleton, at the end of two/four hours after the injection
- Uptake of the radionuclide is monitored with a gamma or single photon emission computed tomographic (SPECT) imaging camera or scintillation camera

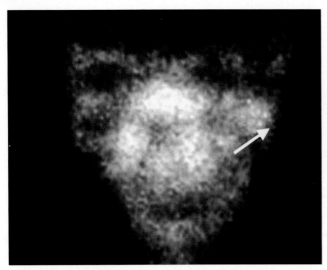

Fig. 3.12: Scintigraphy showing hot lesion in (L) TMJ area for the case of (L) TMJ ankylosis

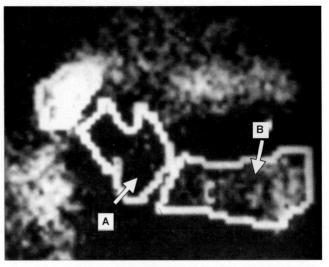

Fig. 3.14: Bone scan of (R) mandibular body after reconstruction with bone graft. A—bone graft rejection, B—viable bone graft

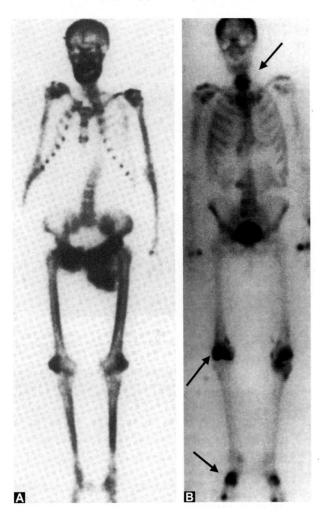

Figs 3.13A and B: Full body scintigraphy: (A) Anterior, (B) Posterior projections showing anterior and posterior structures

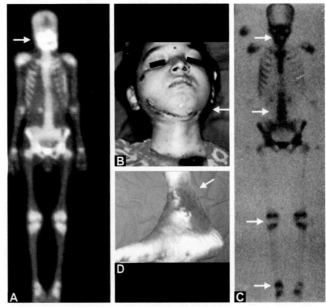

Figs 3.15A to D: Tuberculous osteomyelitis of the bone. An 18-year-old girl with multiple draining sinuses, involving the jaw bone and sternum: (A) Bone scan showing "hot spots" in the jaws, (B) Clinical picture. Four months later, after the start of AKT drugs, patient stopped the medication on her own, (C) Follow-up bone scan with hot spots in the mandible, vertebra, sternum and ankle joint, (D) Two months later patient came back with sinuses at the ankle. The changes were detected early in the bone scan

- In SPECT camera, detectors can rotate 360° around the patient, acquiring up to 128 images in different angulations
- 3D or surface displays are also possible
- Record of radioactivity is shown in the form of images

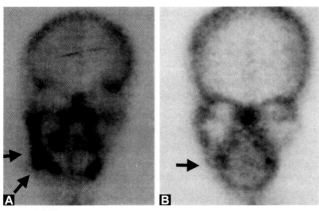

Figs 3.16A and B: Tuberculous osteomyelitis of the (R) mandible: (A) Bone scan showing hot spot, (B) Bone scan showing cold spot after six months AKT drugs

- Tracer uptake record can be seen on computer monitor
- Accuracy of bone scan is now compared to MRI
- But bone scan provides information at very low cost.

Indications of Scintigraphy

1. Dynamic method—for growth assessment of facial skeleton. Comparison of uptake can be done in paired structures
2. To identify skeletal metastases in early stage
3. To survey the presence of occult lesion
4. To locate the presence or extent of multiple osseous lesions
5. To diagnose the presence of neoplasm—benign/malignant
6. To locate abnormal metabolism or growth in the skeleton/jaw bone
7. To assess cessation of growth and fix the time for corrective surgery
8. To study the fate of bone grafts—rejection, vascularity, viability, uptake, etc.

Areas of tracer uptake are known as hot lesions, which suggest normal bone growth, bone stress, repair, osteoblastic activity, increased vascularity, new bone formation, etc.

Cold lesions—are suggestive of decreased metabolic activity, metastases, infection, radiation therapy, vascular compromise, etc.

Clinical Applications

1. Inflammation/infection—osteomyelitis, avascular necrosis
2. Neoplasms—primary bone tumors, osteosarcoma, Ewing's sarcoma, metastasis detection/therapy,

follow-up for early indication of recurrence in the stump
3. Metabolic disorders
4. TMJ afflictions
5. Bone graft follow-up.

Advantages of Scintigraphy

- ^{99m}Tc is easily available
- Inexpensive, noninvasive
- Low radiation dosage
- No adverse effects
- Painless, safe procedure
- High proton yield
- Short-time is required—ideal for children
- No special preparation is required.

Ultrasonography (Figs 3.17 to 3.23)

Ultrasonography (USG) is the refinement of wartime naval sonar system. Used extensively in central nervous system, cardiovascular system, for internal organ studies, (kidney, spleen, etc.), by gynecologists, etc.

3D sonography, color Doppler ultrasonography can be used to assess the flow in the large vessels. Ultrasonography diagnostic imaging system uses high frequencies and a large transducer. Ultrasound generated from transducer penetrates the organ to be imaged. Ultrasound (US) waves emitted from the surface and the skin and body-internal organs reflect incident wave. Ultrasound (US) system receives the reflected wave, calculates the information and forms images. It is sensitive in detecting fluid collection.

Advantages

- Noninvasive
- Economical
- Painless
- Quick
- No adverse reaction
- Mobile equipment—bedside access
- Easier repeatability
- Low cost of storage.

Limitations

- A detailed knowledge of sonostructure is required for interpretation
- Operator dependent
- Bone does not transmit sound—limited use.

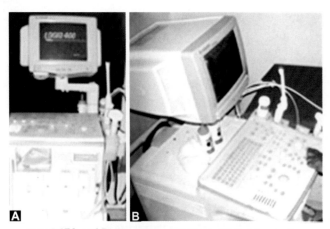

Figs 3.17A and B: The ultrasound diagnostic imaging system

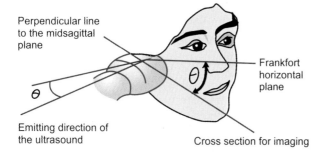

Perpendicular line to the midsagittal plane

Frankfort horizontal plane

Emitting direction of the ultrasound

Cross section for imaging

Fig. 3.18: A transducer application to the facial region for USG

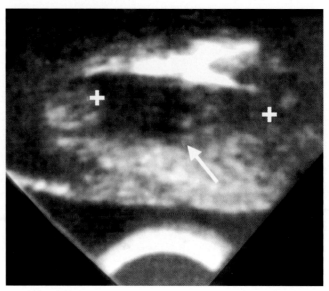

Fig. 3.20: Ultrasonography of parotid gland abscess. Unsharp borders, weak echo and irregular structure

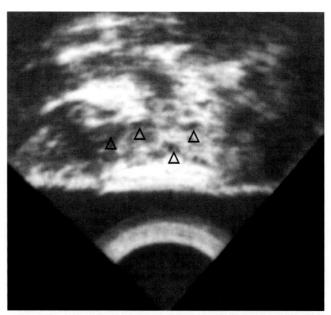

Fig. 3.21: Chronic recurrent sialoadenitis. Small cystic areas are seen

Ultrasonography Procedure

A transducer converts electrical energy into high frequency sound waves, which pass into the tissues of different densities. The vibrational energy is reflected back to the scanning transducer, where the sound waves are converted to images, which are displayed on a monitor.

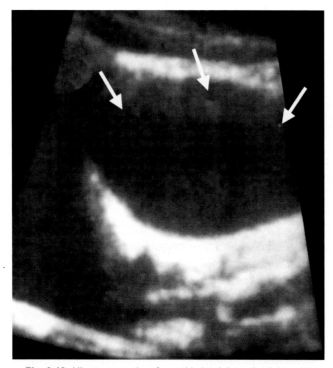

Fig. 3.19: Ultrasonography of parotid gland. Intraglandular cyst. Sharply bordered echo free area

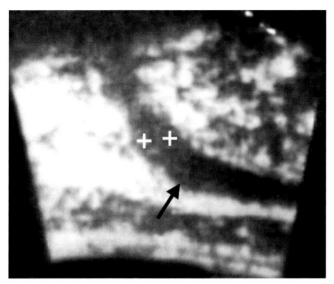

Fig. 3.22: Ultrasound (US) parotid gland duct, intraductal calculus is seen—++, Arrow—efferent duct is dilated

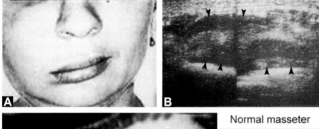

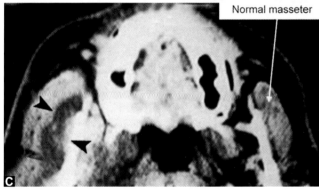

Normal masseter

Figs 3.23A to C: Comparison of ultrasonography and CT scan in facial space infection, (A) Facial swelling on right cheek, (B) Ultrasound (US) scan performed along right mandible. Fluid collection is indicated by hypoechoic area, which is superficial to mandible and just below the masseter muscle. Ultrasound (US) is very sensitive in detecting fluid collection. It is quick and inexpensive. It can be used to diagnose a stage of infection, (Cellulitis or abscess formation), (C) CT scan confirms well defined abscess in submasseteric space

Application

*   Widely used to detect cervical lymph node metastasis
*   Examination of various masses in the neck including abscesses and diseases of salivary glands.

*   Aids in differentiation of solid and cystic masses
*   Valuable for guided aspiration and biopsy.

Computed Tomographic Scan (Figs 3.24 to 3.34)

Computed tomographic scan (CT scan) is considered as 'gold standard' today. The introduction of computerized tomographic scanning technology revolutionized diagnostic radiology, not only because of improved visualization of complex bony anatomy without superimposition, but also because of high contrast dis-crimination of soft tissues.

CT Scan

*   Landmark technique
*   Tomo—slice, graphy—picture
*   Gives cross-sectional information (axial)
*   Allows evaluation of soft tissue and bony structure.

Techniques

*   Plain studies without contrast
*   Simple v/s high resolution
*   Contrast enhanced studies
*   Reconstructions—coronal, sagittal.

Newer Advanced Softwares for CT Scans

*   3D CT—with or without disarticulation of individual bone, rotation in any angle is possible
*   Dental CT—dentascan
*   Multiplanar realtime reconstructions
*   Spiral CT—ultrafast electron gun CT
*   CT angiography
*   Circular, spiral, hypocycloidal are the tube motions employed.

Advantages

*   No special patient preparation
*   Very good speed, quick imaging, reduced patient motion artefact
*   Exact contiguity of images
*   Emergencies, trauma patients, children, oncology—very helpful. Scan time is less than one minute, transfer of information is in few seconds—display in 5 minutes.

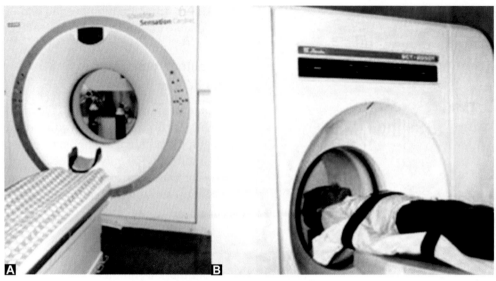

Figs 3.24A and B: CT scan machine

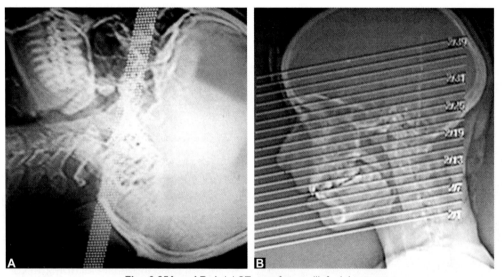

Figs 3.25A and B: Axial CT scan for maxillofacial area

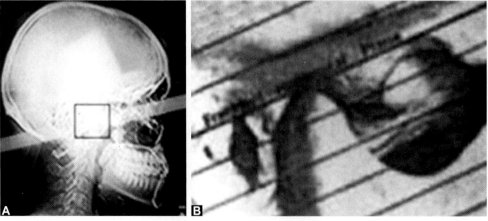

Figs 3.26A and B: Axial CT scan for TMJ

Disadvantages

- Requires a co-operative patient
- Respiratory motion or body motion—degradation of the image

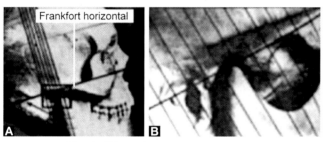

Figs 3.27A and B: Vertical scan for TMJ

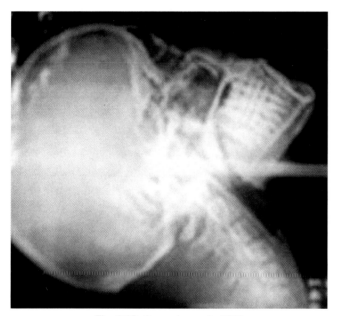

Fig. 3.28: Coronal scan for TMJ

- Medical radiation burden
- Allergic reaction to contrast medium.

The theoretical basis for computed tomography CT began almost 70 to 80 years back. In 1971, Hounsfield's first practical scanner was used for clinical application. In 1973, first scanner in USA generated CT scans of the brain. 1975 onwards rapid improvements in computer soft and hardware allowed widespread use of second and third generation machines. CT uses X-rays to perform it's work. These X-rays come from an X-ray tube, which is placed inside a square machine called the gantry. The part of the patient's body to be scanned goes inside a hole in this gantry. The standard format of the CT scan which is obtained is in axial plane.

Acquisition of Axial CT Scan

Very young patients are lightly sedated and body of the patient is stabilized by strapping. High resolution of axial CT scans with 5 mm axial slices with 4 mm feed from the angle of the mandible to the squamous temporal bone without tilting the gantry (horizontal or zero degree angulation). This will cover the entire maxillofacial area. 2D reconstruction scans are thus recorded on double density floppy and transferred to an independent CT scan viewing console.

Record maintenance: These images are stored on radiographic films or they can be photographed from the monitor screen. CT scans records are kept on 14" x 17" sheets of films, with a multiformat camera, in a 20 images on one format. The patient's name, age, date of examination, etc. are marked on each image.

This standard format of the CT scan (axial images) with restricted orientation and sequential multiple images is abstract, in areas of anatomic complexity and

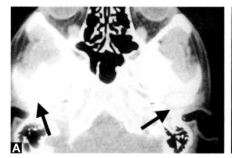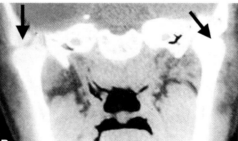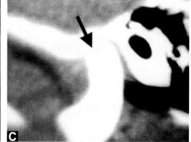

Figs 3.29A to C: (A) Axial CT scan of both normal condyles, (B) Coronal scan for both normal condyles, (C) Sagittal CT scan of (L) condyle in closed mouth position

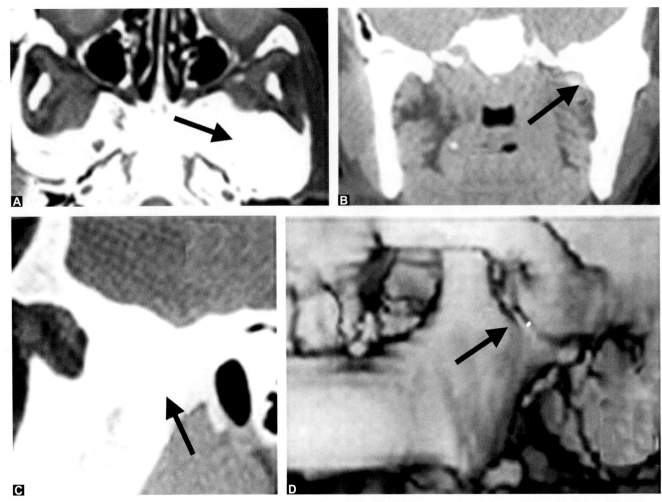

Figs 3.30A to D: (A) Axial CT scan, (B) Coronal CT scan, (C) Sagittal scan, (D) 3D CT scan. All showing ankylosis of (L) temporomandibular joint

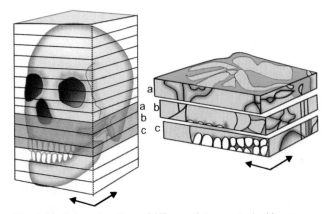

Fig. 3.31: Sequential slices of CT scan data are stacked layer upon layer for obtaining 3D information (3D CT scan)

needs an interpreter, i.e. diagnostic radiologist. These images bear no direct resemblance to the findings of either physical examination or surgery. Axial sections are not optimal, because of the following:

1. Sections lie parallel to the large part of the surfaces of interest.
2. Can miss the areas of interest.
3. During actual surgery, the surfaces exposed, never oriented axially.

Coronal sections are better

1. Requires additional scan time and radiation exposure
2. Coronal view corresponds to the angle of vision used for the clinical examination of the patient

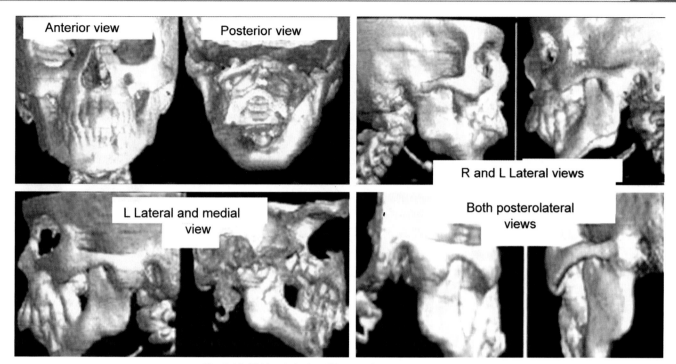

Fig. 3.32: TMJ ankylosis—3D scan pictures in various views

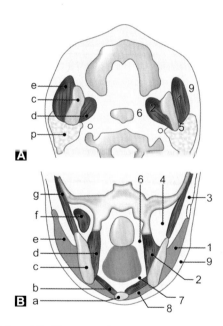

Figs 3.33A and B: Diagrammatic representation of (A) Axial and (B) Coronal images. a—hyoid, b—mylohyoid muscle, c—mandible, d—medial pterygoid muscle, e—masseter muscle, f—lateral pterygoid muscle, g—temporalis muscle, p—parotid gland. 1—masseteric region, 2—medial pterygoid region, 3—superficial temporal region, 4—deep temporal region, 5—parotid space, 6—parapharyngeal space, 7—sublingual space, 8—submandibular space, 9—adipose tissue lateral to masseter

Sagittal sections are also taken, whenever indicated for additional information.

Recently a new system stacks 2D slices sequentially and 3D information can be obtained from routine CT data. The introduction of 3D image display has provided a method of object analysis in three planes of space, obviating the need for mental reconstructions and yielding more spatial information than was previously available.

In 1979, Artzy, Herman and Liu described the technique and in 1982, Marsh and Vannier put forward a program of computer graphics for the production of 3D images from 2D data.

Conceptually, when sequential slices of CT scan data are 'stacked layer upon layer', a three-dimensional matrix of digital information representing the scanned object, results. These images can be rotated, split and anatomic structures can be separated and individual images of different tissue types can be generated. 3D image display data are obtained from high resolution axial computed tomographic scans. HIQ Siemen's scanners can be used. 3D program is located in a second independent console. The Siemen's software program accepts 2D high resolution CT scan data as input and produces a set of 3D reconstruction images

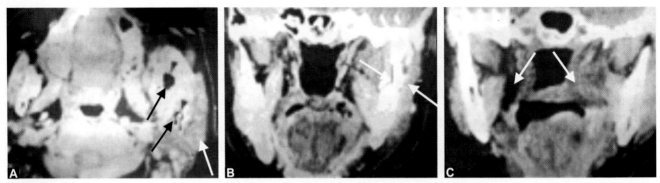

Figs 3.34A to C: CT scan for facial space involvement due to infection: (A) Axial image of (L) parotid (white arrow) and masseteric infection (black arrow indicating fluctuant areas of pus formation), (B and C) Coronal image showing involvement of (L) medial pterygoid region and parapharyngeal space due to odontogenic infection

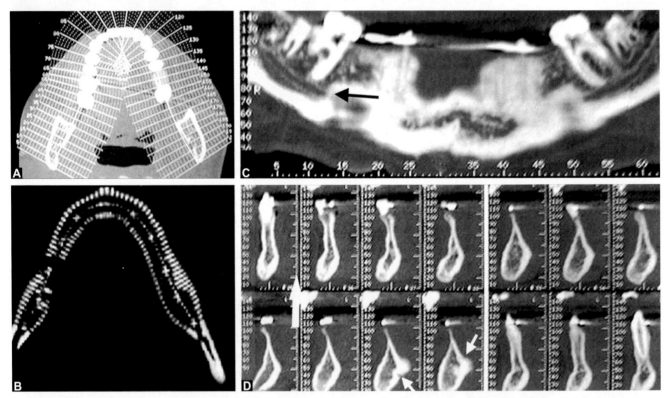

Figs 3.35A to D: Dentascan using specialized software. (A) Axial view of maxilla, (B) Axial view of mandible, (C) Panoramic dentascan reconstruction, (D) Cross sectional images perpendicular to alveolar process of the mandible taken for location of mandibular nerve

as output. Depending on the number of piled sections, the acquisition reconstruction time varies around 20 minutes. The 3D images recorded on 14" x 14" sheets in 8 to 10 on one format or they can be stored on the CD or printed on paper.

The 3D reconstruction images produced, resemble photographs of a skull. This program computes mainly four contours—frontal, rear and both lateral orientations.

Rotation of the original scan data by a selected angle (0° to 90°) permits the reconstruction surfaces from oblique projections and thereby disclosing regions, which are inaccessible to other radiographic procedures.

Several outstanding features make this technique a very useful asset

1. Surgeons can readily assimilate complex anatomic relationships from these images, which look like anatomic dissections.
2. It delineates the abnormal bony morphology.
3. Gives correct representation of the size of the structure to be reviewed, it's relative position and it's relations to other structures and also gives idea about unilateral or bilateral involvement of the lesion, etc.
4. Easy interpretation, efficient in computer line and storage.
5. 3D reconstruction is simple, since preselection views are automatically generated.
6. Facilitates surgical planning.
7. Reduction in operating time.
8. Lesion can be accurately documented and quantified (yields true life-size images).
9. Can be used for quantitative postoperative evaluation and follow-up.
10. Very helpful as effective tool for communication.
11. Excellent teaching aid for the institutions.
12. Radiation exposure does not exceed that of conventional radiography. Radiation is minimum, as pencil beam is used. Minimum secondary radiation.

Dentascan software program (Figs 3.35A to D): The technique of 'Dental CT' also called 'Dentascan' was developed by Schwarz et al in 1987, when they used curved multiplanar reconstructions of the jaw.

The term 'Dental CT' does not represent a particular modality, but rather a specific investigation protocol. The main features of this protocol include the acquisition of axial scans of the jaw with the highest possible resolution together with curved and orthoradial multiplanar reconstructions.

Dental CT has become an established method for imaging of jaw anatomy prior to dental implant placement. In axial plane, the metal artifacts from tooth fillings are kept in the occlusal plane and hence the jaw bone remains undistorted (Unlike medical CT Scan). This allows for accurate display of the vertical as well as the important buccolingual dimensions of the jaw in actual 1:1 life size. The anatomy of the alveolar ridge along with the quality and quantity of bone at the proposed sites of implant placements also can be assessed. Vertical bone height and horizontal bone width can be measured easily from point to point. Selection of the proper length and diameter of the implant can be easily done. Life-sized cross-sectional and/or panoramic images can be obtained.

4 Management of Medically Compromised Patients in Oral Surgery

Knowledge regarding the patient's medical condition is of utmost importance, in patient management and care, pre- and post-surgically. A detailed medical history (as described in chapter 2) will give the practitioner all the necessary and relevant information regarding the patient's general condition as well as physical status.

■ CLASSIFICATION OF PHYSICAL STATUS

In 1962, the American Society of Anesthesiologists (ASA) adopted the ASA Physical Classification. This classification identifies the medical risk to a patient undergoing a surgical procedure. The classification is as follows:

ASA I : A patient without systemic disease; a normal, healthy patient

ASA II : A patient with mild systemic disease

ASA III : A patient with severe systemic disease, that limits activity, but is not incapacitating

ASA IV : A patient with incapacitating systemic disease, that is a constant threat to life

ASA V : A moribund patient not expected to survive 24 hours with or without surgery

ASA E : Emergency operation of any kind, E precedes the ASA number, indicating the patient's physical status

Cardiac Diseases

Although all types of cardiac diseases are at high risk of serious complications, when undergoing surgical procedures under general anesthesia, certain conditions like unstable angina, congestive cardiac failure, valvular septal defects, and myocardial infarction increase the risk four-folds. A history of bypass, angioplasty or valve replacement is of significant importance. Although cardiac disease is not an absolute contraindication, the surgeon should weigh the benefits against the risks, before deciding the choice of anesthesia.

Preoperative Investigations

1. Chest radiograph—posteroanterior view
2. Electrocardiogram
3. Echocardiogram
4. Stress test
5. Blood investigations like lipid profile and bleeding time, clotting time and prothrombin time and index (INR), in case the patient is on long term anti-coagulants.

Preoperative Medication

If the patient is a case of rheumatic heart disease or has undergone valve replacements, a suitable antibiotic prophylaxis must be given. If the patient is on injection Penidura every three weeks, the surgery should be scheduled immediately after the scheduled dose to reduce the risk of infective endocarditis.

Intra- and Postoperative Management

1. All the patients should be monitored intra and post-operatively by means of an ECG, pulse oximeter, and arterial line.
2. A central venous pressure (CVP) cut down may be performed, if necessary.
3. The patient should be maintained on intravenous cardiac drugs till oral feeds are given.
4. Fluid overload should be avoided, especially in cases of congestive cardiac failure. The fluid volume can be judged by the CVP.

Management of the patients, who are on long term anticoagulant and antiplatelet drugs: For the prevention and management of arterial and venous thrombosis (intravascular clot), many patients are advised to take antiplatelet/anticoagulant drugs on long term basis. As per the current information, the patients will have potential precipitation of a thromboembolic event, in case the anticoagulant therapy is withdrawn. There is no need to withdraw the anticoagulant drugs, for non-surgical or minor surgical dental procedures.

If the patient's international normalized ratio (INR) and prothrombin time ratio (PTR) values are within the current recommended therapeutic range. The minor incidents of local postoperative bleeding should be managed with adequate measures.

In case, if PTR and INR values are not within permissible therapeutic levels, then the patient should be shifted to intravenous anticoagulants like heparin.

Indications for Prescribing Anticoagulant Drugs

- Deep vein thrombosis (DVT)
- Pulmonary embolism
- Rheumatic heart disease (RHD) and arterial fibrillation (AF)
- Prosthetic heart valve replacement
- Coronary artery disease (CAD)—myocardial infarction and unstable angina
- Cerebrovascular accidents (CVA)—stroke
  (The use of warfarin in CAD and CVA is controversial).

Oral Anticoagulant Drugs

Coumarins and Indandiones. Acenocoumarol-Acitrom-1, 2, 3, and 4 mg tabs, dicoumarol 50 mg tabs, phenindione, warfarin-uniwarfarin 1, 2, and 5 mg tabs.

Oral anticoagulant drug acts by interfering/antagonizing with the synthesis of vitamin K-dependent clotting factors in the liver (Factors II, VII, IX, and X). Their effect does not become apparent, until the body's existing supplies of prothrombin and other factors mentioned above have been exhausted. Similarly on withdrawal, the anticoagulant activity will not disappear, until the liver has once again produced these factors.

Protocols for Treating the Patients on Anticoagulants

1. Proper history—drug dosage, status of medical condition, PTR and INR level.
2. Proper antibiotic cover.
3. Schedule the appointment within 2 days, once desired range of PTR and INR
   A. PTR 1.5 to 2 and INR 2.0 to 3.0—do not stop or alter the drug dosage
   B. PTR 2.0 to 2.5 and INR 2.5 to 3.5—dosage may be altered
   C. PTR > 2.5 and INR > 3.5—delay invasive procedure, until dosage is decreased.
   Physicians should be consulted regarding the dosage modification.
4. Confirm status of PTR and INR on the day of surgery.
5. Use atraumatic surgical technique. Control postoperative bleeding by local measures.
6. Patients anticoagulant dosage can be regulated back in 48 to 72 hours in consultation with physician.

Antiplatelet Drugs

Aspirin—Colisprin, Ecosprin 75/150 mg tabs; dipyridamole, clopidogrel 75 mg tabs, ticlopidine 250 mg tabs.

These drugs irreversibly acetylate and inhibit the enzyme cyclo-oxygenase in the platelets, thus preventing thromboxane A_2 (TXA_2) synthesis by the platelets and altering platelet function—mainly platelet aggregation. This results in prevention of platelet plug formation and increased bleeding time (BT). These drugs are used in CAD-post MI and in unstable angina, CVA, coronary artery bypass grafting (CABG).

Dose Regulation

Prior to oral surgical procedures, two laboratory tests for screening the patients on oral antiplatelet drugs should be carried out.

i. The Platelet Function Analyzer 100 (PFA 100)—normal value 60 to 120 seconds.

ii. The Ivy Bleeding Time (Ivy BT)—normal value 1 to 6 minutes.

If Ivy BT is more than 20 minutes, then only clinically significant postoperative bleeding is expected. In that case, the Aspirin can be discontinued for 3 to 5 days, which will allow new platelets in sufficient numbers to arrive into the circulation. The life cycle of platelets is 8 to 10 days.

Hypertension

Hypertension is considered to be the elevation of the blood pressure greater than 140/90 mm of mercury.

Uncontrolled hypertension can have the following surgical and anesthetic complications:

1. It reflects on the cardiac status of the patient, thereby increasing the anesthetic risk to the patient.
2. It causes excessive bleeding from the operation site, thereby complicating the surgical procedure, as well as significant blood loss for the patient.

Preoperative Investigations

1. Chest radiograph—posteroanterior view for detecting cardiac enlargement
2. ECG
3. USG of the kidneys
4. Ophthalmic evaluation for papilledema and retinal hemorrhage
5. Renal function tests (blood urea nitrogen, serum creatinine and serum electrolyte).

Preoperative Medication and Management

The patient's blood pressure should be monitored and controlled within the normal permissible limits, prior to the surgical procedure. If the patient is on antihypertensives, the morning dose of medication prior to surgery must be given with sips of water.

Intra- and Postoperative Management

1. The blood pressure should be monitored continuously intra- and postoperatively.
2. The patient's cardiac status should also be monitored on the ECG machine and on the pulse oximeter.

3. Antihypertensives must be continued intra- and postoperatively.
4. If the patient is on diuretics, the patient must be supplemented postoperatively with intravenous potassium supplements.
5. If the procedure is performed under local anesthesia, then local anesthetic without adrenaline or bupivacaine, which does not have any significant effect on the cardiac status is to be used.

Respiratory Diseases

Respiratory diseases can be categorized into obstructive and infiltrative pulmonary diseases. Obstructive pulmonary diseases include, chronic obstructive pulmonary conditions like asthma, chronic bronchitis, pneumothorax and emphysema. Infiltrative diseases are inclusive of diseases that cause inflammatory changes in the alveolar walls. Any respiratory disease is first characterized by dyspnea.

The patient with decrease in the pulmonary reserve poses a great risk for procedures under general anesthesia. The patients should be asked for a thorough history of *beedi*/cigarette smoking as well as past history of tuberculosis. If the patient is suffering from tuberculosis, then details of his drug regimen and duration of treatment is asked. From the surgeon's point of view, the most important aspect is the patient's respiratory reserve and his ability to tolerate general anesthesia. If the patient is treated under local anesthesia, the bronchodilator inhaler should be kept ready for use in case of an emergency.

Preoperative Investigations

1. Chest radiograph—posteroanterior view
2. Pulmonary function tests
3. Blood investigations like arterial blood gases
4. Sputum AFB/Culture
5. Bronchoscopy, if required.

The patient should be counseled to discontinue *beedi*/cigarette smoking prior to the procedure. Any acute infection should be treated by antibiotics. The patient should be on bronchodilators pre, intra, and postoperatively. The patient must carry inhaler for use in case of an emergency.

Intra- and Postoperative Management

1. Arterial blood gas monitoring should also be carried out intra- and postoperatively.
2. Avoid fluid overload.

3. Blood loss should be replaced by whole blood or packed cells to avoid decrease in the oxygen carrying capacity of blood.

Renal Diseases

Patients with renal diseases like renal failure, acute glomerulonephritis, nephrotic syndrome, pose a significant surgical risk. Disturbances in the renal function leads to changes in the acid-base balance, serum calcium and phosphorus levels, fluid retention, and electrolyte concentration. A patient with chronic infection may develop sepsis postoperatively. These patients also have associated hypertension secondary to fluid retention and anemia.

Preoperative Investigations

1. Renal profile—blood urea nitrogen (BUN), serum creatinine, serum electrolytes
2. Creatinine clearance test
3. Serum calcium and phosphorus
4. Urine analysis—physical and microscopic
5. USG of the kidneys
6. Renal Doppler studies
7. Radionuclide scanning for renal clearance time.

Intra- and Postoperative Management

1. Fluid balance, acid-base balance and electrolyte balance, must be closely monitored.
2. Renal profile tests must be performed intra as well as postoperatively.
3. Blood replacement is done by washed packed cells
4. Potassium overload during fluid replacement is to be avoided.
5. The patient should be covered with broad spectrum antibiotics to prevent sepsis. As most antibiotics are excreted through the kidneys, only a few have been proved safe for use. Amoxycillin, doxycycline and minocycline are a few recommended antibiotics.

Hepatic Diseases

A history of chronic alcohol intake, substance abuse, repeated blood transfusions and viral hepatitis is indicative of a probable silent liver disease. The liver is the site of biotransformation of various drugs and anesthetic gases and synthesis of vitamin K. A patient with viral hepatitis should be handled with care to avoid inadvertent transmission of the disease to the operation theatre personnel or another patient. The risk of transmission depends on the type of hepatitis carrier the patient is, i.e. A, B, C, or D. In our practice, the maximum risk is from a hepatitis B or C carrier.

Preoperative Investigations

1. Liver enzymes—serum glutamic oxaloacetic transaminase (SGOT),—serum glutamic pyruvic transaminase (SGPT)
2. Total bilirubin, direct and indirect bilirubin
3. Serum albumin
4. Serum alkaline phosphatase
5. Bleeding time and clotting time
6. Prothrombin time, plasma thromboplastin time and index (INR)
7. USG liver
8. Australia antigen test.

Intra- and Postoperative Management

1. Avoid anesthetic gases that are metabolized in the liver, like halothane.
2. Correction of coagulation deficiencies by IV vitamin K, Fresh frozen plasma transfusions.
3. Careful intra- and postoperative management of blood volume, cardiac output, urine volume and composition.
4. Potassium supplementation during fluid replacement.
5. Appropriate precautions and sterilization techniques to prevent transmission of disease in a carrier of viral hepatitis.

Diabetes Mellitus

Diabetes mellitus is caused by an absolute or relative deficiency of insulin in the body. It can be classified into type 1 (insulin dependent) and type 2 (noninsulin dependent).

Type 1 is more commonly seen in young patients and type 2 in adults. A patient can be classified as a diabetic, when his fasting glucose levels are constantly above 140 mg/dl.

The nature of problems faced by the surgeon during the management of a known diabetic patient are:

1. Optimal blood sugar levels are to be maintained during the procedure, as well as postoperatively to prevent hypoglycemia or hyperglycemia and ketoacidosis. Both the conditions may be life threatening to the patient.

2. The patient is prone to infections and has to be given adequate pre- and postoperative broad spectrum antibiotic coverage to prevent infections.
3. The patient may have additional systemic complications like renal failure, cardiac disorders, ophthalmic problems and generalized vascular disease due to long-standing diabetes.

For surgical purpose a diabetic can be classified in three groups:
1. Sugar levels controlled by diet and oral hypoglycemics.
2. Sugar levels controlled by insulin.
3. "Brittle diabetes", usually of juvenile onset, whose metabolic needs are labile and have sequelae of long-standing disease such as renal failure, retinopathy, and generalized vascular disease.

Elective surgeries can be usually performed without complications in the first two types. In the third type, although the management remains same, a more rigid control is to be exercised intra- and postoperatively.

Preoperative Investigations

1. Chest radiograph—posteroanterior view
2. Electrocardiogram
3. Blood investigations like:
   • Blood sugar fasting and postprandial
   • Glucose tolerance test
   • *Renal profile:* Such as blood urea nitrogen (BUN), serum creatinine (SC), serum electrolytes (SE).
4. Urine analysis for sugar and acetone.

If the patient is on oral hypoglycemics, he must be shifted to insulin on the day of surgery. The general principle for the management of the patient under general anesthesia, is to provide at least 200 gm of carbohydrate with adequate insulin to cover this need.

Intra- and Postoperative Management

1. Check the patient's blood and urine sugar levels on the morning of surgery, with the help of hemoglucose strips and urostrips or glucometer.
2. Prepare a sliding insulin scale to be followed intraoperatively based on the patients sugar levels (Table 4.1).
3. Pre- and postoperative broad spectrum antibiotic coverage.
4. Intra- and postoperative close monitoring of the blood and urine sugar levels.
5. Prevent the patient from going into ketoacidosis or hypoglycemia.

Table 4.1: Sugar levels and insulin dose	
Sugar levels (mg%)	Insulin dose
80–120	Plain 5% dextrose (D)
120–180	4 units in 5% D
180–250	8 units in 5% D
250–300	14 units in 5% D
300 and above	14 units in normal saline

• *Signs of hypoglycemia:* The patient is apprehensive, restless, agitated, the skin is moist and pale, and there is tachycardia. The patient then lapses into coma.

Treatment: In a conscious patient, oral carbohydrates are given to correct the glucose levels. In an unconscious patient intravenous administration of 50 percent glucose solution restores consciousness in 5 to 10 minutes or 1 mg glucagon IM restores consciousness in 15 minutes.

• *Signs of diabetic ketoacidosis:* Vomiting, tachypnea, Kussmaul (deep, rapid breathing at regular intervals) breathing, dehydration and circulatory collapse.

Treatment: Administration of insulin to normalize body metabolism and restoration of body fluids and electrolytes.

6. Shift the patient at the earliest possible to his regular oral feeds and antidiabetic medications.

Thyroid Disorders

Patients having thyroid disorders can be broadly divided into three groups:
(1) Hypothyroid
(2) Euthyroid and
(3) Hyperthyroid.

Out of these, euthyroid patients pose no risk for any surgical procedure. In both hypo and hyperthyroidism, elective surgery is best postponed till the patient is euthyroid.

The signs of hypothyroidism are water and mucopolysaccharide retention, slowing of metabolic processes leading to bradycardia, constipation, lethargy and hypothermia. Untreated hypothyroid patients respond poorly to stress and proceed into myxedema coma.

Hyperthyroidism leads to a hypermetabolic state in the body, resulting in a catabolic state with tachycardia, diarrhea and heat intolerance. If this patient is subjected to stress, he goes into what is known as "thyroid storm", which is a state of metabolic hyperactivity lasting for 24 to 48 hours. There is a severe exacerbation of the signs and symptoms of hyperthyroidism and is usually accompanied by hyperpyrexia. The condition is life threatening and requires control of hyperpyrexia, tachycardia and cardiac failure.

Preoperative Investigations

1. *Thyroid hormone levels:* T3, T4, TSH
2. Serum electrolytes
3. Serum proteins
4. Radionuclide thyroid scan to study the gland.

Intra-and Postoperative Management

1. Monitor the hormone levels intra- and postoperatively.
2. Continuous monitoring of vital parameters, blood pressure, pulse and temperature.
3. Check for signs and symptoms of hypo/hyperthyroidism.
4. Continuous monitoring of the cardiac function, especially during thyroid crisis. Infuse thyroid hormone, if the patient shows signs of hypothyroidism.
5. If the patient is in a thyroid storm, treat by cooling the patient, intravenous infusion of glucose and IV fluids, glucose and corticosteroids.
6. Use narcotic agents and anesthetic medications judiciously in hypothyroid patients, as they can have a profoundly depressing effect.

Adrenal Diseases

Two common adrenal disorders that have to be dealt with during surgical procedures are Cushing's syndrome (overproduction) and Addison's disease (underproduction).

The symptoms of Cushing's syndrome are diabetes, sodium and water retention, potassium excretion, hypertension and fat redistribution. The patient also has a tendency to osteoporosis, poor wound healing and purpura formation. During surgery, attention must be paid to maintaining optimum levels of carbohydrates in the body. Sodium and potassium ion levels and the blood pressure. There may be postoperative problems of bleeding and delayed wound healing.

Underproduction can occur due to adrenal suppression due to exogenous steroids or due to a disease of

adrenal origin (Addison's disease). Usually any patient, who has received steroids for longer than two weeks within a year prior to surgery should be considered as a candidate for adrenal insufficiency.

Preoperative Investigations

1. Renal profile
2. Serum electrolytes
3. Blood sugar fasting
4. Platelet count
5. Coagulation profile.

Patients with adrenal insufficiency should be supplemented with adequate exogenous steroids prior to procedure to help the patient combat with stress.

Intra- and Postoperative Management

1. Continuous monitoring of the vital signs.
2. Adequate intravenous corticosteroid supplementation to prevent adrenal crisis.
3. Maintain fluid and electrolyte balance.
4. Monitor blood sugar levels.

Neurological Disorders

Neurological disorders can be categorized into patients with cerebrovascular disorders, seizure disorders, chronic respiratory disorders and patients with head injury. The main factors of consideration in these patients is to maintain adequate cerebral perfusion intra- and postoperatively and to control any seizure episode during this period. Patients with seizure disorders, usually do not pose a great problem for intraoperative management, except for cases of status asthamaticus, where there can be life threatening complications. The surgeon should weigh the risks and benefits, before the surgical procedure. Patients with cerebellar infarcts, aneurysms, and arteriovenous malformations are very high risk candidates and are absolute contraindications for surgical procedures.

Preoperative Investigations

1. Routine skull radiographs—posteroanterior and lateral views
2. CT scan/MRI brain
3. EEG
4. Liver function tests.

If the patient is an epileptic, adequate control of seizure episodes must be achieved prior to the surgical procedure. The anticonvulsant must be continued till the morning of the surgery. The morning dose is given with sips of water.

Intra- and Postoperative Management

1. The patient should be given intravenous anticonvulsants intraoperatively.
2. Postoperatively the patient should be shifted to his normal dose of anticonvulsants at the earliest possible.
3. Throughout the procedure, hypotension/hypoxia is to be avoided and an adequate cerebral perfusion is to be maintained.

Disorders of Hemopoietic System

Disorders of the hemopoietic system can be grouped into anemias, leukocyte disorders and coagulation factor abnormalities (hemophilia) (Flow chart 4.1). Anemias include iron deficiency anemia, thalassemia, sickle cell anemia; and leukocyte disorders include leukocytosis and agranulocytosis.

Any disturbance in the hemopoietic system:
1. Predisposes the patient to prolonged bleeding during any surgical procedure, which cannot be controlled by routine hemostatics.

Flow chart 4.1: Coagulation pathway or cascade

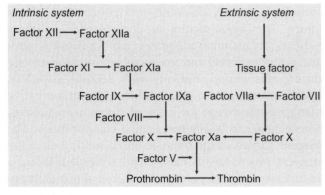

Coagulation factors
- I. Fibrinogen
- II. Prothrombin
- III. Thromboplastin
- IV. Calcium ions
- V. Proaccelerin
- VI. Proconvertin
- VII. Antihemophilic factor
- VIII. Christmas factor/plasma thromboplastin component
- IX. Stuart factor
- X. Plasma thromboplastin antecedent
- XI. Hageman factor
- XII. Fibrin stabilizing factor

2. May cause severe internal bleeding due to blunt injury following intubation, a condition if unnoticed may pose a life-threatening complication.
3. Leukemic and thalassemic patients may be on repeated blood transfusions and may have liver disorder due to excessive deposits of hemosiderin.
4. The rate of postoperative infection and delayed wound healing is also very high, especially in agranulocytosis, leukemia and anemia.

Preoperative Investigations

1. Complete blood count
2. Bleeding time and clotting time
3. Prothrombin time and index (INR)
4. Partial thromboplastin time
5. Coagulation factor assay (in case of factor abnormalities)
6. Platelet count
7. Hemoglobin
8. Liver function tests.

Prior to the procedure, the patient's blood counts must be built up to the normal values by transfusion of whole blood, packed cells, plasma or plasma components and clotting factors.

For a hemophiliac, the factor VIII level should be raised to at least 50 to 70 percent prior to the procedure. Once the blood levels are normal, the patient can be treated as a normal patient with regards to surgical bleeding. Adequate blood must be crossmatched and kept ready for transfusion intraoperatively, if required. In case of leukemics, the patient should be posted for surgery, during his remission phase. The patient should be covered with broad spectrum antibiotics pre- and postoperatively.

Intra- and Postoperative Management

1. Avoid undue trauma to the tissues during any procedure performed.
2. Avoid entering deep tissue spaces blindly, thereby preventing any internal bleeding.
3. Complete hemostasis must be achieved prior to wound closure.
4. Intraoperative transfusion of blood/blood products, if found necessary.
5. Monitoring of hemoglobin, complete blood counts intra- and postoperatively.
6. Maintain adequate blood volume throughout the procedure and at the same time avoid cardiac overload.

7. Monitor the vital parameters closely for any changes in the fluid volume indicated by the pulse and blood pressure.
8. Postoperatively the patient may be maintained on systemic oral coagulants like vitamin K for 3 to 5 days.
9. Cover the patient with adequate broad spectrum antibiotics.
10. Avoid medications that can exacerbate the underlying condition, especially in agranulocytosis.

In view of the rise in blood borne transmission of diseases like AIDS, hepatitis B and hepatitis C, the government has made it compulsory for testing of all the three viruses before stocking the blood in the blood bank. But the decision to transfuse blood and blood products must still be made judiciously weighing the risks and benefits.

Management of a Hemophiliac Patient

Classically hemophilia is of two types: hemophilia A (Factor VIII deficiency) and Hemophilia B (Factor IX deficiency).

The disorder is a sex linked recessive trait. Approximately 50 percent of the female offsprings are carriers of the disorder and 50 percent of the male offsprings have the clotting disorder. These patients have a tendency to bruise easily and have prolonged bleeding.

The successful management of a hemophiliac is dependent on the adequate maintenance of the antihaemophilic globulin. The normal AHG level is 50 to 100 percent. In a hemophiliac, for good hemostasis, the factor level must be 20 percent above normal, though a normal level is also acceptable.

Thromboplastin regeneration time not only determines the factor VIII deficiency, but also distinguishes it from factor IX deficiency.

Factor VIII replacement can be provided through blood, plasma, fresh frozen plasma, and cryoprecipitates. The latter is the replacement choice as it offers only the deficient factor.

Management
1. Build up factor VIII level to 50 to 70 percent
2. Avoid injecting into deep tissue spaces, i.e. avoid block techniques. Use infiltration anesthesia.
3. Atraumatic extraction, surgical procedure.
4. Avoid unnecessary trauma to the soft tissues, avoid suturing if not required.

Immunocompromised Patients

Immunocompromised patients can be grouped into:
- Patients having deficiency in cell mediated, humoral immunity, neutrophils, complements
- Patients on immunosuppressive drugs like chemotherapeutic agents and steroids
- Patients suffering from long-standing debilitating conditions like diabetes and nutritional deficiencies.

These patients are highly susceptible to infections and must be given broad spectrum antibiotic coverage for the same.

Preoperative Investigations

1. Complete blood count
2. Liver function tests
3. Renal function tests
4. Serum proteins
5. Blood sugar levels
6. Urine analysis
7. Routine chest radiograph.

Intra- and Postoperative Management

1. The management will vary according to the condition, the patient is suffering from. Usually it is almost impossible to correct the causative factor and the treatment is usually supportive only.
2. Constant monitoring of the vital parameters.
3. Broad spectrum antibiotic coverage.
4. While handling HIV infected patients, special care must be exercised to prevent the transmission of the disease.

Autoimmune Disorders

The group of autoimmune disorders include systemic lupus erythematosus, scleroderma, collagen disorders, rheumatoid arthritis, Sjögren's syndrome, polyarteritis nodosa, etc. These patients may have significant cardiac, renal and bone marrow impairment, which may contraindicate elective surgery. The patients, whenever possible must be operated during their remission phase. A few of these patients may be on long term corticosteroid therapy, therefore, precautions to prevent adrenal insufficiency must be taken.

A few of these patients have loss of flexibility in the joints, especially the thoracic cage and neck joints, thereby posing problems in intubation and ventilation.

In scleroderma, the patients have a restricted oral opening as well as restricted expansion of the chest wall.

Patients with collagen disorders may also have delayed postoperative wound healing.

Patients Undergoing Radiation Therapy

It is indeed essential to understand the dental and the oral complications of radiotherapy involving the oral cavity and salivary glands. The complications are as follows:

1. *Mucositis:* Mucositis occurs when the radiation field involves oral mucosa. The degree of damage depends upon the type of radiotherapy, the dose and duration of the treatment. It causes considerable amount of discomfort and sometimes dysphagia. It usually subsides in 2 to 3 weeks time.
2. *Loss of taste (hypoguesia):* Hypoguesia occurs because of the damage to the taste buds due to irradiation. However, xerostomia alone can disturb taste sensation. Taste may start to recover within 2 to 4 months. If more than 6000 cGy radiation is given, then the loss of taste is usually permanent.
3. *Xerostomia and infections:* The area of radiotherapy to cancers of the head and neck often involve the major salivary glands. Radiotherapy of tumors of naso- and oropharynx can damage the salivary glands. Salivary secretion diminishes within a week of radiotherapy in practically all patients and the saliva becomes thick. Some salivary function may return after many months. Xerostomia predisposes to infections, particularly periodontal disease, caries, oral *Candida* infection and acute ascending sialadenitis.
4. *Radiation caries and dental hypersensitivity:* Patients frequently take a softer, more cariogenic diet because of dryness and soreness of the mouth and loss of taste. There is a change towards more cariogenic oral flora. Irradiation may also directly damage the teeth, which become hypersensitive, thus making oral hygiene difficult.

    These factors combine to cause rampant dental caries, including areas such as incisal edges and cervical margins which are normally free from caries. The caries begins at any time between 2 and 10 months after radiotherapy, and may eventually result in the crown breaking off from the root. A complete dentition may be destroyed within a year of irradiation.

5. *Osteoradionecrosis and osteomyelitis:* Death of bone of the jaw, particularly the mandible, is a potentially serious complication of irradiation endarteritis. If the soft tissue covering the bone is healthy and undisturbed, there may be no obvious consequences, but infection, often resulting from dental extractions carried out after radiotherapy, can lead to intractable osteomyelitis.

    Irradiation-associated osteomyelitis may occasionally be precipitated by mucosal ulceration caused by denture. As a consequence, some dental specialists refuse to permit patients to wear dentures, specially a full lower denture, after irradiation of the oral mucosa.

    Osteoradionecrosis is however, a less frequent problem now, as megavoltage radiotherapy has less effect on bone than orthovoltage therapy. Osteoradionecrosis appears to develop mainly in patients receiving more than 6000 cGy, particularly to the floor of the mouth and mandible. Osteomyelitis may follow months or years after radiotherapy, but about 30 percent of cases develop within 6 months.

6. *Trismus:* Progressive endarteritis of affected tissues, with reduction in their blood supply, follows radiotherapy. The results may be replacement fibrosis of the masticatory muscles. Fibrosis becomes apparent 3 to 6 months after radiotherapy and can cause permanent limitation of opening.
7. *Dental defects:* Irradiation of developing teeth can cause hypoplasia and retarded eruption.

Management

Treatment Planning

The treatment has to be carefully planned. Oral hygiene measures should be taken. Preventive dental care instituted, and restorative procedures should be carried out. These measures can significantly reduce the caries incidence.

a. *Before radiation:* Extractions before radiotherapy is not always necessary to extract all the teeth before radiotherapy. In any case, clearance before irradiation may not be practicable, because the patient is too old or ill, or the prognosis is too poor. Sometimes the patient has very healthy teeth and good oral hygiene that dental complications after radiotherapy are unlikely.

    The time period between extractions and radiotherapy is a compromise because of the need to start irradiation at the earliest. No bone should be left exposed in the mouth when radiotherapy begins, since, once the blood supply is damaged by radiotherapy, wound healing is jeopardized. Many authors advise an interval of at least 2 weeks between extracting the teeth and starting radiotherapy, but this is not always essential.

b. *During radiotherapy:* Mucositis may be relieved by using warm normal saline mouthwashes and lignocaine viscous 2 percent. Smoking and alcohol should be discouraged. A 0.2 percent chlorhexidine mouthwash maintains oral hygiene and a benzydamine oral rinse or a saliva substitute such as carboxymethylcellulose may provide some symptomatic relief. Trismus may be reduced by instituting jaw-opening exercises with Heister's jaw stretcher three times a day. Antifungal drugs such as nystatin suspension, 100 000 U/ml, as a mouthwash or pastilles used four times daily may be required.

c. *After radiotherapy:* Oral hygiene and preventive dental care should be continued and mucositis managed as outlined above. Dental extractions may precipitate osteomyelitis in the irradiated jaw but, if extractions are unavoidable, trauma should be kept to a minimum, raising the periosteum as little as possible and ensuring that sharp bone edges are removed. Careful suturing is needed and prophylactic antibiotics should be given in adequate doses and continued for 2 to 3 weeks.

Radiation caries and dental hypersensitivity can be controlled with daily topical fluoride applications (sodium fluoride mouthwash, stannous fluoride get or acidulated fluoride phosphate gel). Occasionally full cover acrylic splints are used to protect the teeth (Coffin's caps). Patients should be advised to avoid sweets and sweet confectionery. Instead sugar substitutes such as saccharin or aspartane, may be used, wherever possible. Mouthwashes of sodium bicarbonate may help dissolve the stringy saliva that forms.

Mucosal trauma from dentures may predispose to osteomyelitis and some specialists therefore insist that dentures be abandoned. If dentures are required, they should be fitted at about 4 to 6 weeks after radiotherapy, when initial mucositis subsides and there is only early fibrosis.

Dental Management of Patient Undergoing Chemotherapy

These patients take immunosuppresant drugs and because of that there is leukocytopenia. Hence, all the procedures should be done under antibiotic coverage.

Pregnancy and Lactation

Every female patient in the child-bearing age must be asked for history of pregnancy or missed menstrual cycles. Great care must be taken when dealing with the pregnant patient, since the surgeon has to treat not only the mother, but also prevent any undue harm to the fetus. It is safe to perform procedures under local anesthesia in the second trimester. In the first trimester, there is a risk of stress related abortion as well as teratogenicity, while in the third trimester there is a risk of stress induced early labor. General anesthesia is a contraindication in the third trimester, unless it is a life saving emergency procedure. In the first and second trimesters care must be taken to avoid fetal anoxia.

Again, the risks and benefits must be outweighed prior to the procedure. The mother should be fully explained about the risks before performing any procedure. Teratogenic drugs like tetracyclines, salicylates, and chloramphenicol are best avoided. Amoxycillin, cloxacillin, ampicillin and paracetamol can be safely prescribed.

Food and Drug Administration (FDA) has categorized the potential for drugs to cause birth defects, providing definitive guidelines for prescribing drugs during pregnancy (Table 4.2). They are as follows:

Food and Drug Administration Categories

Category A: Controlled human studies indicate no apparent risk to fetus. The possibility of risk to the fetus is remote.

Category B: Animal studies do not indicate risk. Well-controlled human studies have failed to demonstrate a risk.

Category C: Animal studies show an adverse effect on the fetus but there are no controlled studies in humans. The benefits from use of such drugs may be acceptable.

Category D: Evidence of human risk, but in certain circumstances the use of such a drug may be acceptable in pregnant women despite its potential risk.

Table 4.2: FDA guidelines for the drugs to be prescribed during pregnancy				
Drugs	FDA category	Use in pregnancy	Use in nursing	Possible side effects
Analgesics				
Acetaminophen	B	Yes	Yes	Not reported
Aspirin	C	Not in 3rd trimester	No	Postpartum hemorrhage
Ibuprofen	B	Not in 3rd trimester	Yes	Delayed labor
Naproxen	B/D*	Not in 2nd half of pregnancy	Yes	Delayed labor
Codeine	C	With caution	Yes	Multiple birth defects
Oxycodone	B	With caution	With caution	NRD**
Hydrocodone	C/D*	With caution	With caution	NRD**
Morphine	B	Yes	Yes	Respiratory depression
Propoxyphene	C	With caution	Yes	Not reported
Meperidine	B	Yes	Yes	Not reported
Pentazocine	C	With caution	With caution	Not reported
Antibiotics				
Amoxicillin	B	Yes	Yes	Not reported
Metronidazole	B	Yes	Yes	Not reported
Erythromycin	B	Yes	Yes	Not reported
Penicillin V	B	Yes	Yes	Not reported
Cephalosporins	B	Yes	Yes	Not reported
Gentamycin	C	Yes	Yes	Fetal ototoxicity
Clindamycin	B	Yes	Yes	Not reported
Tetracycline	D	No	No	Discoloration of teeth
Chloramphenicol	X	No	No	Maternal toxicity/fetal death
Chlorhexidine	B	No data	No data	Not reported
Antifungals				
Nystatin	B	Yes	Yes	Not reported
Clotrimazole	B	Yes	Yes	Not reported
Fluconazole	C	With caution	With caution	Not reported
Ketoconazole	C	With caution	No	Fetal toxicity
Local anesthetics				
Lidocaine	B	Yes	Yes	Not reported
Mepivacaine	C	With caution	Yes	Fetal bradycardia
Prilocaine	B	Yes	Yes	Not reported
Bupivacaine	C	With caution	Yes	Fetal bradycardia
Etidocaine	B	Yes	Yes	Not reported
Corticosteroids				
Prednisolone	B	Yes	Yes	Not reported
Sedative/Hypnotics				
Nitrous oxide	Not assigned	Not in 1st trimester	Yes	Spontaneous abortion
Barbiturates	D	Avoid	No	NRD
Benzodiazepines	D	No	No	Cleft lip/palate

Note:

D* indicates caution: If used for prolonged period of time, or high doses.

NRD** : Neonatal respiratory depression.

Category X: Risk of use in pregnant women clearly outweighs possible benefits.

CONCLUSION

Concluding this chapter, a few points need to be highlighted, which will define a basic protocol to be followed during the management of a medically compromised patient.

1. A thorough knowledge of the patient's medical background must be obtained.
2. The surgeon should also have knowledge about the medications taken by the patient and the regularity of the patient in taking the same.
3. A written consent for the surgical procedure has to be obtained from a specialist in the field prior to the procedure.
4. Adequate and necessary preoperative investigations must be performed.
5. The patient should be explained about the risks and benefits of the procedure, with regards to his general condition and a witnessed written condition for the procedure, as well as high risk consent should be obtained from the patient.
6. The operation theatre must be well equipped with functional life support systems and an updated emergency trolley in case of an emergency. The same applies to the postoperative recovery room.
7. The decision of whether or not to operate lies with the surgeon and he must make his choice judiciously weighing the pros and cons with respect to surgical benefits and anesthetic risks.

BIBLIOGRAPHY

1. Daniel M Laskin. Oral and Maxillofacial Surgery, 1st Indian Edition, Vol 1.
2. Killey HC, Seward GR, Ray LW. An Outline of Oral Surgery, 11th revised reprint, Vol 1.
3. Paul H Kwon, Daniel M Laskin. Clinician's Manual of Oral and Maxillofacial Surgery. 2nd Edition.
3. Peterson, Ellis, Hupp, Incker. Contemporary Oral and Maxillofacial Surgery, 4th Edition.

5 Armamentarium Used in Oral and Maxillofacial Surgery

INSTRUMENT USED FOR PICKING UP STERILE INSTRUMENTS

Cheatle's Forceps (Fig. 5.1A)

It is a long angulated instrument that is used for picking up sterile instruments from a tray or linen from the drum. It is stored in a container containing an antiseptic solution like savlon. The solution must be changed everyday.

INSTRUMENT USED FOR PREPARING THE SURGICAL FIELD

Swab Holder (Fig. 5.1B)

It is an instrument with long blades, expanded at the ends, forming an oblong tip. The blades have a central fenestration and transverse serrations.

Uses

1. To hold a swab and clean the area of operation.
2. To swab the throat when there are profuse secretions in an unconscious patient or patients under general anesthesia.
3. To press on the tonsillar bed to arrest hemorrhage
4. To hold the tongue and give anterior traction, thus preventing tongue fall and airway obstruction in an unconscious patient.

INSTRUMENT USED FOR HOLDING THE DRAPES

Towel Clips (Figs 5.1C and D)

There are two types of towel clips:
A. The Pinchter type (The forceps type)
B. Beckhaus towel clip.

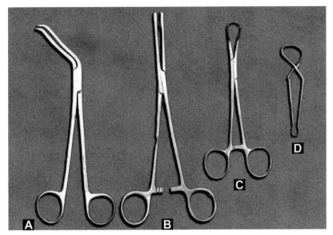

Figs 5.1A to D: (A) Cheatle's forceps, (B) Swab holder, (C) The pinchter type towel clip, (D) Beckhaus towel clip

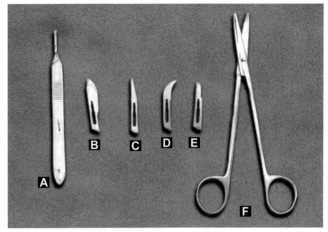

Figs 5.2A to F: (A) Bard Parker blade handle, (B) No. 10 blade, (C) No. 11 blade, (D) No. 12 blade, (E) No. 15 blade, (F) Dissecting scissors

The Beckhaus type of towel clip has a spring joint and the forceps type has a box joint. The tips of the instrument are pointed, curved towards each other and overlap one another.

Uses

1. To hold the corners of the draping sheets during an operation.
2. To hold the tongue.
3. To stabilize the suction tubes, motor cables and other fiber optic instrument cables to the drapes.

INSTRUMENTS USED FOR INCISING THE TISSUES

Scalpel

The instrument used for making an incision is called a scalpel. The scalpel has two parts, a blade and a blade handle.

Bard Parker Blade Handle (Fig. 5.2A)

Various sizes of the handles are available. The most commonly used handle in oral surgery is no. 3. The handle has a receiving slot for the blade. While fitting the blade to the blade handle , it is held with the help of a needle holder or an artery forceps to prevent injury to the operator. The blade is then pushed into the slot till it fits in snugly. The scalpel is always used in the pen grip.

Blades (Figs 5.2B to E)

- No. 10—For making skin incisions
- No. 11—For making stab incisions (for example, to drain an abscess)
- No. 12—For mucogingival procedures
- No. 15—For intraoral surgery.

Dissecting Scissors (Fig. 5.2F)

As the name suggests, dissecting scissors are used to perform soft tissue dissection in the deeper layers. The scissors have a blunt nose for undermining the tissues and a side cutting edge for cutting the tissues.

INSTRUMENTS USED FOR RETRACTING TISSUES

Langenbeck's Retractor (Figs 5.3A and 5.4A)

It has a long handle and an "L" shaped blade. This retractor is most commonly used in oral surgery. It is available in different sizes and blade width. The instrument can be single or double ended. It is used to retract the soft tissues, incision edges, to allow view of the deeper structures.

C-shaped Retractor

This instrument also has a long handle but the blade is "C" shaped. It is more commonly used in abdominal surgeries.

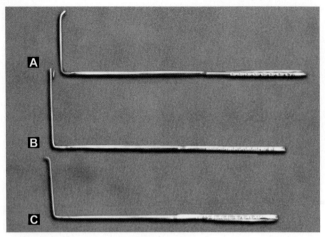

Figs 5.3A to C: (A) Langenbeck's retractor, (B and C) Obwegeser's ramus retractors

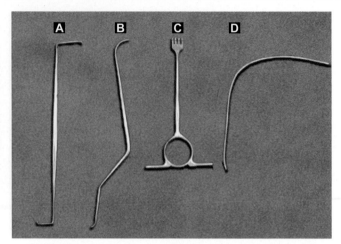

Figs 5.4A to D: (A) Double ended Langenbeck's retractor, (B) Condyle retractor, (C) Cat Paw retractor, (D) Tongue depressor

Austin's Retractor

It is a short right-angled retractor used for retracting the cheek, tongue and the mucoperiosteal flaps.

Obwegeser's Ramus Retractor (Figs 5.3B and C)

The retractor is similar to the Langenbeck's retractor except that the edge of the retracting blade is forked, forming a "V" shaped notch, so as to engage the anterior border of the ramus of the mandible and aid in good tissue retraction.

Uses

1. To retract the soft tissues along the anterior border of the ramus during sagittal split or ramus osteotomy
2. To retract the tissues from the anterior border of the ramus during coronoidectomy procedures.

Condyle Retractors (Fig. 5.4B)

They are special retractors that have an appearance similar to the tongue depressor, but are narrower and the tip of the blade has a 'C' shaped hook that is slipped under the ankylosed mass to retract and protect the medial soft tissues during release of the ankylosis.

Weider's Retractor

It is a broad, heart shaped retractor that is serrated on one side so that it can engage the tongue and firmly retract it medially and anteriorly.

Cat Paw Retractor (Fig. 5.4C)

As the name suggests, the instrument resembles a cat's paw. The blade has prongs that are curved at the tip. It is used to retract small amounts of soft tissue. Excessive force during retraction may lead to perforation or tear in the flap.

Tongue Depressor (Fig. 5.4D)

The tongue depressor is an "L" shaped instrument with a broad smooth blade for depressing or retracting the tongue.

Uses

1. To depress the tongue for visualization of the tonsils and the pharyngeal wall during inspection.
2. To depress the tongue during endotracheal intubation and extubation.
3. To depress the tongue and move it anteriorly to check for airway obstruction and to prevent tongue fall in an unconscious patient.
4. To retract the tongue during surgical procedures in the oral cavity.
5. To retract the cheek.

Seldin's Retractor

It is similar to the periosteal elevator, but the leading edge is dull and not sharp.

It is used only for retracting soft tissues and not for elevating the mucoperiosteal flap.

INSTRUMENTS USED FOR REFLECTING THE MUCOPERIOSTEAL FLAP

Moon's Probe (Fig. 5.5A)

It is a thin, flat instrument that has a small working tip at right angles to the handle. The tip is narrow and sharp.

Uses

To elevate the attached gingiva around the tooth prior to extraction.

Periosteal Elevators (Molt No. 9, Howarth's, Dial's) (Figs 5.5B,C,E and F)

As the name suggests these instruments are used for reflecting the mucoperiosteum. Most of the periosteal elevators have a broad end on one side and a pointed or triangular end on the other.

Uses

1. The pointed end is used to release the interdental papillae.
2. The broad end is used for elevating the muco-periosteal flap from the bone.
3. The broad end can also be used as a soft tissue retractor.

Methods of Reflecting the Periosteum from the Flap

1. *Prying motion:* The pointed end can be used in a prying motion to elevate the soft tissue, for example, reflecting the interdental papillae.

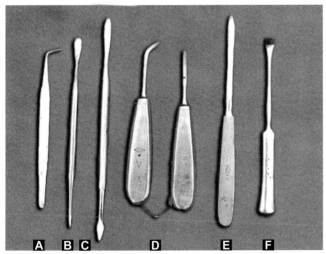

Figs 5.5A to F: (A) Moon's probe, (B to E) Periosteal elevators, (F) Cleft palate raspatory

2. *Push stroke:* It is given with the broad end of the periosteal elevator and is the most efficient stroke to reflect the periosteum from the bone.
3. *Pull stroke:* It is also called the scrape stroke and most likely tends to tear the periosteum.

Cleft Palate Raspatory (Fig. 5.5D)

This broad, flat handled elevator is specially used to elevate the palatal mucoperiosteum while mobilizing the flaps for cleft palate repair.

Hemostatic Forceps (Spencer Wells, Kelly's, Halstead)

These forceps are better known as hemostatic forceps although they are used for catching both arteries and veins. They are used to catch hold of bleeding vessels. The unidirectional, transverse serrations on the blades of the hemostat prevent the vessel from slipping. The vessel is crushed between the blades and hemostasis is achieved. The handle has a catch and the vessel may be held and clamped. Small bleeders may be controlled by just crushing the vessel, whereas bigger vessels may be cauterized or ligated.

Types of Hemostats (Figs 5.6A and B)

- Large
- Straight
- Medium
- Curved
- Small

  A small curved artery forceps is known as a mosquito forceps.

Uses

1. To achieve hemostasis by catching blood vessels. Hemostasis may be achieved just by crushing the vessels or by ligating or cauterizing them.
2. To hold the ends of ligatures.
3. As tissue forceps for holding subcutaneous tissues, aponeurosis (but not skin or nerves)
4. To drain an abscess by Hilton's method
5. To pick up necrotic tissue, granulation tissue, foreign bodies, tooth/root pieces, small fragments of bone, etc.

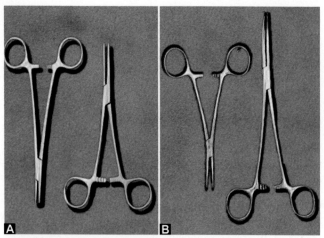

Figs 5.6A and B: (A) Straight hemostats, (B) Curved hemostats

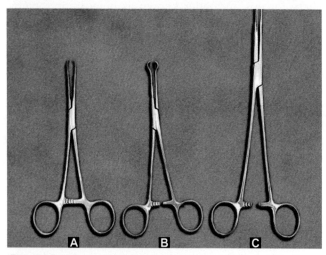

Figs 5.7A to C: (A) Allis tissue holding forceps, (B) Babcock's tissue holding forceps, (C) Lane's tissue holding forceps

INSTRUMENTS USED FOR HOLDING THE SOFT TISSUES

Tissue Holding Forceps

As the name suggests these are used to hold the soft tissues of the body.

Allis Tissue Holding Forceps (Fig. 5.7A)

It is a short instrument, with a catch and the blades have teeth that are delicate.

Uses

1. To hold delicate tissues like the peritoneum, aponeurosis, soft muscles

2. To retract and hold the tissue margins and skin edges.
3. To provide tension for tissue dissection.

Babcock's Tissue Holding Forceps (Fig. 5.7B)

The instrument has fenestrated blades without teeth.

Uses

1. To hold the intestines and delicate structures like peritoneum, fascia, etc.
2. To hold the appendix
3. To hold enlarged lymph nodes or any glandular tissue.

Lane's Tissue Holding Forceps (Fig. 5.7C)

It is a long and stout instrument with sharp teeth on the blades.

Uses

1. To hold tough structures like the skin, coarse muscles.
2. Tissue holding forceps will be described on page 57.

Tongue Forceps

The tongue forceps are of two types:

Swab Holder Variety

It is similar to the swab holder but for the fenestration on the blade which is triangular and the serrations on the blades more coarser. It may cause damage to the tongue.

Towel Clip Type

It is similar to the forceps variety of the towel clip, except in the fact that the tip of one of the blades is expanded into which the tip of the other blade fits.

It is better than the swab holding variety as the tongue is traumatized at only one point.

Uses

1. To hold the tongue during any surgery of the tongue.
2. To arrest hemorrhage from the tongue (When the tongue is pulled forward, the lingual artery is compressed between the tongue and the lower anterior teeth.
3. To prevent tongue fall and airway obstruction in unconscious patients.

Gland Holding Forceps

Swab Holder Variety

It differs from the swab holder in that there are no serrations on the blade.

Kocher's Variety

It is similar to the swab holder but there are two spikes in each blade that are turned to engage the tissues.

Uses

1. To hold the salivary glands, especially the submandibular and the sublingual glands.
2. To hold enlarged lymph nodes.
3. To hold tumors during excision.

INSTRUMENTS USED TO KEEP THE MOUTH OPEN

Mouth Prop (Fig. 5.8A)

Mouth props can be of two varieties: (A) Rubber and (B) Metal.

The function of the mouth prop is similar to the mouth gag, i.e. to keep the mouth open during any surgical procedure performed in the oral cavity. The mouth prop consists of a vertical block having a concave surface on either of its ends to fit on the occlusal surfaces of maxillary and mandibular teeth. The block is placed between the mandibular and maxillary teeth to maintain the mouth open. Usually, there are three or four blocks of varying vertical heights arranged in an ascending order, and connected by a chain. The operator can choose the block according to the required extent of oral opening.

Heister's Jaw Stretcher (Fig. 5.8B)

This instrument is used to forcibly open the mouth. The instrument has two flat blades that are applied between the maxillary and mandibular posterior teeth and are separated by turning a key that is positioned between the two blades.

Uses

1. To force the mouth open when there is trismus due to infection, muscle spasm, hemarthrosis of the temporomandibular joint following trauma.
2. To give postoperative active jaw physiotherapy after surgery for TM joint ankylosis, submucous fibrosis.

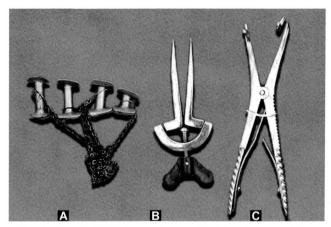

Figs 5.8A to C: (A) Metal mouth prop, (B) Heister's jaw stretcher, (C) Fergusson's mouth gag

When using the above two instruments, care must be taken to prevent luxation of the teeth, especially the anteriors and dislocation of the temporomandibular joint.

Mouth Gag (Doyen's, Fergusson's) (Fig. 5.8C)

This instrument is used to keep the mouth open in a patient under general anesthesia, during surgeries of the oral cavity, tonsils and the pharynx. The flat blades have serrations that rest on the occlusal surfaces of the maxillary and the mandibular teeth. The handle has a catch that is fixed at the required opening.

INSTRUMENTS USED TO DRAIN AN ABSCESS

Lister's Sinus Forceps (Fig. 5.9A)

The instrument has long narrow blades which are serrated transversely for only half an inch at the tip. The instrument does not have a catch. The tip is rounded and bulbous. The shank and the tip are almost at equal length.

Uses

1. To open an abscess by Hilton's method, to break the loculae.
2. To hold a small piece of gauze between the blades to clean a cavity.
3. To dissect out sinus and fistulous tracts in soft tissues.

Hemostatic Forceps

As described earlier.

INSTRUMENTS USED TO REMOVE PATHOLOGIC TISSUE

Curette (Lucas) (Figs 5.9B and C)

The term curette comes from a French word *curer*, meaning "to cleanse". It is primarily an exploratory instrument. These are instruments used to scrape a bony cavity or a soft tissue tract in order to remove any pathological tissue present within them. A curette can be single ended or double ended. The working end may be in the same plane as the shank or at an angulation for adequate access to the pathologic cavity.

Uses

1. It is used to remove tooth particles or debris from the extraction socket.
2. To enucleate cysts, periapical granulomas, intra-osseous tumors.
3. To remove small sequestra which may develop in healing sockets.
4. To remove proliferative or infected clot from the extraction socket.

Volkmann's Scoop (Fig. 5.9D)

This instrument is used to scrape the contents of a cavity. It is similar to a curette, but the concavity of the working edges is more pronounced. It may also be used as a spoon.

Uses

1. To collect the contents from a sinus tract, chronic abscess cavity or a fistula.
2. To scrape or curette bony cavities due to cystic/tumorous lesions or osteomyelitic lesions.
3. To scoop out the cancellous bone for grafting procedures.
4. To introduce graft material, antiseptic powder into the surgical area.

INSTRUMENTS USED TO HOLD THE BONE

Crocodile Bone Holding Forceps (Figs 5.10A and B) Fergusson's Lion Jaw Bone Holding Forceps

They are named so because of the appearance of the beaks sideways. The beaks have toothed margins to allow a good grip on the bone. The Crocodile bone holding forceps has

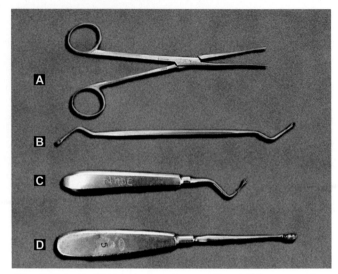

Figs 5.9A to D: (A) Lister's sinus forceps, (B and C) Lucas curettes, (D) Volkmann's scoop

a catch to stabilize the instrument in the required position. In the absence of the above instruments, a *forcep type of a towel clip* may also serve the purpose.

Uses

To hold the bony fragments of the mandible during manipulation of the bony fragments during fracture reduction, resection procedures, after osteotomy cuts, and during fixation of the bony fragments.

Kocher's Toothed Heavy Artery Forceps

This instrument is similar to a long heavy artery forceps, but it has toothed tip.

Uses

1. The instrument is specially designed to hold the coronoid process during coronoidectomy procedure.
2. It can be used like the other bone holding forceps for stabilization of the bony fragment.

Sequestrum Holding Forceps

The instrument appears like the crocodile bone holding forceps, but does not have a catch to prevent crushing of the sequestrum.

Uses

To remove a sequestrum from a chronic osteomyelitic lesion.

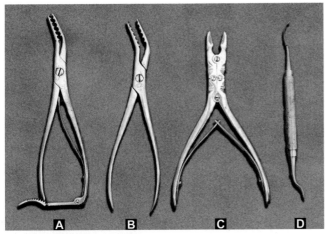

Figs 5.10A to D: (A and B) Crocodile bone holding forceps, (C) Jensen Middleton Rongeurs forceps, (D) Miller and Colburn bone file

INSTRUMENTS USED TO CUT OR REMOVE BONE

Rongeurs Forceps (Blumenthal, Jensen Middleton) (Fig. 5.10C)

The rongeurs forceps have curved handles that have a spring action. The spring increases the force applied and hence efficiency of the instrument. There can be either one spring or a double spring (Jensen Middleton). When the handles are released the instrument automatically opens up. This helps the surgeon to make repeated cuts without making efforts to open the handles. The tip is angulated forward to the handle and has a concave inner surface. The beaks are sharp. They can be either side cutting (Blumenthal) or both side and end cutting. The instrument is used to remove large amounts of bone at a time using multiple, small bites.

Uses

1. To nibble sharp bony margins following simple or surgical extraction of teeth, surgical procedures
2. To peel off thinned out bone present over cystic or tumorous lesions.
3. To trim sharp bony ridges during alveoloplasty procedures.

Miller and Colburn Bone File (Fig. 5.10D)

As the name suggests, the bone file is used to smoothen any sharp bony margin present in the surgical field. The instrument has a long curved working end and a short oval working end. The working ends have horizontal serrations. The instrument is used unidirectionally using a pull stroke. A push stoke usually causes burnishing and crushing of the bone. The working edges must be cleaned regularly to prevent clogging by bone debris, thereby reducing the efficiency of the instrument.

Bone Cutter

A bone cutter is similar to a rongeurs forceps as far as the working principle is concerned. The instrument is activated by spring action. The edges of the blades are sharp and have a side cutting action.

Uses

1. To trim sharp bony margins following extractions, minor oral surgical procedures.
2. To trim sharp ridge projections during alveoloplasty procedure.

Osteotome (Fig. 5.11A)

The osteotome is similar to a chisel, but the edge of the working tip is bibeveled.

It splits bone rather than cut or chip the bone as with the chisel.

Uses

1. Various osteotomy procedures
2. Biopsy of bony lesions
3. Removal or recontouring of the bone.

Chisel (Figs 5.11B to D)

Chisels are unibevelled instruments for cutting bone. They have a heavy round handle and a long flat working tip. The edge of the working tip has a bevel on one side. The working edge is sharp and is flat. To plane the bone, the bevel is kept facing the bone. To cut the bone, the bevel is kept facing away from the bone.

Uses

1. To remove chips of bone as in transalveolar extractions
2. To split the tooth in difficult extractions.

Bone Gouge (Fig. 5.11E)

The bone gouge has a round handle and a blade that has a sharp working tip that is concave on the inner side. The working tip is half round and has a long working area.

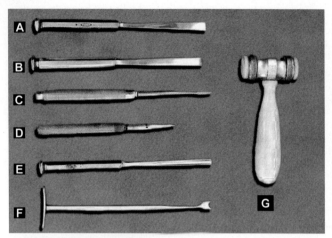

Figs 5.11A to F: (A) Osteotome, (B to D) Chisels, (E) Bone gouge, (F) Nasal rasp, (G) Mallet

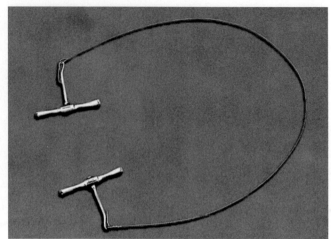

Fig. 5.12: Gigli's saw

Uses

1. To remove cancellous graft material during grafting procedures
2. To make a window in the anterior wall of the maxillary sinus for access to the maxillary sinus during Caldwell Luc procedure.
3. To remove irregular pieces of bone.

Nasal Rasp (Fig. 5.11F)

It is used to fracture the anterior nasal spine and separate nasal septum from the maxilla during LeFort I or premaxillary osteotomy procedures. The instrument has a flat, thin blade with a sharp edge. The edge has a slit that engages the anterior nasal spine.

Mallet (Fig. 5.11G)

A mallet is made up of steel, lead or wood. It is similar to a hammer and is used for giving controlled taps on the chisel, bone gouge or osteotome. To be effective, the mallet should be used with a loose, free swinging movement of the wrist that gives maximum speed to the head of the mallet without introducing the weight of the arm or the body to the blow. The kinetic energy of a body is calculated as $KE = 1/2MV2$, where KE or kinetic energy stands for the energy possessed by the moving body, M stands for the mass of the body and V stands for the velocity of the body.

Usually a six inch mallet is used for minor oral surgical procedures.

Hand Piece, Burs and Saws

It is a quicker method of bone removal by drilling the bone at high speeds. Burs are rotary instruments that cut the bone. They are made up of either stainless steel or carbide. They are available in different lengths, shapes (Fissure, round, tapering fissure) and sizes.

Uses

1. To round of sharp margins after extractions, minor surgical procedures.
2. To aid in bone removal or splitting the tooth, during disimpaction procedure.
3. To round of sharp ridges during alveoloplasty procedures.
4. To perform osteotomy cuts.
5. To release bony ankylosis.
6. To make a bony window for access to cystic cavities, tumours.
7. To perform resection of the maxilla, mandible.

Gigli's Saw (Fig. 5.12)

The armamentarium for the use of Gigli's saw are:
1. Gigli's saw
2. Two handles
3. Introducer
4. Guide

The Gigli's saw is made by twisting a few pieces of wires together, so that it acquires a sharp, barbed, cutting edge when moved to and fro along it's long axis.

At the end there is a ring to which the hook of the handle can be fitted. In Maxillofacial surgery, the saw was usually used to cut the mandible (hemimandibulectomy procedures).

Care must be taken to protect the soft tissues, while using this instrument.

INSTRUMENTS USED TO SUTURE THE TISSUES

Mayo-Hegar Needle Holder (Fig. 5.13A)

The needle holder is a straight instrument with a short working tip. The blade of the needle holder is shorter and stronger than that of the hemostat. The working tip has cross hatched serrations with a single vertical serration to grip the needle. The handle has a catch. Usually a six inch needle holder is used in Oral Surgery. The instrument is held between the ring finger and the thumb and the index and the middle finger support the needle holder.

Suture Cutting Scissors (Dean's) (Fig. 5.13B)

They are used for cutting the suture ends. They can be straight or curved, and angulated or nonangulated. The angulation may be at the joint or at the tip to facilitate access to the posterior areas of the oral cavity. They have long delicate handles and a short cutting edge.

Tissue Holding Forceps

Tissue Holding Forceps (Micro Adson, Gillie's, Adson's) (Figs 5.13C and D)

A. Plain
B. Toothed

They are used to hold the tissues during the process of dissection or suturing. Plain tissue holding forceps have serrations on the inner aspect of the tip to aid in a better grip.

Uses

1. The plain forceps having no tooth at the tip and are used for holding delicate structures like the peritoneum, fascia, delicate muscles and facial skin
2. The plain forceps are also used to hold blood vessels or nerves.
3. The toothed forceps are used to hold tough structures like the aponeurosis and coarse muscles,

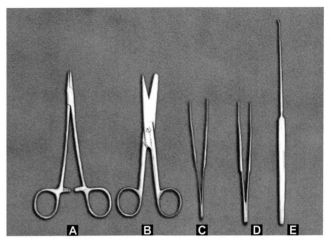

Figs 5.13A to E: (A) Mayo-Hegar needle holder, (B) Dean's suture cutting scissors, (C and D) Adson's tissue holding forceps, (E) Skin hook

keratinized tissues. They are never used to hold the skin.
4. They are also used to hold the needles while suturing.

MISCELLANEOUS INSTRUMENTS

Skin Hook (Fig. 5.13E)

Skin hook is a thin, long instrument, with a delicate curved tip. This tip engages the tissues.

Uses

1. To stretch the edges of the skin incision during suturing to prevent dog ear formation.
2. To retract small amount of soft tissue or edges.

INSTRUMENTS USED TO MAINTAIN A CLEAN SURGICAL FIELD

Suction Apparatus (Fig. 5.14A)

The commonly used suction apparatus is the vacuum pump suction apparatus. It is electrically operated with the help of a motor. It can be mounted on a trolley and moved around. A single or two bottles can be connected.

Suction Tip (Frazier, Nuober) or Cannula (Fig. 5.14B-I)

These are the instruments which are introduced into the surgical field for maintaining a clean field by sucking

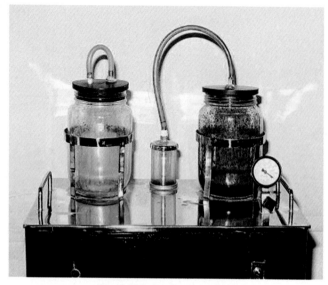

Fig. 5.14A: Suction apparatus

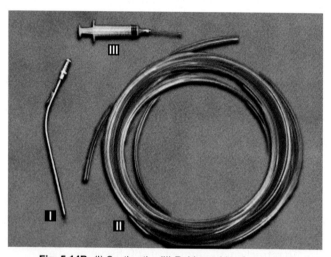

Fig. 5.14B: (I) Suction tip, (II) Rubber tubing for suction, (III) Disposable syringe and needle

away blood, flushing solution, debris, cystic fluid, pus, and secretions. Frazier suction tip has a blade in the handle for better control and a hole to control the suction speed. A stillet is provided to clean the lumen if there is clogging. The tip may be straight or angulated. A no. 4 or no. 5 tip is commonly used in oral surgery.

Suction Tubing (Fig. 5.14B-II)

It is connected to the suction apparatus at one end and the suction tip on the other end. It can be made up of

India rubber or Silicone polymer. The latter is better as it is transparent and can be autoclaved.

INSTRUMENTS USED FOR THE TREATMENT OF FRACTURES OF THE JAW BONES

Rowe's Disimpaction Forceps (Fig. 5.15A-I)

A pair of Rowe's Disimpaction forceps is used for disimpacting the maxilla in LeFort fractures. It consists of one straight and one curved blade. The blades are padded for atraumatic purpose. The straight blade is passed into the nostril and the curved blade enters the mouth and grips the palate. The operator stands behind the patient and grasps the handles of each of the forceps and manipulates the fragments into position.

Uses

1. To disimpact the maxilla in fresh LeFort fractures, malunited fractures.
2. To check for free movements of the maxilla after LeFort osteotomy procedure.

Hayton William's Forceps

This forceps has two widely divergent curved beaks that engage the maxilla behind the tuberosity. It is usually used in conjunction with the Rowe's disimpaction forceps to mobilize the maxilla.

Walsham's Forceps

It is used to manipulate the fractured nasal fragments. The forceps has a padded blade and an unpadded blade that are curved. The unpadded blade of the Walsham Forceps is passed up the nostril, and the nasal bone and the associated fragment of the frontal process of the maxilla are secured between the padded blade externally and the unpadded blade internally. The fragments are then manipulated in their correct position.

Asche's Forceps (Fig. 5.15A-II)

The Asche's septal forceps is used to reduce the fractures of the nasal bone and to align the nasal septum. The blades are passed on either side of the nasal septum and the vomer and the perpendicular plate of the ethmoid are ironed out. If possible the septal cartilage is then

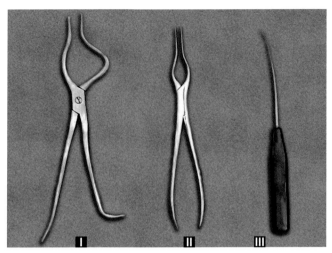

Fig. 5.15A: (I) Rowe's disimpaction forceps, (II) Asche's nasal bone reduction forceps, (III) Bone awl

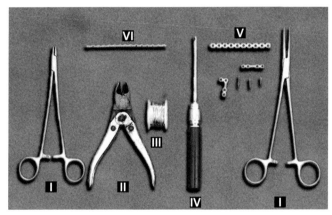

Fig. 5.15B: (I) Wire holder, (II) Wire cutter, (III) Wire spool, (IV) Screw holder, (V) Bone plates and screws (VI) Erich's arch bar

grasped and repositioned in it's groove in the vomer. To reduce the nasal bone fracture, one blade is inserted in the nostril, holding the medial aspect of the nasal bone and the other blade is kept externally holding the lateral aspect of the nasal bone.

Wire Holder (Hayton William) (Fig. 5.15B-I)

A wire holder is similar to a needle holder, except that it has a heavy tip, which may be devoid of the vertical serrations.

Wire (Fig. 5.15B-III)

Usually a 26 gauge wire spool is used in oral surgical procedures.

Uses

1. To stabilize dentoalveolar fractures.
2. To perform intermaxillary ligation.
3. To splint the arch bar to the teeth.
4. Fixation of fractures by transosseous wiring.
5. Indirect fixation of fractures by suspension wiring.

Bone Plates (Fig. 5.15B-V)

Bone plates are usually made up of stainless steel or titanium. They are available in various sizes, lengths and shapes. In oral surgery the thickness of the plates varies from 1.5 mm, 2 to 2.5 mm. 2.5 mm plates are usually used for the mandible, whereas the former two are used for the maxilla. Depending on the requirement, they are available in different lengths, 2 hole, 3 hole, 4 hole, 6 hole, etc. and in different shapes—orbital, "L" shaped, "T" shaped, etc.

Erich's Arch Bar (Fig. 5.15B-VI)

It contains a thin stainless steel strip that has hooks incorporated on it. It is malleable and can be adapted to the contour of the maxillary or mandibular arch and fixed to the teeth by wires.

Uses

1. To stabilize dentoalveolar fractures.
2. To stabilize mandibular or maxillary fractures, that are to be treated by closed reduction.
3. To provide means for intermaxillary ligation.

Tracheostomy Set

A tracheostomy set consists of:
1. Tracheostomy tube
2. Sharp hook
3. Blunt hook
4. Tracheal dilator.

Tracheostomy Tube

The main function of this tube is to allow air entry through a tracheostomy wound. The tube may be made of metal or Portex. A metal tracheostomy tube cannot be left in position for more than 48 hours. The Portex tubes are disposable and can be maintained for indefinite periods. The tracheostomy tube has an inner and an outer tube. If the inner tube is blocked, it can be removed and cleaned and the outer tube can be left in position. The curvature of the tube is such that it does not damage the trachea. There are rings at the base of the inner tube that can either be used to pull the inner tube or to stabilize the tracheostomy tube with loose cords tied around the neck. The Portex tubes have a cuff that can be inflated to stabilize the tube in position in the trachea, especially during the administration of general anesthesia. A cuff kept inflated for a long time may cause pressure necrosis of the trachea. The tube is withdrawn when there is no further evidence of airway obstruction.

Blunt Hook

The blunt hook is used for retracting the isthmus of the thyroid upwards while performing a low tracheostomy.

Sharp Hook

This instrument is used for stabilizing the trachea, while making a stab wound on it, as during respiratory obstruction, the trachea tends to move rapidly up and down. The sharp hook is inserted just below the cricoid cartilage.

Tracheal Dilator

This instrument is meant for dilation of the stab incision given over the trachea, to facilitate introduction of the tracheostomy tube. The blades of the instrument are opened when the handles are brought together.

Nerve Hook

Nerve hook is similar to a bone awl except that it has a relatively blunt tip with a broad curve at the tip. The tip has an eye through which a suture can be passed.

Uses

It is used in neurectomy procedures to tie the nerve for identification.

Aneurysmal Needle (Fig. 5.16)

Similar to the nerve hook, the aneurysmal needle has a blunt tip. The tip has an eye, through which a suture can be passed. The needle is used to pass a suture around a larger blood vessel and ligate it.

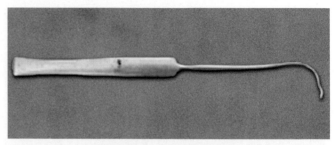

Fig. 5.16: Aneurysmal needle

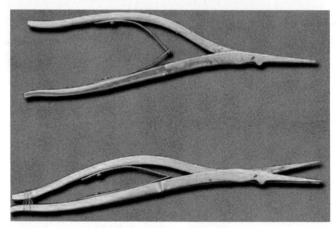

Fig. 5.17: Smith's bone spreader

Bone Spreader (Fig. 5.17)

Smith's bone spreader has three blades that are separated by spring action when the handles are compressed. It is used to separate the bony fragments after completion of the osteotomy cuts, like in downfracture of maxilla after LeFort I osteotomy or during sagittal spilt osteotomy procedure.

▌ DRAINS USED IN ORAL AND MAXILLOFACIAL SURGERY

Drainage is the provision of removal of contents of body organs, cavities or tissues by mechanical means.

Need for Establishing Drainage

1. Obliteration of dead space.
2. Removal of material which is foreign or harmful to the body tissues.
3. To evacuate fluid/blood/urine collection in any body cavity.

Indications for Drainage

1. Abscess cavities with thick, shaggy walls that must collapse and heal from the deepest portions.
2. Surgical defects where postoperative collection of blood/inflammatory fluids is expected.
3. Urinary retention
4. Gastric lavage in case of poisoning, intraoperative ingestion of blood during general anesthesia.
5. Osteomyelitic lesions where drainage is established for inflammatory exudate and necrotic tissues.

Functions

1. To allow for pus, fluid collection, blood to escape from the body cavities.
2. To allow for local introduction of antibiotics, antimicrobials.

Types of Drains (Figs 5.18A and B)

1. Simple rubber catheter (Penrose drain)
2. Corrugated rubber drain
3. Infant feeding tube
4. Foley's catheter
5. Nasogastric (Ryles) tube

Penrose Drain

It is a simple rubber tube, open at both ends, that can be used for drainage of abscess cavities, hematomas, etc.

Nasogastric Tube (Ryle's Tube) (Figs 5.18A and B-IV)

Nasogastric tube is a long hollow tube with one blunt end with multiple openings and an open end. It is made up of polyvinyl chloride. The blunt end is passed through the nostril into the stomach. To check the position of the tube air is pushed into the tube with the help of a syringe and the air entry into the stomach is checked with the help of a stethoscope. Only after confirmation of the presence of the tube into the stomach, the feeds are started. The tube is fixed to the nose with the help of sticking plaster.

Uses

1. To provide feeds to the patients who cannot take oral feeds.
2. To provide gastric lavage postoperatively to flush out blood, fluids ingested intraoperatively.
3. To provide gastric lavage in case of poisoning.

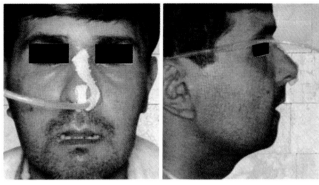

Fig. 5.18A: Patient with nasogastric tube (Ryle's tube)

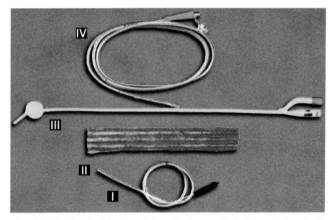

Fig. 5.18B: (I) Infant feeding tube, (II) Corrugated rubber drain sheet, (III) Foley's catheter, (IV) Ryle's tube

Foley's Self-retaining Catheter (Fig. 5.18B-III)

It is a self-retaining catheter used for evacuating the bladder. The self-retaining mechanism is in the balloon near its tip. At the other end of the catheter two tubes are present. The wider tube is meant for draining the urine, while the narrower tube communicates with the balloon and is meant for inflating and deflating the balloon. The catheter is passed through the urethra in either sex, into the bladder. The position is confirmed by the free passage of urine through the wider tube. Then the catheter is anchored within the bladder by inflating the balloon via the smaller tube, by injecting water. When the catheter is to be withdrawn, the water is aspirated through the narrower tube. The catheter is available in various sizes. The commonly used size for males is no. 16 and for females is no. 14.

Indications in oral and maxillofacial surgery

1. For evacuation of the bladder in long cases under general anaesthesia
2. For evacuation of the bladder in unconscious patients.

3. For patients with postoperative urinary retention
4. For non ambulatory patients with multiple fractures
5. Foley's catheter may also be used as a retention stent in comminuted zygomatic complex fractures. The balloon is inflated within the sinus to offer support to the bony fragments and left in position for 5 to 7 days till initial stabilization.

Infant Feeding Tube (Fig. 5.18 B-I)

Infant feeding tube is made up of nontoxic, radio-opaque, polyvinyl chloride. It is a long tube with a blunt tip with multiple openings for facilitating drainage. The other open end has a stopper that can be closed.

The drain is inserted into the dead space and can be either removed externally through the incision line or through a separate incision away from the incision line. Most operators prefer the latter. A negative pressure can be established within the space by attaching and aspirating a 20 cc syringe to the open end. The syringe must be emptied at regular intervals. The drain is fixed to the skin by sutures. It can be removed in 3 to 5 days depending on the amount of drainage. It can also be used for local instillation of antibiotic solutions in deep wounds.

Corrugated Rubber Drain (Fig. 5.18 B-II)

It is a sheet of rubber with corrugations on its surface. It is usually used as a drain following abscess drainage. Multiple holes are usually made in the drain to prevent the drain from getting obstructed. The drain is inserted with one end in the cavity and the other end is kept out of the skin or mucosa. The drain is secured by sutures and is left in place for three to five days.

INSTRUMENTS USED FOR THE EXTRACTION OF THE TEETH AND ROOT REMNANTS

Elevators

The dental elevators are used to luxate the teeth from the socket prior to application of the forceps. In addition to luxation of the teeth, the elevators also expand the bony socket facilitating tooth extraction. They are also used to remove root remnants from the extraction socket.

The elevator has three components:
1. Handle
2. Shank
3. Blade.

The handle is usually large in size to facilitate a good grip on the instrument while working. It may be 180° to the shank or at right angles to the shank. The latter are known as crossbar elevators. The crossbar elevators can generate tremendous amount of force.

The shank connects the handle to the blade. The shank should be strong enough to withstand and transmit the forces applied to the handle.

The blade of the elevator is the working tip of the elevator which is used to transmit forces to the tooth, root and bone. Blades can vary in size and shape and depending on that the elevators are classified as:
1. The straight or the gouge type
2. The triangular type
3. The pick type

Work Principles of Elevation (Fig. 5.19)

There are three work principles applicable to the elevators. They are:
1. *Lever principle:* This is the most commonly used principle. The elevator is a lever of the first order. In this the fulcrum is between the effort and the resistance. In order to gain mechanical advantage, the effort arm must be longer than the resistance arm.
2. *Wedge principle:* The wedge elevator is forced between the root and the bone, parallel to the long axis of the tooth. The wedge is a movable inclined plane which overcomes a large resistance at right angles to the applied effort. It is usually used in conjunction with the lever principle.
3. *Wheel and axle principle:* The wheel and axle principle is actually a modified form of lever principle. The effort is applied to circumference of a wheel which

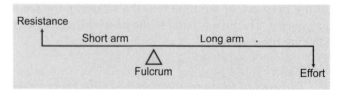

Fig. 5.19: Lever principle of elevation

turns the axle so as to raise a weight. The principle is used with wedge and sometimes with the lever principle. The principle is applicable to the crossbar elevators.

Indications for the Use of Elevators

1. To luxate multirooted teeth prior to forceps application.
2. To luxate, remove teeth that cannot be engaged by the beaks of the forceps, e.g. Impacted teeth, malposed teeth, badly carious teeth.
3. To remove fractured root stumps, apical tips.

Rules to be Followed While Using the Elevators

1. Never use the adjacent tooth as the fulcrum, unless that the adjacent tooth is also to be extracted.
2. Never use the buccal or lingual plate as the fulcrum.
3. Always use finger guards to protect the soft tissues if the elevator slips.
4. Support the shank of the elevator with the index finger to control the forces applied to the elevator.
5. Always elevate from the mesial side of the tooth.
6. The concave or flat surface of the elevator faces the tooth/ root to be elevated.

Commonly Used Elevators

Straight Elevators (Coupland, London Hospital Pattern) (Fig. 5.20A-I)

They are the most common types used for the luxation of teeth. The blade has a concave surface on one side, that faces the tooth to be elevated. Sometimes the blade can be at an angle to the shank, allowing the instrument to reach the posterior areas of the oral cavity easily. Common examples of these elevators are, the Miller and the Pott's elevator.

Hockey Stick or London Hospital Elevator (Fig. 5.20A-II)

This elevator is similar to the Cryer's elevator, with the working blade at an angulation to the shank, but the blade is straight, rather than triangular, and has a convex and a flat surface. The flat surface is the working surface and has transverse serrations on it for better contact with the root stump. When viewed, the instrument looks like

a Hockey stick and hence the name. The principles and functions are similar to the Cryer's elevator.

Apexo Elevators (Fig. 5.20A-III)

These are straight elevators that resemble the Cryer's elevators, but have a biangulated and sharp, straight working tip. They are paired elevators for the mesial and the distal roots. Their uses and work principles are same as for the Cryer's elevators. They can also be used to remove the maxillary root stumps.

Cryer's Elevator

Cryer's elevator is a straight elevator with a triangular blade. The working tip is angulated, with one convex and another flat surface. The flat surface is the working side. It is based on the lever and the wedge principle.

Uses

1. For extraction of root stump of mandibular molars when one root is removed and the other is to be removed.
2. For extraction of mandibular molar root stumps when both the roots are present but one is fractured at a lower level than the other or when the bifurcation is intact.

   Two separate elevators are available for the mesial and distal roots. The working blade is introduced into the empty socket and moved towards the remaining root piece. In this technique the interradicular bone is fractured prior to removal of the root stump.

Winter's Elevator

Winter's elevator is a crossbar elevator. The shank is at right angles to the handle. The working tip is at an angle to the shank. The blade has a convex and a flat surface. The flat surface is the working surface and is placed facing the tooth to be elevated. It works on the wheel and axle principle.

Uses

To luxate the mandibular molar teeth.

Winter Cryer's Elevator (Fig. 5.20B)

As the name suggests, the elevator is a crossbar elevator with a triangular blade. The uses and the applications of this instrument are similar to the Cryer's elevator. It works on the wheel and axle and wedge principles.

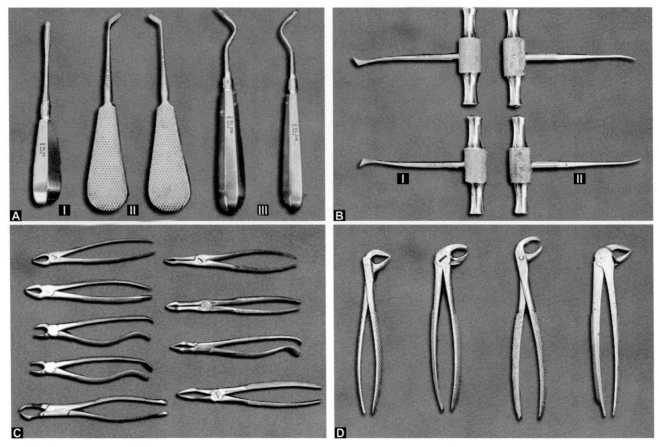

Figs 5.20A to D: (A) (I) Straight elevator, (II) London hospital hockey stick pattern elevators, (III) apexo elevators, (B) (I) Winter Cryer's elevators, (II) Winter's crossbar elevators, (C) Maxillary extraction forceps, (D) Mandibular extraction forceps

Extraction Forceps

They are designed to deliver the teeth from the sockets. Each forceps has two handles, a joint and two beaks. All the forceps have crosshatching on the handles to allow a firm grip and have serrations on the inner side of the beaks to allow a better grip on the tooth. The beaks are applied along the long axis of the tooth, below the CE junction in mandibular teeth, and above the CE Junction in maxillary teeth. A firm grip on the tooth is established prior to giving any forceps movements.

Maxillary Extraction Forceps (Fig. 5.20C)

In all the maxillary extraction forceps the handles and the beaks are at 180° to each other, i.e. in a straight line.

Maxillary anterior forceps: They have identical beaks that are closed, straight, flat and broad. They are used for extraction of the maxillary incisors and the canines.

Basic forces
Maxillary central incisors: Labial movement, mesial rotation.

Maxillary lateral incisors: Labiopalatal movements, removal in the labial direction.

Maxillary canine: Labio-palatal movements, removal in the labial direction.

Maxillary premolar forceps: They have identical beaks that are concave on the side facing the operator. The beaks are broad and open. They are used for extraction of the maxillary premolars. The curvature of the blade is to give access to the premolars placed posteriorly in the arch. Rotational and buccal movements are given for the maxillary second premolar, while only buccopalatal movements are given for the first premolar.

Basic forces
First premolar: Buccopalatal movements and removal in the buccal direction.

Second Premolar: Bucco-palatal movements and removal in the buccal or palatal direction.

Maxillary Molars (Right and Left)

The beaks of these forceps are not identical. One beak is rounded and the other one is pointed. The pointed beak engages the groove between the buccal roots and the other beak engages the palatal surface above the CEJ. The beaks also have a curvature towards the operator like the premolar forceps. When viewed, if the pointed beak is to the left of the operator it is a right sided forceps and vice versa.

Basic forces: The first and the second molars are extracted by giving buccopalatal movements and removal in the buccal direction.

The third molar is extracted by giving buccal movements and distal rotation.

Maxillary Cowhorn forceps: These forceps have unidentical beaks, one of which has a single pointed tip and the other a bifid pointed tip. The single pointed tip engages the furcation between the two buccal roots and the other tip engages the palatal root. It is a paired forceps. The beaks are curved towards the operator. While viewing the concave surface of the beaks, the bifid beak will be on the right for the maxillary right sided forceps and vice-versa. They are used for maxillary teeth, where there is extensive destruction of the crown, but the trifurcation of the roots is intact.

Maxillary anterior root forceps: They have identical, straight, slender and closed beaks. They are used primarily for the extraction of the root stumps of the maxillary anterior teeth.

Maxillary posterior root forceps: They are similar to the anterior root forceps, but like the premolar forceps, they have a curvature towards the operator for access posteriorly. They are used for removing single molar root pieces and premolar root stumps.

Bayonet forceps: They have identical, pointed, angulated and closed beaks. The length of the beaks vary from long to short. According to the thickness of the beaks they can be classified into thick beak and thin beak bayonet forceps. The thick beak bayonet forceps is used to remove maxillary posterior root stumps that are not separated, while the thin beak forceps are used to remove single roots.

Mandibular Forceps (Fig. 5.20D)

The mandibular forceps are designed such that the handles and the beaks are at right angle to each other to facilitate easy access to the mandibular teeth.

Mandibular anterior forceps: The mandibular anterior forceps have identical broad, short, closed beaks. The joint is a rivet joint unlike most forceps that have a box joint. They are used for extracting mandibular anterior teeth.

Basic forces: Central and lateral incisors : Labiolingual and mesiodistal movements and removal in the labial direction.

Cuspid: Labio-lingual movement and removal in the labial direction.

Mandibular premolar forceps: The mandibular premolar have identical broad open beaks that are longer than the beaks of the anterior forceps. They are used for extraction of the mandibular premolar teeth.

Basic forces: Both the premolars are extracted with buccolingual and mesiodistal movements.

Mandibular molar forceps: They have identical, broad, open beaks with a pointed tip. They are used for the extraction of mandibular molar teeth.

Basic forces: All the molars are extracted by buccolingual movements and removal in the buccal direction.

Mandibular Cowhorn forceps: The mandibular Cowhorn forceps have identical, open, short, pointed beaks that resemble the horns of a cow. The beaks are round and taper to a point. The forceps grips the tooth at the bifurcation between the mesial and distal roots. When pressure is applied and the beaks are closed using the buccal and the lingual plates as the fulcrum, the tooth is luxated or literally squeezed out of the socket, provided the root morphology is favorable. They are used to remove grossly carious mandibular molars with extensive destruction of the crown.

Mandibular root forceps: These forceps have identical, slender beaks that are closed. The beaks are longer than that of the premolar forceps to enable the forceps to take a deep grip on the root stump. It is used for removal of root stumps of all the mandibular teeth.

▮ SURGICAL DIATHERMY (CAUTERY, ELECTROCAUTERY) (FIG. 5.21)

There are two basic types of cautery:
1. Mono or unipolar
2. Bipolar

Monopolar Diathermy

It basically consists of:
1. High frequency AC generator (over 20,000 Hz)
2. Regulator
3. Foot control
4. Indifferent electrode
5. Active electrode

The AC electrode generates a high frequency alternate current, the intensity of which is controlled by the regulator. The indifferent electrode is a flat steel plate which is put in contact with the patient's back, thigh or buttocks. The contact between the patient's skin and the indifferent electrode may be improved by, either shaving that area or by using a conductive jelly. The electrode is usually wrapped with a wet cloth to improve conduction.

The active electrode or the tip touches the hemostat in which the bleeder is held. When the foot control is pressed, current is generated and discharged through the active electrode.

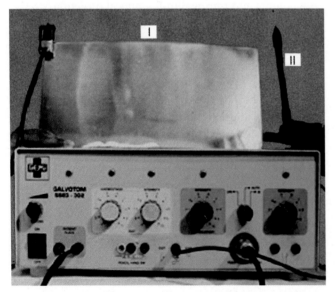

Fig. 5.21: Surgical diathermy (electrocautery machine): (I) Indifferent electrode plate, (II) Active electrode tip

Principles

The large, flat steel plate or the indifferent electrode acts as the earth. The active electrode is a fine tip. Due to the large difference in the size of the two electrodes, a high current density is generated around the active electrode, resulting in a heating effect. By changing the intensity of the current, various functions are possible.
1. Coagulation
2. Cutting
3. Fulguration

Coagulation: Bleeding from the small vessels, viz the capillaries, arterioles, can be controlled. The subcutaneous bleeders and oozing vessels from the incision lines are first clamped with a hemostat and then the cautery is applied. Bleeding from thin walled veins and large arteries cannot be controlled by cauterization. They have to be ligated and then divided.

Cutting: An incision can be made by increasing the current and using a cutting tip. It is used for incising soft tissues with diffuse capillary network so that the small bleeders get coagulated as cutting occurs. It is never used for taking skin incisions.

Fulguration: Fulguration burns the tissue margins. This is useful in resecting small growths, e.g. papilloma, leukoplakia, so as to prevent recurrence.

Precautions

1. Care must be taken to ensure intimate contact between the patient and the indifferent electrode. Avoid point contact.
2. Avoid placement of the indifferent electrode near bony ridges.
3. If ether, cyclopropane are used for general anesthesia, risk of sparking is high.
4. Operator using the tip should wear rubber footwear so as to avoid accidental burn.
5. Avoid contact of the tip with retractors or other metal instruments which will conduct electricity.
6. Do not use near isolated vascular pedicles or nerves.

Bipolar Diathermy

This consists of an AC generator foot switch. It does not have an indifferent electrode. The AC is of low power. The active electrode is in the form of forceps, the two tips of which serve as the two electrodes. As the

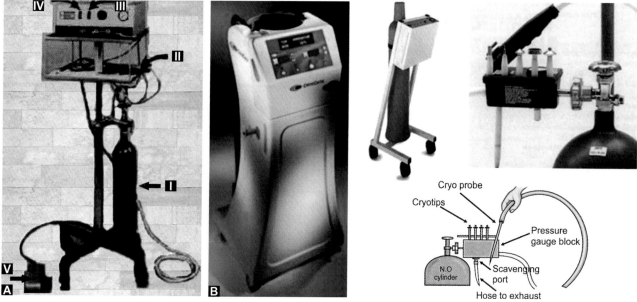

Figs 5.22 (A and B): (A) Old cryosurgery unit: (I) Nitrous oxide cylinder, (II) Cryoprobe, (III) Warming cycle light, (IV) Freezing cycle light, (V) Foot switch, (B) New cryosurgical units

current generated is smaller, the bipolar diathermy can be used only for coagulation, but not for cutting. When the two ends of the forceps are brought together, a circuit is created, producing a localized current. Bipolar diathermy reduces the risk of burns, and interference with other instruments such as ECG units pacemakers. It also reduces the risk of spark ignition of anesthetic gases.

CRYOSURGERY (FIGS 5.22A AND B)

It is the technique of using extreme rapid cooling to freeze and thereby destroy tissues. Rapid cooling to temperatures below freezing point produces a localized destructive effect than slow freezing which causes generalized tissue necrosis.

The effects of rapid freezing on the tissues are:
1. Reduction of intracellular water.
2. Cellular shrinkage.
3. Increased concentration of intracellular solutes.
4. Cell membrane damage.
5. Formation of intracellular ice crystals.
6. Formation of extracellular ice crystals.

The apparatus consists:
1. Bottles for storage of pressurized liquid gases. Liquid nitrogen gives a temperature of $-196°C$, while liquid carbon dioxide, or nitrous dioxide give a temperature between $-20°C°$ and $-90°C$
2. A pressure and temperature gauge
3. *A probe:* The probe is connected to the bottles via a tubing through which the pressurized gas can be directed at the tissue to be destroyed.

Following freezing, the tissues are thawed and refreezed. Alternate cooling and thawing destroys the tissues. The time and temperature for cryotherapy is determined by the depth and extent of the tumor.

It is applied in the treatment of malignancies, vascular tumors, aggressive tumors like ameloblastoma.

Suturing Materials and Techniques

Any surgical procedure involves the creation of a wound and subsequent closure by repositioning and securing the surgical flaps by suturing to allow optimum healing.

A suture is a strand or thread of material used to approximate tissues and also to ligate blood vessels. To suture is the act of sewing or bringing tissues or flap edges together and holding them in apposition until normal healing takes place. Sutures also help the wound to withstand normal functional stresses and to resist wound reopening.

HISTORICAL BACKGROUND

The first description of sutures used in operative procedures is recorded by Edwin Smith Papyrus dated 16th century BC. The first great Arabian, Rhazes started his life as a story teller and later on he turned to medicine in 900 AD. He was credited with first employing "kitgut" to suture abdominal wounds, which was the natural material for a lute player to choose (The Arabic word kit means a dancing master's fiddle, the musical strings of which were made up of sheep intestines). The word gradually evolved into "catgut" or "surgical gut." Many different materials have been used as ligatures and sutures through centuries, e.g. horse hair strands, pig's bristles, gold/silver wires, silk, silkworm gut, linen, cotton (flax), and the tendons and intestinal tissues of various animals.

By 1900, the catgut industry was firmly established in Germany, due to the use of sheep intestine in their sausage industry. In 1902, Claudius established iodine sterilization of the suturing material. The development of synthetic absorbable sutures began in 1931, with the production of an absorbable synthetic fiber of polyvinyl alcohol.

Classification

Sutures can be broadly divided into:
1. *Absorbable:* All suture materials that are digested by the body enzymes or are hydrolyzed by the tissue fluids are absorbable. They can be further classified into **natural and synthetic.**
2. *Nonabsorbable:* Sutures that cannot be digested by tissue enzymes and are encapsulated or walled off are nonabsorbable. Nonabsorbable suture materials can also be classsified into **natural, metallic and synthetic.**

These can be further divided into monofilament and multifilament type in each category.

a. *Monofilament type:* It is made up of a single strand, resists harboring micro-organisms and ties smoothly. It is to be handled delicately without any damage to the strands to avoid breakage postoperatively.

b. *Multifilament type:* It consists of several filaments twisted or braided together into a single strand. This gives good handling and tying characteristics. As this type of suture can harbor bacteria, it is not suitable in the presence of contamination and infection.

They can also be classified as natural and synthetic (Table 6.1).

3. *Coated or Non-coated:* Some sutures like polyester sutures are usually coated with a biologically inert nonresorbable compound. This highly effective lubricant provides a thin coating, which dramatically reduces the surface friction of the braid, which aids the thread in passing more easily through the tissues. This coating, however, makes knot security an issue, as the material will easily untie if not secured with a surgeon's knot.

4. Surgical threads are also classified by the thread diameter. Thread materials range in diameter or thickness from 1-0 to 10-0, with the higher number of zeros, corresponding to the thinner, more delicate thread.

In dentistry, a 3-0 thread diameter is usually used to secure flaps, when a mattress suturing technique is used and then a 4-0 thread is used closer to the flap edges to co-apt tension free flap edges. Thicker sutures are used for approximation of deeper layers, wounds in tension prone areas and for ligation of blood vessels.

Requisites for Suture Materials

1. *Tensile strength:* In selection of a thread 'Tensile strength" is an important quality. Depending on the elasticity of the material, the strength will vary. Flexible materials will have a greater ability to stretch and bear stress. Adequate material strength will prevent suture breakdown and the use of proper knots for the material used will prevent untying or knot slippage.

2. *Tissue biocompatibility, low tissue irritation and reaction:* Sutures made from organic material will evoke a higher tissue response than synthetic sutures.

Tissue reaction is also directly proportional to the amount and size of the suture material used.

3. *Low capillarity:* Multifilament type suture materials soak up tissue fluid by capillary action providing a rich medium for proliferation of microbes and in turn, increasing the chances of inflammation and infection.

4. *Good handling and knotting properties:* Ease of tying and a thread type that permits minimal knot slippage also influence the thread selection.

5. *Sterilization without deterioration of properties:* Most of the suture materials available in packages are sterilized by dry heat and ethylene oxide gas.

PRINCIPLES OF SUTURE MATERIAL SELECTION

The selection of suture material by a surgeon must be based on a sound knowledge of the healing characteristics of the tissues which are to be approximated, thickness of the tissues to be sutured, the physical and biological properties of the suture materials, the condition of the wound to be closed as well as the biological forces exerted on the healing wound, (e.g. muscle pull, swelling) and the probable postoperative course of the patient and the interaction between the suture material and the tissues.

1. *Rate of healing of tissues:* When a wound has reached maximal strength, sutures are no longer required. Therefore:

a. Various suture materials can be chosen for intraoral and extraoral use. The surgeon should select a suture that will lose its tensile strength at about the same rate that the tissues gain strength.

b. Tissues that ordinarily heal slowly such as skin, fascia and tendons should usually be closed with nonabsorbable sutures.

c. Tissues that heal rapidly such as muscles, periosteum may be closed with absorbable sutures.

2. *Tissue contamination:* Foreign bodies in potentially contaminated tissues may convert contamination to infection. Therefore, monofilament absorbable or nonabsorbable sutures are used in potentially contaminated wounds.

3. *Cosmetic results:* Where cosmetic results are important, close and prolonged apposition of wounds and

Table 6.1: General information about suture materials

	Suture	Classification	Raw material	Absorption rate	Tissue reaction	Contraindication	Warnings	Uses
1.	Surgical gut	Natural, monofilament, absorbable	Collagen derived from sheep or bovine intestine			Being absorbable, should not be used when prolonged approximation of tissue under stress is required		Suture subcutaneous tissues, ophthalmic surgery, oral surgery Can be used in the presence of infection
	Plain			70 days	Moderate		Absorbs quickly	
	Chromic			90 days	Moderate, but less than plain gut		Tendency to fray	
2.	Linen	Natural, multifilament, nonabsorbable	Staple flax fibers	Not applicable	Minimal	Poor tensile strength, cannot be used for suturing under tens on	None	Ligation of superficial vessels. Mucosal suturing without stress
3.	Surgical silk	Natural, multifilament, nonabsorbable	Filament spun by the silkworm larva to form its cocoon	Not applicable	Moderate	Cardiovascular surgery	None	General, plastic and ophthalmic surgery, ligating body tissues
4.	Surgical cotton	Natural, multifilament, nonabsorbable	Staple Egyptian cotton fibers	Not applicable	Minimal	None	None	Most body tissues for ligating and suturing
5.	Surgical steel	Natural, multifilament, nonabsorbable	Alloy of iron, nickle and chromium	Not applicable	Low	Should not be used with a prosthesis of another alloy	May corrode and break at points of bending, twisting and knotting	Abdominal wall and skin closure, sternal closure, retention, tendon repair, orthopedic and neurosurgery
6.	Coated Vicryl (Polygalactin 910)	Synthetic, monofilament/multifilament, absorbable	Copolymer of lactide and glycolide coated with polygalactin 370 and calcium stearate	60–90 days	Mild	Being absorbable, should not be used when prolonged approximation of tissue under stress is required	Safety not proved in neural and cardiovascular tissues	Ligate or suture tissues where an absorbable suture is desired
7.	Polydiaxonone	Synthetic, monofilament, absorbable	Polyester polymer	210 days	Slight	Being absorbable, should not be used when prolonged approximation of tissues under stress is required	Absorbs slowly	Abdominal and thoracic closure, subcutaneous tissue, rectal and colon surgery, orthopedic and plastic surgery. Can be used in the presence of infection
8.	Nylon	Synthetic, monofilament/multifilament, nonabsorbable	Polyamide polymer	Degrades at a rate of 15–20% per year	Extremely low	None	None	Skin closure, retention plastic, ophthalmic surgery, and microsurgery
9.	Polypropylene	Synthetic, monofilament, nonabsorbable	Polymer of propylene	Not applicable	Minimal transient acute inflammatory reaction	None	None	General, plastic, cardiovascular surgery, skin closure ophthalmology
10.	Collagen	Natural, monofilament, absorbable	Homogeneous dispersion of pure collagen fibrils from the flexor tendons of beef	56 days	Minimal	After 10 days only 10% of the tensile strength remains, hence cannot be used where tissue healing is slow	None	Ophthalmic surgery

avoidance of irritants will produce the best results. Therefore:

   a. Use the smallest, inert monofilament suture material such as polyamide or polypropylene.

   b. Avoid skin sutures and close subcuticularly wherever possible with Monocryl or Vicryl or Prolene.

   c. Under certain circumstances, to secure close apposition of skin edges, skin closure tape may be used.

   d. Dermabond liquid stitches provide a quick, effective and sutureless approximation of skin. It also acts as a barrier to prevent external microbial infection and gives excellent cosmetic results.

4. *Microsurgical procedures:* The tissues most commonly approximated under microscope are arteries, veins, nerves, tendons, etc. The most commonly used suture is 10-0 Polyamide Monofilament.

5. *Cancer patients:* Hypoproteinemia and chemotherapy can breakdown the wound. Synthetic nonabsorbable sutures are used. If the patient is to be irradiated in the postoperative period, monofilament polypropylene should not be used. Instead, polyester should be used.

6. ***Wound repair in patients following irradiation:*** In these patients, not only the normal healing process is delayed, but the tolerance to trauma of irradiated tissues is markedly reduced.

   a. Use extremely careful and gentle surgical technique.

   b. Avoid tension sutures and mattress sutures as they further increase the degree of ischemia.

   c. Plan closure in layers.

   d. Avoid continuous and constant pressure in irradiated tissues.

   e. For fascial layer use nonabsorbable sutures, polypropylene is ideal.

7. *Nutritional status:* When a patient is undernourished and hypoproteinemic, nonabsorbable sutures should be used, as tissues need to be kept in approximation for a longer period. Use of absorbable sutures may result in wound dehiscence.

8. *Suture size:* The size of the suture material should be properly selected, depending on the tensile strength of the tissues to be approximated and whether or not there will be flap tension or freely mobile tissues.

Biological Response of the Body to Suture Materials

The first response of the body as in any healing process is invasion of the tissue site by neutrophils. If uncomplicated by infection or trauma, the acute cellular tissue response to the suture material changes in about three days after implantation. The original population of neutrophils is replaced predominantly by monocytes, plasma cells, and lymphocytes. Small sprouts of fragile vessels infiltrate the area, and eventually fibroblasts and connective tissue proliferate. Enzyme histochemistry has demonstrated that all the cellular changes are accompanied by the presence of a variety of enzyme patterns. Cellular enzyme activity is an important factor associated with all foreign body reactions. The level of lysosomal enzyme synthesis and function in macrophages is associated significantly with their phagocytic activity.

Assuming the same technique, tissue and other relative factors, the tissue response to all the sutures is relatively the same for the first five to seven days. After this the response is more related to the type of suture material. Plain catgut elicits a more intense response with macrophages and neutrophils, while all the nonresorbable materials show a less intense, relatively acellular response. All sutures passing through the mucous membrane or skin provide a "wick" or pathway through which bacteria can track down and gain access to the underlying tissues. The longer the suture remains, the deeper the epithelial invasion of the underlying tissues. When the suture is removed the epithelial tract remains. These cells may eventually disappear or remain to form keratin and epithelial inclusion cysts. The epithelial pathway may also result in the typical "railroad scar" formation.

SUTURE NEEDLES

The surgical needles are of two types:
1. Eyed and
2. Eyeless (Fig. 6.1A).

Suture needles usually are also classified according to their curvature, radius and shape (Figs 6.1 B and C).

The surgical needle comprises of three parts:
1. Needle eye or swagged end (press fit)
2. Needle body
3. Needle point.

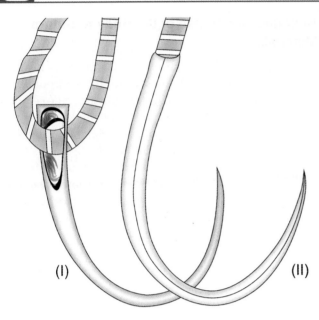

Fig. 6.1A: (I) Eyed suturing needle; (II) Eyeless (swaged) suturing needle

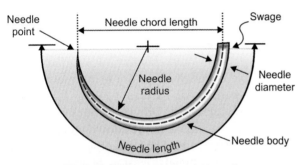

Fig. 6.1B: Anatomy of a surgical needle

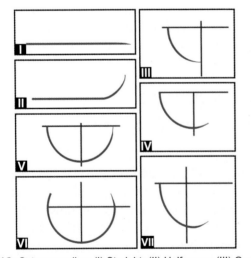

Fig. 6.1C: Suture needles: (I) Straight; (II) Half curve; (III) One-fourth circle; (IV) Three-eight circle; (V) Half circle; (VI) Five-eight circle; (VII) Compound curvature

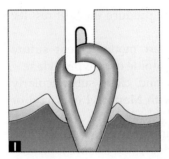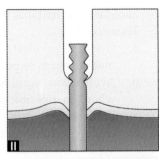

Fig. 6.1D: Advantages of eyeless needle. (I) Tissue disruption caused by double suture strand with eyed needle; (II) Minimum tissue disruption by single suture strand swaged to needle

Needle Eye

The eye can be closed or swaged. The closed eye is similar to the eye of the household needle. The shape of the eye may be round, oblong or square. Eyed needles must be threaded and present the disadvantage of pulling a double thread through the tissues and therefore are also known as traumatic needles. When the suture is attached to the needle via a hole drilled through the end of the needle, and the end is swagged during manufacture, it is called a swaged suture. These are also known as atraumatic needles.

Advantages of Eyeless Needles

1. Less trauma to the tissues, since a single strand of suture material has to be drawn through the tissues and this creates a smaller hole (Fig. 6.1D).
2. Each patient has the benefit of a new, sharp, guaranteed sterile needle.
3. No chances of accidental unthreading of the needle and losing it while suturing.
4. Faster and more efficient procedure.
5. Needles are made up of high quality steel.
6. Tru-tempering process gives uniform strength.
7. By merely quoting the Code Number, the surgeon indicates the type, size, length of the suture as well as the details of the needle.
8. Nurse working hours are saved—no need of ordering, cleaning, sterilizing and threading the eyed needles.

Needle Body (Fig. 6.2)

The body or the shaft section is usually referred to as the needle grasping area. The cross-sectional configuration of the body may be round, oval, side flattened rectangular, triangular or trapezoidal.

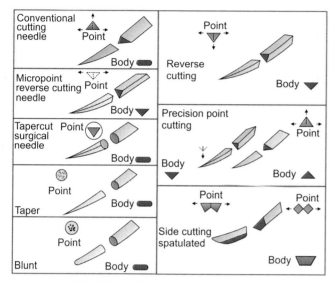

Fig. 6.2: Needle points and body shapes

The longitudinal shape of the body may be straight, half curved, curved (1/4th, ½, 3/8th or 5/8th) or compound curved. The half circle curved needles are the most commonly used needles in oral surgical procedures.

Needle Point (Fig. 6.2)

The point is the extreme tip of the needle to the maximum cross-section of the body. The tip can be cutting, round or blunt. Cutting needles have at least two opposite cutting edges. They are ideal for suturing keratinized tissues like the skin, palatal mucosa, buccal and alveolar mucosa. Cutting edges can be conventional, reverse or side cutting. They are triangular in cross-section.

Round/tapered needles are used for suturing soft and nonkeratinized tissues like muscle, fascia, and neural sheath.

◼ NONABSORBABLE SUTURES

These surgical threads are fabricated either from natural, metallic or synthetic materials.

Perma-Hand Surgical Silk

It is derived from the cocoon of the silk worm larvae. It is basically a protein like keratin of hair and skin and is covered initially by an albuminous layer. This layer is removed by a process of degumming prior to making of sutures. The suture is braided round a core and coated with wax to reduce capillary action. The material has high

tensile strength, which is totally lost after two years. Silk being a foreign protein, tissue reaction is much greater than to the synthetic nonabsorbable sutures; but is less in intensity than surgical gut. Encapsulation of the silk with a fibrous capsule usually occurs in 14 to 21 days. Handling properties are best of all suture materials and it knots easily and securely. It is sterilized by gamma irradiation. It is the most universally used material in Dentistry, as it is relatively inexpensive.

Perma-Hand Surgical Silk is available as eyeless needled sterile suture in sizes 7-0 to 1-0.

Reels as nonsterile sutures are available in sizes 5-0 to 3-0.

Linen

It is made from flax and is cellulose material. It is a natural cellulose polymer. It is twisted to form a fiber to make a suture. Tissue reaction is similar to silk and the material handles and knots well. It gains 10 percent in tensile strength when wet and is fairly unique in this respect. It is very extensively used for tying pedicles and as ligatures.

Cotton

It is derived from the hair of the seed of the cotton plant. Like linen, it is twisted to form a suture. Tissue reaction is like silk and linen and tends to be a polymorphonuclear cellular type. It is weaker as compared to linen. Handling is not as good as silk.

Polyamides

These are better known as Nylon. They are chemically extruded, and generally available in monofilament form. Passage through the tissue is easy, because of low co-efficient of friction and tissue reaction is minimal. Tensile strength loss after 1 year implantation is approximately 25 percent. The fiber tends to be stiff for handling, although this has been improved by the addition of fluid to the suture in the packet. Nylon has a memory and hence knot security is lower than Terylene. It can be available in the braided form also. Monofilament sutures are available in sizes ranging from 10-0 to 2-0.

Polyesters

These fibers are better known as Terylene and Dacron. They are chemically extruded from a polymer and braided to form sutures. They have extremely high tensile strength, which tends to be retained indefinitely; hence it has become the suture of choice in cardiovascular surgical procedures. Teflon or e-PTFE (expanded polytetrafluoroethylene) coating to these polyester threads reduces the tendency to cut through the tissues. However, this coating causes flaking in the tissues. Therefore, Ethicon introduced Ethibond sutures which are polyester coated with polybutylate. It provides excellent bonding and does not flake in the tissues and does not increase the suture diameter.

Polypropylene

This fiber is better known as Prolene. It is a monofilament and is chemically extruded from a purified and dyed polymer. It has an extremely high tensile strength, which it retains indefinitely on implantation and has an extremely low tissue reactivity. It can extend up to 30 percent before breaking and is useful to accommodate postoperative swelling and thereby helps to prevent tissue strangulation. It slides through the tissues readily and is sterilized by ethylene oxide. It is non-biodegradable. It is available is sizes from 8-0 to 1-0. It can be used for dental implant surgery, bone graft procedures, etc.

Stainless Steel

Stainless steel has an enviable reputation among non-absorbable sutures for strength and low tissue reaction. But it needs a very exacting technique, as it can pull or tear out the tissues and necrosis can result due to too tight a suture. Barbs on the end can tear gloves, breaking sterile technique or traumatizing surrounding tissues. Kinks in the wire can render it practically useless.

■ NATURAL ABSORBABLE SUTURES

Surgical Gut

It is a natural polymer built up from molecules of amino acids. It is derived from the submucosa of sheep intestines or the serosa of beef cattle intestines and is over 99 percent pure collagen. It is absorbed by a process of enzymatic digestion by proteolytic enzymes derived from lysozymes contained within polymorphs and macrophages. Absorption rate depends on size and also on the type of the gut whether it is plain or chromicised, and is usually completed within 60 to 120 days. Tensile strength loss of the suture material is however faster than absorption. Plain surgical gut loses its tensile strength in 15 days, while chromic surgical gut loses it within 30 days. Surgical gut is supplied in a sterile fluid to keep the gut hydrated and supple. It is sterilized by gamma irradiation. Allergic reaction to surgical gut is rare now and in olden days it used to be due to iodine sterilization or due to impurities such as mucopolysaccharides, which were found due to improper cleaning process of the animal intestines.

When used intraorally, it loses most of its tensile strength in 24 to 48 hours, unless it is coated with a chromic compound that extends absorption up to 7 to 10 days and extends loss of tensile strength for up to 5 days. Surgical gut sutures may break more rapidly in patients with a very low intraoral pH. A decrease in intraoral pH may be found in metabolic disorders, Sjögren's syndrome, chemotherapy, radiation therapy, some medications like antipsychotics, diuretics, antihypertensive agents, antipsoriasis medications and steroid inhalers. Surgical gut is contraindicated in these situations. It is available with eyeless needles as well as standard sutures, in sizes 5-0 to 2-0.

■ SYNTHETIC ABSORBABLE SUTURES

All these sutures are superior to natural absorbable sutures and more reliable in their performance. These sutures are manufactured in the laboratory and from carbohydrates. These are polymers. A polymer is made up of a large number of molecules called monomers, linked together to form a chain. In synthetic absorbable sutures, the linkage is broken by hydrolysis. Therefore, allergic reactions are eliminated and early absorption in hypoproteinemic conditions is possible. These can be either monofilament or braided, coated or non-coated. They can be natural in color or can be colored violet by D and C Green (Drugs and Cosmetics clearance). They are twice as strong as compared to natural absorbable sutures and lose their tensile strength slowly; thus helping to hold the tissues together during the critical period of wound healing. Different synthetic absorbable sutures support the wound for different time periods. They do not leave behind any foreign body after total absorption, which is by a simple process of hydrolysis and evoke minimal tissue reaction. They have excellent handling characteristics, but require a special square knotting procedure. They are sterilized by ethylene oxide. Their shelf life is five years and should be stored away from heat. They can be suitably selected for different tissue layers in various surgical procedures, depending on whether they are required for short, medium or long term wound healing. They are available in full range, in varying sizes from 10-0 to 1-0 and swagged to different types of needles.

COATED VICRYL - POLYGLACTIN 910 BRAIDED SUTURE MATERIAL

1. *Polyglycolic acid:* It is formed by the monomer, glycolic acid and linking it together to form a polymer, polyglycolic acid; and this comes from the family of sugars.
2. *Polyglactin:* It is a copolymer of lactide and glycolide. Lactic acid belongs to the same family as milk products.

   In Vicryl polyglactin 910, a lactic acid monomer has been introduced in a ratio of one part to every nine parts of glycolic acid. Coated Vicryl is twice as strong as chromic catgut and retains its tensile strength up to 28 days. Thus, it scores over natural absorbable sutures during the critical period of wound healing. The coating consists of 50 percent polyglactin and 50 percent calcium stearate. In polyglactin 910 suture the formulation is 90 percent glycolide, 10 percent lactide, while polyglactin coating is 35 percent glycolide and 65 percent lactide. The chemical similarity between the two materials ensures that the coating will bond permanently on to the basic braiding. Calcium stearate is an absorbable organic lubricant. With Vicryl suture, knots do not "lock" prematurely and snug down as desired. Coated vicryl can be used wherever an absorbable suture or ligature is required. The sterilization is by ethylene oxide process. The shelf life is five years. It should be kept away from moisture and direct heat. Coated Vicryl is available as dyed violet and as undyed beige color, in sizes ranging from 10-0 to 2-0 on different types of needles.
3. *Vicryl plus:* Polyglactin 910 coated, braided synthetic absorbable antibacterial suture.

   Vicryl plus antibacterial suture is the world's first and only antibacterial suture, which offers protection against bacterial colonization of the suture. It contains Triclosan which is a broad spectrum antibacterial agent and effective against the most common pathogens associated with surgical site infections. Its main advantage is that it provides defense against unwanted bacteria by a zone of inhibition that stops bacterial growth. It should not be used for ophthalmic, cardiovascular and neural tissues.
4. *Vicryl Rapide—Polyglactin 910 coated: braided synthetic absorbable suture:* It is identical to coated Vicryl suture. The rapid absorption quality is achieved by exposure of coated Vicryl to gamma irradiation, resulting in material with low molecular weight than coated vicryl. This is available only undyed (beige). It loses all its strength between 10th and 12th days and gets totally absorbed within 42 days. These sutures are intended for use in closing mucosa and skin, where only short term wound support (less than 10 days) is required. Shelf-life of Vicryl Rapide sutures is five years. It is available in sizes 3-0 to 1-0.
5. *Monocryl-Polyglecaprone 25—monofilament synthetic absorbable suture:* It is composed of a copolymer of 75 percent glycolide and 25 percent caprolactone and is available undyed as well as dyed violet. It is the most pliable, flexible monofilament suture with excellent handling properties. The major benefit of this material is its predictable loss of tensile strength over three weeks period. This is due to systematic hydrolysis of the suture material. It is absorbed in 90 to 120 days. It is sterilized with ethylene oxide and ideal for subcutaneous closure. Monocryl is available in natural golden color as well as in violet color and in sizes from 5-0 to 1-0.
6. *Polydioxanone (PDS) and PDS II—Polydioxanone monofilament synthetic absorbable suture:* PDS (Polydioxanone) sutures are formed by polymerizing the monomer-para-dioxanone, in the presence of a catalyst to form a strong but soft, pliable filament, which is broken down by hydrolysis in the presence of moisture.

   The PDS II sutures are an improved version of the initial PDS sutures, which give wound support beyond the four weeks period. Total mass is absorbed between 180 and 210 days. It is available in sizes 1-0 to 6-0.

   Precaution: Adhesive should not be allowed to enter the wound, otherwise foreign body reaction will delay the wound healing.

Principles of Suturing

1. The needle should be grasped at approximately 1/3rd the distance from the eye and 2/3rd from the point.
2. The needle should enter the tissues perpendicular to the tissue surface.
3. The needle should be passed through the tissues along its curve.

4. The suture should be passed at an equal depth and distance from the incision on both sides.
5. The needle always passes from the movable tissue to the fixed tissue.
6. The needle always passes through the thinner tissue to the thicker tissue.
7. The needle always passes from the deeper tissue to the superficial tissue.
8. Tissues must never be closed under tension. Undermining the tissues must be done prior to suturing in such cases.
9. The suture should be tied only to approximate the tissues, not to blanch.
10. The knot should never lie on the incision line.
11. Sutures should be placed at a greater depth than the distance from the incision, so as to evert the wound margins.
12. Sutures on the skin are usually removed in 5 days and intraoral sutures in 7 days. If there is tension while suturing, the sutures may be kept for 10 days.

Surgical Knot Tying

Surgical knot tying is vital to the art of suturing. It is essential for knot security and to prevent untimely knot untying, that the appropriate surgical knot be used for the specific suture material being secured. Knot security can be assessed by measuring the force required to slip or break a knotted loop of suture material. The type of knot that is used for each material is determined by the mode in which each type of thread is manufactured. A knot can be tied using an instrument, like the needle holder or with the hand.

Secure/Square Knot

Standard Square or Reef knotting method (Fig. 6.3A): It is a special knotting technique, once tied, the knots are secure. The first throw is placed in precise position for the knot, using a double loop. The second throw is tied using horizontal tension. Additional two throws are desirable. Totally there should be four throws and the ends should be cut long.

Surgeon's Knot (Fig. 6.3B)

It is formed by two throws of the suture around the needle holder on the first tie and one throw in the opposite direction in the second tie.

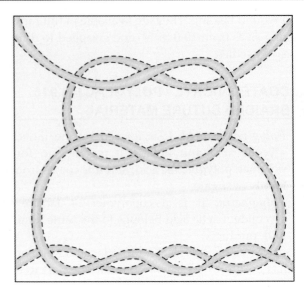

Fig. 6.3A: Square knot

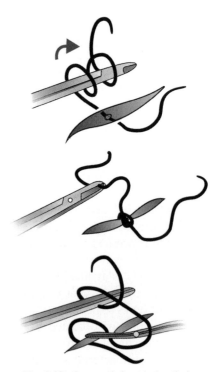

Fig. 6.3B: Surgeon's knot being tied

Synthetic resorbabale and nonresorbable suture materials can be used to prevent untimely knot untying.

Granny's Knot or Slip Knot (Fig. 6.3C)

When using silk, chromic catgut or plain catgut suture material, a slip (Granny's) knot can be used. It involves a tie in one direction followed by a second tie in the same direction and a third tie in the opposite direction to square the knot and hold it securely.

SUTURING TECHNIQUES

Interrupted Suture-Sling Suture (Fig. 6.4)

The suture is passed through both the edges at an equal depth and distance from the incision, needle penetration

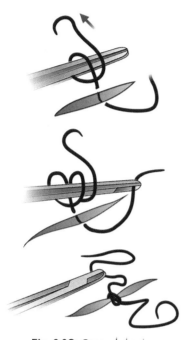

Fig. 6.3C: Granny's knot

should be 3 mm from the wound edges and the knot is tied. It is the most commonly used suture.

Advantages

1. It is strong, and can be used in areas of stress.
2. Successive sutures can be placed according to individual requirement.
3. Each suture is independent and the loosening of one suture will not produce loosening of the other.
4. A degree of eversion can be controlled.
5. If the wound becomes infected or there is an hematoma formation, removal of a few sutures may offer a satisfactory treatment.

Continuous Over and Over Suture (Fig. 6.5A)

Initially, a simple interrupted suture is placed and the needle is then reinserted in a continuous fashion such that the suture passes perpendicular to the incision line below and obliquely above. The suture is ended by passing a knot over the untightened end of the suture. It provides a rapid technique for closure and distributes the tension uniformly over the suture line. It also offers a more water tight closure.

Continuous Locking Suture (Fig. 6.5B)

This technique is similar to the continuous suture, but locking is provided by withdrawing the suture through

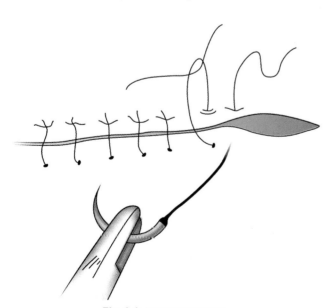

Fig. 6.4: Interrupted suture

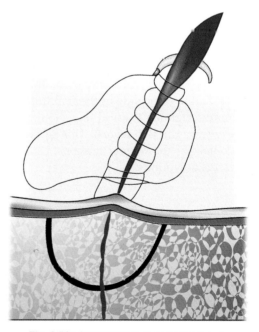

Fig. 6.5A: Continuous over and over suture

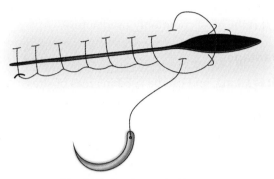

Fig. 6.5B: Continuous locking suture

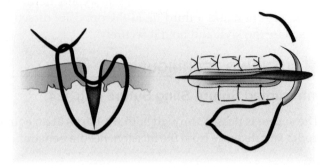

Fig. 6.7: Vertical mattress suture

its own loop. The suture thus passes perpendicular to the incision line. The locking prevents excessive tightening of the suture as the wound closure progresses.

Mattress Suture

These sutures may be horizontal or vertical. These are used in areas, where tension free flap closure cannot be accomplished. Mattress sutures are used to resist muscle pull, evert the wound edges and to adapt the tissue flaps tightly to the underlying structures (e.g. bone grafts, tissue grafts, dental implant, regenerative membrane, etc.)

Horizontal Mattress Suture (Fig. 6.6)

The needle is passed from one edge of the incision to another and again from the latter edge to the first edge in a horizontal manner and a knot is tied. The distance of needle penetration from the incision line and the depth of penetration of the needle is the same for each entry point, but horizontal distance of the points of penetration on the same side of the flap differs (needle penetration through the surgical flap should be at least 8 mm away from the flap edges). This suture provides a broad contact of the wound margins, e.g. closure of extraction socket wounds.

Vertical Mattress Suture (Fig. 6.7)

It is similar to the horizontal mattress, except that, all factors remaining constant, the depth of penetration varies, i.e. when the needle is brought back from the second flap to the first, the depth of penetration is more superficial. It is used for closing deep wounds.

Figure of 8 Suture (Fig. 6.8)

The figure of 8 suture can be used for the extraction socket closure as well as for adaptation of the gingival papilla around the tooth.

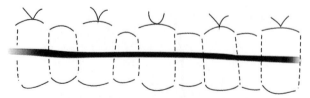

Fig. 6.6: Horizontal mattress suture

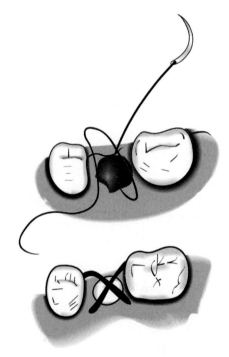

Fig. 6.8: Figure of 8 suture

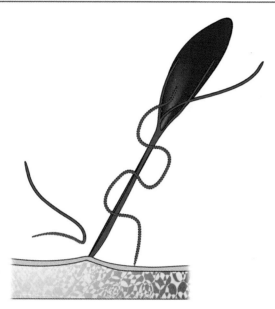

Fig. 6.9: Continuous subcuticular sutures

Subcuticular Sutures (Fig. 6.9)

The subcuticular layer of tough connective tissue if sutured will hold the skin edges in close approximation when cosmetic results are desired. Continuous short lateral stitches are taken beneath the epithelial layer of the skin. The ends of the suture come out at each end of the incision and are knotted. This type of suturing leaves a cosmetic scar.

■ SUTURE REMOVAL

The suture is grasped with an instrument and lifted above the epithelial surface. The scissors are then passed through one loop and transected close to the surface. The suture is then pulled out.

Skin sutures are usually removed after a period of 7 to 10 days depending upon the area, and mucosal sutures are removed between 5 and 7 days.

■ MECHANICAL WOUND CLOSURE DEVICES

Ligating Clips

These can be resorbable or nonresorbable. Ligating clips are made from stainless steel, tantalum or titanium or polydioxanone. They are designed for the ligation of tubular structures.

Surgical Staples

Surgical staples can be used for skin closure and closure of the abdominal layers. Skin staples are made up of stainless steel, and are placed uniformly to span the incision line. They have minimal tissue reaction. They can be used for routine skin closure anywhere in the body. Their use is contraindicated when it is not possible to maintain at least 5 mm distance from the stapled skin to the underlying bone and blood vessels.

Tissue Adhesives

After tight closure of the subcutaneous tissues, the skin layer can be closed with the help of tissue adhesive like N-butyl-cyanoacrylate, which on tissue contact polymerizes into a hard substance that keeps the wound margins together.

Dermabond Topical Skin Adhesive

It is a 2-octyl cyanoacrylate with a long carbon side chain structure that is combined with plasticizers - nontoxic, flexible, transparent bond. It has three dimensional strength and is three to four times stronger than N-butyl-cyanoacrylate. This adhesive is applied to the dry skin over the wound by a proper technique in multiple thin layers (at least three). It sets within three minutes and offers sutureless skin approximation. It has no length restrictions and wounds do not need to be linear. It provides a waterproof clear dressing resulting in excellent cosmetic result.

■ BIBLIOGRAPHY

1. Doctor HG. Surgeons and Sutures, 2nd revised edition 1999.
2. John McFarland (Ed). Sutures in wound Repair - Mr. Ian Capperauld Book on Post-graduate Surgery lectures - 3, Butterworths 1975;9-24.
3. Macht SD, Krizek TJ. Sutures and suturing current concepts. J Oral Surgery 1978;36:710-2.
4. Somerville NJ. Wound Closure Manual, Ethicon Inc. USA 1985;1-101.

7 Asepsis and Sterilization

INTRODUCTION

The concept of asepsis and its role in the prevention of infection was put forward nearly two centuries ago. The general principles for asepsis were laid down by Hungarian obstetrician, Ignaz Semmelweiss in Europe, in early 1850s; and Oliver Holmes in USA. These principles were accepted after Joseph Lister's studies on prevention of wound infection, carried out in between 1865 to 1891. Lister, working on antisepsis; initially used phenol (dilute carbolic acid) for contaminated wounds; later applied it in all surgical wounds; also in operating room by nebulization of the solution. Further developments occurred, with the introduction of steam sterilization, surgical masks, sterile gloves, sterile gowns and sterile drapes, etc.

The studies showed that, despite employment of new methods of sterilization and aseptic techniques, micro-organisms are introduced in surgical sites. These are implicated as the cause of many postoperative infections. However, as suggested by many clinicians, the most postoperative infections result from the following: faulty surgical technique, inadequate asepsis and disinfection. The success of prevention and control of infection in healthcare areas is largely dependent on the aseptic technique of all personnel, who perform invasive procedures, the sterility of all items directly concerned in such procedures and the disinfection of all surfaces and items in the immediate vicinity.

DEFINITIONS OF VARIOUS TERMINOLOGIES

Cleaning: It is a process which removes visible contamination, but does not necessarily destroy micro-organisms. It is a necessary prerequisite for effective disinfection or sterilization.

Asepsis: It is the avoidance of pathogenic organisms. It is the term used to describe methods which prevent contamination of wounds and other sites, by ensuring that only sterile objects and fluids come into contact with them, and that the risk of air-borne contamination is minimized.

Aseptic technique: It aims at excluding all micro-organisms. Surgical technique is aseptic, when sterile instruments and clothing and "no touch technique" is employed. It is the term used to describe methods which prevent contamination of wounds and other sites, by ensuring that only sterile objects and fluids come into contact with them; and that the risks of air-borne contamination are minimized.

Antisepsis: It is the procedure or application of an antiseptic solution, or an agent which inhibits the growth of micro-organisms, while remaining in contact with them, but does not necessarily imply sterility. The examples are scrubbing up and preparation of operative sites.

Antiseptic: It is a chemical, applied to living tissues, such as skin or mucous membrane to reduce the number of micro-organisms present, by inhibition of their activity or by destruction.

Disinfection: It is a process which reduces the number of viable pathogenic micro-organisms to an acceptable level, but may not inactivate some viruses and bacterial endospores.

Disinfectant: It is a chemical substance, which causes disinfection. It is used on nonvital objects to kill surface vegetative pathogenic organisms, but not necessarily spore forms or viruses.

Sterilization: It is the process of destruction or removal of all microbial forms.

Classification of Instruments and Equipment in Surgery

A. *Critical:* Instruments which penetrate mucous membrane or contact bone, the bloodstream or other normally sterile internal tissues, e.g. surgical instruments, scalpel, blades, surgical dental burs, needles, periodontal scalers, etc.

   Single use sterile disposable devices should be used whenever applicable.

B. *Semicritical:* Instruments which contact mucous membrane, but do not penetrate the soft tissues, e.g. mouth mirrors, dental handpieces, etc.

   It is heat sterilize or high level disinfectant.

C. *Noncritical:* Instuments which contact intact skin. For example, X-ray heads, face bows, pulse oximeter, blood pressure cuff, etc.

Clean and disinfect using a low to intermediate level disinfectant

Clearance of used instruments and equipment from the operatory and preparation for reuse is a process itself. It consists of five steps:
1. Transport of used items
2. Cleaning and disinfection
3. Preparation and packing
4. Sterilization
5. Storage.

Correct cleaning, packaging, sterilizer loading procedures, sterilization methods or high level disinfection methods should be followed to ensure patient safety.

◼ TRANSPORT OF USED ITEMS

Disposable items should be discarded into suitable container, syringes are destroyed and needles burnt and cut, and discarded into separate sharps container.

The rest of the used instruments should be transported in a separate tray from the operatory to the instrument cleaning area. Dental health care workers (DHCW) incharge of transport can be exposed to micro-organisms from contaminated instruments and devices through percutaneous injury or contact with nonintact skin of the hands or contact with mucous membranes of the eye, nose or mouth due to water splash. Contaminated instruments should be handled carefully to avoid percutaneous injuries.

Instrument Processing Area

Dedicated separate area should be available. This helps in quality control and ensures safety. The instrument processing area should have following sections:
1. Receiving, cleaning and decontamination
2. Preparation and packing
3. Sterilization
4. Storage.

Ideally, partitions should separate the sections to control traffic flow and contain contamination generated during cleaning. Processing space should be adequate for the volume of work anticipated and the items to be stored. DHCWs should be provided with ongoing training and regular monitoring for quality control.

Receiving, cleaning, decontamination: The DHCW should wear puncture resistant, heavy duty utility gloves, mask, protective eyewear, or face shield and gown or apron, while handling or manually cleaning contaminated instruments and devices. Reusable instruments should be received, sorted, cleaned and decontaminated in one section of the processing area. Initial cleaning removes organic and inorganic contamination. Removal of debris and contamination is achieved by scrubbing with a detergent and water or by an automated process (e.g. ultrasonic cleaner or washer-disinfector), using chemical agents.

If visible debris is not removed, it will interfere with microbial inactivation and can compromise the disinfection or sterilization process.

If manual cleaning is not done immediately, the instruments should be placed in a puncture resistant container filled with detergent, a disinfectant or an enzymatic cleaner. Soaking them in this manner will prevent drying of blood and body fluids. Use of a liquid chemical sterilent/high level disinfectant (e.g. glutaraldehyde) as holding solution is not recommended.

■ CLEANSING OF INSTRUMENTS

Cleansing Agents

Soaps and detergents: They are commonly used for the removal of debris from the instruments. Soaps are salts of fatty acids; and detergents are synthetic compounds. Both the groups act by reducing surface tension along the instrument surface, leading to emulsification of contaminants which are removed in the rinsing phase.

Soaps: They are effective at pH 9 or higher and even in a weak acidic environment, or in one containing soluble salts of calcium and magnesium, precipitation of soap will occur.

Detergents: They are compatible with calcium and magnesium ions and maintain their efficiency in neutral or slightly acidic solutions. Some detergents possess bactericidal activity against some specific gram-positive organisms. For example, sodium lauryl sulfate is effective against *Strep pneumoniae*. The spectrum of antibacterial activity of detergents is too narrow to classify them as disinfectants.

Other fat solvent solutions: Such as acetone, ether, and xylene, are sometimes used in cleaning. These solutions are sometimes expensive, caustic to living tissues and probably less effective in overall cleaning ability than soaps and detergents. Some disinfectant solutions such as aldehyde and phenols are also used in cleaning of instruments. These solutions should be thoroughly rinsed from the instrument surface prior to their use, as they are toxic to living tissues.

Lawrence and Block (1668) reported that proteins and other polymolecular structures, particularly when dry, serve as a protective covering for micro-organisms and prevent penetration of sterilizing medium. All surgical instruments must be cleansed of the debris including blood, saliva and necrotic material. This debris prevents contact of the sterilizing medium with the instruments, such as heat, chemicals or gas. Instruments such as bone files and bone burs should be thoroughly cleaned; as solid particles are wedged into small crevices. The various methods by which it can be achieved are mentioned: (i) scrubbing by hand usually with a stiff wire brush, (ii) ultrasonic cleaning devices. Rubbo and Gardner (1965) reported that these devices act by converting electrical energy into vibratory sound waves, which pass through a soap solution containing the instruments.

In nutshell:

1. " Sterile" does not mean safe and clean.
2. An item heavily loaded with microbiological material will be more difficult to sterilize than one lightly contaminated.
3. Medical devices/instruments must be thoroughly cleaned to reduce organic material or bioburden before sterilization and as soon as possible after use. This is the most effective stage of any decontamination procedure, which should accompany or precede all disinfection procedures.
4. Dried biological material is much more difficult to remove than fresh deposits. Blood with its content of iron, acid and sodium chloride is highly corrosive.
5. Improperly cleaned instruments if sterilized may be free of living micro-organisms, but they will be smeared with endotoxins—"the corpses of bacteria", which can trigger very strong inflammatory reactions in the body.
6. Presoak the instruments after use in water or an enzyme solution. This prevents drying of saliva and blood.

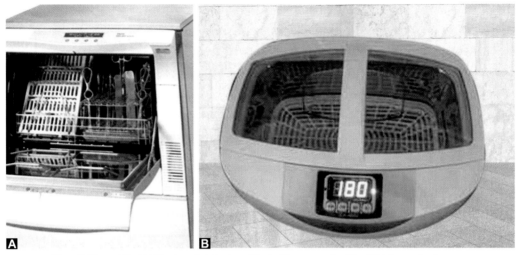

Figs 7.1A and B: (A) Washer disinfector with air filter, spray facility, (B) Ultrasonic cleaners

7. Manual scrubbing or washing in still/stagnant water increases the microbial count; hence should be avoided.

8. Automated washer disinfectors offer the safest, most reliable option, provided they are suitably monitored and maintained.

9. As an alternative to washer disinfectors (dishwasher), ultrasonic cleaning bath is recommended (Figs 7.1A and B).

10. Use of single use disposable items and equipment whenever possible.

11. Consider items difficult to clean (endofiles, broaches and burs) as single use disposables and discard them after each use.

Mechanism of Action

The disinfectant and antiseptics act on micro-organisms by one or more of the mechanisms listed in Table 7.1.

Drug Concentration and Therapeutic Index

In general, antiseptic effect increases with a rise in concentration. Alcohol is an exception, and shows maximum antiseptic activity in a 70 percent concentration. The potency of a particular concentration

Table 7.1: Mechanisms of action of disinfectants and antiseptics
- Coagulation of bacterial proteins
- Alteration in the properties of bacterial cell wall
- Binding of sulfhydryl groups essential for enzyme action
- Competition with essential substrates for the important enzymes in bacterial cell

is meaningful, only in relation to tissue toxicity (therapeutic index). The presence of debris and necrotic tissue reduces the penetration of these agents, thereby lowering their concentration. In the same way, tissue proteins reduce the concentration of halogen-containing and metallic antiseptics by adsorption, while anionic surfactants like soaps reduce the effective concentration of cationic surfactants by chemical neutralization.

Temperature and Duration of Contact

A limited rise in environmental temperature and prolonged contact can enhance antiseptic activity. A rise in temperature by 10°C generally doubles the antibacterial activity of chemical agents; whereas it increases that of moist heat a hundred-fold.

PACKAGING OR WRAPPING INSTRUMENTS FOR AUTOCLAVING (FIGS 7.2A TO G)

Packing instruments before sterilizing prevents them from becoming contaminated after sterilization till it is opened and used. Instruments must be clean, but not necessarily dry. Closed (nonperforated) containers (closed metal trays, capped glass vials) and aluminum foils cannot be used, because they prevent the steam from reaching the inner sections of the packs. Cassettes, drums, trays with opening on all sides may be used.

Packaging used for autoclaving must be porous, to permit steam to penetrate through; and reach the instruments. The materials used for packaging could be fabric or sealed biofilm/paper/muslin cloth pouches,

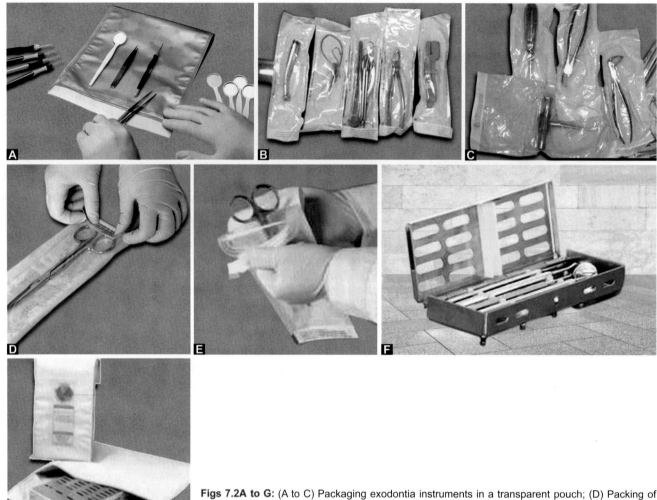

Figs 7.2A to G: (A to C) Packaging exodontia instruments in a transparent pouch; (D) Packing of instrument in a sterilization pouch; (E) Assistant delivering the sterile instrument; (F) Instruments packed in a metal cassette; (G) Instruments packed in a metal tray and enclosed in a pouch

nylon bags and tubings, sterilization wrap, and paper-wrapped cassettes. The bag or wrap is heat-sealed or sealed with tape. Pins, staples, and paper clips are not advisable; as they make holes in the wrap; and may allow micro-organisms to pass through subsequently.

The instruments are assembled into sets or trays and wrapped, packaged or placed into container system for sterilization. Hinged instruments should be processed open and unlocked.

An internal chemical indicator should be placed in every package, in addition, an external indicator (e.g. chemical indicator tape) should be used when the internal indicator cannot be seen from outside package. For unwrapped loads, an internal chemical indicator should be placed in tray or cassette with items to be sterilized (Figs 7.3A and B).

In case, the pack of instruments is to be stored and not used shortly after sterilization, the autoclave cycle should end with a drying phase. The instruments stored in damp conditions result in tarnish, corrosion or rusting.

Marking of Packs

Packs should have some external indication, showing that the pack has been processed. Autoclave tapes on packs change color after exposure to sterilization cycle. That does not prove sterilization, hence, it should be used in conjunction with the test for cycle sterilization. Each pack must be labeled with the contents, date of sterilization, autoclave number, and load number. This will help in locating processed items in case of recall.

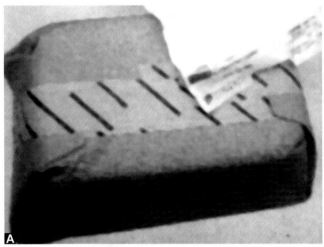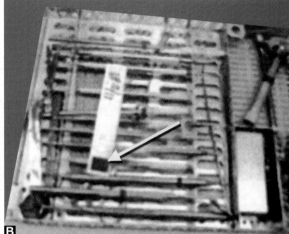

Figs 7.3A and B: (A) External chemical indicator, (B) Internal chemical indicator

METHODS OF STERILIZATION

Sterilization can be defined as the use of a physical or chemical procedure to destroy all forms of micro-organisms including bacteria, spores, fungi, and viruses. The term sterilization can only be applied to instruments, and not to skin, where only antisepsis can be achieved. A general principle is that all items used to penetrate soft tissue or bone, enter into or contact the blood stream or other normally sterile tissues, should be sterilized and be sterile at the point of use. A sterility requirement for medical products means that the theoretical probability that a living organism will be present on an object after the sterilizing process is equal to or less than one in a million, so-called sterility assurance level (SAL) = 10 degree.

There are several ways of achieving sterilization. Sterility may be achieved by: (1) Heat (2) Chemical (3) Ionizing radiation. Most commonly used methods are as follows: (i) by steam; or moist heat, at a raised atmospheric pressure, in an autoclave, (ii) by dry heat/hot air, at normal atmospheric pressure, in a dry oven, (iii) by use of ethylene oxide, (iv) by low-temperature steam and formaldehyde (LTSF) and (v) by irradiation.

Principles

1. All used instruments should be thoroughly cleaned; all deposits of blood and debris should be removed before sterilization.
2. It is essential for the sterilizing agent (heat, steam and/or gas) to be in contact with every surface of each item to be sterilized for the specified period of time at the specified temperature.
3. All sterilizing equipment must be regularly serviced and maintained by suitably qualified engineers. Appropriate test must be applied to check temperature, humidity, pressure, and gas content when appropriate; and which proves the elimination of bacteria and spores.
4. The manufacturer's instructions should be strictly adhered to for its operation and maintenance.

Heat is the most common and one of the most effective, simplest methods of sterilization. Heat may be transmitted through air, water, or oil. Heat method can be utilized in two forms: (i) moist heat, and (ii) dry heat.

Moist/Steam Heat Sterilization: Autoclave (Figs 7.4A to D)

Steam sterilization involves heating water to generate steam in a closed chamber (Autoclave—in which drums and trays with the materials to be sterilized can be kept inside) producing moist heat that rapidly kills micro-organisms. There is a mass heat transfer as the steam condenses. Use of saturated steam under pressure is the most practical, quickest, safest, effective, economic method of sterilization, known for the destruction of all forms of microbial life, because of its: (i) high penetrating capacity, and (ii) it gives up a large amount of heat (latent heat) to the surface with which it comes into contact, and on which it condenses as water. The advantages are: (i) the results are consistently good,

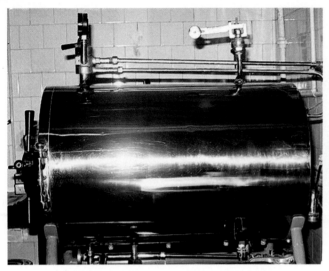

Fig. 7.4A: Horizontal autoclave for big institutes

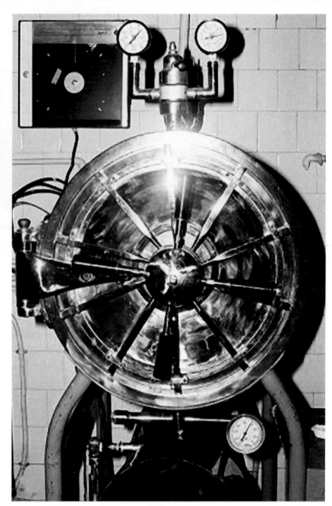

Fig. 7.4C: Front view of the big horizontal autoclave

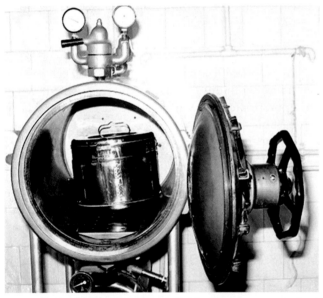

Fig. 7.4B: Autoclave with door open. Inside drums, trays can be kept with the material to be sterilized

and reliable, (ii) the instruments can be wrapped prior to sterilization. (iii) time efficient. (iv) good penetration. The main disadvantages are: (i) blunting and corrosion of sharp instruments, and (ii) damage to certain rubber goods.

There are two types of autoclaves or steam sterilizers available:

1. Downward (gravitation) displacement sterilizer: This is nonvacuum type autoclave.
2. Steam sterilizers (autoclave) with pre- and post-vacuum processes—Class B type

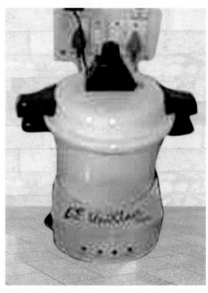

Fig. 7.4D: Small autoclave for the clinic

Steam Sterilizers (Autoclave) with Pre- and Post-Vacuum Processes

The sterilization process is composed of three main phases:

1. *Pretreatment phase/heat-up cycle:* All air is virtually expelled by a number of pulses (atleast three) of vacuum and the introduction of steam, so that the saturated steam can affect the goods during second phase.
2. *Sterilizing phase/sterilization cycle:* The temperature increases sufficiently up to the degree at which sterilization is to take place. Actual sterilizing period, is also called "Holding Time", starts when the temperature in all parts of the autoclave chamber and its contents (The Load) have reached the sterilizing temperature. This should remain constant within specified temperature band, throughout the whole sterilization phase (Plateau/Holding time).
3. *Post-treatement phase/depressurization cycle and drying cycle:* In this phase either the steam or the revaporized condensed water is removed by vacuum to ensure that the goods are dried rapidly.

Precautions

Trapped air pockets in the load prevent steam penetration during sterilization of porous material such as textiles and hollow items with long narrow lumina. A single vacuum pulse is inadequate for wrapped/hollow/porous loads. Several, (at least three) prevacuum pulses are needed to define preset vacuum level.

There are three major factors required for effective autoclaving: pressure, temperature and time.

Pressure: It is expressed in terms of psi (pounds per square inch) or kpa (kilopascals; kpa = 0.145 psi).

Temperature: To achieve required pressure, the temperature must be reached and maintained at 121°C (250°F). With the increase in temperature and pressure, superheated steam is formed. The exposure to this superheated steam brings about the sterilization. This steam which is lighter than air rises to the upper portion of the autoclave as more steam is formed, it eliminates air from autoclave. The purpose of complete elimination of air is to help superheated steam penetrate the entire load in the autoclave and remain in contact for the appropriate length of time.

Time: Wrapped loads (paper wraps or a thin cloth) require a minimum of 20 to 30 minutes after reaching full temperature and pressure. By selecting the correct temperature and time cycle, a wide variety of materials can be sterilized by this method: dressing packs, surgical instruments, laboratory equipment, culture media and pharmaceutical products. Liquids can be sterilized by autoclave, provided that the contents do not get inactivated by the high temperatures.

Higher temperatures and greater pressures shorten the time required for sterilization. At 15 psi pressure, the temperature of steam can reach 121°C. The time required to kill all living organisms at this temperature is 15 minutes. At 126°C for 10 minutes, and at 134°C for 3 minutes sterilization can be completed. The time required for sterilization for a particular item also varies with the amount of material and the thickness of the wrap. Perkins (1969) has discussed the instrument wrapping techniques and the placement of the packs in the autoclave.

The superiority of steam over hot air as a method of sterilization is due to the following: (i) Moist heat acts by denaturation and coagulation of enzymes and proteins; whereas dry heat acts by destructive oxidation of cell constituents. Moist heat kills more rapidly and at much lower temperature than dry heat. (ii) With the condensation of a large amount of latent heat to the surface. With steam condensation, besides emission of large amount of heat, there is a great contraction in it's volume. This results in production of negative pressure, and brings more steam to the site. Soon the temperature of the surface is raised to that of the surrounding steam. Thus, steam acts more quickly in heating exposed articles than hot air. (iii) Steam penetrates better than hot air. This is, partly due to its density, which is half that of air; and partly due to negative pressure.

Presently, two types of autoclaves are available: (i) Porous load autoclaves—to achieve complete sterilization, 121°C at 20 psi are maintained for 20 minutes. The articles which can be sterilized by this method include: towels used for draping, suture materials, cotton rolls rubber gloves, etc. (ii) Small portable bench model type autoclaves—for complete sterilization, 136°C at 32 psi are maintained for five minutes. The steam entering the top of the chamber penetrates the material in a top to bottom flow.

Sterilization cycles that operate at a high temperature for shorter times and are indicated for unwrapped and solid instruments which need to be used immediately. Standard sterilizing conditions— three to ten minutes at 273°F. It invariably results in residual air in the autoclave chamber.

To avoid or minimize corrosive action of steam on metals, the use of following agents have been reported. Crawford and Oldenburg (1967) recommended the addition of ammonia to the autoclave. Accepted Dental Therapeutics (1977) recommends use of dicyclohexylammonium nitrate or cyclohexylamine and decylamine. Bertolotti and Hurst (1978) recommend 2 percent sodium nitrate.

Tests for Efficiency for Heat Sterilization—Sterilization Monitoring

The mechanical, chemical and biological parameters are used to evaluate both the sterilizing conditions and the procedure's effectiveness.

Mechanical techniques for monitoring sterilization include assessing cycle time, temperature and pressure by observing the gauges or displays on the sterilizer and noting these parameters for each lot. Some tabletop sterilizers have recording devices that printout these parameters. Correct readings do not ensure sterilization, but incorrect readings can give first indication of a problem with sterilizer.

Spore testing: Biological indicator—should be done once a week to verify proper functioning of the autoclave with the help of *Geobacillus stearothermophilus* strips or vials (Fig. 7.5A).

Thermocouple: This is a thermometric testing, and a reliable gauge of efficiency. One recording is taken from a thermocouple placed inside a test pack of towels and a second one from the chamber drain. Comparison between the two recordings gives a good guide regarding the speed at which the steam penetrates the load.

Brown's test: These are ampoules that contain a chemical indicator; which changes its color; from red through amber to green at a specific temperature.

Autoclave tape: This is a tape printed with sensitive ink that undergoes a color change at a specific temperature. This test forms the basis of the Bowie-Dick test for high-vacuum autoclaves. Two pieces of strips are stuck onto a piece of square paper and placed in the middle of the test pack. With the application of temperature of 134°C for 3.5 minutes, there is a uniform development of bars throughout the length of the strips. This shows that the steam has passed freely and rapidly to the center of the load (Figs 7.5B and C).

STORAGE OF STERILE GOODS

Crump (1966) reported that the storage of instruments is also a problem. The pattern of storage varies from place to place. They are either stored in drawers, or in containers, in packs or sterile trays. The maintenance of sterility during transportation and storage is of utmost importance.

Packs should be stored with the following considerations:

i. Instruments are kept wrapped until ready for use.
ii. To reduce the risk of contamination, sterile packs must be handled as little as possible.
iii. Sterilized packs should be allowed to cool before storage; otherwise condensation will occur inside the packs.
iv. To prevent contamination from rodents, ants, and cockroaches, the store must be subjected to adequate pest control.

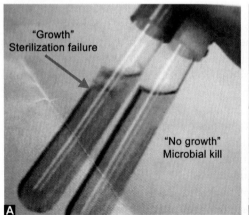
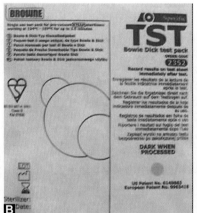
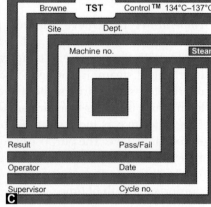

Figs 7.5A to C: (A) Biological indicator. If the repeat BI test is positive, the sterilizer should not be used, until it has been repaired, and declared as satisfactorily working with BI tests in three consecutive empty chamber sterilization cycle, (B and C) Autoclave function testing

v. Materials should be stored at least 8" off the floor and 18" from the ceiling.

vi. Sterile packs must be stored and issued in correct date order. The packs, preferably, are stored in drums which can be locked. Preset trays and cassettes are useful, as the instruments can be organized as per the procedure.

Dry Heat Sterilization

Dry heat sterilization involves heating air with transfer of heat energy from the air to the instruments. It is an alternative method of sterilization of instruments, particularly, the sharp instruments. The basic action is dehydration and oxidation of micro-organisms. Dry heat has less penetration, and is less effective than moist heat. The advantage is that, the instruments do not rust if they are dried prior to their placement in the sterilizer and there is relatively low cost of equipment. The disadvantage is that the process is time consuming and high temperature may damage the material to be sterilized. It is achieved by two methods:

1. Dry heat oven type sterilizer (static air): It has coils and heat rises within 60 to 120 minutes at 320°F or 160°C.
2. Dry heat: Rapid heat transfer (forced air) at high velocity within 12 minutes at 375°F/190°C. For wrapped items and within 6 minutes at 375°F for unwrapped items.

Hot Air Oven (Figs 7.6A and B)

It is used to sterilize items which do not get damaged by high temperatures, such as laboratory glassware, glass syringes and instruments. Hot air is a poor conductor of heat and has poor penetrating capacity. It does not penetrate grease, oil, and powders; and equipment containing these substances should be sterilized by other methods. High temperature damages fabrics and melts rubber/plastic, hence should not be sterilized by this method.

Temperature and time: This method of sterilization completely depends upon a combination of time and temperature. The sterilization is complete, if, the two factors are achieved throughout the load. The following of temperatures and times are used (Table 7.2).

Kelsey (1969) reported that the long time required for sterilization, is because of poor heat conduction by air and poor penetration of dry heat. The only advantage of this method is the maintenance of sharp edges of

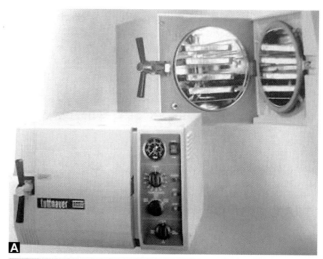

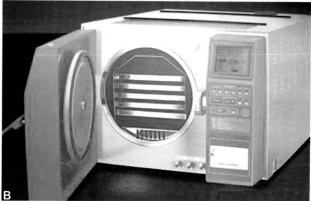

Figs 7.6A and B: Hot air sterilizer with automatic control of temperature (0 degree to 200 degrees)

Table 7.2: Relation of temperature and time		
Temperature		Time (minutes)
°C	°F	
160	320	120/60
170	340	60
150	300	150
140	205	180

cutting instruments, such as chisels. Hence sharp instruments are preferably sterilized by exposure to dry heat. Autoclaving will reduce their sharpness and lead to rusting. Custer and Coyle (1970) found that carbon steel instruments can loose their hardness because of dry heat.

The instruments must be clean and dry prior to wrapping. The wrapping material must be heat resistant. Aluminum foil, metal, and glass containers may be used in dry heat oven. The instruments should be loosely wrapped; otherwise they may puncture the wrapping. Paper and cloth packs must be avoided because they may char. The instruments sterilized with wrapping should be kept/stored in sterile condition; if not to be used immediately.

Spore testing should be done once a week to verify proper functioning of the sterilizer with the help of *Bacillus atrophaeus* strips.

Glass Beads Sterilizer (Fig. 7.7)

This method employs a heat transfer device. The media used are glass beads, molten metal or salt kept in a cup or crucible. The temperature achieved is of 220°C. The method employs submersion of small instruments such as endodontic files and burs, rotary instruments into the beads; and are sterilized in 10 seconds provided they are clean.

Oliet et al (1958) reported that temperatures vary in different areas of the sterilizer. A warm-up time of at least 20 minutes is recommended to ensure uniform temperatures in these sterilizers. Grossman (1974) recommended the use of salt media sterilization, because the accidental introduction of metal or glass clinging to the endodontic instruments into the root canal may cause blockage.

Some handpieces can be sterilized by dry heat. The handpieces should be carefully cleaned and lubricated with special heat resistant oils. Other handpieces which have sealed bearings or which have been pressure lubricated with appropriate oils can be autoclaved. The instructions given by respective manufacturers

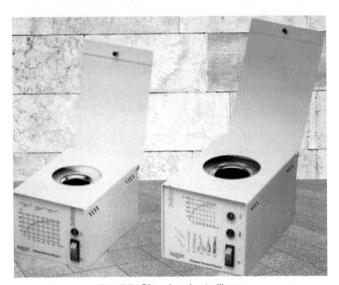

Fig. 7.7: Glass beads sterilizers

regarding the cleaning, lubrication and sterilization are of importance and should be followed.

Ethylene Oxide Gas Sterilization

Ethylene oxide gas is an alkaline, non-corrosive agent, highly penetrative that infiltrates packaged medical devices to kill bacteria, spores and viruses. Eto is toxic and flammable/explosive at low temperatures (flash point of −20°C) so it is used on products that could get damaged or cannot withstand high temperature processes used to sterilize objects sensitive to temperatures greater than 60° such as plastics, optics and electricals. It destroys micro-organisms by alkylation; and causes denaturation of nucleic acids of micro-organisms. It is highly toxic, irritant, mutagenic and potentially carcinogenic, and should not be used where heat sterilization of an object is possible. It is highly flammable, but when mixed with carbon dioxide this danger is minimized.

It is an excellent sterilizer of heat sensitive items. It is ideal for electric equipment, flexible fiber endoscopes and photographic equipment. As it is highly toxic it causes blister on contact with living tissues. The duration that the gas should be in contact with the material to be sterilized is dependent on temperature, humidity, pressure, and the amount of material.

Roberts and Rendell-Baker (1972) reported that, once exposed to the gas, some objects such as plastic require 1 to 7 days to degas. This process may be hastened by warming the objects during the degassing phase. It is mainly used in industries for presterilizing single-use medical devices.

The advantages are: (i) it penetrates extremely well, even through plastics, (ii) it can be used at a low temperature, (iii) it leaves no residue, (iv) it is a deo dorizer, (v) it is comparatively nontoxic, and (vi) many heat sensitive articles, e.g. plastic, rubber, can be sterilized. The disadvantages include: (i) high cost of the equipment, and (ii) toxicity of the gas, and the need for venting it, (iii) explosive and inflammable, and (iv) longer period of aeration.

Sterilization by Low-Temperature Steam and Formaldehyde (LTSF) (Chemical Vapor Sterilization/Unsaturated Chemical Vapor Sterilization)

This method uses a combination of dry saturated steam and formaldehyde to kill bacteria, spores and most viruses. The destruction of micro-organisms is due to the double action; by the heat and chemical—formaldehyde. Formaldehyde acts by alkylation of the nucleic acids, which are responsible for synthesis of proteins. It takes longer time than an autoclave; and shorter time than dry heat method. The required combinations of temperature and pressure are 127 to 132°C/270°F at 20 to 40 psi for 30 minutes. The advantages of this method are: (i) lack of corrosion of instruments, (ii) shorter duration of sterilization cycle, and (iii) the sterilization is achieved at a low temperature (73°C), hence, it is suitable for heat-sensitive equipment and items with plastic components which might get damaged by other processes. The disadvantage is that it requires provision of adequate ventilation to expel chemical vapors released from the chamber at the end of the cycle. This type of chemical sterilizer is also called Harvey sterilizer or Chemiclave. It uses chemical solution containing 0.23 percent formaldehyde, 72.38 percent ethanol (ethylmethyl, Ketone solution), acetone, ketone, water and other alcohols. It is suitable for handpieces, burs—carbon steel and diamond, orthodontic wires, bands, pliers, etc.

Irradiation

Radiation used for sterilization is of two types: (i) ionizing radiation, e.g. X-rays, gamma rays, and high-speed electrons and (ii) nonionizing radiation, e.g. ultraviolet light, and infrared light. These forms of radiation can be used to kill or inactivate micro-organisms.

Ionizing Radiation

It is effective for heat labile items. Bellamy (1959) reported that it has great penetrating properties. It is commonly used by the industry to sterilize disposable materials such as needles, syringes, swabs, culture plates, catheters in bulk, suture material, cannulas, and pharmaceuticals sensitive to heat, and various types of plastic materials including disposable plastic heart-lung machines. The lethal action of this radiation is believed to be due to its effect on the DNA of nucleus and on the other vital cell components. There is no appreciable rise in temperature. High energy gamma rays from cobalt-60 are used to sterilize such articles.

Nonionizing Radiation

Two types of nonionizing radiations are used for sterilization, ultraviolet and infrared.

Ultraviolet rays

It is absorbed by proteins and nucleic acids and kills micro-organisms by the chemical reactions it sets up in the bacterial cell. It has low penetrating capacity and its main application is purification of air in operating rooms; viz, to reduce the bacteria in air, water and on the contaminated surfaces. All forms of bacteria and viruses are vulnerable to ultraviolet rays below 3000 atmospheric pressure. Excessive exposure of skin can produce serious burns. Care must be taken to protect the eyes while using UV radiation for sterilization. Now, UV chambers are available for storage of sterilized packages (Fig. 7.8).

Infrared rays

It is another form of dry heat sterilization. It is a convenient method of sterilizing a large number of syringes sealed in metal container, within a comparatively short span of time.

It is most commonly used to purify air, such as in the operating room. Infrared is effective, however, it has no penetrating ability. It is largely limited in medical field to air sterilization and the preparations of immunizing agents by bacterial or viral attenuation.

Boiling Water

Water maintains and conducts heat extremely well. Boiling water produces a temperature of 100°C at normal atmospheric pressure. It requires 10 minutes

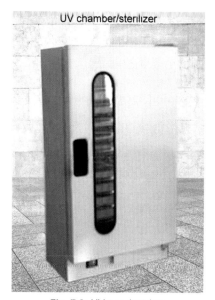

Fig. 7.8: UV ray chamber

exposure to this temperature, to kill many bacteria and some viruses (including HIV and HBV). However, prolonged time of 24 hours is required to kill bacterial spores, and even this prolonged time will not kill many viruses. Hence, boiling water is not recommended for sterilization of tissue penetrating instruments. Cutting instruments should not be sterilized by boiling as they loose their sharpness.

Oil

Hot oil baths have been used for sterilization of metallic instruments. At a temperature of 175°C, submersion for 15 minutes is required for sterilization. The disadvantages of using oil include: poor penetration, poor sporicidal activity, presents a fire hazard, and is difficult to remove from instruments such as handpieces without recontamination. It should not be used for hypodermic syringes or needles because of the danger of oil embolization.

■ DISINFECTION

Disinfection (high level disinfection) is the term used for destruction of all pathogenic organisms, such as, vegetative forms of bacteria, mycobacteria, fungi and viruses, but not bacterial endospores, from inanimate surfaces, such as walls, furnishings, and equipment; and antisepsis is the term applicable to living tissues such as skin and mucous membrane.

Methods of Disinfection

Disinfection by Cleaning

Cleaning with a detergent and clean hot water is an excellent mode of disinfection. It removes almost all pathogens including bacterial spores.

Disinfection by Heat

Heat is a simple and reliable disinfectant for almost anything except living tissues. The hot water used in the process of physical cleaning greatly enhances the quality of disinfection. Mechanical cleaning with hot water provides an excellent quality of disinfection for a wide variety of purposes.

Low Temperature Steam

This method kills most vegetative micro-organisms and viruses by exposure to moist heat. The typical conditions are exposure to steam at a temperature of 73°C for a period of 20 minutes below atmospheric pressure. By this method items can be easily cleaned as the coagulated protein residues can be easily removed. This makes it a useful procedure to render dirty instruments safe to handle prior to sterilization.

Disinfection by Boiling Water

Refer to Boiling Water in Sterilization.

Disinfection by Chemical Agents (Figs 7.9 and 7.10)

They are used to disinfect the skin of a patient prior to surgery, and to disinfect the hands of the operator. No available chemical solution will sterilize instruments immersed in it. Secondly, there is a risk of producing tissue damage if residual solution is carried over into

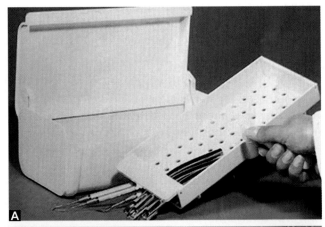

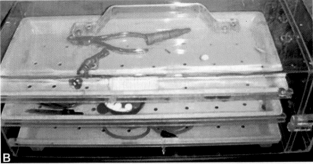

Figs 7.9A and B: Chemical sterilization box

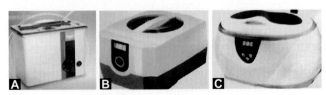

Figs 7.10A to C: Ultrasonic cleaners

the wound while it is being used. The chemicals used are: aldehydes, diguanides, phenolics and halogen derivatives.

Aldehydes

i. *Formaldehyde:* This is a broad spectrum antimicrobial agent which is used for disinfection. It is a hazardous substance, flammable and irritant to the eye, skin and respiratory tract. This is used up to 50°C and has limited sporicidal activity. It is used for large heat-sensitive equipment such as ventilators and suction pumps excluding rubber and some plastics.

ii. *Glutaraldehyde:* It is toxic, irritant and allergenic. It is a high level disinfectant. It is applicable where heat cannot be used. It is active against most vegetative bacteria (including *M. tuberculosis*), and some viruses (including HIV and HBV), fungi and bacterial spores. It is frequently used for heat sensitive material. A solution of 2 percent glutaraldehyde (Cidex), requires immersion of 20 minutes for disinfection; and 6 to 10 hours of immersion for sterilization .

Diguanides

Chlorhexidine is active against number of bacteria; including *Staph aureus* and some gram negative bacteria, but not spores, fungi and viruses. It can be prepared in alcohol or with cetrimide. It gets inactivated in the presence of soap, pus, plastics, etc. It is mainly used for cleaning skin and mucous membrane; 0.5 percent chlorhexidine in 70 percent alcohol; or chlorhexidine with cetrimide (Cetavlon or Savlon), or a 4 percent solution with detergent (Hibiscrub) as a preoperative scrub. As a 0.2 percent aqueous solution or 1 percent gel it can be used for suppression of plaque and postoperative infection.

Halogens

Hypochlorites: They are active against bacteria, spores, fungi, and viruses, including hepatitis B virus. They are readily inactivated by blood, pus and dilution. Sodium hypochlorite solution (household bleach) 1:10, freshly prepared solution, is an effective surface disinfectant.

▌ DISINFECTANTS

A disinfectant may be classified, on the basis of their properties, into the following: bactericidal, sporicidal, viricidal and fungicidal. They are usually used for decontamination of inanimate objects. The increase in their efficiency is related to increased toxicity. Certain limitations have to be considered prior to embarking on their use.

i. *Inactivation:* The presence of debris, blood or pus, inactivate the agents; hence, the instruments and the surfaces to be disinfected should be thoroughly cleaned.

ii. *Concentration:* Many agents retain their effectiveness in concentrated forms; and some agents at certain temperatures.

iii. *Stability:* Certain agents are not stable; particularly when used in dilute forms, and get deteriorated on storage. These agents are required to be prepared freshly. Such dilute solutions loose their efficacy and become contaminated and grow bacteria and yeasts.

iv. *Adequate contact:* Disinfection requires an appropriate period of exposure to the agent.

v. *Neutralization:* Substances such as soaps and detergents may neutralize the actions of the disinfectants.

Alcohols—Low Level Disinfectant

Ethanol and isopropyl alcohols are frequently used as antiseptics. Alcohols possess some antibacterial activity, against some gram-positive and gram negative bacteria, especially against *M. tuberculosis*. Alcohols act by denaturing proteins. They are not effective against spores and viruses. Spaulding (1939) found that to have maximum effectiveness, the alcohol must have a 10 minutes contact with the organisms. Solutions of 70 percent alcohol are more effective than higher concentrations, as the presence of water speeds up the process of protein denaturation as reported by Lawrence and Block (1968). The alcohols do not function as disinfectants when instruments, handpieces, or other equipment are simply wiped with them, since they evaporate quickly. Instruments made of carbon steel should not be soaked in alcoholic solutions, as they are corrosive to carbon steel. Rubber articles absorb alcohol, and prolonged soaking can cause a reaction when the article subsequently comes in contact with living tissue.

Alcohols can dissolve cements holding instruments, and plastics may harden or swell in their presence.

Aqueous Quarternary Ammonium Compounds

Benzalkonium chloride (Zephiran) was commonly used both as an antiseptic and a disinfectant. Neugeboren et al (1972) reported that the spectrum of their antibiotic activity is similar to alcohols, being limited largely to gram-positive organisms and some gram negative organisms. It is not effective against spores, viruses and *M. tuberculosis*. Hotchkiss (1946) reported that the molecule is a strong surfactant that increases the bacterial permeability of bacterial cell wall and permits escape of phosphorous and nitrogen. It also denatures intracellular proteins.

The effectiveness of these compounds depends on strength, activity and duration of contact. In many circumstances these goals are not achieved. Certain studies have reportedly implicated quaternary ammonium compounds contaminated with certain pathogens, such as, *Pseudomonas, Enterobacter* and other gram-negative organisms with outbreaks of nosocomial (hospital-acquired) infections.

Phenolic Compounds—Intermediate Level, Broad Spectrum Disinfectant

Phenol itself is toxic to skin and bone marrow. The phenolic compounds were developed to reduce their side effects but are still toxic to living tissues. These compounds, in high concentration, are protoplasmic poison, and act by precipitating the proteins and destroy the cell wall.

Lawrence and Block (1968) reported that their spectrum of activity includes lipophilic viruses, fungi and bacteria but not spores. The newer synthetic combinations seem to be active against hydrophilic viruses; hence these are approved by ADA for use as surface or immersion disinfectant.

These compounds are used for disinfection of inanimate objects such as walls, floors and furniture. They may cause damage to some plastics, and they do not corrode certain metals, such as brass, aluminum, and carbon steel. It has unique action, that it keeps working for longer period after initial application, known as "Residual Activity".

Aldehyde Compounds—High Level Disinfectant

i. Aqueous solution of formaldehyde (formalin)
ii. Glutaraldehyde (cidex) are effective disinfectants.

Formaldehyde

It is not popular because of its pungent, suffocating odor and because 18 to 30 hours of contact is necessary for cidal action.

Glutaraldehyde

Stonehill et al (1963) reported that glutaraldehyde kills vegetative bacteria, spores, fungi and virus by alkylation on a 10-hour contact. The Center for Disease Control includes it in the list of effective agents against hepatitis viruses. It is also toxic and irritating and, hence, not used on certain surfaces such as furniture, walls and floors. It can be safely used on metal instruments (for less than 24 hours), rubber, plastics and porcelain. It is activated by addition of sodium bicarbonate, but in its activated form it remains potent only for 14 days. Recommended for the immersion of instruments using 2 percent W/V solution (cold soak—10 hours).

■ ANTISEPTICS

An antiseptic is a chemical disinfectant (usually bacteriostatic in the concentration it is used) that can be diluted sufficiently to be safe for application to living tissues (intact skin, mucous membranes, and wounds) while still retaining its antimicrobial property. They are less toxic than the disinfectants or the agents used for sterilization. Notable antiseptic agents include: alcohols, aqueous quaternary ammonium compounds, hexachlorophene, and iodophor compounds.

Alcohols

Two types of alcohols are available: (1) Ethyl alcohol, (2) Isopropyl alcohol. They are frequently used for skin antisepsis as surface disinfectant prior to needle puncture. They are good organic solvents. Their benefit is derived primarily in their cleansing action. The alcohols must have a prolonged contact with the organisms to have an antibacterial effect. This contact is prevented due to its rapid evaporation.

Alcohol is sometimes used as a rinse following a surgical scrub. Its effectiveness lies in the solvent action and not in its antibacterial properties. Ethanol (Ethyl alcohol) is employed in the concentration of 70 percent as a skin antiseptic. It has poor activity against bacterial spores, fungi, and viruses. Isopropyl alcohol is an inflammable secondary alcohol with an unpleasant burning taste. It is about twice as toxic as ethyl alcohol. It is slightly more potent a germicide than ethyl alcohol; and has a marked degreasing action. It is used in the concentration of 60 to 70 percent v/v, for disinfection of skin. The alcohols do not have reliable sporicidal, viricidal, or fungicidal action; hence, they are not useful for sterilizing surgical instruments.

Aqueous Quarternary Ammonium Compounds

Benzalkonium chloride (Zephiran) is the most commonly used antiseptic. Its spectrum of activity is primarily gram-positive bacteria. It is well tolerated by living tissues. It is not widely used because of its narrow spectrum of activity.

Hexachlorophene Compounds

These compounds are used for many years for surgical scrubs and preoperative preparation of the surgical site. They are effective against gram-positive organisms; less effective against gram negative organisms and fungi; and are not effective against viruses, spores, and *M. tuberculosis*. Skin cleansing with an agent causes reduction in surface bacteria. The bacteria in crevices and follicles begin multiplying immediately. The studies by Best et al (1950) and Lowbury and Lilly (1960) have shown that repeated scrubs allow hexachlorophene build-up on the skin. This caused a reduction in skin bacterial count. Harber et al (1967) reported that hexachlorophene solutions are susceptible to bacterial contamination. Smylie et al (1959) have shown that, hexachlorophene, to be fully effective, must be applied to dry skin, because the combination of water and protein will precipitate it. Despite the disadvantages, these compounds are valuable solution for surgical preparation in patients sensitive to iodine.

Iodophor Compounds—Intermediate Level, Broad spectrum

It is used for surgical scrub, soaps and surface antisepsis. It can discolor surfaces and clothes. Usually effective within 5 to 10 minutes. Many studies have shown, that, iodophor compounds are the most effective antiseptics. Iodine is complexed with organic surface-active agents, such as, polyvinyl-pyrrolidone (Betadine, Isodine). Their activity is dependent on the release of iodine from the complex. The surface agent is film forming; this prevents the solution from staining clothes or skin. Boswick et al (1961) have shown that skin sensitivity to the iodine is not a major problem, because of its complexing action.

These compounds are effective against most bacteria, spores, viruses, and fungi. These are the most commonly used surface disinfectants along with hypochlorite. Concentrated solutions have less free iodine. Iodine is released as the solution is diluted. An appropriate dilution is 1: 213 parts of iodophor (Iodine-Povidone-Iodine) and distilled water, respectively.

The advantages are: (i) low toxicity, (ii) prolonged residual effect, (iii) inexpensive and (iv) odorless. Geraci (1963) reported that these compounds build up on the skin after successive scrubs, and that this provides long lasting antibacterial activity.

Chloride Compounds

Available as two types: (1) sodium hypochlorite (household bleach) (2) chlorine dioxide.
1. Sodium hypochlorite—rapid action (3 minutes) surface disinfectant, highly corrosive and has strong odor. A solution of 1 part of 5 percent sodium hypochlorite with nine parts of water is used.
2. Chlorous acid and chlorine dioxide is high level disinfectant in 3 minutes.

▌ OPERATING ROOM PROCEDURES (FIGS 7.11 AND 7.12)

The ceiling, walls, and floors are regularly disinfected, especially following a contaminated case. The operating rooms should have two sets of doors. The operating theatre should provide a safe, efficient and user-friendly environment; being at the same time, free from bacterial contamination, as far as possible. The access to operation theatre and the recovery area is restricted to operation theatre personnel, who are required to don (wear) special scrub dress before entering the operating room area. The scrub suit comprises of a pair of pants/skirt/pyjama and a shirt/blouse. A surgical cap is used to cover the hair completely. A mask is then placed and tied over the nose and mouth. Theatre shoes or shoe covers may be used. Conductive shoes are helpful, as these prevent build up of static electricity, which can

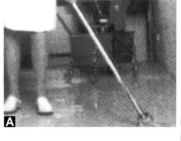
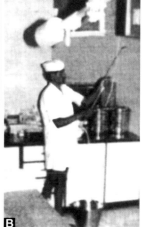
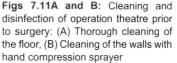

Figs 7.11A and B: Cleaning and disinfection of operation theatre prior to surgery: (A) Thorough cleaning of the floor, (B) Cleaning of the walls with hand compression sprayer

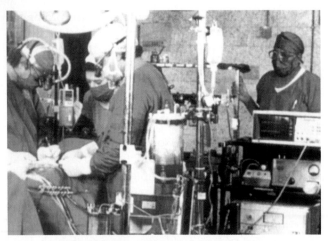

Fig. 7.12: Operation theatre dressing code

Table 7.3: Parameters and the optimum levels for effective fumigation		
Sr. no.	Parameters	Optimum levels for effective fumigation
1.	Relative humidity	Over 70%
2.	Temperature	30-40°C
3.	Formaldehyde levels	5 ppm or more

cause spark and subsequent explosion involving the volatile inflammable anesthetic gaseous agents. The shoes also lessen the chance of patient electrocution. The various electrical devices surrounding and attached to the patient, in the operating theatre are potential sources of electrical shock. Arbeit et al (1972) reported that one tenth of a milliampere of a 60 cycles per second current can produce ventricular fibrillation. The surgeon, with the conductive shoes, becomes an alternative pathway for aberrant currents. Sterile clothing, masks, gloves, and special shoes or shoe covers are worn during the operation.

Once the patient is prepared and draped, only those personnel, who have scrubbed, gowned and gloved may work at the surgical site. The backs of those who are gowned are considered nonsterile, and also the areas below the waist; unless the gowns are long and back gowns are worn. Hence, one must be careful to keep the arms above the waist, when not operating. The mask and surgical cap are not sterile, hence should not be touched. Some of the hospitals have the operating light's handles, which are detachable and sterilizable, which can be adjusted by the surgeon. Other lights must be adjusted by other members of the nonscrubbed staff.

The operation theatres are disinfected (Figs 7.11A and B) by fumigation. Fumigation can be achieved by the use of fumigators as well as potassium permanganate reaction technique. Fumigation is initiated after setting up of the instrument (STERI-TRAX) in place. The chemical used is 40 percent formalin. Fumigator is set for 30 minutes (Table 7.3).

Relative Humidity

Relative humidity (RH) plays a major role in fumigation. A minimum of 70 percent is essential. Higher the humidity, better is the disinfection. Water used in the fumigator along with the fumigant (Formalin) helps to achieve and maintain the desired RH.

Temperature

Evaporation of gaseous fumigant is more at the higher temperature. The use of fumigator makes the temperature factor less important since it allows the formation of mist in the operation theatre.

Formaldehyde Levels in the Air in the Operation Theatre

The dose of formalin is usually decided by the size of the room. As a general rule, about 180 ml is used for a room of the size 1000 cubic feet (= 10 x 10 x 10 feet).

Masks (Figs 7.13A and B)

Disposable masks made of synthetic fibers are better; and contain filters made of polyester (e.g. Bard Vigilon) or polypropylene (e.g. Filtron).

Surgical antifog masks with flexible nosebands are available which follow facial contours and retain a high efficiency of filtration. Masks provide protective function for the wearer against blood-borne viruses, as part of a policy of universal precautions. Full face visors offer better protection.

Eye Protection (Fig. 7.14)

It is advisable to wear eye protection, during any procedure which is likely to generate droplets of blood or other body fluids. It also protects mucous membrane of the eyes of the wearer from blood-borne viruses. A variety of light weight antifog goggles, glasses and visors are available which do not obstruct vision.

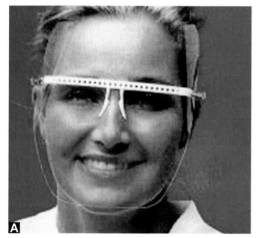

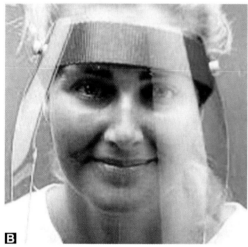

Figs 7.13A and B: Full cover transparent shield for face

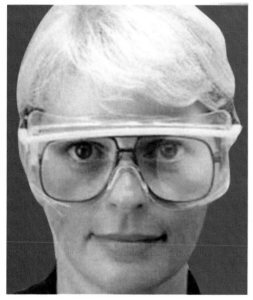

Fig. 7.14: Eye protection during surgery

Hair/Beard Cover

Long hair must be tied up; and all hair must be completely covered by close fitting cap made of synthetic material. Beards should also be completely covered.

Footwear

There is little evidence that floor plays a significant role in spread of infection in hospital. Staff members should wear clean, comfortable, antislip and antistatic shoes. Footwear should fit well and avoid producing "bellows effect." Construction should be significantly robust to protect the feet from sharp injury.

Antiseptic Environment

The principle is to minimize bacterial contamination, especially, in the vicinity of operating table; the concept of zones is useful, and must be employed.

- Outer, or general access zone—e.g. patient reception area and general office.
- Clean, or limited access zone—e.g. the area between reception and general office, dispersal area, corridors and staff room.
- Restricted access zone—e.g. for those properly clothed personnel engaged in operating theatre activities, anesthetic room, etc.
- Aseptic or operating zone—e.g. the operating theatre.
- *Airflow:* The air may be filtered, or allowed to flow past an ultraviolet radiation device to reduce bacterial counts. Operating theatres have two types of air flow: (i) conventional and (ii) unidirectional. The normal turbulent airflow through theatre is necessary to maintain humidity, temperature, and air circulation. Besides, an increased rate of air change is necessary to reduce the number of contaminated particles over the patient. Air is pumped into the room through filter and passed out of vents in the periphery of operating room and does not return to operating room.

Hand Scrub Techniques

Hand scrub is the first step towards aseptic surgical technique. Several studies have shown that it is the single most important and successful method of controlling the spread of infection in the hospital environment.

Wise et al (1959) have shown that 20 to 30 percent of surgeon's gloves get punctured by the end of operation. Cole and Bernard (1964) have documented the outpouring of bacteria from the surgeon's hands, through the punctured gloves into the wound. The gloves are likely to get punctured, or ripped, while working with wires or instruments. It is therefore, imperative to have clean hands inside the gloves.

The purpose of hand scrub is two-fold: The first is to remove the superficial contaminants and loose epithelium. This is achieved by the mechanical action of the brush. The second purpose is to reduce bacterial count on the skin. Selwyn and Ellis (1972) reported that the use of the iodophor scrubbing solutions, results in the effectiveness of the scrub in reducing the surface bacterial count. About 20 percent of skin bacteria are inaccessible, residing in the follicles, crevices, and lipids of the skin. The residual antiseptic scrub solution also helps in keeping the surface bacterial count low. Many techniques of hand scrub have been suggested.

All jewellery be removed before washing. The nails should be checked for cleanliness. All gross subnail contamination should be removed. The scrubs can be prepacked impregnated with soap solutions or can be reusable with a soap dispenser. Nails should be scrubbed first thoroughly with a brush. The arms are wetted to a few inches above the elbows.

The scrubbing begins at the tip of one finger of one hand. The scrubbing is continued along the skin surfaces of fingers, and the interfinger webbing. The scrubbing is continued until all the surfaces of the hand are completed. Then the hands are cleaned along the forearms and the scrubbing is progressed towards the elbow extending 2″ above the elbow. In the similar manner the other hand is scrubbed beginning at the fingertips and scrubbing towards the elbow.

A scrubbed area should not be touched again, because of the possibility of contamination from an unscrubbed area. Dunphey and Way (1973) recommend that scrubbing procedure may be done for approximately 10 minutes. After the scrubbing of both the arms the brush is discarded and the arms are rinsed of excess soap. The rinse should be done with arms elevated above the elbow height to enable the water to drain from the fingertips progressing down the arms and the elbows. The arms are not rubbed during the rinse. Only the superficial excess soap is removed. Dobson and Shulls (1967) have shown that the residual soap provides about three hours of antibacterial action.

The surgeon approaches the scrub nurse for the sterile drying towel. The technique of drying begins at the fingertips of one hand and progresses down the arm. Then, with the opposite side of the towel, the other arm is dried in a similar manner.

Hand Disinfection (Figs 7.15 and 7.16)

There are some proprietary preparations available for preoperative washing of hands of surgeons and assistants which have a bactericidal effect and which do not cause excessive drying of skin. The preparations available are:

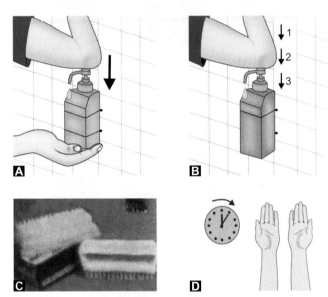

Figs 7.15A to D: Surgical hand disinfection: (A) Disinfectant soap solution is dispensed on the palm, 3 ml per push, (B) Three such pushes give adequate quantity for hand scrub, (C) Rub into hands, grooves and up to elbows for 5 minutes and scrub with the brush, (D) You are ready to put on gloves

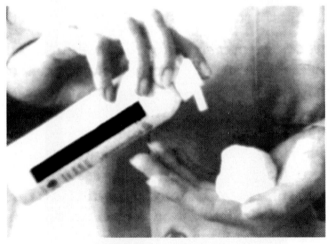

Fig. 7.16: Hand disinfection

i. Hibiscrub and Phisomed—contains 4 percent chlorhexidine gluconate.
ii. Betadine—contains 7.5 percent Povidone-Iodine.
iii. Three percent PCMX, and
iv. Soap containing disinfectants like hexachlorophene.
v. Seventy percent Hibisol (2.5% chlorhexidine in 70% alcohol) lotion may be applied as an extra precaution.

Washing must be continued for 5 minutes in running water. This is followed by drying of hands and forearms.

Gloving

All protective barrier techniques should be employed. *Hand gloves:* They help to protect the operator from infection by bacteria and viruses from patient's blood. They may be washed, worn, and sterilized and worn again for more than one operation, provided that they have not been punctured or damaged. Gloving is essential to protect both the surgeon and the patient from blood-borne viruses and to prevent wound becoming contaminated with the surgeon's skin flora.

There are two types of gloves:
i. *Latex gloves:* It is a clear and the most common type of glove.
ii. *Brown milled rubber gloves:* These are thinner than latex gloves; and provide a better tactile sensation. However, they are more fragile and require more frequent changes during the operation. The "hand to glove", and "glove to glove" technique of donning the gloves should be employed. Double gloving affords extra protection, but at the expense of reduced sensitivity and dexterity, and possible discomfort.

Preparation of the Surgical Site (Fig. 7.17)

Hair in the area of surgery is removed, preferably, just prior to scrubbing the skin. Shaving the area at night before produces small abrasions on the skin and resident bacteria multiply as a result of injury. This problem can be overcome by decreasing the time interval between the shave and the skin preparation. A lubricating ointment should be applied to patient's eyes, and they are covered. The external auditory meatus is plugged and blocked, if bleeding in the vicinity is anticipated.

The scrubbing should begin in the center of the site to be prepared, and move outward concentrically, away

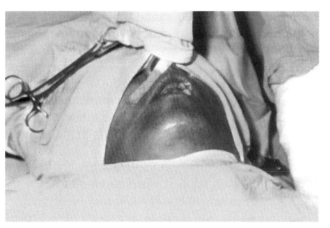

Fig. 7.17: Preparation of surgical site and draping the patient

from the site of operation. This avoids contamination of already scrubbed site of surgery.

Studies by Zinner et al (1961), Scopp and Orvieto (1971), and Cutcher et al (1971) have shown remarkable reduction in bacteremia during tooth extraction following preparation with iodophor or phenol-alcohol mouth rinses. These transient bacteremias are not of importance in normal patients, however, this preparation is very important in the following categories of patients:
i. History of rheumatic heart diseases: Prosthetic heart valves, prosthetic hip replacement,
ii. Shunts for dialysis,
iii. Patients on immunosuppressive therapy
iv. Other debilitating diseases.

It is important to reduce contamination by the patient's own normal flora, and the resistant bacteria acquired from hospital environment. This significantly reduces the incidence of postoperative infections.

Much depends upon the type of surgery to be performed. For all extraoral procedures, a presurgical scrub is recommended. The skin in and around the site is prepared. The solutions used are Cetavlon and Betadine (Povidone-Iodine). For intraoral surgery, a circumoral preparation should precede, to prevent transfer of resident skin flora to intraoral site. The same solutions may be used. Mouth can also be disinfected by the use of 0.2 percent chlorhexidine just prior to surgery.

The iodophor compounds are by far the most effective solutions for skin preparation. Prigot and Roc (1962) have shown that they do not interfere with wound healing.

Draping the patient: The purpose of draping a patient is to isolate the field of surgery from other parts of body that have not been prepared for surgery, and also from nonsterile equipment (Fig. 7.17). Patient should be draped with sterile towels. Patient's hair should be covered with sterile head cover. Another towel should cover chest and shoulders. The suction tubing is clipped to this towel so as to prevent it from falling down and from touching nonsterile nondisinfected surfaces. The site of needle puncture in oral mucosa, preferably dried and an antiseptic applied, such as chlorhexidine 0.5 percent or povidone-iodine solution may be applied.

Disposable items: Many disposable items are supplied in sterile packs by their respective manufacturing companies. These are sterilized by methods such as gamma radiation. The sterility of such products can be relied upon; if the supplier is from a reputable manufacturer; and the wrapper seal is not broken. The single use surgical blades and suture needles are recommended (Figs 7.18A to D).

Other Precautions

Preoperative gingival/periodontal care: It is necessary that, the interdental embrasures are rendered free of plaque, food debris, and, if calculus is present, it is desirable that the patient should undergo preoperative scaling and the patient is given oral hygiene instructions. This helps in keeping the bacterial population to a minimum.

Use of antimicrobial mouth rinse: The use of an antimicrobial mouth rinse preoperatively reduces the number of bacteria considerably. The action is a combination of

mechanical removal and antisepsis. The recommended rinses contain diguanides like chlorhexidine.

Use of antibiotic prophylaxis: The clinician relies on the use of antibiotics prophylactically to reduce the incidence of postoperative infection. It is prudent that clinician should employ adequate aseptic procedures and perform meticulous surgical procedure obviating the need of using antibiotic prophylactically. Antibiotics should be avoided when there is no real and specific indication as it causes bacterial resistance and superinfection.

Handpieces: Ham et al (1970) evaluated sterilization of handpieces. The sterilization of handpieces is frought with many difficulties. The saliva, bone debris, bacteria and other contaminants get sucked inside the handpiece during their usage. Amongst the handpieces that are available in market, only a few are autoclavable. Autoclaving of handpieces leads to increase in corrosion, rendering subsequent cleaning more difficult. The handpieces, after their sterilization, require lubrication prior to their usage. This lubrication may further lead to contamination. Immersion in boiling oil has been advocated; however, the oil that collects on the innerside of handpieces is difficult to be removed; which ultimately, lands up into the surgical sites. Disinfection of handpieces is not adequate (Figs 7.19A to C).

Formalin disinfection: Equipment, which is seriously contaminated such as anesthesia apparatus is cleaned by this method.

Common Disinfectants

Chlorhexidine (Hibitane): There are several commercial preparations. It is used for skin and body tissue disinfection. It is used with isopropyl alcohol to enhance its efficiency for skin. It can also be used with cetrimide to have detergent activity.

Phenolics: These are not used for skin or tissues. It is used for areas with significant soiling. It should not be used in food preparing areas.

Glutaraldehyde: Used for disinfection of heat-sensitive instruments, e.g. endoscopes. It should not be used for environmental cleaning.

Isopropyl alcohol preparation: They are used for disinfecting skin, e.g. venipuncture.

Povidone-iodine: Solutions containing a detergent are employed for preoperative skin preparations.

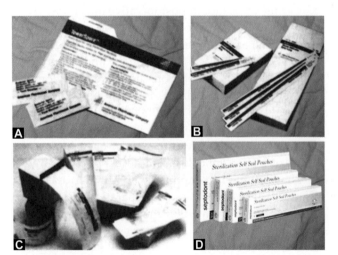

Figs 7.18A to D: Disposable items—presterile packs

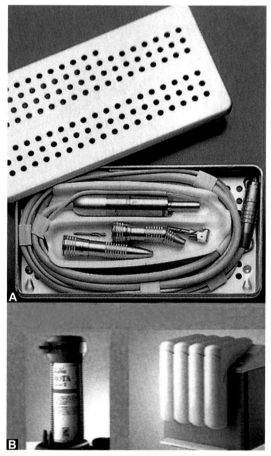

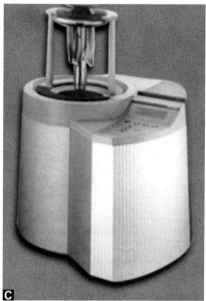

Figs 7.19A to C: (A) Handpieces, tube, motor is placed in the cassette for sterilization, (B) After use handpieces are cleaned with spray rotor for removing the deposits with pressurized air, (C) A Universal machine to clean, lubricate disinfect and sterilize handpieces

Hypochlorites (Chloros, Domestos): These act by release of chlorine. It is readily inactivated by organic matter, pus, etc. It is useful for food preparation, feeding bottles and rubber teats. It is useful in areas where there are hazards of viral hepatitis.

BIBLIOGRAPHY

1. Accepted Dental Therapeutics. Chicago- ADA – 1977.
2. Arbeit SR, Parker B, Rubin IR. Controlling the electrocution aazard in the hospital. JAMA 1972;220:1581.
3. Cole W, Bernard H. Inadequacies of present methods of surgical skin preparation. Arch Surg 1964;89:215.
4. Crawford JR, Oldenburg TR. Practical methods of office sterilization and disinfection. J Oral Med 1967;22:133.
5. Kelsey JC. Sterilization and disinfection: objectives and perspectives. Ann R Coll Surg Engl 1969;44: 214.
6. McLundie AC. Sterilization in general dental practice. BDJ 1968;124:214.
7. Rubbo S, Gardner JF. A Review of Sterilization and Disinfection. London; Llyod-Luke Medical Bools Ltd, 1965.

8 Infection Control

INTRODUCTION

This chapter contains detailed guidelines on control of cross infection.

OBJECTIVE

Elimination or reduction in spread of infection from all types of micro-organisms. It is the duty of every dental practitioner to care for all patients, including those with infectious diseases. The clinician also has a professional responsibility for implementing effective infection control to protect other patients, and a responsibility for safe practice for all members of the dental team. Sir William Osler once remarked that "Soap and water and common sense are the best disinfectants." Despite the advent of numerous disinfectants, thereafter, the basis of infection control still remains the same as the above mentioned procedure.

INFECTION

Infection is the deposition of organisms in the tissues and their growth resulting in a host reaction. In case the response of host is minimal or nil, it is usually termed as "colonization." The acquisition of a strain

of *Staphylococcus aureus*, which grows in anterior nares without causing any tissue reaction, and the person is not aware that he is a carrier, is an example. On the other hand, the same strain may cause an infection at the angle of lips (angular cheilitis) in the same person.

The number of organisms required to cause an infection is termed "the infective dose". The infective dose is dependent on:
1. Virulence of the organism.
2. Susceptibility of the host.
3. Other important and relevant factors are age, pre-existing disease and drug therapy, etc.

INFECTION CONTROL

Infection control involves two basic factors:
1. Prevention of spread of micro-organisms from their hosts (patients and clinicians).
2. Killing or removal of micro-organisms from objects and surfaces.

CROSS INFECTION

Cross infection is defined as the transmission of infectious agents among patients and staff within a clinical environment. In dentistry, the source of infection may constitute: (1) patients suffering from infectious diseases, (2) patients, who are in the prodromal stage of certain infections and (3) healthy carriers of pathogens.

Pathways of Cross Infection

There are six common pathways: (1) patient to practitioner, (2) practitioner to patient, (3) patient to patient, (4) clinic to community, (5) clinic to practitioner's family and (6) community to patients.

Patients suffering from acute illnesses, usually do not seek dental treatment. The likely source of infection, is usually a person, who is in the prodromal phase of an infection attends the clinic. The patient at this stage, may appear healthy, but the saliva and blood may be infectious. The diseases which can spread easily in this manner are viral infections such as measles, mumps and chickenpox.

Healthy carriers, who are important factors in the transmission of disease can be classified as follows:
1. *Convalescent carriers:* In this stage, the patient suffers an acute illness and apparently recovers. However, the blood and secretions serve as persistent reservoirs of the infective organisms. Such individuals can be identified on the basis of past history of infection.
2. *Asymptomatic carriers:* These persons, may have a subclinical infection; and are unaware of it. They give no history of past infection, hence cannot be diagnosed easily. These individuals may carry infective organisms in saliva and blood.

The classic example is that of hepatitis B virus infection. It may manifest with or without symptoms, and the clinician may be faced with either convalescent or asymptomatic carriers of hepatitis B virus infection.

▮ ROUTES OF TRANSMISSION

Transmission of infection within a dental surgery may occur via several routes: (i) direct contact of tissues with infective biological fluids such as blood and oral secretions; (ii) indirect contact: with contaminated instruments, equipment, or environmental surfaces; (iii) inhalation of aerosolized infective droplets/particles, (iv) direct inoculation into cuts and abrasions of unprotected skin or mucosa via contaminated sharps or instruments.

Infection through any of these routes requires that all three of the following conditions be present, "the chain of infection":
1. Pathogen (i) sufficient infectivity, and (ii) sufficient dose.
2. Exposure portal through which the pathogen may enter the host.
3. Susceptible host.

Dental patients and dental healthcare workers (DHCWs) may be exposed to a variety of micro-organisms via blood or oral or respiratory secretions. These micro-organisms may include the following: (i) Bac-teria: staphylococci, streptococci, *M. tuberculosis*, and (ii) Viruses: Herpes simplex virus types 1 and 2, cyto-megalovirus, Hepatitis B virus (HBV), hepatitis C virus (HCV), human immunodeficiency virus (HIV), and (iii) other bacteria and viruses specifically those associated with upper respiratory tract infections. Some of the infectious agents of concern in dentistry and their possible routes of transmission are summarized in Table 8.1.

▮ INFECTIOUS DISEASES OF CONCERN IN DENTISTRY

Bacterial Infections

Tuberculosis: This disease is caused by *M. tuberculosis*. It is transmitted by inhalation, ingestion and inoculation. The two main infections seen are in the form of tuberculous cervical lymphadenitis and pulmonary infection. Immunization with BCG vaccine adequately covers dental staff. In addition, gloves and masks should be worn. The inhalation, sedation and anesthesia equipment must always be treated with high level disinfectants. It is worth remembering that *M. tuberculosis* is highly resistant to heat and chemical disinfectants, as it has a thick lipid coat.

Syphilis: This is caused by *T. pallidum.* Transmission in a dental setup is not reported, probably, because the organism is highly labile. However, regular wearing of gloves offers adequate protection.

Gonorrhea: It is caused by *N. gonorrhoeae.* It is more common sexually transmitted disease. There is no report of such a transmission episode in dental care setup. However, gloves offer adequate protection.

| **Table 8.1: Some infectious agents of concern in dentistry and their routes of transmission** ||
Micro-organisms	Major transmission route
Bacteria	
N. gonorrhoeae	Inoculation
T. pallidum	Inoculation
M. tuberculosis	Inoculation/Inhalation
Strep. pyogenes	Inhalation
Viruses	
Cytomegalovirus	Inhalation
Hepatitis viruses	
Hepatitis B	Inoculation
Hepatitis C	Inoculation
Hepatitis D	Inoculation
Herpes simplex 1 and 2	Inoculation
Human immunodeficiency virus (HIV)	Inoculation
Measles virus	Inhalation
Mumps virus	Inhalation
Respiratory viruses	
Influenza virus	Inhalation
Rhinovirus	Inhalation
Adenovirus	Inhalation
Rubella virus	Inhalation

Legionellosis: It is caused by gram negative bacteria, which usually reside in warm and stagnant water reservoirs. They cause life threatening pneumonias in elderly. The majority of infections are subclinical, while a minority causes pneumonia (Legionnaire's disease) and a flu-like illness (Pontiac fever). The organism is water-borne and is transmitted via aerosols. These factors indicate that there is a possibility that legionellosis may spread via water in the dental unit water systems, which are frequently aerosolized. There is evidence to indicate that Legionella species multiply in dental unit water systems, which sometimes remain unused for days.

The dental unit water systems should be flushed with fresh water before and after use and particularly prior to the treatment of the first patient in the morning to eradicate any contaminants. The dental staff should be informed of the long term risk of legionellosis.

Viral Infections

Herpes virus infection: There are at least six herpes viruses: Herpes simplex (types 1 and 2), varicella zoster (VZV), Epstein-Barr virus (EBV), cytomegalovirus (CMV) and human herpes virus 6 (HHV6). A single exposure is sufficient for infection with these DNA viruses, which often results in the development of a life-long latent infection.

Herpes simplex virus: This is the most common herpes virus transmitted to dental clinical staff. The major signs of primary herpes infection are acute illness with fever and malaise, cervical lymphadenopathy, and ulcerative gingivostomatitis. Sometimes a recurrent infection, in the form of herpes labialis, occurs. This begins with discomfort at the site of infection and the appearance of clusters of small vesicles that soon rupture, followed by coalescence into a large ulcer. Ninety percent of orolabial herpes simplex lesions are caused by type 1 (HSV-1) and 10 percent by (HSV-2); herpes simplex virus infections of the fingers (herpetic whitlow) can be caused by direct contact with either a herpetic lesion or infected saliva. Patients who are immunocompromised, e.g. HIV positive, or those who are immunosuppressed, and those with cancer therapy, may have more frequent and prolonged episodes of herpes infections, and are a relatively common source of cross infection.

Transmission occurs by direct contact of abraded skin or intact mucosa with infected lesions or secretions. Transmission of infection to dental staff can result in primary herpetic stomatitis or herpetic whitlow. The latter is a painful infection on a finger characterized by vesicles, which precede skin breakdown and subsequent crusting. Treatment with acyclovir, taken when the premonitory signs are present, decreases the symptoms and duration of viral shedding and, possibly the number of recurrences in some patients. Wearing of gloves provides adequate protection against the virus.

Varicella zoster virus: This virus is the causative agent of both chickenpox and shingles; the former is the primary disease and the latter is the secondary disease, caused by the reactivation of the latent virus residing in sensory ganglia. Chickenpox is the mild form, and is mainly seen in children. Shingles can be painful and debilitating, especially if trigeminal ganglion is involved.

Chickenpox is highly contagious and spreads via air borne route. The non immune dental staff may contact the disease via inhalation of aerosols from a patient, who is incubating the disease, attends the clinic. Masks and gloves offer some protection.

Cytomegalovirus (CMV): This virus has the characteristic ability to cause latent infections. The fetus, preterm neonates and immunocompromised patients are at risk of serious disease. Congenital CMV syndrome is the most important, affecting the live-births leading to encephalitis, microcephaly, and mental retardation.

A possible link between risk for congenital defects in neonates of healthcare workers and CMV infection has been suggested, as CMV infection occurs in medical personnel to a great extent than nonmedical personnel. There is no documentary evidence of transmission of CMV to dental staff. However, female staff of child-bearing age should note that CMV is transmitted in body fluids, particularly saliva; and most of the individuals shedding CMV are healthy and unidentified. Routine use of gloves and masks is a good protective measure.

Epstein-Barr virus (EBV): The virus causes glandular fever (infectious mononucleosis), particularly in young adults. The virus may remain latent in oropharyngeal or salivary epithelium. The major mode of its spread is by kissing; it may also be transmitted by blood. The virus is present in saliva, and the dental staff is at no risk of EBV infection. Masks and gloves offer adequate protection.

Human herpes virus 6 (HHV6): This is the new addition to the herpes family. It causes a generalized rash (exanthem subitum) in the affected individual. It is present in saliva of some population, however, occupational hazards to medical or dental staff has not been reported.

Influenza, rhino and adenoviruses: These viruses commonly cause respiratory tract infections. The route of transmission of these viruses is by droplets. The members of dental staff are at risk from these infections. However, there is little documentary evidence to substantiate this relation. Masks and gloves offer good protection.

Rubella (German measles): This virus belongs to the family of Toga viruses and has worldwide distribution. It affects developing fetus by causing cataract, deafness and hepato-splenomegaly, etc. At risk is non immune female staff of child bearing age. The virus is transmitted by droplets. Female staff should be warned of the possible dangers of the virus to the fetus. Rubella vaccine, a constituent of combined MMR (measles, mumps, rubella) vaccine, should be given to such members of staff.

Coxsackie virus infections: The diseases caused by this virus are: (a) hand, foot and mouth disease and (b) herpangina. These diseases are of importance in dentistry, because (i) they cause oral ulcerations, and (ii) they possibly can spread in the dental clinic. These infections may remain subclinical and may occasionally lead to myocarditis or encephalitis. The virus is found in saliva. It can spread via direct contact or aerosols. Gloves and masks offer protection.

Human T-lymphotropic virus 1 (HTLV-1): This is a RNA retrovirus (same family as HIV). It has been reported in IV drug users. This virus plays a role in adult T cell leukemia and tropical spastic paraparesis. The route of its spread is via blood while sexual transmission and IV drug abuse have been implicated. In dental practice it can spread due to contaminated sharps and needle prick injuries.

Hepatitis B virus (HBV): This is a DNA virus which causes acute hepatitis. It has a long incubation period (45 to 180 days, mean 75 days). During the acute infection, and in carriers of HBV, viral particles released from the liver are present in circulation. Hepatitis B surface antigen (HbsAg) is identified by serological tests as the main indicator of active infection. A second antigen, HbeAg, which is derived from core particles of the virus present in the liver. It indicates continuing activity of the virus in the liver and the presence of HbeAg in the blood correlates with high levels of infectivity.

Patients with history of multiple blood transfusions, IV drug abuse, chronic hepatic disease, chronic renal failure, etc. should be subjected to routine hepatitis profile. The mode of transmission is by sexual intercourse, blood transfusion, contaminated needles, and sharp instruments; and from mother to child. There are no important dental or oral manifestations in HBV infection.

All members of the dental team should be vaccinated against hepatitis B and maintain this vaccination schedule.

Hepatitis C virus (HCV): It is a RNA virus, now recognized as the major cause of non-A, non-B hepatitis. The mode of transmission is similar to HBV infection; being predominantly bloodborne and infection is common in injecting drugs users and recipients of unscreened blood and/or blood products. The acute phase of HCV infection is usually asymptomatic and only approximately 10 percent of individuals have overt hepatitis. Following primary infection, however, the majority (about 80%) proceed to become persistent carriers of the virus and, as with HBV infection, there is a long term risk of chronic liver disease with cirrhosis and hepatocellular carcinoma.

Human immunodeficiency virus (HIV): HIV is a RNA retrovirus. The virus infects the major cellular component of immune system and the CNS; especially the T-helper cells. The majority of the manifestations seen in HIV infection are due to affection of this immune system.

The mode of transmission of HIV is quite similar to that of HBV; through sexual contact, blood or blood products, and from mother to child.

Infection with HIV has oral manifestations. Hence with HIV exposure, testing may be useful to ascertain the possible future occurrence of oral manifestations of HIV infection. This requires more frequent oral examinations. It is imperative that HIV testing be done in conjunction with a physician and with patient's informed consent.

Human immunodeficiency virus (HIV-1, HIV-2): The two viruses are very similar and their modes of spread and clinical effects are identical. Although there is some evidence that disease progression is slower in HIV-2 infection. Recent work has shown that an HIV-infected individual produces very high levels of virus, 10-10 virus particles per day, and is consequently potentially infectious to others for life. At ambient temperatures, the virus is protected from desiccation and may persist in dried blood or secretions for several days. The major cellular component for HIV is the CD4 antigen which is present on helper.

Revised Classification of HIV-associated Oral Lesions (1990)

Group I: Lesions Strongly Associated with HIV Infections

  i. *Candidiasis*: Erythematous, hyperplastic, and pseudo-membranous
 ii. Hairy leukoplakia (EBV)
iii. HIV-gingivitis
 iv. Necrotizing ulcerative gingivitis
  v. HIV-periodontitis
 vi. Kaposi's sarcoma
vii. Non-Hodgkin's lymphoma.

Group II: Lesions Less Commonly Associated with HIV Infection

  i. Atypical ulceration (oropharyngeal)
 ii. Idiopathic thrombocytopenic purpura
iii. Salivary gland diseases:
    a. Dry mouth due to decreased salivary flow rate
    b. Unilateral or bilateral swelling of major salivary glands

 iv. Viral infections (other than EBV):
    a. Cytomegalovirus
    b. Herpes simplex virus
    c. Human papilloma virus (warty like lesions):
       • Condyloma acuminatum
       • Focal epithelial hyperplasia
       • Verruca vulgaris
       • Varicella-zoster virus:
         — Herpes zoster virus
         — Varicella.

Group III: Lesions Possibly Associated with HIV Infection

  i. Bacterial infections excluding gingivitis/periodontitis:
    a. *Actinomycosis*
    b. *Enterobacter cloacae*
    c. *Escherichia coli*
    d. *Klebsiella pneumoniae*
    e. *Mycobacterium avium intracellulae, and*
    f. Tuberculosis.
 ii. Cat-scratch disease
iii. Exacerbation of apical periodontitis
 iv. Fungal infection other than candidiasis: Cryptococcosis, geotrichosis, histoplasmosis, and mucormycosis.
  v. Melanotic hyperpigmentation
 vi. Neurologic disturbances: Facial palsy, and trigeminal neuralgia
vii. Osteomyelitis
viii. Sinusitis
 ix. Submandibular cellulitis
  x. Squamous cell carcinoma
 xi. Toxic cell epidermolysis.

Signs and Symptoms of HIV Disease

The WHO report on AIDS (1990), describes the various signs and symptoms of HIV disease/AIDS, as follows:

Earlier Signs of HIV Infection

(i) Unexplained weight loss of more than 10 percent of body weight. (ii) Unexplained fever lasting more than one month. (iii) Unexplained chronic diarrhea. (iv) Shingles (caused by herpes zoster virus). (v) Oral thrush (infection by a fungus, *C. albicans*). (vi) Oral hairy leukoplakia. (vii) Persistent generalized lymphadenopathy (PGL). Persistent increase (more than three months) in the size of the lymph nodes in several sites of the body; such as neck, axilla and groins.

Late Signs of HIV Infection

Approximately 30 to 40 percent of seropositive patients will develop AIDS within seven years after infection. The manifestations appear when the immune system is severely damaged. AIDS is responsible for two main categories of disease: (i) opportunistic infections, and (ii) certain tumors.

Opportunistic infections: The clinical signs vary according to the organism responsible and the organs affected. The principal organs affected are the lungs, gastrointestinal tract, brain and skin. The following is a list of the main signs of opportunistic infections more specifically diagnostic of AIDS.

a. *Lungs:* Cough, shortness of breath, and chest pain.
b. *Gastrointestinal tract:* Difficulty in swallowing, nausea, vomiting, abdominal pain, severe weight loss (malabsorption), and chronic severe diarrhea.
c. *Brain:* (i) Headache, impaired mental function, fits, peripheral and central paralysis, inco-ordination and coma, (ii) Visual defects.
d. *Skin/mucocutaneous:* (i) Perioral and oral ulceration, and (ii) Genital and perianal ulceration.

Certain Tumors

a. *Kaposi's sarcoma:* Generalized Kaposi's sarcoma is frequently associated with AIDS. It affects about 15 percent of patients with AIDS in Africa. It presents in the form of purple or red/brown cutaneous plaques or nodules. These lesions are found not only in the skin, but also found in the mucosal lining, such as in the mouth, and in the lungs and gut. A characteristic clinical appearance is of one or more erythematous or violaceous macules or swellings with or without ulceration. It is predominantly seen in the palate or in the gingiva.
b. *Lymphomas:* The risk of lymphoma (tumors of the lymph nodes, skin, gut and brain) is about 100 times greater in patients with AIDS than in normal subjects. The commonly seen tumor is non-Hodgkin's lymphoma. It presents in the form of a firm, elastic, reddish or purplish swelling, with or without ulceration. The most common sites are gingiva and palate. If universal precautions are undertaken, the infection control procedures will not change, due to patient's positive history of HBV or HIV. Referral to

patient's physician for serological confirmation may be considered, if the results of such tests will help the dental practitioner in the management of the patient's overall dental needs.

■ GENERAL PRINCIPLES

Universal Precautions

Infection control strategies reduce the risk of transmission of infectious diseases caused by bloodborne pathogens such as HBV and HIV. All infected patients cannot be identified on the basis of medical history, physical examination and laboratory investigations, hence, the philosophy is that to consider all patients to be infected with pathogenic organisms. Hence, it is recommended that certain basic infection control procedures must be followed routinely for all patients, referred to as ''universal precautions.''

Universal precautions, for dental team, entail:
1. Employment of various personal protective barrier techniques, such as gowns, face masks, protective eyewear, gloves, etc. which reduce the risk of exposure to potentially infectious material. In addition, precautions should be taken against injury from sharp instruments.
2. *Immunization:* The CDC recommends that all members of the dental team, who are exposed to blood or blood contaminated articles, should be vaccinated against hepatitis B, with a booster dose after three years.
3. Routine handwashing.

Handwashing and Care of Hands

It is an important and effective way of preventing spread of infectious organisms from one person to another. In a clinical set up, hands must always be washed: (i) at the beginning of each session, (ii) between patient contacts, (iii) before putting on sterile gloves, (iv) immediately after skin contact with blood or other body fluids, (v) after touching inanimate objects, (vi) before touching eyes, nose, face or mouth, (vii) before leaving the clinic, (viii) before eating, drinking, smoking, or inserting contact lens, (ix) after any break in the routine or chain of asepsis such as answering the telephone or retrieving an instrument. Soap dispensers and taps should be operated by the elbows or wrists, and not with gloved hands or bare hands.

Hand wash technique: (i) Remove all jewellery (watch, ring, bracelet), (ii) Clean fingernails with a plastic or wooden stick, (iii) Scrub hands, nails and forearm with a liquid germicidal agent, (iv) Rinse hands thoroughly with running water, (v) Dry hands with towel.

The hands should be thoroughly washed with an antimicrobial hand wash, using a recommended procedure prior to wearing gloves. A combination of liquid soap and an antimicrobial agent; is more effective than bar soap alone. Gloves should be removed as soon as patient contact is over.

Hand care: Gloving is an important aspect of hand care. Some of the "skin reactions" to gloving are caused by bacterial irritation rather than a true allergic response. The bacteria on the skin beneath the gloves thrive in a moist and warm environment and may produce enough waste products to irritate the skin. It is recommended to dry hands thoroughly after washing before gloving. Torn, cut or punctured gloves must be removed immediately. Any obvious sores, abrasions and cuts must be covered with protective adhesive waterproof dressings (elastoplast) prior to donning gloves. Personnel with exudative or suppurative lesions or dermatitis should refrain from direct patient care and equipment, until the lesions are healed completely. Handcream must be used at the end of the session, to prevent drying and cracking of skin. Fingernails should be short, trimmed and clean.

Personal Protection: Protective Attire

Barrier Technique

The use of barrier technique is very important; which includes clinic attire, face mask, protective eyewear, and gloves (Figs 8.1 and 8.2).

Clinic attire: All personnel involved in direct patient care must wear freshly laundered uniform or high necked, long cuffed, sleeved cover gowns while performing surgery. The American Dental Association (ADA) guidelines recommend changing garments at least daily and more frequently and when visibly soiled or contaminated. All protective clothing should not be worn outside of the clinic areas, such as corridors, canteens and elevators. All disposable protective barriers should be discarded prior to leaving surgery or the operative area.

Face masks: These must be worn by all the members of the staff during patient care. Masks should be changed when sneezing occurs, when damp, and in between

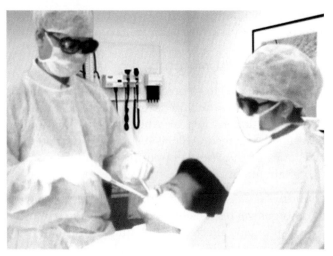

Fig. 8.1: Use of protective clinic attire

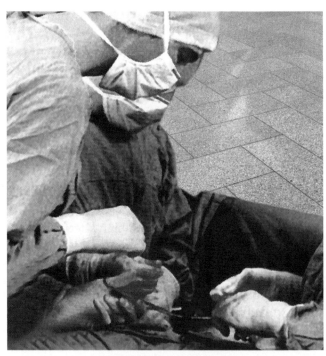

Fig. 8.2: Use of sterile gloves

patients. The maximum time for wearing masks should be not more than one hour, since it becomes dampened from respiration, causing degradation in its filterability. A chin length plastic face shields must be worn, in addition to face masks, for greater protection against splatter.

Head caps: Hair should be properly tied. Long hair (which extends below collar level) must be either covered or restrained away from face. In case, hair contamination is expected, hair cover/caps must be used.

Protective eyewear: Eyewear with solid side-shields or chin-length face shields must be used when splashing and splattering of blood, saliva or pus is expected. This occurs from sprayed debris, particularly when rotary cutting instruments are used.

Gloving: It is an effective barrier to reduce risk of transmission of disease. Gloving is mandatory for all types of patient care. All staff must wear gloves during patient contact (blood, saliva, mucous membrane). It has been shown that working with bare hands results in the retention of micro-organisms, saliva and blood under the fingernails for several days. There is evidence to indicate that dental staff, who do not wear gloves contract herpes simplex infections, HBV infection and possibly HIV infection. Recent studies also show that gloves will minimize needle stick injuries.

The disposable gloves are made of latex or polyvinyl. Sterile gloves are required during surgical procedures (Fig. 8.2). For other procedures nonsterile gloves should be worn. Overgloves or paper towels must be used for opening drawers, cabinets, etc. The contamination caused by pushing up glasses, touching the face and hair, rubbing the nose, adjusting the mask, etc. should be avoided. If contact must be made, a barrier (such as paper towel) should be used, or gloves removed and a new pair used before proceeding. The efficacy of gloves as a barrier/protection is greatly diminished if they are perforated. It is important that the dental practitioner ascertains the quality of the gloves prior to their purchase and uses those with good quality assurance. The frequency of changing of gloves is a topic of debate. It has been shown that approximately 80 percent of gloves may get perforated during surgery and one-half of them become permeable to bacteria after several hours of use; therefore, it is advisable to change gloves at least hourly for long procedures, even on the same patient.

The standard recommendation is that a new pair of gloves is used for each new patient. New gloves be worn for surgical cases or any other treatment, which results in blood or saliva contamination. The American Dental Association has condemned the reuse of gloves, because this practice results in defect in the glove material, which will diminish its value as an effective barrier, and adequate removal of previous patient pathogen cannot be uniformly guaranteed.

Rarely, allergic reactions to gloves may develop in some members of staff or patients. This may be due to latex (polyisoprene) or antioxidants such as mercaptobenzothiazole, and these individuals can safely use polyurethane or vinyl gloves. In addition, skin creams; a spray on microfilm on the skin or a cotton glove liner may be of some value. The dental practitioner should be aware of some drawbacks related to the usage of gloves, namely: (i) difficulties in handling small instruments such as endodontic instruments (lessens with practice), (ii) loss of fine sense of touch (minimized by gloves with a good fit), (iii) inflammability, and hence the danger of working close to open flames, and (iv) possible effect on setting time of some impression materials (eliminated by correct purchasing or glove removal).

Refreshments: Eating, drinking, or application of cosmetics in clinical areas including clinical laboratories, is not recommended.

Prevent Environmental Contamination (Fig. 8.3)

Uncovered jewellery should not be worn during dental procedures. A wristwatch worn under the cuff of the cover gown, and thus is protected by it, is acceptable. Pens/pencils should be cleaned and disinfected if contamination has occurred. Food and beverages must not be kept in patient care, laboratory and sterilization areas. All procedures and manipulations of potentially infective materials should be performed carefully to minimize droplets, splatters and aerosols, whenever possible. Use of rubber dam and high volume evacuation (HVE) is recommended.

Spills of blood and body fluids: Gross inorganic material should be removed with an absorbent material, using a glove, followed by disinfection. In case there is a blood contamination on the floor, a disposable impervious shoe covering should be used. Spraying solution directly

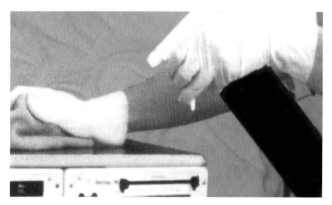

Fig. 8.3: Environmental cleaning and disinfection

on to a spill should be avoided in order to decrease the risk of splatter exposure.

Environmental cleaning and disinfection (Fig. 8.3): At the end of treatment session of each patient and at the completion of each session of daily work, dental unit surfaces and countertops should be cleaned. These surfaces should be disinfected with a suitable chemical *germicide*. The chemical germicides are of two types:

Intermediate level disinfectants: A "hospital disinfectant", which is labeled as "tuberculocidal" (mycobactericidal) is recommended for disinfecting surfaces that have been soiled by patient material. These disinfectants include phenolics, iodophores, and chlorine-containing compounds. Because mycobacteria are among the most resistant groups of micro-organisms, germicides effective against mycobacteria should be effective against many other bacterial and viral pathogens. A fresh solution of sodium hypochlorite (household bleach) prepared daily is an inexpensive and effective germicide. Concentrations ranging from 500 to 800 ppm of chlorine are effective on environmental surfaces that have been cleaned of visible contamination. Caution should be exercised, since chlorine solutions are corrosive to metals, especially aluminum.

Low level disinfectants: A "hospital disinfectant" which is not labeled as for tuberculocidal activity (e.g. quaternary ammonium compounds) are appropriate for general cleaning purposes such as floors, walls, and other surfaces. Intermediate and low level disinfectants are not recommended for reprocessing critical and semicritical dental instruments.

All environmental surfaces should be disinfected between patients and at the beginning and end of the day. Use of 70 percent alcohol, quaternary ammonium compounds or antiseptic agents for surface disinfection within the clinical and surgical area are considered to be inadequate.

Disposable blood/saliva impermeable barriers, such as plastic wrap or aluminum foil must be used to cover the surfaces from direct or indirect contact, whenever possible. Areas difficult to clean and disinfect include: light handles, light controls, chair switches, evacuation controls, three-way syringe, saliva ejector, etc. Floor should be cleaned daily.

Protective barriers must be worn during cleaning. Heavy-duty puncture resistant rubber gloves, face mask and protective eyewear must be worn during surface cleaning and disinfection.

The "spray-wipe-spray" technique, for cleaning, should be employed to clean and disinfect all "high touch areas", is as follows:

1. Spray the surface and/or equipment with cleaner/disinfectant.
2. Dry the surface with paper towel and discard.
3. Spray the surface and/or equipment with cleaner/disinfectant and leave in contact for 10 minutes.
4. Set up for next clinical procedure.
5. Clean the chair with soap and water.

This technique is performed in three stages. The first "spray" stage is a cleaning stage. In the second stage the surfaces are "wiped" cleaned. The third stage is to "spray" the areas again and leave them in contact for 10 minutes. This is the disinfecting stage.

Bulletin boards used for displaying posters, schedules and other information, etc. should allow for easy cleaning of wall surfaces and should be located outside of splatter zone. Patient's charts and radiographs should not be handled in the operating areas to avoid contamination. Chart entries can be made after gloves are removed and hands washed to prevent contamination with blood/saliva.

Use of Sharp Instruments and Needles (Figs 8.4A to C)

Sharp items such as needles, blades and wires; contaminated with patient's blood or saliva should be considered potentially infective; and handled with care to prevent injuries. All sharp items should be disposed of in designated puncture resistant containers. Orthodontic wires and bands are also considered sharps, and disposed off accordingly. Unsheathed needles should not remain on the instrument tray or in the operating field. An uncapped needle and syringe should not be passed from assistant to surgeon, and vice versa.

Patient Management

It is safer to accept that all patients should be handled as if they were an infection risk, or as carriers of blood-borne pathogens (Universal precautions).

Use of *antimicrobial mouthrinse* 0.2 percent chlorhexidine is required before and after treatments. Rubber dam and high volume evacuation must be used during dental procedures whenever possible.

Identification of risk (Patient screening): The medical history of each patient should be obtained and updated

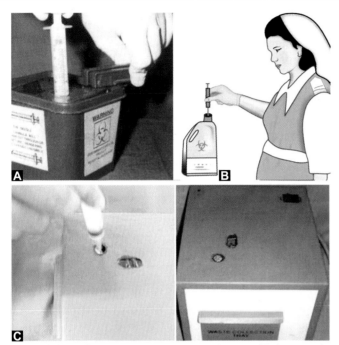

Figs 8.4A to C: (A) Needle and syringe hub cutter, (B) Storage of sharps for disposal, (C) Needle destroyer

at each visit. While taking history, the clinician should identify the infectious diseases of concern, and appropriate questions such as medications, recurrent illnesses, hepatitis status, unintentional weight loss, lymphadenopathy, oral soft tissue lesions or other infections should be included. All patients should be asked routinely about a history of TB and symptoms suggestive of TB. Persons with known active pulmonary TB, or those who warrant a high index of suspicion of TB, should not be provided elective dental care. Dental treatment should be postponed until the medical chart shows that the patient is undergoing treatment and compliance with TB medication is documented. A high index of *suspicion* of pulmonary TB should be maintained in a patient with any of the following; recent history of productive cough lasting in excess of three weeks, bloody cough, fever, complaints of fatigue, chills and night sweats.

The following procedures should be performed in the patient's presence: (i) sterile trays and the handpiece opened, (ii) suction tips and saliva ejector placed on the hoses, (iii) paper cup placed on its stand. The patient should be discouraged from bringing family members into the operatory area.

Sterilization and Disinfection of Instruments

Refer to Chapter 7 on Asepsis and Sterilization.

Disinfection of dental equipment

i. *Handpieces (rationale for sterilization of handpieces):* The internal surfaces of handpieces become contaminated with blood and debris, etc. This retained material is expelled intraorally during subsequent use. Restricted access to internal surfaces limits its cleaning and disinfection. Surface disinfection is not adequate.

The handpieces which are not autoclavable should be subjected to a disinfection regimen. The handpiece is wrapped in gauze soaked with a recommended disinfectant and kept in a sealed plastic bag for a recommended time. Prior to use, the residual chemical residue may be removed by rinsing with sterile water or wiped with gauze soaked in alcohol.

Other methods: (i) Disinfectant sleeves: These are readily available disposable disinfectant sleeves. It contains a combination of alcohol and two synthetic phenols, which is sealed for 10 minutes. (ii) Handpiece condom: It is a thin disposable sheath made of latex. It covers the entire handpiece.

ii. *Dental unit water systems (DUWSs):* The dental unit water systems (the tubes that connect the high-speed handpiece, air/water syringe and ultrasonic scaler to the water supply) have been shown to harbor a wide range of micro-organisms including bacteria, fungi, and protozoas. These organisms gain an entry along with water. When the system is switched off, a negative pressure is created, resulting in retraction of water. These micro-organisms colonize and replicate on the inner surfaces of the waterline tubings, resulting in microbial accumulations termed "biofilms". These biofilms, once formed serve as a reservoir for amplifying free floating micro-organisms in the water exiting the waterlines. Heating dental unit water to increase patient comfort may further augment biofilm formation. If dental unit waterlines, systems not maintained properly, these microbial accumulations can contribute to occasional odors and visible particles of biofilm material exiting the system.

Smith et al (1999) reported that the source of bacterial contamination within the dental unit water supply is thought to be because of micro-colonies of proliferating bacteria, fungi and protozoa on the inner surface of the water lines. Non pneumonic legionellosis of the Pontiac fever type may occur in dental personnel or their patients and cause symptoms clinically indistinguishable from other flu like episodes.

Water quality improvement: The ADA Council on scientific affairs recommends to improve the design of dental equipment, so that water delivered to patients during nonsurgical dental procedures contains no more than 200 colony forming units/ml (cfu/ml) of bacteria at any point of time in the unfiltered output of dental unit. Marais and Brözel (1999) reported that distilled water was ineffective in controlling bacterial counts and biofilm. Electrochemically activated water was effective for this purpose.

This problem can be taken care of by employing the following:

1. *Antiretraction valves:* These valves are fitted to the DUWSs. Retraction valves may cause aspiration of potential infected material back into the handpiece and waterlines. Antiretraction valves (one-way flow check valves), should be installed to prevent aspiration and to prevent transfer of potentially infected material.
2. *Bacterial filter:* Filters are fitted in water lines of handpieces and 2-way syringe hoses.
3. *Chemical disinfection regimens:* The DUWSs are flushed with a disinfectant, e.g. sodium hypochlorite solution. This reduces bacterial population. Presently, some units have integrated disinfecting system.
4. *Aspirators:* They should be cleaned and flushed after every patient; and flushed with a disinfectant at the end of the day. The liquid waste is drained directly into the drains.
4. *Surgery design and zones:* The working area of the clinic is divided into various zones. These zones are (i) high and (ii) low contamination zones. The surgery arranged accordingly. The aim is to restrict contaminated items to as small an area as possible.
   a. *High contamination zone (Zone A):* This area is of a high contamination potential. This zone is an area around the patient which includes the dental unit, waste disposal bag, instruments and materials, etc. The staff or the dental surgery assistant should remain within this area.
   b. *Low contamination zone (Zone B):* This comprises of the remainder of the clinic.

Disposal of Waste/Infected Materials (Fig. 8.5)

Waste materials can be (i) biohazardous and (ii) nonbiohazardous.

Biohazardous material includes: (i) waste items soaked with blood or other body secretions, (ii) waste capable of causing infectious disease, (iii) waste that is capable of having a poisonous effect, (iv) human tissue removed during surgery, (v) teeth and incidental tissue, (vi) blood-soaked material (cotton roll, gauze, pellets, etc.), (vii) bloody gloves.

Nonbiohazardous material includes: (i) matrix band, (should be disposed in sharp container), (ii) masks, caps, gloves, patient's napkins, (iii) impression materials, X-ray packets, surface covers.

The following procedure is adopted for disposal of medical waste:

The bags used for collection and disposal of different waste are color-coded for ease of identification. In a clinical set-up, the medical waste is collected in a small bag. After completion of the procedure the bag is closed and sealed. The waste bag is disposed in yellow plastic trash bags. All other waste, such as, gloves, masks, paper towels and paper barriers should be placed in blue plastic bags. Sharp objects are collected in separate pucture-proof containers, and taken for incineration. Liquid waste is poured into a drain and flushed with water.

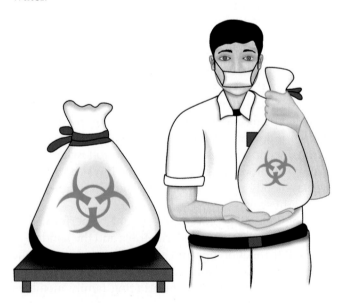

Fig. 8.5: Biohazardous waste disposal

In a hospital set-up, the contaminated or infected waste includes instruments, dressings, syringes, blood-stained beddings, and clothing which has been in direct contact with infectious patients. It also includes the gloves, masks and caps worn in contact with the infected patients or those under isolation. These articles are collected in orange plastic bags, and two bags should be used for safety. It should be transported directly to a special chilled infection store for final removal to the incinerator. All handling of infected waste must be done by staff who are trained, experienced and well aware of hazards of the job and take appropriate precautions.

Handling Biopsy Specimens

Specimens incorrectly collected and transported substi-tute a danger to members of staff and laboratory per-sonnel. Hence, should be put in sturdy containers with a secure lid to prevent leaking during transportation. It is absolutely essential to label the specimens clearly and accurately. Avoid contaminating the exterior of the container. In case, contamination occurs, use another container. Use appropriate transport media and re-frigeration if necessary. Avoid delay in dispatching to laboratory. Haemolytic streptococci on a dry swab may survive only for as short time as 30 minutes; while gono-cocci survive only for seconds. In case of doubt about the need for urgent transport, the microbiologist should be consulted. High risk specimens, as in hepatitis are subject to special precautions.

Swabs: While taking the specimen, rotate the swab to ensure even distribution of micro-organisms on the collecting material. Swabs selected from infected sites should be transferred slowly and carefully to the swab container, so as to avoid contamination of the rim.

Prosthodontics

The following factors must be considered: (i) impression trays: Clean the tray immediately after separating impression from cast unless otherwise, if advised by the doctor. Clean and soak the tray in an approved disinfectant solution, (ii) instruments, articulators and custom trays: All items must be cleaned and sterilized (spatulas, shade guides, acrylic burs, wax knives, etc.) (iii) custom impression trays, base plates and occlusion rims and all prostheses must be disinfected, following manufacturer's recommendation, after construction and before use on the patient. Following each clinical session

and before returning to dental laboratory, articulators, casts, mounts, base plates must be disinfected by spraying with 1:10 chlorine solution, (iv) alginate impression: (a) the patient must rinse mouth with an antiseptic rinse prior to making an impression, (b) rinse the impression under running tap water to remove saliva and other debris, (c) immerse the impression in an approved disinfectant solution (1:10 chlorine) for 30 seconds and rinse again under tap water, (d) immerse again in the approved disinfectant for 10 minutes, wrap in a towel soaked in disinfectant and place in a bag, (v) final impression: follow the procedure mentioned for alginate impression.

Dental Radiography

The staff working in radiology department, usually, is not aware of the medical history of the patients referred for radiography. Hence, it is essential to take certain precautions. The major concern arises from saliva contamination of working areas and equipment. The X-ray tube head, exposure selector, and timer button are likely to get contaminated with saliva.

Intraoral Techniques

(i) Put on gloves, (ii) Place all film holders, and/or film packets required for the patient in a special tray, (iii) Carry out the requested/needed radiographic examination, (iv) Place the contaminated film packet and film holders in the special trays.

After completion of the radiographic examination: (i) The film holding devices may be rinsed under running water to remove saliva. Any metallic part may be autoclaved. Plastic attachment may be placed in chlorhexidine solution. (ii) Film packets are wiped with gauze to remove excess saliva and placed in the special tray. (iii) Wipe the X-ray tube head, exposure selector, timer button, and film packets with detergent chloros. (iv) Transfer the tray with film packet to the darkroom. (v) The films are processed. The film packets are collected in the tray; to be discarded into yellow bag.

Other Precautions
Rubber Dam Isolation

The advantages are: (i) it reduces aerosols and droplets that may be contaminated with infectious micro-organisms, and (ii) it eliminates splatter.

Minimizing Dental Aerosols and Splatter

Aerosols and splatter is generated by high speed handpieces, air-water syringes and ultrasonic scalers. The magnitude of aerosol and splatter can be reduced by the use of rubber dam and high speed evacuation.

Needle Stick Injury

Measures for Prevention

This can be prevented by: (i) ensuring that the needles and surgical blades are sheathed/covered, when not in use, (ii) keeping full control of sharp instruments; and retaining full concentration while handling such instruments, (iii) keeping gloved fingers behind the cutting edges of surgical blades and elevators or the points of probes or needles, (iv) adequate retraction of tissues with appropriate instruments, (v) placing needles in sharp safe box, (vi) taking care when clearing away the surgical sharps, wires, etc. (vii) overgloving or using double gloves, whenever indicated.

Postaccidental Management—Chemo-prophylaxis

The measures to be undertaken are as follows: (i) remove the gloves, (ii) wash the site of injury under running water with soap and water, (iii) avoid scrubbing; and encourage bleeding and then protect, (iv) it is controversial, whether or not, to apply antiseptic preparations like spirit or povidone iodine. Some workers do not advise to use antiseptic preparation, as their effects on local defenses are not known, (v) inform the patient about the incident, (vi) usually, it is necessary to take blood specimens of both the patient and the injured person; and tested for HBV and HIV.

In case, the patient is seropositive, has AIDS, or refuses the test, the health care workers (HCWs) should be:

1. Counseled about the risks of infection and evaluated clinically and serologically as soon as possible after exposure. A baseline HIV test should be carried out immediately since seroconversion will not have occurred immediately after injury.
2. Advised to report and seek medical evaluation for any febrile illness that may occur within 12 weeks of exposure.
3. The HIV test should then be repeated approximately 6 to 12 weeks after contamination, and on a periodic basis if seronegative.
4. Advised to follow recommendations for preventing transmission of HIV infection.
5. During this period, advise from HIV counselors is of utmost importance; regarding domestic relations and procedures at workplace.
6. The practitioner should be immediately evaluated by a physician.

If the patient is known or suspected HBV carrier, the prophylactic requirement will depend upon the immune status of the clinician. Those clinicians: (i) who never had vaccination should receive hepatitis B immunoglobulins (HBIg) within 48 hours of exposure and a course of HB vaccination should begin as soon as possible, and (ii) those who have been vaccinated, the management, would much depend upon, the antibody response. If the antibody titer is more than 100 mU/ml within the previous year, no further action is necessary. If blood testing was not done within the year, or, if there is low antibody titer, a booster dose of vaccine, followed by retesting of antibody titer may be necessary. Those who fail to respond to the vaccine should be given protection with HBIg.

Presently, there is no prophylaxis for HCV infection. The management, would consist of monitoring liver functions and testing for anti-HCV antibodies. There is little evidence to suggest that such cases may respond favorably, if treated at the earliest sign of infection with interferon-α.

HIV Infection Control

It can be described under two headings: (1) Measures at the time of surgery, and (2) Measures for health care workers.

Measures at the Time of Surgery

The protocol to be followed in the operation theatre, is as follows:

Special precautions: When dealing with HIV positive or "high risk " patients, special precautions are to be taken, which are as follows:

1. *Operation theatre:* The following factors may be considered: (i) the patient should be posted at the end of operation list to allow for sufficient time for adequate cleaning of the theatre following surgery, (ii) it is advisable to cover the operating table with waterproof sheet, (iii) the patient should be allowed to recover fully in operating room, so as to restrict

contamination to operating room, and to avoid contaminating recovery room.

2. *Personnel:* (i) members of staff with laceration or abrasions on their hands are excluded from the theatre, (ii) non essential personnel should not be allowed inside the theatre; or their number is kept to a minimum, (iii) a member of staff; nurse/technician may be stationed outside operation theatre as an additional circulating member; to fetch anything, viz. drugs, equipments; required by the operating team. This prevents infections spreading to the rest of the area of theatre complex. (iv) all members of staff not actually involved in the surgery should have following attire, wherever possible: (a) disposable foot covers, (b) disposable cap and face mask, (c) disposable plastic gowns and gloves and (d) protective eyewear, (v) all members of staff, included in actual surgery; in addition to the attire mentioned above should have following: usual hand scrubbed and autoclaved gown and two pairs of disposable (single use) sterilized latex gloves. The contamination of skin from glove perforation can be reduced approximately 5-fold by wearing double gloves. It is usually comfortable if the larger sized glove is worn first (inside; in proximity with the skin) and smaller glove is worn outside (as an overglove), (vi) in case, the mask or cap of any of the member of operating team is splattered with blood it should be immediately changed.

3. *Surgery technique:* (i) a 'no touch' technique is employed, wherever possible; to minimize risk of sharp injury, (ii) scissors or cutting diathermy must be used in preference to blade/scalpel, (iii) sharp instruments should not be handed over to the surgeon and vice versa; instead they are placed in a receiver or kidney tray and then transferred across. This reduces the risk of sharp injury, (iv) emphasis is laid on meticulous surgery and adequate attention to achieve good hemostasis. This reduces the risk of inadvertent injury to the operators; in case there is unexpected bleeding.

4. *At the end of surgery:* (i) patient should be allowed to recover from anesthesia in operation theatre; and not taken to recovery room. Patient is transferred directly to the ward, (ii) in case of spillage of blood or body fluids, the area should be mopped up by a person experienced in the job, using gloves and old linen/paper towels or newspapers and sent for incineration in plastic bags. The area should then be covered with 1 percent 'sodium hypochlorite' (Household bleach) for thirty minutes. The solution is cleaned up with absorbent material (thick quality blotting paper) and placed in the contaminated waste container. The floor should then be wiped with soap and water followed by 1 percent sodium hypochlorite solution, (iii) the members of operating team should remove their shoe covers and gowns before removing gloves. The gloves should be discarded and sent along with the infected waste for proper disposal.

5. *Operation theatre waste disposal:* (i) all disposable sharps should be put in a rigid puncture proof plastic container, properly labeled and sent for incineration. Needles to be capped after shredding, (ii) all non-sharp waste (like gauze pieces, IV bottles, tubings, etc.) should be put in a large plastic bag, labeled and sent for incineration.

6. *Reusable instruments:* (i) the instruments which can be autoclaved should be autoclaved before washing. The instruments are allowed to cool. They are washed with soap and water with brushes. They are rinsed thoroughly with running water and reautoclaved, (ii) the nonautoclavable instruments are immersed in 2 percent glutaraldehyde solution for one hour. The solution is discarded. The instruments are cleaned with warm water and detergent. They are rinsed and left to soak in 2 percent glutaraldehyde for three hours, (iii) The suction bottles should contain 30 ml of 2 percent glutaraldehyde or 60 ml of 1 percent sodium hypochlorite solution. At the end of surgery they should be carefully emptied out, rinsed and auto-claved, (iv) the ventilator tubes should be rinsed with running tap water for 5 minutes. Subsequently, immersed in 2 percent glutaraldehyde solution for two hours.

7. *Laboratory specimens:* They should be put in 10 percent formalin filled jars with a tight leakproof cork, and then put in a plastic bag which is tightly closed and sealed, properly labeled (biohazardous) and transported to the laboratory.

8. *Operation theatre:* The operating room need not be closed down or fumigated after performing surgery in a seropositive patient. The operation table, floor and walls should be thoroughly cleaned with 1 percent sodium hypochlorite solution.

9. *Equipment and surfaces:* The equipment and surfaces which are difficult to disinfect, and may get contaminated, should be covered/wrapped in/by aluminum foils; or by disposable plastic covers.

Universal precautions: These are the usual aseptic precautions which should be observed for all the patients during any surgical procedure. These comprise of: (i) proper handwashing, (ii) surgical attire used for operation theatre, (iii) Covering the operation table with waterproof or disposable sheet, and (iv) all the steps mentioned above should be undertaken in all cases, regardless of the HIV status of the patients.

Measures for Health Care Workers

The transmission of HIV infection from patient to HCW has been reported. The published data abroad showed that, the risk of acquiring HIV through needle stick injury is approximately 0.4 percent and through exposure of mucous membrane is 0.04 percent. Needle stick injury, is the most common cause of contracting HIV infection in HCWs. The risk of acquiring HIV infection can be negligible, if the HCWs observe adequate safety measures.

The infectivity of HIV virus is less than that of HBV. Seroconversion after needle stick injury with HBV infected blood is 6 to 30 percent as against HIV, which is 0.4 percent. The precautions required for attending patients which HIV/AIDS infection and HBV infection are identical.

The transmission of HIV infection can also take place in healthcare setting from patient to patient. However, the bloodborne spread from infected patient to other patient is of minimal concern, whenever sufficient medical and surgical equipments are available and careful attention is paid to the sterilization of instruments and other procedures to minimize the risk of blood contamination, i.e. observing universal safety precautions.

As a general principle, if certain strict precautions are followed, the chances of transmission of HIV infection and other infections through bloodborne agents in health care setting can be avoided. In this unit, we would deal with these precautionary measures to be followed by HCWs in health care settings.

Need for HIV infection control: The majority of people infected with HIV look and feel healthy for a number of years. The disease has a long latent period (5 to 10 years) in the development of full blown disease or with clear cut clinical manifestations; hence these patients are

asymptomatic. Secondly, during the early phase, known as "window period", antibodies are not demonstrated; despite presence of high degree of viremia (infective virus in blood). This period may last from 4 to 12 weeks after exposure to virus. During this period, the patient is highly infectious, however, he will be taken as a normal individual, as antibodies are not demonstrated. In view of these facts it is advisable for the HCWs, to consider all patients as potentially infected with HIV and take "universal precautions" regardless of the HIV infection status. These precautions include: handwashing, careful handling of sharp objects, proper sterilization, disinfection or disposal of instruments after use, appropriate use of gloves, masks and gowns, etc.

Inform the patient about the incident. Usually, it is necessary to take blood specimens of both the patient and the injured person; and tested for HBV and HIV. The operator should be given hepatitis prophylaxis since the risk of developing hepatitis after contamination with blood from a high risk patient is greater than the risk of HIV infection.

HIV-postexposure prophylaxis (PEP)/chemo-prophylaxis for health workers: The guidelines for use of postexposure chemo-prophylaxis to prevent HIV infection; adopted in UK health departments and USA.

Postexposure prophylaxis is recommended when there has been significant exposure to material known or strongly suspected, to be infected with HIV. The significant routes of exposure are percutaneous inoculation, exposure of broken skin or contact with mucous membranes including the eye.

For convenience of description, it can be described in the following way:

(i) Exposure has occurred, with the mucous membrane or skin with evidence of chapping, dermatitis, abrasion, or open wound; and the volume of blood is small (e.g. few drops, short duration): There is negligible risk; risk or drug toxicity may outweigh benefit of PEP regimen, if source HIV titer is high or unknown, (ii) exposure has occurred, with similar conditions, however, to a larger volume of blood (e.g. several drops, major blood splash; and/or duration of several minutes or more); then the basic PEP regimen is recommended; if the source has high HIV titer then expanded regimen is recommended, (iii) the exposure is percutaneous; however, is less severe (e.g. solid needle, superficial scratch), then the basic PEP regimen is recommended; or if the source has high HIV titer, then expanded regimen is required, and (iv) the exposure is

Table 8.2: HIV-postexposure chemo-prophylaxis for health workers		
Type	Drugs	Regimen
Basic (28 days)	Zidovudine + Lamivudine	600 mg/day (300 mg bid, 200 mg tid or 100 mg 4 hourly) + 150 mg
Expanded (28 days)	As above +Indinavir or Nelfinavir or Nevirapine	800 mg 8 hourly, 750 mg tid, or 200 mg bid

percutaneous; however, is more severe (e.g. large bore hollow needle, deep puncture, visible blood on device or needle used in source patient's artery or vein); then expanded regimen is recommended (Table 8.2).

WASTE DISPOSAL IN A HEALTH CARE SETTING

Classification

WHO classification of waste is as follows:
• General nonhazardous,
• Sharps,
• Chemical and pharmaceutical,
• Infectious, and
• Other hazardous medical wastes.

Aims of Waste Treatment

The aims include: (i) disinfection, (ii) reduction in the bulk volume, (iii) making surgical waste unrecognizable, and (iv) rendition of the dangerous recyclable items unusable.

Segregation (Fig. 8.6)

Segregation is the key to management of hospital waste. It allows sorting out of different categories of waste and placing them in different containers or bags. The advantages are: (i) reduction in total treatment cost, (ii) general waste does not become infectious, (iii) reduction

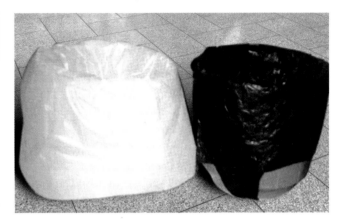

Fig. 8.6: Segregation of waste materials

in the chances of infecting HCWs, (iv) segregation of different wastes on the basis of classification; and as per the guidelines. The bags should be labeled; bearing the international biohazard symbol. All the waste, after segregation, must be stored in color coded containers. The following is the color coding prescribed by Biomedical Waste (Management and Handling) rules, 1998; (Table 8.3).

Disposal of Hospital Waste (Table 8.4 and Fig. 8.7)

Household noninfective waste: It is to be collected in thick polythene bags or plastic cans and discarded like household waste.

Sharp infected hospital waste: It is to be collected separately in puncture resistant, or plastic containers containing 1 percent sodium hypochlorite, which can be closed or sealed. Needles and syringes should be disinfected and destroyed mechanically before disposal.

Infected hospital waste: The infected waste from the wards, operation theatre, OPD and laboratories should be collected in metallic containers decontaminated by autoclaving and then disposed off at garbage disposal

Table 8.3: The color coding to be employed in waste disposal			
Color coding	Type of container	Waste category	Treatment options as per schedule 1
Yellow	Plastic bag	Categories: 1, 2, 3, and 8	Incineration/deep burial
Red	Disinfected container/ plastic bag	Categories: 3, 6 and 7	Autoclaving/microwaving/chemical treatment
Blue/white translucent	Plastic bag/ puncture-proof container	Categories: 4 and 7	Autoclaving/microwaving/chemical treatment and destruction/shredding
Black	Plastic bag	Categories: 5, 9 and 10 (solid)	Disposal in secured landfill

Table 8.4: Types of waste and the methods of disposal	
Waste	*Method of disposal*
Liquid waste, bloody body fluids, suction fluids, excretions and secretions	Buried in deep pit, and covered with bleaching powder and lime
Solid wastes and dressings	Incineration
Laboratory and pathology wastes	Deep burial

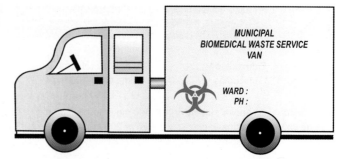

Fig. 8.7: Collection of biohazardous wastes from institutions and sending it to common community incinerator

sites in the hospital; which is subsequently transferred to the municipal disposal sites on daily basis. The metal containers should be thoroughly cleaned and disinfected after emptying the waste.

The staff engaged in disposal of hospital waste should be made aware of the risks involved, adequately trained in safe handling and experienced in this regard.

Disposal of Infected Waste

It is done by the following methods: (i) incineration—it is a sophisticated method of burning the waste, (ii) deep burial with bleaching powder or lime.

9 Antimicrobial Therapy

INTRODUCTION

Antimicrobial agents include antibacterial, antiviral and antifungal agents. Antimicrobial therapy is an integral part of dental practice. This chapter deals with the antimicrobial agents commonly used in orofacial infections. There is a plethora of antimicrobials available now.

The clinician should be conversant with these drugs and basic principles of using them effectively. In order to have a clear understanding, we must know the different terminologies used.

An antibiotic is a chemical substance produced by a micro-organism, which has the capacity, in dilute solutions, to inhibit the growth of or kill other organisms.

A chemotherapeutic agent is a drug which is manufactured entirely by chemical synthesis, e.g. sulfonamide, trimethoprim and many of antitubercular drugs. The term chemotherapy is also now used for the drug treatment of malignant neoplasms (Tables 9.1 and 9.2).

Table 9.1: Factors determining the efficiency of antimicrobial agents*

1. Host defense
2. Source of infection
3. Tissue(s) affected
4. Margin of safety
5. Bacterial susceptibility/resistance to the agent being used

*Adapted from Pharmacology and Pharmacotherapeutics, from Satoskar and Associates. Revised 16th edn,1999.

CLASSIFICATIONS

1. On the basis of preparation:
   i. **Naturally occurring**, e.g. from fungi, e.g. penicillins, cephalosporins, erythromycin, tetracycline, chloramphenicol, and aminoglycosides, etc.
   ii. **Synthetic**, e.g. sulfonamides.
2. On the basis of family:
   i. Penicillins
   ii. Cephalosporins

Table 9.2: Mechanisms of action of antimicrobial agents*	
Sr. no. *Actions*	*Antimicrobial agents*
1. Inhibition of cell wall synthesis	Penicillins, cephalosporins, bacitracin, vancomycin
2. Inhibition of the cytoplasmic membrane	Polymyxin, colistin, polyene, antifungal antibiotics
3. Inhibition of protein synthesis and impairment of function of ribosomes	Aminoglycosides, tetracyclines, chloramphenicol, macrolide antibiotics, and lincomycin
4. Interference in transcription/translation of genetic information	Quinolones, metronidazole
5. Antimetabolite actions	Sulfonamides, trimethoprim
6. Binding to viral enzymes essential for DNA synthesis	Vidarabine and acyclovir

*Adapted and modified, from Pharmacology and Pharmacotherapeutics; from Satoskar and Associates. Revised 16th edn 1999.

   iii. Sulfonamides
   iv. Tetracyclines
   v.   Aminoglycosides
   vi. Macrolide
3. On the basis of spectrum of activity:
   i.   *Narrow:* Penicillins
   ii. *Broad:* Ampicillins, tetracyclines.
4. On the basis of effect:
   i.   *Bacteriostatic:* Erythromycin, tetracycline, sulfonamide, etc.
   ii. *Bactericidal:* Penicillins, cephalosporins, etc.
5. On the basis of their effect on gram positive or gram negative bacteria:
   i.   *Antibiotics acting on gram positive bacteria:* Penicillins, cephalosporins, erythromycin, bactrim, tetracycline, gentamycin, etc.
   ii. *Antibiotics acting on gram negative bacteria:* Penicillin acts on gonococci.
6. On the basis of systems:
   i.   *Urinary tract:*
    • *Nalidixic acid:* Acts on kidney and urinary bladder
    • *Furadantin:* Acts on bladder
   ii. *Skin:* Neomycin, bacitracin, polymyxin.
   iii. *Orally (locally):* Neomycin, streptomycin.

■ PRINCIPLES OF ANTIBIOTIC THERAPY

There are many antibiotics available now; it is prudent for a clinician to have guiding principles in applying a rational regimen in a patient. For the convenience of description, the principles can be divided into the following groups:

Selection of Antimicrobials

1. *Clinical evaluation and diagnosis for antimicrobiological etiology:* This is to ascertain that the infection is due to micro-organisms susceptible to the available antimicrobials. The use of antibiotics, as nonspecific antipyretics should be disapproved.
2. *Study of culture and sensitivity:* In order to identify the causative organism and whenever possible; samples of pus, saliva, blood and urine should be taken. The causative organisms are cultured and tested against a range of antibiotics for maximum sensitivity. Successful therapy depends upon the nature of causative organisms and their sensitivity patterns, e.g. in case of osteomyelitis caused by penicillin-resistant *Staphylococcus aureus*; the following antibiotics may be used; flucloxacillin, or cephalosporin.
3. *Age of the patient:* Certain drugs like chloramphenicol, may cause serious toxic effects in infants; hence should not be used.
4. *Pregnancy and neonatal period:* Many of the antimicrobial agents cross placental barrier. They should be used only when it is really necessary. Penicillins, cephalosporins, erythromycin, (except estolate which is hepatotoxic), lincomycin, clindamycin, azithromycin, and probably sulfonamides (for short-term use) can be safely used.
5. *Severity of the disease:* In general, antimicrobial therapy should be considered for patients with established orofacial infections. Empirically, a bacteriostatic agent should be used. In cases of severe infections a combination of antibiotics effective against a wider spectrum may be employed.

6. *Nature of the drug:* It is preferable to use bactericidal drug, but not essential. However, bactericidal drugs are essentially used in the management of infective endocarditis and immunocompromised patients.

7. *Possibility of drug resistance:* In case the infection is caused by staphylococci resistant to penicillin, an alternative should be prescribed.

8. *History of previous allergic reactions to a microbial agent:* Two aspects must be reviewed:
   • Previous allergic reactions, and
   • Previous toxic reactions.
   An alternative drug must be used in case of allergic reactions.

9. *Risk of toxicity of the drug:* The antibiotics, in general are safe drugs, however, patients should be warned of possible side effects. The risk is much more particularly in the presence of hepatic and renal damage. The mechanisms of clearance of drugs has to be considered. There are two ways the drugs can be cleared: (i) by renal excretion and (ii) by nonrenal mechanisms (Table 9.3).

10. *Cost of therapy:* Presently many effective drugs are available. Newer drugs are added from time to time; which are usually more expensive, but not necessarily more effective. Proper selection of the suitable drug is imperative.

11. *Use of narrow spectrum antibiotic:* It minimizes the risk of superinfection with resistant organisms.

Antimicrobial Combinations

Use of combinations of 2 to 3 antimicrobial drugs, routinely, is not recommended. However, the drugs are combined under certain situations for the following reasons:

1. To have an additive synergistic effect against an organism.
2. In mixed infections when bacteria are sensitive to different drugs.
3. To achieve delay in development of resistance.

Table 9.3: Mechanisms of clearance of antimicrobials	
Renal excretion	*Nonrenal excretion*
Penicillins	Erythromycin
Cephalosporins (except cefoperazone)	Doxycycline
	Chloramphenicol
Fluoroquinolones	
Aminoglycosides	
Amphotericin B	

4. To decrease the incidence of adverse reactions to an individual drug, another drug is added so that the doses of individual drug can be reduced and possible toxic effects can be avoided.

5. When the infection is severe and body defense is inadequate and where the diagnosis is difficult. The combination therapy widens the spectrum of activity. However, once a diagnosis is made, an appropriate regimen must be instituted.

6. *To reduce the chances of superinfections:* Prolonged therapy with broad spectrum antibiotic, such as tetracycline, is sometimes combined with antifungal agents to prevent superinfections due to fungi such as monilia.

7. *To reduce cost of therapy:* In susceptible organisms, cotrimoxazole works out to be cheaper than amoxicillin or cephalosporin.

The bactericidal drugs act on multiplying bacteria; and hence; if a bacteriostatic drug is used with a bactericidal agent, inhibition of bacterial multiplications may occur. This reduces the efficacy of bactericidal agent.

Combining penicillin with chlortetracyclines produces antagonistic effect: In general, when a bacteriostatic agent is added to bactericidal agent, one of the following may result:

1. *Antagonism:* If the bacteria are highly sensitive to bactericidal drug.

2. *Additive effect:* If the bacteria are relatively resistant to bacteriostatic drug.

Combining certain bacteriostatic drugs may have additive effect; sometimes may have synergistic effect as with combination of sulfamethoxazole and trimethoprim. Combining bactericidal drugs may cause synergistic effect, especially with drugs with different mechanism of action, e.g. combination of penicillin with aminoglycoside results in synergism against susceptible *E. coli, Klebsiella, Proteus, Pseudomonas.* This occurs because penicillin helps in entry of aminoglycoside through microbial cell wall, e.g. combination of ampicillin and clavulanic acid acts synergistically, the latter drug inhibiting beta-lactamase production by the organism and thus protects penicillin.

The risks involved in combination therapy are following:

1. Increased risk of superinfection by resistant organisms.

2. Emergence of organisms resistant to multiple drugs used.

3. Increased risk of adverse reactions.
4. Sense of false security; which may lead to incomplete evaluation and inadequate therapy for the patient.
5. Increase in the cost of therapy.

In general, antibiotics should not be combined unless it is documented by sensitivity testing and antagonism has been excluded.

Antimicrobial Prophylaxis

The situations where prophylaxis is indicated are as follows:
1. For preventing endocarditis following minor surgical procedures or tooth extraction.
2. In patients with compound musculoskeletal injury, penetrating wounds, skull injuries or rhinorrhea and otorrhea.
3. Deep punctured wounds that are at high risk for infection.

Routine prophylaxis in cases of minor surgical procedures is not necessary. Indiscriminate use of antimicrobial agents on the contrary can be hazardous. Such a procedure may cause allergic and adverse reactions, leads to emergence of resistant organisms and causes superinfection due to other nonresistant organisms. However, they are useful when used as specific agents to prevent or to destroy specific organisms. Prophylaxis for short periods is more likely to be successful than given for long periods. Prolonged therapy also leads to emergence to resistant organisms.

Bacterial Resistance

It can be (i) natural or (ii) acquired.

■ REMOVAL OF SOURCE OF INFECTION

Antimicrobial therapy is not a substitute for surgery. All sources of infections must be adequately dealt with. The offending tooth must be either extracted or endodontically treated, collection of pus must be drained, foreign bodies and infected nonvital tissues such as sequestra must be removed.

On an outpatient basis and in clinical emergency situations, such as septicemia or Ludwig's angina, antimicrobial agents are prescribed empirically. As soon as the results of culture and sensitivity are available the treatment should be reviewed.

Principles of Antibiotic Administrations

The principles comprise of the following:
1. Dosage and duration of drug.
2. Route and frequency of administration.

Dosage

Dose must be adequate to produce a concentration of antibiotic at the site of infection greater than that required for inhibiting the causative organism.
- In renal failure, the dosage of drugs excreted by renal route may require change of drug or reduction in its dosage (e.g. aminoglycosides, vancomycin); whereas those drugs eliminated by hepatic route (e.g. erythromycin) can usually be given in normal dosage.
- In severe infections, a loading dose or a large initial dose is useful.

Duration

Antibiotics once prescribed should be taken at least for a period of 4 to 5 days. In severe infections prolonged use may be necessary.

The antibiotic once prescribed should not be changed until an adequate time lapse, i.e. 48 to 72 hours, for evidence of effectiveness or otherwise.

After the infection is successfully resolved, treatment should be continued for a period of 48 to 72 hours.

Route and Frequency of Administration

The antibiotics used by oral route should be acid stable (e.g. penicillin V, amoxicillin) and should be absorbed from gastrointestinal tract.

Use of Narrow Spectrum Antibiotic

It minimizes the risk of superinfection with resistant organisms.

Antibiotic Prophylaxis

Successful prophylaxis is possible when the pathogens are sensitive to drug(s) prescribed (Table 9.4).

Collaboration between Clinician and Bacteriologist

It is an important aspect of antimicrobial therapy especially in severe infections. Frequent discussions are to be encouraged.

Table 9.4: Micro-organisms commonly found and implicated in orofacial infections			
Dental caries	Periodontal disease	Apical abscess	Other diseases
Strep. mutans group	Porphyromonas gingivalis	Streptococci species	A. israelii
Crown caries	Adult periodontitis	Strep. intermedius	Actinomycosis
Strep. salivarius	Rapidly progressing periodontitis	Strep. angiosus	C. albicans
Root caries	Prevotella intermedia	Strep. constellatus	Candidiasis
Actinomyces species	Adult periodontitis	Bacteroides species	
Root caries	Juvenile periodontitis		
Lactobacilli	Acute necrotizing ulcerative gingivitis		
Fissure caries	Severe gingivitis		
	Fusobacterium		
	Acute necrotizing ulcerative gingivitis		
	Actinobacillus actinomycetecomitans		
	Juvenile periodontitis rapidly		
	Progressing periodontitis		
	Borrelia vicenti		
	Periodontitis		

BETA-LACTAM ANTIBIOTICS

Antibiotics of this group are:

(i) Penicillins and (ii) semisynthetic derivatives of penicillin, and (iii) cephalosporins.

a. *Structure:* These substances and their derivatives have a molecular structure based on a nucleus of two fused rings, one of which is the beta-lactam ring. This structure is common to all antibiotics in this group.

b. *Antibacterial activity:* Beta-lactam antibiotics act by inhibiting cell wall synthesis of susceptible bacteria. They are effective mainly during the growth phase when cell walls are being synthesized.

c. *Bacterial resistance:* The bacteria can develop enzymes known formerly, as, penicillinase. These enzymes can destroy the beta-lactam ring in the nucleus of penicillins and it's derivatives thereby rendering them ineffective. Cephalosporins are generally more resistant to the effect of beta-lactamases.

d. *Toxic effects:* The principal adverse effect of penicillin is allergy. Allergy established to one type of penicillin is likely to cause similar reaction to other penicillins and it's derivatives.

e. *Excretion:* These antibiotics are excreted unchanged through kidneys.

Penicillins

Penicillin was discovered in 1929, however, the clinical trials were performed in 1940. It is derived from a mould, *Penicillium notatum*. It was the first antibiotic drug to be used; and is still the best.

Classification

1. Naturally occurring penicillins: Crystalline penicillin (penicillin G), phenoxymethyl penicillin (penicillin V)
2. Semisynthetic penicillins:
   a. Short-acting, e.g. ampicillin, amoxicillin, amoxicillin with clavulanic acid, piperacillin and methacillin. They have special properties and uses. They are stable to gastric acids, make oral administration reliable and are resistant to beta-lactamase.
   b. Long-acting, e.g. procaine penicillin, procaine penicillin fortified and benzathene penicillin.

Penicillin is linked with procaine to provide a sustained release preparation which gives an effective level of penicillin over a period of 24 hours.

Administrations

Route of administrations: The oral route is the safest and the most frequently employed. In cases where the

intramuscular injections are given in surgeries which should be adequately equipped to deal with emergencies which may arise following such injections. In situations where IV administrations is indicated the patient should be hospitalized.

Subsequent to parenteral administrations, or doses in excess of one gram taken orally, the patients should be kept under observation for at least 30 minutes until it is established that no immediate side effects are likely to occur.

Broad spectrum with IV administration: Administration of penicillins through IV route achieves much higher serum levels. The spectrum of bactericidal activity is much greater following IV use of penicillins; because of higher serum levels achieved.

Oral Administration

Since the levels of penicillin G achieved following oral administrations are not reliable, it is no longer administered by this route.

The semisynthetic penicillin that is phenoxymethyl-penicillin and ampicillin are well absorbed following oral administration. However, should be administered at least one hour before meals or three hours after meals to obtain maximum effect. Amoxycillin is well absorbed orally and can compete with food for absorption. It can be administered independently of food taken. The absorption of orally administered drugs is not reliable, following administrations of atropine or atropine-like substances used in dentistry, as premedications; for either sedation or general anesthesia. Under such circumstances parenteral route should be employed.

Length of Course

Antibiotics once instituted, should be continued for at least 4 to 5 days to prevent reinfection/recurrence of disease and to completely eradicate the disease.

Broad spectrum effect with clavulanic acid: Clavulanic acid is derived from *Streptomyces clavuligerous*. It acts by inhibiting beta-lactamase enzymes. The result of combining with amoxycillin is to broaden antibacterial spectrum of amoxycillin to include organisms that are resistant to amoxycillin because of their beta-lactamase production, e.g. species of staphylococci, nonhemolytic streptococci (including *Strep. faecalis*), and some gram negative bacteria like *Hemophilus*, *E. coli*, *Klebsiella* and *Proteus* species.

Measurements of Penicillin (Units and Micrograms)

A standard method of expressing the potency of penicillin was adopted in 1944 using crystalline sodium penicillin G as the standard. It is expressed in 'International units'(iu).

250 mg penicillin equals approximately 4,00,000 iu.

Toxic Effects

Penicillin is remarkably free of toxic effects even in large doses administered over long periods. However, hypersensitivity reactions, in the form of allergy and anaphylaxis are reported. In case of allergy to one type of penicillin, there is likelihood that the person is allergic to other penicillins and in some cases to cephalosporins.

There is an inherent risk with all antibiotics of superinfection by a resistant organism. Allergy is the most common side effect of penicillin therapy. It may manifest in the form of skin rashes, dermatitis, serum sickness. These effects can be controlled by withdrawal of penicillin and use of antihistaminics.

Anaphylaxis

Anaphylaxis can occur and is a life threatening situation. It is sudden in onset, characterized by coughing, tonic spasms, gasping, cyanosis, weak pulse and rapid drop in blood pressure.

Other Effects

Pregnancy: The absolute safety of any of the penicillins or their semisynthetic derivatives taken during pregnancy is not established. Penicillin should be employed only if there is an infection caused by a susceptible organism. The first choice is amoxycillin.

Lactation: Penicillin appears in breast milk as similar levels to serum levels. Phenoxymethylpenicillin is preferable because of lower concentration in breast milk than serum.

Oral contraceptives: Penicillin may render oral contraceptives ineffective. However, it has been reported that ampicillin did not reduce efficiency of oral contraceptives in the limited number of cases studied.

Cephalosporins

Cephalosporins have similar structure to penicillin but have a different source.

Mode of action: They are bactericidal. They act by inhibiting the cell wall synthesis in growing bacteria. They should not be used with other bacteriostatic agents which inhibit protein synthesis such as tetracycline, erythromycin and lincomycin, etc.

Spectrum of activity: They are effective against most species of staphylococci and streptococci except some species of *Strep. faecalis.*

Indications: Cephalosporins are bactericidal antibiotics and effective against most gram positive cocci, including most division III streptococci (enterococci) and most staphylococci. Cephalosporins provide an alternative drug in cases where penicillins are contraindicated.

Cephalosporins because they are bactericidal, may be used as an alternative drug to penicillin for prophylaxis against infective endocarditis.

Classification: Cephalosporins are arbitrarily classified by generations; which is based on general features of spectrum of activity.

First generation: Cephalosporins of this generation are effective against gram positive micro-organisms, most gram positive cocci except enterococci. Methicillin resistant *Staph. aureus* and *Staph. epidermidis.* They are also active against *E. coli, Klebsiella,* pneumoniae and

P. mirabilis: This generation of cephalosporins includes cephalothin and cephalexin.

Second generation: This generation of cephalosporins has greater activity against gram positive micro-organisms than first generation cephalosporins. This generation of cephalosporin includes cefotaxime.

Third generation: These cephalosporins have less activity against gram positive organisms than first generation and more activity against Enterobacteriaceae, including beta-lactamase producing strains.

Tetracyclines

The tetracyclines are a large family of antibiotics that were discovered as natural products by Benjamin Minge Duggar and first described in 1948. Benjamin Duggar made his discovery of the world's first tetracycline antibiotic, aureomycin, in 1945.

The first of these compounds was chlortetracycline, which was introduced in 1948, under the name of aureomycin (because of the golden yellow color of

S. aureofaciens colonies producing it) followed by oxytetracycline and tetracycline. Tetracyclines had marked contrast from penicillin and streptomycin, in being active orally and were effective against a wide range of micro-organisms; hence are called "broad-spectrum antibiotic". All tetracyclines are slightly bitter solids, which are weakly water soluble, but their hydrochloride salts are more soluble. The aqueous solutions are unstable. The tetracyclines developed later on have high lipid solubility and greater potency.

Classifications

Tetracyclines are classified as broad spectrum antibiotics.

A. **On the basis of chronology of development,** as well as for convenience of description, they may be divided into 3 groups:
   1. **Group I:** (1) tetracycline, (2) chlortetracycline, and (3) oxytetracycline
   2. **Group II:** (1) demeclocycline, (2) methacycline, and (3) lymecycline
   3. **Group III:** (1) doxycycline, and (2) minocycline
B. **On the basis of occurrence:** Tetracyclines can also be divided on the basis of occurrence in the following way:
   a. **Naturally occurring:**
      (1) tetracycline, (2) chlortetracycline,
      (3) oxytetracycline, and (4) demeclocycline
   b. **Semisynthetic:**
      (1) doxycycline, (2) minocycline,
      (3) meclocycline, (4) lymecycline,
      (5) methacycline, and (6) rolitetracycline

Mechanism of Action

Tetracyclines are primarily bacteriostatic; the drugs inhibit protein synthesis by binding to the 30S subunit of microbial ribosomes in susceptible organism. Subsequent to this binding, attachment of charged aminoacyl-tRNA to the mRNA-ribosome complex is interfered with. This results in failure of growth of peptide chain.

They prevent introduction of new amino acids to the nascent peptide chain. The action is usually inhibitory and reversible upon withdrawal of the drug. Resistance to the tetracyclines results from changes in permeability of the microbial cell envelope. In susceptible cells, the drug is concentrated from the environment and does not readily leave the cell. In resistant cells, the drug is not actively transported into the cell or leaves it so rapidly that inhibitory concentrations are not maintained. This is often plasmid controlled. Mammalian cells do not actively concentrate tetracyclines.

Mechanism of Resistance

There are three types of tetracycline resistance:
1. Tetracycline efflux.
2. Ribosomal protection.
3. Tetracycline modification.

Antibacterial Spectrum

The tetracyclines inhibited practically all types of pathogenic micro-organisms except fungi and viruses; hence the tetracyclines are "broad spectrum antibiotics". They are active against the following micro-organisms:

(1) Gram positive and gram negative bacteria, (2) spirochetes: including *T. pallidum*, (3) myco-plasmas, (4) rickettsiae, (6) *Candida albicans*, (7) *My-coplasma pneumoniae*, (8) *Chlamydia trachomatis*, (9) *Borrelia recurrentis*, (10) *Yersinia pestis* (11) *Vibrio cholerae*, (12) *Campylobacter fetus*, (13) *Brucella species*, (14) *Streptococcus pneumoniae*, and (15) *Neisseria gonorrhoeae*.

Pharmacokinetics

The earlier tetracyclines are incompletely absorbed from GI tract; absorption is better if taken on empty stomach. Doxycycline and minocycline are completely absorbed irrespective of food.

Formation of Metal Chelates

Stable chelate complexes are formed by the tetracyclines with many metals, including calcium, magnesium, and iron. Such chelates are usually very insoluble in water. The affinity of tetracyclines for calcium causes tetracyclines to get incorporated into newly forming bones and teeth as tetracycline-calcium orthophosphated complexes. Deposits of these antibiotics in teeth cause a yellow discoloration. Tetracyclines are widely distributed in the body tissues. They are concentrated in liver and spleen, and binds to connective tissue in bone and teeth. They bind to mitochondria. The CSF concentration of tetracyclines is ¼ that of plasma. Most tetracyclines are excreted in urine. The dose has to be reduced in renal failure, except doxycycline.

The tetracyclines cross the placental barrier into the fetus. They are also secreted in the milk of lactating mothers in sufficient amounts to affect the infant. The possible effects of these agents on bones and teeth of the child should be considered before their use during pregnancy or in children under 8 years of age.

Indications

It is first-line therapy for Rocky Mountain spotted fever (*Rickettsia*), Q fever (*Coxiella*), psittacosis and Lymphogranuloma venereum (*Chlamydia*), and to eradicate nasal carriage of meningococci. Tetracycline tablets were used in the plague outbreak in India in 1992. Doxycycline is also one of many recommended drugs for chemoprophylactic treatment of malaria for travelers to areas of the world where malaria is endemic.

Cautions, Contraindications, Side Effects

The tetracycline antibiotics group:
1. Can stain developing teeth, even when taken by the mother during pregnancy
2. Can cause permanent teeth discoloration (yellow-grey-brown); when taken during infancy and childhood to eight years of age
3. Gets inactivated by Ca^{2+} ion, and hence not to be taken with milk, yogurt, and other dairy products
4. Gets inactivated by aluminum, iron, and zinc, and hence not to be taken at the same time as indigestion remedies
5. Gets inactivated by common antacids and over-the-counter heartburn medicines
6. Causes skin photosensitivity; and hence exposure to the sun or intense light is not recommended
7. Causes drug-induced lupus and hepatitis
8. Can induce microvesicular fatty liver
9. Can cause tinnitus
10. May interfere with methotrexate by displacing it from the various protein binding sites
11. Can cause breathing complications as well as anaphylactic shock in some individuals
12. Should be avoided during pregnancy as it may affect bone growth of the fetus
13. Passes into breast milk and is harmful to breastfed infants, and should therefore be avoided during breastfeeding if possible.

In 2010, the FDA added Tetracycline to its Adverse Event Reporting System (AERS). The AERS contains a list of medications under investigation by the FDA for potential safety issues. The AERS cites a potential link between the use of tetracycline products and Stevens-Johnson syndrome, toxic epidermal necrolysis and erythema multiforme.

Other Uses

Since tetracycline is absorbed into bone, it is used as a marker of bone growth for biopsies in humans. Tetracycline labeling is used to determine the amount of bone growth within a certain period of time, usually a period of approximately 21 days. Tetracycline is incorporated into mineralizing bone and can be detected by its fluorescence. In double tetracycline labeling, a second dose is given 11 to 14 days after the first dose, and the amount of bone formed during that interval can be calculated by measuring the distance between the two fluorescent labels.

Tetracycline is also used as a biomarker in wildlife to detect consumption of medicine or vaccine containing baits.

In genetic engineering, tetracycline is used in transcriptional activation. Tetracycline is also one of the antibiotics used to treat ulcers caused by bacterial infections. In cancer research at Harvard Medical School, tetracycline has been used to reliably cause regression of advanced stages of leukemia in mice, by placing it in their drinking water.

Administration

The most commonly used dosage form is oral capsule. The capsule should be taken ½ an hour before or 2 hours after food. Oral suspension and dry syrup are banned in India to avoid their usage by children. It is not recommended for IM route as it is very painful and has poor absorption from the site. It can be used by IV route, slowly, only in severe cases.

Preparations

1. Oxytetracycline: Terramycin 250, 500 mg capsules
2. Tetracycline: Achromycin, hostacycline, resteclin, 250, 500 mg capsules
3. Demeclocycline: Ledermycin, 150, 300 mg capsules
4. Doxycycline: Tetradox, biodoxi, doxt, novadox, 100 mg capsules
5. Minocycline: Cyanomycin 50, 100 mg capsules.

Precautions

1. Avoid administering to pregnant and lactating women, and infants and children up to 12 years of age.
2. Avoid administering along with common antacids, as they get inactivated.
3. Avoid administering along with milk and milk products, as it gets inactivated by Ca^{2+} ion,
4. Avoid administering along with indigestion remedies as it gets inactivated by aluminum, iron, and zinc.

Adverse Reactions

1. *Allergy:* Tetracyclines can cause skin rashes, urticaria, pruritus. They can cause skin photosensitivity; and hence exposure to the sun or intense light is not recommended. Very rarely they can cause breathing complications as well as anaphylactic shock.
2. *Gastrointestinal tract:* They can cause epigastric pain, nausea, vomiting, and diarrhea
3. *Superinfection:* Tetracyclines are the most common antibiotics responsible for causing superinfection, because they cause marked suppression of the normal intestinal flora.
4. *Antianabolic effect:* When administered in large doses and for prolonged periods, tetracyclines can produce an anabolic effect resulting in increased excretion of urinary nitrogen and certain amino acids, leading to weight loss
5. *Liver:* Tetracyclines can induce microvesicular fatty liver (hepatitis), if taken in large doses over a short period of time.

    Tetracyclines should be avoided in pregnancy in the interest of both mother and fetus, as it may affect bone growth of the fetus
6. *Kidney:* In patients with renal impairment, tetracyclines may cause an aggravation of azotemia
7. *Teeth and bones:* Tetracyclines chelate calcium, resulting in the formation of a tetracycline orthophosphate complex and therefore, are deposited in areas of calcification in bones and teeth. Administration of tetracyclines to pregnant women may leads to yellow staining of teeth of infants. It may lead to defective enamel formation and hypoplasia of teeth. Pigmentation of teeth may occur and there is increased risk of caries. These drugs should be

avoided in infants and in children up to the age of 12 years.

8. *Benign intracranial hypertension:* Some infants, may develop increased intracranial pressure, which manifests in the form of bulging of the anterior fontanelle, headache, photophobia and papilledema in adults.

9. *Miscellaneous:* Intravenous administration of tetracyclines may cause local thrombosis, or thrombophlebitis of the injected vein. These drugs may interfere with blood coagulation, especially in those having a bleeding tendency; this effect probably is secondary to chelation of calcium.

Erythromycin

1. Erythromycin is the principal member of macrolide group of antibiotics. Other macrolides currently available are azithromycin and roxithromycin, both are available for oral administration.

2. Erythromycin is a broad spectrum antibiotic. It is effective against most gram positive cocci, including many penicillinase resistant strains of staphylococci and *S. aureus*, and many gram negative bacteria encountered in dental infections.

Preparation

It is available in forms of oral, IM or IV administrations.

Mode of Action

Erythromycin is generally considered to be a bacteriostatic agent, though in some circumstances, it has bactericidal effect. It acts by inhibition of protein synthesis.

Pharmacology

i. *Oral preparation salts:* Erythromycin is available as stearate or estolate salt. The stearate salt is acid-labile, but less readily absorbed than the estolate form. The estolate form is well absorbed, but in adults is associated with cholestatic hepatitis.

ii. *Intramuscular preparations:* Erythromycin (base or plain) is utilized for intramuscular injections.

iii. *Intravenous preparations:* Erythromycin lactobionate is used for intravenous administration slowly, in conjunction with intravenous infusion.

Absorption

Erythromycin is absorbed from upper part of small intestine. Food may delay absorption, and, it is recommended that erythromycin be given one hour before meals.

Excretion

Erythromycin is excreted unchanged, in bile via liver. Approximately, a quarter of the total dose is excreted through kidneys. Impaired liver, or to a lesser extent, impaired kidney function, could increase toxic effects of erythromycin. Hence, patients with hepatic or renal dysfunction who are taking erythromycin should be observed for adverse effects.

Toxic Effects

Allergy to erythromycin is rare: Allergic reactions reported are skin rash and other skin symptoms. Anaphylaxis is reported.

Gastrointestinal effects: These include nausea, vomiting and diarrhea, etc.

Cholestatic hepatitis: Erythromycin has been associated with cholestatic hepatitis in adults only. It is almost always related to the use of estolate forms.

Interactions

i. *With antihistaminics and sympathomimetics:* Erythromycin in conjunction with astemizole causes increased levels of astemizole, leading to serious arrhythmias. Erythromycin, concurrently used with terfenadine may produce serious prolongation of QT interval (ECG). There is a potential for arrhythmia with sympathomimetic drugs. Hence such combinations are contraindicated.

ii. *With theophylline:* Erythromycin when given with high doses of theophylline, may produce theophylline toxicity; including arrhythmias. Further, theophylline may reduce the serum concentration of erythromycin to subtherapeutic levels.

iii. *With carbamazepine:* Erythromycin when administered along with carbamazepine may increase the risk of carbamazepine toxicity.

iv. *With warfarin:* Patients taking erythromycin and warfarin concurrently, there is increase in prothrombin time, leading to an increased risk of bleeding.

v. *With benzodiazepines:* There is an increase in half-life of some benzodiazepines including midazolam and triazolam.

vi. *With oral contraceptives:* Erythromycin may affect the action of oral contraceptives.

Use during Pregnancy and Lactation

There are no teratogenic effects reported with the use of erythromycin. Erythromycin appears in breast milk. No adverse effects have been reported on infants fed by mothers taking erythromycin.

Concomitant Use of Other Antibiotics

As the mechanism of action of erythromycin is different from that of penicillin and cephalosporins, these antibiotics may be less effective when used together.

Lincomycin and clindamycin appear to compete with erythromycin, hence these antibiotics should not be used along with erythromycin.

Sulfonamides and Trimethoprim

Sulfonamides were first introduced in 1935. These agents are bacteriostatic; and get inactivated by presence of pus. Sulfonamides act by inhibition of bacterial synthesis of folic acid from para-aminobenzoic acid (PABA).

Absorption, Distribution and Excretion

* Sulfonamides are well absorbed after oral administration and widely distributed through all body fluids.
* They cross placental barrier and also appear in breast milk.
* They are excreted through kidneys by glomerular filtration with preferential water reabsorption. The concentration of sulfonamides in urine is greater than that in blood. This leads to formation of crystals of sulfonamides; termed as crystalluria; and leads to renal damage. This can be avoided by excessive fluid intake and by administering substances which increase urine alkalinity.

Toxic Effects

Allergic reactions: They include skin rashes, exfoliative dermatitis, S-J syndrome, polyarteritis nodosa and peripheral neuritis and photosensitivity.

Hemopoietic system: Prolonged therapy can lead to macrocytic anemia, due to inhibition of conversion of folic acid to folinic acid; rarely depression of bone marrow or selective blood dyscrasias like acute hemolytic anemia, agranulocytosis and aplastic anemia.

Renal damage: Crystallization of sulfonamides may lead to renal damage. The signs include blood stained urine, renal pain and reduced urinary flow.

Prolonged therapy should be accompanied by regular blood investigations including a differential white cell count.

Pregnancy and Lactation

Sulfonamides, including the combination with trimethoprim may cause kernicterus by displacing bilirubin from plasma albumin in babies during their initial month of intrauterine life. Sulfonamides may cause increase in incidence of fetal malformations.

The drugs also are present in breast milk and may lead to diarrhea, rash, jaundice, or kernicterus. Sulfonamides or trimethoprim, or their combinations are not recommended for use in pregnancy or lactation.

Oral Contraceptives

Sulfonamides and trimethoprim may render oral contraceptives ineffective.

Sulfadiazine

It penetrates blood-brain barrier and achieves high levels in CSF. It is commonly used for prophylaxis to post traumatic meningitis. A loading dose of 3 g is followed by 1 g, 6 hourly for 7 to 10 days. The drug can be administered by IV route; 1 g, 6 hourly. Caution should be exercised by taking a fluid intake of at least two liters/day to avoid crystalluria and renal damage.

Cotrimoxazole (Combination of Sulfamethoxazole and Trimethoprim)

This agent inhibits the conversion of folic to folinic acid which is important for bacterial synthesis of DNA and RNA. In this way, two bacteriostatic agents join to form a bactericidal combination, cotrimoxazole (bactrim or septran).

Spectrum of activity: It is active against *Strep. pyogenes* and most staphylococci and hemophila.

Indication: Useful in acute exacerbation in post irradiation osteomyelitis secondary to osteoradionecrosis. It is also used in mixed actinomycotic infections along with penicillin.

Preparations: It is available for oral administration.

Adult: 80 mg of trimethoprim and 400 mg of sulfamethoxazole tablets are available. Two tablets are taken 12 hourly.

Child: 20 and 100 mg respectively. The tablets can be dissolved in water; and, therefore, useful in patients with intermaxillary fixation.

Quinolones

Mechanism of Action

Inhibit synthesis of bacterial DNA.

Nalidixic Acid

Spectrum of activity: It is effective against gram negative bacteria, especially *E. coli*; *Shigella* and many strains of *Proteus*; and less effective against *Aerobacter* and *Klebsiella* species.

Absorption, distribution and excretion: It is easily absorbed from gastrointestinal tract. It remains bound to plasma proteins; and excreted through kidney.

Adverse reactions: Include nausea, vomiting and diarrhea. Allergic reactions include pruritus, rash, urticaria, fever, eosinophilia and photosensitivity. CNS manifestations include headache, malaise, drowsiness and myalgia. Overdosage may lead to convulsions in children.

Dosage: It is available as 250 and 500 mg tablets and syrup. The dose is 4 g daily in 4 divided doses. It should not be prescribed in cases of cerebral arteriosclerosis, parkinsonism, impairment of hepatic and renal functions. It should be avoided during pregnancy and young children.

Fluoroquinolones

They are chemically related to nalidixic acid; and have fluorine in their chemical structure and hence the name. The commonly used fluoroquinolones are: acrosoxacin, enoxacin, cinaxon, norfloxacin, ciprofloxacin, ofloxacin, pefloxacin, lomefloxacin and sparfloxacin.

Antibacterial spectrum: They have broad spectrum of activity; and are bactericidal against most gram positive and gram negative organisms. It is effective against staphylococci including methicillin resistant *Staph. aureus* (MRSA); and against streptococci including *Strep. pneumoniae*. They have good activity against Enterobacteriaceae (*E. coli*, *Klebsiella* and *Proteus mirabilis*), including many organisms which are resistant to penicillins, cephalosporins and aminoglycosides.

Absorption, distribution and excretion: They are adequately absorbed from gastrointestinal tract and distributed in body fluids. Most of them, except pefloxacin are excreted by kidney.

Therapeutic uses: These drugs, except norfloxacin, are useful in treating systemic and serious infections. Norfloxacin, because of it's low serum levels is not useful in systemic infections; is effective in infections of urinary and gastrointestinal tracts.

Adverse reactions: Generally, these drugs are well-tolerated.
1. GI tract toxicity includes nausea, vomiting, diarrhea, anorexia and abdominal discomfort.
2. CNS toxicity includes confusion, nervousness, agitation and hallucinations.
3. Allergic reactions are rare.

■ ANTIVIRAL ANTIBIOTICS

Viruses are of two types:
1. Deoxyribonucleic acid (DNA) viruses, e.g. herpes simplex; varicella zoster; smallpox; hepatitis B; human cytomegalovirus.
2. Ribonucleic acid (RNA) viruses, e.g. rubella, measles, dengue, HIV.

Antiviral compounds can be classified as follows:
1. Compounds interfering with nucleic acid synthesis, e.g. idoxuridine, acyclovir.
2. Thiosemicarbazones, e.g. methisazone.
3. Natural substances, e.g. interferon.
4. Miscellaneous agents, e.g. amantadine, antiviral antibiotics, gamma globulin.

Acyclovir (Cyclovir, Zovirax)

Acyclovir is a guanosine analog and a potent antiviral drug with low toxicity. It is useful in treating infections with:
1. Herpes simplex virus types (I and II)
2. Varicella zoster virus.

Action: It inhibits viral DNA synthesis, in patients with herpes zoster. Acyclovir does not reduce intensity of postherpetic neuralgia.

Dosage: Oral 200 mg five times a day for seven days or by IV infusion.

Both herpes simplex and varicella zoster viruses produce their effects by replicating in them. To be effective, treatment must be started soon after onset of lesions or during the prodromal phase of illness. Most of herpes lesions are mild and heal without any problem.

The treatment of the cases of herpes virus can be described in the two following ways:

1. *In immunocompetent individuals:* The treatment is used for those who have early lesions and for those in whom the lesions are widespread.
2. *In immunocompromised individuals:* In these cases it may lead to dissemination of infection; hence treatment should begin at any stage of infection.

Oral acyclovir is partially absorbed with bioavailability of 15 to 30 percent.

Adverse reaction: The drug is generally well tolerated and is less toxic. With IV administration it may cause thrombophlebitis, elevation of blood urea and creatinine, CNS toxicity includes delirium, tremors, abnormal EEG and psychiatric disturbances. The drug should be avoided in pregnancy.

Preparations: Acyclovir is available as cream, 3 percent eye ointment, tablets and powder for preparing infusion.

Valacyclovir and Famciclovir

These are prodrugs for cyclovir and pencyclovir, respectively and are used for similar purposes.

Ganciclovir

Ganciclovir is an analog of guanine; and is a virustatic. It is available in the form of IV infusion. Its use is limited to immunocompromised cases with cytomegalovirus (CMV) infections because of its toxicity. Its adverse reactions include neutropenia, thrombocytopenia, gastrointestinal and gonadal toxicity.

Aminoglycosides

Aminoglycosides group of antibiotics includes gentamycin, vancomycin, streptomycin, kanamycin, neomycin, and tobramycin. These are bactericidal and similar in structure; and are effective against many gram negative bacteria, especially those, resistant to penicillins. These are potentially toxic and are administered parenterally. These drugs are used in the treatment and prevention of severe infections.

Aminoglycosides are known to have toxic effect on vestibular and cochlear (auditory) branches of VIII cranial nerve; and on kidneys. This toxicity is due to accumulation of the drug secondary to impaired renal function. These are bactericidal and act by inhibition of protein synthesis.

Gentamycin

Administration: It is preferably administered by intramuscular injection, as there is a better control on absorption and avoids high serum concentrations.

Spectrum of activity: Gentamycin is effective against a wide range of gram positive and negative bacteria including penicillinase resistant staphylococci.

The combined effects of ampicillin and gentamycin are effective against a wide spectrum of gram positive bacteria including streptococci and staphylococci; and gram negative bacteria. Gentamycin and ampicillin should be administered separately. In solutions containing both ampicillin and gentamycin, the gentamycin is destroyed.

Indications: In orofacial region, gentamycin is indicated in severe anaerobic infections. In the past, the main indication used to be for prophylaxis to infective endocarditis.

Dose and route of administration: Gentamycin is administered either by intravenous infusion or by intramuscular injection. When administered intravenously, it should be infused to avoid high serum concentration and possible toxic effects from rapid administration. Intramuscular route is preferable as it gives more reliable serum concentration.

- Adult dose is 3 to 7 mg/kg/day in 2 to 3 divided doses.
- Child dose is 1 to 3 mg/kg/day in 2 to 3 divided doses.

Toxic effects:

1. It causes ototoxicity (vestibular and cochlear), if the serum concentrations exceeds 10 mg/ml, transient tinnitus has been reported.
2. When used for a period exceeding a week, nephrotoxicity may occur.
3. Allergic reactions are reported. In such cases its use is contraindicated; and an alternate drug may be used.

Pregnancy and lactation: There is no established evidence that its use in pregnancy is safe. There are no reports of whether or not gentamycin appears in breast milk. Hence, it is not recommended to use gentamycin in lactating mothers.

Vancomycin

Vancomycin has similar properties to gentamycin. It is bactericidal; and effective against most gram positive bacteria including many strains of streptococci; as well as a number of gram negative bacteria.

Indications

- Severe orofacial infections
- Patients who are allergic to penicillin
- Patients with risk for endocarditis.

Dose and route of administration: It is administered by slow, intermittent intravenous infusion.
- Adult dose is 500 mg (IV infusion) every six hourly or 1 g every 12 hourly
- Child dose is up to 44 mg/kg/day in divided doses by IV infusion.

Adverse reaction: It includes allergic reactions including anaphylaxis, deafness, tinnitus, hypotension and irritation at the site of injection. Rapid administration may lead to pruritus, generalized flushing and erythematous macular rash.

Pregnancy and lactation: Safe use is not yet established. It is not recommended to be used in pregnant women, unless expected benefit outweighs the potential risks. Vancomycin is excreted in breast milk and its use in nursing mothers is not recommended.

ANTIMYCOTIC AGENTS

A relatively few antimycotic agents with minimal toxicity and side-effects are available as compared to a plethora of antibiotics. The principal antimycotic agents used in oral mycoses fall into two main groups. These agents are used for treatment of different forms of oral candidiasis.
1. *Polyenes:* Nystatin and amphotericin B.
2. *Azoles:* Imidazoles and triazoles.

Polyenes

They are commonly used for treatment of oral candidiasis.

Amphotericin B

Mode of action: It acts by inhibiting fungal growth through an interaction with ergosterol. It exerts either a fungicidal or fungistatic effect, depending on the concentration used.

Polyenes bind more effectively to ergort than to other mammalian sterols.

Spectrum of activity: It includes most fungi that cause disease in humans, including Candida species.

Absorption: Amphotericin B is poorly absorbed from gastrointestinal tract.

Administration: It is usually administered intravenously or used topically.

Adverse effects: The most common adverse effect of systemic use is nephrotoxicity. Hypokalemia and mild anemia are also common. Other rare effects include acute hypersensitive reactions, including anaphylaxis.

Drug interactions: Amphotericin B may potentiate nephrotoxicity of other agents such as aminoglycosides and cyclosporins; Its use with glucocorticoids may lead to electrolyte disturbances, particularly hypokalemia.

Preparations and dosage: The available preparations for oral delivery are ointment, suspension, cream and lozenges.
- Oral systemic dose for adults is 100 to 200 mg 6 hourly. Lozenges can be given 8 hourly to a maximum of 80 mg/day
- *Oral suspension:* 1 ml 8 hourly, retained in the mouth (after food), in contact with the lesions
- *IV infusions:* Administered at 0.25 mg/kg/day for both adults and children.

Nystatin

Mode of action: It is the most popular agent for treating superficial infections of *C. albicans.*

It should be used topically, however, it may be used orally for the treatment of mucocutaneous infection caused by *C. albicans.*

Nystatin is similar to that of amphotericin B. It has both fungicidal and fungistatic activity depending upon its concentration.

Adverse effects: It causes systemic toxicity.

Preparations: Nystatin is available in the form of creams, tablets, suspensions, oral rinses, gels and pastilles.

Ointment is used for the treatment of angular cheilitis. Tablets (5,00,000 IU) used for the treatment of oral candidiasis. Suspension is used for young children and noncompliant patients. Oral rinse is relatively ineffective, because of short contact time with oral lesions. The oral rinse contains sugar and increases the risk of dental caries. Pastilles and lozenges can be sucked slowly and therefore have a longer duration of action. These forms of administration, by the virtue of sweetened formulations, result in better patient compliance, and prolonged retention. This results in a better fungicidal action than suspension. Pastilles are ideal for treatment of *Candida* associated denture stomatitis. However, because of their sucrose content, there is increased risk of developing dental caries. A slow released form offers rapid clinical improvement in cases of oral candidiasis. This form, is to be kept in mouth and not swallowed, is sugar free and offers prolonged contact time. It is more effective than pastilles; the effect lasting for up to a week after treatment.

The various topical preparations of nystatin in the treatment of oral candidiasis can be summarized as follows:
- Dissolved vaginal pessaries (1,00,000 IU) one pastille four times a day
- Ointment/cream to be applied to commissures three times daily
- Oral suspension (1,00,000 units/ml) four times daily, continued for several days after healing.

Azole Antifungal Agents

These agents are classified into two groups:
1. *Imidazoles:* Clotrimazole, econazole, fenticonazole, isoconazole, ketoconazole, miconazole, sulconazole and tioconazole.
2. *Triazoles:* Fluconazole and itraconazole.

Azoles are becoming popular in the management of oral candidiasis. The agent, fluconazole is the drug of choice in treatment of oropharyngeal candidiasis in HIV infection.

Mode of action: Azoles act by inhibiting the cytochrome p-450 enzymes that are involved in synthesis of fungal cell membranes. Clotrimazole, econazole, fenticonazole, isoconazole, miconazole, sulconazole and tioconazole are all used for local treatment. Miconazole can also be given by mouth for oral and intestinal infections.

Ketoconazole, fluconazole and itraconazole are used for both local and systemic candidiasis.

Clotrimazole

Clotrimazole is primarily a fungistatic, with a broad spectrum of activity both anticandidal and antistaphylococcal. It is mainly used for superficial infections of oral cavity, skin and vagina caused by Candida. As a cream it is useful in the treatment of angular cheilitis due to its dual action.

Adverse reactions: Mild and rare; in the form of local skin irritation, nausea and vomiting.

Preparations: It is available in the form of cream, and lozenges: 1 percent cream is applied three times daily while lozenges are available in 10 mg units, dissolved in the mouth five times a day

Miconazole

Like clotrimazole, it has broad spectrum of activity against fungi including *C. albicans* and also against staphylococci. Hence it is useful in the treatment of angular cheilitis. It can be given topically, intravenously or intrathecally. It is effective in all types of oral candidiasis. Systemic use of miconazole has been taken over by less toxic drugs such as ketoconazole and fluconazole.

Adverse effects: Rare with topical use. The most common effect after intravenous use is thrombophlebitis. Drugs of azole group are known to enhance anticoagulant effect of oral anticoagulants such as warfarin.

Preparations: It is available in the form of tablets, oral gel, intravenous injections, topical and vaginal preparations. Cream is used in the treatment of angular cheilitis.

It has been formulated into a lacquer, which is effective in treatment of *Candida* associated denture stomatitis (Dumicoat 50 mg/g). Application of the contents of one bottle to upper surface of upper denture after thorough cleansing and drying, repeated twice at intervals of one week, is recommended. A single application of miconazole lacquer over fitting surface of denture, as a slow delivery, is capable of reducing the numbers of *Candida* on denture surfaces for a substantial period of time.

Ketoconazole

Mode of action: It is effective against a wide spectrum of fungi including *Candida*.

Absorption: Unlike other imidazoles, it is readily absorbed after oral administration.

Indications: Its main indication is secondary oral candidiasis; such as chronic mucocutaneous candidiasis.

Adverse effects: The most common adverse reactions are gastrointestinal intolerance with nausea and vomiting. Hepatotoxicity is rare. It causes depression of testosterone biosynthesis, which manifests as painful gynecomastia, loss of libido and sometimes loss of hair. It is also a potential teratogen.

Interactions: It interacts with many drugs. With nonsedative antihistamine, such as terfenadine and astemizole, and can lead to arrhythmias, and tachycardia. With cyclosporin, there can be profound immunosuppression and life threatening renal dysfunctions. Concomitant use of rifampicin, decreases ketoconazole concentrations.

Preparations: It is available in the form of tablets, suspensions and creams. Two percent cream is applied to commissures three times a day in chronic hyperplastic candidiasis. Systemic dose is 200 to 400 mg daily.

Fluconazole

Fluconazole is water-soluble and does not require a low gastric pH for absorption. It is poorly bound to plasma proteins and is eliminated by kidney.

Mode of action: It has a broad spectrum of antifungal activity. It differs from other azoles in that it has an excellent absorption from gastrointestinal tract; and is weakly protein bound in serum. Unlike other azoles, it is not metabolized in humans, and is excreted largely through kidney approximately 80 percent unchanged. It has a high systemic absorption and is now considered a drug of choice for candidiasis in HIV disease, in 200 mg weekly doses.

Adverse effects: Fluconazole is well tolerated. The adverse effects such as nausea, headache, and gastrointestinal discomfort are usually mild. It may cause elevation of liver enzymes and an allergic rash. It should be avoided in pregnancy, as it may cause embryotoxicity.

Interactions: Interactions are lesser than the agents mentioned earlier. Being a structural analog to other azoles, it also shows similar interactions. Nonsedative antihistaminics such as terfenadine and astemizole should not be administered along with fluconazole. Fluconazole can lead to high serum concentrations of many drugs by decreasing their metabolism in liver. Hence, decreased clearance of cyclosporin may result in significant immunosuppression, leukopenia and renal dysfunction. Similarly, interactions with other drugs such as phenytoin, warfarin and hypoglycemics, fluconazole can produce toxic concentrations in serum, prolonged prothrombin times.

Preparations: It is available in capsule and intravenous formulations. The adult dose for treating oropharyngeal candidiasis is 50 mg daily for 7 to 14 days; and 50 mg daily for 14 to 30 days for esophageal candidiasis.

Itraconazole

Itraconazole is water insoluble and lipophilic drug, and requires a lower pH for ionization than ketoconazole. It is highly protein bound and excreted in bile. It is well absorbed after oral administration and has a wide spectrum of activity, including species. It is effective in various superficial mycoses including oral candidiasis due to *C. albicans*, *C. krusei* and *C. glabrata*. As the last two are resistant to fluconazole, itraconazole is the drug of choice in treatment of fluconazole resistant *Candida*.

Adverse effects: Generally, it is well-tolerated. Gastrointestinal disturbances are rare.

Interactions: Similar to fluconazole.

Preparations: It is available in capsule and oral solution forms. The adult oral dose is 100 mg daily for fifteen days for oropharyngeal candidiasis.

Disadvantages of using azoles:

1. *All azoles are fungistatic:* This factor should be considered in treating chronic infections in immunocompromised patients.
2. None of azoles is entirely beneficial.
3. They are expensive.
4. Hepatotoxicity may be common to all of them and the potential for endocrine toxicity exists particularly at higher doses.

Resistance: The emergence of resistance to triazoles, particularly to fluconazole is a serious clinical problem in patients with HIV disease.

Metronidazole

It is effective in anaerobic infections and acute necrotizing ulcerative gingivitis (ANUG). Metronidazole is used with one of the penicillins, usually, amoxycillin to treat acute orofacial infections with an anaerobic component of causative micro-organisms. Metronidazole, can also be used in combination with cephalosporins for treating anaerobic infections where there is penicillin allergy or any other contraindication.

Spectrum of activity: It is very effective against a wide range of gram positive and negative bacteria including Bacteroides, Clostridia and Spirochaetes.

Indications: ANUG has been successfully treated with metronidazole. It has also been successfully used in chronic destructive periodontal disease and juvenile peridontitis.

Administration, absorption and distribution: Metronidazole is absorbed from gastrointestinal tract. It competes with food for absorption. It is widely distributed through body fluids after administration. It crosses placental barrier and appears in breast milk.

Excretion: Metronidazole is excreted in urine, which may be colored red-brown. Impaired renal and hepatic function can prolong presence of the drug in serum. It is also excreted in saliva and breast milk in similar concentrations to plasma.

Toxic effects and contraindications:

1. Studies in humans have shown no evidence of carcinogenicity, however, teratogenic effects are possible.
2. Blood dyscrasias are reported. Blood investigations are recommended if the therapy exceeds ten days. Metronidazole should be avoided in patients with blood dyscrasias.
3. *CNS pathology:* Metronidazole affects patients with CNS pathology such as depression or psychosis. The reported effects are convulsions, dizziness, vestibular symptoms, hypotension and hallucinations, etc. Metronidazole is contraindicated in patients who are taking phenytoin.
4. Metronidazole may enhance the effects of warfarin and prolong coagulation time. In such patients, the assistance from physician is obtained to supervise warfarin therapy.

■ LINCOMYCIN AND CLINDAMYCIN

Lincomycin was first described in 1963 and later its derivative clindamycin. Clindamycin is more active and has less side effects. The oral preparations of clindamycin has replaced oral lincomycin. Lincomycin is reserved for parenteral administrations.

Antibacterial activity: The spectrum of activity of both the antibiotics is similar; however, clindamycin is more active. These antibiotics are bacteriostatic; and act by inhibiting protein synthesis. Both antibiotics are effective against most gram positive bacteria; and against many gram negative bacteria including *Bacteroides*, Anaerobic Streptococci and Clostridia.

Distribution: These antibiotics are well distributed, however, they do not penetrate CSF. They appear in breast milk and cross placental barrier. Their distribution includes bone and because of their presence in bone it has been suggested that these antibiotics are suitable for treating bone infections. These antibiotics form a second line of treatment in osteomyelitis.

Administration: Clindamycin is well absorbed when given orally and may be administered independently of food. Lincomycin, does not compete well with food and hence should be administered one hour before; or two hours after meals; for achieving maximum absorption. Intramuscular and intravenous preparations exist.

Excretion: It is either through the kidneys; or following liver metabolism through bile or urine. Renal or hepatic disease may prolong the presence of these antibiotics.

Toxic effects:

1. The main toxic effects are related to gastrointestinal tract; which include nausea, vomiting and diarrhea. Candidiasis may occur and neither antibiotic may be used in presence of *Candida* infections.
2. Hematological reactions include neutropenia, leucopenia, agranulocytosis and thrombocytopenic purpura. In cases, where, treatment is prolonged for more than six days, necessary investigations should be carried out for detecting blood dyscrasias.
3. Pseudomembranous colitis is characterized by diarrhea, abdominal pain, fever, and blood and mucus feces. The antibiotic should be stopped.

Pregnancy and lactation: These antibiotics are safe during pregnancy and lactation. In lactation, alternative drugs appear in low concentrations in breast milk.

GUIDELINES FOR ANTIBIOTIC PROPHYLAXIS

The American Heart Association (AHA) and the American Dental Association (ADA) recently modified their recommended protocols for antibiotic prophylaxis against bacterial endocarditis. In addition, the ADA and the American Academy of Orthopedic Surgeons, (AAOS) also issued a new recommendation against routine use of antibiotic prophylaxis in patients with prosthetic joint replacements.

These changes reflect improvements in understanding of these disease processes and changing attitudes towards the use of antibiotics (Tables 9.5 to 9.7).

Table 9.5: Cardiac conditions associated with endocarditis		
Prophylaxis recommended		*Prophylaxis not recommended*
High risk category	*Moderate risk category*	*Negligible risk category*
• Prosthetic cardiac valves	• Most other congenital cardiac malformations	• Isolated secundum atrial septal defect ASD
• Previous bacterial endocarditis	• Acquired valvular dysfunction, e.g. rheumatic heart disease (RHD)	• Surgical repair of ASD or patent ductus arteriosus (PDA)
• Complex cyanotic congenital heart disease (CHD)	• Hypertrophic cardiomyopathy	• Previous coronary bypass graft surgery
• Surgically constructed systemic pulmonary shunts or conduits	• Mitral valve prolapse (MVP)	• MVP without valvular regurgitation
		• Physiologic, functional or innocent heart murmurs
		• Previous Kawasaki disease
		• Previous rheumatic fever
		• Cardiac pacemakers and implanted defibrillators

Table 9.6: Dental procedures and endocarditis prophylaxis
Endocarditis prophylaxis recommended for:
• Dental extractions
• Periodontal procedures including surgery, scaling and root planning, probing and recall maintenance
• Dental implant placement and reimplantation of avulsed teeth
• Endodontic (root canal) instrumentation or surgery only beyond the apex
• Subgingival placement of antibiotic fibers or strips
Initial placement of orthodontic bands but not brackets
Intraligamentary local anesthetic injections
Prophylactic cleaning of teeth or implants where bleeding is anticipated
...ocarditis prophylaxis not recommended for:
...storative dentistry (operative and prosthodontic) with or without retraction cord
...al anesthetic injections (nonintraligamentary)
...anal endodontic treatment; post placement and build-up
...ent of rubber dams
...rative suture removal
...t of removable prosthodontic or orthodontic appliances
...al impressions
...tments
...radiographs
...liance adjustment
...ary teeth

Table 9.7: Prophylactic regimens for dental, oral, respiratory tract , esophageal procedures		
Situation	*Antibiotic*	*Regimen*
• Standard general prophylaxis	Amoxicillin	Adults, 2.0 g; children, 50 mg/kg orally one hour before procedure
• Cannot use oral medications	Ampicillin	Adults, 2.0 g IM/IV; children, 50 mg/kg IM/IV within 30 minutes before procedure
• Allergic to penicillin	Clindamycin	Adults, 500 mg; children, 20 mg/kg orally one hour before procedure
	or	
	Cephalexin, Cephadroxil	Adults, 2.0 g; children, 50 mg/kg orally one hour before procedure
	or	
	Azithromycin or Clarithromycin	Adults, 500 mg; children, 15 mg/kg orally one hour before procedure
• Allergic to penicillin and unable to take oral medications	Clindamycin	Adults, 600 mg; children, 15 mg/kg IV one hour before procedure
	or	
	Cephazolin	Adults, 1.0 g; children 25 mg/kg IM/IV within 30 minutes before procedure

10 Minor Oral Surgical Procedures

MINOR ORAL SURGERY

The first dictum of medicine and surgery is—'*Primum Non Curarum*—first do no harm'. Minor oral surgery comprises of those surgical procedures, which can be comfortably completed by a dentist in not more than 30 minutes. Minor surgical procedures will include carrying out complicated surgical extractions (combination of tooth sectioning, mucoperiosteal flap reflection, bone removal prior to the use of a forceps or elevators), elimination of small lesions in the oral cavity, which are in the hard or soft tissues.

BASIC PURPOSE OF SURGERY

The basic purpose of any surgery is as follows:
• Elimination of disease
• Prevention of disease
• Removal of damaged or redundant tissue
• Improvement of function and esthetics.

PRINCIPLES OF ORAL SURGERY

• Developing a surgical diagnosis
• Basic necessities for surgery
• Aseptic technique
• Incision planning
• Flap design
• Tissue handling
• Hemostasis
• Dead space management
• Decontamination and debridement
• Suturing
• Edema control
• Postoperative infection control
• Patient's general health and nutrition
• Follow-up.

Developing a Surgical Diagnosis

The decision to perform a surgery depends upon the several diagnostic steps. Before undertaking the surgery, the clinician should perform following steps:

- First identify the clinical problem
- Carry out thorough logical reasoning and use the available data
- Establish the relationship between the individual problems
- Obtain the pre-surgical evaluation data
  - Patient's physical, laboratory and imaging examination data
  - Possible etiological factors for the lesion development
  - The thorough history of lesion.

Clinical Characteristics of Lesion

- Location
- Shape
- Sharpness of boundaries
- Color
- Consistency
- Texture
- Mobility or fixation
- Local induration or inflammation
- Erosion or ulceration
- Pulsation
- Fluctuation
- Regional lymphadenopathy
- Radiological changes.

The oral cavity is an excellent barometer of general systemic health. Oral abnormalities can be extensions or manifestations of underlying systemic disease. Therefore, the surgical decision should be undertaken after ruling out systemic problems.

History of Lesion

- Chief complaint—pain, edema, swelling, regional lymphadenopathy, decreased sensation (hypoesthesia) and altered sensation (paresthesia)
- Duration of the lesion
- Change in any senses—taste, smell, hearing, vision
- Change in size, degree of fluctuation, erythema, erosion, etc.

Transalveolar Extraction (Open or Surgical Extraction)

Transalveolar extraction is the method used for recovering the roots, that are fractured during routine extraction of teeth (routine closed extraction method) for a variety of reasons. It consists of removal of some amount of the bone investing the roots, if required, and using the forceps or elevators to deliver a tooth/root.

Indications for transalveolar surgical extraction

- Any tooth, which offers a lot of resistance for elevation technique
- Retained roots, which cannot be grasped by the forceps or delivered with an elevation technique
- Previous history of difficult or attempted and failed extraction technique
- Any large restoration with root canal therapy—brittle teeth
- Hypercementosis/ankylosis of a tooth
- Germinated/dilacerated tooth
- Radiographic evidence of complicated/difficult root pattern or roots with unfavorable or conflicting lines of withdrawal
- Sclerosis of the bone
- Teeth associated with pathology—periapical granuloma, cyst, tumor, etc.
- Impacted teeth, embedded teeth.

Pre-extraction clinical assessment

- Presence of infection
- Access to the tooth:
  - Oral opening of the patient—adequate
  - Restricted—due to trismus, TMJ disorders, muscle fibrosis, etc.
- Hypomobility of the tooth—hypercementosis, ankylosis
- *Condition of the crown:*
  - Marked attrition—usually with calcified pulp chamber, brittle tooth
  - Presence of extensive caries, large restorations
  - Previous history of endodontic treatment
- Tooth alignment in the arch
- Age of the patient—old age—sclerosis
- Embedded roots.

Indications for preoperative radiographs

- History of difficult or attempted, failed extraction
- A tooth which is abnormally resistant to elevation or forceps extraction (hypercementosis, ankylosis, dilacerated roots, extra long roots, curved roots)

- Any teeth or roots in close relationship to either the maxillary sinus or inferior dental canal or mental nerve
- Any teeth with history of trauma (fractured crown or roots or alveolar bone)
- Any partially erupted, unerupted tooth, missing tooth, supernumerary tooth, retained root, lingually placed tooth, impacted tooth
- Heavily restored tooth or pulpless tooth—brittle, possible presence of periapical pathology
- Any condition, which predisposes to dental or alveolar abnormalities like: osteitis deformans (hypercementosis of the roots), osteoradionecrosis, osteopetrosis, etc.

Pre-extraction Radiological Evaluation (Fig. 10.1A)

Relationship with associated vital structures

- Maxillary sinus
- Inferior alveolar canal
- Mental nerve
- Adjacent teeth roots.

Configuration of roots

- Number of roots
- Width—greater below CE junction than at the CE junction
- Size of roots
- Curvature of roots, divergence of roots
- Length—thin, tapered roots
- Resorption of roots
- Shape of the individual root
- Hypercementosis, ankylosis, root caries
- Previous endodontic therapy.

Condition of surrounding bone

- Density of bone surrounding the tooth
- Dense bone—condensing osteitis, sclerosis will increase the difficulty.

Multiple Extractions

Single sitting procedure for multiple adjacent teeth with slight modification of routine extraction pattern facilitates a smooth transition from a dentulous to an edentulous state.

- Soft tissue reflection is extended slightly to form a small envelop flap, exposing a crestal bone prior to extractions
- After extractions, the ridge is checked for any sharp bony spicules or undercuts
- Alveolectomy/plasty   suturing.

Order of Multiple Teeth Extractions

- Maxillary posterior teeth except first molar
- Maxillary anterior teeth except the canines
- Maxillary first molar
- Maxillary canine
- Mandibular posterior teeth except the first molar
- Mandibular anterior teeth except the canines
- Mandibular first molar
- Mandibular canine.

Difficult Extraction/Breakage of the Root

- Reposition the patient
- Visualize the root directly or with the help of a mouth mirror
- Irrigate the socket forcibly
- Suction the area
- Probe with an explorer, endofile or an apexo elevator
- Sometimes it is prudent to leave very small root tip behind, but the risk/benefit ratio should be in patient's favor.

Surgical Extractions (Complicated Extractions)

- Unplanned extractions—an event that can convert an uncomplicated extraction into a complicated one
- Proper pre extraction assessment of a difficult case

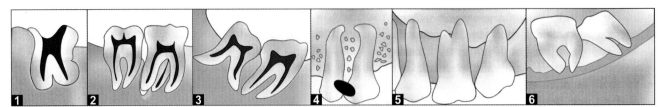

Fig. 10.1A: Preoperative radiograph is helpful to detect these conditions: (1) Hypercementosis, (2) Extra-roots, (3) Dilacerated roots, (4) Curved, long root, (5) Roots in the maxillary sinus, (6) Approximity to the inferior alveolar nerve

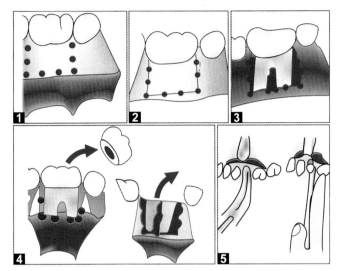

Fig. 10.1B: Postage stamp technique of transalveolar extraction: (1) Reflection of mucoperiosteal flap and bur holes are made, (2) Connected bur holes to create a window, (3) Exposing the roots, (4) Sectioning the crown and roots for easy removal, (5) Transalveolar extraction of a root piece by planning small envelop flap

- Any premonition or suspicion that the tooth/bone will break—think and plan
- Properly planned surgical extraction is always less traumatic (people attack the tooth—the hardest structure in the body, but hesitate, when it comes to soft tissue incision)
- Do not shy away from complicated extraction
- Proceed as predicted with fewer surprises.

Postage Stamp Technique for Transalveolar Extraction (Fig. 10.1B)

- Helps in controlled removal of bone, preventing uncontrolled fracture of the alveolar process
- Allows judicious use of elevators and forceps
- Allows tooth sectioning in a controlled manner, facilitating predictable result instead of an apical root fracture.

Three Basic Principles

- Obtain adequate access which makes difference between success and failure
- Create an unimpeded path of removal
- Use controlled force.

Basic Necessities for Surgery

The main requirements for any surgery are adequate visibility and assistance. Adequate visibility will depend on the following:

- Adequate access
- Adequate light source
- A clean surgical field (free from excessive bleeding).

Adequate Access

Adequate access will require:
- Comfortable patient
- Adequate oral opening
- Proper retraction of the tissues by assistant
- High volume suction, hemostasis of the operating field.

Patient

- Comfortable, mentally and physically
- Alleviation of fear, assurance
- Informed consent
- Minimum amount of draping
- Rinsing with antiseptic mouth wash.

Equipment

- The instrument kit should be prepared and sterilized
- Effective light source and suction.

Assistant

Four handed surgery with the help of a skilled assistant. The assistant should be familiar with the procedure being performed to anticipate the surgeon's needs.

Surgeon's and Assistant's Preparation

- Wearing of protective eye glasses
- Wearing mask
- Wearing surgical cap
- Wearing gloves.

Aseptic Technique

Aseptic technique has been explained in detail in Chapter 7 on Asepsis and Sterilization.

Planning of an Incision

Planning of an incision is a basic step in any surgery. The incision is defined as 'a cut or a wound deliberately made by an operator in the skin or mucosa using a sharp instrument such as a surgical blade, cautery, etc. so that the underlying structures can be exposed adequately for surgical access. Thorough anatomical knowledge is essential. Incision is placed parallel to the structures without causing damage to the vital structures. Extraoral incisions should be planned along the 'Langer's lines' of the normal skin tension or creases, so that minimum scar formation will be seen. Intraoral incision should be planned to prevent subsequent scar contraction or fibrosis, which will prevent normal functioning of the oral soft tissues.

The sharp blade of a proper size and shape should be selected. Essential for clean, single stroke incision without much tissue damage.

- Incision should be placed on the sound bone, or away from the surgical area to ensure the prevention of wound dehiscence
- Either pen (intraoral incision) (Fig. 10.1C) or table knife (extraoral incision) grasp is used with proper support and pressure to produce uniform atraumatic clean incision, with predictable depth
- The skin or the mucosa to be incised, should be stabilized with finger pressure to guide the passage of the blade
- A firm continuous stroke should be used. Repeated strokes increase both the amount of tissue damage and the bleeding, thereby impairing the wound healing. Long continuous strokes are preferable to short interrupted ones
- No sharp angles, the change in direction is accomplished by a gradual curve. Sharp angles tend to produce slough due to poor circulation and may lead to extensive scarring.

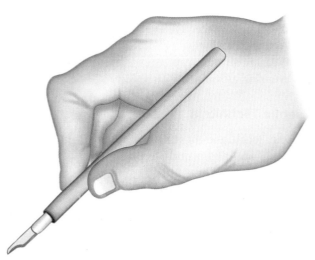

Fig. 10.1C: Pen grasp for intraoral incisions

Incisions in the Oral Cavity

- It is desirable to incise through attached gingiva and over a healthy bone. The suture line should have adequate bone support underneath for uneventful healing
- Incisions placed near the teeth for extractions should be made in the gingival sulcus
- Incisions involving the reflection of the mucoperiosteal flap are direct, straight line or curvilinear taking the shortest distance vertically through the tissues
- Indirect incisions are used to access the areas like soft palate, tongue, cheeks, lips, floor of the mouth, etc.
- Integrity of the interdental papillae should be maintained as far as possible
- Blood supply to the incision should be adequate
- Incisions should be at right angles to mucosa to prevent shelfing edges, that might cause necrosis of the undermined part.

Contraindications for Placement of Incision Lines

Avoid placing incisions

- Over the canine prominence—soft tissue defect will be created due to bony fenestration
- Vertical incision in the mental nerve region
- On the palate—near the greater palatine vessels
- Through incisive papillae
- Over bony lesions—dehiscence
- Over freni
- Vertical incisions on the lingual side of the mandibular arch.

Types of Incisions

Horizontal: It is seldom used because of natural contour of maxilla and mandible. These types of incisions are directed along the gingival margin either mesially or distally.

- Internal bevel incision—starts at distal area from the margin and is aimed at bony crest. This is also known as first incision.
- Crevicular incision—starts at the bottom of the pocket and is directed to the bony margin. This is known as second incision. These incisions are mainly used in periodontal flap surgeries.

Vertical: Vertical or oblique incisions are most desirable and are also called as releasing incisions, on one or both the sides of the flap. It may be single resulting in triangular type of flap.

- Double vertical incisions on both sides of the flap will result in trapezoidal flap
- The incisions should extend beyond mucogingival line reaching the alveolar mucosa to allow the release of a flap for reflection
- Vertical incisions should be placed at obtuse angle to the horizontal incision and should leave interdental papillae intact.

Semilunar (curved, elliptical): This type of incision is used, when it is desirable to maintain the attached gingiva intact around the teeth and for endodontic surgery. The horizontal component of this flap rests on the alveolar bone. The gap of 5 mm must be present from the base of the gingival sulcus to the incision.

Flap Design

The preparation of adequate mucoperiosteal flap is of paramount importance. Standard surgical protocols should be followed while designing a flap or reflecting it to preserve the integrity and function of the soft tissues. The properly designed flap may bring about minimum morbidity like pain, swelling, etc. postoperatively, but it will definitely prevent the potential morbidity (including complications) associated with damage due to inadequate exposure.

While taking intraoral incision for flap designing, convenience, access, avoidance of injury to the vital structures, maintaining the integrity of the interdental papilla, etc. should be thought about.

Main Complications of Flap Surgery

- Flap tearing
- Flap necrosis
- Flap dehiscence.

Flap tearing: The incision should be clean, sharp and should penetrate the entire mucoperiosteum, if the flap is being reflected over the bone. The flap should be reflected as one unit. The flap should be large enough to prevent tearing or for avoiding the need to modify during surgery. Adequate size of the flap is a must for proper instrumentation and visual access. The length of the flap should be no more than twice the width of the base.

Flap necrosis: Ideally, the base of the flap should be wider than the reflected free margins to allow for the adequate blood supply to the reflected tissues. Flap should have margins that either run parallel to each other or preferably converge from the base to the apex of the flap. Whenever possible, the axial blood supply should be included in the base of the flap. For example, palatal flap can be based on greater palatine artery (pedicled flap).

Flap dehiscence: This is seen in the immediate post-operative phase after suturing is done. This means separation of the flap margins or gaping of a wound. This is prevented by designing a flap in such a way that the sutures will be placed over the solid healthy bone. Poor tissue handling, too tight suturing, hematoma formation, infection, suturing under tension may lead to dehiscence.

Principles of Flap Designing

Intraoral surgical flaps are made to gain surgical access to the area to be operated or to move tissues from one place to another.

Indications

For basic oral surgical procedures to allow complete visualization of the operative field and to access osseous tissues, whenever required.

Types of Flaps (Fig. 10.1D)

A. • Full thickness—mucoperiosteal flap
   • Partial thickness
B. • Envelope flap
   • Two sided triangular flap
   • Three sided rhomboid flap
   • Semilunar flap.
C. • Labial, buccal flaps
   • Palatal, lingual flaps

Envelope Flap (Fig. 10.1E)

- The most common type of flap.
- The incision is made to any length (depending on the amount of exposure needed) intraorally around the necks of the teeth along the free gingival margin on the buccal or lingual aspect including the interdental papillae

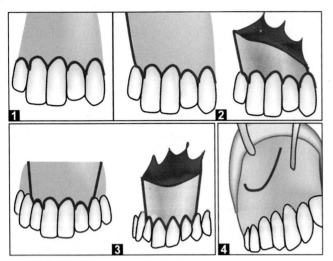

Fig. 10.1D: Types of flaps. (1) Gingival margin crevicular incision, (2) Two-sided triangular flap, (3) Three-sided rhomboid flap. Note that the base should be wider than height, (4) Semilunar flap

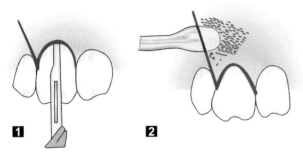

Fig. 10.1E: Incision and reflection of the mucoperiosteal flap with periosteal elevator

- The entire mucoperiosteal flap is raised by using periosteal elevator to a point to the apical one-third of the tooth
- This is mainly used for the surgical extraction of a tooth or roots.

Two-sided triangular flap: In addition to the envelope flap, a vertical releasing incision is used in order to have better access to the area. This vertical releasing incision is made on one side of the envelope flap (at the proximal or distal end) going divergent towards the buccal vestibule forming an obtuse angle at the free gingival margin. The vertical incision should be made in the interproximal area, as the tissues here are thick. To avoid periodontal defect, the incision should never lie directly on the facial aspect of the tooth. Once the incision is taken, then the

two sided triangular flap is reflected towards the base of the flap by using periosteal elevator.

Three-sided rhomboid flap: This is the modification of the earlier flap to improve the visibility and access. An additional vertical incision is added in the opposite direction from the earlier release. Here, care should be taken that the base of the flap must be wider than the apex to ensure good blood supply.

Semilunar flap: Whenever the periapical area is required to be exposed to carry out periapical surgery, this flap is designed. Again the base of the flap should be broader than the apex and the suture line should not lie on the bony defect.

The incision is taken at least 5 mm away from the free gingival margin. This flap is useful to avoid damage to interdental papilla and to prevent periodontal post surgical defects. In case of crowding of the teeth, the suturing is not a problem with this flap. The only disadvantage of this flap is that it often lies on the bony defect.

Tissue Handling

Respect the tissue and the tissue will respect you (remember this adage).

Gentle handling, no excessive pulling or crushing, proper retraction with judicious force, avoidance of extreme temperature, minimum use of electrocautery, avoidance of the use of chemical agents are the key factors for satisfactory wound healing. During cutting of the bone by using electrical engine and handpiece and bur, continuous saline irrigation should be done to avoid generation of heat. Selection of the proper instruments is also important to minimize the tissue trauma.

Hemostasis

Hemostasis should be achieved during surgery for the following reasons:
- To minimize the intraoperative total blood loss
- Increase visibility
- To increase the speed of the surgery and to cut down the total operating time
- To minimize the postsurgical hematoma.

(Hematoma decreases the vascularity, increases the wound tension, acts as a culture media and makes it susceptible for the development of postoperative wound infection.

Hemostasis can be Achieved by

Intermittant pressure: With cotton/gauze sponges or with hemostat clamping. Pressure is usually applied for 20 to 30 seconds for smaller tiny vessels, while large vessels require about 5 to 10 minutes of continuous pressure.

Use of electrocautery: For this judicious thermal coagulation, the area around the vessel should be dried thoroughly. Avoid unnecessary burning the tissue.

Suture ligation: Whenever large vessel is severed, the ends are grasped with a hemostat. Nonabsorbable suture (linen) is used to ligate the ends of the vessels.

Placement of compression dressing over the wound: Many times there is oozing over a large area and hemostasis is difficult. A cotton pad or folded ribbon gauze is stabilized over the wound and secured with tie over sutures and left in place for 2 to 3 days.

Use of vasoconstrictor agents: Such as epinephrine, commercial thrombin or collagen Gelfoam, etc.

Dead Space Elimination

Dead space is the area that remains devoid of tissue after closure of the wound. It is created as a result of removal of tissue in the depths of a wound or by not suturing in multiple layers (single layer approximation). This dead space is usually filled with hematoma.

How to Avoid a Dead Space

* Multiple layer suturing from the depth to the surface
* Use of pressure dressing over the wound in the postoperative period for 12 to 18 hours
* Use of surgical packing of the defect. Whenever proper approximation of the margins is not possible the strip or the ribbon gauze impregnated with an antibacterial medication can be used
* Use of drains alone or along with the pressure dressings
* Nonsuction drains or suction drains can be used.

Decontamination and Debridement

* Irrigation during surgery
* Irrigation at the end of surgery
* Careful debridement of necrotic tissue, foreign bodies, severely injured tissues
* Antibiotic prophylaxis

In intraoral wounds, patients should be instructed to use frequent medicated mouthwashes after every food intake.

In extensive oral surgical wounds, the patient should be fed through Ryle's tube till the wound heals to avoid oral contamination.

Suturing

Suturing has been described in detail in Chapter 6 on Suturing Materials and Techniques.

SURGICAL MANAGEMENT OF IMPACTED TEETH

* **An unerupted tooth**—is a tooth that is in the process of eruption and is likely to erupt based on clinical and radiographic findings.
* **Malposed tooth**—A tooth unerupted or erupted which is in an abnormal position in the maxilla or in the mandible
* **An embedded or impacted tooth**—is the tooth that has failed to erupt completely or partially to its correct position in the dental arch and its eruption potential has been lost.

The word impaction is from Latin origin—*impactus.*
Impaction is cessation of eruption of a tooth caused by a physical barrier or ectopic positioning of a tooth. An impacted tooth is one that is erupted, partially erupted or unerupted and will not eventually assume a normal arch relationship with the other teeth and tissues.

■ CLASSIFICATION OF IMPACTED TEETH

Impacted teeth seen in the following order of frequency:
1. Mandibular third molars
2. Maxillary third molars
3. Maxillary canine
4. Mandibular premolar
5. Maxillary premolar
6. Mandibular canine
7. Maxillary central incisors
8. Maxillary lateral incisors.

Causes of Impaction of Teeth

Inadequate Space in the Dental Arch for Eruption

Phylogenic theory: Due to evolution, the human jaw size is becoming smaller and since the third molar tooth is last to erupt, there may not be room for it to emerge in the oral cavity.

Mendelian theory: Here genetic variations play a major role. If the individual genetically receives a small jaw from one of the parents and/or large teeth from the other parent, then impacted teeth can be seen, because of 'lack of space'.

Causes of impaction of a tooth can be divided into local and systemic causes (Table 10.1).

Indications for Removal of Impacted Teeth

- Recurrent pericoronitis/pain/infection/caries—pericoronitis is the inflammation of the gingiva surrounding a crown of a partially erupted tooth
- Deep periodontal pocket associated with partially erupted tooth
- Prior to orthodontic treatment—to control the tooth crowding in the mandible
- Prevention of root resorption and caries—caries of the impacted tooth crown and the adjacent tooth can be seen due to an inability to access and clean the area. Root resorption of the distal root of the adjacent second molar is seen in the 21 to 30 years of age group. Root resorption of lateral incisor may be seen associated with an impacted maxillary or mandibular canine
- Management of cysts and tumors, abscess of odontogenic origin (associated lesions).
- Prevention of pathological fractures
- Preparation of orthognathic surgery—prior to sagittal split osteotomy of ramus in order to avoid bad split—inadvertent fracture of the mandible, lower third molars are extracted. Maxillary third molars are removed during LeFort I osteotomy procedure
- Management of preprosthetic concerns—before the fabrication of the prosthesis, impacted teeth should be removed
- Impacted teeth in the line of fracture
- Prophylactic removal.

Table 10.1: Local and systemic causes of impaction of tooth	
Local causes	*Systemic causes*

• Obstruction for eruption
   — Irregularity in position and presence of an adjacent tooth
   — Density of the overlying and surrounding bone
	• Prenatal causes—heredity

• Lack of space in the dental arch—crowding, supernumerary teeth	• Postnatal—rickets, anemia, tuberculosis, congenital syphilis, malnutrition
• Ankylosis of primary or permanent teeth	• Endocrinal disorders of thyroid, parathyroid, pituitary glands like hypothyroidism, achondroplasia, etc. Here the primary retention of teeth is seen due to lack of osteoclastic activity, which does not provide resorption of the bone overlying the developing tooth
• Nonabsorbing, over-retained deciduous teeth	• Hereditary-linked disorders—Down's syndrome, Hurler's syndrome, osteopetrosis. Cleidocranial dysostosis, cleft palate, etc. Here failure of the overlying bone to resorb and develop an eruption pathway is absent
• Nonabsorbing alveolar bone	
• Ectopic position of tooth bud	
• Dilaceration of roots (trauma)	
• Associated soft tissue or bony lesions	
• Habits involving tongue, finger, thumb, cheek, pencil, etc. (Secondary retention—ankylosis of teeth. Infra-occlusion of the tooth is seen due to arrested eruption, after initial emergence without any obvious barrier such as a tooth, tissue or habit to block eruption)	

Risk of Nonintervention

- Crowding of dentition based on growth prediction
- Resorption of adjacent tooth and periodontal status
- Development of pathological conditions such as infection, cyst, tumor.

Risk of Intervention

Minor transient: Sensory nerve alteration, alveolitis, trismus and infection. Hemorrhage, dentoalveolar fracture and displacement of tooth.

Minor permanent: Periodontal injury, adjacent tooth injury, temporomandibular joint injury.

Major: Altered sensation, vital organ infection, fracture of the mandible, maxillary tuberosity, injury and litigation.

Benefits of Nonintervention

- Avoidance of risk
- Preservation of functional teeth
- Preservation of residual ridge.

Benefits of Intervention

- In relation to age—in young patients, less morbidity.
- In relation to different therapeutic measures. Local measures against alveolitis, pain, swelling and trismus, etc.

Classification of Impacted Teeth

Maxillary and mandibular third molars are classified radiographically by angulation, depth and arch length or relationship to the anterior aspect of the ascending mandibular ramus.

Classification is helpful for the following:

- Describes the general position of the impacted third molar
- Aids in estimating the difficulty in removing the tooth.

Difficulty Index

- Very difficult   : 7 to 10
- Moderately difficult   : 5 to 7
- Minimally difficult   : 3 to 4

From Table 10.2 difficulty index can be arrived at as follows:

Table 10.2: Difficulty index for removal of impacted lower third molars	
Classification angulation	*Difficulty index value*
Mesioangular	1 easiest to remove
Horizontal/transverse	2
Vertical	3
Distoangular	4
Depth	
Level A	1
Level B	2
Level C	3
Ramus relationship/space available	
Class I	1
Class II	2
Class III	3

Distoangular impaction   4
Level B   2
Class II   2

Eight is the total difficulty score. Very difficult extraction.

Winter's Classification (Fig. 10.2A)

Angulation: According to the position of the impacted third molar to the long axis of the second molar. The Winter's classification is suggested:

1. Mesioangular
2. Horizontal/transverse/ Inverted
3. Vertical
4. Distoangular
5. Buccoangular
6. Linguoangular

These may occur simultaneously in:
a. Buccal version
b. Lingual version
c. Torsoversion

- Mesioangular impaction is the most common finding
- Forty three percent of mandibular impacted third molars are mesioangular
- Sixty three percent of maxillary impacted third molars are mesioangular.

Depth (Fig. 10.2B): As per the relationship to the occlusal surface of the adjoining second molar of the impacted maxillary or mandibular third molar, the depth can be judged.

1. *Position A:* The highest position of the tooth is on a level with or above the occlusal line.

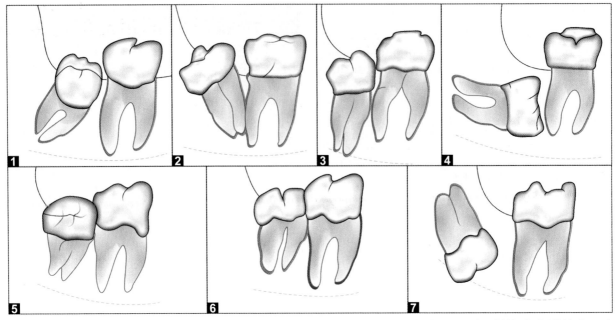

Fig. 10.2A: Winter's classification of impacted mandibular third molars: (1) Mesioangular (2) Distoangular, (3) Vertical, (4) Horizontal, (5) Buccoangular, (6) Linguoangular, (7) Inverted

2. *Position B:* Highest position is below the occlusal plane, but above the cervical level of the second molar.
3. *Position C:* Highest position of the tooth is below the cervical level of the second molar.

The deeper the impacted tooth, the more overlying bone is present and the more the angulation of impaction deviates from parallel to the long axis of the adjacent tooth, the more difficult it is to remove the impacted tooth.

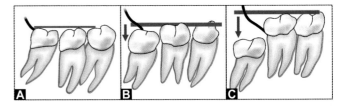

Fig. 10.2B: Classification of impacted mandibular third molars according to the depth of impaction

Pell and Gregory Classification (Fig. 10.2C)

Relationship of the impacted lower third molar to the ramus of the mandible and the second molar (based on the space available distal to the second molar).

- *Class I:* Sufficient space available between the anterior border of the ascending ramus and the distal side of the second molar for the eruption of the third molar
- *Class II:* The space available between the anterior border of the ramus and the distal side of the second molar is less than the mesiodistal width of the crown of the third molar. It denotes that the distal

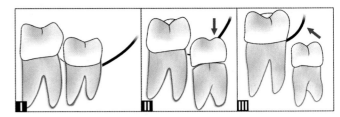

Fig. 10.2C: Pell and Gregory classification

portion of the third molar crown is covered by the bone from the ascending ramus
- *Class III:* The third molar is totally embedded in the bone from the ascending ramus because of absolute lack of space.

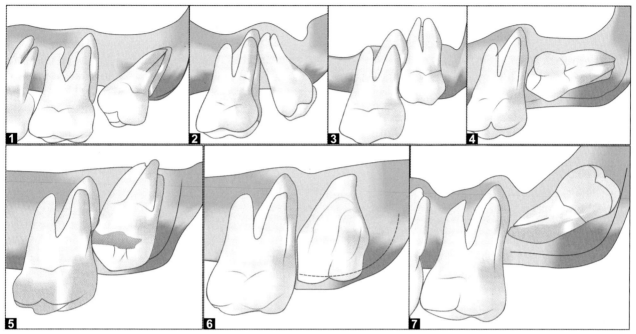

Fig. 10.2D: Classification of impacted maxillary third molars: (1) Mesioangular, (2) Distoangular, (3) Vertical, (4) Horizontal, (5) Buccoversion, (6) Linguoversion, (7) Inverted

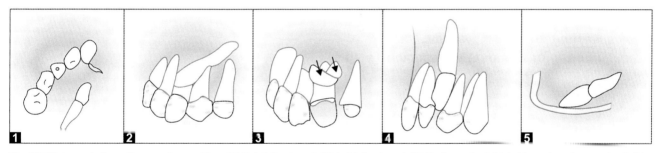

Fig. 10.2E: Impacted maxillary canine position: (1) Palatally placed, (2) Labially placed, (3) Partly on the labial side and partly on palatal side, (4) Canine locked between the roots of adjacent teeth, (5) Canine in the edentulous maxilla

Maxillary Third Molars' Classification (Fig. 10.2D)

1. Angulation and depth classification is same as mandibular third molars.
2. Classification of the maxillary third molar in relation to the floor of maxillary sinus.
   a. Sinus approximation (SA)—no bone or a thin bony partition present between impacted maxillary third molar and the floor of the maxillary sinus.
   b. No sinus approximation (NSA)—2 mm or more bone is present between the sinus floor and the impacted maxillary third molar.

Classification of Impacted Maxillary Canines (Fig. 10.2E)

- Labial or palatal placement of impacted maxillary canine
- *Intermediate position:*
  - Crown between the lateral incisors and premolar.
  - Crown above the root tip with labial/palatal orientation of the lateral incisor or premolar.
- *Aberrant position:* Impacted maxillary canines lie in the maxillary sinus or nasal cavity.

- *Class I:* Palatally placed maxillary canine
  a. Horizontal
  b. Vertical
  c. Semivertical
- *Class II:* Labially or buccally placed maxillary canine
  a. Horizontal
  b. Vertical
  c. Semivertical
- *Class III:* Involving both buccal and palatal bone, e.g. crown is placed on the palatal aspect and the root is toward the buccal alveolar process
- *Class IV:* Impacted in the alveolar process between the incisors and first premolar.
- *Class V:* Impacted in the edentulous maxilla.

Classification for Impacted Mandibular Canine (Table 10.3)

Table 10.3: Classification for impacted mandibular canine	
Labial	*Aberrant*
• Vertical	• At inferior border
• Oblique	• On the opposite side
• Horizontal	

Factors Responsible for Increasing the Difficulty Score for Removal of Impacted Teeth

- As per the angulation
- As per the depth
- As per the space available for the eruption
- Crown size—large bulbous crown increases the difficulty
- Configuration of the roots of the impacted tooth—the point of application of the elevator and the path of delivery of the impacted tooth depends mainly on the configuration of the roots.
  a. *Length of the roots*—longer the roots, more difficult the extraction.
  b. *Root development*—if the root development is (less than one-third) insufficient, then the tooth is more difficult to remove. It moves like a ball in the socket and difficult to elevate.
  c. *Curvature of the roots*—dilacerated, curved, divergent roots are difficult to remove. Fused conical roots are easy.
  d. *Root size*— thin, slender roots are difficult to remove. Stout, bulbous, hypercementosed roots also increase the difficulty.
- Bone texture and density—depends on the age, sex and systemic problems. Younger patients have

spongy, elastic pliable bone, while older group of patients may exhibit sclerozed bone.
- Size of the follicular sac—presence of large follicular sac makes the extraction easier, as the amount of bone removal is less. Nonexistent or narrow follicular sac around the crown will require bone cutting around the crown (difficult extraction).
- Space or contact in relation to mandibular second molar—If the impacted tooth is locked against the crown of the second molar and there is no space for elevation, then sectioning of the tooth should be planned.
- Relationship to the inferior alveolar neurovascular bundle—proximity of the roots to the neurovascular bundle increases the possibility of the damage/injury to the nerve during extraction. Temporary altered sensation of the lower lip can be experienced by the patient (paresthesia/anesthesia) which can last for few days/few months. Radiological assessment is important. Dentascan or CBCT can show exact location of the nerve.
- Nature of covering tissue:
  – Soft tissue impaction
  – Partial bony impaction—covered by soft tissue, as well as partially by the bone.
  – Fully bony impaction.
- Access to the operative field, inability to open the mouth wide, a large uncontrollable tongue, small orbicularis oris muscle (oral sphincter).
- Sever gag replex-increases difficulty.

Radiological Examination

Intraoral X-ray

- Intraoral X-rays are possible, if tooth is in the alveolus and not in the ramus
- Possible if oral opening is adequate
- If there is no gagging
- Useful to study the relation with adjoining tooth
- Useful to study the configuration of the roots and status of the crown (caries, size, etc.)
- Useful to record the relationship with inferior alveolar canal
- For bucco or linguoversion 'tube shift' method should be used or occlusal film is taken.

The position and depth of the tooth can be assessed by taking intraoral X-ray or even lateral extraoral X-ray and tracing can be done, which was originally advocated by George Winter.

Three imaginary lines are drawn which are known as Winter's lines (Fig. 10.2F).

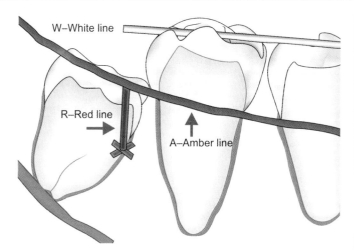

Fig. 10.2F: Winter's lines: W-White line, A-Amber line, R-Red line

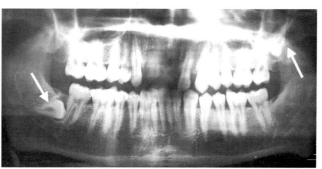

Fig. 10.2G (1): Extraoral X-rays for detection of impacted teeth: OPG-lower right and upper left third molars are impacted

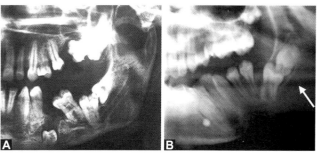

Fig. 10.2G(2): (A) Multiple impacted teeth, (B) Kissing molars

- *White line* corresponds to the occlusal plane. The line is drawn touching the occlusal surfaces of first and second molar and is extended posteriorly over the third molar region. It indicates the difference in occlusal level of second and third molars.
- *Amber line* represents the bone level. The line is drawn from the crest of the interdental septum between the molars and extended posteriorly distal to third molar or to the ascending ramus. This line denotes the alveolar bone covering the impacted tooth and the portion of tooth not covered by the bone.
- *Red line* is drawn perpendicular from the amber line to an imaginary point of application of the elevator. It indicates the amount of bone that will have to be removed before elevation, i.e. the depth of the tooth in bone and the difficulty encountered in removing the tooth.

If the length of the red line is more than 5 mm then the extraction is difficult. Every additional millimeter renders the removal of the impacted tooth three times more difficult (more than 9 mm—below the level of the apices of the second molar).

Extraoral X-rays (Figs 10.2G 1, 2, 3)

For mandibular teeth
- OPG
- Lateral oblique view mandible

For maxillary teeth
- OPG
- PA view Water's position

Indicated in
- Patients with restricted oral opening/trismus excessive gagging

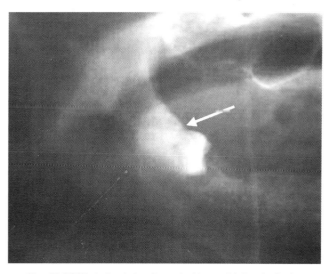

Fig. 10.2G(3): Lateral view-impacted lower third molar in the edentulous jaw

- Impacted tooth in an aberrant position
- For ruling out associated pathology
- To study the relationship of the tooth to inferior alveolar nerve (Fig. 10.2H) and (Figs 10.2-I: 1, 2, 3)/Table 10.4 inferior border. For maxillary teeth—relationship to the maxillary sinus.

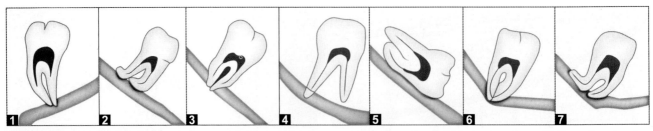

Fig. 10.2H: Radiological prediction for inferior alveolar nerve proximity: (1) Darkening of root, (2) Deflection of root, (3) Narrowing of root, (4) Dark and bifid apex, (5) Interruption of white line of the canal, (6) Diversion of canal, (7) Narrowing of canal

■ SURGICAL REMOVAL OF IMPACTED TEETH

1. Asepsis and isolation
2. Local anesthesia/sedation + LA/general anesthesia
3. Incision—flap design
4. Reflection of mucoperiosteal flap
5. Bone removal
6. Sectioning (division) of tooth
7. Elevation
8. Extraction
9. Debridement and smoothening of bone
10. Control of bleeding
11. Closure—suturing
12. Medications—antibiotics, analgesics, etc.
13. Follow up.

Isolation of Surgical Site

- Scrubbing + painting of skin and oral mucosa. Scrubbing solutions used first on skin only.
  - Cetrimide + absolute alcohol or cetrimide + povidone + iodine
  - Cetrimide + absolute alcohol + chlorhexidine.
- Cleaning solutions—used on skin only to remove residual soap solution
  - Normal saline
  - Alcohol—spirit
- Painting solution—act topically to inhibit further growth of microbes
  - Povidone-iodine 5 percent for skin, 1 percent for oral mucosa

Fig. 10.2-I(1): Narrowing of canal

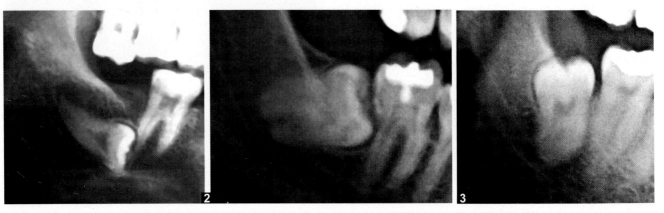

Fig. 10.2-I(2 and 3): (2) Interruption of the white line of the canal, (3) Darkening of root

Table 10.4: Radiological prediction of injury to the inferior alveolar nerve: Depends on the relationship of the root to the canal (Figs 10.2H and I)		
Related, but not involving the canal	*Related to changes in canal*	*Related with changes in canal*
Close proximity of the root to the canal, but intervening bone separates the both (i) separated (ii) adjacent, (iii) super imposed. Trace the outline of the root as well as the canal, which will show no disturbance	i. Darkening of the root (radiolucent)	i Interruption (loss of lines)—the dense roof and floor of the canal is seen as two white radio-paque lines (Tram lines).
	ii. Dark and bifid root	
	iii. Narrowing of the root	
	iv. Deflected root	Either of these two lines or both may be disrupted to indicate deep grooving of the roots
	a Density of the root is altered, when the root impinges on the canal	
	b When the canal crosses the root apex, it can be identified by the double periodontal membrane shadow of the bifid root apex	ii. Converging (narrowing) canal— when canal crosses root apex, there is reduction in its diameter. Hour glass appearance indicates partial encirclement of the canal
	c. If sudden narrowing of the root is noted where the canal crosses, it indicates the deep grooving or perforation of the root or involvement of the root with the canal	iii. Diverted canal—The canal appears diverted, when it changes its direction. This is due to an upward displacement of the canal passing through the root
	d. The root may be seen deflected buccally, lingually or mesially distally, when it reaches the canal	

– Chlorhexidine gluconate—7.5 percent for skin, 0.2 percent for rinsing oral cavity.

Drape the patient with sterile drapes to cover upper part of the face to isolate the oral cavity.

Local Anesthesia

- For mandibular molars and canines—pterygomandibular nerve block
- For maxillary molars—posterior superior alveolar nerve block and palatine nerve block or infiltration
- For maxillary canines—infraorbital nerve block + palatal infiltration of incisive canal and bilateral palatine nerve blocks.

Good infiltration is a must to provide hemostasis and to define the tissue planes.

- Saline adrenaline in concentration of 1:400000
- Plain saline (in case of hypertensive patients)
- LA solution with adrenaline.

Incision (Flap Design)

The mucoperiosteal flap for removal of impacted tooth is required to be designed well for adequate access and for elimination of obstruction to the pathway of removal. The incision for this mucoperiosteal flap will have an anterior limb and a posterior limb connected with or without an intermediate limb.

For Mandibular Molars (Fig. 10.2J)

Anterior releasing incision should begin from the vestibule upwards towards midway of the CEJ of second molar at an angle. If third molar is deep and surgery requires more removal of bone, this incision should be placed anterior to the second molar. The incision is then continued in the gingival sulcus (over the alveolar crest, if tooth is fully embedded) up to the distal aspect of third molar. Distal releasing incision is started from the distal most point of third molar across external oblique ridge into the buccal mucosa. This incision should not be taken on the lingual aspect of the ridge, as the lingual nerve can be found at or above the crest of the alveolar ridge, in approximately 17 percent of the population. However, the normal position of the lingual nerve is 2 mm inferior to the crest and 0.5 mm lingual to the lingual cortex of the mandible in the third molar region. The length of this mucoperiosteal flap and the number of teeth included will be determined by the amount of exposure necessary to gain the visibility of the region and the experience of the clinician.

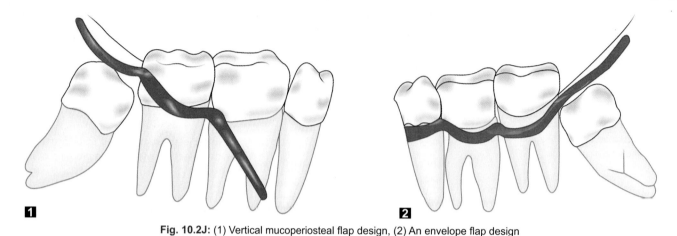

Fig. 10.2J: (1) Vertical mucoperiosteal flap design, (2) An envelope flap design

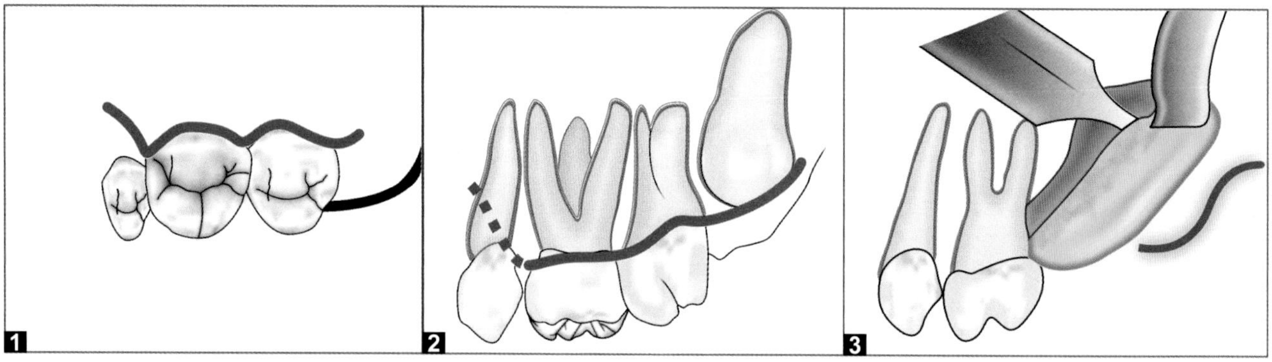

Fig. 10.2K: Mucoperiosteal flap design for the removal of impacted maxillary third molar. Dotted line indicates possible extension of the incision for additional access

The incision should not be extended too far upward distally to avoid:

i. Intraoperative brisk bleeding from the buccal vessels and anastomosing branches from lingual and facial arteries.
ii. Postoperative trismus due to cutting through the fibers of temporalis muscle.
iii. Herniation of buccal pad of fat into the surgical field.

The sharp point of periosteal elevator is used to carefully elevate a mucoperiosteal flap beginning at the point of the incision behind the second molar. The elevator is brought forward to elevate the periosteum around the second molar and down the releasing incision. The other flatter end of the periosteal elevator is then used to elevate the periosteum posteriorly to the ascending ramus of the mandible.

For Maxillary Molars (Fig. 10.2K)

The anterior releasing incision is started anterior to second molar from the vestibule and till the mesial interdental papilla of the second molar. The incision should follow the gingival sulcus of second molar and continue over the tuberosity area from the distal most point of second molar.

For Maxillary Canines

If the canine is *buccally* placed:
• Flap with anterior releasing incision
• Trapezoidal flap
• Semilunar flap.

If the canine is *palatally* placed—the incision is taken in the gingival sulcus on the palatal side from the mesial aspect of the first molar of the same side. Releasing incision is given obliquely across the palate and should be deflected away from the palatine foramen. If *unilateral*—an incision is restricted to the canine region of the opposite side. If bilateral—an incision is extended to the first molar of the opposite side.

For Mandibular Canines

If buccally placed then crevicular incision from the midline is taken up to first molar. Anterior releasing incision is given close to the midline. Care should be taken to protect the mental nerve. If the canine is placed on the lingual side, then lingual envelope flap is taken.

Bone Removal

Aim

i. To expose the crown by removing the bone overlying it.
ii. To remove the bone obstructing the pathway for removal of a tooth.

How much Bone is to be Removed?

Adequate amount of bone should be removed to enable the elevation. But the extensive bone removal can be minimized by sectioning the tooth.

Two Ways of Bone Removal (Fig. 10.2L)

a. High speed, high torque handpiece and bur technique
b. Chisel and mallet technique.

Bur technique: Either no. 7/8 round bur or a straight no. 703 fissure bur is used. Either of these burs can be used for bone removal or for sectioning of a tooth. Burs should be always used along with copious saline irrigation to avoid thermal trauma to the bone.

First step: The bur is used in a sweeping motion around the occlusal, buccal and distal aspect of the mandibular third molar crown to expose it and to have its orientation.

Second step: Once the crown has been located, the buccal surface of the tooth is exposed with the bur to the cervical level of the crown contour and a buccal trough or gutter is created. The buccal trough should be made in the cancellous bone. It is important that the adequate amount of trough is created to remove any bony obstruction for exposure and the delivery of the tooth, especially around the distal aspect of the crown. The distolingual portion of the tooth should be exposed without cutting through the lingual bony plate to prevent damage to the lingual nerve.

For the canine removal, the gutter/trough is created around the surface of the crown free from the contact with the neighboring/overlying teeth. The bone removal around the crown is done till CE junction and to expose the crown beyond the greatest width.

Important precautions while drilling the bone

• Protect overlying soft tissues by retraction with either periosteal elevator or Langenbeck retractor
• Continuous irrigation either with 1 percent povidone-iodine or with normal saline to reduce the thermal necrosis of bone

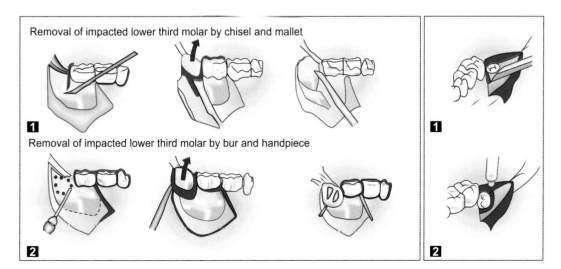

Removal of impacted lower third molar by chisel and mallet

1

Removal of impacted lower third molar by bur and handpiece

2

1

2

Fig. 10.2L: (1) Removal of impacted lower third molar by chisel and mallet, (2) Removal of impacted lower third molar with bur and handpiece

Chisel and mallet technique

- Historical importance
- Very rarely used
- Less bone necrosis than bur technique
- Can cause inadvertent fracture of the bone
- The jaw bone should be supported, while using this technique.

First step: For mandibular/maxillary molars, the first step is the placement of vertical stop cut, which is made by placing a 3 mm or 5 mm chisel vertically at the distal aspect of the second molar with bevel facing posteriorly (5 to 6 mm height). The aim is to prevent the force transmission anterior to the direction of the bone removal.

Second step: At the base of the vertical stop (limiting) cut, the chisel is placed at an angle of 45° with the bevel facing upwards or occlusally, and oblique cut is made till the distal most point of third molar. This will result in the removal of a triangular piece of buccal plate distal to second molar. Additional triangular piece of bone is removed at the junction of vertical and oblique bone cut to gain the entry of the elevator tip. Finally the distal bone must be removed, so that when the tooth is elevated, there should be no obstruction at the distobuccal aspect.

In case of canine removal, bone is cut till the level of CEJ and to expose the entire crown.

Lingual Split Bone Technique (Fig. 10.2M)

- It is described originally by Sir William Kelsey Fry
- Later popularized by T Ward
- Quick and clean technique
- Creates a saucerization of the socket, thereby reduces the size of the residual blood clot
- Used for mandibular third molar removal, especially those which are placed lingually
- Support the mandible at the inferior border.

Steps

1. Vertical stop cut is made by placing the chisel with the bevel facing posteriorly, distal to the second molar.
2. With the chisel bevel downward, a horizontal cut is made backward from the lower end of the vertical limiting stop cut.
3. The buccal bone plate is removed above the horizontal cut.
4. The distolingual bone is then fractured inward by placing the cutting edge of the chisel along the dotted line A. Bevel side of the chisel is facing upward and cutting edge is parallel to the external oblique ridge. The chisel is held at 45° to the bone surface.
5. Finally small wedge of bone, which then remaining distal to the tooth and between the buccal and lingual cut, is excised and removed.

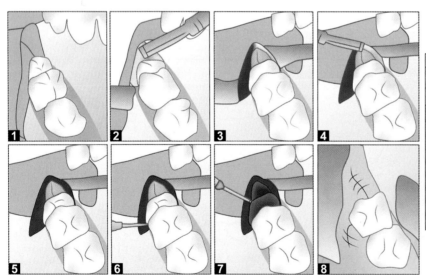

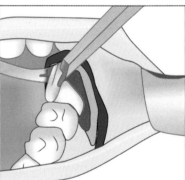

Lingual split being done

Fig. 10.2M: Lingual split bone technique

6. A sharp straight elevator is then applied and minimum force is used to elevate the tooth. As the tooth moves upward and backward, the lingual plate gets fractured and facilitates the delivery of the tooth.
7. After the tooth is removed, the lingual plate is grasped with the hemostat and freed from the soft tissue and removed.
8. Smoothening of the edges is done with bone file. Wound irrigated and sutured.

Tooth Sectioning, Elevation and Extraction

- Reduces the amount of bone removal (conserves the bone) required prior to elevation of the tooth
- Reduces the risk of damage to the neighboring teeth
- Planned sectioning permits the parts of the tooth to be removed separately in an atraumatic manner by creating space into which it is displaced and the remaining crown or root segments removed.
- The direction in which the impacted tooth should be sectioned is dependent on the angulation of the impacted tooth, based on the line of draw of the segments
- Can be performed either with a bur or chisel. Bur use is preferable. Mallet blows may give psychological discomfort to the patient
- The bur is used in a controlled fashion to avoid damage to the vital structures and surrounding teeth and soft tissues
- The tooth is usually sectioned one-half to three-fourths with the bur and then it is completely sectioned with the elevator.

Horizontal Impaction (Fig. 10.2N-1)

Same as that for distoangular impaction.

Mesioangular Impaction (Fig. 10.2N-2)

Distal half of the crown is sectioned off from the buccal groove till the CEJ; from buccal to lingual and extended into the furcation. A straight elevator is placed in the cut and rotated to fracture the distal portion of the crown which is removed. Then a straight elevator is placed on the mesial aspect of the third molar below the cervical area. A purchase point can be prepared into the crown at the mesiobuccal line angle with a small round bur, if the access to the elevator is not possible. Then a cryer or crane pick elevator can be used to elevate the tooth, engaging the purchase point.

Vertical Impaction (Fig. 10.2N-3)

Sectioning is similar to mesioangular disimpaction procedure.

Distoangular Impaction (Fig. 10.2N-4)

Most difficult to remove, because of its pathway of delivery into the ascending ramus. Large amount of distal bone removal is required. The crown is sectioned from the roots just above the cervical line after sufficient bone is removed from the occlusal and distobuccal aspect. The entire crown is removed to improve the visibility and access to the roots. If the roots are divergent, they are further sectioned into two pieces and delivered individually. If the roots are convergent the simple use of straight elevator is sufficient.

Elevation

- *Coupland elevator*—placed at the base of the crown.
- *Winter Cryer's*—may be used in wedging action/buccal elevation. Buccal elevation may be done in molar and canines by drilling a purchase point in the roots just below CEJ.

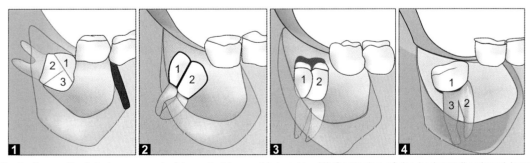

Fig. 10.2N: Sectioning method during removal of impacted lower third molar: (1) Sectioning of the horizontally placed lower third molar, (2) Sectioning of the mesioangularly placed lower third molar, (3) Sectioning of the vertically placed lower third molar, (4) Sectioning of the distoangularly placed lower third molar

- Wedging action is useful, when molar crown is split vertically down to bifurcation of roots.

Important precautions: Support the inferior border and lingual cortex of the bone in the mandibular impaction. Support to the palatal bone in the maxillary third molar or canine impactions during elevation should be given. Support the neighboring tooth to prevent luxation of the same.

Debridement and Smoothening of Bone Margins

- Irrigation of the socket
- Curetting to remove any remaining dental follicle and epithelium
- Look for pieces of coronal portion (especially in carious teeth/sectioned teeth), check for remnants of bone/granulation tissue, bleeding points
- Check for caries (root/crown)/erosion/damage to the adjacent teeth
- Round off the margins of the socket with large vulcanite round bur or bone file

- Irrigate the socket again
- Control bleeding before suturing.

Closure

3-0 black silk is used. Interrupted sutures given and maintained for 7 days. Complete surgical procedure for the removal of lower impacted third molar is shown in (Fig. 10.2O).

In case of molars, suture distal to second molar should be placed first and should be water tight to prevent pocket formation.

In case of palatally impacted canines, incisive papilla should be sutured carefully to reduce postoperative bleeding.

■ COMPLICATIONS

Intraoperative Complications

During Incision

For molars, facial vessel or buccal vessel may be cut. For lower canines–mental vessels and for upper canines—

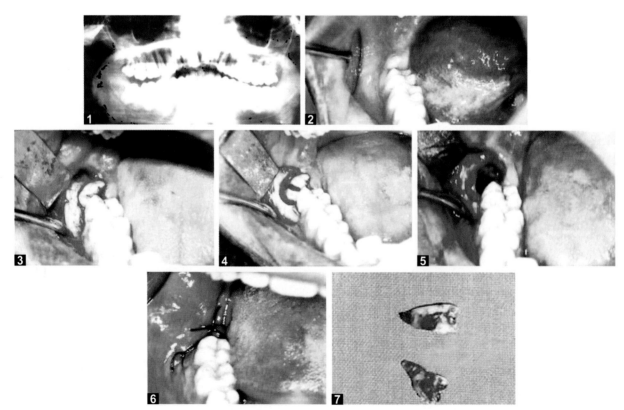

Fig. 10.2O: Surgical procedure for removal of lower right impacted third molar: (1) OPG of mesioangularly impacted lower right third molar, (2) Intraoral clinical picture, (3) Incision and mucoperiosteal flap reflection, (4) Sectioning of a tooth, (5) Surgical extraction done, (6) Suturing, (7) Extracted tooth

incisive canal or greater palatine vessels may be damaged.

During Bone Removal

Damage to the second molar, damage to the roots of overlying teeth, slipping of the bur into the soft tissues, fracture of the mandible when using chisel and mallet.

During Elevation

- Luxation of neighboring/overlying tooth
- Fracture of the adjoining bone
- Fracture of the tuberosity
- Slipping of the tooth into pterygomandibular/temporal spaces , sublingual pouch and/maxillary sinus.

- Damage to nasal wall/overlying teeth/lingual, inferior alveolar or mental nerve.

During Debridement

- Damage to inferior alveolar nerve/lingual nerve.
- Damage to maxillary sinus.

Postoperative Complications

Pain, swelling, trismus, hypoesthesia, sensitivity, loss of vitality of neighboring teeth.
- Pocket formation.
- Sinus tract formation, oroantral fistula, oronasal fistula.

SURGICAL ENDODONTICS

Apicoectomy, apical surgery, endodontic surgery, root resection, root amputation are the terms which are used for surgery involving the root apex to treat the apical infection. It is the cutting off of the apical portion of the root and curettage of periapical necrotic, granulomatous, inflammatory or cystic lesions. In spite of good endodontic treatment, if periapical lesions are not resolved, then apical surgery is undertaken.

Indications

- Apical anomaly of root tip—dilacerations, intracanal calcification, open apex
- Presence of lateral/accessory canal/apical region perforations
- Roots with broken instruments/overfillings
- Fracture of apical third of the root
- Formation of periapical granuloma/cyst
- Draining sinus tract/nonresponsive to RCT
- Extension of root canal sealant cement/filling beyond the apex
- Teeth with ceramic crowns
- When patient with chronic periapical infection, will not be available for follow-up.

Contraindications

- Presence of systemic diseases—leukemia, uncontrolled diabetes, anemia, thyrotoxicosis, etc.
- Teeth damaged beyond restoration

- Teeth with deep periodontal pockets and grade III mobility (Pre-existing bone loss)
- When traumatic occlusion cannot be corrected
- Short root length
- Acute infection which is nonresponsive to the treatment
- Root tips close to the nerves, e.g. mental nerve, inferior alveolar nerve or in maxilla close to the maxillary sinus.

Procedure (Figs 10.3A to E)

Three accepted procedures can be used:
1. Root canal filling and immediate apicoectomy and curettage.
2. Root canal filling is done several days/weeks/months earlier followed by apicoectomy and curettage.
3. Increase in the periapical lesion even after root canal filling and draining sinus. May be due to faulty filling which is redone and then followed by root amputation and curettage.

Steps

- Asepsis and isolation
- Local anesthesia with infiltration technique
- Incision design
- Mucoperiosteal flap—either semilunar or submarginal envelope flap with extension of at least one tooth on either side

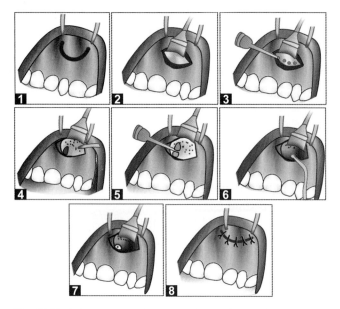

Fig. 10.3A: Apicoectomy and curettage-Surgical procedure: (1) Semilunar incision, (2) Reflection of mucoperiosteal flap, (3) Creating a bony window with bur, (4) Bony window complete to expose the root apex area, (5) Sectioning of the root tip horizontally, (6) Removal of sectioned root tip and periapical curettage, (7) Preparation of the retrograde filling, (8) Suturing

- Submarginal envelope flap is known as Ochsenbein-Luebke flap design. It is indicated when the esthetics of the gingival margin cannot be compromised (maxillary teeth with crowns). A scalloped incision is made below the attached gingiva with one or two releasing incisions. Contraindication for this flap—periodontal breakdown, large periapical lesion, a short root.
- Raise the mucoperiosteal flap with periosteal elevator
- Retract the flap away with Langenbeck retractor
- Identify the apex in the intact buccal plate—create a bony window with surgical bur over the root apex area. Care is taken not to damage the adjoining roots (make bur holes with round bur and then join them with tapered fissure bur). Locate the apex
- Section the root tip horizontally (not more than one-third the length of the entire root). No bevel angle is advocated for sectioning (0 to 10 degrees)
- Remove all periapical granulation tissue with angulated curettes
- Use hot burnisher to seal the root tip
- Close flap and suture it.

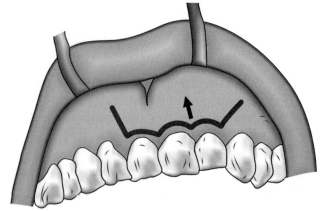

Fig. 10.3B: Ochsenbein-Luebke submarginal envelope flap for apicoectomy

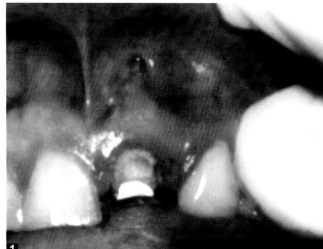

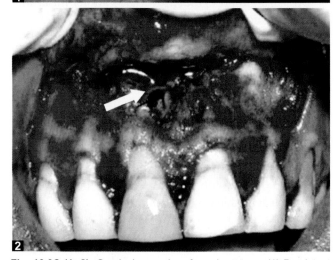

Fig. 10.3C (1, 2): Surgical procedure for apicoectomy (1) Persistant sinus tract after root canal filling, (2) Mucoperiosteal flap reflected to expose the periapical lesion. Note the perforation of the buccal cortex

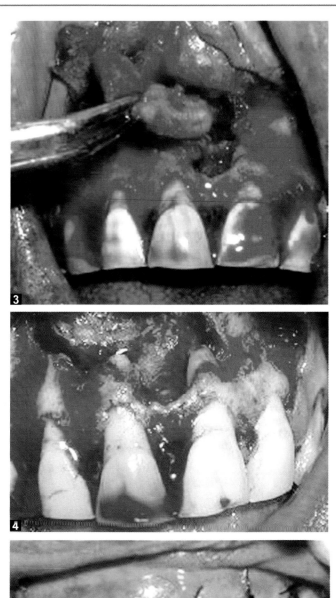

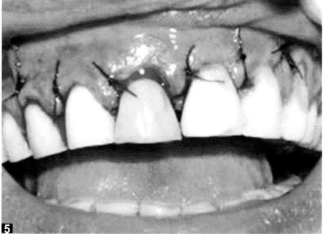

Fig. 10.3C (3, 4, 5): (3) Bony window widened and cystic lesion enucleation is being carried out, (4) All the apices of three anterior teeth involved in the lesion are exposed for apicoectomy procedure. (root canal filling is done prior to surgery), (5) Suturing

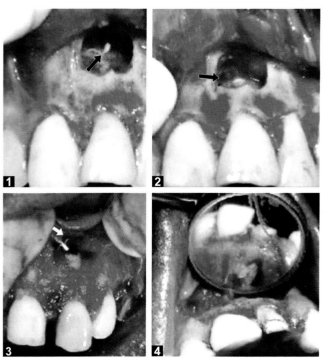

Fig. 10.3D: (1) Overfilled root canal beyond the root apex, (2) After burnishing of the filling at the root apex, apicoectomy was done, (3 and 4) Retrograde filling with amalgam

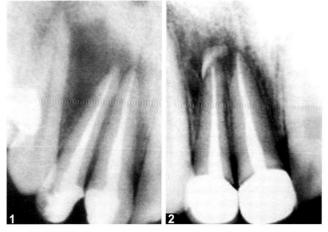

Fig. 10.3E: (1) Preoperative periapical X-ray of a periapical lesion involving (R) Central lateral incisors, (2) Follow-up X-ray after two years

Retropreparation (Fig. 10.3F)

The ultrasonic tip is used for retropreparation. The tip is placed at the apical opening of the canal and guided gently deeper into the canal as it cuts. Once the retropreparation is completed the prepared cavity is inspected. The gutta-percha at the base is recondensed with small 0.5 mm microplugger.

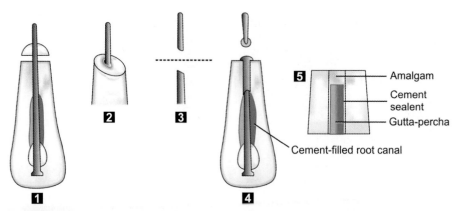

Fig. 10.3F: (1) Apicoectomy of one-third of the length of the root, (2) Overfilled gutta-percha point and preparation of bevel between 0 and 10 degrees, (3) Cutting off of excess gutta-percha point, (4) Preparation for retrograde filling using amalgam, (5) Final retrograde filling

The aim of placing root end filling material is to establish an apical seal that inhibits the leakage of residual irritants from the root canal into the surrounding tissues.

A wide variety of retrograde filling materials have been used—gutta-percha, amalgam, gold foil, titanium screws, glass ionomer, zinc oxide-eugenol, cavit, composite resin, polycarboxylate cement, silver points, etc.

In the defect in the periapical region hydroxylapatite can be packed to enhance the bony healing.

Complications

Intraoperative

- Bleeding—control with local application of adrenaline pack 1:1000, pressure pack/Gelfoam
- Damage to the neighboring root
- Entry into sinus/inferior alveolar canal.

Postoperative

- Abscess formation
- Fenestration, sinus tract formation
- Increased mobility of the tooth.

■ BIBLIOGRAPHY

1. Archer WH. Oral and Maxillofacial Surgery. 5th Edition. Philadelphia: WB Saunders Co; 1975.

2. Bluestone LL. The Impacted Mandibular Bicuspid and Canine. Dent Items Int 1951;73:341.

3. Dunbeck WE. The Impacted Lower Third Molar. New York: Dental Items Int Publishing Co; 1945.

4. Field HJ. The Impacted Upper Cuspid. Dent Cosmos 1935;77:378.

5. Gorlin R, Goldman HM. Thoma's Oral Pathology, 7th Edition. St Louis: CV Mosby Co; 1970.

6. Hitchin AD. The Impacted Maxillary Canine. BDJ 1956;100:1.

7. Killey HC, Kay LW. The Impacted Wisdom Tooth, 2nd Edition. Edinburgh: Churchill Livingstone; 1975.

8. Laskin DM. Indications and Contraindications for Removal of Impacted Third Molars. DCNA 1969;13:919.

9. Laskin DM. Evaluation of the Third Molar Problem. JADA 1974;82:824.

10. Lewis JES. Modified Lingual Split Technique for Extraction of Impacted Mandibular Third Molars. J Oral Surg 1980;38:578.

11. Pell GJ, Gregory CT. Report on 10-years study of Tooth Division Technique for Removal of Impacted Teeth. Am J Orthod – Oral Surg (Oral Surg Sect) 1942;28:660.

12. Thoma KH. Oral Surgery, 5th Edition. St Louis: CV Mosby Co; 1969.

13. Ward TG. Split Bone Technique for Removal of Lower Third Molars. BDJ 1956;101:297.

14. Baumann L, Rossman SR. Clinical Roentgenologic and Histopathologic Findings in Teeth with Apical Radiolucent Areas. Oral Surg 1956;9:1330.

15. Shafer WG, Hine MK, Levy BM. Textbook of Oral Pathology, 4th Edition. Philadelphia: WB Saunders Co; 1983.

SECTION 2

General Anesthesia and Sedation in Oral and Maxillofacial Surgery

11 Introduction to General Anesthesia and Sedation

The history of maxillofacial surgery coincides with the development of endotracheal anesthesia by S. Rowbothom Ivan McGill, Britain, who had been the pioneer of maxillofacial and major oral surgery in the world and British anesthesiologists have made these more complex operations safe. Horace Wells used N_2O for exodontia, but the advent of ether in 1846, overshadowed the weaker anesthetic. In 1860, Colton repopularized N_2O for dentistry. Frederic Hewitt invented a gas and O_2 machine in 1887. In 1910 McKesson introduced intermittent flow machine, which provided control of O_2 and N_2O on demand.

In the past, complications have occurred, when dental chair anesthesia was common. Now with the introduction of new anesthetic agents, the techniques of anesthesia have changed, reducing the morbidity and mortality.

Pain is a major factor that brings patients to the dental clinic. The control of pain and anxiety is therefore, an essential part of the dental practice. To accomplish this objective, various techniques are used, including local anesthetics, and various types and combinations of sedative and general anesthetic agents. The choice of the most appropriate modality for a particular situation is based on the nature, severity and duration of the procedure; the age and physical and psychological status of the patient, the level of fear and anxiety. Dental patients are ambulatory, the procedures are usually shorter, the depth of anesthesia or level of sedation is often less, and it is the fear and apprehension of the patient, rather than the nature of the procedure, that frequently dictates the use of these techniques.

Drugs that depress the central nervous system, produce a progressive dose-related effects. Small doses produce light sedation. In this state, the patient remains conscious, with some alteration of mood, relief of anxiety, drowsiness, and sometimes analgesia. As the dose is increased, or as other drugs are added, greater central nervous system depression occurs, resulting in deepening of sedation and sleep from which the patient can be aroused. Finally, when consciousness is lost and the patient cannot be aroused, light general anesthesia begins. General anesthesia can be deepened by additional drug administration. Thus, depending on the patient's need, the correct procedure of sedation/general anesthesia can be chosen.

We now see that anesthesia in dentistry undergoing tremendous changes. The renaissance in office based anesthesia holds great promise for all of dentistry, allowing dentists to perform at a level of care that could not have been provided under ordinary clinical conditions.

PROBLEMS OF GENERAL ANESTHESIA IN A DENTAL CHAIR

- Sharing the airway between anesthetist and the surgeon/dentist
- Airway is contaminated with blood, good throat packing is essential
- Sitting position of the patient
- Patient exhibits anxiety prior to surgery
- Dysrhythmias are common
- Atmospheric pollution by N_2O may be severe.

- Anticipated difficult intubation in case of maxillo-facial surgery
- Ambulatory surgery—the brief nature of dental procedures means that majority of patients may be managed on an ambulatory basis. Modern anesthetic drugs permit rapid recovery of consciousness and early discharge. Thus, when in the opinion of anesthetist patients are ready for discharge, they must be accompanied by a responsible adult.

The details of these problems and the anesthetic techniques are discussed in the following chapters.

12 Preanesthetic Evaluation

The majority of dental procedures are done in the dental office, usually without supplemental sedation or anesthesia. Complicated procedures and uncooperative or phobic patients may require anesthetic care in the operating room. Procedures for healthy adult patients can usually be facilitated with routine anesthetic care. Anesthesia for the mentally retarded, combative or pediatric patient presents a unique challenge.

Administration of an anesthetic agent always begins with preoperative evaluation of the patient and proper planning of the procedure.

PURPOSE OF PREOPERATIVE PREANESTHETIC EVALUATION

1. To obtain pertinent information about the patient's medical history and physical as well as mental condition.
2. To determine the need for a medical consultation and the kind of investigations required.
3. To educate the patient about anesthesia, postoperative care, treatment of pain in the hope of reducing anxiety and thereby facilitating recovery.
4. To choose the anesthetic plan to be followed, guided by the risk factors uncovered by medical history.
5. To obtain informed consent.

The ultimate goal of preoperative medical assessment of a patient is to reduce the morbidity of anesthesia as well as surgery.

Two functions of preoperative evaluation are closely related. Acquisition of a pertinent medical history and information about physical and medical conditions, which affect all the decisions about investigations, consultations and discussions of care and plans with the patient.

Routine Preoperative Anesthetic Evaluation

History

1. Current problems
2. Other known problems
3. Treatment/Medicines for the problems: dose, duration and effectiveness
4. Current drugs use: reason, dose, duration, effectiveness and side effect
5. History of drug allergies
6. History of use of tobacco—smoking or smokeless tobacco or alcohol cosumption, frequency, quantity and duration
7. Prior anesthetic exposure: type and any adverse effects

8. General health and review of organ systems
    i. Cardiovascular system (hypertension, heart disease, angina, activity level)
    ii. Respiratory system (cough, cold, sputum, asthma, upper respiratory tract infection)
    iii. Central nervous system (headache, dizziness, visual disturbances, stroke, seizures - epilepsy)
    iv. Gastrointestinal system (nausea, vomiting, reflux, diarrhea, weight change)
    v. Renal system (abnormal function)
    vi. Hepatic system (jaundice, hepatitis)
    vii. Endocrine system (diabetes mellitus, thyroid dysfunction, pheochromocytoma)
    viii. Hematologic system (Excessive bleeding, anemia, any particular blood disorder or dyscrasias).
    ix. Musculoskeletal system (back or joint pain, arthritis)
    x. Reproductive system (menstrual history) Pregnancy.

Physical Examination

It broadly includes:
1. Vital signs
2. Airway
3. Heart
4. Lungs
5. Extremities
6. Neurologic examination.

The history and physical examination complement one another. The examination helps to detect abnormalities not apparent from the history. While the history helps to focus the examination on the organ systems that should be examined closely. Examination of healthy asymptomatic patients should minimally consist of measurement of vital signs and examination of the airway, heart, lungs, and extremities using standard techniques of inspection, palpation, percussion and auscultation.

The preanesthetic evaluation means to increase this awareness of a situation or condition. It is not necessary to understand the causes of the condition or the indicated therapy for it. For instance, when the patient comes for dental treatment, the pulse should be examined to detect arrhythmias or when a patient gives history of dyspnea the dentist should be aware of its presence. If the overall evaluation indicates the need for further examination, the patient should be sent to a physician for more thorough examination, diagnosis and treatment.

Pulse rate and Blood pressure (BP) should be checked to find out about any irregularity of pulse or whether there is any deviation from the normal values of both. If there is rise in blood pressure from the normal values of 120-140 systolic and 60-80 of diastolic in adult, the patient might need treatment to bring it to normal value and hence should be referred for further evaluation and management to physician.

The importance of examining the airway cannot be overemphasized. The oral cavity should be inspected closely for the presence of caries, crowns, loose teeth or dentures and particularly protruding upper incisors. The extent of mouth opening is assessed together with the degree of flexion of the cervical spine and extension of the atlanto-occipital joint. Micrognathia (a short distance between the chin and the hyoid bone), a large tongue, limited range of movement of the temporomandibular joint or cervical spine, or a short neck suggest that difficulty may be encountered in endotracheal intubation.

There are numerous causes of difficult laryngoscopy related to patients. The anatomical features associated with difficult laryngoscopy are:
• Short muscular neck
• Protruding incisors (buck teeth)
• Long and high arched palate
• Receding lower jaw
• Poor mobility of mandible
• Increased anterior depth of mandible
• Increased posterior depth of mandible (reduces jaw opening, requires radiographs)
• Decreased atlanto-occipital distance (reduces neck extension, requires radiographs).

Many of these factors are normal anatomical variations, but there may also be congenital or acquired deformities.

Congenital deformities: Many of the syndromes like Down, Pierre Robin's, Treacher Collins', Marfan's are associated with airway abnormalities such as a small mouth, large tongue and cleft palate.

Acquired factors can affect jaw opening, neck movements or the airway itself. Reduced jaw movements is a common cause of difficult laryngoscopy. Trauma and infection can cause reflex spasm of the masseter and medial pterygoid muscles (trismus). This typically occurs with dental abscess and fractures of the mandible and is usually relaxed by anesthetic agents. In contrast, reduced jaw movements associated with temporomandibular joint ankylosis is usually fixed.

Any local soft tissue swellings or mass can also reduce jaw movements.

Soft tissue edema of the face/upper airway from dental abscesses, other infections, drug hypersensitivity, burns and trauma can cause considerable anatomical distortion with life threatning airway obstruction. Foreign bodies, tumors and scarring after infection, burns and radiotherapy can also cause difficult laryngoscopy.

Hence, preoperative examination of the airway is essential (Figs 12.1A and B). Many additional clinical tests to predict difficult laryngoscopy have been described. One of these is "Mallampati" test which is a simple classification of the pharyngeal view obtained during maximal mouth opening and tongue protrusion

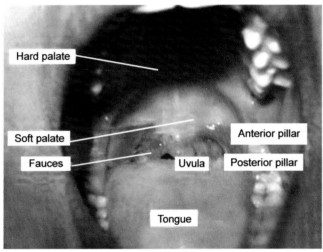

Fig. 12.1A: Oral cavity

(Fig. 12.1B). In practice, this test suggests a higher incidence of difficult laryngoscopy if the posterior pharyngeal wall is not visualized. The predictive value of this test may be strengthened if the thyromental distance (thyroid cartilage, prominence to the bony point of the chin during full head extension) is less than 6.5 cm (Figs 12.2A and B).

Cardiovascular system: The most frequent diseases of the heart of concern are congenital heart diseases, valvular heart diseases, coronary artery diseases, arrhythmias and defects of the conductive system and congestive heart failure.

The dentist should suspect a congenital heart disease if there is general retardation of growth and maturation, accompanied by cyanosis of the lips and nail beds. The fingers may or may not be clubbed, depending on the severity of defects.

The most common clinical manifestation of coronary artery diseases are angina pectoris, coronary thrombosis and myocardial insufficiency. The usual symptoms are substernal or precordial pain, anginal atttacks and dyspnea.

Valvular defects are usually recognized by the presence of characteristic murmur. Rheumatic fever is in itself responsible for a high percentage of valvular defects and any patient giving a previous history of this disease should be thoroughly questioned as to his ability to carry out normal activities without undue stress.

The most common symptoms of congestive heart failure are dyspnea on mild exertion, prominent and

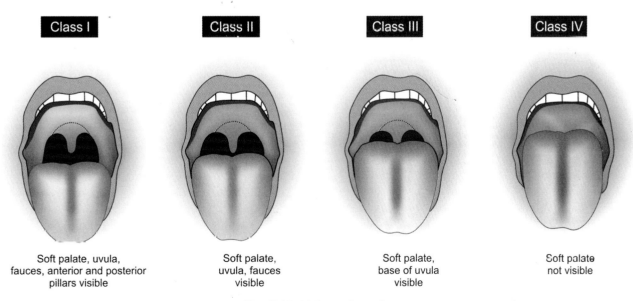

Class I	Class II	Class III	Class IV
Soft palate, uvula, fauces, anterior and posterior pillars visible	Soft palate, uvula, fauces visible	Soft palate, base of uvula visible	Soft palate not visible

Fig. 12.1B: Mallampati's grading

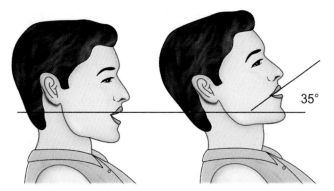

Fig. 12.2A: Atlanto-occipital extension

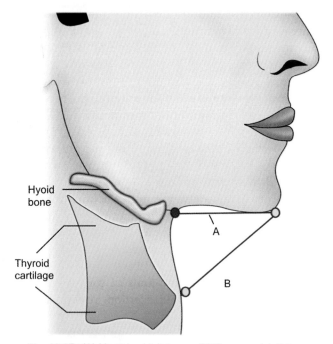

Fig. 12.2B: (A) Mentohyoid distance, (B) Thyromental distance

distended neck veins due to increased venous pressure, short spells of coughing due to pulmonary congestion and possibly edema of ankles.

Hypertension or high blood pressure is not a disease but a symptom of some underlying disease. Hence, it needs proper evaluation.

Hypertension may produce cardiac changes due to strain on the heart muscles and subsequent hypertrophy. Diastolic pressure in excess of 110 mm Hg is associated with an increased risk of myocardial ischemia. Gross hypertensive responses, with ECG evidence of ischemia on some occasions are likely to occur in response to noxious stimuli during anesthesia in these patients. Episodes of marked hypertension,

ischemic ST changes on ECG and the combination of hypotension and tachycardia are associated with an increased incidence of postoperative myocardial infarction.

Thus, the dentist should always be cognisant of the importance of the patient's cardiac status while performing preanesthetic evaluation. A large percentage of the fatalities that occur during anesthesia in the dental office should well be due to underlying cardiac disease. In these particular patients, the margin of acceptable error and safety is greatly reduced.

Diseases of the lungs are of the utmost importance because of their implications on gaseous exchange.

The most commonly encountered conditions of the ventilatory mechanisms are upper respiratory tract infections, bronchitis, bronchiectasis, obstruction, asthma and pulmonary emphysema. Auscultation of the chest should be done by dry or wet sounds. These patients need further evaluation and detailed examination by the physicians.

In physical examination, one should not forget to examine skin and mucous membrane for pallor to find out anemia, jaundice in case of impaired liver function and hepatitis, petechiae seen in blood dyscrasias, physical trauma and subacute bacterial endocarditis.

Laboratory Tests

Routine preoperative laboratory studies for all patients undergoing anesthesia and surgery include a determination of hemoglobin and hematocrit values. Total and differential white blood cell count and urinalysis.

What further investigations need to be carried out depends on many factors including patient's age, disease state, proposed surgery or preoperative drug therapy. Obviously specific laboratory tests should be done when the history and physical examination suggest dysfunction of an organ system. For example, a chest X-ray, electrocardiogram and blood chemistry (glucose, blood urea nitrogen and electrolytes) are indicated in any patient with symptoms or signs of pulmonary or cardiac disease or a history of diabetes, hepatic or renal disease. Patients with a history of a bleeding disorder should have tests for estimation of bleeding time, prothrombin time and partial thromboplastin time. More sophisticated tests such as liver or pulmonary function tests, arterial blood gas analysis, computed tomography or magnetic resonance imaging may be indicated by history and physical examination.

It is customary for all patients above the age of 40 years, undergoing general anesthesia, to have an electrocardiogram, chest X-ray and blood chemistry including blood sugar, serum electrolytes, creatinine, blood urea nitrogen, in addition to the routine tests, even if they are asymptomatic. Although, it is recognized that the yield of these tests in terms of identification of an unsuspected disease is very small, they serve as useful baseline values for comparison, should the patient develop unexpected complications in the intra-and postoperative period.

American Society of Anesthesiologists (ASA) have introduced a grading system as a simple description of the physical status of a patient requiring anesthesia and surgery. Despite its apparent simplicity, it remains one of the few prospective descriptions of the patient, which correlates with the risk of anesthesia and surgery (Table 12.1).

The advantages of this classification are two-fold. First, it allows anesthesiologists and others to compare outcomes (complications or death) within

Table 12.1: ASA physical status scale	
Class I	- A normally healthy individual
Class II	- A patient with mild-to-moderate systemic disease
Class III	- A patient with severe systemic disease that is not fully incapacitating, but with some functional limitations
Class IV	- A patient with severe systemic disease, that is a constant threat to life
Class V	- A moribund patient who is not expected to survive 24 hours, irrespective of treatment
Class VI	- Added as a suffix for emergency operation

their own institutions. In the final analysis, outcome is one important measure of how well the physicians are providing care. Second and perhaps more important, it provides anesthesiologist with a quick summary of the physical status of a patient on a daily basis. Hence, at the conclusion of the preoperative evaluation the anesthesiologist should assign each patient to one of the categories.

13 Preoperative Anesthetic Preparation and Premedication

Preoperative preparation is the beginning of anesthetic process. A good or adequate preoperative preparation improves clinical outcome, increases patient's satisfaction and helps to reduce adverse outcomes or events subsequently.

BASIC PLAN OF PREOPERATIVE ANESTHETIC PREPARATION

The basic plan of preoperative preparation is as follows:
A. Patient's counseling or psychological preparation
B. Premedication
C. Preoperative instructions for
   • Fasting guidelines,
   • Administration of current medication or pre-existing drug therapy.

The important considerations here are—requirements of surgery, techniques of anesthesia–local or general and patient's underlying medical condition.

Patient Counseling/Psychological Preparation

Good psychological preparation is often as effective as pharmacological preparation. Majority of the patients undergoing surgical procedures have high levels of apprehension and anxiety. During preoperative visit anticipated surgical events, risks and limitations, benefits and alternatives of anesthetic procedure should be discussed with the patient and his relatives. The information should provide answers to patient's all questions, also should provide reassurance.

Procedure Done under Local Anesthesia with or without Sedation

It is important to explain to the patient, symptoms and signs of local anesthetic toxicity. Patient can alert the surgeon early in such an event.

Local anesthetic toxicity (signs and symptoms)

1. Tingling and numbness initially around lips, slowly spreading over to rest of the body.
2. Bitter, metallic taste or sensation in mouth.
3. Ringing in ears.
4. Lightheadedness.
5. Tremulousness.
6. Dysarthria.
7. Confusion.

Hypersensitivity Reactions

They can be in the form of allergy, anaphylaxis, toxicity and idiosyncracy.

Allergic and idiosyncratic reactions are extremely rare with present amide type of local anesthetic agents, i.e. lignocaine and bupivacaine. Allergic reactions to additives and preservatives in local anesthetic preparations are known. If it occurs in dental chair, it could be disastrous. Skin sensitivity test may predict the susceptible individual. All patients undergoing treatment under local anesthesia, ideally should undergo skin sensitivity test.

The test is conducted as follows:

It can be tested during preoperative visits or on the day of surgery. But, there has to be at least 2-3 hours time gap between the test and the procedure.

For percutaneous testing, solution of a 1:100 dilution of additive free 1 percent lignocaine (0.5% for bupivacaine) is first injected intradermally to raise a 1 mm bleb. If this is uneventful, a 1 mm bleb of undiluted 1 percent lignocaine (0.5% for bupivacaine) is used 10 minutes later. If, this is uneventful, 2 cc of the local anesthetic is used. A positive test is a wheal of greater than 0.8 cm. If significant flare occurs to a specific drug, then an alternative drug should be used. This testing does not exclude allergy to preservatives and/additives used in the LA solution. A patient with known allergies or positive skin testing, it is safer to use preservative, additive free preparation.

Consent

Written, informed, valid consent for anesthesia as well as for surgery to be obtained prior to procedure. Also, special consent for medical problems due to medical diseases and for tracheostomy, if difficult intubation or airway is suspected. An adult who is mentally stable, well-oriented, not under influence of drugs or alcohol can sign the consent form himself. In case of mentally subnormal individuals, one of his parents or guardians should be signing the consent. Again, in case of minors, one of the parents or guardians should sign the consent. And lastly, in case of patients from an orphanage, the chief of the orphanage has to sign the consent form.

Premedication

Premedication can be defined as 'preliminary medication', drugs with specific pharmacological actions, administered preoperatively with specific goals to achieve (Table 13.1).
1. Selection and dosage of the premedication drugs will depend on the following:
   a. Age of the patient.
   b. Weight of the patient.
   c. Physical status and type of anesthesia used.

Table 13.1: Objectives of premedication
1. Relief of apprehension or anxiety
2. Sedation
3. Analgesia
4. Amnesia of perioperative events
5. Antisialagogue effect
6. Reduction of stomach acidity and volume
7. Prevention of nausea and vomiting
8. Vagolytic actions
9. Fascilitation of anesthetic induction
10. Prophylaxis against allergies.

Table 13.2: Routes of administration for premedication	
Enteral	*Parenteral*
Oral	Sublingual
Rectal	Intranasal
	Intramuscular (IM)
	Intravenous (IV)

2. Timing of the premedication is decided depending on initial onset, peak effect and duration of action and the route of administration (Table 13.2).

Oral administration: It is the most commonly used route of drug administration. It is a popular mode of administration in children. Various formulations are tablets, capsules, syrups, linctuses, gels and lozenges, etc.

Advantages

- It is easiest, safest, most economical and convenient mode.
- It obviates the need of syringes, needles and trained personnel.

Disadvantages are namely:

- Its dependence on patient compliance
- Considerable time is taken between administration of drug and attainment of therapeutic effect
- Potentially erratic and incomplete absorption from the gut
- Inability to titrate the drug level
- Inability to alter the sedation on demand and
- May have prolonged action.

Rectal administration: It is extremely valuable route to sedate young children, who otherwise spit the orally introduced drug. If the rectum is loaded, it becomes cumbersome to administer the drug and also the absorption becomes erratic. Midazolam and ketamine like drugs may be given by this route.

Intranasal administration: Rapid absorption of drug takes place from the highly vascular nasal mucosa. It avoids first pass effect of liver. Concentrated solutions are needed to be used. Midazolam, ketamine, and fentanyl like drugs may be given by this route.

Sublingual administration: Area underneath the tongue has vascular mucosa. Rapid absorption of drug takes place. This route also avoids first pass effect of liver. Again concentrated solutions are required.

Intramuscular administration: Its advantages include rapid onset of action, maximal effect seen within 30 minutes, more reliable absorption of drug than enteral routes. The disadvantages include the prolonged effect of action, trained personnel required for administration, and all known risks associated with injection. Many children and few adults have phobias of needles. Most premedication can be given by this mode.

Premedicant Drugs (Table 13.3)

Benzodiazepines: Most popular agents selected for premedication. They produce sedation, amnesia and

Table 13.3: Premedicant drugs		
Group	*Drug*	*Side effects*
Benzodiazepines	Diazepam Midazolam Oxazepam Lorazepam	None in normal dosage
Opioid	Pethidine Morphine Fentanyl Pentazocine	Respiratory depression Sickness
Barbiturates	Pentobarbitone Quinal barbitone	Restlessness in presence of pain
Phenothiazines	Chlorpromazine Promethazine Trimeprazine	Pallor, hypotension Restlessness in presence of pain
Butyrophenones	Haloperidol Droperidol	Restlessness in presence of pain. Extrapyramidal effects
Anticholinergic	Atropine Glycopyrrolate Scopolamine	Dry mouth, Restlessness in presence of pain
α_2-adrenoceptor agonist	Clonidine Dexmedetomidine	Hypotension, Bradycardia

excellent anxiolysis, but no analgesia. In the presence of pain, there could be 'antanalgesia' like effect. At times it can cause agitation and restlessness. Usually in clinical dose range it does not produce respiratory depression, but with combination with opioid, rapid injection, large doses or in sensitive individuals, it can give rise to arterial desaturation.

Midazolam: It is sedative, anxiolytic and excellent amnestic agent. It is water soluble, rapidly metabolized drug. It is 3 to 5 times more potent than diazepam. When given intramuscularly, the onset of action is seen within 5 to 10 minutes, with peak effect seen in 30 to 60 minutes. The usual adult dose is 0.05 to 0.1 mg/kg of body weight. The IV dose is 2 to 5 mg, in 0.5 mg increments, till desired effect is seen. Mental function returns to normal within 4 hours of administration. Since it is water-soluble, it does not produce phlebitis. Intranasal dose is 0.6 mg/kg. It can also be given sublingually, orally and rectally.

Diazepam: It is considered as "gold standard" with which other drugs are usually compared. The anxiolytic, amnestic and sedative effects of diazepam, made it popular. Ninety percent of the oral dose is absorbed in 30 to 60 minutes in adults and 15 to 30 minutes in children. It is metabolized by hepatic microsomal enigma style system to active metabolites. Hence, prolonged effect may be observed in cases of liver cirrhosis or in the elderly. Enhanced effects are also observed in chronic renal failure patients and in patients with low serum albumin. Diazepam is dissolved in organic solvent. Hence, causes pain on intravenous injection and after IM injection, absorption of the drug is unpredictable. With concomitant opioid administration may produce respiratory and cardiovascular depression. Diazepam also reduces seizure threshold for regional anesthetics clinically. Though it is not proved experimentally.

Flumazenil: Drug antagonizes sedative and to certain effect amnestic effect of midazolam. Dose is 0.1 to 0.5 mg. It is a short-acting drug and requires to be given in infusion form.

Other Sedative and Hypnotic Agents

Barbiturates: They have been used in preoperative sedation since long ago. They are inexpensive and have both parental and oral preparation. They do not provide analgesia, in fact, in the presence of pain, they may produce deterioration or even antianalgesic effect. Also, there is possibility of cardiorespiratory depression. Barbiturates should be avoided in porphyria. With all these limitations, they have largely been replaced by benzodiazepines, e.g. secobarbital dose 50 to 200 gm orally, pentobarbital dose 50 to 200 gm orally, the initial action occurs in 15 to 20 minutes and peak action in 45 minutes and the duration lasts for 2 to 4 hr.

Butyrophenones: Droperidol falls in this group of drugs. It is mainly used as antiemetic. It also produces sedation and calms the patient. But, at times there could be dysphoria and restlessness. Dose IV or IM 2.5 to 7.5 mg.

Phenothiazine: These drugs produce sedation, anticholinergic effects and also have antiemetic properties. They are always used with opioid analgesic agents. Commonly used drugs in this group are promethazine, perphenazine, chlorpromazine, etc. "Lytic cocktail" once popular combination for dental anesthesia, consisted of 50 mg pethidine, 25 mg promethazine, 10 mg chlorpromazine. With advent of new drugs this combination is now abandoned.

Promethazine (Phenergan): Dose is 10 to 25 mg orally in similar doses given IM or IV. It is used for its antisialagogue, antihistaminic and sedative effect. It is especially useful in children. It is also a powerful tranquilizer and a antiemetic agent.

Trimeperazine tartrate (Vellargan): Dose 3 to 4 mg/kg 2 hours preoperatively. Available as syrup for oral administration to children, although now largely surpassed by benzodiazepine.

Diphenhydramine: It blocks histamine receptors and has sedative antiemetic and anticholimytic properties, with an oral dose of 50 mg. The effect lasts for 3 to 6 hours. It is mainly used as premedicant in patients with known allergies.

Analgesic Agents

Opioids: The opioids have sedative and analgesic action rather than anxiolytic. They have higher incidence of side effects as compared to benzodiazepines. Respiratory depression, postoperative nausea and vomiting are fairly common. They are also known to cause cardiovascular depression. They tend to produce spasm of sphincter of Oddi, which can rapidly lead to upper quadrant pain. Opioid may cause flushing, dizziness and miosis (pupillary constriction).

Morphine: Morphine is well absorbed after IM injection with onset of analgesia after 15 to 30 minutes. Peak effects are seen in 45 to 90 minutes, with analgesia lasting for 4 hours. Morphine may cause orthostatic hypotension, pruritus, respiratory depression, nausea and vomiting. It is habit forming and addictive drug.

Fentanyl: It is 50 to 125 times more potent than morphine. The incidence of respiratory depression is high. This drug has to be used with caution. The dose is 1 to 2 µgm/kg. It has rapid onset within 30 to 60 seconds and shorter duration of action (30 to 60 minutes). It can be used intranasally, orally and also transdermally as patches.

Pethidine: The dose is 50 to 100 mg IM/IV. The effect of single dose lasts for 2 to 4 hours. It increases heart rate and causes orthostatic hypotension. It is 1/10th as potent as morphine.

Pentazocine: 1/30th as potent as morphine. IM/IV rarely causes respiratory depression. It also raises heart rate and systemic blood pressure.

Buprenorphine: It is highly potent drug. Dose is 3 to 6 µgm/kg, IM/IV. Respiratory depression is very common.

Anticholinergic Agents

Anticholinergic agents used for premedication include atropine, glycopyrrolate and scopolamine. Actions common to anticholinergic agents are:
1. Vagolytic effects
2. Antisialagogue actions
3. Sedation and amnesia.

Vagolytic effects: Atropine, glycopyrolate and scopolamine increase heart rate by blocking acetylcholine action on muscarinic receptors in SA node. Atropine is more effective than glycopyrrolate and scopolamine in increasing heart rate and is very useful in preventing intraoperative bradycardias resulting from vagal stimulation or stimulation of carotid sinus. Atropine is also very effective in preventing vasovagal attacks.

Antisialagogue actions: It includes drying of salivary, gastric, tracheobronchial and secretions of sweat glands. Glycopyrrolate is more potent and longer-acting drying agent and is less likely to increase heart rate. Scopolamine is more effective antisialagogue than atropine. In the presence of heart disease or cardiac arrhythmias glycopyrrolate is a better drug than atropine, as an anticholinergic premedicant. All three drugs take about 20 to 30 minutes for drying action. Hence, should be given 30 minutes prior to planned procedure.

Sedation and amnesia: Glycopyrrolate does not cross blood-brain barrier and hence does not cause sedation or amnesia. Both atropine and scopolamine cross blood-brain barrier. Atropine can cause delirium in elderly. Scopolamine has good amnesic and sedative action. So, in elderly subjects, it is better to use glycopyrrolate instead of atropine. Scopolamine is not freely available yet.

Side effects

1. Pupillary dilatation and cycloplegia. This could be harmful in glaucoma patients.
2. Tachycardia and cardiac arrhythmias.
3. Delirium, confusion, and restlessness.
4. Inspissations of existing secretions in trachea and bronchi.
5. Increase in body temperature.

Dose: Atropine—0.12 mg/kg.
Glycopyrrolate—0.044 mg/kg.

In children, atropine is better than glycopyrrolate. In elderly glycopyrrolate is more useful than atropine. In young adults depending upon basal pulse rate—if low pulse rate, then atropine is preferred, if pulse rate is high (more than 100/min) glycopyrrolate is preferred. In the presence of fever, anticholinergic premedication should be avoided. Instead, other drying agents like promethazine can be used.

Aspiration Prophylaxis

Several pharmaceutical agents have been used to alter gastric pH and fluid volume. They include histamine receptor (H_2 receptor) blocking agents, gastrokinetic drugs, clear antacids and anticholinergic agents.

Histamine receptor blocking agents: Cimetidine, ranitidine and famotidine are the commonly used H_2 receptor blockers. These drugs raise the gastric pH by blocking histamine-mediated secretions of gastric hydrogen ion. The drug regimen started night before surgery is usually more effective in raising gastric pH than single dose preoperatively, on the day of surgery. As with most of the drugs, parenteral administration produces more rapid onset of action than the oral route. Although, these drugs reduce acidity, they have no effect on volume of gastric secretions or stomach emptying time. Cimetidine is known for drug interactions and side effects. Other drugs have largely replaced it's use. Ranitidine is equally effective, has fewer side effects and has longer duration of action.

Doses

Cimetidine (adult dose): 150 to 300 mg orally or parenterally 60 to 90 minutes prior to surgery and repeated 8 hourly.

Ranitidine (adult dose): 50 to 100 mg orally, 50 to 100 mg parenterally, on the night before surgery and 1 hour prior to surgery. Action lasts for about 9 to 10 hours. Ranitidine is known to prolong sedative effect of midazolam. But, a single dose of either drug usually does not exhibit clinically significant adverse effects.

Famotidine: 40 mg at bedtime and 40 mg on the morning of surgery. Onset occurs in 1 hour and persists for 10 to 12 hours. The drug is administered orally.

Gastrokinetic drugs (Metoclopramide): It is a dopamine antagonist, that stimulates upper GI motility, increases gastroesophageal sphincter tone and relaxes pylorus and duodenum. It has been shown to reduce gastric fluid volume and reduce risk of aspiration. At times it can precipitate extrapyramidal reactions. Also rapid injection can cause abdominal cramping.

Dose: Orally 10 mg 30 to 60 minutes prior to surgery. Parenterally 5 to 20 mg given over 3 to 5 minutes, 15 to 30 minutes prior to surgery.

Antacids: These are used to neutralize the pH of gastric fluid already present in stomach. A single dose of clear antacid given 15 to 30 minutes prior to anesthesia is effective in raising gastric fluid pH above 2.5. Particulate or colloid antacid suspensions are more effective than nonparticulate (clear) antacid in elevating gastric pH above 2.5. But in the event of aspiration of gastric contents into lungs, particulate antacids are known to cause major injury to lung parenchyma. 30 ml of 0.3 mg sodium citrate solution is commonly used for this purpose.

All routine minor and major surgeries do not require aspiration prophylaxis.

Indicated conditions include obesity, pregnancy, diabetic patients, alcoholics, patients on long term steroid therapy, ascites, hiatus hernia, patients with history of gastroesophageal reflux, etc.

Antiemetics: Some anesthesiologists include anti-emetics with premedication as routine practice. While some believe in giving just prior to emergence or during recovery period. For routine dental surgery, sedative techniques and anesthesia, do not require regular antiemetic administration. But, for major maxillofacial surgeries, it is advisable to give antiemetics as during surgical procedure some amount of blood enters stomach that can irritate the stomach mucosa and induce vomiting postoperatively. The drugs used as antiemetics include, droperidol, metoclopromide, phenothiazine like prochlorperazine and ondansetron.

Prochlorperazine is the most common. Phenothiazine is used to prevent nausea and vomiting. Ondansetron is given 4 mgm IV or 8 mgm orally preoperatively. The effect lasts for 4 to 8 hours.

Premedication for Outpatient Dental Surgery

All patients need to receive anticholinergic agent either atropine or glycopyrrolate 30 minutes prior to the procedure and diazepam 0.25 mg/kg orally on night before surgery to reduce anxiety. For short procedure under local anesthesia, diazepam can be given orally in similar doses 60 to 90 minutes prior to the procedure to allay anxiety. For procedures which require longer periods of drilling, etc. instead of diazepam, midazolam may be given (0.05 to 0.1 mg/kg) IM 30 minutes prior to surgery. If patient is already in pain, then preoperatively pethidine (1.5 mg/kg), fentanyl 100 mg, pentazocine 0.5 to 0.6 mg/kg may be added to midazolam. But this does delay the recovery time.

Premedication for Major Maxillofacial Surgery

Along with atropine or glycopyrrolate, pethidine and promethazine (50 + 25 mg) should be given 30 minutes prior to surgery. Instead of pethidine, pentazocine or buprenorphine (3 mg to 6 mg/kg) or fentanyl may be given. Promethazine helps in drying secretions, sedation and act as antiemetic. It also prevents histamine release after opioids.

Premedication for Children

The vagus activity is predominant in children. Also the air passages being small, presence of secretions can have deleterious effects. So anticholinergic premedication becomes mandatory. But most of the children have fears or phobias of needle pricks. So, syrup trimaperazine or promethazine or midazolam intranasally or orally (0.6

mg/kg) should be given. Once sedated, anticholinergic agents should be given IM/IV.

Ketamine hydrochloride is also a popular drug for children. But, it is mainly used as sedative. Hence, it is discussed with sedative techniques.

Preoperative Instructions

Fasting Guidelines (Table 13.4)

Clear fluids: Apple juice, coconut water, water, tea and coffee without milk.

Nonclear fluids: Milk (breast milk, formula milk), orange juice, etc.

Concurrent Medication or Pre-existing Drug Therapy (Table 13.5)

Antihypertensives: All antihypertensives except MAO inhibitors should be continued till the day of surgery. The usual morning dose should be given with sip of water and postoperatively as soon as orals would be resumed. If oral route is not available in such instances other route or different drug can be given parenterally, which should be started on consultation with physician. Sudden withdrawal of these drugs can precipitate hypertensive episode during preoperative period.

Angina prophylaxis: These drugs should also be continued in perioperative period. Or else, it can precipitate ischemic episode. If oral route is not available, transdermal patch of glyceryl trinitrate is to be placed on chest wall or forehead. Effect usually lasts for almost 24 hours.

Psychotropic drugs: Many of these drugs potentiate effects of anesthetic agents. Major tranquilizers and tricyclic antidepressants have anticholinergic side effects. In the presence of catecholamines and under anesthesia, they potentiate ventricular tachyarrhythmias. Also, sudden withdrawal can precipitate severe reactions. Hence,

	Table 13.4: Fasting guidelines for surgery		
	Age	Clear fluids	Nonclear fluids/ solids
1.	Child— < 6 months	2 hr prior	4-6 hr prior
2.	Child — 6 to 36 months	2-3 hr prior	6 hr prior
3.	Child — >36 months	2-3 hr prior	6-8 hr prior
4.	Adults	2-3 hr prior	6-8 hr or not after midnight

the drugs to be continued till the day of surgery with extreme caution in mind. Avoid adrenaline in local infiltration.

Lithium is known to potentiate action of muscle relaxants used in anesthesia. They should be omitted 48 to 72 hours prior to surgery. Patients should be shifted on some other drugs on consultation with psychiatrist.

MAO inhibitors also should be discontinued 2 to 3 weeks before surgery. They adversely react with opioid analgesics and can give rise to cardiovascular instability. These patients too, should be shifted on some other drugs on consultation with psychiatrist.

Antiparkinsonism drugs: Drugs like levadopa, potentiates ventricular arrhythmias. Hence, it is prudent to omit these drugs 24 hours prior to surgery. If stopped for longer period, there would be reappearance of Parkinson symptoms and there is definite risk of aspiration. So, the drugs need to be restarted as soon as possible in postoperative period.

Anticonvulsants: These drugs also to be continued till the day of surgery. Sudden withdrawal of drugs can precipitate convulsions in postoperative period. Most of the drugs are fairly safe. If oral route is not available in postoperative period, patient should be switched over to injectable drugs. Phenobarbiturate and eptoin can potentiate sedative actions of anesthetic agents.

Alcohol: It should be stopped prior to surgery. There is possibility of acute alcohol withdrawal symptoms in postoperative period. Patients should be given good dose of benzodiazepine sedation.

Antidiabetic or hypoglycemic agents: All oral antidiabetic drugs to be stopped on the day of surgery. Restarted as soon as patient switches back to orals. If oral route is not available, patient should be switched over to crystalline insulin and managed on 'sliding scale.'

In case of insulin dependent diabetic, morning dose to be omitted and managed on 'sliding scale' with intravenous insulin, on consultation with physician.

Concurrent Drug Therapy (Table 13.5)

Antituberculous therapy: Aminoglycosides potentiate action of muscle relaxants. These drugs to be omitted on the day of surgery, to be restarted in postoperative period.

Antibiotics: All antibiotics can safely be given.

Table 13.5: Concurrent drug therapy		
To be continued	*To be discontinued*	*To be modified*
• Antiarrhythmics • Antiasthmatic	• Diuretics—on the morning of surgery	• Insulin • Oral anti-coagulants
• Antibiotics • Antiepileptic • Antihypertensive	• Oral antidiabetic —same • Aspirin—one week prior	• Steroid cover
• β blocker		
• Calcium channel blocker	• Monoamine oxidase (MAO) inhibitor— 2 weeks prior	
• Cardiac drugs		
• Eye drops (Timodal)	• Oral contraceptive pills—1 month cycle	
• Sedative/tranquilizer/ anxiolytics		
• Immunosuppressants		

Steroids: Long term steroid therapy calls for replacement during anesthesia, either with short-acting hydrocortisone or long-acting dexamethasone.

Contraceptive pills and other hormones: Estrogen containing pills have additive effects under anesthesia on antithrombin III and can precipitate thrombotic episode. Ideally, estrogen containing pills should be stopped at least 4 weeks before major elective procedure. But for minor surgery, routine of contraceptive pills need not be disturbed.

Hormone replacement therapy (HRT): The hormones content of these pills are very low. It does not require any alteration in schedule of this drug.

Progesterone (Postponement) pill: Needs no alteration in schedule of this drug.

Other Instructions

Smoking: Ideally should be stopped 4 to 6 weeks prior to the surgery to decrease the incidence of postoperative pulmonary complications. Stopping 1 to 2 weeks before the surgery also benefits the patient by enhancing the ciliary activity of respiratory mucosa and by reduction in the sputum volume. Not smoking for 12 to 24 hours prior to the surgery may benefit the patient by eliminating circulating nicotine and carbon monoxide from the blood. Nicotine causes tachycardia and peripheral vasoconstriction. With high levels of carbon monoxide in blood, patients are susceptible for hypoxic episodes.

Dentures: Chances of aspiration of loose dentures or slipping from the position can cause obstruction of the airway.

Cosmetics: Lipsticks, nail varnishes and other cosmetics may interfere with observation of cyanosis or pallor and may also interfere with estimation of oxygen saturation. Patients are instructed to defer their use.

Artificial limbs: Should be removed as metal component of the artificial limb may induce electrical burns.

Artificial eyes and contact lenses: Dislodgements can cause corneal abrasions or injury to surrounding delicate structures of eye. Removal is a must.

Hearing aids: Should be kept in place so as to maintain effective communication with the patient.

Emptying the bladder: Prior to surgery, ensure that the patient's bladder is emptied. Patient should be accompanied by a responsible adult, who will also escort him home, specially important in ambulatory surgery.

14 Anesthetic Equipment

Chapter Outline

- ❖ Anesthesia and Resuscitation Equipment
- ❖ Monitoring Equipment
- ❖ Oxygen Therapy Equipment
- ❖ Intravenous Infusion Equipment

With advancing technology, not only the procedure of anesthetizing a patient, but even monitoring a patient during general anesthesia has vastly been simplified over the years with the introduction of newer equipment. The practice of anesthesia has shifted from purely clinical to a clinical cum technologically based art. Many a times due to mechanical fault with the anesthetic equipment, or a failure to recognize a technical snag by the anesthesiologist, or improper handling of the anesthetic equipment or misuse of the equipment, or the physical principles of which the anesthesiologist did not understand, we have seen a patient being lost. Hence, it is essential for the anesthesiologist to have a thorough knowledge of the physical and mechanical aspects of the anesthetic equipment, their functioning and maintenance, so that in the event of mechanical failure or fault, he can use his skill and continue with safe and smooth anesthesia. The art of anesthesia is essentially not only clinical but also practical.

At the same time, one should not forget that most of the anesthetic equipment that are used to give general anesthesia are basically part of the equipment that are also needed for resuscitation of a patient in the event of any catastrophe, that might even occur during the surgical procedures under local anesthesia. For this reason any person who deals with patients under local anesthesia should have a basic knowledge of anesthetic equipment.

The basic equipment that an anesthesiologist needs for general anesthesia falls into four groups: Anesthetic and resuscitation, monitoring, oxygen therapy and intravenous infusion equipment.

ANESTHESIA AND RESUSCITATION EQUIPMENT

Anesthesia Machine

Anesthesia machine is an equipment, by which the operator can deliver a desired concentration of a mixture of anesthetic agents (gases as well as liquids) in an inhalational (gaseous) form with oxygen and/or air, which serves as a vehicle to carry this mixture to the outlet of the equipment (Figs 14.1A and B).

In its simplest form an anesthesia machine consists of a metallic frame, having a facility to connect central pipelines as well as cylinders of gases like oxygen, nitrous oxide, air, etc. flow meters, vaporizers and a facility to deliver high flow of oxygen (oxygen flush or emergency oxygen knob) in the event of any leak or an emergency situation. It also has a working platform to keep various drugs and small equipment, and at times, a tray on the top to keep various monitors.

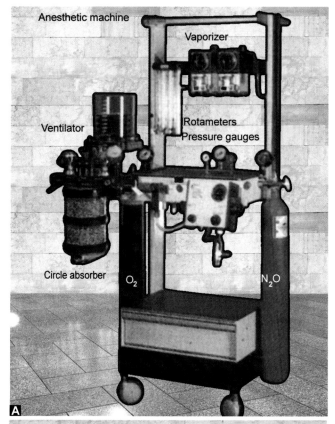

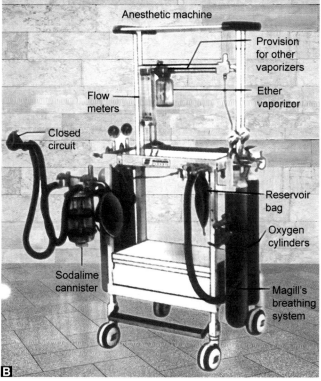

Figs 14.1A and B: Anesthetic machines

Anesthesia machines can be of either intermittent flow or continuous flow variety. In the intermittent flow machines (e.g. Walton 5 machine), there is a demand valve, i.e. gases flow only on demand of the patient. However, these machines are obsolete nowadays. In continuous flow machines (e.g. Boyle machine), oxygen, nitrous oxide, air, etc. have individual flow meters for setting desired flow of each gas. Vaporizers are meant for setting desired percentage output concentration of the liquid anesthetic agents like halothane, isoflurane, etc. (ether and trilene in older models of the machines). Flow meters for gases and vaporizers for liquid anesthetic agents are gas/agent specific and the one meant for a particular gas or anesthetic agent cannot be used for the other. They are highly specific, precise and most expensive constituents of the anesthesia machines.

Most dangerous hazard (but fortunately rare, due to constant vigilance of anesthesiologists) that can occur with the use of an anesthesia machine, is the delivery of a hypoxic gas mixture (gases with an oxygen percentage less than that of air, e.g. when an oxygen cylinder is getting over and the patient receives gases other than oxygen). This can lead to hypoxic brain damage and coma, even cardiac arrest and death can occur. To avoid this hazard most of the newer anesthesia machines have devices, which in the event of delivery of a hypoxic gas mixture activate an alarm either auditory or visual, which tells the operator that a hypoxic gas mixture is being delivered, so that immediate action can be taken.

Anesthesia machines have been evolved from simple pneumatic devices to complex computer based integrated systems with numerous controls, displays, indicators and alarms. The prevailing trend is to incorporate and integrate ventilators and vigilance aids, such as airway pressure monitors, respirometers, respiratory gas monitors, pulse oximeters, electrocardiograms and automatic blood pressure monitors into the machine (state of the art technology).

Breathing System (Circuit)

Breathing system is an assembly of equipment, that not only carries anesthetic mixture from the outlet of anesthesia machine to the patient, but also allows to monitor and control patient's breathing (Fig. 14.1B).

The essential components of any breathing system, in addition to various connectors and adapters, consist of a bag mount with a reservoir bag (1.5 to 2 liter capacity), long (one meter) corrugated rubber or plastic tubing/s (breathing tube/s) and an expiratory valve, ordinary spring loaded/nonrebreathing valve, which is connected to a mask or an endotracheal tube attached to the patient.

It is the excursions (rhythmical inflation and deflation) of the reservoir bag, that allows visual monitoring of adequacy or inadequacy of patient's own breathing and the reservoir bag also allows one to assist or control (take over) patient's breathing, in case the breathing is inadequate. Corrugated tubings are flexible and help to prevent kinking and if made up of plastic, are light in weight and thereby cause less drag on the mask or endotracheal tube. An expiratory valve can be simple spring-loaded valve (e.g. Heidbrink valve) or a nonrebreathing valve (NRV) as seen on most of the resuscitation bags (e.g. Ambu, Laerdale, Penlon, etc.). A nonrebreathing valve allows to control patient's breathing for longer periods, without increasing patient's inspired or arterial carbon dioxide tension and it also allows a smooth transition from spontaneous to controlled breathing or vice versa. At the same time, these systems (open systems) are less economical than the closed systems (described below), there is also increased heat and moisture loss from the patient's body and they increase theatre pollution. Theatre pollution with open systems can be reduced by using scavenging system, that gets rid of exhaled gases entering into the operation theatre atmosphere.

Breathing system can be reusable or disposable. It can have a single simple corrugated tubing (e.g. Magill's system) or can have a coaxial tubings, i.e. one tubing within the other (e.g. Bain's system) or can have double tubings, inspiratory and expiratory (e.g. closed circuit). It can allow entire exhaled gases to vent to the atmosphere (e.g. Magill's system with NRV) or allow minimal/partial rebreathing (e.g. Magill's system with Heidbrink valve or Bain system) or it can allow exhaled gases from the patient to be reused (rebreathed) after getting rid of carbon dioxide from the exhaled gases (e.g. circle absorber/carbon dioxide absorber/closed system). Each has its own advantages and disadvantages. However, closed system is economical as low flow of anesthetic gases are required, there is less heat and moisture loss from the patient's body and operation theatre pollution is almost nil, as compared to open systems.

Anesthetic Mask

Mask is an integral part of any anesthetic breathing system/circuit during the induction phase (beginning) of anesthesia or any resuscitation procedure. A mask allows administration of gases from the breathing system, without introducing any invasive apparatus (e.g. endotracheal tube) into the patient's airway. It is placed on the patient's face covering his/her mouth and nose (face-mask) or only on the nose (nasal-mask). Face-masks are designed to fit the patient's face perfectly without any leaks, whereas nasal masks are designed to fit snugly around the nose without any leaks (Fig. 14.2). Nasal masks are smaller in size than face masks and generally used only for conservative dentistry for dental chair anesthesia.

- *Parts:*
  - Connector or mount
  - Body
  - Edge or seal
- *Sizes:* 1, 2, 3, 4, 5.

The mount is usually constructed of hard rubber, but may be made up of plastic or metal. It is the mount to which a breathing system/circuit is attached. The body

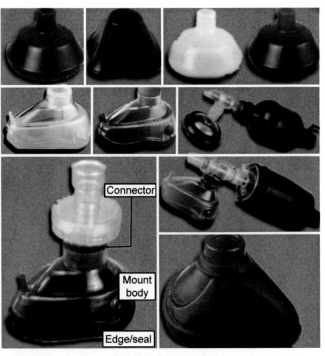

Fig. 14.2: Face masks

of the mask may be made up of rubber, neoprine, plastic or silicone. Some masks have transparent body which is useful, as it allows observation of the patient for vomitus, secretions, blood, lip color and condensation of exhaled moisture. The edge or seal is the part of the mask, that comes in contact with the face. It is anatomically shaped and to achieve a snug fit on the face, it is fitted with an air-filled cuff, which also has a soft cushioning effect or a flap, which takes up the contour of the face. Masks come in variety of sizes and shapes. A variety of masks should be kept readily available, so that the selection of an appropriately fitting mask becomes possible for the operator.

Laryngoscope

Laryngoscope is designed for doing direct laryngoscopy (directly viewing the vocal cords) and to pass an endotracheal tube into the larynx under vision.
- *Parts:* Handle, blade with light bulb.
- *Sizes (for the blades):* Neonate (infant), pediatric (child), adult and extra large.

The handle is a hollow cylinder containing two 1.5-volt batteries. During use it forms generally a right angle with the blade, but it may form an acute or an obtuse angle in some varieties of laryngoscopes. The blade may be attached to the handle with a hook on connection or secured by a screwed connection. The blades are interchangeable. Laryngoscope blades can be curved (e.g. MacIntosh Laryngoscope—most popular) or straight (e.g. Magill Laryngoscope—useful for neonates and small children) (Figs 14.3 and 14.4). The blade includes base, tongue plate, flange, web, tip and a bulb socket. The base is slotted to engage the hinge pin of the handle. The tongue plate or spatula serves to manipulate the tongue and other soft tissues to visualize the larynx. The flange is parallel to the tongue plate and connected by a web. It helps to deflect the interfering soft tissues and to guide the endotracheal tube. The tip of the blade is blunt and thick to prevent trauma to the soft tissues. It elevates and secures the epiglottis directly (with straight blade) or indirectly (with curved blade). The bulb socket is meant for fitting the light bulb. It has an electrical connection to the hook on the base. As the blade is locked on the handle (at 90 degrees), electrical connection is made complete and the bulb is illuminated.

Method of insertion: (Figs 14.5 and 14.6). The patient should be supine, with flexion of the lower cervical spine and extension of the head at the atlanto-occipital level.

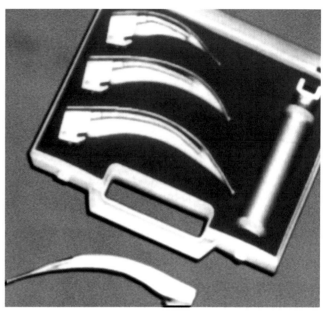

Fig. 14.3: Laryngoscope blades

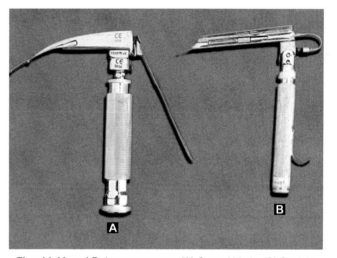

Figs 14.4A and B: Laryngoscopes: (A) Curved blade, (B) Straight blade

The head should rest on a small pillow or a ring. This position, popularly known as 'sniffing the morning air position', brings the passage from the incisor teeth to the larynx in a straight line. The mouth of the patient is then opened by the right hand of the operator and the locked blade (handle and blade at right angle to each other) of the laryngoscope is introduced between the upper and the lower sets of teeth from the right side of the mouth. The blade is then advanced into the mouth towards the glossoepiglottic fold in such a way, that the tongue is pushed to the left side in the patient's mouth. The blade

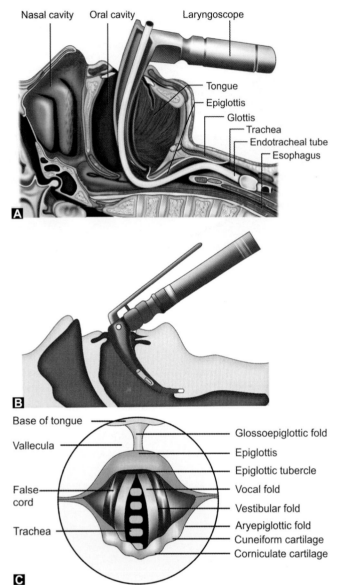

Figs 14.5A to C: Supine position for intubation with laryngoscope. View of the larynx at laryngoscopy

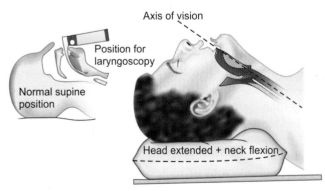

Fig. 14.6: Laryngoscopic vision in supine position and with extension at atlantoaxial level and flexion of lower cervical spine

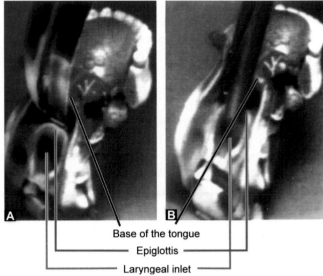

Figs 14.7A and B: Laryngoscopy: (A) Curved blade, (B) Straight blade

is advanced till the epiglottis is visualized. The tip of the curved blade is advanced up to the junction of the base of the tongue with the epiglottis and the blade is then lifted upward and forward along the axis, as to carry the base of the tongue and the epiglottis forward. The laryngeal inlet will now come into the view. The tip of the straight blade is passed posterior to the epiglottis, so as to pick up the epiglottis with the tip of the blade and the blade is then lifted anteriorly, thereby elevating the epiglottis directly to expose the laryngeal inlet (Figs 14.7 and 14.8).

Endotracheal Tubes

Endotracheal tube is a specially designed tube with one end straight and the other being obliquely cut (beveled end) (Figs 14.9A to E). Beveled end enters the trachea through the laryngeal inlet. It is used for the surgical procedures in which it is not feasible to administer anesthetic gases via mask, procedures which are long-lasting, procedures in which there are chances of having blood, secretions, pus, vomitus, etc. in the oral cavity or where patient needs to be given muscle relaxants and controlled breathing. It is always passed with direct laryngoscopy under vision after anesthetizing the patient, except in cases, where patients are unable to open mouth, e.g. temporomandibular (TM) joint ankylosis or when a difficult intubation is expected.

- *Sizes:* 2, 2.5, 3, 3.5, 4,……10, 10.5 (internal diameter in mm).

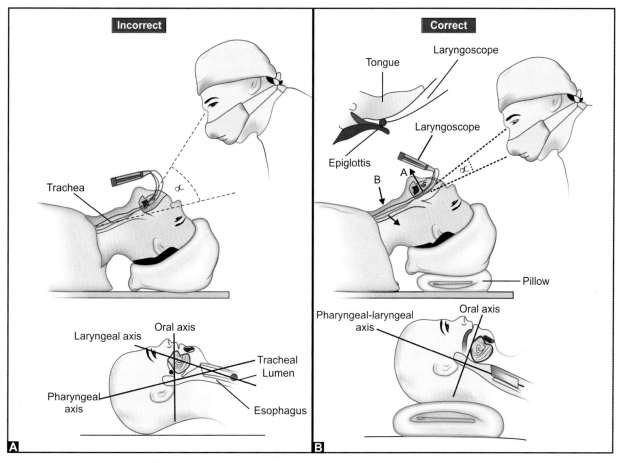

Figs 14.8A and B: Incorrect and correct procedures for laryngoscopy

Endotracheal tubes may be plain or cuffed. They can be made up of plastic (generally PVC), red rubber or latex. They may be disposable or reusable. The cuffs may be of low volume-high pressure or high volume-low pressure types. Endotracheal tubes may be introduced orally or nasally. When a nasal tube is required, one designed for the purpose is more appropriate. These are available in both disposable and reusable forms, and are characterized by a longer bevel giving a softer tip, a streamlined cuff and no side port.

When the anesthesiologist is not in the immediate proximity to the patient's head, the precurved disposable oral (south pole) or nasal (north pole), ring Adair Ellwyn (RAE) tubes have been found to be useful. This type permits the breathing circuit to be led away from the patient and minimizes the potential for kinking and obstruction under the drapes, as it presents a low profile, while emerging from oral or nasal cavity. Other precurved endotracheal tubes are Oxford (L-shaped) tubes used for cleft-palate surgery

and Tehran (S-shaped) tubes used nasally for difficult intubation, especially in cases of TM joint ankylosis or retrognathic/micrognathic jaw surgeries.

Another variety called armored tubes are made of latex and embedded (reinforced) with spiral rings made of nylon or metal (flexometallic) and are nonkinkable. They may be used orally or nasally. A metal or plastic stylet is required to be used during intubation for oral route but not for nasal route. For laser surgery various 'laser-resistant' tubes are available. Each has its own advantages and disadvantages.

Airways

The purpose of introducing an airway is to lift the tongue and epiglottis away from the posterior pharyngeal wall and prevent them from obstructing the space above the larynx. It is therefore useful in maintaining a patent airway in any unconscious or heavily sedated patient, where tongue fall occurs due

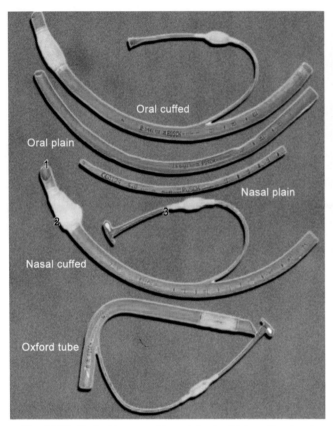

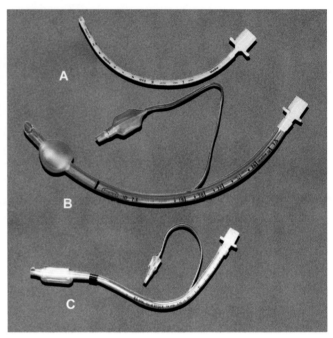

Fig. 14.9C: Disposable endotracheal tubes: (A) Pediatric oral uncuffed tube, (B) Nasal cuffed tube and (C) Oral cuffed tube

Fig. 14.9A: Red rubber reusable endotracheal tubes. Nasal and oral tubes. Parts of a tube: (1) Bevel, (2) Cuff, (3) Pilot balloon

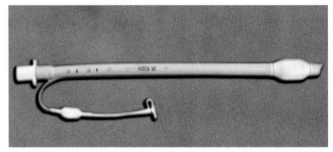

Fig. 14.9D: Flexometallic (armoured) tube

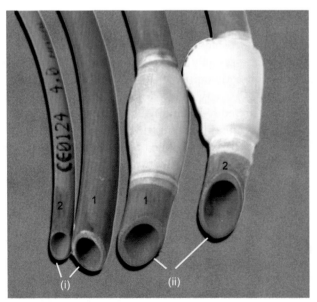

Fig. 14.9B: Bevels of reusable endotracheal tubes. (i) Plain and (ii) Cuffed: (1) Oral tube, (2) Nasal tube

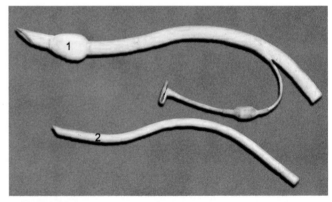

Fig. 14.9E: Tehran tubes for difficult intubations: (1) Cuffed tube, (2) Plain tube

to relaxation of the muscles of the floor of the mouth and pharynx. It is made up of metal, rubber or plastic. It can be passed orally (oropharyngeal airway) or nasally (nasopharyngeal airway).

Oropharyngeal (Oral) Airway (Placed from Lips to Pharynx)

- *Parts:* Flange, bite portion, air/suction channel (curved portion)
- *Sizes:* 1, 2, 3, 4.

The bite portion lies between the teeth/lips and the flange lies outside the lips. The flange prevents an airway from slipping into the mouth and it also serves as a means to fix the airway in place. The pharyngeal end rests between the posterior wall of the oropharynx and the base of the tongue, and by pressure along the base of the tongue, pulls the epiglottis forward.

In addition to maintaining an open airway, it may be used to obtain a better mask fit, to prevent a patient from biting and occluding an orotracheal tube, to protect the tongue from being bitten, to facilitate oropharyngeal suctioning through the air or suction channel or to provide oxygen through the same channel.

Methods of insertion: There are two methods. After lubrication with a jelly, it is introduced between the teeth (upper and lower incisors) after opening the jaw with one hand.

1. With concave side facing the upper lip, then advanced gently till the junction of the bite portion and the curved section is near the incisors, the airway is then rotated through 180 degrees and slipped behind the tongue, so that it lies posterior to the tongue.
2. With concave side toward the tongue, while depressing and pushing forward the tongue with a tongue depressor (tongue blade), the airway is advanced and gently allowed to slide behind the tongue.

Pharyngeal and laryngeal reflexes should be depressed before placement of an oral airway to avoid coughing or laryngospasm. Unlike other maneuvers to maintain a patent airway, including chin lift, jaw thrust, and tracheal intubation, insertion of an oral airway does not cause movement of the cervical spine. Selection of the correct size is very important, as too small an airway may cause the tongue to kink and push part of it against the roof of the mouth, causing obstruction, and too large an airway may cause obstruction by displacing the

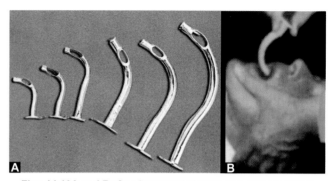

Figs 14.10A and B: Oropharyngeal airways and method of their insertion

epiglottis posteriorly and may traumatize the larynx. The correct size can be estimated by holding the airway next to the patient's mouth in such a way that the tip of an airway rests cephalad to the angle of the mandible. The correct size will allow to feel the expiratory blast (flow) while the airway is *in situ* (Figs 14.10A and B).

Nasopharyngeal (Nasal) Airway (Placed from the Nose to the Pharynx)

- *Parts:* Flange or a movable disc attached to a tube
- *Sizes (diameter)*
  - 7.0/7.5 for adult males
  - 6.5/7.0 for adult females
  - Same/one size smaller than an appropriate endotracheal tube for children.

It resembles a shortened endotracheal tube with a flange or a movable disc at the proximal end to prevent its migration into the nose. An ordinary endotracheal tube which is cut short, can also be used as a nasopharyngeal airway. A safety pin is used as a flange. The flange lies outside the nostril and the tube in the nasal cavity. The pharyngeal end of the tube may be straight or beveled and it lies below the base of the tongue, but above the epiglottis (Figs 14.11 and 14.12).

Nasal airways are used after oral, pharyngeal or maxillofacial surgery to keep the airway patent or to maintain the airway and administer anesthesia during conservative dentistry. It is preferable in patients with loose teeth or in patients with trauma or pathology of the oral cavity or when patient cannot open his mouth.

Method of insertion: It should be lubricated thoroughly along its entire length. Each nostril should be inspected for its size and patency. Vasoconstrictors may be applied before insertion to reduce bleeding. The airway is held in the hand on the same side, as it is to be inserted with the

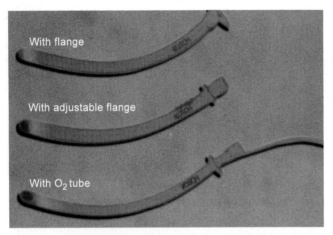

Fig. 14.11: Nasopharyngeal tubes (airways)

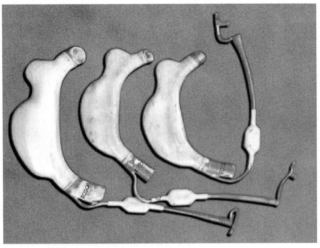

Fig. 14.12: Special cuffed nasopharyngeal airways

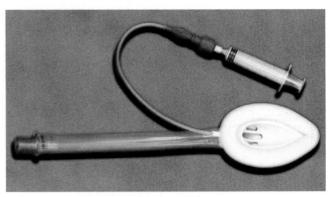

Fig. 14.13: Laryngeal mask airway

bevel against the septum and inserted perpendicular, in line with the nasal passage. It is then gently advanced posteriorly. If the resistance is felt during insertion, the other nostril or the smaller size should be used.

A nasal airway is better tolerated in the patient with intact airway reflexes than an oral airway. The airway length may be advanced by sliding it in or out till the pharyngeal end rests below the base of the tongue but above the epiglottis. If it is inserted too much inside, laryngeal reflexes may be stimulated and if it is too much outside, airway obstruction may not be relieved. The correct placement will allow to feel the expiratory blast (flow).

Contraindications to the use of a nasopharyngeal airway include patients with hemorrhagic disorders, coagulopathy, a history of epistaxis requiring medical treatment or patients on anticoagulants; or patients with basilar skull fracture, and any pathology, sepsis or deformity of the nose or nasopharynx.

Laryngeal Mask Airway (LMA)

Laryngeal mask airway (LMA) is a device which is midway between mask and endotracheal tube. Just as mask makes an airtight seal around the face, LMA makes an airtight low-pressure seal around laryngeal inlet after inflation of the cuff (Fig. 14.13).
- *Parts:* Mask, tube at an angle of 30 degrees, black line on tube to face upper incisors and pilot balloon.
- *Versions:* Plain, reinforced, and intubating, pre-sale LMA.
- *Sizes:* 1, 1.5, 2, 2.5, 3, 4, 5.

It is to be autoclaved before every use. Deeper level of anesthesia is required for insertion to avoid laryngospasm. It can be passed with/without use of muscle relaxants.

Method of insertion: With patient in position as for laryngoscopy and with cuff deflated, it is held like a pen and with its aperture facing anteriorly, it is pressed against hard palate and advanced till it goes beyond the base of the tongue. Cuff is inflated and then connected to the breathing circuit.

Advantages
- No laryngoscopy required
- Less postoperative sore throat
- Useful in failed intubation to ventilate the patient
- Intubating LMA is useful in intubating patients with difficult airway.

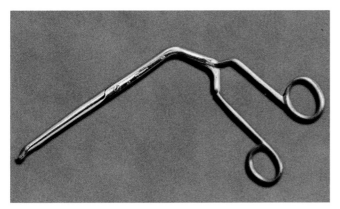

Fig. 14.14: Magill's forceps

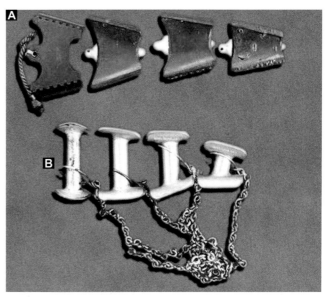

Figs 14.15A and B: Mouth props: (A) Rubber, (B) Metallic

Disadvantages
• Does not prevent aspiration
• Can cause gastric distention.

Magill's Forceps

Magill's forceps is an instrument, which is most often used for guiding an endotracheal tube, from the pharynx into the larynx during nasal intubation. It is also used to pack the throat with a roller gauze during oral and pharyngeal surgery, to pick up a broken or dislodged tooth lying in the oral cavity or to pass a Ryles (nasogastric) tube. It is L-shaped and it has no catch. It is available in two sizes—adult and pediatric (Fig. 14.14).

Mouth Prop (Bite Block)

The mouth prop is a small rounded or rectangular piece of instrument made up of metal, plastic or rubber (Figs 14.15A and B).

A mouth prop is placed between the occlusal surfaces of upper and lower molar teeth, following introduction of an endotracheal tube to prevent them from occluding an endotracheal tube and to avoid biting the tongue and to keep the mouth open for suctioning. As a mouth prop/bite block does not extend into the pharynx, it is usually less irritating than an oral airway. A variety of bite blocks have been developed. Some have a channel for endotracheal tube passage; some have string, so that it can be easily retrieved. The curved portion of an oral airway can be removed or shortened, modifying the remaining portion as a bite block. A barrel of a plastic syringe fitted around the endotracheal tube or a roll of gauze piece can be used as a makeshift bite block.

The mouth prop is generally used by the surgeons for many surgical procedures to keep the mouth open or stretch open the already relaxed jaw. It is also used to forcibly open a clenched jaw (trismus), or when patient's airway is at stake (blood or vomitus in the pharynx), or to place an airway, when patient's breathing is obstructed or when the patient is biting on an endotracheal tube.

Resuscitation Bag

Resuscitation bag is an assembly of equipment consisting of a self-inflating bag, a non-rebreathing valve and a facemask (Figs 14.16 and 14.17). As it is useful for ventilating a patient in emergency situation, it should always be available in the operation theatre as handy as possible. If any problem occurs with anesthesia machine or a breathing system, which cannot be diagnosed or corrected quickly, a resuscitation bag will allow the user to ventilate the patient with room air (with or without oxygen) till the problem is solved. It is also useful and should be available during patient transport. It can also be used for administering anesthesia in the absence of an anesthesia machine, e.g. in rural set-up or field situations.

There are varieties of resuscitation bags available in the market. Some have a reservoir bag for oxygen; the others have small-corrugated tubing for the same purpose. Each of them has a nipple for connecting an oxygen source. They are generally reusable, but even disposable resuscitation bags are also available.

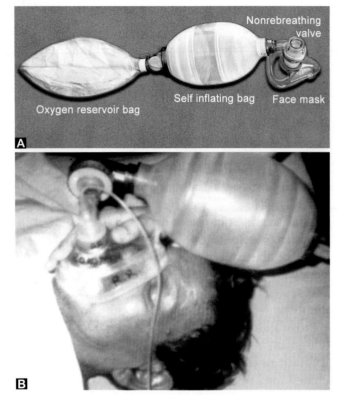

Figs 14.16A and B: Resuscitation bag and its use on the patient

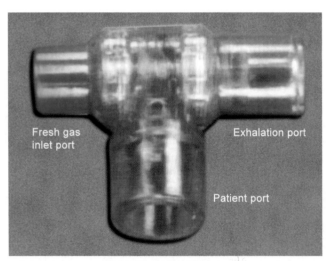

Fig. 14.17: Nonrebreathing valve

- *Sizes:* Three sizes are available; for infant, child and adult.

After proper positioning of the patient, the mask has to be placed on the patient's face and the bag can be intermittently compressed and released while watching the inflation and deflation of the patient's chest. The exhalation blast can be heard or felt from the expiratory port of the nonrebreathing valve.

■ MONITORING EQUIPMENT

Under anesthesia, it is the duty of an anesthesiologist to maintain the vital parameters of the patient within normal limits. Hence, it becomes his moral responsibility not only to monitor vital parameters of the patient, but also to diagnose and treat the conditions which make them deviate from their normal range. Not all, but few of the important monitors that are helpful for this purpose, are discussed below in brief.

Blood Pressure Monitor

Blood pressure monitor is available in various forms:
- Simple sphygmomanometer/aneroid dial
- Noninvasive automatic blood pressure monitor (NIBP)
- Invasive direct arterial blood pressure monitor (IABP)

Blood pressure is generally monitored on the right or left upper arm. It is necessary to monitor patient's blood pressure as most of the anesthetic agents are vasodilators and/or myocardial depressants, giving rise to hypotension.

Cardioscope

Cardioscope not only allows to monitor the electrocardiogram (ECG) of the patient, but it also allows to monitor patient's heart rate, rhythm, the type of arrhythmias and ST-segment changes (important to diagnose myocardial ischemia) (Fig. 14.18). It has minimum three leads and maximum 12 leads. Generally, a three lead ECG is monitored under anesthesia. These leads are attached on the anterior chest wall, one near the right shoulder, one near the left shoulder and one near the lower end of sternum on the right side. Drugs used for anesthesia have effects on rate, rhythm and contractility of the heart and hence it is vital to monitor these parameters under anesthesia. It also alarms the anesthesiologist about cardiac arrest well in advance as generally slowing of the heart rhythm or intractable arrhythmias occur before cardiac arrest. Cardioscope with a defibrillator is useful as it allows to defibrillate the heart on the spot, if the need arises.

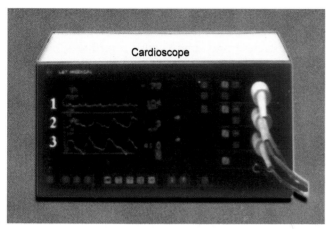

Fig. 14.18: Triple channel monitor: (1) Electrocardiogram (ECG), (2) Direct arterial pressure, (3) Central venous pressure

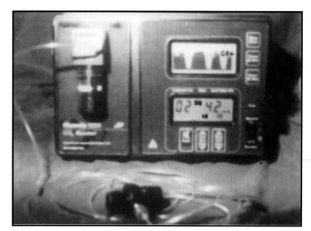

Fig. 14.20: Capnograph (ETCO$_2$ monitor)

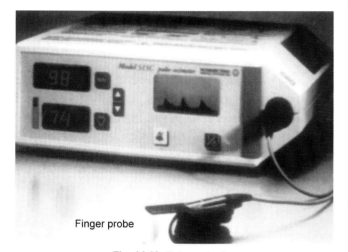

Fig. 14.19: Pulse oximeter

Pulse Oximeter

Pulse oximeter is noninvasive equipment that allows to monitor continuously the oxygen saturation of the patient and also the heart rate. It has a small probe which can be attached on any of the fingers or toes or on the ear lobule. Hypoxia can occur under anesthesia if the patient breathes an hypoxic mixture of gases or the breathing circuit gets disconnected and it is not noticed in time. It is important to know that hypoxia can lead to brain death, coma and even cardiac arrest. Pulse oximeter is therefore a useful monitor to prevent such complications and protect the patient from such catastrophe (Fig. 14.19).

Capnometer/Capnographs

Basically capnometer is an equipment that continuously records the carbon dioxide tension (in mm Hg or %) of the expired gas mixture (only numerical values as in capnometer or numerical value with graphical recording as in capnograph) (Fig. 14.20). It is popularly known as an End Tidal CO$_2$ monitor (ETCO$_2$). It is a noninvasive monitor having a probe or an adapter that can be attached to an endotracheal tube, a face-mask or a nasal catheter. It allows the anesthesiologist to monitor whether the patient is breathing adequately (if on spontaneous breathing) or whether the patient is being ventilated adequately (if he is on controlled breathing). In addition, it also allows the anesthesiologist to know many things, e.g. if the endotracheal tube has inadvertently entered the esophagus, the breathing circuit has got disconnected, the breathing circuit is functioning well and not allowing too much rebreathing, etc.

Respiratory Gas Monitor

Respiratory gas monitor is an equipment that allows the anesthesiologist to monitor the contents and the concentration of the inspired as well as expired gas mixture and thereby the concentration of the anesthetic gases, oxygen and carbon dioxide of the inspired gases. It is a noninvasive monitor having a probe or an adapter that can be attached to an endotracheal tube, a face-mask or a nasal catheter. This helps preventing delivery of a hypoxic gas mixture and also high concentration of anesthetic gases. It is something more than a capnometer and obviates the need to use a capnometer.

OXYGEN THERAPY EQUIPMENT

It is a well-known fact that patients under general anesthesia as well as in the postoperative period are prone to hypoxia due to some specific reasons. Under anesthesia, it is a routine practice to give a mixture of anesthetic gases containing at least 30 percent oxygen. Postoperatively, it is very easy to give an oxygen enriched room air via a T-piece system (one of the breathing systems) to those patients who have endotracheal tube *in situ*. However, for those patients, breathing spontaneously without having face-mask or endotracheal tube *in situ*, it is very important to have equipment that can deliver oxygen enriched air. For both type of patients, oxygen cylinder and oxygen flow/meter are needed. For those having no endotracheal tube *in situ*, either an oxygen mask or a catheter is required (Figs 14.21 and 14.22).

Oxygen Cylinder

Oxygen cylinders are available in various sizes. They are black in color with a shoulder painted white. Those meant to be used on anesthesia machines have a flushed valve whereas those used in the wards have a bull-nose

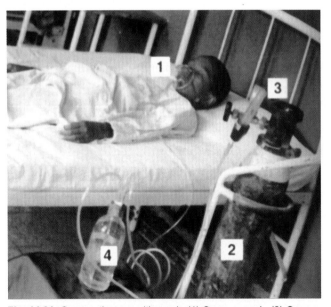

Fig. 14.21: Oxygen therapy with mask: (1) Oxygen mask, (2) Oxygen cylinder, (3) Oxygen flowmeter, (4) Wolfe's bottle for humidifying oxygen

valve. It is not possible to use a flushed valve cylinder in the wards. On the ward cylinder, oxygen flowmeter can be attached and there is also a facility to attach a humidifier to the flowmeter.

Oxygen Flowmeter

Oxygen flowmeter allows the operator to deliver a desired flow of oxygen to the patient. Generally, 3 to 4 liters per minute of flow is given, but it varies from patient to patient, depending upon the type of oxygen delivery system (poly mask, venti mask, nasal cannula, nasal catheter, T-piece, etc.), type of surgery done, age of the patient and general condition of the patient.

Oxygen Mask

These are generally facemasks of different varieties. Poly mask is a semioval-shaped mask, available in two sizes, for children and for adults. It is a loosely fitting mask around the mouth and nose through which moderate flow of oxygen (3 to 6 liters) can be delivered. Too little oxygen flow will allow rebreathing and too high flow may obstruct exhalation. Oxygen percentage cannot be judged and not more than 35 percent can ever be given. Venti masks are designed to work on Venturi principle. Here the delivered oxygen flows through a jet and entrains room air from the surrounding entrainment port while it approaches the patient. Various flow rates of oxygen with its approximate delivered oxygen concentrations are written on the device and hence it becomes easy for the operator to choose the mask and deliver the desired concentration of oxygen.

There are some oxygen facemasks that have a reservoir bag for oxygen, and some have even directional valves. Recommended flow rate is 10 to 15 liters/min of oxygen. With reservoir bag, one can deliver up to 65 percent oxygen and if they have directional valves also, then one can deliver even up to 90 percent oxygen.

Nasal Catheter/Prongs

Nasal prongs are the most simplest, most commonly used and easily available devices (Figs 14.22A and B). But, not more than 1 to 3 liters of oxygen per minute can be delivered, as high flow makes the patient uncomfortable due to wheezing sound and a feeling of dry mouth. If a nasal catheter is used, its tip should be advanced up to the fold of the soft palate. If it is introduced too far, it can produce gaseous distension

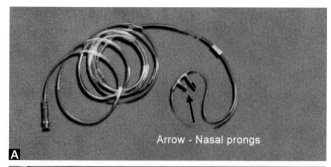

Arrow - Nasal prongs

A

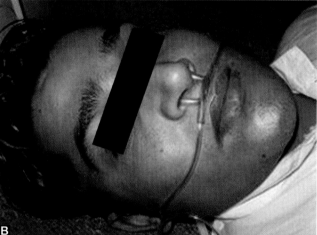

B

Figs 14.22A and B: (A) Nasal prongs for oxygen therapy, (B) Combined (Oxygen therapy + ETCO$_2$ monitoring) nasal prongs

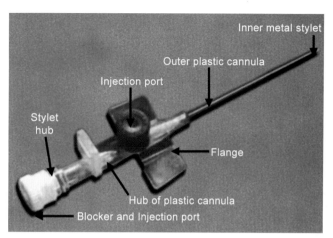

Fig. 14.23: Intravenous cannula

of the stomach. Nasal prongs (two short plastic prongs that fit into the external nares) are preferred by some as they are comfortable for the patients. Concentration of delivered oxygen is generally low and can never be judged. Generally with oxygen flow rate of 1 to 2 liters/min, these devices provide 24 to 28 percent oxygen.

INTRAVENOUS INFUSION EQUIPMENT

Infusion equipment includes intravenous cannulation devices like scalp needles and cannulae (available from small-25G to big-16G sizes), three ways, infusion sets and infusion fluids.

Scalp Needle

Scalp needle is a modified hypodermic needle. To the stainless steel needle (a beveled needle without a hub), a plastic flange and a thin tube has been attached. At the end of the tube is a port (hub) to which a syringe nozzle, a three-way or an infusion set can be attached. When nothing is to be injected, the port can be kept closed by a

blocker, which is attached to the port. The flange allows better fixation of the needle to the hand and the tubing makes injection of drugs comfortable and painless for the patient, as one does not manipulate the fixation site on the vein while injecting the drug. However, when patient moves the cannulation site, especially on the joints, there is a possibility of counter puncturing of the vein, as the stiff, sharp metal needle cannot mould to the changing counter of the cannulation site.

Intravenous Cannula

Intravenous (IV) cannula is a plastic cannula with a hub into which fits a metal stylet, which has a bevel at one end, and a hub at the other end (Fig. 14.23). While puncturing the vein, the entire set (with the beveled end of the stylet) enters the vein. As soon as the stylet punctures the vein, blood is observed entering the hub of the stylet. The whole set is then further advanced about 1 to 2 mm so that even the cannula enters the vein, the stylet is then kept steady and only the cannula is advanced further into the vein. The stylet is then removed and only the plastic cannula remains in the vein. This device is more useful and comfortable as compared to hypodermic needle or a scalp needle, as it prevents counter puncturing of the vein while taking an intravenous line and also post insertion when patient moves the site of cannulation.

Bivalve (Three Way)

Bivalve or three-way is a device that is attached to the needle before attaching an infusion set. This device has three ports. One is attached to the IV needle, one to the

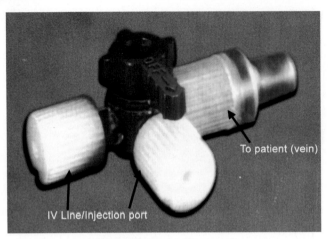

Fig. 14.24: Bivalve (three way)

infusion set and the third port remains free, which can be closed or blocked when not in use. It is this third port, which allows administration of drugs or any other fluid either simultaneously, or singularly depending upon which way the shaft of the three-way has been turned (Fig. 14.24).

Infusion Set

Infusion set consists of a plastic tubing having one sharp end that can enter the infusion bottle (fluid) and the other that will fit the hub of a needle, cannula or a three-way. Closer to the end that fits a bottle, in a chamber called Murphy's chamber, which has a dropper through which the infusion fluid drips into Murphy's chamber. This chamber should be half-filled with air and half with the infusion fluid. This will allow one to see the rate at which the fluid is given to the patient. This can be an ordinary dropper or a microdropper. With ordinary dropper, 15 drops make 1 ml (cc); while with a microdropper 50 drops make one ml of a solution. Micro drip set is useful in children and for continuous infusion of some drugs. The set has a drip controller, which allows on/off as well as the drip rate to be set.

Before connecting the set to the needle, the fluid should be allowed to run so as to fill the entire set and half of Murphy's chamber with the fluid so that no air enters the venous line.

Intravenous Fluids

A variety of fluids are available. The ones, which are generally used under anesthesia are: 5 percent dextrose (glucose), normal saline (0.9% sodium chloride solution) and Ringer's lactate solution. These are called crystalloids. Others known as colloids, e.g. Haemaccel, hetastarch, etc. are used when blood loss needs to be replaced and blood is not available.

15 Pharmacology of Commonly Used Anesthetic Drugs

Induction of anesthesia is usually accomplished by either intravenous (IV) route or the inhalational (gaseous) route, however, in specific circumstances it may be administered by intramuscular, oral and rectal route. Intravenous route is commonly used for older children and adults. Inhalational route is commonly used for smaller children who are scared of needle pricks. Drug which has short duration of action is commonly used for dental anesthesia as most of the cases are day-care patients.

INTRAVENOUS (IV) INDUCTION AGENTS

Drugs used for intravenous (IV) induction produce full anesthesia in one arm-brain circulation time. IV drugs should be given slowly to minimize adverse cardiovascular effects like bradycardia and hypotension. They also cause respiratory depression and sometimes even apnoea. Recovery is rapid with IV induction drugs due to rapid distribution of these drugs to fat and areolar tissues leading to fall in serum concentration. Theatre pollution is avoided with IV induction drugs. These drugs can also be used for maintenance of anesthesia by infusion technique, i.e. *total intravenous anesthesia* (TIVA). Lower induction doses are required in the

premedicated patients, severe anemia, malnourished patient, liver and kidney diseases. Side effects of these drugs get exaggerated in these patients. *Contraindications* for IV induction agent are airway obstruction, TM joint ankylosis, submucous fibrosis and predicted difficult intubation (In cases where oral opening is not adequate for laryngoscopy) (Table 15.1).

INHALATIONAL INDUCTION AGENTS

Inhalational induction is slower. It is dependent on the inspired anesthetic agent and its concentration, alveolar ventilation, the blood-gas partition coefficient and cardiac output. If solubility in blood (blood-gas partition coefficient) is less, then anesthetic agent is more potent and onset of anesthesia is faster. To be acceptable, the smell of the anesthetic agent should be pleasant and not too pungent. They are commonly used for maintenance of anesthesia. To use inhalational agent, carrier gas is required, e.g. oxygen or oxygen and air. Vaporizers are required to give inhalational agent. *The classical description of the stages of general anesthesia refers to the clinical changes observed during ether anesthesia. With the newer anesthetic agents, these signs are not observed due to speed of induction and loss of consciousness.*

	Penthothal	Methohexitone	Propofol	Ketamine
	Table 15.1: Comparison of action of IV induction drugs			
Group	Thiobarbiturate	Oxybarbiturate	Alkyl phenol	Phencyclidine
• Respiratory system	Depresses	Depresses	Depresses	Stable
• Cardiovascular system	Depresses	Depresses	Depresses and hypotension	Stable or increase in heart rate and BP
• Pain on injection	—	Occurs	Occurs	—
• Thrombophlebitis	—	Occurs	Occurs	—
• Central nervous system excitability	—	Convulsion may be there	—	Convulsion may be there
• Salivation	Less	Less	Less	High
• Laryngeal reflexes	Activated	Activated	Depressed	Preserved in lighter plane
• Recovery	Slow, somnolence	Rapid and clear	Rapid and clear	Hallucination, nausea, vomiting
• Contraindication	Porphyria	Convulsion	Egg allergy	Convulsion, hypertension, heart disease
Doses—adult	4–5 mg/kg	1–2 mg/kg	1–2.5 mg/kg	1–2 mg/kg

Minimum Alveolar Concentration

The minimum alveolar concentration (MAC) of an anesthetic agent is to produce lack of reflex response to skin incision in 50 percent of patients.

Volatile anesthetic agents are rapidly removed from the body via lungs and little evidence of metabolism can be demonstrated following short exposure (Table 15.2).

Ideal Inhalational Agent

The following properties are desirable in an inhalational anesthetic agent (Table 15.3):
- It must be possible to obtain pure compound.
- It should be stable (it should not be broken down by light or alkali).
- It should not undergo metabolism in the body and should be free of organ toxicity.
- It should not form flammable mixture with air, oxygen or nitrous oxide.
- It should have low blood gas partition coefficient.
- It should be reasonably potent, allowing the use of high concentration of oxygen.
- No long term adverse effect, if breathed in low concentration for a prolonged period (occupational hazard to theatre personnel).
- It should be pleasant to smell.
- Cardiovascular side effect should be minimal.
- It should possess analgesic property, in addition to hypnotic property.
- It should be readily reversible.

- No teratogenic effect should be there.
- It should not be carcinogenic.

Ether (CH₃CH₂-O-CH₂CH₃)

Ether (CH_3CH_2-O-CH_2CH_3)

It is known as diethyl ether. Originally prepared in 1540 by Valerius Cordus, who called it sweet oil of vitriol. It is a colorless volatile liquid of molecular weight 74, specific gravity of 0.719 and boiling point 35°C. Its blood gas partition coefficient is 15, MAC for anesthesia is 3.04. Ether vapor is inflammable in air and explosive with oxygen. Therefore, it cannot be used when the cautery is being used for surgical procedures. It is largely unaltered in the body, 85 to 90 percent being eliminated by lungs. The clinical signs of stages of anesthesia described by Guedel were during ether anesthesia.

It stimulates the sympathetic system yielding to increase the heart rate and to depress the vagus nerve. Blood pressure falls in the deeper planes of anesthesia. A functioning of sympathetic nervous system is essential for maintenance of normal blood pressure during ether anesthesia. Respiratory movements first increase due to stimulation of respiratory center and later on it decreases as the anesthesia deepens. It stimulates salivation, therefore atropine premedication is essential. Its vapor is irritant to respiratory tract producing cough and laryngeal spasm. On induction, it induces analgesia followed by excitement and then anesthesia. It increases the CSF pressure. Blood sugar level rises with ether anesthesia, therefore it should be used cautiously in

Table 15.2: Clinical signs of anesthesia (specially with ether anesthesia)

Stage	Eyes			Respiration			Airway reflexes abolished	CVS		Muscle tone	Remarks
	Reflexes abolished	Pupil size	Movement	Rate	Muscle tone (Inter-costal)	Muscle tone (Diaphragm)		Heart rate	Blood pressure		
I Analgesia	None	N	N	N	N	N	None	↑	N	N	Good for venipuncture, labor pains, dental analgesia
II Excitement	Eyelash, eyelid	Dilated	Divergent	Irregular	↑	↑	Swallowing	↑↑	↑	↑↑	Tachycardia, tachypnoea, aspiration risk +
III Surgical planes											
Plane 1	Conjunctival	N	N	N	N	N	Vomiting and pharyngeal	↑	N	↑	Risk of aspiration +
Plane 2	Corneal	N	N	↓	↓	N	Laryngeal	N	↓	↓	Risk of aspiration + airway obstruction due to tongue fall
Plane 3	Pupillary light	Dilated	None	↓↓	↓↓	↓	Carinal	↓	↓↓	↓↓	Ideal to intubate, surgical stage needs IPPR
Plane 4	All	Fully dilated	None	Nil	↓↓↓	↓↓↓	All	↑ or ↓	↓↓↓	↓↓↓	Respiratory arrest and CVS collapse
IV Death	Respiratory arrest Medullary paralysis (Due to overdosage of an anesthetic drug)										Active cardiopulmonary resuscitation

N—normal, ↑—increase, ↑↑—moderate increase, ↑↑↑—significant increase, ↓—decrease, ↓↓—moderate decrease, ↓↓↓—significant decrease

Agents	MAC	Blood/gas (Partition coefficient)	Boiling Point °C	Remarks
Ether	1.92	12	36	Flammable, explosive, slow induction recovery, increased salivation, PONV +, irritant to RS
Halothane	0.75	2.3	50	Myocardial depression, arrhythmias, hepatitis, pleasant induction
Enflurane	1.68	1.9	56	Epileptogenic
Isoflurane	1.15	1.4	48	Stable CVS, pungent odor, coughing salivation +, PONV +
Sevoflurane	2.00	0.69	58	Rapid, pleasant induction and rapid recovery, good for day cases, no PONV
Desflurane	6.00	0.42	23	Irritant to RS, unstable at room temperature
Nitrous oxide	1.04	0.47	−89	Non-irritant, analgesic, amnesic, PONV+

Table 15.3: Differences between commonly used inhalational agents

diabetic patients. Postoperative nausea and vomiting occurs in 50 percent of the patients. It can be administered either by open ether technique, face-mask anesthesia or via endotracheal tube using anesthesia machine. It has a wide margin of safety.

Ethyl Chloride (C₂H₅Cl)

Prepared by Valentine in 17th century. For many years it was used only as local analgesic. Carlson of Gothenburg, Sweden used it as local spray to ease the pain of dental extraction in 1894 and succeeded unexpectedly in producing general anesthesia as the vapor was inhaled. It is a clear fluid with ethereal odor. Boiling point is 12.5°C, mol wt is 64. It is eliminated unchanged from the lungs. The safety margin is small owing to its low volatility and relatively low blood gas partition coefficient (2.0). Its actions are decreased in the heart rate due to vagal stimulation, hence atropine premedication is a must. Heart muscles are directly depressed and cardiac arrest/respiratory arrest has been reported. Adrenaline increases myocardial irritability during ethyl chloride anesthesia. Postoperative nausea and vomiting is a common feature. It is not used nowadays as there is possibility of potential danger of cardiac arrest.

Halothane (Fluothane)

It is synthesized in 1951. It is 2-bromo-2-chloro-1,1,1-trifluoroethane. It is a colorless liquid with molecular weight 197, boiling point of 50 degree C, blood gas partition coefficient is 2.5 and MAC of 0.87 percent. It

is neither flammable nor explosive. As an anesthetic agent, it is 4 to 5 times potent than diethyl ether. It has a characteristic odor, pleasant to smell and it is nonirritant to respiratory tract. For induction of anesthesia 2 to 4 percent concentration is required and 1 to 2 percent for maintenance of anesthesia. Blood pressure falls in proportion to the concentration of the vapor inhaled. Hypotension is due to sympathetic blockade, central vasomotor depression and direct depression of myocardium and smooth muscles of blood vessels. Ganglionic blocking drugs must be given with extreme caution during halothane anesthesia. Increased myocardial excitability can lead to ventricular premature contraction, tachycardia and ventricular fibrillation. Factors which increase the likelihood of arrhythmias are hypercarbia, sensory stimulation in light plane of anesthesia and injection of adrenaline. Cardiac arrest has been reported following adrenaline infiltration during halothane anesthesia. Bradycardia may occur along with hypotension. There is increase in CSF pressure and respiratory center is depressed. Respiratory rate increases and depth of respiration decreases with halothane anesthesia, it causes bronchodilation, therefore can be used safely in patients with bronchospasm, emphysema and chronic bronchitis.

It causes moderate relaxation of skeletal muscles, hence requirement of nonpolarizing muscle relaxant is decreased. If used in obstetric patient, it causes uterine atony and postpartum hemorrhage. Postoperative nausea, vomiting is not severe as compared to ether anesthesia. Shivering and tremors have been reported postoperatively.

It can be used as induction agent in children, part of balanced anesthesia technique for maintenance of anesthesia. It can be used with simple vaporizer like Goldman vaporizer or highly specific vaporizer like fluotec, which gives exact concentration of vapor at any temperature, pressure and gas flows (liters/min).

Nitrous Oxide

Nitrous oxide is the only inorganic gas used for anesthesia. It was first prepared by Priestley in 1772. Anesthetic properties were suggested by Sir Humphrey Davey in 1799. Colton demonstrated its effects to Horace Wells in 1844, who used it in dentistry and had one of its own tooth extracted painlessly.

It is manufactured by heating ammonium nitrate in an iron retort to 240°C.

$$NH_4NO_3 \rightleftharpoons 2 H_2O + N_2O$$

The issuing gas is collected, purified and compressed into metal cylinders at 51 atm (750 lbs/sq. inch). Impurities in nitrous oxide = nitric oxide and nitrogen dioxide.

Both these substances are toxic to body and can cause disturbances in breathing and circulation leading to cardiac arrest.

Physical properties: Colorless, odorless gas, boiling point = –89°C. Blood gas-partition co-efficient is 0.47. Neither flammable nor explosive, but supports combustion of other agents.

Pharmacological actions: It is good analgesic but not potent anesthetic. It does not potentiate other agents but the effects are simply additive. It is eliminated unchanged mostly via lungs. It is stable and unaffected by soda lime. Respiratory effects are decreased tidal volume and respiratory rate increases. There is a decrease in ventilatory response to CO_2. Cardiovascular effects are myocardial depression and increase in pulmonary vascular resistance. Closed cavity pressure may increase because it is highly diffusible gas, e.g. middle ear surgery, bowel obstruction.

Side effects: Nitrous oxide is usually regarded as nontoxic anesthetic agent provided it is administered with sufficient concentration of oxygen. Sometimes it causes postoperative nausea and vomiting. Its chronic use causes bone marrow depression, vitamin B_{12} and folate metabolic disturbances. It should be avoided in first trimester of pregnancy to avoid its teratogenic effect. It augments respiratory depressant effect of thiopentone and opiates.

Premixed N_2O and O_2: Pressurized nitrous oxide and oxygen (50:50%) at a maximum cylinder pressure of 2000 lbs/sq. inch is available for analgesic purposes. The apparatus is known as Entonox apparatus. It is used in dental anesthesia, obstetric analgesia and relief of pain during dressing of surgical wound.

Zones of N_2O:
Four zones of N_2O anesthesia have been described:
1. *Moderate analgesia:* (6-25%) Nitrous oxide inhaled. Twenty-five percent of nitrous oxide is more potent than 10 mg morphine.
2. *Dissociative analgesia:* (26-45%) Thirty percent gives rise to psychological symptoms and lack of ability to concentrate. This is more severe at 45 percent concentration.
3. *Analgesic anesthesia:* (46-65%) Near complete analgesia. Patient may respond to commands.
4. *Light anesthesia:* (66-80%) Complete analgesia and amnesia, not possible to communicate with the patient.

▌ MUSCLE RELAXANTS

A muscle relaxant is used to facilitate tracheal intubation at the start of anesthesia. During the maintenance of anesthesia muscle relaxation may be required to facilitate surgery and intermittent positive pressure ventilation (IPPV).

Muscle relaxant can be either of the following:

Depolarizing: Depolarizes the neuromuscular end plate, e.g. suxamethonium (Scoline). Depolarizing muscle relaxant does not require reversal agent. It gets metabolized with pseudocholinesterase enzyme and its effects wear off. It is rapidly acting and has short duration of action.

Nondepolarizing: Competitive antagonism at neuro-muscular junction, e.g. pancuronium, vacuronium, atracurium and rocuronium. Nondepolarizing muscle relaxant requires reversal with anticholinesterase drugs (Table 15.4).

Reversal of Anesthesia

The only component of anesthesia that is truly reversible at the conclusion of general anesthesia is the effect of the nondepolarizing muscle relaxant.

The timing of the last dose of muscle relaxant is important and if it is too near to the conclusion of

| Table 15.4: Muscle relaxants, doses and duration of action* ||||
Muscle relaxants	Initial dose (mg/kg)	Duration of action (min)	Remarks
Depolarizing			
Suxamethonium	1–2	5–10	Muscle pains+, hyperkalemia, arrhythmia, prolonged action in patients with deficiency of pseudocholinesterase enzyme
Nondepolarizing			
Pancuronium	0.1	20–40	Tachycardia, hypertension, avoid in renal failure
Vecuronium	0.1	10–20	Bradycardia, avoid in renal failure
Atracurium	0.5	20–40	Histamine release may be there, metabolized by self-degradation (Holfman elimination)
Rocuronium	0.6	20–30	Rapid onset of block, intubation faster, excreted by kidney

*Action of nondepolarizers is prolonged in acidosis, hypokalemia, hypocarbia, hypothermia, patients on aminoglycoside, antibiotics and myasthenia gravis

surgery, adequate time must be allowed before reversal is attempted.

Nondepolarizing muscle relaxant is reversed by anticholinesterase drugs, e.g. neostigmine sulfate (0.05-0.07 mg/kg). The atropine sulfate (anticholinergic) is administered along with this to prevent the muscarinic effects of neostigmine like bradycardia, profuse salivation and bronchospasm. The status of the neuromuscular block can be checked by the use of peripheral nerve stimulator.

16 Sedation Techniques for Dentistry

Traditionally dentistry has been carried out under local anesthesia. However, sedation is required for uncooperative children, adult patients with simple genuine fear and phobia of dental treatment, and for medically compromised patients (cardiovascular disease, asthma, chronic epilepsy, spasticity, parkinsonism) and also for those having persisting fainting attacks or gagging. As for general anesthesia, only patients who satisfy ASA I and II criteria should be considered for sedation.

Since the early work of Langa with nitrous oxide and Jorgenson using intravenous agents, a variety of sedative techniques for dentistry have been described. Patients can remain fully conscious or can almost become anesthetized, when different techniques of deep sedation or ultralight anesthesia are used.

DEFINITIONS

Conscious Sedation

It is a state of mind obtained by IV administration of combination of anxiolytics, sedatives and hypnotics and/or analgesics that render the patient relaxed, yet allows the patient to communicate, maintain patent airway and ventilate adequately.

Deep Sedation

Deep sedation is a depressed level of consciousness with some blunting of protective reflexes, although it remains possible to arouse the patient. The ideal sedative medication for use during dental practice would provide for an easily titratable level of sleepiness (sedation), predictable amnesia and decreased anxiety (anxiolysis), while providing for a rapid recovery with minimal side effects.

SEDATION TECHNIQUES

The plethora of sedative techniques, which have been described, confirm that the ideal technique does not exist. Oral, rectal, and intramuscular techniques of sedation are referred to as premedication.

Premedication is given preoperatively to produce narcosis and the latent period may range from 15 to more than 30 minutes. The term sedation is used to describe techniques in which clinical actions develop more rapidly and this term is commonly applied to inhalational and intravenous techniques.

Intravenous Sedation

The first generally accepted intravenous (IV) sedation regime was devised by Professor Jorgenson of

California, who advocated the use of diluted solution of pentobarbitone, pethidine and hyoscine by slow IV injection in the management of mentally handicapped patients. This technique while effective, often produces quite deep levels of sedation with prolonged recovery. This was followed by the use of small incremental doses of methohexitone (Brevital) after an initial loading dose of the same drug to produce ultralight anesthesia. With this technique patient's comfort was obtained at the expense of the integrity of the respiratory and cardiovascular systems—a potentially dangerous situation.

For many years diazepam was the IV agent of choice, but concerns about active metabolites and recirculation leading to prolonged recovery and pain on injection with venous sequelae have led to it being superseded by midazolam, which is more potent and shorter-acting. Midazolam is an excellent anxiolytic with a powerful anterograde amnesic effect. It must be titrated very carefully and slowly until the patient reaches a sedation 'endpoint', characterized by a delayed response to questions and commands and some slurring of speech. Verbal contact must be maintained. For most patients, this will require 0.07 to 0.14 mg/kg which will provide useful sedation for about 45 minutes. Midazolam has no analgesic properties and local anesthetic injections will be required for painful procedures. In sedative doses, midazolam causes minimal cardiovascular depression, but respiratory depression can be marked. Patients must be monitored carefully and use of pulse oximetry to monitor oxygen saturation is highly recommended. Oxygen should be administered via nasal cannulae at 1 to 2 liters per minute (LPM) to prevent hypoxia. Patients must fulfill set criteria for recovery before being discharged. Patients must be accompanied home by a responsible adult. Ideally, the sedative agent should be given in the morning and the patient may resume normal activities on the following day. Flumazenil, is a specific benzodiazepine antagonist available to treat any inadvertent overdose of benzodiazepines.

Advantages of Intravenous Sedation

1. Highly effective technique
2. Rapid onset of action
3. Titration is possible
4. Patent vein is a safety factor
5. Control of salivary secretions possible
6. Nausea and vomiting less common
7. Gag reflex diminished
8. Motor disturbances (epilepsy, cerebral palsy) diminished.

Disadvantages of Intravenous Sedation

1. Venepuncture is necessary.
2. Venepuncture complications (infiltration, hematoma, thrombophlebitis) may occur.
3. More intensive monitoring required.
4. Delayed recovery.
5. Escort needed.

Since IV sedation techniques may produce major depression of cardiorespiratory parameters, it is not to be administered to the patient by any person, except those who have had training in anesthesiology.

Drugs Commonly Available for IV Sedation

1 Sedative, hypnotics and antianxiety drugs
   a. Benzodiazepines—diazepam, midazolam
   b. Barbiturates—methohexitone
2. Nonbarbiturate hypnotics
   a. Propofol
   b. Ketamine
   c. Innovar (droperidol and fentanyl combination)
3. Antihistaminics—promethazine
4. Narcotic agonists—pethidine, pentazocine, fentanyl.

Other Commonly Used Sedative Techniques

Propofol: It is the most recent IV anesthetic agent, which is introduced into the clinical practice. Propofol has been used for induction and maintenance of anesthesia, as well as for sedation for short dental procedures done under local anesthesia. Propofol by continuous infusion, provides a readily titratable level of sedation and a rapid recovery, once infusion is terminated, irrespective of the duration of the infusion. Generally, at propofol infusion rate greater than 30 mg/kg/min, patients are amnesic. In comparison with midazolam used to maintain sedation, propofol provides equal or better control and more rapid onset and offset. Sedative dose of propofol is 10 to 50 mg/kg/minute. IV propofol is well-suited for day care set-up as it possesses significant antiemetic activity at low doses and recovery from anesthesia is rapid without hangover effect. Full orientation generally returns within 5 to 10 minutes after stopping the infusion.

Ketamine hydrochloride: Ketamine is a phencyclidine derivative. It is a nonbarbiturate hypnotic, which produces dissociative type of anesthesia. It produces sedation, amnesia and intense analgesia. It has a very high margin of safety. It has a good tissue compatibility (no irritation of veins). Since the intraoral muscles, particularly, those of the tongue, do not become relaxed under the effect of ketamine, the airway remains unobstructed. This unique characteristic is ideal for dentistry. Airway obstruction, if occurs, is usually due to mechanical causes, such as excessive salivation due to the use of ketamine or pressure on the lower jaw by the operator. Despite alleged retention of the protective pharyngeal and laryngeal reflexes, tracheal soiling and aspiration has been reported following induction of anesthesia with ketamine. The addition of sedative premedication increases the incidence of aspiration especially, when ketamine is used in anesthetic doses (1–2 mg/kg IV or 8–10 mg/kg IM).

Dramatic increases in heart rate and blood pressure are produced by intravenous ketamine, which can be modified by premedication with benzodiazepines, especially midazolam in the titrated dose of 0.07 mg/kg IV.

Ketamine should be avoided in patients with hypertension and ischemic heart disease. Ketamine causes clinically insignificant transient dose related respiratory depression. Main disadvantage of ketamine is that, it increases intracranial and intraocular pressure. There is increased incidence of nausea and vomiting with the use of ketamine. During the operative procedure, purposeless muscle movements of the extremities, myoclonic movements and athetoid or fibrillary like motion of the mouth and tongue are frequently seen. Patient shows some rigidity of the jaw muscles and mouth may have to be forcefully opened with Fergusson's mouth gag. This side effect of ketamine may interfere with the operative procedure and may be objectionable to the dental surgeon.

Ketamine is known to produce emergence phenomenon in the form of vivid dreams, hallucinations and illusions. The frequency of emergence reactions in children is only 0 to 5 percent, considerably less than that in adults. IV benzodiazepines decrease the incidence of dreams, when administered prior to induction of ketamine anesthesia. Since the elimination half-life of ketamine is 2 to 3 hours, recovery from anesthesia is delayed.

In an attempt to reduce the side effects and the recovery times ketamine should be used in low doses to produce sedation and analgesia (0.1–0.5 mg/kg IV or 2–4 mg/kg IM). The current practice of administering intermittent bolus doses of ketamine may be improved through the use of continuous infusion techniques (10–20 micrograms/kg/min).

Propofol and ketamine combination: Addition of small dose of ketamine (10–30 micrograms/kg/hr) to propofol (0.5–1.5 mg/kg/hr) might provide the ideal sedative combination in dentistry, producing titratable sedation, intense analgesia, increased hemodynamic stability, less respiratory depression and a low incidence of psychomimetic side effects.

Fentanyl—sedative/hypnotic combination: Fentanyl is an ideal narcotic for use in dental practice. Its duration of action is short (30 to 45 minutes). It is suitable for outpatient dental practice. It does not cause hypotension. Bradycardia, respiratory depression, nausea, vomiting and muscle rigidity can occur, when it is used in higher doses. For sedation it can be given IV in the dose of 1 to 2 microgram/kg along with any sedative/hypnotic drug like midazolam, methohexitone or propofol.

Neurolept analgesia: The term describes a state of indifference and immobilization, where patient becomes analgesic, deeply sedated and partially or wholly amnesic, but yet remains capable of obeying commands and answering simple questions. This state is produced by the agent innovar, a combination of droperidol and fentanyl. Droperidol, a tranquilizer and a powerful antiemetic will be effective for upto 6 hours, whereas the narcotic component fentanyl has a limited activity of a maximum of 45 minutes. This sedative technique is unsuitable for outpatient dental practice, because of its prolonged activity.

Pethidine and promethazine combination: Pethidine (narcotic) in 50 mg doses and promethazine (phenergan) in 25 mg doses are drawn into the same syringe and diluted to a concentration of 5 mg/ml of pethidine and 2.5 mg/ml of promethazine. 1 to 2 ml of this mixture is administered IV at one time till adequate level of sedation is achieved. Duration of sedation is normally for 60 to 90 minutes and the patient is drowsy for several hours and recovery is delayed.

Inhalational Sedation

In 1966, Langa popularized the descriptive term **relative analgesia** for painful dental surgery. The term originates from the concept that the first stage of anesthesia in Guedel's classification might be subdivided into three planes; the first two were relative analgesia and the last was complete analgesia. Nitrous oxide concentrations of 6 to 25 percent, 26 to 45 percent and 46 to 55 percent correspond to the three planes. In the first plane, there is moderate sedation and some analgesia (moderate analgesia), in the second plane the sedation is described as dissociation and there is a greater element of analgesia (dissociative analgesia) and in the third there is total analgesia (analgesic anesthesia), preceding to loss of consciousness. Nitrous oxide concentrations of 66 to 80 percent, give light anesthesia, where there is complete analgesia and amnesia and it is not possible to communicate with the patient.

The term relative analgesia, however, is misleading because for complete dental work, relative analgesia is not necessary. Langa believed that the nitrous oxide concentration (20 to 30%) should be sufficient in most patients to carry out treatment without local anesthesia, but the more recent view is that control of pain should be obtained essentially by local anesthesia and any analgesic effect of the nitrous oxide serves only to remedy minor deficiencies in the local block. Accordingly, a better descriptive term is 'inhalational sedation' if nitrous oxide is used in this way.

Indications

1. Uncooperative children of reasoning age.
2. Mildly apprehensive adult patients.
3. Medically compromised patients.
4. Patients with gagging problem.

Cardiovascular diseases: In patients with angina pectoris, congestive cardiac failure, severe cardiac dysrhythmias, myocardial infarction and high blood pressure inhalational sedation have been employed with great success, because nitrous oxide has analgesic, amnesic and sedative properties, helping the patient to relax and thus reducing the work load of the myocardium and providing the patient and myocardium with the oxygen enriched gas mixture.

Asthma: Any type of stress in these patients is a potential cause of an acute exacerbation of asthma and thus the use of inhalational sedation is frequently warranted in these patients.

Epilepsy: Nitrous oxide is not an epileptogenic agent and therefore may be employed in patients with a history of chronic seizure activity as long as hypoxia is avoided.

Hepatic dysfunction: Nitrous oxide does not undergo biotransformation and therefore be used without additional risk and with a high probability of success in a patient with hepatic dysfunction.

Gagging: Gagging is a potential problem during many dental procedures. Nitrous oxide sedation has proved to be a highly effective method of eliminating or at least minimizing severe gagging especially during short procedures.

Contraindications

1. Patients with extreme anxiety.
2. Nasal obstruction, sinus problem, common cold, habitual mouth breathing.
3. Upper respiratory tract infections.
4. Patients with serious psychiatric disorders.
5. Chronic obstructive pulmonary disease (COPD). These patients have chronically elevated carbon dioxide blood levels, and the stimulus for breathing in these patients is a lowered blood oxygen content. Oxygen enriched mixture of gases with inhalational sedation technique, raises the oxygen saturation of the blood and removes the stimulus for involuntary breathing leading to respiratory apnoea in the patients.
6. First trimester of pregnancy.

Advantages

1. Easy to administer.
2. Onset of action is rapid.
3. Nitrous oxide has bland, pleasant, nonirritating odor.
4. Rapid uptake and elimination of nitrous oxide ensures that no hangover effect is experienced.
5. Recovery is fast.
6. Titration is possible.
7. There is a wide margin of safety.
8. There is cardio-respiratory stability.
9. Nausea and vomiting–uncommon.
10. Reflex integrity is maintained.
11. No preparation of patient is required.
12. No need for any escort.

Disadvantages

1. Equipment is expensive.
2. In the absence of scavenging system, exposure to nitrous oxide may cause occupational hazards to dental and nursing staff. The abortion rate is higher in practicing female dental assistants, when this technique is used. Methods that aid in minimizing exposure of the office personnel to nitrous oxide levels are as follows:
   a. Testing the equipment for leaks.
   b. Venting of waste gases outside the building.
   c. Use of scavenging nasal hoods.
   d. Use of airsweep (portable electric fan).
   e. Minimizing conversation with patient (avoid mouth breathing).
   f. Monitoring of air with infrared (IR) nitrous oxide analyzer to prove the effectiveness of the control measures, at least 2 to 3 times in a year.

Reasonable concentration of nitrous oxide appears to be approximately 50 parts per million (ppm).

Techniques of Administration

Nitrous oxide-oxygen sedation will always begin and end with the patient receiving 100 percent oxygen. The patient should be advised to avoid a heavy meal prior to the use of nitrous oxide-oxygen sedation. The patient is requested to void if necessary, prior to treatment. If the patient is wearing contact lenses, they should be removed as gas leak around the bridge of the nose may produce drying of the eyes. Review baseline vital signs prior to sedation. During sedation keep verbal communication with the patient and monitor vital signs and oxygen saturation using pulse oxymeter and ECG.

Position the patient in comfortable, reclining position in dental chair. Start the flow of oxygen at 5.0 liters per minute (LPM) and place the nasal-mask over the patient's nose. Remind the patient to breathe through the nose. Nasal-masks are available in a variety of sizes. The size is checked and the one being used should fit the patient's nose. With a well fitting nasal-mask and an oxygen flow of 5 LPM—most of the patients are comfortable and the reservoir bag remains partially inflated and it deflates and inflates to a degree with each breath. Once an adequate minute volume of gas

flow has been determined for the patient the titration of nitrous oxide may begin. Initially nitrous oxide is given in the concentration of 10 percent for a few breaths, then increased slowly till patient experiences some sensory disturbance, such as tingling sensation in fingers, toes, lips or tongue and tinnitus. At this point the concentration of nitrous oxide is decreased slightly as this is probably just beyond the desirable point and proceed with local anesthetic injection. The administration of 35 to 40 percent (or less) nitrous oxide in oxygen normally produces the euphoria and the tranquilization necessary to allow dental procedure, provided that supplementary local anesthetic is used. At the completion of treatment nitrous oxide flow will be terminated and patient is permitted to breathe 100 percent oxygen for not less than 3 to 5 minutes to minimize the possibility of developing diffusion hypoxia.

As it is a common practice to permit most patients to leave the office unescorted to operate a motor vehicle, there must be some valid criteria in determining the degree of recovery. Response of the patient to questioning will be the primary determinant of recovery from sedation. Vital signs like heart rate, blood pressure and respiratory rate are valuable adjuvants in the determination of recovery from sedation. Lastly, patient's motor coordination is evaluated using Trieger test where patient is asked to carefully connect all the dots on the figure preoperatively and postsedation. Scoring of the test is based on the number of dots that are completely missed, time required to complete the test and the general quality of the lines. Within 90 seconds after the cessation of the administration of 25 percent nitrous oxide in oxygen, full recovery of psychomotor function is evident.

Clinical Indicators of Oversedation

1. Patient uncomfortable.
2. Persistent closing of mouth.
3. Spontaneous mouth breathing.
4. Patient responds sluggishly to command.
5. Patient becomes uncooperative.
6. Patient laughs, cries, or feels giddy.
7. Patient has uncoordinated movements.
8. Patient talks incoherently.

Short Anesthesia in a Dental Chair

■ INTRODUCTION

The term "dental anesthesia" usually encompasses the administration of a local anesthetic agents (LA) or sedation techniques or general anesthesia (GA), to individuals for the extraction of teeth, minor oral surgical procedures or conservative dentistry either in dental surgeries, clinics, or dental hospital outpatient departments. Extensive oral and maxillofacial surgery is carried out normally by oral and maxillofacial surgeons on hospital inpatients and the anesthetic consideration for this treatment are similar to those of general anesthesia for ENT surgery.

Local anesthetic blocks are safer than general anesthetic techniques and patients should be encouraged to have dental work performed under local anesthesia. Some patients, however, find cooperation difficult or impossible, because of fear and anxiety. A sympathetic approach coupled with behavioral management techniques, hypnosis or simple sedation can be very successful in helping some of these patients. General anesthesia should only be used, if there are very strong indications.

The estimated mortality rate of dental anesthesia is 1:260,000, which compares favorably with the extrapolated mortality rate of GA of 1:10,000. Much of this difference results from the fact that dental anesthesia is of very short duration and the patients are usually fit and healthy. However, the fact, that the deaths have also occurred mostly in young, fit patients undergoing a brief, comparatively trivial procedure, has been a major cause of concern. The majority of outpatient dental anesthetics have been given by nonspecialist anesthesiologists, either medically or dentally qualified and in surgeries which are often poorly equipped for the purpose, particularly with regards to electrical monitoring devices. The only way to prevent this occurrence is to reduce the necessity for GA to as low a level as possible by public education and preventive dentistry and the service to be provided by trained anesthesiologists in a properly equipped environment and with skilled assistance in order to reduce the risk to the patient to the absolute minimum. **The dental surgeon should never act as both operator and anesthetist at the same time.**

The central role of the anesthesiologist is to protect the patient from the pain and stress of surgical intervention and to preserve physiological homeostasis during the perioperative period. The word 'anesthesia' is derived from Greek, meaning 'insensible'or without any feeling.

DEFINITION OF GENERAL ANESTHESIA

It is a controlled state of unconsciousness, accompanied by partial or complete loss of protective reflexes, including the inability to independently maintain an airway or respond purposefully to verbal command. The process should be reversible. It is the condition induced by pharmacological or other means, which results in all of the following effects:

1. Loss of awareness.
2. No recall of events at the conscious level, although it is possible, that events may still be retained in the subconscious, from which they may be recalled under certain circumstances.
3. Lack of overt muscular response to surgical stimulation. An exception is the respiratory musculature, which usually responds to surgical stimulation by an increase in respiratory rate and tidal volume.
4. Minimal autonomic response to surgical stimulation, although this cannot be totally abolished.
5. All the protective reflexes like pharyngeal and laryngeal reflexes are suppressed.
6. Patient is noncommunicative and it is not possible to arouse the patient.

HISTORY

History has demonstrated that it has been members of the dental profession, who have consistently been in the forefront in the research and development of new techniques and medications for the management of pain and anxiety. Horace Wells (a dentist) and William T.G. Morton (dentist and physician), in 1840, were the founders of anesthesia and the first to employ nitrous oxide (Wells) and ether (Morton) for the management of pain during surgical procedures. Prior to this time dental treatment was performed without the aid of any form of anesthesia. The advent of ether in 1846, overshadowed the weaker anesthetic like nitrous oxide (N_2O).

G.Q. Colton (who had introduced the gas to Wells originally) repopularized N_2O for dentistry on 31st March 1868, in London. In 1868, Edmund Andrews of Chicago suggested the addition of 20 percent oxygen to reduce the danger of hypoxia. In 1887, Frederic Hewitt, who advocated sound teaching and practice in the use of anesthetics in dental surgery invented a 'gas' and oxygen machine. This and others were superseded in 1910, when E.I. McKesson of Toledo introduced his intermittent flow machine, which provided the control of oxygen and N_2O on demand by the patient and became very popular. These earlier models were followed by the Walton series of the British Oxygen Company and later the AE machines. Considerable doubts have been expressed regarding the accuracy of traditional intermittent or demand flow machines and is now of historical interest only.

In the area of intravenous medications, the dental profession again laid the way, with the introduction of the IV barbiturates in the late 1930's, Victor Goldman and Stanley Drummond-Jackson in England, and Adrian Hubbell in the United States, pioneered the techniques of IV general anesthesia for ambulatory oral surgical patients.

EQUIPMENT

Anesthetic Machine

A standard continuous flow anesthetic machine is used in most situations. Modern machines have an oxygen failure alarm and a shut off mechanism for N_2O plus a link between the oxygen and N_2O rotameters, so that hypoxic gas mixtures cannot be delivered. If the oxygen and N_2O rotameters, can be controlled independently, then an oxygen monitor must be connected to the fresh gas outlet.

Machines such as quantiflex MDM are designed for providing inhalation sedation and will not deliver less than 30 percent oxygen. Continuous flow machines have the advantages of economy, simplicity, reliability, familiarity to junior anesthetists, accuracy, and flexibility.

Dental Chair

Whichever position is adopted for anesthesia, it must be possible to put the chair into a horizontal or even head low position immediately in an emergency. If the chair is electrically powered, there should be a manual release to achieve this in the event of a power failure. The chair should have an adjustable headrest to allow the head to be correctly positioned and the arm-rests should be easily removable. In the hospital outpatient or day stay unit, if the supine position is to be used, an operating table can be used.

Breathing Circuits and Masks

Various breathing circuits can be used in dental anesthesia in combination with nasal masks. There are two principle dental anesthetic masks in use—the Goldman and the McKessan. Though, a full face mask may be needed at first, it is easy to use the Goldman mask from the beginning in younger children, because it will at least partially overlap the mouth. The Goldman nasal mask can be very satisfactorily combined with co-axial circuit and has the benefit of low resistance to breathing with ease of connection to a scavenging system. The Goldman mask with an integral Heidbrink valve was designed for use with continuous flow equipment and has an inflatable cuff in the manner of the conventional face mask. The McKesson mask with a spring loaded expiratory valve has twin narrow-bore supply tubes for use with on demand machines. More recently, the silicon rubber Dupaco masks have become available and are suitable for both inhalation, sedation and conventional anesthesia.

Nasopharyngeal Airways

A selection of soft nasopharyngeal airways should be available, which are necessary to improve the nasal airway during anesthesia.

Mouth Props and Gags

The device used most commonly to keep the mouth open during anesthesia is the mouth prop. The McKesson type comes in various sizes and is suitable for most patients. Mouth gags of the Fergusson type are used less commonly, because of the possibility of causing trauma inside the mouth if incorrectly applied. It is useful to have a gag available for emergencies.

Mouth Packs

The mouth pack is inserted with the object of constructing a diaphragm/partition between the site of operation and the lower airway. Dental packing material may be either gamjee-cotton wool inside a stockinette sleeve or ribbon gauze (8 cm x 120 cm) or a synthetic sponge material.

Correct placement is essential: The pack should not push the tongue back against the posterior pharyngeal wall and should prevent any debris from passing into the lower pharynx or larynx. The anesthetist must observe the reservoir bag and ensure that the airway is not compromised during placement of the pack. It should prevent mouth breathing. A small tail from the pack must always protrude out of the mouth to alert staff of its presence. It may need to be changed during the course of anesthesia, if it becomes fully soaked. At the end of the procedure, the pack is removed.

Monitors and Resuscitation Equipment

For safe practice of dental anesthesia, use of cardioscope, noninvasive blood pressure apparatus and pulse oxymeter is highly recommended. A defibrillator must be available in any situation, where GA is to be administered.

A full range of tracheal tubes with all the accessories for tracheal intubation, plus two working laryngoscopes must be immediately available. A full range of emergency drugs with needles and syringes must be available in the surgery, along with all the equipment required for setting up an intravenous infusion. All anesthesiologists must be familiar with the recommended resuscitation equipment and drugs and should be able to perform tracheal intubation.

▊ INDICATIONS FOR GENERAL ANESTHESIA

1. Young children, especially when multiple extractions in different quadrants of the mouth is planned. Extensive conservative dentistry work in young children, combined with the extractions in one sitting.
2. Uncooperative patients, either those who are mentally subnormal or who have physical infirmity, enough to become uncontrollable under local analgesia, e.g. spastics.
3. Patients, who are too apprehensive to cooperate with local anesthesia methods.
4. Acute infective conditions, except where there is edema of the floor of the mouth or Ludwig's angina, and in whom acute sepsis has not led to trismus with limitation of the opening of the mouth. Due to the low pH of infected tissues, local analgesia will not relieve pain. Where severe infection is present treatment is best carried out as an inpatient.
5. Allergy to local anesthetics—true allergy to local anesthetics is very rare. The preservative methyl-

paraben present in some local anesthetic solutions can provoke allergic reactions. Patients who claim to be allergic, should be questioned carefully, since it is much more common for patients to describe vasovagal fainting reactions, or flushing and palpitation as a result of absorption of adrenaline from the anesthetic solution.

6. Failure of action of local anesthetic agent.
7. Failure of sedation.

DAY STAY SURGERY

Multiple extractions, conservative dental treatment, extraction of impacted third molar teeth, enucleation of simple cyst and other small operations, which are of short duration, taking only 20 to 40 minutes, are suitable to be carried out on a day stay basis. The main advantage of day stay surgery for the patient, is a rapid return home, avoiding admission to hospital, while the advantage to the hospital or health authority is considerable saving in cost. In selecting patients for treatment on a day stay basis, certain strict criteria must be met:

1. Patients must be fit and healthy and free from cardiopulmonary disease satisfying ASA categories I and II.
2. Surgery must not be expected to last more than 1 hour.
3. There should be no significant risk of complications like excessive bleeding or vomiting, which would require admission to hospital.
4. Recovery from anesthesia should be rapid and proper recovery facilities should be available.
5. Patients must be accompanied home by responsible adults and home circumstances should be suitable for continuing postoperative care.

Most hospitals have inpatient facilities for dental emergencies and patients with recognized risk factors must be admitted for treatment.

POSITION IN DENTAL CHAIR: HORIZONTAL/SITTING

There has been considerable controversy regarding the most appropriate position for patients during dental anesthesia. Traditionally, outpatient dental treatment under GA was performed with the patient seated upright in the dental chair. Until Bourne in 1957, drew attention to the dangers of the unrecognized fainting attack occurring immediately prior to or during induction of anesthesia. He postulated, that many of the cases of cerebral damage or deaths related to dental anesthesia could be explained by hypotension, bradycardia or cardiac arrest associated with a fainting and recommended a routine adoption of supine position.

In the supine position, there is a greater risk of airway obstruction due to the tongue and soft palate falling backward. There is greater risk of pharyngeal soiling with the blood and regurgitation of stomach contents and there is reduction in expiratory reserve volume.

Cardiovascular changes during dental anesthesia do not appear to be influenced by posture. Tachycardia and hypotension occur with both intravenous and inhalational techniques and there are no significant differences between sitting and supine positions.

In order to achieve the best balance of respiratory and cardiovascular conditions, the position commonly adopted for outpatient dental anesthesia is the semisupine. Patient's head should be slightly extended and the mandible should be horizontal and parallel to the floor, when the mouth is open.

PREOPERATIVE CONSIDERATIONS

A routine should be established, that prevents any oversight in the preparation of the patient for the surgery. Advice, preferably written, to be given before hand to ensure:

1. The patient has had nothing to eat or drink for at least 4 hours prior to the appointment.
2. The patient should be instructed to wear clothing, that is not tight around the neck or waist and have sleeves that are easily drawn up above the elbow in case IV agents are used.
3. Cosmetics are not used.
4. Valuables are not brought to the surgery.
5. An escort attends with the patient.
6. Arrangements for transport home have been made.

Before the patient is taken up for the procedure, written informed consent for anesthesia and surgery should be obtained. The identity of the patient is confirmed. Bladder should be emptied to avoid micturition during anesthesia. In order to ensure rapid recovery and early ambulation, premedication is avoided. When the patient is positioned in a dental chair, a waterproof apron should be placed around the patient's neck to protect his clothing. An attempt to assess the patency of nasal airway should be made, since if this is blocked, endotracheal intubation may be required. Anesthetist should make note of presence of crowns, bridges, loose teeth, dentures or soft tissue lesions. Any removable appliances should be removed, as they may cause airway obstruction when the patient becomes unconscious.

INDUCTION OF ANESTHESIA

The traditional way of anesthetizing patients for exodontia/minor surgery, means that the airway is shared with the surgeon without tracheal intubation. The method has continued because of the combined skills of anesthesiologist and dental surgeons, the speed at which surgery is carried out, the light levels of anesthesia, and the youth and fitness of the patients. Most of the patients anesthetized are between 3 and 8 years of age. One of the only indications in the adults for GA is the acutely abscessed tooth. Other adults requiring GA are mentally handicapped, challenged people.

Anesthesia can be induced using an inhalation or intravenous technique. Inhalation induction is commonly used for younger children, especially, if intravenous access is likely to be difficult. Older children and adults will usually accept an intravenous needle.

Inhalational induction, is usually commenced by holding the nasal mask close to the patient's face and cupping the hand below the chin to direct the gas mixture towards the mouth and nose. A high initial gas flow of the nitrous oxide and not less than 30 percent oxygen should be used. After a few breaths, the volatile agent like halothane is administered and the concentration increased by 0.5 to 1 percent increments, again after every few breaths. The nasal mask should be applied as soon as the patient will accept it and the mouth should be closed to discourage mouth breathing.

Halothane remains a popular agent, because of smooth, rapid induction. It has a nonirritant relatively pleasant smell. However, there is 30 percent incidence of dysrhythmias during halothane anesthesia. A concentration of 3 to 4 percent may be necessary briefly during induction, but once the jaw has relaxed sufficiently to insert a mouth prop, the concentration can be reduced to 1 to 2 percent for maintenance of anesthesia. Enflurane is an useful alternative to halothane. Because of lower potency of enflurane, higher concentrations are required to produce adequate levels of anesthesia. Incidence of dysrhythmias is 10 percent during enflurane anesthesia. Isoflurane has shown to be inferior to halothane in outpatient, pediatric, dental anesthesia. Isoflurane has a pungent smell and is irritant to the tracheobronchial tree; therefore, gaseous induction may be complicated by high incidence of coughing, salivation, laryngospasm and episodes of oxygen desaturation. Once sufficient jaw relaxation occurs, to allow insertion of a mouth prop, deeper levels of anesthesia are not required, especially, when very brief procedure is anticipated.

Children above the 'age of reason' (6 years) may be offered IV induction. There will be rare exceptions for IV induction, such as mentally handicapped adults and patients with extreme phobia of needles. The prior application of a eutectic local anesthetic cream mixture (EMLA, Astra Pharmaceuticals) to the back of the hand, at least 1 hour prior to procedure makes venipuncture virtually painless and more acceptable.

The long elimination half-life of thiopentone (9 hours) makes it unsuitable for outpatient anesthesia, although an exception can be made in a patient of epilepsy, who is not stable on antiepileptic treatment. The advent of methohexitone provided an agent, which is both rapid and short-acting than thiopentone with an elimination half-life of 97 minutes. It is used in the dose of 1.5 mg/kg in adults and 2 mg/kg in children. Following induction, there is usually a fall in blood pressure of about 15 percent, as a result of reduction in peripheral vascular resistance. A compensatory tachycardia results and the blood pressure is restored, once the mouth prop is inserted and surgery commences. Disadvantages of methohexitone are pain on injection, involuntary muscle movements, hiccoughs and respiratory depression. Methohexitone should be avoided in patients with epilepsy. It still remains popular in USA, because of its low cost and proven history. Propofol is the most expensive drug and the most recently introduced in the Indian market. It is rapidly metabolized and the patient is clear headed and back to normal cerebration within a very short time. Doses of 2 to 2.5 mg/kg are satisfactory in adults. But children need more dosage upto 3 to 3.5 mg/kg. Propofol causes greater degree of cardiorespiratory depression than other intravenous agents. It also produces pain on injection.

MAINTENANCE OF ANESTHESIA

Once the mouth prop and pack have been inserted, surgery can commence. If the procedure is to take a little longer, then the anesthesia is maintained using the nasal mask delivering oxygen (minimum 30%), nitrous oxide and a low concentration of the volatile agent. The anesthesiologist's prime responsibility is to maintain a clear airway by holding the mandible forward and upward to prevent the tongue falling backwards. There is a significant incidence of hypoxia and to a lesser extent hypercarbia during pediatric dental extractions, using the conventional nasal mask technique. Children with large adenoids and/or tonsils or a large soft palate may obstruct their nasal airway, as soon as they become unconscious, especially when lying flat (supine). It is difficult to sustain an adequate depth of anesthesia, if the patient is a persistent mouth breather. A nasopharyngeal airway may be essential in some of these patients. Brain laryngeal mask airway (LMA) has been recommended after both inhalational and IV induction, because episodes of hypoxia are less frequent. However, surgical access may be limited using an LMA. The LMA is particularly useful for minor oral surgical procedures such as raising a small flap, extraction of unerupted teeth, which is likely to take little longer time. Endotracheal intubation must be used to provide reliable oxygenation in certain indicated patients or whenever the surgery is expected to last longer or intraoral persistent bleeding is expected throughout the procedure.

The anesthesiologist must monitor the patient's condition by observing the color of the lips and mucosal surfaces and watching the movement of the reservoir bag in the circuit. It may be possible to feel the carotid pulse in a child using the little finger on the facial artery underneath the mandible. In an adult because of the potential for cardiorespiratory complications, the electrocardiogram, noninvasive blood pressure and oxygen saturation must also be monitored.

ENDOTRACHEAL ANESTHESIA

Formal endotracheal intubation, is now undertaken much more commonly than in the past. Mentally handicapped patient, extended surgery (beyond 15 to 20 min), obstruction of nasal airways or difficulty in maintaining an airway are indications for endotracheal intubation. Endotracheal intubation may be achieved during inhalation anesthesia or by the use of an IV induction agent followed by intermediate acting, nondepolarizing muscle relaxant such as atracurium or vecuronium. Suxamethonium should be avoided in ambulant outpatients, because of postoperative muscle

pains. A nasotracheal tube is always to be preferred, as it allows access to both sides of the mouth without movement of the tube and the throat can be packed more securely. Provided the procedure outlasts the action of neuromuscular blocking drug and the patient can be retained in the recovery area for a reasonable period of time. It may be unnecessary to use anticholinesterases. Controlled ventilation confers the added advantage of cardiac stability. The use of opioid is accompanied by an increased incidence of nausea and vomiting postoperatively. All children should be examined before discharge, particularly if nasal tube has been used, as bleeding from disrupted adenoids may sometimes be troublesome.

RECOVERY

At the end of the surgery, the mouth prop is removed, but the new packs secured with long threads are left in place over the sockets. Patient should be laid in the lateral position during recovery. Even after very short procedures, fall in oxygen saturation can occur in the recovery period as a result of residual respiratory depression, inadequate reversal, airway obstruction or the diffusion of nitrous oxide into the alveoli. The airway and breathing must be monitored continuously and suction used to keep the mouth clear of blood, if necessary. Oxygen should be given until the patient has opened the eyes and expelled the mouth packs.

Patients should remain in the recovery area for at least 2 hours before being discharged into the care of a responsible adult, who must accompany them. The patient should be fully conscious, alert, fully oriented in time and space with no hangover effect at the time of discharge. Vital parameters must be stable. Patient should be able to stand and walk unsupportedly. There should not be any bleeding from the operated site. Postoperative nausea and vomiting and pain should be minimal.

Four quadrant multiple extractions are likely to cause more severe and lasting pain and postoperative analgesia is indicated. This can consist of preoperative mild oral analgesics such as liquid paracetamol, rectal paracetamol at the end of surgery before awakening or oral liquid analgesics, when the child has recovered from anesthesia. Intramuscular injections of nonsteroidal anti-inflammatory drugs (NSAIDs) are painful and opiates are probably unnecessarily powerful, especially in a day care set up and should be avoided.

Written postoperative instructions must be given, which emphasize that the patient must not drive or operate machinery for the rest of the day and that alcohol must be avoided.

COMPLICATIONS OF DENTAL ANESTHESIA

Hypoxia

Even when 30 percent oxygen is given during dental anesthesia, arterial hypoxia is likely to occur unless a perfect airway is maintained. This can be difficult, when the surgeon exerts pressure during extractions on the lower jaw and the mandible will need repositioning constantly. Airway obstruction can also occur as a result of malposition of mouth pack, tongue falling back, and enlarged tonsils and adenoids. If it is difficult to obtain a clear nasal airway, then insertion of a soft, well-lubricated nasopharyngeal airway will usually solve the problem.

Laryngospasm

If it occurs during induction, it may be necessary to reduce the inspired concentration of volatile agent and give more oxygen to prevent hypoxia. Intraoperatively, it can occur due to the combination of the surgical stimulus and too light a level of anesthesia or as a result of blood or saliva irritating the vocal cords. The surgery must stop and the pharynx should be cleared with suction. Oxygen must be administered under pressure with a face mask, if necessary. If the laryngospasm does not correct itself then endotracheal intubation may be required.

Mouth Breathing

Mouth breathing will dilute the anesthetic gases and the patient may become too lightly anesthetized and will start to struggle. The pack should be correctly positioned to seal off the mouth. Nasopharyngeal airway may be required.

Contamination of Trachea

Every effort should be made to protect the airway. Complete obstruction of the larynx or trachea has catastrophic consequences. Teeth, crowns, portion of fillings have all been retrieved in the past. In the semisupine position aspiration may be more likely and in the supine position regurgitation of stomach contents may occur more readily necessitating use of an artificial airway.

Apnea

Apnea may be due to the following:
a. Respiratory obstruction.
b. Breath holding in light anesthesia.
c. Deep anesthesia.
d. Severe hypoxia.
e. Grave cardiovascular depression requiring resuscitation.
f. **Fainting—fear, anxiety and occasionally pain in the patients presenting for outpatient dental anesthesia, can cause significant autonomic nervous system overactivity. High circulating catecholamine levels and an increased sympathetic component can give rise to a labile blood pressure and tachycardia. Parasympathetic overactivity can cause bradycardia and sweating and predispose to fainting. Fainting is triggered by emotional factors and as a result of stimulation of the limbic cortex and hypothalamus, produces reflex vasodilatation mainly in muscles.**

Bradycardia occurs due to increased parasympathetic activity and decreased venous return due to vasodilatation. The fall in cardiac output and severe hypotension causes a rapid loss of consciousness, which can usually be corrected by putting the patient in a head low position or elevating the legs to restore the venous return. In the dental chair the patient may be actively prevented from falling and if the fainting is not recognized, soon enough severe brain damage and even death may result. Careful monitoring of the pulse and blood pressure throughout the procedure is therefore vital.

Hypotension

Causes of hypotension may include the following:
a. Induction of anesthesia in the dental chair, whether it is by inhalational or intravenous route.
b. Pressure on the carotid sinus area, when supporting the lower jaw.
c. Bradycardia and hypotension due to surgical stimulation of vagal reflexes
d. Severe hypoxia.

Cardiac Dysrhythmias

There is a high incidence of cardiac dysrhythmias during dental and oral surgeries. Nodal rhythm and ectopic beats, both unifocal and multifocal, are common. Tachycardia is very common with heart rates over 120 beats per minute during tooth extraction especially in children. Parasympathetic responses can also occur. Important factors in the etiology of dysrhythmias include high preoperative catecholamine levels (fear, anxiety and pain), surgical stimulation in a lightly anesthetized patient and the presence of airway obstruction with hypoxia. Halothane sensitizes the myocardium to the action of circulating catecholamines and its use is associated with 30 percent incidence of dysrhythmias. Enflurane and isoflurane produce dysrhythmias in about 10 percent patients.

An effective method of preventing cardiac disturbances is to infiltrate the tissues around the tooth with a local anesthetic solution, which does not contain adrenaline. This can be done easily after a brief induction and reduces considerably the depth of anesthesia required for any procedure. Additionally, it provides an element of postoperative pain relief.

Nausea and Vomiting

Incidence of nausea and vomiting is high, after any oral procedure and proper preoperative preparation of the patient, selective use of anesthetic agents (Propofol), avoidance of opioids and anticholinesterases, and prophylactic use of antiemetics (metaclopromide ondansetron) will reduce the incidence.

18 Tracheal Intubation for a Patient Undergoing Oral and Maxillofacial Surgery

INDICATIONS FOR TRACHEAL INTUBATION

1. Multiple extractions in one sitting
2. Multiple minor surgical work
3. Mentally retarded patients
4. All extensive maxillofacial surgeries

For a patient undergoing any of the above procedures under general anesthesia, intubation of the trachea becomes mandatory, for the management of airway, as well as for the administration of gases. The reasons are as follows:

1. Patient's airway is shared by the anesthetist and the surgeon.
2. Airway needs to be protected from aspiration of blood coming from the operative area as well as any foreign bodies like broken teeth, etc.
3. There are chances of regurgitation and aspiration of gastric contents.
4. For surgery lasting for long hours.

ARMAMENTARIUM REQUIRED FOR INTUBATIONS

Laryngoscope

Laryngoscope is required for visualization of the vocal cords. The laryngoscope blades in common use, for the right handed person are straight or curved. There are four sizes of the blades available. Depending on the size and age of the patient, appropriate sized blade is chosen (*See* Figs 14.3 and 14.4).

Endotracheal Tubes (Figs 18.1A to F)

For the purpose of securing airway, different types of endotracheal tubes are available in different materials.

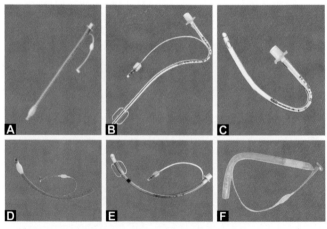

Figs 18.1A to F: Endotracheal tubes: (A) Flexometallic (armoured) tube, (B) Nasal cuffed north pole tube, (C) Oral plain south pole tube, (D) Cuff oral red rubber tube, (E) Cuff oral/nasal PVC disposable tube, (F) Oxford red rubber cuff tube

The size of the tube selected depends again on the age of the patient. The sizes of the endotracheal tubes are no. 0 to no. 11 ranging from neonate to adult. The tubes are either plane or with cuff. The commonly used tubes are either rubber or portex cuffed tubes. Special tubes are also available for nasal intubation.

After insertion of endotracheal tube, the cuff is inflated for protection of the airway from aspiration of gastric contents or blood from operation site. It also prevents air leak.

Procedure for Endotracheal Intubation

Intubation can be achieved in following ways:
1. After induction of general anesthesia (by IV or inhalation method).
   a. Oral—orotracheal intubation.
   b. Nasal—nasotracheal intubation.
2. Awake intubation
   a. Blind oral
   b. Blind nasal
   c. Retrograde—rail road technique
   d. By use of fiberoptic scope.

Induction of general anesthesia: Patient is taken on operation table (who has been fasting, at least for 4 hours). After usual checkup of vital parameters, an IV line is started. Patient is given IV induction agent till he looses consciousness, after that a muscle relaxant is given through the IV route to facilitate laryngoscopy and intubation. Before insertion of laryngoscope, patient is preoxygenated using face mask and ventilation with a bag.

The patient's head is kept on a pillow and then head is extended by gentle traction on upper teeth. This gives flexion at cervical spine (35°) and extension at the atlanto-occipital joint (15°).

Ideal Position for Intubation (Figs 18.2A to E)

The handle of the laryngoscope is held in the right hand and the tip of the curved laryngoscope blade is inserted into the right corner of the mouth and advanced along the side of the tongue toward the right tonsillar fossa, so that the tongue lies in the recess on the left side of the laryngoscope blade. The blade is inserted behind the base of the tongue and the tongue along with mandible is lifted up when tip is lying in the vallecula.

Depending upon the site of surgery, the tube is passed through the nose or mouth. The tip of the tube

is passed beyond vocal cords under direct vision, till the cuff lies just beyond the cords. The tube is connected to breathing circuit by proper connections. The position of the tube is confirmed by auscultation of both the sides of chest by using stethoscope, when the patient is being ventilated (for checking equal air entry). The tube is fixed to the corner of the mouth by the use of adhesive tapes, if it is passed orally and to the circumference of the nostril, if it is passed through the nose, and secured over the bridge of the nose.

Thus, intubation can be achieved orally—orotracheal intubation or nasally—nasotracheal intubation (Figs 18.3 and 18.4).

Awake Intubation

Awake intubation is indicated in certain cases, where oral opening is restricted or due to anatomical deformity, the larynx cannot be visualized, e.g. TM joint ankylosis,

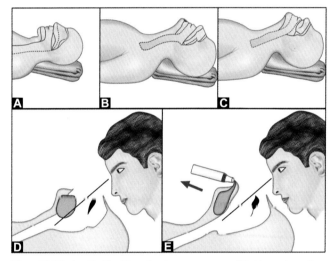

Figs 18.2A to E: Position for laryngoscopy: (A) Normal supine, (B) Head extended (HE), (C) HE + neck flexion, (D) Axis of vision, (E) Laryngoscopic vision (C to E) Extension at atlantoaxial level and flexion of lower cervical spine)

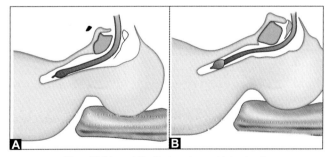

Figs 18.3A and B: Oral and nasal tube *in situ*

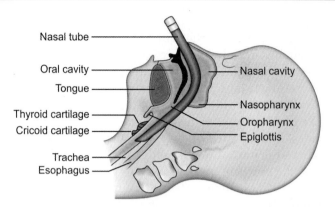

Fig. 18.4: Nasal tube *in situ*

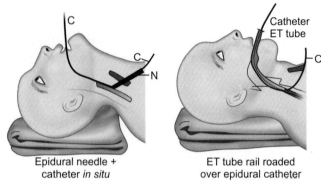

Fig. 18.5: Retrograde oral intubation technique. C: Catheter; N: Needle; ET Tube: Endotracheal tube

large oral cysts or tumors, marked hypoplasia of the mandible, facial deformity after burns or trauma.

Drugs used for sedation during awake intubation: Agents commonly used for this purpose are those belonging to the benzodiazepine group (diazepam, midazolam), short-acting narcotics (fentanyl) or the infusion of propofol.

Antisialagogue administration: The reduction in secretions increases effectiveness of topical local anesthetic agent. The drugs used are atropine or glycopyrrolate.

Local anesthetic techniques: It is necessary to use topical anesthesia for the airway.
- Lignocaine 4 to 10 percent (spray or viscous gel) is used.
- Surface anesthesia to nasal mucosa is achieved by packing the ribbon gauze soaked in local anesthetic solution.
- Surface anesthesia of oropharyngeal and laryngeal region is achieved by gargles, spray, lozenges and ultrasonic nebulizer.
- Cricothyroid puncture is used to anaesthetize the tracheal mucosa.
- Regional nerve blocks used are maxillary nerve block, glossopharyngeal nerve block and superior laryngeal nerve block.

Blind nasotracheal intubation: It should be performed gently, preferably with the patient breathing spontaneously. Patient should be explained the entire procedure, so that maximum cooperation can be obtained.

One of the major problems with a blind nasotracheal intubation is the incidence of nasal bleeding, it can also create a false route in the posterior pharyngeal wall.

Retrograde method (Railroad technique) (Figs 18.5 and 18.6): Provided there is access to cricothyroid membrane, retrograde method in the conscious or sedated patient, using catheters or wires may provide a simple solution, whenever there is intubation difficulty.

Fiberoptic intubation (Figs 18.7A and B): Latest state of the art, fiberoptic instruments are being used with increasing frequency in anesthesia. In this technique either a conventional railroading over fiberoptic scope is used or a guidewire is passed through suction channel to railroad the tracheal tube.

Complications Associated with Tracheal Intubation

During intubation:
- Direct trauma to the teeth, luxation of teeth due to laryngoscope blade.
- Fracture and/or subluxation of cervical spine.
- Hemorrhage (nasal).
- Trauma to the eyes due to the laryngoscope.
- Surgical emphysema of the neck and mediastinum.
- Pharyngeal damage.
- Aspiration of gastric contents and foreign bodies.
- Accidental intubation of esophagus.
- Misplacement of the tube.

After intubation:
- Obstruction of the airway
  - Outside the tube
  - By the tube itself
  - Within the tube
- Rupture of the trachea and bronchus.
- Aspiration of stomach contents.
- Displacement of tube.

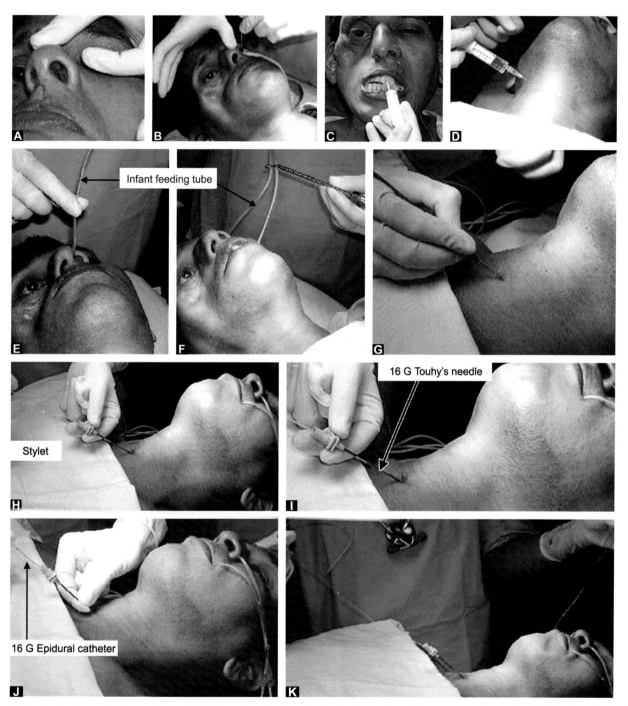

Figs 18.6A to K: Steps of retrograde nasal intubation (Rail-Road method). (A) Inspection of the patency of the nostril, (B) Packing the nostril with roller gauze strip soaked in LA solution with adrenaline, (C) LA viscous solution pushed to achieve surface anesthesia of the pharynx, (D) Transtracheal LA injection through cricothyroid puncture, (E) Infant feeding tube being introduced through the nostril, (F) Infant feeding tube is brought out from the oral cavity, by encouraging the patient to push out the tube by tongue movements, (G) Small incision over cricothyroid membrane, (H and I) Introduction of 16 gauge Touhy's needle with stylet *in situ*, in trachea, (J) Epidural catheter is being introduced through Touhy's needle, while securing the needle at the entry point, (K) Epidural catheter emerging from mouth through cricoid membrane, trachea and laryngeal aperture

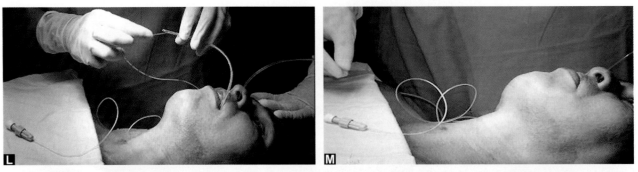

Figs 18.6L and M: (L) Epidural catheter is being threaded through the eye into the lumen of infant tube. (M) Epidural catheter is brought out through nostril from the oral cavity with the help of infant feeding tube from nostril to oral cavity

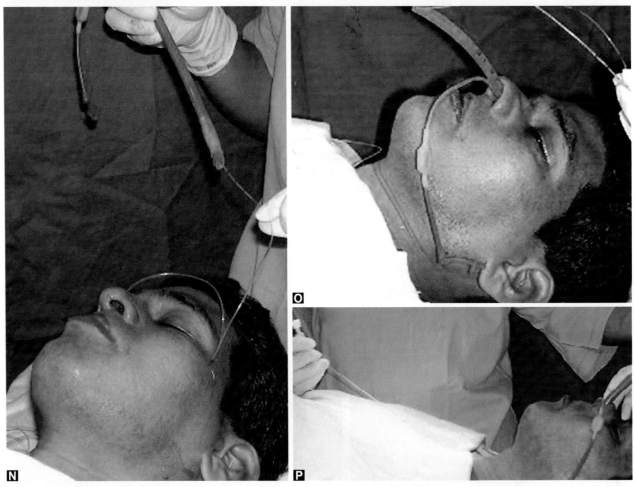

Figs 18.6N to P: (N and O) Rail-roading of endotracheal tube over epidural catheter. (P) Epidural catheter held taut till endotracheal tube reaches the level of cricothyroid membrane. After that, the epidural catheter has to be held loosely

At extubation:

- Difficulty of impossible extubation.
- Tracheal collapse.
- Airway obstruction.
- Aspiration of stomach contents.

Following endotracheal intubation anesthesia—early recovery phase (0-24 hrs)

- Sore throat
- Damage to nerves
- Edema—glottic, supraglottic/subglottic

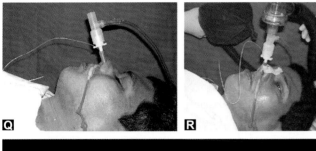

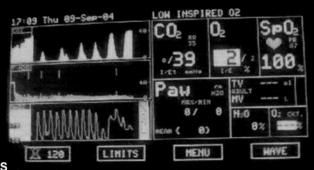

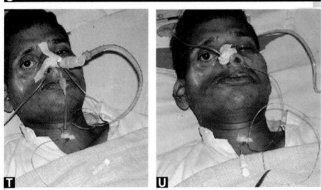

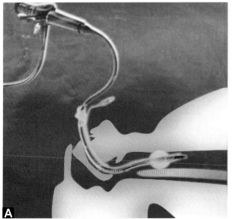

Figs 18.6Q to U: (Q) Successful retrograde intubation (Rail roading), (R) Confirmation of endotracheal tube placement, (S) Monitoring the patient, (T) Patient in the recovery room, (U) Patient extubated, but epidural catheter kept *in situ* (For any emergency in immediate recovery period)

- Retroarytenoid edema
- Hoarseness and voice changes
- Vocal cord paralysis.

Intermediate recovery phase (24 to 72 hrs): Infection

Late (72 hrs +) recovery phase:
- Laryngeal ulcer, granuloma and polyp
- Synechia of vocal cords, laryngotracheal membranes and webs.
- Laryngeal fibrosis
- Tracheal stenosis
- Stricture of nostrils
- Mouth and pharyngeal damage
- Associated nonairway damage

Complications at Endotracheal Intubation

Direct trauma: These injuries include bruised or lacerated lips and tongue, chipping of teeth or inadvertent extraction, luxation of teeth, lacerations of the pharynx, submucosal hemorrhage and tears of vocal cords. With nasal intubation, there can be trauma to the turbinates followed by epistaxis. Careful suction and packing of the nostrils, if required should be done.

The incidence of dental complications of tracheal intubation has been quoted as 1 in 1000. Careless movement of the head may produce serious lesions such as fracture, luxation of the cervical spine with spinal cord compression or section.

Hemorrhage occurs following intubation by nasal route. Extensive hemorrhage requiring blood transfusion may occur, if there is damage to the middle turbinate. Gentle and patient maneuver of the tube will prevent this complication. Trauma to the eye may occur by inadvertently rubbing the cornea with operator's

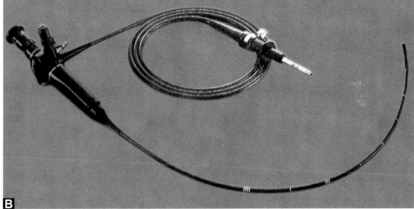

Figs 18.7A and B: (A) Intubation using fiberoptic laryngoscope, (B) Fiberoptic laryngoscope

hand or the handle of laryngoscope (ointment and cover with tape). Tearing of the mucosa lining the pyriform fossae, may lead to surgical emphysema of the neck and mediastinum, it can lead to the development of tension pneumothorax, when patient is ventilated under mask.

Nasal intubation can cause trauma to the nasopharynx and may lead to retropharyngeal abscess or mediastinitis (infection).

The risk of aspiration of stomach contents is particularly high in patients with full stomach, poorly functioning cardiac sphincter or loss of protective reflexes.

Esophageal intubation is potentially hazardous complication, if it remains undetected. The tube may be also misplaced in one of the main bronchus, preventing air exchange on the other side.

Complications During Intubation

Obstruction of the tube: Biting on the tube, if patient is in lighter planes or just before extubation. In case of recycled tubes, kinking of the tube is very common. Complete or partial blockage (inside the lumen of the tube) can result from blood clot, tissue, dried secretions, dried tube lubricants, foreign bodies, etc.

Rupture of trachea or bronchus can occur due to sharply beveled tubes or sharp tipped stylets, over-inflation of the cuff, use of excessive force or repeated attempts at intubation. Ignition of the tube is a complication of laser surgery.

Complications following intubation

1. Sore throat is a common and benign sequelae of tracheal intubation. Damage to the hypoglossal nerve may occur due to pressure from laryngoscope blade.

2. Glottic edema may occur in supraglottic, retro-arytenoid and subglottic regions. It is more common in children.

3. Hoarseness is quite common, but vocal cord paralysis is not a common sequelae.

4. Infection may occur at any point, along the route of the tube. Nasotracheal intubation can be followed by sinusitis. Treatment may require local mouthwashes to parenteral antibiotics, depending on the severity of the infection.

5. Laryngeal polyp formation due to growth of granulation tissue has a low incidence and it is not related to the type of tube, route of intubation or duration of intubation.

6. Synechia of cords, laryngotracheal membranes and webs, laryngeal fibrosis, tracheal stenosis, stricture of nostril are other complications.

19 Complications of General Anesthesia

Chapter Outline

❖ Anesthetic Complications
❖ Postoperative Anesthetic Complications

With an aging population and advances in surgical care and technology, we find ourselves treating increasingly sicker patients, who are undergoing more complex procedures. The anesthetic agents and adjuvants are among the most potent and rapidly acting drugs used in medicine. These anesthetic agents and the techniques impair a variety of essential body functions, in addition risk the major organ systems. Thus, these medications and techniques leave the patient open to the risk of anesthesia related complications in the perioperative period.

Complications following anesthesia and surgery may be categorized into those related to the:
1. Surgical procedure
2. Patient's medical condition and
3. Anesthetic procedure.

ANESTHETIC COMPLICATIONS

Anesthetic complications may occur in the: (a) preoperative period, (b) during operation, or (c) in the postoperative period (Table 19.1).

Preoperative Period (Related to Prior Drug Therapy)

Some of the examples are given below:

Table 19.1: Complications of anesthesia	
1. Preoperative period	• Related to prior drug therapy
2. During operation	• Related to anesthesia drugs used
	• Anesthesia technique
	• Intubation technique
	• Equipment failure
	• Positioning
	• Medical condition
	• Surgical pathology
	• Blood transfusion
3. Postoperative period	• Related to anesthetic drugs
	• Anesthesia technique
	• Intubation technique
	• Pain
	• Infection
	• Medical condition
	• Surgery

Anticholinesterases: For example echothiopate eye drops, anti-cancer drugs, oral contraceptives give rise to prolonged apnea following suxamethonium administration due to reduced plasma cholinesterase.

Antihypertensives: For example β-blockers diminish cardiac reserve, *diuretics* cause hypovolemia with reduced body potassium, which may enhance neuromuscular block and give rise to arrhythmias, if patient is on digoxin.

Steroids: They cause depression of cortex and predispose to stress induced hypotension.

■ COMPLICATIONS

Coughing

Occurs in patients in light planes of anesthesia.

Causes: Irritation by artificial airways, secretions, blood and regurgitated gastric material. This is more common in patients with chronically inflamed upper airways, like in smokers or in patients with upper respiratory tract infection (URTI).

Management: Coughing under anesthesia can be controlled by deepening of anesthesia and/or by giving muscle relaxants.

Hiccup

Intermittent spasm of the diaphragm.

Causes

1. Afferent impulse from the abdominal or thoracic viscous via the vagus.
2. Coeliac and abdominal autonomic plexus stimulating sensory phrenic nerve endings.

Management

a. Deepen the level of anesthesia
b. Use of muscle relaxant
c. Nasopharyngeal stimulation with a catheter may work in some cases.

Wheezing

Causes

1. Reflex stimulation under light anesthesia
   • Tracheal intubation
   • Carinal stimulation
   • Surgical stimulation while operating on upper abdomen, anus, cervix.
2. Endotracheal tube (ETT)
   • ETT inserted too far
   • Kinked or partially blocked ETT
   • Overdistended ETT cuff
3. Anaphylactic reaction

4. Aspiration
5. Pneumothorax
6. Drugs—β-blockers like propranolol

Management

1. Rule out mechanical obstruction.
2. IPPV (Intermittent positive pressure ventilation) with increased inspired oxygen concentration.
3. Treat the cause.
4. Deepen the level of anesthesia with inhalation agent like halothane.
5. Aminophylline IV 250 to 500 mg slowly.
6. Salbutamol IV 250 mg/2.5 mg inhalation.
7. Adrenaline IV (1–3 ml of 1:10,000) severe anaphylaxis.
8. Steroids IV 200 mg 4 hourly.
9. Ketamine (if other drugs fail).

Cyanosis

Common causes of cyanosis

• Misplaced ETT
• Disconnection
• Airway obstruction
• Oxygen supply failure
• Cardiac arrest

Management

1. Check pulse—if absent, treat as for cardiac arrest.
2. Check gas flow settings on rotameters.
3. Increase inspired oxygen setting.
4. Monitor oxygen saturation (SaO_2), end tidal CO_2 (ET CO_2) and ECG.
5. Check—does chest move normally?
   If does not move, blow down ETT.
   a. Lungs easy to inflate—fault in the ventilator, gas supply or in the breathing circuit.
   b. Lungs impossible or difficult to inflate—there is a fault with the:
      • ETT
        — in bronchus—withdraw the tube slightly
        — in esophagus or pharynx
        — check $ETCO_2$
        — blocked or kinked
        — inspect with laryngoscope, check the patency with a catheter
        — herniated cuff –to rule out deflate cuff.
      • Chest
        — Rule out bronchospasm, pneumothorax, hemothorax and fluid in alveoli

If chest moves, fault may be in
  i.   Chest
  ii. Circulation
  iii. Oxygen source

Cardiac Arrhythmias

Causes

1. Hypercarbia.
2. Hypoxia.
3. Induction drugs.
4. Inhalation agents.
5. Laryngoscopy.
6. Surgical stimulus.
7. Light plane of anesthesia.
8. Adrenaline infiltration.
9. Use of bone cement.
10. Release of tourniquet
11. Electrolyte disturbances.

Management

• Confirm that ventilation and oxygenation are adequate.
• Rule out the causes one by one.
• Use antiarrhythmic drugs, two percent lignocaine, etc.

Fluctuations in Blood Pressure

Hypertension

Causes

1. Light anesthesia
2. Hypoventilation
3. Hypercarbia
4. Infiltration of adrenaline
5. Rise in intracranial tension

Management

• Treat the cause.
• If severe, use vasodilators, nitroprusside, nitroglycerine, etc.

Hypotension

Causes

Anesthetic drugs
• Induction
• Inhalation
• D-tubocurarine

• Opioid
• Intermittent positive pressure ventilation (IPPV)

Surgical
• Blood loss
• Head-up position.

Medications
• β-blockers

Management

1. Volume load
2. IV atropine
3. IV vasopressor like mephentermine, vasoxyl, dopamine

Hypoxemia

Causes

1. Equipment failure
   • Oxygen delivery
   • Circuit disconnection/misconnection
2. Hypoventilation
   • Depressed ventilation
   • Obstructed airway
   • Wrong ventilator settings
3. Ventilation perfusion mismatch
   • Endobronchial intubation
   • Esophageal intubation

Management

1. Ventilate the patient with self-inflating bag till the problem is sorted out.
2. Rule out any disconnections/misconnections.
3. Check the position of ETT.
4. Find out the site of obstruction and appropriate action.

Carbon Dioxide Status

Hypercarbia

Causes

1. Hypoventilation
   • CNS depression
   • Muscle weakness due to muscle relaxant
   • History of chronic obstructive pulmonary disease (COPD)
2. Accumulation of carbon dioxide in circuit
   • Nonfunctioning nonrebreathing valve
   • Exhausted soda lime
   • Low fresh gas flow

Management
- Assist ventilation.
- Correct the cause.

Hypocarbia

Cause: Hyperventilation
Management: Reduce IPPV

Change of Body Temperature

Hypothermia

Causes
- Heat loss due to
  - radiation
  - conduction
  - convection
  - evaporation from body

Management: Warm the patient.

Hyperthermia

Causes

1. Anticholinergic blockade of sweating
2. Infection
3. Thyrotoxicosis

Malignant Hyperthermia

Malignants hyperthermia is a very rare complication of general anesthesia with a high mortality, unless it is detected and treated early. Symptoms are high fever, tachycardia, tachypnea, cyanosis.

Cause: Triggering agent—inhalation anesthetic agents or suxamethonium.

Management

1. Stop anesthesia and disconnect patient from the anesthesia machine
2. Ventilate with 100 percent oxygen.
3. Start cooling the patient (ice packs).
4. Treat arrhythmias.
5. Treat acidosis and hyperkalemia.
6. Maintain urine output with IV fluids.
7. Give dantrolene if available. It is a specific treatment which lowers mortality.

Laryngospasm

Signs

In partial spasm, the patient makes a typical 'croaking sound' during inspiration. When the spasm is complete, the patient makes no sound at all. Both are accompanied by respiratory obstruction-suprasternal, supraclavicular indrawing, intercostal and subcostal recession, see-saw respiration and the use of accessory muscles.

Causes

1. Reflex response to intubation.
2. Saliva, blood, gastric contents contact with glottic structures.
3. Inhalation of irritant vapor, e.g. diethyl ether.
4. After extubation.

Prevention of Laryngospasm is the Real Objective

1. Before extubation, laryngoscopy under deep plane of anesthesia.
2. Extubate under deep level of anesthesia, or
3. Extubate when the patient is responding to verbal commands.

Management

1. Ventilating with 100 percent oxygen under positive pressure with bag and mask.
2. Intubate with a small dose of suxamethonium, if impossible to ventilate.
3. Suck the oropharynx.

Life threatening Upper Airway Obstruction

Signs

1. Tracheal tug or inspiratory stridor.
2. Rocking movement of the chest.
3. Vigorous abdominal movement.
4. Alae nasi moving.
5. Suction of suprasternal notch and intercostal spaces.
6. Tachypnea.
7. Cyanosis.

Management

1. Give 100 percent oxygen.
2. Insert 2 large bore IV cannulae (10 to 14 G) through cricothyroid membrane.
   Connect one cannula to anesthetic machine and push emergency oxygen flush for a short period to produce inflation.

NB: Check that the patient's expiration is through the glottis, otherwise disconnect the cannula to allow each expiration.

Connections: IV cannula ⇒ 10 ml syringe barrel ⇒ 8 mm cuffed ETT ⇒ catheter mount ⇒ anesthetic machine.

Pulmonary Aspiration in the Anesthetized Patient

It is said that the gastric fluid volume is 25 ml or more or the pH is less than 2.5, are needed to produce the acid aspiration syndrome.

Signs

- Tachypnea, bronchospasm.
- Tachycardia, cyanosis, respiration rhonchi crepitation.

Management

1. Place patient in head low position and on side.
2. Laryngoscopy and suction (consider bronchoscopy if solid matter inhaled).
   a. Intubate with a cuffed tube.
   b. Endotracheal suction in head low position.
   c. Intermittent positive pressure ventilation with oxygen.
   d. Treat bronchospasm with IV aminophylline 500 mg or salbutamol 250 mg.
   e. Methylprednisolone 2 gm IV slowly.
   f. Pass nasogastric tube and aspirate stomach contents. Give 30 ml sodium citrate.
   g. Chest X-rays.
   h. Chest physiotherapy.
   i. If surgery is essential, consider regional technique. *Consider IPPV if clinical diagnosis is aspiration.*

Cardiac Arrest during Anesthesia (Absent Carotid Pulse)

Management

1. Stop all anesthetic agents. Administer 100 percent oxygen. Note the time.
2. Call for help. Get a defibrillator.
3. Commence external chest compression (ECC) over lower sternum—80 to 100 compressions per minute.

4. Ventilate via endotracheal tube (ETT).
   Check oxygen supply, machine, ventilator, breathing circuit, and ETT are safe.
   If in doubt change or replace ETT, manually ventilate with another simple breathing system or use another anesthetic machine to provide oxygen from a cylinder.
5. Monitor ECG.
   The details of the CPR management are given in Chapter 20 on Cardiopulmonary Resuscitation.

Severe Drug Reactions

Diagnosis

- Flushing and urticaria
- Hypotension
- Bronchospasm.

Management

1. Adrenaline dilute 500 mg in 5 ml (1:10,000) and give 1 to 5 ml slowly IV.
   Hydrocortisone 200 to 500 mg or 2 g, methylprednisolone IV are of uncertain value.
2. Raise the legs.
3. Administer oxygen and ventilate.
4. Start IV fluids.
5. Aminophylline 250 mg IV slowly.
   Salbutamol 250 μg IV slowly or
   2.5 mg nebulized.
6. Antihistaminics, e.g. chlorpheniramine 10 to 20 mg IV.

Complications due to Improper Patient Position

Nerve Injury

Many complications have been associated with improper patient positioning during surgery. These include nerve damage as a result of ischemic injury and compression neuropathy, e.g. radial, ulnar, common peroneal, optic and facial nerves.

Prevention

1. Evaluation of patient's postural limitations during preanesthetic evaluation.
2. Padding pressure points of susceptible nerves during surgery.
3. Avoid flexion/extension of a joint beyond its limit.

Air Embolism

Causes

1. Faulty IV technique
2. Disconnection of CVP line and if CVP is low.
3. Opening of veins at subatmospheric pressure (sitting position).

Management

1. Immediate flooding of the wound with saline.
2. Compression of the neck veins.
3. Lower the operative site below the level of heart.
4. Stop nitrous oxide. Give 100 percent oxygen.
5. Aspirate air through CVP catheter if *in situ*.
6. CPR if required.

Awareness during General Anesthesia

Cause: This is associated with the use of muscle relaxants during which a patient may be paralyzed while awake at the time of intubation or surgery.

1. This can occur when an insufficient dose of induction agent is given. While waiting for the nondepolarizing relaxant to take effect, there is a drop in the blood level of IV anesthetic. An inhalation agent should be introduced early to reduce the risk of awareness.
2. Incorrect delivery from a faulty anesthesia machine, dilution of the breathing mixture with the emergency oxygen accidentally left on, entrapment of air into the circuit, empty vapourizer, or in case of total intravenous anesthesia (TIVA), empty syringe pump.
3. Certain surgeries during which awareness is commonly encountered—cesarean section, with restriction of drugs to prevent depression of fetus, cardiopulmonary bypass with great dilution of anesthetic drugs, very light anesthesia in a very high risk case or during bronchoscopy.

Prevention

1. A thorough preoperative check up of the machine and the ventilator.
2. Check the level of inhalation agent in the vapourizer.
3. Monitoring of end expiratory concentration of the agent is essential along with clinical signs, to gauge the proper depth of anesthesia.

POSTOPERATIVE ANESTHETIC COMPLICATIONS

Postoperative Nausea and Vomiting

Predisposing Factors that Increase Nausea and Vomiting

1. Female gender
2. Young
3. Obesity
4. Pregnancy
5. Abdominal distention
6. Intracranial hypertension
7. Drugs: Premedicants—opiates, NSAIDs, antibiotics Anesthetics—ether, nitrous oxide
8. Presence of pain, hypoxia, hypotension, hypoglycemia in the postoperative period.
9. Types of surgery—middle ear, eye, gastrointestinal surgery.

Prevention

1. Treat the underlying cause.
2. Keep patient in supine position.
3. Antiemetics:
   - Promethazine 12.5 to 25 mg IM/IV (antihistaminics).
   - Metoclopramide 10 to 20 mg orally (PO-per oral route)/IV(dopamine antagonist)
   - Cimetidine 300 mg IV (acid prophylaxis)
   - Ranitidine 50 mg IV (acid prophylaxis)
   - Sodium citrate 30 to 60 ml orally (nonparticulate antacid).

Postoperative Hypertension

Causes

1. Pain
2. Hypoxia
3. Hypercarbia
4. Shivering
5. Emergence delirium
6. Full bladder
7. Excess catecholamines–anxiety, pheochromocytoma
8. Malignant hyperpyrexia

Management

1. Treat the cause.
2. If the cause cannot be identified and treated, then

- Chlorpromazine 2 to 5 mg IV. Repeat as necessary. If tachycardia (more than 90/min), then give propranolol IV slowly.
3. If hypertension still persists, consider sodium nitroprusside infusion, with intra-arterial monitoring.

Postoperative Respiratory Inadequacy

Causes

1. CNS depressant
   - Opioids
   - Anesthetic agents
   - Benzodiazepines
2. Muscle relaxants
   Nondepolarizing effects potentiated with
   - Aminoglycoside antibiotics
   - Excess of neostigmine
   Depolarizing
   - Pseudocholinesterase deficiency
   - Type II block
   Biochemical events
   - Hypocapnia
   - Hypokalemia
   - Acidosis
   - Hypothermia

Management

1. *If patient still intubated,* ventilate with oxygen.
2. *If patient extubated,* ventilate with 100 percent oxygen via face mask and consider reintubation.
3. Assess neuromuscular block with nerve stimulator. If residual block is revealed, give IV atropine and neostigmine. Do not exceed a total of 5 mg neostigmine.
4. *Assess* if patient has come out of the effect of inhalation agent.
5. If benzodiazepine is given, give flumazenil 20 µg IV over 15 seconds, then 100 µg every 60 seconds as required.
6. If a narcotic is given, give naloxone (0.4 mg diluted to 4 ml, given in 0.1 mg increments).
7. If patient is sedated, give IV doxapram (upto 100 mg).
8. Keep patient on ventilator.
9. Monitor:
   Blood gases
   - Electrolytes
   - Temperature
   - Neuromuscular block
   - Neurological examination

- Serum cholinesterase
- X-ray chest

Failure to Wake-up

Causes

1. An overdose of anesthetics
   - Opioids
   - Benzodiazepines
   - Premedication
2. Cerebral hypoxia
3. Hypercarbia
4. Endocrine causes—hypoglycemia, hyperglycemia, hypothyroidism
5. Liver failure
6. Kidney failure
7. Hypothermia

Management

1. If ventilation inadequate, ventilate with 100 percent oxygen.
2. Wait and watch.
3. Use specific antagonist.
4. If hypothermia, warm the patient.
5. Correction of
   - Fluid, electrolyte and acid-base balance
   - Hypoglycemia.

Postoperative Infection

Spread of infection can occur from:
1. Use of contaminated anesthesia equipment.
2. Introduction of vascular cannulae.
3. Intubation.
4. Mechanical ventilation.

Prevention of infection in patients

1. Before and after each case, hands should be washed with soap and water.
2. Gown and mask should be worn. The use of gloves to avoid patient contact.
3. Strict aseptic technique.
4. Use of disposable items.
5. Cleaning and sterilization of reusable equipment.
6. Use of bacterial filters in breathing circuit.

Postoperative Restlessness

Causes

1. Hypoxemia
2. Pain

3. Drug effect
4. Psychological set-up of patient

Management

1. Rule out hypoxemia
2. Treat the cause.

Respiratory Obstruction

Causes

Upper airway obstruction
1. Falling back of tongue
2. Secretions, blood, tooth, foreign body
3. Throat pack

Lower airway obstruction
1. Bronchospasm
2. Aspiration

Management

1. Clear the airway
2. Ventilation with bag and mask

3. Intubation SOS
4. Oxygenation
5. Tracheostomy SOS
6. Treat bronchospasm, aspiration

Postoperative Shivering

Causes

1. Following halothane anesthesia
2. Hypothermia
3. Reaction to blood transfusion

Management

1. Oxygenation
2. Warm the patient
3. Stop the blood transfusion

The incidence of perioperative complications has come down due to the:

1. Availability of monitoring equipment, and
2. Improved anesthetic and surgical care.

20 Cardiopulmonary Resuscitation

Cardiac arrest is the most serious complication faced by a medical personnel. A prompt diagnosis and immediate cardiopulmonary resuscitation (CPR) can prevent many deaths.

CARDIAC ARREST AND ITS TREATMENT

In cardiac arrest, circulation ceases or stops and vital organs are deprived of oxygen. It can be broadly defined as "inability of the heart to sustain an effective output."

Etiology

Causes of cardiac arrest are varied and many.

1. *Cardiac disease:* Coronary artery disease, valvular lesion, cardiomyopathies, heart blocks.
2. *Hypoxia:* Due to respiratory obstruction or disease.
3. *Hypotension:* Due to massive blood loss.
4. *Hypoglycemia:* In diabetic patients or in children/adults due to preoperative conditions.
5. *Fainting:* Most common during anesthesia in dental chair.
6. *Effect of drugs:* Intravascular injection of adrenaline, sensitivity to local anesthetic agent.
7. *Electrolytic changes:* Intravenous administration of calcium, rise of serum potassium in diabetic acidosis or renal failure.
8. *Vagal reflex mechanism:* During intubation, surgical stimuli provoking bradycardia.
9. *Terminal stages of any disease:* Diabetic coma, malignancy, etc.

Diagnosis of Cardiac Arrest

1. *Pulse:* Absence of pulse in major vessels like carotid or femoral.
2. *Respiration:* Cessation of respiration, absence of breath sounds.
3. *Auscultation of the heart:* Absence of heart sounds.
4. *Pupils:* Pupils may be dilated with a sluggish or no reaction to light.
5. *Skin color:* There may be pallor or cyanosis.
6. *General condition:* An unconscious person not responding to stimuli.

Treatment of Cardiac Arrest

Cardiac pulmonary resuscitation (CPR) is most effective, when started immediately and should be initiated by any person present at the time of cardiac arrest/when the patient collapses.

Management of CPR depends on whether the arrest has occurred in the hospital or outside the hospital and on the availability of a single or double rescuer.

Outside the hospital, it is the *basic life support* (BLS). Inside the hospital it *is BLS plus advanced care life support* (ACLS) and *postresuscitation life support, in short called as* **cardiac pulmonary cerebral resuscitation (CPCR)**.

Basic Life Support

Aim: The major objective of BLS is to maintain oxygenation in lungs, brain and heart with rescue breathing and cardiac compression by which oxygen is transported to tissues before the ACLS.

Procedure: The three parts sequence (ABC).

Maintain

- Airway
- Breathing
- Circulation

Each part of ABC begins with an assessment phase to determine patient's response, presence of pulse and state of respiration.

Airway

When the victim is unresponsive, one has to first position the patient and assess the airway.

Position of the victim: The victim must be made to lie supine, on a firm flat surface. If the head is higher than the feet, then the blood flow to the brain may be reduced and also the airway management is easier, when the patient is supine.

Position of the rescuer: The rescuer should be at the victim's side at a distance equal to the width of the victim's body and at the level of the victim's shoulder.

Triple maneuver
1. Open the mouth—clear the airway
2. Head tilt and chin lift
3. Jaw thrust.

Opening the airway: In an unconscious patient, muscle tone is often impaired resulting in obstruction of the pharynx, by base of the tongue and soft tissue of the pharynx. Since the tongue is attached to the lower jaw, moving the lower jaw forward will lift the tongue away and open the airway.

Head tilt and chin lift (Figs 20.1A and B)
1. Place one hand on the victim's forehead and apply firm backward pressure to tilt the head back.

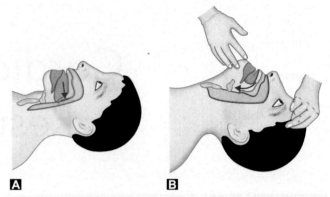

Figs 20.1A and B: Opening the airway with chin lift and head tilt: (A) Airway obstruction due to tongue fall in supine position, (B) Obstruction relieved with chin lift and head tilt

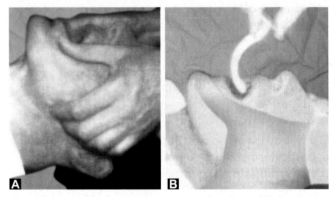

Figs 20.2A and B: Opening the airway by jaw thrust: (A) Jaw thrust, (B) Insertion of oral airway

2. Place the fingers of the other hand under the bony part of the chin.
3. Lift the chin forward and support the jaw.

Jaw thrust (Figs 20.2A and B)
1. Grasp the angle of the victim's lower jaw and lift with both hands, one on each side, displacing the mandible forward, while tilting the head backward.
2. If there is a foreign material or vomitus in the victim's mouth, it should be removed quickly.
3. One should be careful about loose dentures, which may pose a serious problem in mouth to mouth breathing.
4. A Guedel's or Safar's airway, laryngeal mask airway, esophageal gastric tube, if available may be used.

Foreign Body Airway Obstruction

Back blows: It should be given on the middle of the back of the patient (4 times). This produces the cough impulse.

Hemlich maneuver: Consists of manual thrust with the patient breathing, rescuer behind the patient and compressing the patient's chest 6 to 10 times.

Finger sweep method: For unconscious patient, with foreign body, this can be used both in adults and children.

Breathing: One must first determine the presence or absence of breathing by,
- Placing the ear near the victim's mouth or nose
- Looking for chest wall movement
- Auscultation of chest for breath sounds.

Expired air resuscitation

- Mouth to mouth breathing
- Mouth to nose breathing
- Mouth to airway breathing.

Mouth to mouth breathing *(Fig. 20.3):* A quick and effective way to provide oxygen to the victim. The rescuer uses his expired air oxygen to supply to the victim.
1. Open the airway with triple maneuver.
2. Close the victim's nostrils with the thumb and index finger.
3. Take a deep breath and form a seal with lips around the victim's mouth before exhaling.
4. Two slow breaths (of 1/2 to 2 seconds per puff) are given to provide good chest expansion, decreasing the possibility of gastric distention at the same time.

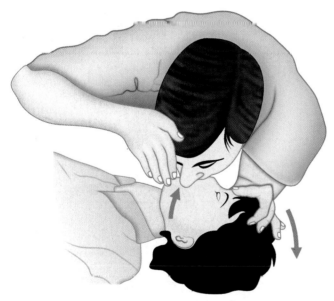

Fig. 20.3: Mouth-to-mouth rescuer breathing

Mouth to nose breathing: When mouth to mouth breathing is not possible, because of difficulty in opening the mouth or a seal cannot be formed.
1. Tilt the victim's head back with one hand over the victim's forehead.
2. Close the victim's mouth.
3. Lift the victim's lower jaw with the other hand.
4. Take a deep breath, form a seal with lips around victim's nose and blow.
5. Victim is then allowed to exhale.

Mouth to airway breathing: Open the airway with the triple maneuver.
1. Close the victim's nostrils with the thumb and index finger.
2. Take a deep breath and form a seal with the lips around the victim's mouth before exhaling.
3. Two slow breaths (of 1/2 to 2 seconds per puff) are given to provide good chest expansion, decreasing the possibility of gastric distention at the same time.

Mouth to Barrier Device

Some rescuers may prefer to use a barrier device, during expired air resuscitation. Two such devices available are masks and face shields. Most masks have a one-way valve, so that exhaled air does not enter rescuer's mouth. A barrier device ideally should have low resistance for gas flow or the user may get tired from excessive respiratory effort.

If rescue breathing is necessary, position the barrier device over the victim's mouth and nose ensuring adequate air seal. The breaths are given in the same sequence at the same rate as described earlier.

Mouth to Mask Breathing

This device includes a transparent mask with a one-way valve mouthpiece. Some devices have an oxygen adapter that permits the administration of supplemented oxygen.

Mouth to mask breathing is reliable form of ventilation, since it allows the rescuer to use two hands to create a seal.

Technique
- Place the mask around the patient's mouth and nose. Positioning of the mask should be proper so that an airtight seal can be obtained.
- Seal the mask by placing the heal and thumb of each hand along the border of the mask and compress

firmly to provide a tight seal around the victim's mouth and nose.

- Place the remaining mask along the bony margin of the jaw.
- Lift the jaw while performing a head tilt.
- Follow the same sequence as for mouth to mouth breathing.

Circulation Check

The carotid artery is the most easily palpable in a groove between the trachea and large strap muscles of the neck. The carotid pulsations are felt, while all other pulses may not be palpable. If no pulse is palpated one should start external cardiac compression to establish circulation.

External Cardiac Compression (Figs 20.4A to C)

In this technique the rescuer applies pressure over the lower half of the sternum, at the rate of 80 to 100 per minute. These compressions provide circulation as a result of a generalized increase in intrathoracic pressure, due to direct compression of the heart between the sternum and the vertebrae. When the compressions are accomplished by rescue breathing, the blood supplied to the organ is likely to carry oxygen.

- Position the victim, supine on a firm surface.
- Locate the lower margin of the victim's rib cage.
- Locate the lower part of the sternum, by moving the fingers along the notch, where the rib meets the sternum in the center of the chest wall.
- Place the heel of one hand, on the lower half of the sternum, with the other hand on top of the first hand, in such a way that the long axis of the rescuer's hand is placed on the long axis of the sternum. This helps in keeping the force of compression on the sternum (Figs 20.5A to C).
- The fingers are kept interlocked at the chest.
- The rescuer's elbow should be locked into a position, such that the arms are straightened and shoulders are placed directly over the hand, so that the thrust of each compression is straight down on the sternum.
- For the normal sized adult, the sternum should be depressed approximately ½ to 1½ inches by the force provided by the rescuer's body weight.
- Optimal sternal compression is the one, which can generate an adequate carotid pulse.

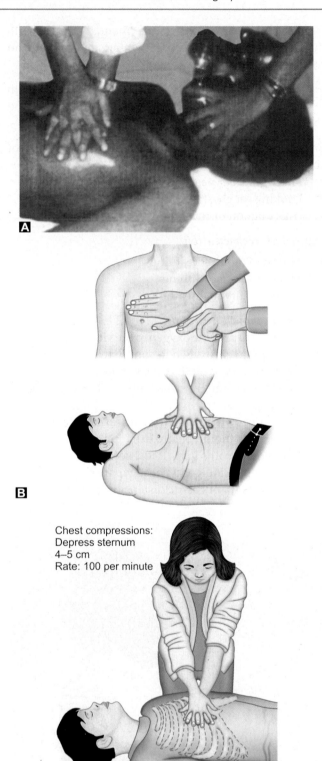

Chest compressions:
Depress sternum
4–5 cm
Rate: 100 per minute

Figs 20.4A to C: External cardiac massage: (A) Clinical picture, (B and C) Diagrammatic representation

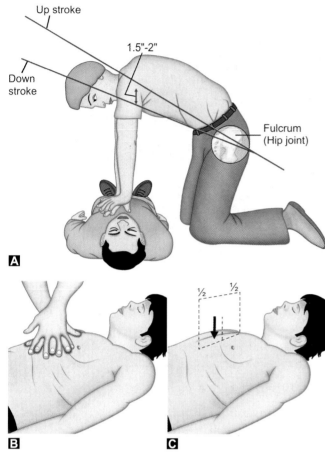

Figs 20.5A to C: External cardiac massage: Chest compression showing the proper position of the rescuer (with shoulder over the victim's sternum and elbows locked)

- The rescuer should release the pressure, after each compression to allow blood to flow into the chest and heart.
- Duration of each compression should be 50 percent of the compression release cycle with a chest compression rate of 80 to 100 per minute.

Assessment of the patient during CPR
Inspection
- Chest rise
- Depth of compression
- Position of rescuer's hands

Palpation
- Check for return pulse
- Assess peripheral pulse

Auscultation
- Breath sounds
- Heart sounds

Standard approach to unconscious patient in one rescuer CPR

- Determine unconscious position of the victim's spine
- Open the airway and deliver slow air breaths
- Perform 18 compressions at the rate of two ventilations
- After 5 cycles of compression re-evaluate the patient
- Check for return of the carotid pulse
- If absent, resume CPR

With two rescuer CPR, the ratio of compression and ventilation is maintained at 5:1.

Advanced Cardiac Life Support

The emergency care provided by BLS helps to restore circulation; advanced cardiac life support (ACLS) helps to evaluate and restore the spontaneous circulatory function. In addition to BLS skills, ACLS includes use of adjunctive equipment and techniques available in a hospital set-up assisting ventilation and circulation, such as ECG monitoring with arrhythmia recognition and defibrillation (Figs 20.6A and B), establishment of IV access and drug therapy.

Key Points

Advanced cardiac life support (ACLS) primary survey: Continue ABC of BLS and defibril-late first.

First ABCD of ACLS
- A — Airway
- B — Breathing
- C — Circulation
- D — Defibrillation

Second ABCD of ACLS
- A—perform endotracheal intubation
- B—assist ventilation
- C—circulatory support, gain IV access, attach monitor, identify rhythm, measure blood pressure, provide appropriate medication
- D—differential diagnosis, find and treat the cause

Drug Therapy

During cardiac arrest, drug therapy is secondary management to the more fundamental interventions. Airway management, ventilation, chest compression and defibrillation, if appropriate, should take precedence over medication.

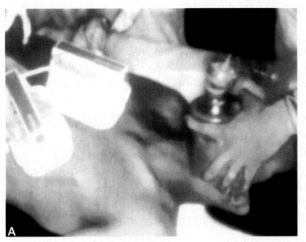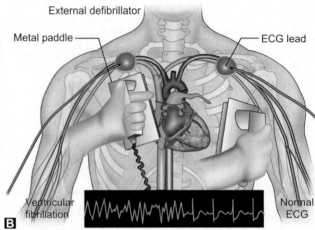

Figs 20.6A and B: External defibrillation: (A) Clinical picture, (B) Diagrammatic representation

Drugs used are as follows:

1. Adrenaline
2. Atropine
3. Xylocaine
4. Calcium
5. Sodium bicarbonate

Adrenaline

Only vasopressor drugs are accepted uniformly for CPR since 1940. It is still the drug of choice even today.

Action: Alpha-adrenergic properties. Increase peripheral resistance, which leads to increase in aortic diastolic pressure causing increase in coronary pressure and myocardial blood flow.

Dose: Empirical dose is 10 mcg/kg body weight repeated every 5 minutes.

Atropine sulphate

Action: Enhances sinus node automaticity and atrioventrical condition by the vagolytic effect. Atropine is indicated in asystole and when bradycardia coexists with hypotension.

Dose: Adults, 0.5 mg IV every 3 to 5 minutes up to a total of 0.4 mg per kg. Children, 0.2 mg per kg, minimum of 0.1 mg per kg to a maximum of 0.5 mg per kg body weight.

Lignocaine or xylocaine

Indications

1. Ventricular tachycardia (VT).
2. Ventricular premature contraction (VPC).

Dose: 1 mg/kg body weight followed by 0.5 mg/kg body weight, followed by infusion (maximum 3 mg/kg body weight).

Calcium: Indicated in hypocalcemia, hypercalcemia, Ca-channel blocker overdose, etc.

Dose: 10 mg/kg body weight.

Sodium bicarbonate
Specific indications

1. Metabolic acidosis.
2. Prolonged duration of arrest.
3. Hyperkalemia.

Side effects

1. Hyperosmolarity
2. Hypernatremia
3. Hypercapnea
4. Paradoxical intracellular acidosis

Dose: 1 mg/kg body weight initially, half dose repeated every 10 minutes. If blood gases are known, dose can be calculated as 0.3 x base deficit x wt in kg (where x means multiplied by).

Other Drugs Used in CPR

Drugs	Dose
Dopamine	5 to 10 mcg/kg body weight.
Dobutamine	2 to 5 mcg/kg body weight.
Calcium chloride	5 to 10 mcg/kg body weight.
Amrinone	0.75 mg/kg body weight.

Vasopressors

Norepinephrine	Infusion—0.1 mcg/kg body weight.
Phenylephrine	50 to 200 mcg/kg body weight.

Vasodilators

Nitroglycerine	Infusion 0.25 to 0.5 mcg/kg body weight
Sodium nitroprusside	0.25 to 0.5 mcg/kg body weight

Postcardiac Arrest Complications

1. Complications of CPR
   Rib re, gastric laceration or rupture, splenic rupture, pneumothorax.
2. Ischemic injury
   a. Renal
   b. Cerebral
   c. Hepatic and others.

Outcome of Resuscitation

- Depends on many factors like age of the patient, the cause line factor witnessed or unwitnessed, the rhythm and the ischemia time, etc.
- Neurological recovery is 50 percent.
  - If the arrest time is less than 6 minutes, and CPR time is less than 15 minutes—the outcome is satisfactory.
  - If arrest time exceeds 6 minutes and CRP time exceeds 15 minutes chances of survival are almost nil.

S
E
C
T
I
O
N

3

Temporomandibular Joint Disorders

21

Temporomandibular Joint: Afflictions and Management

ANATOMY OF THE TEMPOROMANDIBULAR JOINT

The temporomandibular joint (TMJ), also known as the craniomandibular joint/articulation is peculiar to mammals. It is the articulation between the squamous part of the temporal bone and the head of the mandibular condyle (Figs 21.1A and B). The mandibular articulation is labeled as a bilateral diarthrodial or freely movable joint. It is also considered as complex joint, because it involves two separate synovial joints (right and left), in which there is a presence of intracapsular disk or meniscus and both the joints have to function in co-ordination. The TMJ articulation consists of a mandibular or glenoid fossa, an articular eminence or tubercle, a condyle, a separating disk, a joint fibrous capsule and an extracapsular check ligaments.

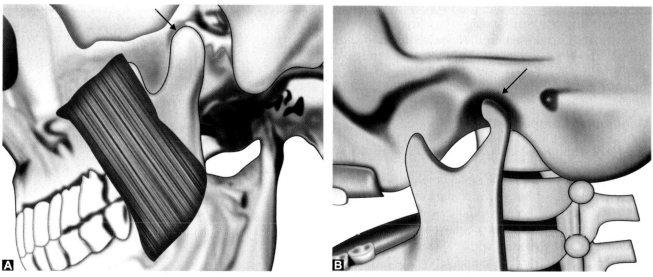

Figs 21.1A and B: Craniomandibular articulation

Articulatory System

The articulatory system comprises of the following:
a. Temporomandibular joint (TMJ)
b. Masticatory and accessory muscles.
c. Occlusion of the teeth.

The function is governed by sensory and motor branches of the third division of the trigeminal nerve (mandibular nerve) and a few fibers of the facial nerve. The occlusion of the teeth plays an important role in the function of the TMJ. Normally, the greatest part of the force of mastication is borne by the dentition of the jaws, but in case of occlusal disharmony, a great deal of force can be shifted to the joint itself.

Mandibular (Glenoid) Fossa (Cranial Component)

Limits: Anteriorly, the articular eminence or tubercle, and posteriorly, a small conical postglenoid tubercle.

Articular eminence: It is a small prominence on the zygomatic arch. It is strongly convex anteroposteriorly and somewhat concave mediolaterally.

Postglenoid tubercle: It separates the articular surface of the fossa laterally from the tympanic plate. And the tympanic plate separates the TMJ from the bony part of the external auditory canal.

Glenoid fossa: It has an anterior articular area formed by the inferior aspect of temporal squama. Its surface is smooth, oval and deeply hollowed out and the bone is very thin at the depth of the fossa. This roof of the glenoid fossa creates a partition between middle cranial fossa and the joint. The fossa is lined by a dense avascular fibrocartilage. In cross section, the fossa and the eminence form a 'lazy S' posteroanteriorly. Squamotympanic fissure separates it from tympanic plate, which forms a posterior wall of the glenoid fossa (Fig. 21.2).

Mandibular Component

Mandibular Condyle

The articular part of the mandible is an ovoid condylar process (head) with narrow mandibular neck. It is broad laterally and narrower medially. The mediolateral dimension varies between 13 to 25 mm and anteroposterior width varies between 5.5 to 16 mm. The majority of human condyles (58%) are slightly convex superiorly, with a radius of curvature

greater than the distance from the medial to lateral poles. Twenty five percent of condyles may be flat superiorly and approximately 12 percent are pointed or angular in shape and 3 percent are bulbous or rounded in shape (Figs 21.3A to D). The surface of the articular eminence that most closely approximates the condyle is consistently congruent with the surface of the condyle. The two condyles of a patient may be asymmetric. A combination of flat condyle on one side with a convex condyle on the other side is most common. The articular part of the condyle is covered by *fibrocartilaginous tissue*

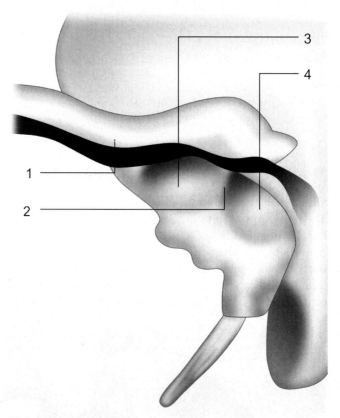

Fig. 21.2: Cranial component of the articulatory system of temporomandibular joint: (1) Articular eminence, (2) Postglenoid tubercle, (3) Glenoid fossa, (4) External auditory canal

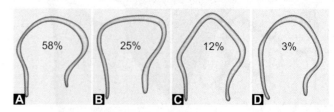

Figs 21.3A to D: Shapes of the mandibular condylar head

and *not with hyaline cartilage*, as in most other joints in the human body.

Temporomandibular Joint Capsule

Temporomandibular joint capsule is a thin sleeve of fibrous tissue investing the joint completely. It is a funnel shaped capsule, which blends with the periosteum of the mandibular neck and it envelops the meniscus. It is attached above anteriorly to the anterior border of the articular eminence and posteriorly to the lip of the squamotympanic fissure and to the anterior surface of the postglenoid process and also to the circumference of the cranial articulating surface and below to the neck of the condyle, on the lateral as well as on the medial aspect. Inside this fibrous tissue capsule, there is a lining of silky synovial membrane (Fig. 21.4).

Ligaments

Lateral or Temporomandibular Joint Ligament (Fig. 21.4)

Temporomandibular joint capsule is reinforced by this main stabilizing ligament. It extends downward and backward from the articular eminence to the external and posterior side of the condylar neck. Its posterior fibers are united with the capsular fibers. This ligament is composed of collagenous fibers that have specific length

and poor ability to stretch, hence it maintains the integrity and limits the movement of TMJ. It mainly limits the anterior excursion of the jaw as well as prevents posterior dislocation, hence it is called as *'check ligament'* of TMJ. But in certain situations, if the joint movements consistently function against ligament, then the ligament elongates and this can create change in the joint biomechanics and can lead to certain pathologic changes.

Accessory Ligaments (Fig. 21.5)

Accessory ligaments make no contribution to joint activity.

Sphenomandibular ligament: A flat band arising from the sphenoid spine and the petrotympanic fissure, runs downward and medial to the TMJ capsule and gets inserted on the lingula of the mandible. It is a remnant of Meckel's cartilage. Sphenomandibular ligament is an important landmark during surgery, as internal maxillary artery and auriculotemporal nerve lies between it and the mandibular neck.

Stylomandibular ligament: It is dense, thick band of the deep cervical fascia extending from the styloid process to the mandibular angle (Figs 21.4 and 21.5).

Articular Disk or Meniscus (Figs 21.6A and B)

The TMJ is a diarthroidial synovial paired joint. This means that there are two joint movements, which occur

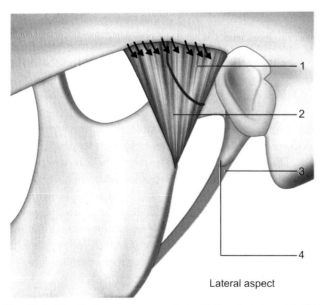

Fig. 21.4: Mandibular component of the TMJ articulation: (1) TMJ capsule, (2) Lateral or TMJ ligament, (3) Stylomandibular ligament, (4) Styloid process

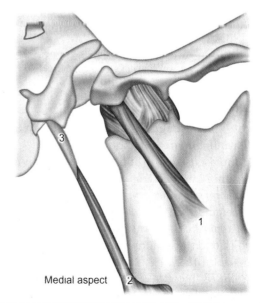

Fig. 21.5: Accessory ligament of TMJ articulation: (1) Sphenomandibular ligament, (2) Stylomandibular ligament, (3) Styloid process

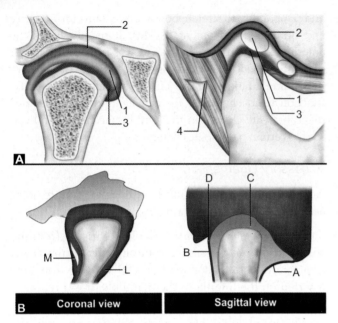

Figs 21.6A and B: (A) TMJ articular space compartments: (1) Articular disk or meniscus, (2) Temporodiskal or superior compartment, (3) Condylodiskal or inferior compartment, (4) Retrodiskal tissue. (B) Attachment of the disk and capsule to the condylar head. L and M—Lateral and medial capsular attachments. A—Anterior band, B—Bilaminar zone, C—Intermediate band, D—Posterior band of the disk

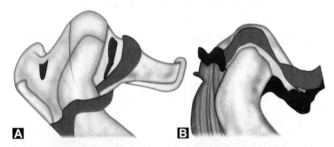

Figs 21.7A and B: Rees described the shape of the meniscus as Jockey's cap, which overlaps the condylar head

in separate compartments of this synovial joint and that one joint cannot operate without the other.

The meniscus or an intervening disk divides the articular space into two compartments:

1. *Lower or inferior compartment*—condylodiskal complex between the condyle and the disk.
2. *Upper (temporodiskal) or superior compartment* between the disk and the temporal bone or glenoid fossa (Figs 21.6A and B).

The *disk* is biconcave in the sagittal section. The superior surface is concavoconvex to match the anatomy of the glenoid fossa and inferior surface is concave to fit

over the condylar head. A detailed study by Rees in 1954 reported that the shape of the articular disk or meniscus is like a school boy's or jockey's cap which overlaps the condylar head (Figs 21.7A and B).

The disk blends medially and laterally with the capsule, which is attached to the medial and lateral poles of the condyle. Anteriorly, the disk is attached to the *articular eminence* above and to the articular margin of the condyle below. It is also confluent anteriorly with the capsule as well as with the fascia of the superior head of the lateral pterygoid muscle. Posteriorly, the disk is attached to the posterior wall of the glenoid fossa above and to the distal aspect of the neck of the condyle below. This area is called as the *posterior bilaminar zone* or *retrodiskal tissue* which has a rich neurovascular supply. Sensory branches of auriculotemporal nerve are abundant here.

The upper joint space always extends farther anteriorly than the lower joint space, which is smaller and more tightly reinforced by the disk attachments, whereas the upper joint space is larger and not as well-reinforced.

The volume of the upper joint space is about 1.2 ml and of the lower joint space is about 0.9 ml.

The disk is a firm but flexible structure. Rees in 1954, described three zones—*posterior band, intermediate zone and anterior band.* The anterior band is moderately thick (about 2 mm), but narrow anteroposteriorly. The thickest and widest is the posterior band (3 mm), whereas the intermediate band is the thinnest (1 mm). The interposition of the thin intermediate zone between the two thicker zones gives the meniscus more flexibility and enables it to alter shape from concave to convex during forward movement.

Histologically, the disk is a meshwork of firmly woven avascular fibrous connective tissue and it is also noninnervated with possible exceptions around its periphery. These collagen fibers impart flexibility to the disk. The disk is designed to transmit the forces generated through the condyle to the articular eminence. *It promotes lubrication, energy absorption and joint range of motion. It acts as a main shock absorber enabling the articulating bones to move against each other with minimum friction and heat production. Disk has a very little potential* for repair after insult. The pliable disk is able to support stabilization of the condyle against the articular eminence.

The posterior attachments of the disk are complicated. This region of the disk is known as bilaminar zone, because it contains two strata of fibers with loose areolar connective tissue filling the space between them. The superior stratum is attached to the tympanic plate and is comprised of elastin rather than collagen, which allows the disk to translate forward with the condyle. It also has got fat and blood vessels. The inferior stratum consists of a fairly compact, inelastic sheets of collagen fibers that attach to the posterior surface of the condyle.

The posterior attachment tissues are highly innervated by the auriculotemporal nerve. Histological examination of this tissue reveals that it is not designed for loading. Above the posterosuperior aspect of the condyle and anterior to the bilaminar zone, the disk is very vascular and this region is called the *vascular knee (genu vasculosa).* The anterior extensions of the disk at its attachment to the superior belly of the lateral pterygoid is also vascular.

The articular surfaces of the condyle and eminence are covered by dense fibrous connective tissue. This connective tissue layer is thickest on the anterior and superior surfaces of the condyle and on the posterior slope and crest of the articular eminence. *The absence of hyaline cartilage on the articulating surface has been wrongly interpreted as indicating that the joint is not a stress bearing joint.*

The hyaline cartilage present in the head of the condyle is the growth center of the condylar process and lies beneath the articular surface (a thin band of cells— the intermediate or proliferative zone). In older joints, this layer may not be very distinct, but the cells of this zone are capable of proliferative activity throughout life and play an important part in the remodeling and repair of the articular surface.

The synovial tissue—is a connective tissue membrane, which lines the joint cavities or spaces and secretes synovial fluid for lubrication of the joint. The upper and lower joint spaces are bathed in a viscous synovial fluid. This fluid is an ultrafiltrate of blood plasma plus a mucin. It is composed chiefly of highly polymerized hyaluronic acid, which is responsible for its viscous quality and is capable of absorbing tremendous shearing forces applied to the joint. The synovial membrane is the innermost layer of the fibrous capsule and unlike avascular articular tissue, it has got excellent regenerative capacity.

Function of the synovium (besides lubrication) is to provide *nutrition, phagocytosis and immunological response* (Synovitis—proliferation of the synovial cells with the concomitant release of prostaglandins and large quantity of collagenase—pain).

Blood Supply

Lateral aspect is supplied by superficial temporal branch of the external carotid artery. Rich vascular supply to the deep and posterior aspect of retrodiskal capsular part by deep auricular, posterior auricular and masseteric branches of the internal maxillary artery. Vascular supply to the lateral pterygoid muscle also supplies to the head of the condyle by penetration of numerous nutrient foramina vessels. The venous pattern is more diffuse, forming a plentiful plexus all around the capsule.

Nerve Supply

The mandibular nerve, the third division of the fifth cranial nerve innervates the jaw joint. Three branches from the mandibular nerve send terminals to the joint capsule.

1. The largest is the auriculotemporal nerve which supplies the posterior, medial and lateral parts of the joint.
2. Masseteric nerve
3. A branch from the posterior deep temporal nerve, supply the anterior parts of the joint.

Movements (Fig. 21.8)

The mandible can be depressed, elevated, protruded or retruded. Lateral excursions can also be carried out. There is a variation of normal patterns of motion in different individuals, which are caused by many factors, including the following:

1. Condyle head size, shape and inclination.
2. Glenoid fossa depth and angulation.
3. Articular eminence height and degree of inclination.
4. Length and laxity of ligaments comprising the joint capsule.
5. Degenerative joint disease state resulting either from local causes or from systemic diseases.
6. Strength, length, position and tonicity of muscles of mastication and the suprahyoid musculature.
7. Neuromuscular control of the muscles (Both the afferent proprioceptor and the efferent motor impulses through the 5th and 7th cranial nerves can be affected by stimuli from the hypothalamic nuclei to the cerebral cortex and vary according to the emotional status of the patient).

The movements of TMJ are manifold. It is ginglymus, diarthroidial type of joint, as it is capable of rotating around more than one axis and is capable of hinge/rotatory movement

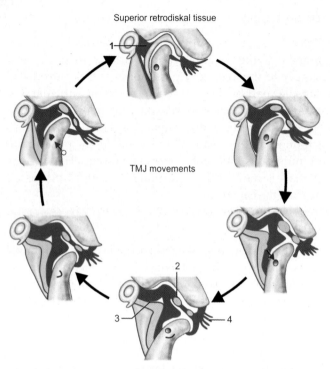

Fig. 21.8: TM joint movements: (1) Superior retrodiskal tissue, (2) Posterior band of the disk, (3) Retrodiskal tissue, (4) Superior head of the lateral pterygoid muscle

(ginglymoid) and also capable of gliding/translatory movement (diarthroidial). Some amount of vertical motion is also possible. By alternate action of the homologous joints, it allows lateral motion and by combination of all, circumduction. Rotation and some slight translation takes place in the lower joint space between the condyle and the articular disk. Translation of the condyle disk complex takes place in the upper joint space.

The disk is attached to the condyle both medially and laterally by the collateral ligaments. These ligaments allow rotation of the disk across the articular surface of the condyle in an anteroposterior direction, while restricting medial and lateral movements. The condylar head can rotate within the encompassing disk (condyle disk complex) and together with disk, it translates against the articular eminence. At rest, the condyle articulates on the intermediate zone of the disk and is maintained in this position by constant interarticular pressure provided by the elevator muscles.

During mouth opening, when the condyle disk complex translates down the articular eminence, the disk rotates posteriorly on the condyle.

The superior retrodiskal lamina, which is composed of loose connective tissue and elastic fibers, allows the condyle disk complex to translate forward without damage to the retrodiskal tissues. During full mouth opening, the superior retrodiskal tissue is fully stretched and offers a posterior retractive force on the disk, limiting the further sliding of the disk. Simultaneously, there is contraction of the fibers of the superior head of the lateral pterygoid muscle. Further gliding and hinging of the condyles brings them in contact with the most anterior parts of the disks as the mouth fully opens.

In closure, movements are reversed. Each head glides back and hinges on its disk. Here the lateral pterygoid muscle relaxes, to allow the disk to glide back and up into the mandibular fossa. During opening and closing, the disk and the condyle move together because of two features—the morphology of the disk and intra articular pressure. If there is any change in intra-articular pressure or in the morphology of the disk, then condyle disk movements can be altered leading towards dysfunction of the complex co-ordinate.

Muscle function: The functions of the muscles of mastication in jaw movements are co-ordinated and balanced by normal muscle tone. Abnormal contraction of any one individual muscle, disrupts the synchronous function that produces co-ordinated movements. The muscles of mastication (medial and lateral pterygoid, masseter, buccinator, mylohyoid, temporalis and anterior belly of the digastric) are assisted by the suprahyoid and digastric muscles, especially in the jaw opening movements. The tongue, with motor innervation accomplished by the hypoglossal nerve, is a strong muscular structure, whose action and position affects jaw movements.

Jaw opening (depression): It is dominated by digastric muscle contraction, which depresses the body of the mandible. This action is assisted by the suprahyoid, sternohyoid and geniohyoid muscles. The lateral pterygoid muscle is believed to be the 'trigger' for opening and contracts to pull the condylar head downward and forward on the articular eminence.

Jaw closure (elevation): It is accomplished by the simultaneous contraction of the masseter, medial pterygoid, and temporalis muscles.

Protrusive movement: It requires equal and simultaneous contracture of lateral and medial pterygoid muscles.

Retrusion: It is brought about by posterior fibers of temporalis muscle, assisted by middle and deep parts of the masseter, digastric and geniohyoid muscles.

Lateral movements: These are carried out by unilateral contracture of medial and lateral pterygoid of each side acting alternatively.

The TMJ is thus classified as a complex, multiaxial, synovial, bicondylar and ginglymodiarthrodial type of joint. It is highly specialized unique joint and has got many distinctive characteristics:

1. Articular surfaces of TMJ are not covered by a hyaline cartilage, but by an avascular fibrocartilage (This is attributed to the membranous ossification by which the mandible, temporal bone and clavicle are formed. Clavicular end of sternoclavicular joint is also covered by avascular fibrocartilage).

2. The right and left articulations are connected by the mandible, the movements are coupled. The individual movement of one articulation directly affects the other.

3. Mandible is stabilized by three functionally linked articulations—the dentition and the two TMJs. Any discrepancy of the dentition will affect the movements of the TMJ.

4. The function of this unique joint is also dependent on delicate neuromuscular balance.

5. The TMJ is the only joint to have a rigid end point of closure, produced as a consequence of teeth contacting.

6. The TMJ is in close proximity to the upper part of the cervical spine. Functionally, the cervical spine, the TMJ and occlusion of teeth are interrelated. Abnormality of any of these components can alter the function.

7. The joint functions as a regional adaptive growth center for the growth and development of the mandible and the middle third of the face, in response to changes in the 'functional matrix' of surrounding masticatory muscle and other soft tissues (In case of restricted stimulus from the soft tissues, as a result of trauma or infection or neuromuscular congenital anomalies, condylar growth response will be restricted. It will also affect the growth and development of facial structure).

The clinicians must recognize dissimilarities between the TMJ and other articulations in contemplating corrective or replacement surgery:

1. The functional stresses on the TMJ are more subtle, than those on most other joints, but they can be easily modified by extraneous factors and are more influential in determining the morphology of the articular elements.

2. Reconstruction of many other articulations is often impossible with anything but alloplasts. But, it is not true with the TMJ.

3. The TMJ has more intimate proximity to vital structures than any other articulation (Except portions of the vertebral column).

▌ TEMPOROMANDIBULAR JOINT DISORDERS

Classification

  i. Intra-articular origin or intrinsic disorders.

  ii. Extra-articular origin or extrinsic disorders.

    Extrinsic factors are those not directly associated with the TMJ, whereas intrinsic factors relate to those conditions existing within the confines of the capsule of the joint.

Disorders due to Extrinsic Factors

Masticatory muscle disorders

a. Protective muscle splinting.

b. Masticatory muscle spasm (MPD syndrome).

c. Masticatory muscle inflammation (myositis).

Problems that result from extrinsic trauma

a. Traumatic arthritis

b. Fracture

c. Internal disk derangement

d. Myositis, myospasm

e. Tendonitis

f. Contracture of elevator muscle—myofibrotic contractures

Because of these extra-articular factors, the function of the TMJ may be hampered.

Whenever, there is a restriction of normal oral opening or inability to open the mouth fully, the term trismus is used. Trismus is brought about by extra-articular causes and it is also labeled as false ankylosis.Trismus is also defined as a condition in which muscle spasm or contracture prevents opening of the mouth (due to infection or other conditions which alter muscle structure).

Causes of trismus

1. *Due to infection:* Orofacial infections around the joint area can bring about trismus or limitation of oral opening. Odontogenic acute infections like pericoronitis, Ludwig's angina, submasseteric and infratemporal abscess, etc. Chronic infections

affecting the jaws also can bring about trismus. Tuberculous osteomyelitis of ramus and/or body mandible, etc.

2. *Trauma:* Fracture of the zygomatic arch may impinge on the coronoid process and restrict the oral opening. Fracture of the mandible also can bring about trismus, because of pain and tenderness or muscle spasm.

3. *Inflammation:* Myositis or muscular atrophy can bring about trismus.

4. *Myositis ossificans:* Following trauma, a hematoma can be formed within the fibers of the masticatory group of muscles especially in the masseter, which can progress into ossification and the muscle stiffness. Clinical and radiographic examination will confirm the presence of these changes.

5. *Tetany:* Typical carpopedal spasm along with trismus can be seen due to hypocalcemia.

6. *Tetanus:* Following acute infection by *Clostridium tetani*, the typical lockjaw symptom can be seen associated with other symptoms, because of persistent tonic muscle spasm.

7. *Neurological disorders:* Epilepsy, brain tumor, bulbar paralysis, embolic hemorrhage in medulla oblongata can bring about trismus.

8. *Psychosomatic trismus:* It is also known as trismus hystericus. Due to extreme fear, anxiety associated with hysterical fits.

9. *Drug induced trismus:* Strychnine poisoning can bring about spasms leading to trismus.

10. *Mechanical blockage:* Elongation, exostosis, osteoma, osteochondroma of coronoid process will cause mechanical blockage and interfere with the normal mandibular movements.

11. *Extra-articular fibrosis:* Chronic cervicofacial sepsis, postradiation therapy, ossification of sphenomandibular ligament, bands of scars and burns of the face and neck region, oral submucous fibrosis will lead toward progressive trismus.

A classical clinical example of trismus is seen occasionally, following the injection of the inferior alveolar nerve block with local anesthetic agent. Bleeding, created by needle puncture in the medial pterygoid muscle, produces a hematoma followed by fibrosis and subsequent trismus. In most cases the hematoma is spontaneously resolved and normal jaw function returns within a week or two. In some of the cases, under sedation or general anesthesia, manipulation of the jaw, with jaw stretcher may be required to break-up the adhesions and restore the function.

Disorders due to Intrinsic Factors

1. *Trauma*
   a. Dislocation, subluxation
   b. Hemarthrosis
   c. Intracapsular fracture, extracapsular fracture
2. *Internal disk displacement*
   a. Anterior disk displacement with reduction
   b. Anterior disk displacement without reduction.
3. *Arthritis*
   a. Osteoarthrosis (degenerative arthritis, osteoarthritis)
   b. Rheumatoid arthritis
   c. Juvenile rheumatoid arthritis
   d. Infectious arthritis
4. *Developmental defects*
   a. Condylar agenesis or aplasia—unilateral/bilateral
   b. Bifid condyle
   c. Condylar hypoplasia
   d. Condylar hyperplasia
5. *Ankylosis*
6. *Neoplasms*
   a. Benign tumors: osteoma, osteochondroma, chondroma
   b. Malignant tumors: Chondrosarcoma, fibrosarcoma, synovial sarcoma.

Dislocation, Subluxation, Hypermobility of Temporomandibular Joint

During normal or unstrained opening of the mouth, the condylar heads translate forward to a position under the apices of the articular eminences. If oral opening proceeds to its maximum capacity, the condylar heads move to the anterior slope of the articular eminences in many normal individuals. Excursion of the condylar heads beyond these limits may be viewed as abnormal and termed as dislocation. In contrast to the fracture dislocation of the condylar head, here the intact condylar head is displaced out of glenoid fossa, much anteriorly beyond articular eminence, but still remains within the capsule of the joint. As far back as 3000 BC in Egypt, Hippocrates first reported a dislocation of the mandible. His method of reduction has survived the ages and is still being used in modern times. Mandibular condylar dislocation is uncommon, compared to the other joints in the body. Its incidence is reported to be 3.1 percent.

The dislocation can be unilateral or bilateral: *Anterior mandibular dislocation* can be classified as:

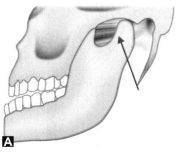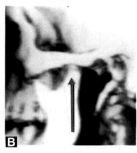

Figs 21.9A and B: (A) Acute dislocation of TM joint, (B) Three-dimensional scan showing the position of condylar head beyond articular eminence. (Acute dislocation)

1. Acute
2. Chronic recurrent (habitual) subluxation
3. Long-standing.

The term luxation is also used for acute dislocation and the terms, *subluxation or hypermobility or habitual chronic recurrent dislocation* is substituted for the term dislocation, when it is incomplete (Figs 21.9A and B).

Causes of Acute Dislocation

a. Extrinsic forces or iatrogenic causes
b. Intrinsic or self-induced forces

Anterior acute dislocation of the condyle occurs, in which the normal anatomic relationships within the joint have been completely disrupted, with the condyle fixed anterior to the articular eminence. Relocation of the condyle in its normal position in the glenoid fossa does not occur voluntarily. It can occur as a single acute event or as chronic recurrent episodes.

Extrinsic or iatrogenic causes: Acute dislocation is common and can be brought about by a blow on the chin, while mouth is open. Injudicious use of mouth gag during general anesthesia or excessive pressure on the mandible, during dental extraction can lead to acute dislocation. It can be post traumatic, spontaneous or associated with psychiatric illness.

Intrinsic or self-induced forces as excessive yawning, vomiting, singing loudly, blowing wind instruments, laughing loudly or opening mouth too wide for eating or hysterical fits can also bring about episode of acute dislocation. There is associated spasm of the lateral pterygoid muscle, as well as spasm of the other muscles of mastication and therefore, the condylar head gets locked into the abnormal anterior position in the infratemporal fossa and cannot be manipulated back to close the mouth. In this situation, unassisted reduction becomes impossible.

Predisposing factors: Laxity of ligaments, capsule and abnormality of skeletal form. Previous injuries, occlusal disharmonies can bring about laxity of the capsule. Flattened eminence and shallow fossa, systemic diseases like Parkinson's disease, epilepsy, Ehlers-Danlos syndrome, etc. can be the predisposing factors. The use of antipsychotic drugs may cause extrapyramidal reactions and dislocation.

Clinical picture of acute dislocation: Dislocation is a dramatic event. It may be unilateral or bilateral. History of the patient may be diagnostic.

Unilateral acute dislocation: It is characterized by difficulty in mastication and swallowing. Speaking may be difficult and profuse drooling of saliva can be present in the early stages. A deviation of the chin toward contralateral side is seen. The deviation produces a lateral cross and open bite on the contralateral side (Figs 21.10 and 21.11).

The mouth is partly open and the affected condyle cannot be palpable. In obese person, absence of condyle from the glenoid fossa may not be apparent, but in others a definite depression will be seen and felt in front of the tragus (Fig. 21.11).

Bilateral acute dislocation: It is associated with pain, inability to close the mouth, tense masticatory muscles, difficulty in speech, excessive salivation, protruding chin. The mandible is postured forward and movements are restricted. There is a gagging of the molar teeth with the presence of anterior open bite. Difficulty in swallowing and drooling of saliva is seen. Patient will complain of pain in the temporal region rather than the joint and may be extremely apprehensive. The distinct hollowness can be felt in both the preauricular regions. Associated muscle spasm contributes to the fixed position of the condyles (Figs 21.12 and 21.13).

Management: The major problem in reduction of dislocation is overcoming the resistance of the severe muscle spasm. Therefore, initially attention is given to reduce tension, anxiety and muscle spasm. This can be achieved by (i) reassuring the patient, (ii) tranquilizer or sedative drugs, (iii) pressure and massage to the area, and (iv) manipulation. Recurrent episodes of acute dislocations are both painful and frustrating to the patient. These may occur at any time and force the patient to seek expert assistance to reduce the dislocation. Longer the time span, the more difficulty in reduction procedure.

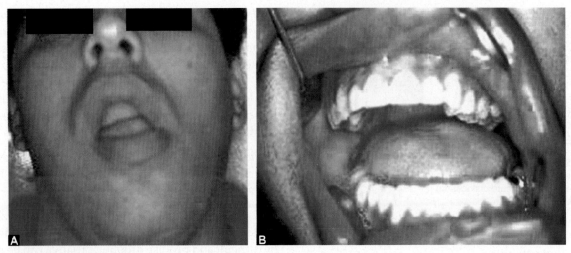

Figs 21.10A and B: Unilateral acute dislocation of (R) TM joint. (A) Extraoral picture showing inability to close the mouth and deviation of the mandible on the unaffected side, (B) Intraoral picture showing the deviation of the mandible

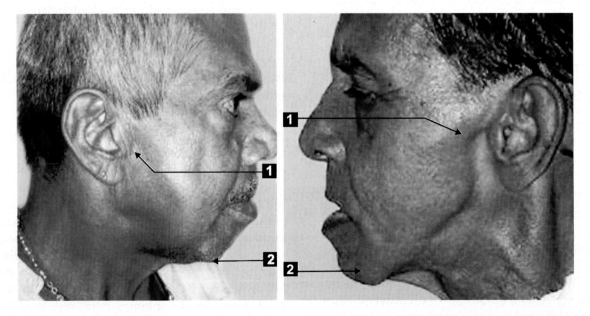

Fig. 21.11: Unilateral acute dislocation of TMJ. Note the preauricular area depression (1) and (2) laterognathia of the mandible

Depending on the amount of associated muscle spasm and pain experienced by the patient plus patient co-operation, the acute dislocation can be reduced by the operator as follows:

1. Manipulation without any form of anesthesia.
2. Manipulation with local anesthesia.
3. Manipulation under general anesthesia/sedation with muscle relaxants.

Manipulation procedure: Remains the same irrespective of the type of anesthesia used. Under local anesthesia, the patient will be seated in a dental chair, while under general anesthesia the patient is made to lie on the operation table in a supine position. First of all, the patient should be given assurance about the procedure and asked to relax completely in a dental chair. Normally, the dislocation is maintained by muscle spasm secondary to painful stimuli arising from the capsule. Few drops of local anesthetic solution may be injected in the glenoid fossa which will eliminate the pain factor and spontaneous reduction may be brought about due to elimination of a neural reflex (Fig. 21.14).

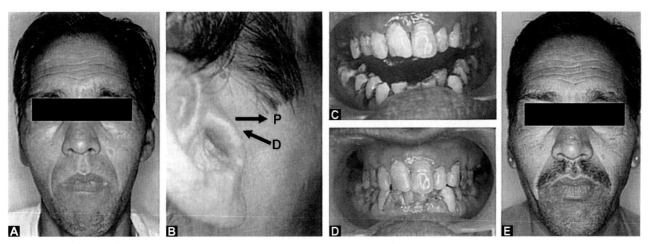

Figs 21.12A to E: Acute bilateral dislocation of TMJ: (A) Clinical frontal face of a patient having acute bilateral TMJ dislocation. Elongated face, (B) Depression in preauricular area. Prominence of dislocated head seen, (C) Anterior open bite with posterior molar gagging seen, (D) Original occlusion of patient, after reduction, (E) Normal face after reduction. D = Depression, P = Prominence

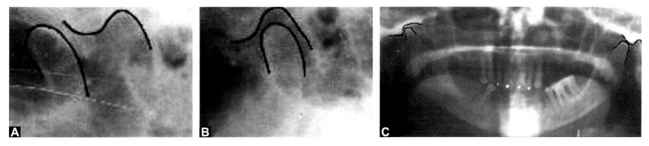

Figs 21.13A to C: (A) Transcranial view of (L) TMJ showing acute dislocation, (B) After reduction, TMJ in closed position, (C) OPG showing bilateral acute dislocation of TMJs

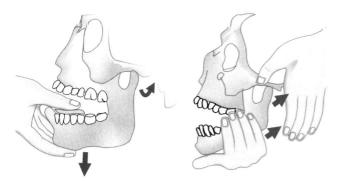

Fig. 21.14: Manipulation procedure for reduction of acute TMJ dislocation

Otherwise, the operator has to stand in front of the patient and he has to grasp the mandible with both the hands, one on each side to reverse the process of dislocation. The thumbs of the operator should be covered with gauze to prevent injury during manipulation, as sudden reduction can take place trapping the thumbs of the operator by the teeth. The thumbs are placed on the occlusal surfaces of the lower molars and fingertips are placed below the chin. Operator has to exert full body pressure and give downward pressure on the posterior teeth to depress the jaw and at the same time the fingertips are placed below the chin to elevate it by giving upward pressure. The downward pressure overcomes spasm of the muscles, plus it brings the locked condylar head below the level of articular eminence and then the backward pressure is given to push the entire mandible posteriorly. This will allow the condylar head to go back into its original position. After this reduction procedure, the mouth is closed and patient is asked to keep the oral opening restricted. Immobilization can be carried out, by giving barrel bandage to the patient for the period of 10 to 14 days and patient is kept on semisolid diet. This will allow to give rest to the joint. Anti inflammatory, analgesic drugs should be prescribed for the period of 3 to 5 days. The patient is warned to avoid excessive oral opening and support the chin, while yawning in future. The term 'long-standing' is applicable to those cases, which remain unusually dislocated for longer than one month. Frequently, this follows extraction of teeth or tonsillectomy under general anesthesia, where the jaw is excessively forced open. Dislocation may then remain unnoticed, if not examined postoperatively. Long-standing dislocations are occasionally encountered due to passive acceptance of the condition by the patient. In these cases, with passage of time, additional muscle spasm and fibrotic changes occur in the ligaments and muscles, thus increasing the severity of the problem.

Long-standing acute dislocation, which does not respond to the above procedure can be reduced by administering general anesthesia. If manual reduction fails, then open surgical procedure can be opted as a last resort.

Open reduction consists of opening the joint through preauricular incision and direct vision manipulation can be done. If this also fails, then eminectomy or condylectomy procedure can be carried out, so that future locking of the condylar head can be avoided.

Chronic Recurrent or Habitual Dislocation or Subluxation (Figs 21.15 to 21.17)

The term should be reserved for repeated episodes of dislocation, where there is *abnormal anterior excursion of the condyles beyond the articular eminence, but the patient is able to manipulate it back into normal position.* So here the condylar head moves, unassisted, forward and backward over the articular eminence.

This *recurrent, incomplete, self-reducing, habitual dislocation is termed as hypermobility or chronic subluxation* of the TMJ. The triad of ligamentous and capsular flaccidity, eminential erosion and flattening and trauma is well recognized in the genesis of chronic recurrent subluxation.

In such predisposed individuals, the acts of yawning, vomiting, laughing may precipitate subluxation. It is also seen in severe epilepsy, dystrophia myotonia and the Ehlers-Danlos syndrome. It can be also seen in professionals like teachers, speakers or musicians. It can be very embarrassing in public appearances to these patients. In recurrent subluxation, patient enters into vicious cycle. With each episode of subluxation, there is further stretching of the capsular ligament, which aggravates the condition and leads to further recurrence.

Ehlers-Danlos syndrome: This is a rare inherited disorder of the connective tissue, in which recurrent dislocation of the TMJ is seen. Four cardinal symptoms are as follows:
1. Hyperelasticity of the skin.
2. Fragility of the skin.
3. Hypermobility of the joints.
4. Fragility of the blood vessels.

Chronic subluxation with pain: Excessive excursive movement or hypermobility of the mandibular condyle. It is not necessarily painful. But in some of the patients, sudden sharp and severe pain occurs when the mouth is opened widely. Occasionally, the problem is of such

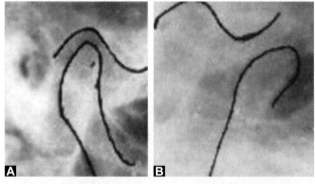

Figs 21.15A and B: Chronic subluxation of TMJ. Transcranial X-rays of (R) TMJ in closed and open position showing hypermobility of TMJ

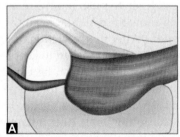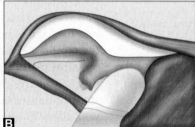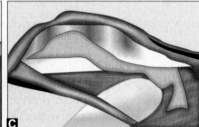

Figs 21.16A to C: Habitual or recurrent dislocation or subluxation of TMJ: (A) Normal relationship of the condylar head and disk in rest position, (B) Maximum translated position. Rotation of the disk is seen posteriorly, (C) Subluxation of the condylar head, trapping of the disk forward, with disk space collapse above the head. Self reducing condition

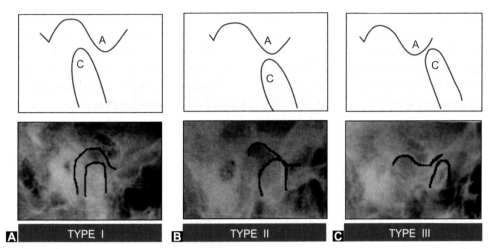

Figs 21.17A to C: Classification patterns of condylar mobility. A—Articular eminence, C—Condyle: (A) Type I—Condyle placed behind articular eminence at maximal mouth opening, (B) Type II—Condyle just under the articular eminence at maximal mouth opening, (C) Type III—Condyle situated anteriorly to the articular eminence at maximal mouth opening

a magnitude, that the patient becomes reluctant to masticate food.

In literature, over a span of at least 100 years, there are descriptions of numerous and varied procedures designed to correct this abnormality. The plethora of surgical procedures available suggests that not only this problem is difficult to manage, but the majority of procedures described in the literature have proved less than successful over a period of time.

The review of the different management procedures is as follows:

1   *Intermaxillary fixation or limiting the oral opening by giving elastics:* Total immobilization of the jaw for the period of 3 to 4 weeks gives rest to the joint. But patient has to be kept on liquid diet. By applying prefabricated splint to the maxillary and mandibular arches, elastic guidance can be given to restrict oral opening or if the patient is co-operative, he/she is advised to restrict the oral opening on his/her own and instructed to eat food with the spoon or advised to take small morsels of food, thereby restricting the oral opening.

2. *Use of sclerosing solution injections into the joint space:* Sodium psylliate provided consistently best results. But is no longer available. Sodium morrhuate has been used as a sclerosing agent, but has failed to produce good results. Sodium tetradecyl sulfate, which was developed for mildly sclerosing varicose veins and hemorrhoids, can be used with caution, as allergic or anaphylactic reactions have been reported. The injection of these sclerosing solution brings about fibrosis in the capsule, but the results are short lived. Hence, the use is not recommended.

In the absence of effective sclerosing agent, chronic subluxation associated with severe pain and not responding to conservative line of treatment becomes a surgical problem.

In 1976, *Miller and Murphy* divided surgical procedures to correct recurrent condylar dislocation into five categories:

1. Capsule tightening procedure.
2. Creation of a mechanical obstacle or block.
3. Direct restraint of the condyle
4. Creation of a new muscle balance.
5. Removal of mechanical obstacle.

Capsule tightening procedures: These procedures were apparently effective over a short period.

a. *Capsulorrhaphy*—consists of shortening the capsule by removing a section and suturing it to make it tight.
b. *Placement of a vertical incision* in the capsule and then drawing it tight by overlapping the edges and suturing.
c. *Reinforcement of the joint capsule* by turning down a strip of temporal fascia and suturing to the capsule.

Creation of a mechanical obstacle (Figs 21.18A and B) A number of procedures have been suggested for creating an obstacle, in the region of articular eminence, so that it can effectively block the excessive anterior excursion of the condyle.

a   *Lindermann* performed an osteotomy on the eminence and turned it down in front of the condylar head to prevent its forward movement.

b.   *Mayor* advocated a placement of a graft (taken from the zygoma) over the eminence to increase the size and height.

c.   *Placement of silastic block or vitallium mesh implants to add the height of eminence.*

d.   *Dautry* advocated an osteotomy on the zygomatic arch and depressing it in front of the condylar head to serve as an obstacle to abnormal forward translation.

e.   *Findlay* reported the use of L shaped pins anchored in the zygomatic process of the temporal bone and projecting it anterior to the condyle.

In the long term results it was noticed, that all types of mechanical devices used to restrain the forward excursion of the condyle have certain disadvantages. Hence not used frequently, because of poor rate of success.

Direct restrain of condyle: Procedures directed towards restraining the condyle from abnormal forward movements have been attempted for over half a century.

a.   Temporalis fascia turned down and sutured to the lateral surface of the articular capsule.

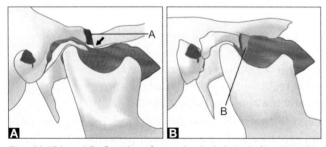

Figs 21.18A and B: Creating of a mechanical obstacle for preventing hypermobility. (A) Dautry's zygomatic arch osteotomy, (B) Mayor's grafting technique on the eminence

b.   Piece of fascia lata threaded through a hole in the zygomatic arch and second hole in the condyle. The fascia was then tightened, until half of the preoperative opening existed.

These techniques are complicated and have questionable long term results.

Creation of new muscle balance

a.   After taking intraoral incision, from the tip of the coronoid to retromolar area, the temporalis tendon and periosteum is divided, at and below the coronoid tip and masseter muscle is also partly elevated from the lateral surface of the ramus. This vertical wound is then sutured into a tight horizontal manner. The same procedure is repeated on the opposite side. This procedure brings about scar formation or fibrosis and thereby restricts the oral opening.

b.   Medial pterygoid muscle also can be shortened (medial pterygoid myotomy procedure).

Removal of mechanical obstacles: Techniques involving surgical removal of obstacles, which are believed to block or restrict the condyle from returning to its normal position in the glenoid fossa, have been directed towards the meniscus, condylar head, and articular eminence.

a.   *Removal of torn meniscus or meniscectomy:* Torn meniscus, which was thought as the obstacle, is removed. This technique became very popular, but unfortunately the undesirable results like protracted pain, grating, roughening of the condylar head, and an occasional ankylosis were noticed.

b.   *The high condylectomy:* The shortened head of the condyle will have less tendency to lock in front of the articular eminence. Here, it involves excision of the superior portion of condylar head, above the attachment of the lateral pterygoid muscle, so that the balance of the muscle function is not disturbed (Figs 21.19A to F).

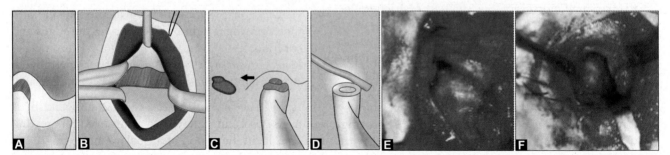

Figs 21.19A to F: High condylectomy procedure: (A to C) Excision of the superior portion of condylar head above the attachment of lateral pterygoid muscle, (D) Smoothening of the rest of the head with bone file, (E) Condyle exposed surgically, osteophyte is seen, (F) High condylectomy and contouring of condylar head (Intra operative pictures–E and F)

c. *Eminectomy:* In 1951, Myrhaug first reported this procedure. The rationale for this procedure is to allow the condylar head to move forward and backward free of obstruction, by the excision of the articular eminence, instead of attempting to restrict the forward movement of the condylar head (Figs 21.20 to 21.22).

Indications

1. Recurrent episodes of dislocations.
2. Chronic hypermobility associated with severe pain.
3. Irreversible TMJ pain associated with clicking or grating.

Eminectomy (Figs 21.20 and 21.21 and 21.22)

This procedure is relatively simple to perform. The main advantage is that the main joint cavity is not opened and avoids injury to meniscus and capsule. It can be performed under local anesthesia bilaterally with gratifying results.

The basic step in this procedure consists of undermining and turning the skin and subcutaneous flap upward making small horizontal incision over the zygomatic arch in the region of articular eminence in front of the tragus. The articular eminence is located approximately 1.5 cm anterior to external auditory meatus. This distance is measured and the location of eminence is marked with marking ink prior to the incision. The eminence is next exposed by a T incision, the horizontal portion being over and parallel to the arch and vertical portion extending to the apex of the eminence. The periosteum is then reflected to expose the entire lateral portion of the eminence. A series of bur holes are drilled with a small round bur at the base of the eminence, in a line parallel to the arch. The bur is directed downward at approximately 10 degrees from horizontal plane. The bur holes are next connected with fissure bur, extending the cut as far inward as the shank of the bur will permit. After this the eminence is sectioned and separated with broad osteotome. Base of the articular eminence is then smoothened with a sharp bone file (The foramen spinosum is located at the mesial

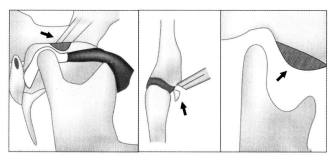

Fig. 21.20: Diagrammatic picture of eminectomy procedure

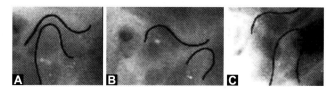

Figs 21.21A to C: Transcranial X-rays of TMJ: (A) Preoperative view in closed position, (B) Preoperative view in open position showing subluxation of condylar head, (C) Postoperative view after eminectomy in open position. Patient's complaint of severe pain in open position was relieved after eminectomy

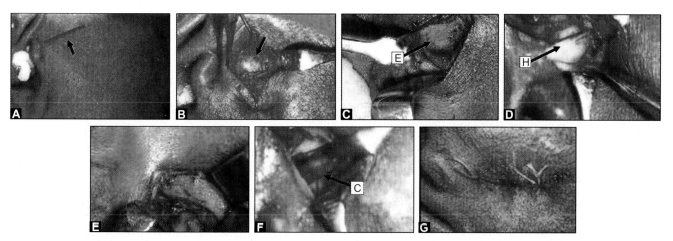

Figs 21.22A to G: Surgical procedure of eminectomy: (A) Extraoral incision parallel to zygomatic arch, (B) Surgical dissection, (C) Exposure of articular eminence, (D) H—Horizontal cut with the bur at the lower portion of the eminence, (E) Eminectomy completed (F) C—Free condylar head movement checked (G) Closure

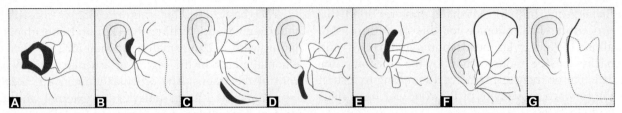

Figs 21.23A to G: Surgical approaches to TM joint and associated structures: (A) Posterior auricular incision, (B) Endaural approach, (C) Risdon's incision, (D) Hind's incision, (E) Preauricular incision, (F) Popowich incision, (G) Thoma's preauricular incision

aspect of the articular eminence. Injury to the middle meningeal artery may be a source of major hemorrhage after eminectomy). The irrigation of the area is then carried out. The tissues then carefully sutured. The application of an effective pressure dressing that is left in place for at least 48 to 72 hours.

SURGICAL APPROACHES TO MANDIBULAR CONDYLE AND ITS NECK (FIGS 21.23 AND 21.24) (TABLE 21.1)

Surgical access to the TM joint is an exacting procedure. It requires technical skill and a thorough knowledge of anatomy of the area. TMJ has got close proximity to the main trunk of the facial nerve with its branches in the temporal and facial areas. It has also got close proximity to the auriculotemporal nerve and the abundant vascular supply. Several approaches to the TMJ have been proposed and used clinically.

Postauricular Approach (Fig. 21.24)

The incision is taken behind the external ear in the crease near the superior aspect of external pinna and extended to the tip of the mastoid process.

This highly cosmetic incision has got several disadvantages. Main problems are small surgical exposure with poor access and visibility, stenosis of the external auditory canal, infection involving the external auditory canal or cartilaginous framework or both, paresthesia (temporary or permanent) of the external pinna and deformity of the auricle.

Endaural Approach (Fig. 21.25)

Short facial skin incision with extension into the external auditory meatus. The incision begins above the level of the zygomatic arch and extends downward and backward into the intercartilaginous cleft between the tragus and the helix and then extends inwards along the roof of the auditory meatus for approximately 1 cm.

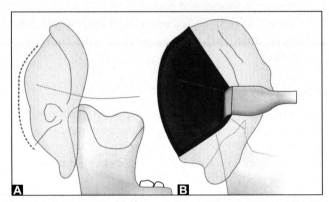

Figs 21.24A and B: Post or retroauricular approach to TMJ. (A) Initial curved incision in the retroauricular crease, (B) Transection of external auditory meatus and retraction of the external ear anteriorly to expose the joint capsule

Advantages: Excellent cosmetics.

Disadvantages: The limited access and possibility of meatal stenosis or chondritis.

Table 21.1: Surgical approaches to TMJ
1.   Submandibular (Risdon's) approach
2.   Postramal (Hind's) approach
3.   Postauricular approach
4.   Endaural approach
5.   Preauricular approach
• Dingman's
• Blair's
• Thoma's
• Popowich's modification of Al-Kayat and Bramley's
6.   Hemicoronal approach
7.   Coronal or bicoronal approach

Submandibular (Risdon) Approach (Fig. 21.26)

Here the incision is taken about 1 cm below the angle of the mandible. It extends forward, parallel to the lower border of the mandible and curves backward slightly behind the angle. Approach to the neck of the condyle

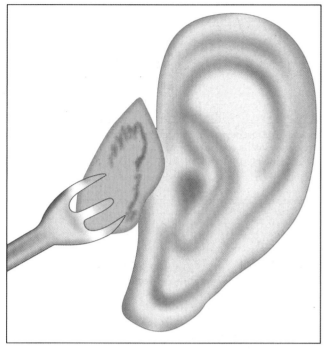

Fig. 21.25: Lamport's s endaural approach to TM joint

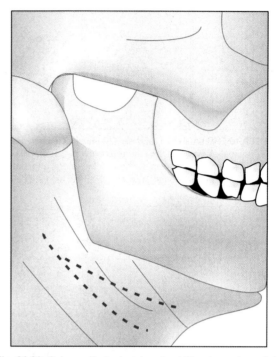

Fig. 21.26: Submandibular incision should be planned parallel to Langer's lines

and ramus is achieved by sharply incising through the pterygomasseteric sling and reflecting the masseter muscle laterally to expose the neck of the condyle and sigmoid notch.

Poor access to the condylar head region. Procedures involving the articular portion of the head and the meniscus cannot be performed by this approach.

Postramal (Hind) Approach (Fig. 21.27)

Indicated for surgeries involving the condylar neck and ramus area. Highly cosmetic procedure. Excellent visibility and accessibility. A skin incision is placed 1 cm behind the ramus of the mandible and extends 1 cm below the lobe of the ear to the angle of the mandible. Communicating fascia between the sternomastoid muscle and the parotid gland and masseter muscle (parotidomasseteric fascia) is carefully separated, to expose the posterior border of the ramus. Perforation of the posterior facial vein and injury to the main trunk of the facial nerve is avoided. Once the posterior border of the ramus has been exposed, the pterygomasseteric sling is incised at the angle and the masseter muscle, parotid gland are reflected upward and laterally to expose the neck of the condyle. After completion of

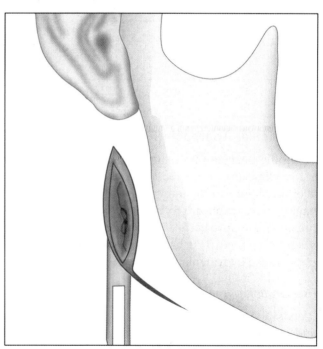

Fig. 21.27: Postramal (Hind's) incision

the surgical procedure, the pterygomasseteric sling is reapproximated and sutured and the wound is closed in layers.

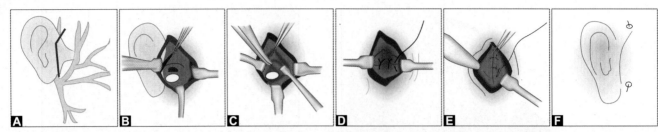

Figs 21.28A to F: Preauricular incision: (A) Initial incision in the preauricular fold, (B) Oblique incision through the superficial layer of temporalis fascia. Periosteal elevator is then inserted below the temporalis muscle to expose the lateral portion of the zygomatic arch, (C) Cut in the capsule to enter the TMJ space and incision through the lateral attachment of the disk, entering the inferior joint space, (D) After surgery, suturing of the capsule, (E) Suturing the wound in layers, (F) Final skin subcuticular suturing

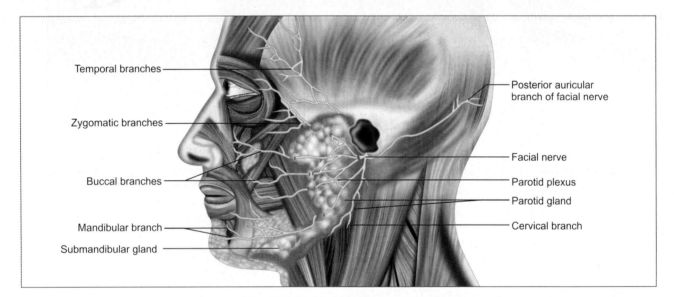

Fig. 21.29: Facial nerve and its branches

Preauricular Approach (Figs 21.28 to 21.31)

This is the most basic and standard approach to the TMJ. Many clinicians have modified this basic incision for avoiding injury to the auriculotemporal nerve and for having better exposure to the TMJ. First, the standard preauricular approach is described. Later, variations are briefly presented. This basic incision is advocated and popularized by Dingman (1951).

Preparation of the Surgical Site

Preparation and draping should expose the entire ear and lateral canthus of the eye. Shaving of the preauricular hair is optional. Cotton soaked with antibiotic ointment may be placed into the external auditory canal.

Marking the Incision

The incision is outlined at the junction of the facial skin with the helix of the ear. A natural skin fold along the entire length of the incision from (the free margin of the attached ear to the scalp) the helix to the upper border of the tragus can be used.

Infiltration of Vasoconstrictor

The preauricular area is very vascular. A vasoconstrictor can be injected subcutaneously, in the area of the incision to decrease the intraoperative bleeding.

Skin Incision

The incision is made through the skin, subcutaneous connective tissue to the depth of superficial layer of temporalis fascia. Any bleeding superficial vessels are cauterized before deeper dissection proceeds.

Dissection to the TMJ Capsule

Blunt dissection with periosteal elevator undermining the superior portion of the incision (that above

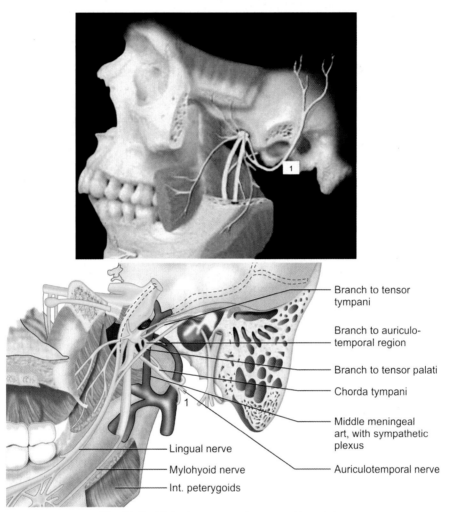

Branch to tensor tympani

Branch to auriculo-temporal region

Branch to tensor palati

Chorda tympani

Middle meningeal art, with sympathetic plexus

Lingual nerve

Mylohyoid nerve

Int. peterygoids

Auriculotemporal nerve

Fig. 21.30: (1) Auriculotemporal nerve and its relation

the zygomatic arch), so that a flap can be retracted anteriorly for approximately 1 to 1.5 cm. This flap is dissected anteriorly at the level of the superficial layer of temporalis fascia.

Below the zygomatic arch, dissection proceeds bluntly adjacent to the external auditory cartilage. Scissor dissection proceeds along the external auditory cartilage in an avascular plane between it and the glenoid lobe of the parotid gland.

With the flap retracted anteriorly, above the zygomatic arch, an oblique incision is made through the superficial layer of the temporalis fascia beginning from the root of the zygomatic arch, just in front of the tragus toward the upper corner of the retracted flap. The fat globules contained between the superficial and deep layers of temporalis fascia are then exposed. At the

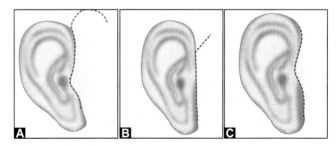

Figs 21.31A to C: Preauricular incisions: (A) Blair's inverted hockey stick incision, (B) Thoma's angulated incision, (C) Dingman's incision

root of the zygoma, the incision can be through both the superficial layer of temporalis fascia and the periosteum of the zygomatic arch. The sharp end of the periosteal elevator is used to expose the lateral surface of the zygomatic arch, till the articular eminence is exposed. The entire TMJ capsule will be then revealed (Fig. 21.28).

Exposing the Interarticular Spaces

Inverted L-shaped incision should be taken in the capsule and with the retraction of this developed flap, the joint spaces can be entered. The opening is extended anteroposteriorly by cutting along the lateral aspect of the eminence and fossa. Vertical incision is taken in the capsule till condylar neck, allows the separation down the periosteal layer.

Closure

The surgical procedure planned for TMJ disorder is carried out. The joint space irrigated well and any hemorrhage is controlled before closure. The wound is closed in multiple layers.

Modifications of Basic Preauricular Incision (Figs 21.31 and 21.32)

All these modifications of basic preauricular incision were made to have better access and visibility, and wider exposure and to prevent injury to the auriculotemporal nerve and the branches of the facial nerve.

1. *Blair and Ivy in 1936 used an 'inverted hockey stick' incision over the zygomatic arch,* which gave easy access and better visibility and also facilitated exposure of the arch along with condylar area.

2. *Thoma in 1958*—recommended an 'angulated vertical incision' which is carried out across the zygomatic arch in the fold, directly in front of the ear, extending down slightly above the ear lobe, to avoid the main trunk of the facial nerve.

3. *Al-Kayat and Bramley in 1979 described a modified preauricular approach to TMJ and zygomatic arch* considering the main branches of the vessels and nerves in the vicinity.

   The facial nerve exits the skull through the stylomastoid foramen. It enters the parotid gland, where it usually divides into two main trunks— temporofacial and cervicofacial. The facial nerve divides at a point between 1.5 and 2.8 cm below the lowest concavity of the bony external auditory canal, according to Al-Kayat and Bramley. These measurements can be used to identify the main trunk (whenever required) and avoid it during TMJ surgery.

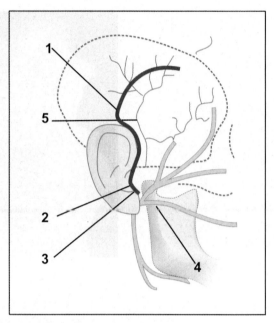

Fig. 21.32: Modified preauricular incision: (1) Skin incision, (2) Tragus, (3) Lower limit of skin incision, (4) Facial nerve branches, (5) Superficial temporal artery

The terminal branches of the facial nerve are classified as temporal, zygomatic, buccal, marginal mandibular and cervical. The location of the temporal branches is of particular importance during TMJ surgery. The temporal nerve branches lie within a dense fusion of periosteum, temporal fascia and superficial fascia at the level of the zygomatic arch. Al-Kayat and Bramley found that the nerve averaged 2 cm from the anterior concavity of the external auditory canal. But in some cases, the nerve is found as near as 0.8 cm and as far anteriorly as 3.5 cm. Protection of the nerve can be achieved by making an incision through the temporal fascia and periosteum down to the arch, not more than 0.8 cm in front of the anterior border of the external auditory canal.

4. *Popowich and Crane in 1982, further modified basic Al-Kayat and Bramley's incision.* A large incision shaped like a question mark, was made in the temporal area and extended in the preauricular area (Fig. 21.32).

A Surgical Approach Via Popowich Incision (Figs 21.33A and B)

This approach to the zygomatic arch and joint gives excellent visibility with safety. The incision is longer and wider than the conventional. The skin incision is

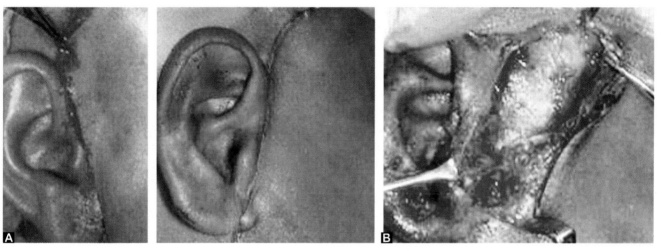

Figs 21.33A and B: (A and B) Popowich and crane incision, (B) Exposure of parotidomasseteric fascia

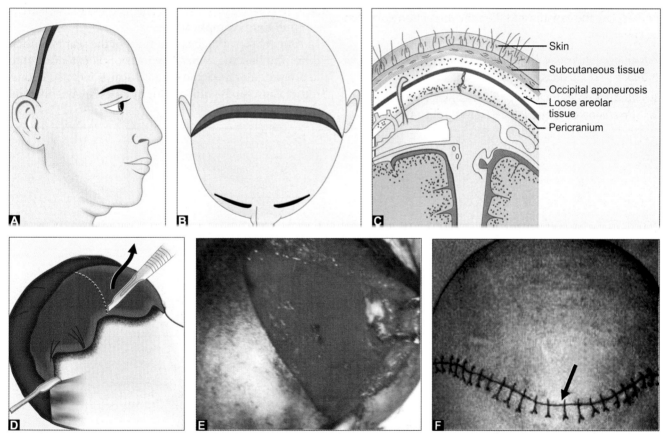

Figs 21.34A to F: Coronal approach: (A) Hemicoronal incision, (B) Bicoronal or coronal incision, (C) Layers of the scalp, (D) Coronal flap reflection to expose the supraorbital rims, further incision can be taken in pericranium to expose the middle third of the face, (E) Surgical exposure for malunited zygomaticomalar complex fracture, (F) Final suturing

question mark shaped and begins about a pinna's length away from the ear, anteroposteriorly just within the hair line, curves backward and downward well posterior to the main branches of the temporal vessels, till it meets the upper attachment of the ear. The rest of the incision is same as the routine preauricular incision. The temporal incision is carried through the skin, superficial fascia to the level of temporal fascia. The facial nerve branches run in the superficial fascia and it is important that the full length of this fascia is reflected with the skin flap. Blunt dissection in this plane is carried out till about 2 cm above the zygomatic arch, where the temporalis fascia splits. Starting at the root of the zygomatic arch, an incision running at 45 degrees upward and forward is made through the superficial layer of the temporalis fascia. The zygomatic arch is exposed after reflecting periosteum, lateral layer of temporal fascia and superficial fascia as one layer. Downward dissection will expose the capsule and then the dissection is carried out as usual.

Advantages of Popowich (1982) modification of Al-Kayat and Bramley's (1979) incision

1. Reduction in incidence of facial nerve palsy.
2. Provision of donor site for temporalis fascia.
3. Decreased hemorrhage (dissection through avascular zone).
4. Improved visibility and easier identification of fascial planes.
5. Reduction in postoperative edema and discomfort.
6. Potential complications of muscle herniation and fibrosis avoided.
7. Good cosmetic results.
8. Avoidance of auriculotemporal nerve anesthesia/paresthesia.
9. Reduction in total operating time.

Coronal Approach (Figs 21.34A to F)

Hemicoronal (unilateral incision) and bicoronal or coronal incision (bilateral incision) is more extensive, but versatile surgical approach to the upper and middle regions of the facial skeleton, including the zygomatic arch and the TM joint areas. It provides excellent access to these areas with minimum complications.

A major advantage is that most of the scar is hidden within the hairline, when the incision is extended into the preauricular area, the surgical scar is inconspicuous. This incision can be utilized for more extensive bilateral involvement.

Ankylosis of the Temporomandibular Joint and its Management

22

Ankylosis is a Greek terminology meaning 'stiff joint'. Here because of immobility of the joint, the jaw function gets affected. Hypomobility to immobility of the joint can lead to inability to open the mouth from partial to complete. The incidence of intra-articular temporomandibular joint (TMJ) ankylosis is difficult to assess. But, in the western literature it is reported as decreasing, due to better understanding of management of condylar fractures and also to the decreased incidence of middle ear infection following the introduction of antibiotics. But in India, the incidence of TMJ ankylosis is still high. The reported age distribution ranges from 2 to 63 years. Onset is usually seen before the age of 10.

CLASSIFICATION OF ANKYLOSIS

1. False ankylosis or true ankylosis.
2. Extra-articular or intra-articular.
3. Fibrous or bony.
4. Unilateral or bilateral.
5. Partial or complete.

Extra-articular and intra-articular types of TMJ ankylosis have been described depending mainly on the anatomic site of the fusion or union. Intra-articular ankylosis indicates union between the articular surfaces of the TMJ, while extra-articular ankylosis results from lesions involving extra-articular structures.

The fusion or union of the articular surfaces of the head of the condyle with the glenoid fossa may be of fibrous or bony, depending on the nature of the tissue (Figs 22.1 and 22.2).

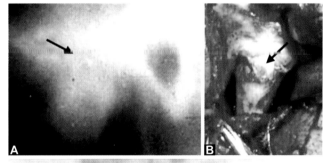

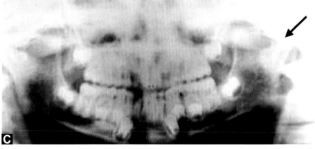

Figs 22.1A to C: Fibrous ankylosis of TMJ: (A) Tomogram of (L) TMJ showing fibrous fusion at the joint space, (B) Surgical exposure showing fibrous union of (L) TMJ. Note the condylar head is not deformed, (C) OPG—Fibrous ankylosis

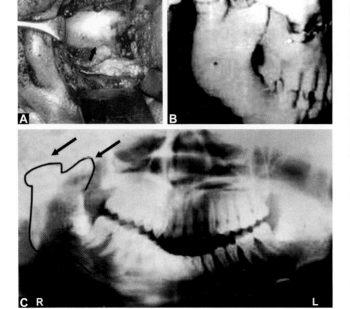

Figs 22.2A to C: Bony ankylosis: (A) Surgical exposure of (L) TMJ showing the bony ankylosed mass, with deformed head of the condyle, (B) 3D CT scan showing (R) TMJ bony ankylosis, (C) OPG—(R) Side Bony ankylosis and deformed condylar head

Table 22.1: Etiopathology of ankylosis of TMJ	
• Trauma	• Congenital
	• At birth, forceps delivery
	• Hemarthrosis (Direct/indirect trauma)
	• Condylar fractures
	— intracapsular
	— extracapsular
	• Glenoid fossa fracture (rare)
• Infections	• Otitis media
	• Parotitis
	• Tonsilitis
	• Furuncle
	• Abscess around the joint
	• Osteomyelitis of the jaw
	• Actinomycosis
• Inflammation	• Rheumatoid arthritis
	• Osteoarthritis
	• Septic arthritis—hematogenous spread
• Rare causes	• Polyarthritis
	• Measles
• Systemic diseases	• Smallpox
	• Scarlet fever
	• Typhoid
	• Gonoccocal arthritis
	• Scleroderma
	• Beriberi
	• Marie-Strümpell disease
	• Ankylosing spondylitis
• Other causes	• Bifid condyle
	• Prolonged trismus
	• Prolonged immobilization
	• Unknown
	• Burns

ETIOPATHOLOGY

The definite cause of ankylosis of TMJ is unknown. Two main factors predisposing to the ankylosis are *trauma and infection* in or around the joint region. In 1968, Topazian reported that 26 to 75 percent of cases of TMJ ankylosis are seen following trauma, while 44 to 68 percent are seen due to infection (Table 22.1).

Joint infection: It may occur secondary to septicemia due to osteomyelitis, septic sore throat, scarlet fever, tuberculosis, meningitis, etc.

Direct spread of infection from adjacent areas may occur in cases of otitis media (infection of middle ear), mastoiditis, osteomyelitis of temporal bone or parotid abscess, soft tissue abscess, skin infections, or severe odontogenic submasseteric, infratemporal abscesses, etc.

Diseases affecting the joints: Such as rheumatoid arthritis, osteoarthritis and ankylosing spondylitis bring about degenerative changes, destruction of the disk followed by the repair process. This can lead to the ankylosis of TMJ.

Any other degenerative disease will also lead towards the destruction of the meniscus along with the narrowing of the joint space, leading to bony contact between the condylar head and roof of the glenoid fossa.

Trauma: A high percentage of TMJ ankylosis are seen following trauma. At birth, TMJ may receive trauma from a forceps delivery. Trauma during intrauterine life leads to congenital ankylosis.

Ankylosis is also generally associated with some form of facial injury at later date involving fracture of the neck or head of the condyle. Direct blow over the joint or at the chin may also cause bleeding into the joint. Any injury with hemorrhage into the joint space will initiate a progression of undesirable changes (clot organization and deposition of bone). If mandibular movement is not encouraged over a prolonged period of time, fusion will result. Comatose patients with associated condylar fracture are prone to develop ankylosis. Prolonged immobilization of condylar fractures, especially in children, where abundant blood supply is more likely to increase the incidence of hemarthrosis following injury leading to ankylosis. Therefore, a maximum period of immobilization of three weeks in the adults and two weeks in the children following reduction of condylar fracture is recommended.

PATHOGENESIS

Trauma will bring about extravasation of blood into the joint space called *hemarthrosis*. This predisposes to calcification and obliteration of a joint space, where immobility of the joint is maintained over a prolonged period. Many times initial fibrous bands lead towards bony consolidation to ossification.

In intra-articular ankylosis, the meniscus undergoes progressive destruction with flattening of the glenoid fossa and the head of the condyle is deformed and thickened, resulting in narrowing or obliteration of the joint space. Many times, bony fusion may extend well beyond the joint space to involve the cranial base and even the sigmoid notch, zygomatic arch, coronoid process. In the severest form, it may include the lateral pterygoid plate and even the spine of the sphenoid bone.

DIAGNOSIS

Diagnosis of TMJ ankylosis is relatively easy and is dependent more upon careful clinical examination, rather than the diagnostic tests. Restricted oral opening or nil oral opening is seen and patient will complain of difficulty in mastication. Protrusive movements are not possible on the involved side. Also partial mobility or complete immobility of the condyle is readily noticed, when one palpates the joint movements. Pain is totally absent. In addition, in a young patient, a nature of facial deformity will help to differentiate between unilateral and bilateral involvement.

CLINICAL MANIFESTATIONS

Clinical manifestations vary according to: *(a) severity of ankylosis, (b) time of onset of ankylosis, and (c) duration.*

1. Early joint involvement—less than 15 years: Severe facial deformity and loss of function.
2. Later joint involvement after the age of 15 years: Facial deformity marginal or nil. But, functional loss severe.

Those patients in whom the ankylosis develops after full growth completion have no facial deformity.

Unilateral Ankylosis (Fig. 22.3)

Seen in a child or in a person where the onset was usually in the childhood.
1. Obvious facial asymmetry.
2. Deviation of the mandible and chin on the affected side.
3. The chin is receded with hypoplastic mandible on the affected side.
4. Roundness and fullness of the face on the affected side.
5. The appearance of the flatness and elongation on the unaffected side.
6. The lower border of the mandible on the affected side has a concavity that ends in a well defined antegonial notch.
7. In unilateral ankylosis, some amount of oral opening may be possible. Interincisal opening will vary depending on whether it is fibrous or bony ankylosis.
8. Cross bite may be seen.
9. Class II angles malocclusion on the affected side plus unilateral posterior cross bite on the ipsilateral side seen.
10. Condylar movements are absent on the affected side.

Bilateral Ankylosis (Fig. 22.4)

1. Inability to open the mouth progresses by gradual decrease in interincisal opening. The mandible is symmetrical but micrognathic. The patient develops typical '*bird face*' deformity with receding chin.
2. The neck chin angle may be reduced or almost completely absent.
3. Antegonial notch is well defined bilaterally.
4. Class II malocclusion can be noticed.
5. Upper incisors are often protrusive with anterior open bite. Maxilla may be narrow.
6. Oral opening will be less than 5 mm or many times there is nil oral opening.

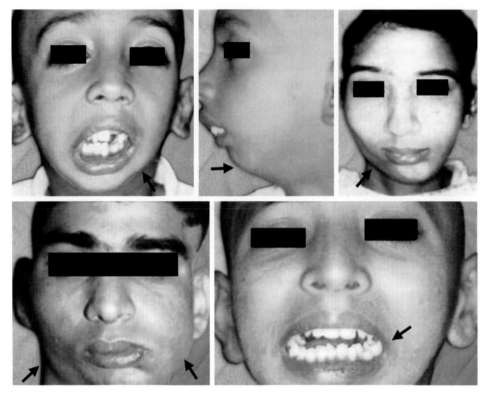

Fig. 22.3: Unilateral ankylosis: Facial and dental features

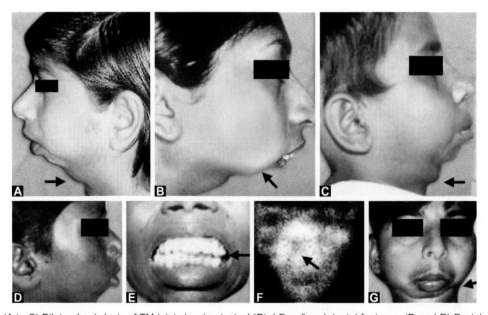

Figs 22.4A to G: (A to C) Bilateral ankylosis of TM joint showing typical "Bird Face" and dental features, (D and E) Facial profile and nil oral opening in bilateral TMJ ankylosis, (F) Scintigraphy showing increased uptake in TMJ areas, indicating active reankylosis process, (G) Severe micrognathia in bilateral TM joint ankylosis case

7. Multiple carious teeth with bad periodontal health can be seen.
8. Severe malocclusion, crowding can be seen and many impacted teeth may be found on the X-rays.

Diagnosis

Diagnosis is based on the following:
1. History of trauma, infection, etc.
2. Clinical findings.
3. Radiographic findings—are important in arriving at a final diagnosis (Fig. 22.5).
   a. *Orthopantomograph*—will show both the joints picture which can be compared in unilateral cases. Presence of antegonial notch can be appreciated which develops secondary to the contraction of the depressor muscles and their action against elevator group of muscles. The antegonial notch becomes more pronounced in severe cases.
   b. *Lateral oblique view*—will give anteroposterior dimension of the condylar mass. Elongation of coronoid process can be seen.
   c. *Cephalometric radiograph*—is taken to evaluate the associated skeletal deformities.
   d. *Posteroanterior radiograph*—will reveal the mediolateral extent of the bony mass. It will also highlight the asymmetry in unilateral cases.
   e. *CT scan*—very helpful guide for surgery. Relation to the medial cranial fossa, the anteroposterior width, mediolateral depth can be assessed. Any presence of fractured condylar head on the

medial aspect of ramus can be located. In cases of reankylosis, the bony fusion can be seen. 3-D CT scan will give life size picture of all aspects of the deformity (Figs 22.6 and 22.7).

Radiographic Findings

Fibrous Ankylosis (Fig. 22.1)

In fibrous ankylosis, reduced joint space and hazy appearance can be seen. But, still the normal anatomy of the head and glenoid fossa can be appreciated.

Bony Ankylosis (Fig. 22.2)

Complete obliteration of joint space. Normal TMJ anatomy is distorted. Deformed condylar head or complete bony consolidation replacing the joint space can be seen. Elongation of the coronoid process on the side of hypomobility will be seen.

Sawhney in 1986, graded TMJ ankylosis into following types (Table 22.2).

Sequelae of Untreated Ankylosis

1. Normal facial growth and development affected.
2. Speech impairment.
3. Nutritional impairment.
4. Respiratory distress (tongue fall in sleep), especially, in bilateral involvement with severe micrognathia.
5. Malocclusion.
6. Poor oral hygiene.
7. Multiple carious and impacted teeth.

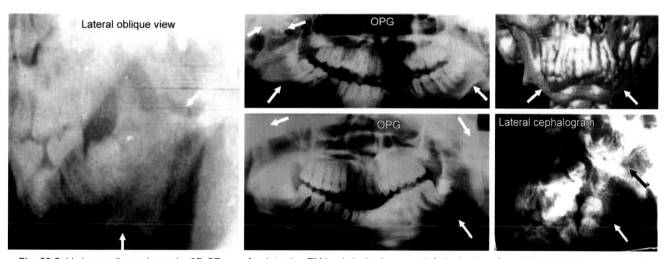

Fig. 22.5: Various radiographs and a 3D CT scan for detecting TMJ ankylosis. Arrows at inferior border of mandible indicating pronounced antegonial notch

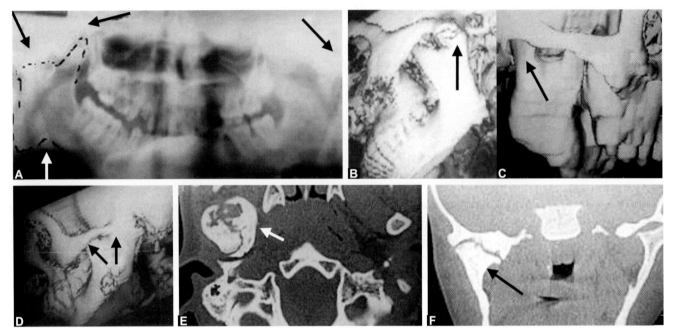

Figs 22.6A to F: (A) OPG bilateral ankylosis, (B) Unilateral ankylosis-3D scan, (C) Normal TMJ in 3D scan, (D) (L) TMJ ankylosis 3D scan showing bony fusion and elongated coronoid process, (E) Axial scan—bony ankylosis, (F) Coronal scan—bony ankylosis

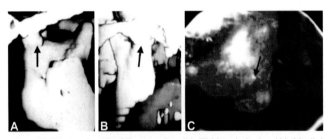

Figs 22.7A to C: 3D CT scan for (L) TMJ ankylosis: (A) Medial rotation 3D scan with disarticulation, (B) Lateral rotation 3D scan with disarticulation, (C) Intraoperative picture of TMJ ankylosis

Table 22.2: Grading of TMJ ankylosis by Sawhney (1986)	
Type I	:	The condylar head is present without much distortion. Fibrous adhesions make movement impossible
Type II	:	Bony fusion of the misshaped head and the articular surface. No involvement of sigmoid notch and coronoid process
Type III	:	A bony block bridging across the ramus and the zygomatic arch. Medially an atrophic dislocated fragment of the former head of the condyle is still found. Elongation of the coronoid process seen.
Type IV	:	The normal anatomy of the TMJ is totally destroyed by complete bony block between the ramus and the skull base

■ MANAGEMENT OF TEMPOROMANDIBULAR JOINT ANKYLOSIS

The treatment of TMJ ankylosis is always surgical. Early surgical correction of the ankylosed joint is highly desirable, if satisfactory function is to be regained.

Surgical strategy adopted depends on the following:
a. Age of onset of ankylosis.
b. Extent of ankylosis.
c. Whether there is unilateral or bilateral involvement.
d. Associated facial deformity.

Aims and Objectives of Surgery

1. Release of ankylosed mass and creation of a gap to mobilize the joint.
2. Creation of a functional joint.
   a. To improve patient's nutrition.
   b. To improve patient's oral hygiene.
   c. To carry out necessary dental treatment.
3. To reconstruct the joint and restore the vertical height of the ramus.
4. To prevent recurrence.

5. To restore normal facial growth pattern (based on functional matrix theory).
6. To improve esthetics and rehabilitate the patient (cosmetic surgery may be carried out at a later date or at second phase).

Surgical Techniques

Number of techniques have been advocated by different surgeons. Critical analysis of all, filters only to three basic methods.

  I : Condylectomy
  II : Gap arthroplasty
  III : Interpositional arthroplasty

Most surgical procedures can be done through a preauricular incision alone.The Popowich's incision is chosen for its obvious advantages. Whenever required, additional submandibular incision can be used for fixation of the graft, etc.

Condylectomy (Figs 22.8A to F)

Condylectomy is advocated in cases of fibrous ankylosis, where the joint space is obliterated with deposition of fibrous bands but there is not much deformity of the condylar head.

Radiologically and clinically after surgical exposure one can see the demarcation between the roof of the glenoid fossa and the head of the condyle. The condylectomy procedure can be carried out via preauricular incision. Horizontal osteotomy cut is carried out with the help of the surgical bur at the level of condylar neck. Vital structures on the medial surface of the condylar neck should be protected, by using special condylar retractor, inserted prior to the bony cut. The condylar head then should be separated from the superior attachment carefully. The rest of the stump should be smoothened out and wound closed in layers. Unilateral condylectomy tends to cause deviation of the mandible towards the operated side on oral opening and if bilateral, anterior open bite will be caused as a result of the loss of height in the vertical rami.

Therefore, when the site of the fused joint is mobilized via condylectomy, then after recontouring by arthroplasty, an alloplastic material can be used to maintain the joint space, satisfactory occlusion and joint movements.

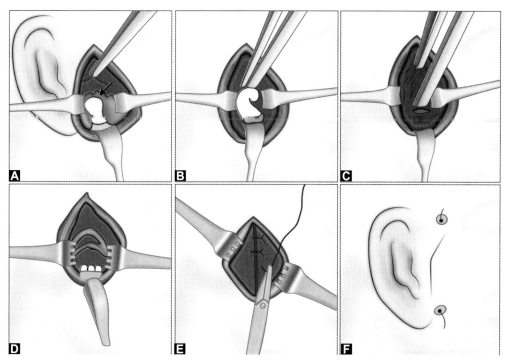

Figs 22.8A to F: Condylectomy—surgical procedure: (A) Exposure of condylar head via preauricular incision, (B) Sectioning of condylar head, (C) Breaking the fibrous adhesions, (D) Condylectomy complete, (E) Suturing the capsule, (F) Final skin suturing

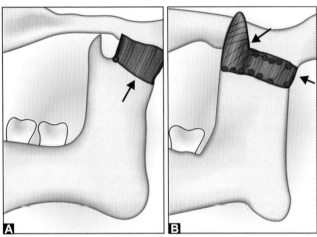

Figs 22.9A and B: Diagrammatic representation: (A) Gap arthroplasty, (B) Gap arthroplasty with coronoidectomy

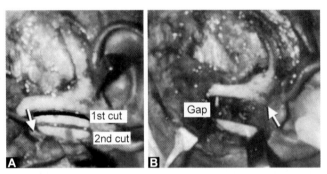

Figs 22.10A and B: Gap arthroplasty surgery: intraoperative pictures: (A) Surgical exposure of left ankylosed TM joint. 1st and 2nd bony cuts are seen. The wedge of bone between the two cuts is removed to create a gap and release the ankylosis, (B) Gap arthroplasty completed to achieve the mobility of the joint

Gap Arthroplasty (Figs 22.9 to 22.11)

In the extensive bony ankylosis, a broad, thick area of bone deposition obliterates the entire joint, sigmoid notch and coronoid process. Identification of the previous joint structure is impossible and mobilization at the level of the joint becomes difficult, if not impossible (one cannot identify the roof of the glenoid fossa, which forms the floor of the middle cranial fossa).

The term *gap arthroplasty* is therefore, used to describe the operation, in which the level of section is below that of the previous joint space and in which, no substance is interposed between the two cut bony surfaces. Section consists of two horizontal osteotomy cuts and removal of a bony wedge for creation of a

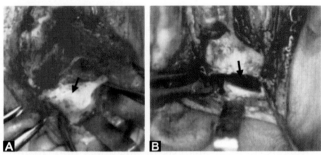

Figs 22.11A and B: Intraoperative photographs: (A) Bony fusion, (B) Gap arthroplasty

gap between the roof of the glenoid fossa and ramus. Here, it is recommended to create a minimum gap of at least 1 cm to prevent reankylosis. **The width of the bone removed is considered crucial.** It is not usually possible to remove the entire block *in toto*, particularly from the medial aspect, which is in close proximity to the internal maxillary artery. Hence, bone is removed carefully by using a large round bur, until the medial bone is thinned out enough to be readily removed by using hand chisel or osteotome. It is important to create a gap of equal dimension both laterally and medially, so that the possibility of medial reankylosis due to bone contact is avoided.

Interpositional Arthroplasty (Figs 22.12 A to H and 22.13 A to H)

Most authorities agree that recurrence of ankylosis is less likely when something is interposed between the two cut bony surfaces. Topazian compared gap and interpositional arthroplasties and reported a 53 percent incidence of recurrence, when the gap arthroplasty method was used.

So, interpositional arthroplasty involves the creation of a gap, but in addition a barrier (autogenous or alloplastic) is inserted between the cut bony surfaces to minimize the risk of recurrence and to maintain the vertical height of the ramus (Table 22.3).

Artificial Replacement of the Joint

Prefabricated condylar prosthesis made of steel, vitallium or titanium have been also used extensively. Fossa liners along with specially constructed TMJ prosthesis reconstruct the entire joint. These are commercially available or custom fabricated.

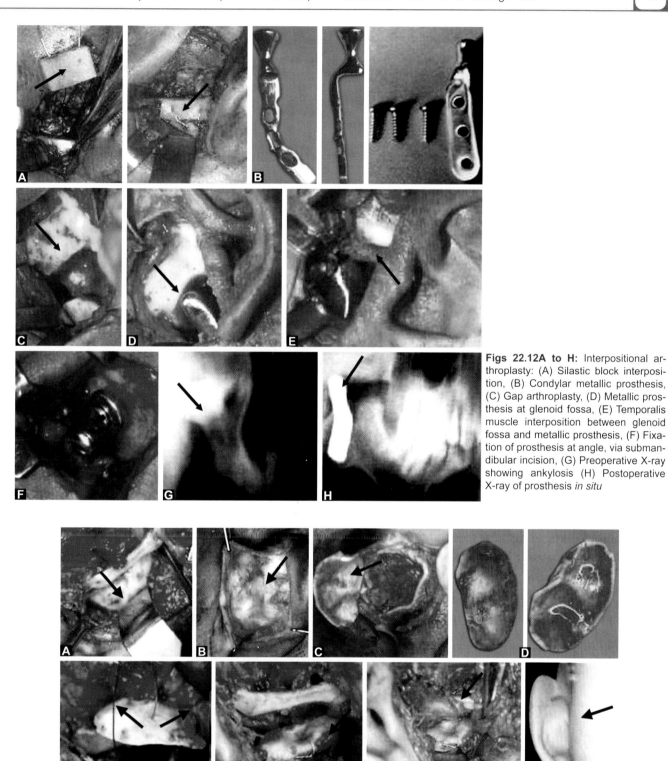

Figs 22.12A to H: Interpositional arthroplasty: (A) Silastic block interposition, (B) Condylar metallic prosthesis, (C) Gap arthroplasty, (D) Metallic prosthesis at glenoid fossa, (E) Temporalis muscle interposition between glenoid fossa and metallic prosthesis, (F) Fixation of prosthesis at angle, via submandibular incision, (G) Preoperative X-ray showing ankylosis (H) Postoperative X-ray of prosthesis *in situ*

Figs 22.13A to H: Use of auricular cartilage graft as an interpositional material: (A) TM joint ankylosis in 8 years old boy, surgical exposure, (B) and (C) Harvesting of auricular cartilage graft, (D) Auricular graft obtained, (E) Fixation of auricular cartilage graft on to the ramus stump with wire, (F) Auricular graft final fixation, (G) Raw surface at glenoid fossa side, covered with temporalis muscle, (H) Contour of the external ear is not changed

Table 22.3: Interpositional materials used		
Autogenous	*Heterogenous*	*Alloplasts*

1. Cartilaginous grafts
   • Costochondral
   • Metatarsal
   • Sternoclavicular
   • Auricular cartilage
2. Temporal muscle
3. Temporal fascia
4. Fascia lata
5. Dermis
	1. Chromatized submucosa of pig bladder
	
	2. Lyophilized bovine cartilage
	
	(Still under research)
		1. Metallic
		   • Tantalum foil/plate
		   • 316L Stainless steel
		   • Titanium
		   • Gold
		2. Nonmetallic
		   • Silastic
		   • Teflon
		   • Acrylic
		   • Nylon
		   • Proplast
		   • Ceramic implants

The Internationally Accepted Protocols for the Management of Temporomandibular Joint Ankylosis

Put forward by Kaban, Perrot and Fisher in 1990
1. Early surgical intervention.
2. *Aggressive resection:* A gap of at least 1 to 1.5 cm should be created. Special attention should be given to the fusion on the medial aspect of the ramus. Old malunited condylar fractured piece can be seen attached on the medial side.
3. *Ipsilateral coronoidectomy and temporalis myotomy:* In most of these cases, there is always association of elongated coronoid process. After carrying out gap arthroplasty, the coronoidectomy on the same side should be carried out either separately or in combination with the gap arthroplasty cut from the same extraoral incision. The coronoid process is cut from the level of sigmoid notch till the anterior border of the ramus. The temporalis muscle attachments are severed by carrying out temporalis myotomy. The oral opening is checked after this procedure by the assistant. If maximum interincisal opening is greater than 35 mm is obtained, then there is no need to carry out contralateral coronoidectomy.
4. Contralateral coronoidectomy and temporalis myotomy is necessary: If maximum incisal opening is less than 35 mm. Then uninvolved side coronoidectomy and temporalis myotomy can be carried out through intraoral incision (Figs 22.14 and 22.15).
5. Lining of the glenoid fossa region with temporalis fascia.

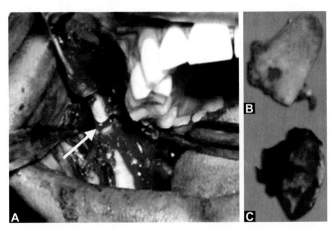

Fig. 22.14A to C: (A) Intraoral coronoidectomy surgical procedure, (B and C) Bilateral coronoid processes excised along with temporalis myotomy

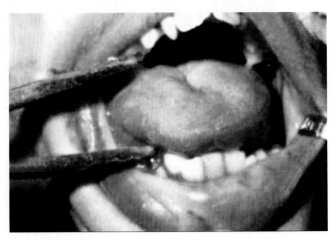

Fig. 22.15: Checking oral opening with jaw stretcher after gap arthroplasty

6. Reconstruction of the ramus with a costochondral graft.
7. Early mobilization and aggressive physiotherapy for the period of at least six months postoperatively.
8. Regular long term follow up.
9. To carry out cosmetic surgery at the later date, when the growth of the patient is completed.

Release of the jaw movements is quite dramatic, upon completion of coronoidectomy. It is also desirable to excise the coronoid rather than release it and allow it to be pulled up superiorly by the temporalis muscle. Unless the coronoid process is removed, there is potential for reankylosis after reattachment.

Lining of the Glenoid Fossa Side by Temporalis Myofascial Flap (Figs 22.16 A to C)

Temporalis fascia along with a varying thickness of temporalis muscle may be harvested as an axial flap based on the middle and deep temporal arteries and veins. The dependable blood supply, the proximity to the TMJ and the ability to alter the arc of rotation by basing the flap inferiorly or posteriorly, makes this a versatile flap for lining the glenoid fossa. It is used as an interpositional material after release of ankylosis of TMJ.

Interposition Arthroplasty Using Autogenous Costochondral Graft (Figs 22.17 and 22.18)

Basic three goals:
1. To replicate structurally normal joint anatomy.
2. To provide functional articulation.
3. To establish an area, where adaptive growth can occur (in children).

Costochondral graft is harvested through the inframammary incision. Either 5th, 6th or 7th rib is harvested. If two ribs are required, some surgeons advocate that an intervening rib should be left. And costochondral junction of the rib is chosen along with some amount of length of the rib. The length of the total graft will depend on the height of the ramus to be restored. A minimum of 1.5 cm of costochondral junction should be included in the graft. This should be carved to simulate condylar head. The graft should be fixed on the lateral aspect of the ramus with the screws or transosseous wires. A minimum gap of 0.5 to 1 cm should be kept between the graft and glenoid fossa side, so that free movement is possible without any friction.

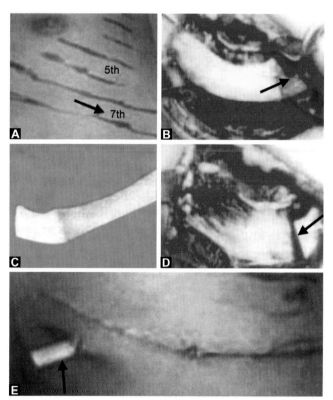

Figs 22.17A to E: (A) Inframammary markings for incision at the 7th rib, (B) Harvesting of the 7th rib. Costochondral junction exposed, (C) Adequate length of costochondral graft, (Rib graft), (D) Rib graft harvested from donor bed, (E) Inframammary incision closed in multiple layers. Skin subcuticular suturing done. Drain is secured

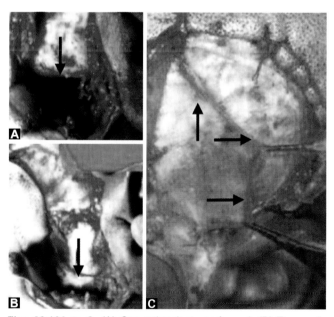

Figs 22.16A to C: (A) Gap arthroplasty performed, (B) Temporalis myofascial flap is used for lining the glenoid fossa, (C) Only temporalis fascia also can be mobilized to cover the glenoid fossa and used as an interpositional autogenous graft

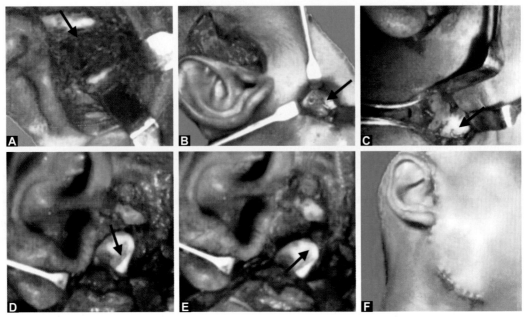

Figs 22.18A to F: (A) Gap osteoarthroplasty, (B) CC graft pushed through small submandibular incision over the lateral aspect of the ramus, (C) Fixation of the CC graft at the angle of the mandible, (D) CC graft carved simulating condylar head, which was placed in the gap, (E) Checking the CC graft movement in open mouth position, (F) Final suturing

Disadvantages

1. Increased operating time
2. Additional surgical site
3. Donor site morbidity – such as pneumothorax, pleural tear and pleuritic pain
4. Graft overgrowth
5. Possible potential for reankylosis.

   Figures 22.19 and 22.20 show the results of surgery for TMJ ankylosis.

Complications during Temporomandibular Joint Ankylosis Surgery

During Anesthesia

a. As the patient cannot open the mouth, awake blind intubation has to be done, where patients co-operation is required, which is very difficult to obtain from younger group of patients.
b. Because of small mandible and altered position of the larynx, intubation poses a problem
c. Aspiration of blood clot, tooth or foreign body during extubation, as thtroat cannot be packed prior to surgery.
d. Danger of falling back of tongue and obstructing airway is always there, after extubation.

During Surgery

a. Hemorrhage due to damage to any of the superficial temporal vessels, transverse facial artery, inferior alveolar vessel and internal maxillary vessels, pterygoid plexus of veins.
b. Damage to external auditory meatus.
c. Damage to zygomatic and temporal branch of facial nerve.
d. Damage to glenoid fossa and thus leading entry into middle cranial fossa.
e. Damage to auriculotemporal nerve.
f. Damage to parotid gland.
g. Damage to the teeth during opening of the jaws with jaw stretcher.

During Postoperative Follow-up

a. Infection
b. Open bite
c. Recurrence of ankylosis.

Frey's Syndrome (Figs 22.21A and B)

Frey's syndrome was described by Frey. He reported the incidence of localized gustatory sweating and flushing following a gun shot wound and suppurative parotitis.

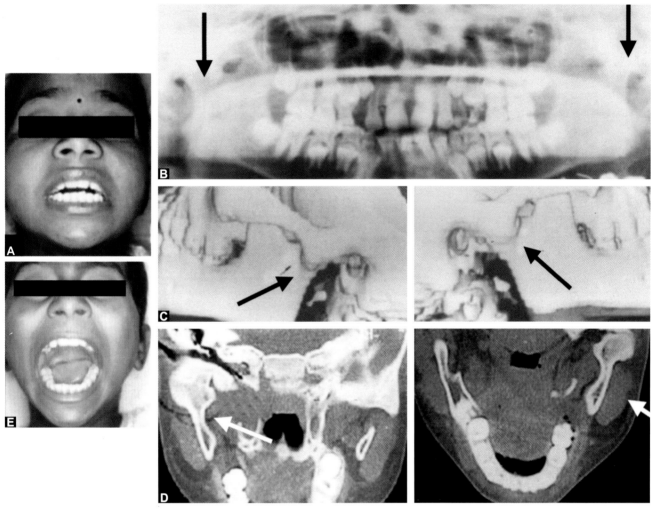

Figs 22.19A to E: An 8 year old girl reported with C/O inability to open the mouth since 3 years. She gave H/O trauma 4 years back: (A) Preoperative interincisal opening was 2 mm, (B) OPG, (C) 3D CT scan, (D) Coronal CT scan—all showing bilateral TMJ ankylosis. Bilateral TMJ surgery with CC graft interpositioning was done, (E) Postoperative oral opening

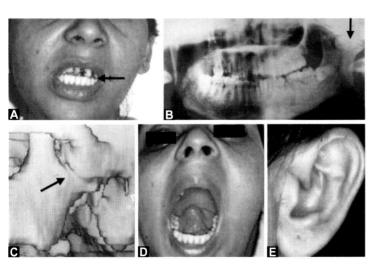

Figs 22.20A to E: A 23-year-old female C/O inability to open the mouth since 6 years. She gave H/O abscess in preauricular area 6 years ago. Gradual decrease in oral opening was noticed by her: (A) Interincisal oral opening—4 mm, (B and C) OPG and 3D CT scan showed (L) TMJ ankylosis. (L) side TMJ gap arthroplasty with bilateral coronoidectomy was done. Auricular cartilage and temporalis myofascial flap was used as interpositional autogenous material, (D) Postoperative oral opening—5 cm, (E) No auricular deformity seen postoperatively

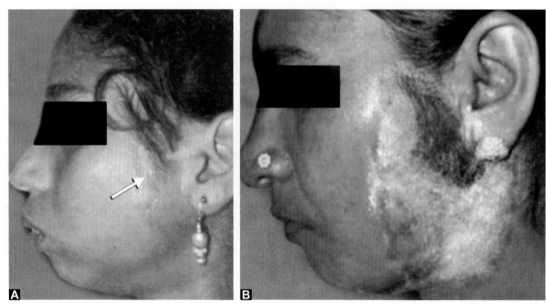

Figs 22.21A and B: Frey's syndrome: Patient C/O severe sweating and burning sensation in (L) preauricular region since last 10 years. Patient gave H/O some surgery in L parotid region 10 years back. A minor starch iodine test is positive

This auriculotemporal nerve syndrome may follow the surgery of the parotid gland and TM joint, a facial wound or parotid abscess.

1. It is characterized by pain in the auriculotemporal nerve distribution.
2. Associated gustatory sweating and occasionally erythema is seen.
3. There is flushing on the affected side of the face accompanied by sweating within the hairline, the periauricular region and beneath the pinna.
4. A minor starch iodine test is positive in these patients (The skin is painted with a solution of iodine, castor oil and absolute alcohol. Corn starch is dusted onto the dried, painted area. A positive test will be evoked after the patient chewed a lemon wedge for 5 minutes).

Treatment Options for Frey's Syndrome

1. *Topical agents*
   a. Commercial antiperspirants—effective only for milder symptoms.
   b. Anticholinergic preparations—topical glycopyr-rolate should be used with caution. Should not be applied on cut or infected skin. Contraindicated in diabetic patient, cardiovascular, CNS system, renal or hepatic diseases.

2. *Radiation therapy*—dose of 50 Gy is needed. Used only in very symptomatic patients, where other treatments have failed or contraindicated.
3. *Surgical procedures*
   a. Skin excision—for localized and relatively small areas.
   b. Auriculotemporal nerve section—results may not be permanent.
   c. Tympanic neurectomy—safe procedure can be done on outpatient basis.

Recurrence of Temporomandibular Joint Ankylosis

Recurrence of TMJ ankylosis is distressing both to the patient and surgeon. Several factors have been said to be responsible for reankylosis.

1. An inadequate gap created between the fragments.
2. Missing on the medial condylar stump and leaving it behind.
3. Fracture of the costochondral graft.
4. Loosening of the costochondral graft due to inade-quate fixation to the ramus.
5. Inadequate coverage of the glenoid fossa surface.
6. Inadequate postoperative physiotherapy.
7. Higher osteogenic potential and periosteal osteo-genic power may be responsible for high rate of recurrence in children.

23 Myofascial Pain Dysfunction Syndrome

Temporomandibular joint (TMJ) disorders are among the most misdiagnosed and mistreated maladies in medicine. Though, a lot of research is constantly being carried out, TMJ problems raise many questions, some of which remain unanswered or debatable, because of the complex nature of this joint.

It has got multifactorial origin or etiology and part of the misunderstanding stems from the inability to point at exact etiological factors. Further confusion is created due to different terms used for the various TMJ symptoms, such as Costen's syndrome, TMJ syndrome, TMJ pain dysfunction syndrome and myofascial pain dysfunction syndrome (MPDS).

It is very important for the clinician to learn to distinguish the many types of TMJ dysfunction, as so many other etiological factors mimic the same symptoms. For example, organic diseases, certain dental conditions, periodontal disease may cause similar symptoms and need to be evaluated.

HISTORY

Historically, TMJ disorders have been described as having their etiologies in either malocclusion, or the patient's psychological status or as being secondary to an intrinsic joint pathology.

Costen (1934), was the first one to indicate an *occlusal etiology in* TMJ pain. He reported association of bite overclosure (due to loss of posterior teeth) with symptoms like ear pain, sinus pain, decreased hearing, tinnitus, dizziness, burning and vertigo and occipital headaches *(Bite raising era)*.

Schwartz (1956), coined the term TMJ *pain dysfunction syndrome* and blamed the *spasm of the masticatory and perimasticatory musculature* leading towards the symptoms. He also noted that many TMJ sufferers had an altered psychologic make up as well. He advocated the use of muscle relaxants, restriction of oral opening for resting the muscles.

Laskin (1969), put forward a provocative paper on *Myofascial pain dysfunction syndrome.* He implicated psychophysiologic theory stating that the psychological stress leads to myospasm (tranquilizers, muscle relaxants).

Mackenzie and Banks and Toller and Poswillo (1975), stressed on the diagnosis and treatment of *intrinsic joint disorders* (different disk surgeries).

Dentists have a historic role in resolving acute pain and restoring oral function. But, when confronted with patients, who appear to be suffering from obscure facial pain and functional jaw problems, they are less comfortable handling these situations. These TMJ disorders are not life threatening, but their treatment relates to improvement in the quality of life. Faulty or painful function disturbs day-to-day activities and body image. These problems sometimes become so significant, that they impair person's emotional stability. Usually, these patients run from pillar to post for the want of relief. Most of the dentists and physicians dismiss their problem as illegitimate, as it is not demonstrable on radiographs or by visual examination.

Epidemiologic study has shown that at least 30 percent of the population suffer from this problem and the ratio of females to male patients is 3:1. The target group for therapy appears to be women between the ages of 15 to 40 years.

The MPDS is a pain disorder, in which unilateral pain is referred from the trigger points in myofascial structures, to the muscles of the head and neck. Pain is constant, dull in nature, in contrast to the sudden sharp, shooting, intermittent pain of neuralgias (chronic pain). But the pain may range from mild to intolerable.

■ CLINICAL CHARACTERISTICS

1. A zone of reference.
2. Trigger points in muscles.
3. Occasional associated symptoms.
4. Presence of contributing factors.

Trigger Points

Trigger points exist as a localized tender areas within taut bands of skeletal muscles and when stimulated by macro- and microtraumatic episodes, they refer a characteristic pain pattern to a distant group of muscles, i.e. zone of reference.

Palpation of trigger points will give rise to a positive 'jump sign'.

■ PATHOPHYSIOLOGY (ETIOLOGY)

The MPDS can be visualized as a vicious cycle of several contributing factors such as :
1. Muscular hyperfunction.
2. Physical disorders.
3. Injuries to the tissues.
4. Parafunctional habits.
5. Disuse.
6. Nutritional problems.
7. Physiological stress.
8. Sleep disturbances.

It is difficult to know the initiating point, since it arises from the multifactorial origin. There are many different groups with various ideas about the disorders. They can be put into following major groups:
1. Psychologic or central etiology.
2. Occlusal or peripheral etiology.
3. The third group is recently considered is due to intrinsic joint disorder etiology.

Psychogenic Cause

It is possible that certain psychologically unbalanced individuals, due to unusual habits, perpetuate muscular disturbance leading to occlusal disharmony and thereby affecting the TM joints.

There is muscle fatigue seen in these individuals brought about by muscle spasm. This fatigue is believed to be related to psychologically motivated, persistent, tension relieving oral habits. Under emotional stress, the skeletal musculature exhibits general and sustained hyperfunction, which leads to the susceptibility to neurotic muscular contraction leading to muscle fatigue.

Persistent Tension Relieving Oral Habits

Pipe smoking, sleeping on stomach with the mandible supported by the forearm, teeth clenching, teeth grinding (bruxism), lip licking, jaw thrusting, nail biting, tongue thrusting, pencil/pen biting, constant chewing of tobacco and chewing gum, etc.

Sleep disturbances in these individuals undergoing stress also aggravate the problem and the habits, because of increased irritability.

Occlusal Disharmony

Occlusal disharmony can be either inherent or acquired or iatrogenic.
- *Inherent malocclusion*—is due to developmental deformities. Gross occlusal diskrepancy can lead to TMJ disorder due to constant microtrauma.
- *Acquired malocclusion*—failure to replace the loss of any tooth or teeth for a prolonged period causes drifting of the teeth leading to occlusal imbalance.
- *Iatrogenic occlusal disharmony*—faulty restorations, with high points and unbalanced vertical dimensions in dentures are the causative factors.

Faulty occlusion also leads to muscle spasm and changes the physiodynamics of TMJ leading to pain.

Loss of vertical dimension or deep bite causes the shift of condyles posteriorly, impinging on the sensitive bilaminar zone- causing constant pain.

All the above factors lead towards either micro- or macrotraumatic episodes leading towards muscle spasm.

1. Pain in MPDS is due to muscle spasm which follows the micro- or macrotrauma injury to musculoskeletal system.
2. Sensory input from the injured area, results in increased tone of musculature, in order to stabilize the affected part.
3. This hypertonicity may lead to muscle fatigue and the accumulation of metabolic byproducts such as lactic acid, prostaglandins, bradykinins, histamine and leukotrienes. The accumulation of these chemical pain mediators, lower the threshold of pain receptors to mechanical and chemical stimuli leading to MPDS.
4. In addition, chronic pain often involves a psychogenic component, which modifies the reaction to pain and complicates the treatment.

SYMPTOMS

The MPDS exhibits varied symptoms. One particular patient may complain of all the various symptoms, whereas in another patient only a single symptom may be present (Table 23.1).

HISTORY OF THE PATIENT

It is important that the patient should be allowed to describe his symptomatology in detail. Intelligent and effective treatment cannot be instituted without an accurate diagnosis. Probably the most beneficial aid (in this disorder) to diagnosis is a complete and standardized history and examination. The history should include questions concerned with:

1. Mode of onset, duration, frequency and quality of pain. Site and reference point of pain.
2. Time of the day, at which pain is most pronounced.
3. Occupation.
4. Sleeping habits.
5. Parafunctional habits.
6. History of previous trauma, prolonged dental work, etc.
7. Family or emotional problems.
8. Associated symptoms.
9. How the pain is lessened or relieved? How the pain is aggravated?

While taking the history, following questions regarding three components should be asked or looked for and the significant points should be noted down (Table 23.2).

Follow-7 R's for occlusal rehabilitation

1. Remove—extract
2. Reshape—grind
3. Reposition—orthodontia/orthognathic surgery

Table 23.1: Various symptoms of MPDS

Cardinal symptoms of MPDS

   i. Pain or diskomfort (unexplained nature), anywhere about the head or neck
  ii. Limitation of motion of the jaw
 iii. Joint noises—grating, clicking, snapping, etc
 iv. Tenderness to palpation of the muscles of mastication
     [Negative recent history of trauma, infection, ear or joint or maxillary sinus pathosis]

Associated symptoms in MPDS

Neurologic	Gastrointestinal tract	Musculoskeletal	Otologic
• Tingling	• Nausea	• Fatigue	• Tinnitus
• Numbness	• Vomiting	• Tension	• Ear pain
• Blurred vision	• Diarrhea	• Shift joint pains	• Dizziness
• Twitches	• Constipation	• Tiredness	• Vertigo
• Trembling	• Indigestion	• Weakness	• Diminished hearing
• Lacrimation	• Dry mouth		

Table 23.2: History of the patient: Three components		
Physical component	*Psychologic component*	*Dental component*
General health	Ethnic background	Supracontacts
Nutrition	Social customs	Incorrect dynamics
Age	Behavior	Improper vertical dimension
Occupation	Emotional health	
Lifestyle	Personal annoyances	
	Parafunctional stress relieving habits	

4. Restore—conservative dentistry
5. Replace—prosthesis
6. Reconstruct—TMJ surgery
7. Regulate—control habit and symptoms.

Physical Examination

Physical examination consists of an evaluation of entire masticatory system along with head and neck region.
* Articular (joint)
* Muscular
* Dental
* Cervical.

Articular or TMJ Function and Range of Motion

a. Amount of oral opening and the excursions
b. Extent of movement
   i. ROM → Range of motion
   ii. AROM → Active range of motion
   iii. PROM → Passive range of motion
c. Palpation for tenderness
d. Grading of click or crepitation—noises evaluation
e. Auscultation (stethoscopic evaluation), if needed.

Palpation: Simultaneous palpation of both the joints, with index finger laterally over the joint and through the external auditory canal in open and closed movements is done (Figs 23.1A and B).

Range of motion

1. It should be inspected for hypomobility or hypermobility and associated pain, if present. Normal vertical range of motion in adults is between 40 to 50 mm. Hypomobility without pain gives early indication of pathology. Measurement of maximum pain free movement is noted. The AROM and PROM tests should be carried out to delineate the source of

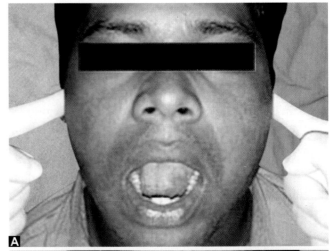

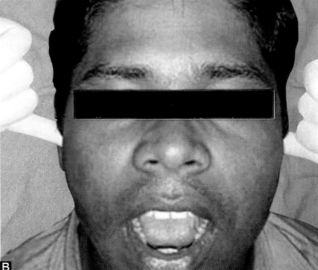

Figs 23.1A and B: (A) Simultaneous palpation of both the joints with index finger laterally over the joints, (B) Palpation of both the joints through the external auditory canal in open and closed position

restriction, whether articular or muscular or both. The AROM tests all anatomic structures. *Limited AROM with pain indicates structural restriction, but PROM tests all inert structures. Restricted movements suggest all contractile elements, i.e. muscle problems.*

2. Direction of opening —opening path and amount of deviation should be noted. Early opening deviation is due to spasm of lateral pterygoid muscle on the side towards which the deviation is seen. Gradual deviation is due to muscle imbalance. Stronger opening muscles on one side overpower the weaker muscles on the opposite side (Fig. 23.2).

3. Protrusive deviation and movement—normal range of protrusive movement is 10 mm.

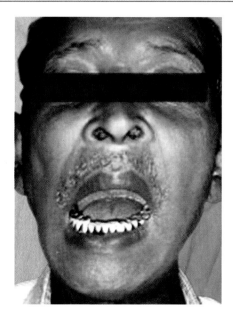

Fig. 23.2: Deviation of the mandible towards right side on oral opening with pain

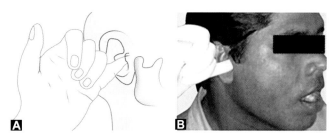

Figs 23.3A and B: Posterior joint palpation

4. Lateral excursions—normal left and right lateral excursion should be around 10 mm. Pain or restriction may indicate one or more of the following conditions—joint inflammation, muscle dysfunction, anteriorly displaced disk, etc.

Areas of tenderness on palpation: It should be noted. In posterior joint palpation, pain unrelated to closure or straight lateral palpation may indicate ear problem or inflammation (Figs 23.3A and B).

Timing of the click: Early, intermediate or wide open zones of condylar excursions are noted and whether it comes during opening, closing or both should be ascertained. Whether a distinct sound-click is felt or audible or whether only crepitus or multiple scraping, grating noises are felt is also noticed.

The joint noises can be heard with a stethoscope: Posterior joint palpation is also made to appreciate the opening and closing cycles of the click.

Muscular Examination

Systemic palpation of the muscles and their tendons is the best way to ascertain both subclinical and clinical existing levels of dysfunction. The areas responsive to palpation have been called 'trigger points'. The muscles are palpated bilaterally and simultaneously with firm but gentle pressure lasting for 1 or 2 minutes. The main

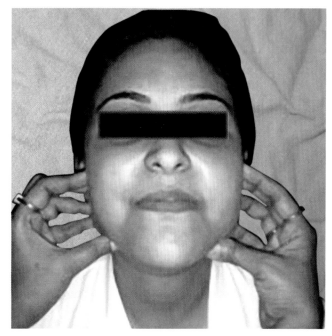

Fig. 23.4: Masseter muscle palpation

pressure is exerted with the middle finger of each hand. The adjacent fingers may be used when the area being palpated is large enough (Fig. 23.4).

Muscle palpation: It is helpful for the following:
1. Location of muscle pathology.
2. Evaluation of muscle tone.
3. Location of trigger points.
4. Evaluation of temperature change.
5. Location of swelling.
6. Identification of anatomic landmarks.

Sequence and sites of muscle palpation: The muscular structures are palpated using the sequence shown in Figures 23.5A to D. The subjective pain pattern should be precisely mapped. During muscle palpation, patient is asked questions regarding unilateral or bilateral pain, tenderness, whether it is mild, moderate or severe.

During palpation eye wincing or palpation associated with bodily withdrawal should be noted. Reference zone of the pain also should be located.

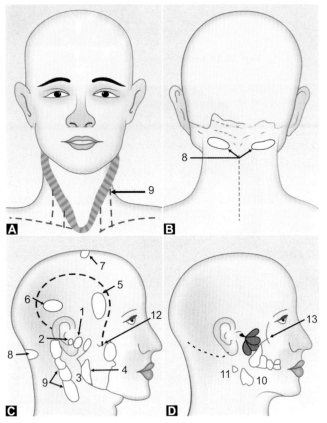

Figs 23.5A to D: Sequence and sites for muscles and joints palpation: (1) Lateral palpation, (2) Posterior joint palpation via ear. *Extraoral muscles* (3 and 4) Masseter, (5) Anterior temporalis, (6) Posterior temporalis (7) Vertex, (8) Neck, (9) Sternocleidomastoid, (10) Medial pterygoid, (11) Posterior digastric. *Intraoral muscle palpation,* (12) Temporalis tendon, (13) Lateral pterygoid

Resistance tests (Figs 23.6A to D): Primary muscle disorders are likely to be responsive to maximal resistance. With the head supported and the mouth open a finger breadth, a gradual buildup of force is generated by the hand of the examiner. The patient is instructed to resist the examiner's initiative to move the jaw. The test is interrupted, if pain is produced. A positive response will include pain that is similar to the original complaint. Biting tests are another method of putting the muscles and TMJs under load.

Dental/Occlusal Evaluation

Gross occlusal diskrepancies, prematurities or interferences should be noted.

Anterior open bite, collapsed bite, cross bite, reduced vertical dimension, etc. should also be noted. Attrition, wear facets, mobility of teeth, missing teeth should be checked. Type of malocclusion, skeletal, dentofacial deformities should be looked for.

Cervical Examination

Here, the neck group of muscles are palpated and neck range of motion should also be checked.

Temporomandibular joint is in close proximity to the upper part of the cervical spine. Functionally, the cervical spine and the TMJ occlusion are interrelated. Any change in one of these can affect the function or position of the other. Patient's posture should be noticed (Figs 23.7A and B).

Shoulder and neck muscles are palpated, as they control anteroposterior and lateral position of the head. Incline the patient's head forward for shoulder and neck examination. Look for tender points.

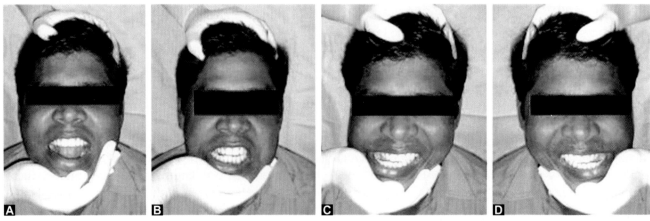

Figs 23.6A to D: Resistance test with a gradual build up of force, in open, protrusive and lateral excursion movements

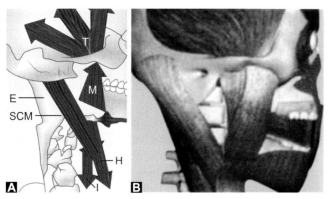

Figs 23.7A and B: Relationship of cervical and masticatory muscles. M—masseter, T—temporalis, SCM—sternocleidomastoid, E—neck extensors, I and H—infrahyoid muscles

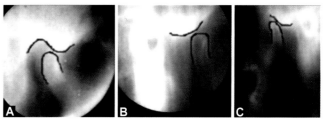

Figs 23.8A to C: (A) Tomogram showing normal relation of the condylar head to the eminence in open position, (B) Tomogram showing hypermobility of the TM joint, (C) Tomogram showing acute dislocation of the condylar head

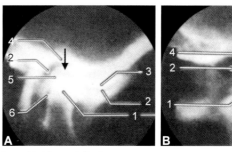

Figs 23.9A and B: Double contrast arthrography of the TM joint. (A) Normal TMJ image in closed position, (B) Open jaw position image indicating anterior displacement of the disk (arrow), 1. condylar head, 2. upper joint space, 3. articular eminence, 4. mandibular fossa, 5. disk. 6. lower joint space

Hyoid bone palpation: Ask the patient to swallow. Irregular contraction can be noted while breathing, speaking or swallowing (digastric is a link between supra and infrahyoid group of muscles). Neck range of motion should also be checked.

Radiographic evaluation: It is helpful in diagnosis of the following:

   i. Intra-articular pathologies.
   ii. Osseous pathological process.
   iii. Soft tissue pathologies.

The use of radiographs should be done judiciously in MPDS patients depending on the patient's signs and symptoms instead of ordering routine set of radiographs.

   i. *Panoramic radiography*
     a. For overall screening of TMJ on both sides simultaneously.
     b. For assessment of articular surfaces of condylar head and glenoid fossa.
     c. For any other osseous deformities.
     d. For evaluation of both the joint spaces.
   ii. *Tomograms:* For elimination of superimposition and to have clear detailed picture of TMJ (Figs 23.8A to C).
   iii. *Transcranial radiographs:* Comparison of both joints in open and closed position is helpful in detecting internal joint pathology. Also shows range of motion of condylar head.

Recent diagnostic methods (Figs 23.9A and B)

   i. *TMJ arthrography*—double contrast arthrography is more useful than single contrast method. Invasive and uncomfortable for patient. It is used in order to examine soft tissue components of the TMJ, especially, the disk. In this newer technique, 0.3 to 0.6 ml of contrast medium is injected into the upper and lower joint spaces to coat the internal surfaces. The contrast medium is subsequently withdrawn and in turn 1.0 to 1.5 ml of air is reinjected. These steps result in a thin contrast medium coating of the TMJ components, allowing good visualization of the shape and position of the disk.

   ii. *Computed radiography (CR)*—it uses an 'imaging plate' instead of the conventional X-ray film. Information from the 'imaging plate' is then fed into a computer for storing and processing into graphic images. Here the assessment of soft and hard tissue can be done.

   iii. *CT scan and MRI*—noninvasive methods of obtaining superior image of dense soft tissue disk, as well as of the hard tissue. Magnetic resonance imaging (MRI) does not use ionizing radiation. The principles of MRI involve taking advantage of the weak resonance energy emitted by the spinning actions of hydrogen nuclei when placed in a strong magnetic field. The signals emitted are then fed into computer for sorting and processing into graphic images.

CT scan provides the most accurate radiographic assessment of the bony components of the joint. Here, the image is obtained in one plane of space, but allows the reconstructions in different views.

iv. *Bone scintigram—nuclear imaging*—the technique involves injection of ^{99}Tc, (Technicium-99), a gamma emitting isotope that is concentrated in areas of active bone metabolism. Approximately after 3 hours of injection of this radioactive isotope, images are obtained using gamma camera.

Single photon emission computerized tomography (SPECT) images can then be obtained to determine active areas of bone metabolism known as" hot spots" or uptake areas. Very sensitive technique. Changes in the bone can be detected much earlier than the radiographs, but difficult to interpret. Interpretation is always based on history and clinical findings.

Psychological Evaluation of a Patient

If the patient is apparently depressed, then the clinical symptoms may be exaggerated. Psychiatrist should be involved, if patient is giving definitive history of stressful living environment or having emotional personality.

Psychological Symptoms

- Frustration
- Maladaptive behavior
- Anxiety
- Pain verbalization
- Depression
- Poor sleep
- Hypochondriasis
- Poor dietary habits
- Anger
- Clenching/bruxism
- Fear
- Medication dependencies.

Internal Derangement of the Temporomandibular Joint

Definition: Internal derangement (ID) is a disruption of the internal aspects of the TMJ, in which an abnormal relationship exists between the disk and the condyle, fossa and articular eminence.

Associated changes: Synovitis, there can be intracapsular scarring or adhesions within the joint, hemorrhage, fibrocartilaginous metaplasia, dystrophic calcifications and osteoarthritis.

Etiology of internal derangement (ID): Multifactorial
i. Microtrauma—overloading from bruxism and other parafunctional habits, hypermobility of the joint.
ii. Macrotrauma—obvious history of trauma and osseous morphologic changes.

A result of disk displacement may be stretching or tearing of the retrodiskal tissues. Degenerative changes may occur in these attached tissues.

Symptoms

- Pain during function
- Limited oral opening
- Masticatory and cervical tenderness.

Internal Derangements

A. • Disk displacement
   • Disk displacement with reduction
   • Disk displacement without reduction
B. Structural incompatibility of the articular surfaces
   • Adhesions
   • Alterations in the form
   • Due to systemic joint disorders like rheumatoid arthritis, etc.

Anteromedial displacement of disk is more common. The prevalence of disk displacement appears to increase with age.

Figure 23.10 shows normal physiomechanical disk to condyle relationship during translation. When there is no internal derangement, the relationships of the mid-disk to condyle remain consistent throughout opening and closing.

Anterior Disk Displacement with Reduction

Here, the disk is dislocated anterior to the condylar head, resulting in pain during translation. There is reciprocal clicking in anterior dislocation with reduction, the patient demonstrates a click on opening and a click, usually less noticeable, on closing. The clicks are not always audible, but the dentist can feel them during posterior joint palpation, as the disk slips on and off the condyle during functional movements.

During opening: Due to disk reduction, a clicking or popping sound ensues as the posterior part of the disk interferes with the condylar translation.

During closing: Reciprocal click occurs again, as the condyle returns to the original position, gliding over the posterior part of the disk (Fig. 23.11).

Anterior Disk Displacement without Reduction

Here, there is a closed lock form, where the disk interferes with condylar translation. Patient will not be able to open the mouth fully. Here, if patient attempts to open the mouth further, pain in the affected joint will

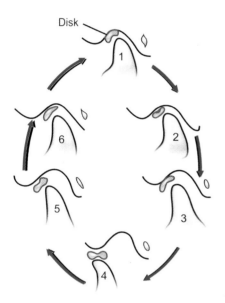

Fig. 23.10: Normal disk movement

be exhibited and deviation of the mandible towards the painful side will be noticed. This is because of the painful side remaining locked and it brings about translatory opening of the opposite side (Fig. 23.12).

If this chronic condition continues, then it will progress towards perforation of the disk.

Following five *clinical findings* will be seen in *disk dislocation without reduction:*

Positive history—sudden change in condylar movements

1. Limited mandibular opening.
2. Unilateral condition, one side condyle cannot translate fully
3. Unrestricted ipsilateral eccentric movement, checked by moving the mandible on the affected side. 10 to 12 mm normal range.
4. Restricted contralateral eccentric movement—less than 8 mm.
5. Loss of joint sounds—earlier history of clicking.

Systemic Joint Diseases Causing Internal Derangement

1. Degenerative type—pathology in the articular surface—osteoarthritis
2. Inflammatory—rheumatoid arthritis, juvenile rheumatoid arthritis, ankylosing spondylitis, Reiter's syndrome, lupus erythematosus. Disorders of immune system, hereditary factors.
3. Infective arthritis—bacterial, viral.

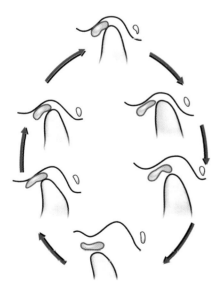

Fig. 23.11: Anterior disk displacement with reduction

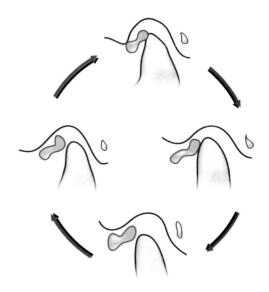

Fig. 23.12: Anterior disk displacement without reduction

OBJECTIVES OF TREATMENT IN MYOFASCIAL PAIN DYSFUNCTION SYNDROME

All the proposed theories revolve around myospasm caused either from the central or the peripheral origin. The treatment of this myospasm involves many different modalities. Definitive therapy always involves elimination of underlying cause (occlusal diskrepancies, stress, etc).

In MPDS, pain is provoked by manual palpation or functional manipulation. It is therefore appropriate to consider diagnostic injection with local anesthetic agent. Diagnostic blocking of a muscle trigger point is extremely helpful, when myofascial trigger point pain is suspected. It is also helpful to anesthetize the TMJ, so true joint pain can be separated from other pains.

Whenever muscle injections are given, a use of vasoconstrictor is contraindicated. Use lignocaine without adrenaline or use bupivacaine.

For TMJ pain, auriculotemporal nerve block is given. The advantage of this nerve block is that, entry into the joint structures can be avoided by blocking the auriculotemporal nerve, before its fibers reach the joint (Figs 23.13A and B).

Technique for Auriculotemporal Nerve Block

Preauricular area is prepared taking routine aseptic measures. Usually 27 or 26 gauge needle is inserted through the skin just anterior to the junction of the tragus and the ear lobe. The needle is then advanced behind the posterior aspect of the condyle in an anteromedial direction to a depth of 1 cm where the 1.5 ml of anesthetic solution is deposited after aspiration. If the true source of pain is the joint, then the pain should be eliminated or decreased within 5 minutes.

Treatment of MPDS

In the literature, there is no universal agreement for the treatment of MPDS. Various treatment modalities have been suggested.

First important task is counselling of the patient and giving the assurance regarding prognosis and planning for symptomatic pain relief. Once the pain is relieved, then the patient's acceptance for further treatment modalities is achieved. Nature of the myofascial pain resulting from parafunctional habits secondary to stress and anxiety should be explained to the patient in detail and patient should be encouraged for behavior modification. Modification of diet and home exercises should be suggested. Initially soft diet should be prescribed along with the medication.

Medications

1. Aspirin   : 2 tabs 0.3 to 0.6 gm/4 hourly
2. Piroxicam   : 10 to 20 mg/3 to 4 times a day
3. Ibuprofen   : 200 to 600 mg/3 times a day
4. Pentazocine   : 50 mg/2 to 3 times a day
5. Valium/Librium : 5 to 10 mg/2 to 3 times a day
6. Methocarbamol   : 500 mg/2 to 3 times a day
7. Amitriptyline   : 10 to 25 mg/3 times a day or at bedtime

- *Nonsteroidal anti-inflammatory drugs*—to reduce inflammation and to provide pain relief, both in the muscles as well as in the joints (for 14 to 21 days.)
- *Muscle relaxants*—are recommended only for short duration, as they produce sedation and addiction.

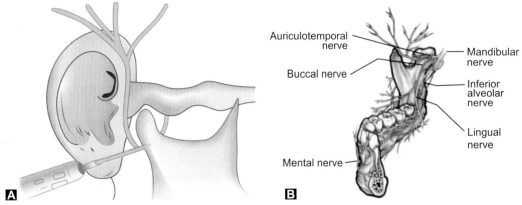

Figs 23.13A and B: (A) Auriculotemporal nerve block, (B) Mandibular nerve and its distributions

Diazepam 2 to 5 mg or cyclobenzapine 10 mg at bedtime can be given for 10 days or meprobamate 400 mg TDS x 7 days.

- *Ethyl chloride spray* or intramuscular local anesthetic injections in the affected muscles can also give relief. The patient is asked to follow the stretch exercises subsequently. Two percent lignocaine or 0.05 percent bupivacaine can be used.

Physiotherapeutic Modalities

Heat application: It increases local circulation, acts as a sedative, lowers muscle tension. Increases permeability of membranes and metabolic activity. Heat application can be given superficial or deep. Heating lamps, moist or dry heating pads or packs, hot moist application of towels can be given for 15 to 20 minutes, 4 times a day.

Ultrasound: It is a effective way to produce heat, deep in the tissues, with the use of ultrasonic waves. Alters blood flow and metabolic activity.

Application to the muscles and joints can be given. 0.7 to 1.0 Watt per cm^2 for 10 minutes every alternate day given by physiotherapist.

Cryotherapy: Ice packs application to the painful area 4 times a day for 20 minutes. Cold compressions lower the thermal gradient in the skin, interrupting massive concentration of histamines, thus lowering pain threshold in the skin.

Spread of pain is interrupted by sudden cold stimulus, it also raises cutaneous pain threshold by counter-irritation.

Massage with counter-irritants and vibrators: Firm friction massage produces temporary ischemia followed by hyperemia. It inactivates trigger points.

Use of vapocoolent spray: Fluoromethane or ethyl chloride spray is applied to painful area for 5 seconds. The muscle is gently stretched after that. The eyes, nose and ears are protected from the spray.

Tetanizing and sinusoidal currents: Fatiguing the muscle helps to recover gradual rhythmic movement.

Electrogalvanic stimulation: Delivers a wide range of intensity (voltage) to activate the injured muscle. It stimulates local circulation, achieves excitability and conductivity without painful heating. Pulse at 80 cycles/second for 10 minutes followed by exercise for 5 minutes is used.

Transcutaneous electronic nerve stimulator (TENS): It interferes with the sensation of pain in the brain and increases blood flow to the site.

Active stretch exercises: It includes opening and closing of mouth 10 times as a warm up against resistance. It can help to restore the normal range of motion, by flexibility and strengthening the muscles. Each of these physiotherapy modalities can be very helpful to reduce the pain and increase the range of motion along with the medication.

Stress Management

Managing daily stress is one of the best ways to help restore harmony between the muscles and TMJ. Biofeedback technique teaches the patient how to relax. Other methods like acupressure, acupuncture, yoga, hypnosis, zen therapy, transcendental meditation, deep breathing relaxation, etc. also can help to relieve the stress.

Biofeedback instrument provides audio as well as visual output allowing the patient to hear and see increased muscle activity and then relax.

Intra-articular Injections

Hydrocortisone intra-articular injections can be used to treat the inflammation within the joint. Two percent lignocaine 0.5 cc can be mixed with hydrocortisone for relieving the pain.

These injections should not be used routinely. But the injections can be used selectively, once in a month with other supportive and corrective treatments.

The technique of TMJ intra-articular injection (Figs 23.14A and B): The preauricular area must be prepared in routine aseptic manner. Patient is asked to carry out opening and closing movements. Joint movements are palpated by the operator and a mouth prop should be kept between the last posterior teeth to keep the mouth wide open. This makes the joint cavity more accessible for the injection. A 2 ml Luer-lok syringe is fitted with 1 ml solution of hydrocortisone + 0.5 ml of 2 percent lignocaine and is fitted with a 25 gauge 1.5″ long needle. When the mouth is fully opened and the condyle is placed anteriorly, the pathway of the needle in the joint cavity is easy. The direction of insertion of the needle is inward, forward and upward till it strikes the roof of the glenoid fossa at a depth of 2 to 3 cm. The needle is withdrawn about half a centimeter and 1 ml solution

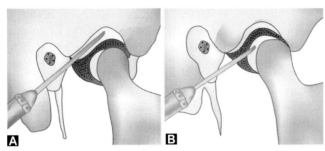

Figs 23.14A and B: Intra-articular injection technique for temporomandibular joint

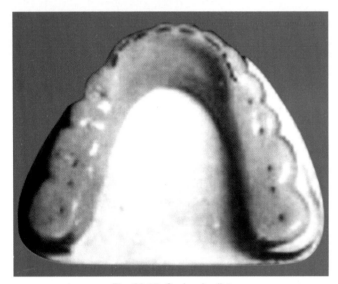

Fig. 23.15: Occlusal splint

is injected after aspiration, slowly in the upper joint cavity. After changing the direction further downward rest of the solution is injected in the lower joint cavity. Patient should be covered with routine antibiotic/anti-inflammatory regime.

Occlusal Splints (Fig. 23.15)

They can be used for the following:
    i. To temporarily disengage the teeth.
    ii. To create a balanced joint-tooth stabilization of the mandible.
    iii. To reduce spasm, contracture and hyperactivity of musculature.
    iv. To improve/restore the vertical dimension.
    v. To serve as safety or protective appliance.
    In majority of cases two types of occlusal splints are used. The splints should be removed while eating.

1. Stabilization splint

Twelve to eighteen hours use is advocated up to 4 to 6 months. These are fabricated over the maxillary teeth, covering the occlusal and incisal surface. Similar to Hawley's plate, but occlusal coverage is added. The splint is made up of acrylic. A flat platform is added perpendicular to the mandibular incisors, so that the splint will disengage the teeth and relax the muscles. The splint should be worn as instructed and patient should be recalled for check up at 2 weeks interval. Follow up is done until the occlusion is stabilized and muscles are free of tenderness. If patient does not have relief at the end of 3 months, reevaluation of the original diagnosis should be done.

This splint reduces the load on the retrodiskal area and thereby relieves the pain. It can be also used to eliminate occlusal interferences associated with bruxism.

Instead of acrylic material, prefabricated commercially available resilient splints are also available for protection of teeth from trauma or from forces of bruxism (Figs 23.16 and 23.17).

2. Relaxation Splints

Relaxation splints are used for disengagement of teeth and for only short period (up to 4 weeks). They are fabricated over the maxillary incisor teeth. A platform is added to disengage mandibular anteriors.

Temporomandibular Joint Arthrocentesis

This is a simple treatment for limited mouth opening accompanied by severe pain.

Progress of internal derangement of TMJ is as follows:
- First stage—clicking is accompanied by normal maximal mouth opening (MMO).
- Next stage—progression of the first stage to this stage. Here clicking will gradually stop with varying degrees of restriction in oral opening (closed lock). This stage is attributed to a nonreducible, anteriorly displaced disk acting as an obstacle for the translation of the condyle (Fig. 23.12).

Literature shows that the treatment options for closed lock were initially, conservative treatment and if it failed, then surgical contouring and repositioning of the disk. Later on, arthroscopic lysis and lavage and use

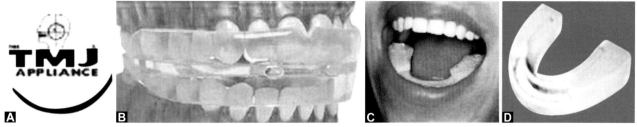

Figs 23.16A to D: (A and B) Prefabricated TMJ appliance. The TMJ appliance • Immediate application • No fitting required • One size for all adults • Shorten base for children • Joint decompression • Limits bruxing • Treats myofunctional habits • Double mouthguard • Zero chair time. (C and D) TMD appliance—It is made up of thermoplastic material, which allows custom fitting to the lower teeth and the correct bite. Low profile design allows for easy speech when in place. Aerofoil shaped splint over the lower back teeth reduces TM joint symptoms by decompressing the temporomandibular joints

Design features of the T4B®

- No impressions or custom fitting
- Single size for all patients
- Distal end may be trimmed if required
- High grade silicone material for maximum flexibility and comfort
- Used one hour daily plus overnight

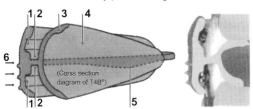

Cross-section photo above shows relationship of the T4B® with teeth and fixed appliances.

1. Appliance channels to accommodate brackets and orthodontic archwire
2. Tooth channels.
3. Tongue tag for the proprioceptive positioning of tongue tip as in myofunctional and speech therapies.
4. Tongue guard stops tongue thrusting when in place and forces patient to breathe through nose.
5. Splint (patented aerofoil-shape) achieves gentle decompression of the temporomandibular joints.
6. Lip bumpers discourage over-active mentalis muscle activity.

Fig. 23.17: Special features of the temporomandibular joint appliance

of hydraulic pressure in the upper joint compartment were applied for ID and found effective in closed lock cases in establishing normal MMO.

Simple arthrocentesis does not require arthroscope.

Arthrocentesis (Lavage or Irrigation of the Upper Joint Cavity)

Objectives

   i. Improve the disk mobility.
   ii. Eliminate joint inflammation.
   iii. Remove the resistance to condyle translation. Return to normal function.
   iv. Early physiotherapy.
   v. Eliminate pain.

Indications for arthrocentesis: All patients who had proved refractory to conservative treatment (medication, bite appliance, physiotherapy and manipulation of the joint).

Arthrocentesis technique (Figs 23.18A to C): Patient is made to lie supine with the head turned. Preauricular area is prepared as usual. With palpating index finger on the affected side, the TMJ movements are palpated. Two points are marked over the skin indicating the articular fossa and eminence. Auriculotemporal nerve block injection given using 0.5 ml of 2 percent lignocaine solution.

A 19 or 18 gauge, 1.5 inch long needle is then inserted into the superior joint compartment corresponding to the posterior mark. This first needle is inserted about 1 inch in depth and stabilized. Then another 19 or 18 gauge 1.5 inch long needle is inserted at the second mark corresponding to articular eminence. A 10 cc syringe is filled up with Ringer lactate solution and connected to the first needle. The solution is pushed to distend the joint space. This solution should flow freely out of the second needle like a fountain. The position of both needles are manipulated till such free flow is established. Before injection, it is made sure that

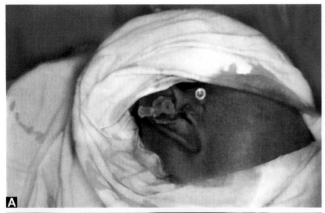

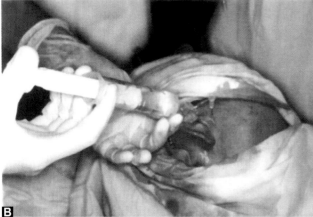

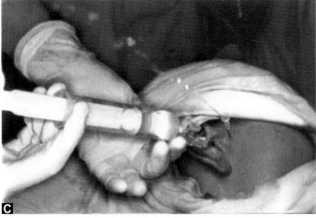

Figs 23.18A to C: Arthrocentesis procedure for TM joint: (A) Insertion of first and second needles at posterior aspect of superior joint compartment and articular eminence respectively, (B) Ringer lactate solution is pushed in the first needle to distend the joint space, (C) Fountain like flow from the second needle during lavage

patient's mouth is fully stretched open and mouth prop is inserted to maintain it, during the entire procedure.

Initially, the solution which will flow out of second needle will be blood tinged or turbid, but as more

solution is pushed through the first needle, (up to 200 ml) the flow of clear solution will be noticed. On termination of procedure, 1 ml of hydrocortisone is injected into the joint space, followed by removal of the needle.

Hypothesis

Due to lavage, the pain mediators prostaglandin E_2 and leukotriene B get washed out, reducing the inflammation and pain. Speculation is that because of synovitis the sliding of the disk is prevented by its adherence to the fossa. This persistent inability of the disk to slide can be readily reversed by simple lavage. This nonreducing disk might result from adhesive forces originating from an increase in synovial fluid viscosity or from a vacuum effect created between the disk and fossa. The injected fluid distends hydraulically, the joint space and enables the disk to slide and thereby re establishes normal MMO.

Postarthrocentesis Medication

Tablet naproxen sodium 275 mg three times daily and diazepam 2.5 to 5 mg at bedtime to be taken for 2 weeks in association with the use of a bite appliance at night. Patient should be kept on soft diet. Patient should start physiotherapy program on the following day to establish normal MMO. The procedure can be repeated after a gap of one week at least three to four times with one week's interval. Eighty percent of the patients show improvement in pain, MMO and clicking or grating disappears in at least 50 percent of cases.

Advantages

- Simple technique
- Minimum armamentarium
- Less invasive
- Inexpensive
- Highly effective
- Therapeutic benefit.

Temporomandibular Joint Arthroscopy

Temporomandibular joint arthroscopy consists of the insertion of a specially designed fiberoptic endoscope into a joint compartment for observation (diagnostic) and therapeutic purpose. The TMJ arthroscopy was made popular by Ohnishi in 1975, with the development of a 1.7 mm diameter needle type arthroscope.

Techniques

i. Basic single puncture diagnostic technique.
ii. Double puncture technique for therapeutic, as well as, surgical purpose.

Patient selection: After all conservative methods have failed.

i. Disk dysfunction
ii. Osteoarthrosis
iii. Synovial disease
iv. Hypomobility due to disk problems
v. Hypermobility associated with severe pain.

Contraindications

i. Regional infection
ii. Presence of tumor
iii. Usual medical contraindications to surgery.

Instrumentation (Figs 23.19 to 23.21)

i. Arthroscope 1.7 to 2 mm diameter
ii. Fiberoptic light source and cables
iii. Videocamera and cable
iv. Monitor
v. Videorecorder.

Percutaneous puncture instruments

i. 2 cannulas
ii. Sharp trocar
iii. Blunt obturator.

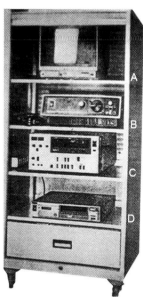

Fig. 23.19: Equipment for arthroscopy. (A) Monitor, (B) Xenon light source, (C) Control box, (D) Video recorder

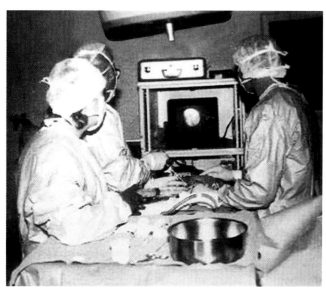

Fig. 23.20: TMJ arthroscopy in progress

Hand instruments (Fig. 23.21)

i. Biopsy forceps—for synovial membrane or fibro-cartilage.
ii. Biopsy scissors—for adhesions.
iii. Probe—curved, blunt.

Irrigation system

i. Ringer lactate solution
ii. IV delivery system
iii. 2 connecting tubing
iv. 2 three-way stop cocks
v. Luer-Lok syringe

Sterilization: The arthroscope may be sterilized with ethylene oxide gas or formalin chamber or chemical sterilization can be done. Nonoptical parts and all other accessories should be autoclaved.

Arthroscopic Techniques

Anesthesia: For diagnostic arthroscopy, local anesthesia with or without sedation is sufficient. For therapeutic or surgical purpose general anesthesia is indicated.

Position of the patient and instrumentations: Patient is placed in a dorsal supine position on the operation table. Head is rotated so that the affected side is superior. Patient is prepared and draped in usual surgical aseptic manner.

A TV monitor along with power instruments, camera control, light source are all positioned in such a

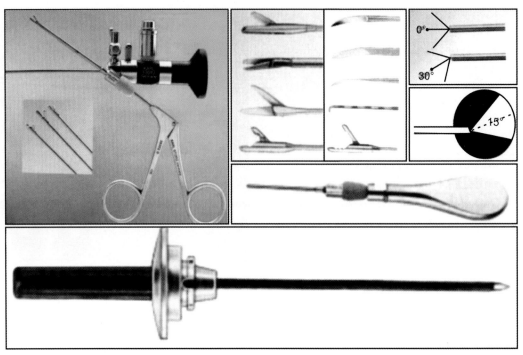

Fig. 23.21: Instrumentation for arthroscopy. Arthroscope camera, trocar, cannula, biopsy forceps, scissors, probes, blades, etc

way, that operator will have direct view of the monitor. Mandibular movements palpated and the mandible must be distracted by the assistant's padded thumb on the occlusal surfaces of lower molars and the index, middle and ring finger along the inferior border of the mandible and then maintained in the distracted position by inserting a mouth prop.

Marking: A line is drawn from the mid-tragus of the ear to the lateral canthus of the eye. First point is marked 10 mm anterior to the tragus and 2 mm inferior to the canthus tragus line. This corresponds to the maximum concavity of the glenoid fossa, the target for the first puncture (while marking and palpating this point, superficial temporal artery pulsations also to be checked).

Another point is marked 20 mm anterior to the midportion of the tragus and 10 mm below the canthus tragus line. This corresponds to the peak of the eminence. This second marking is made for the second puncture in double puncture technique.

Anesthesia: Around 1 to 3 cc of local anesthetic solution with adrenaline is injected into the superior joint space by using 18 or 19 gauge 1.5 inch long needle. The needle should be inserted from an inferior, posterior and lateral approach aiming for the midportion of the posterior slope of the articular eminence. Local anesthetic is used for anesthesia and hemostasis, plus it distends the upper joint space, for easier introduction of the arthroscope and for clearer observation.

Single puncture technique (Figs 23.22(A) and 23.23): Mainly used for examination of the joint. The sharp trocar is inserted into the cannula and inserted at first marking point to create a puncture wound. The trocar and cannula should be kept perpendicular to the skin surface and directed anterosuperiorly (10° angle to the horizontal plane) aiming at the roof of the glenoid fossa. The depth of cannula can vary from 5 to 10 mm. Then the trocar can be withdrawn as soon as the resistance felt is ceased, blunt obturator is inserted and the cannula is advanced to the center of the joint. The average depth for insertion ranges from 25 to 45 mm. The blunt obturator is then removed and the backflow of the fluid will be noticed. Then the joint lavage is carried out to remove blood or any puncture debris by flushing 20 to 25 cc of Ringer lactate solution. After the adequate lavage, the cannula is held in position and the arthroscope is inserted. Once the scope is in position, the joint is systematically examined.

Arthroscopy is proceeded from the known to unknown. Thus, first the structure should be identified for orientation and then the scope can be moved to obtain

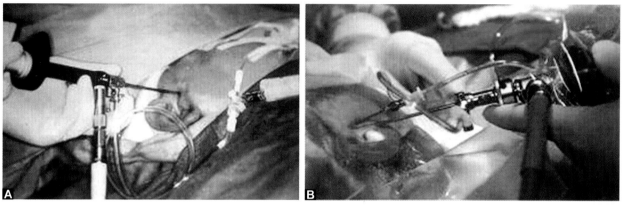

Figs 23.22A and B: Arthroscopic technique (A) Single puncture technique, (B) Lavage by injecting lactated Ringer's solution into the inflow system

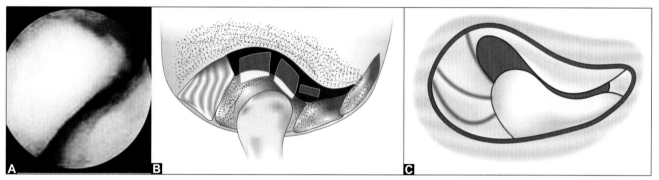

Figs 23.23A to C: (A) TMJ diagnostic arthroscopy, (B) Normal condyle disk relation, (C) Arthroscopic view of condyle and disk

an entire view of the joint. Rotation or forward and backward movements or side to side movements of the scope can be carried out for complete visualization of the joint cavity.

Double puncture technique (Figs 23.24 to 23.26): The arthroscope or operative instruments or an outflow cannula can be introduced via a second marking point entry. This puncture facilitates examination of the anterior space and joint lavage can be carried out without much extravasation of the fluid.

After initial examination and diagnosis is done through the arthroscope, lavage is carried out. If proper instruments are available, then arthroscopic surgery like incision, shaving or resection of tissue can be done. Operating arthroscope consists of a double channel sheath for introduction of operating instruments to be used under direct vision.

Surgical hand instruments
1. Probe—used for palpation and hooking the disk, wall of the cavity and loose bodies.
2. Knives— for cutting the adhesions.
3. Yag-Laser— to burn, coagulate or vaporize the tissue.

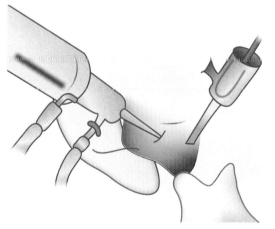

Fig. 23.24: Double puncture arthroscopy

4. Forceps—used to grasp the loose bodies, tissues to be sent for biopsy of the synovial membrane/fibrocartilage.
5. Intra-articular shaver system—electrically driven, rotating cutting, suction device.
6. Suturing needle—for disk, synovial membrane.

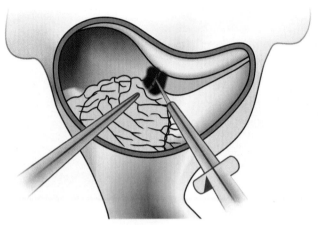

Fig. 23.25: The lysis, lavage and manipulation technique as performed in the superior joint space. An arthroscopic knife is used to incise the adhesion between the posterior slope of the eminence and the remodeled retrodiskal tissue. The lysis is carried out under direct vision

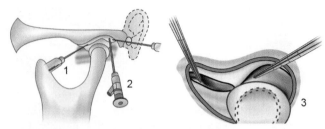

Fig. 23.26: Double puncture arthroscopy (1-2) cannulae in position (3) Surgical lysis in progress

Uses of arthroscopic technique

- i. Lavage—arthrocentesis
- ii. Lysis of adhesion
- iii. Disk mobility improvement
- iv. Sclerotherapy or disk suturing for hypermobility
- v. Retrodiskal cauterization
- vi. Shaving of the articular surfaces
- vii. Biopsy
- viii. Documentation by still or cine photography or video recording.

Complications: Drawbacks and possible complications

- i. Inadequate findings
- ii. Costly equipment
- iii. Otologic findings—complete or sensory hearing loss and severe vertigo
- iv. Facial paralysis
- v. Instrument breakage
- vi. Iatrogenic damage to the disk.

Arthroscopic Anatomy (Fig. 23.23)

To visualize the joint structures into clear focus, the arthroscope is first placed at the maximum depth permissible and then gradually withdrawn. Sweeping motion along the horizontal plane allows the visualization of the disk. The angle viewing scope can be rotated through 360° arc.

Synovium: It appears as soft, folded, translucent material. In a normal joint the synovial capillaries have a spider web appearance. A red/white line demarcates the junction between the synovium and the disk.

Disk: It is a milky white structure with a smooth surface.

Articular eminence: It is seen as a rounded protuberance covered with fibrocartilage. It is a highly reflective white surface, but color and texture will vary in the degenerated joint.

Glenoid fossa: It has a round concave shape and covered with the same type of fibrocartilage on the articular eminence. Bone is not seen in the healthy TMJ. The appearance of gray or brown denuded bony surface indicates pathology.

Arthroscopic examination: It is divided into two zones.

1. *Anterior zone* comprises of synovial tissue, the anterior slope of the eminence with its fibrocartilage and anterior portion of the disk.
2. *Intermediate zone (avascular zone)* comprised of articular cartilage covering the articular eminence and meniscus.
3. *Posterior zone* comprised of synovial tissue and glenoid fossa. Examination always begins in the posterior zone with the condyle in the forward position. Operator can detect synovial inflammation, adhesions, edema, perforation or prolapse of disk.

Postoperative Care

The puncture wound dressing is done with topical application of antibiotic ointment and covered with small adhesive tape. Analgesics, anti-inflammatory, muscle relaxants can be prescribed. After 24 hours, dressing can be removed and physiotherapy can be instituted.

Surgical Treatment of Temporomandibular Joint Dysfunction Disorders

First introduced by Humphrey in 1956. Since then, numerous philosophies of treatment and surgical modalities have evolved. But, the surgery should be undertaken only after all noninvasive conservative therapies have failed. Some of these surgical techniques, such as high condylectomy (excision of the condyle), aim at bypassing the obstacle, whereas others, such as partial or total diskectomy or disk recontouring and repositioning, eminectomy are designed to eliminate the obstacle by removing it or correcting the displacement. All these methods have met with considerably high success rates. The procedures on condyle included condylotomy, osteoplasty (condylar shave or high condylectomy). Eminectomy can also be done. Theoretically, these procedures reduce the intra-articular pressure by increasing the joint space, which in turn reduces load on the rich neurovascular retrodiskal tissues.

Condylar shave and arthroplasty: It consists of removing several millimeters of the articular surface. Recontouring should be done.

Condylectomy is the excision of the condyle. This procedure had mixed results and multiple complications, particularly an open bite, malocclusion and deviation of the mandible on opening.

Eminectomy: It may be performed to increase an access to the joint space for reconstruction of the disk, as well as to diminish the obstacle in the pathway of translocation.

Disk surgery: Autogenous grafts like dermis, temporalis fascia, myofascial flaps, auricular cartilage or homologous tissues like lyophilized cartilage, dura or collagen have been used after removal of the disk. Alloplastic materials like Silastic, Proplast, Teflon have also been used after diskectomy. Fragmentation of alloplastic material may result in foreign body giant cell reactions and lymphadenopathy. Subsequent resultant bone degeneration with pain dysfunction is often noticed.

Success rate of open joint surgery is generally 70 to 80 percent better than disk surgery.

SECTION 4

Orthognathic Surgery

Introduction to Orthognathic Surgery, Diagnosis and Treatment Planning

24

Variety is a spice of life and the human face is certainly no exception to this adage. Variations in facial proportions within normal limits make a human face interesting. Various facial patterns lend a unique identity to the person. It is the harmony and symmetry of each segment, which contributes towards the total beauty of the face. Any deviation from the normal facial development definitely brings about an unpleasant facial appearance, with a disturbance in both esthetics as well as function.

These dentofacial deformities can induce severe psychological problems in the affected individuals. A study conducted by the National Research Council of USA reveals that dentofacial deformities affect 20 percent of the population, out of which 5 percent of the population have major severe skeletal deformities. In our day to day practice, we come across various developmental dentofacial deformities and these should be considered/studied in relation to all three planes of space to have proper understanding of the deformity (Fig. 24.1).
1. Anteroposterior plane
2. Vertical plane
3. Transverse plane.

Types of Severe Skeletal Dentofacial Deformities

Types of severe skeletal dentofacial deformities can be broadly grouped into following categories (Tables 24.1 to 24.8).
1. Mandible Excess : *Mandibular prognathism*
   Deficiency : *Mandibular retrognathism*
2. Maxilla Excess : *Vertical maxillary excess (VME)*
   Deficiency : *Vertical maxillary deficiency (VMD)*
3. Combination
   • Bimaxillary protrusion
   • Nasomaxillary hypoplasia associated with prognathic mandible
   • Nasomaxillary hypoplasia associated with cleft lip and palate
4. Facial asymmetry
   • Asymmetric prognathism of the mandible
   • Unilateral condylar hyperplasia
   • Hemifacial hypertrophy (rare).

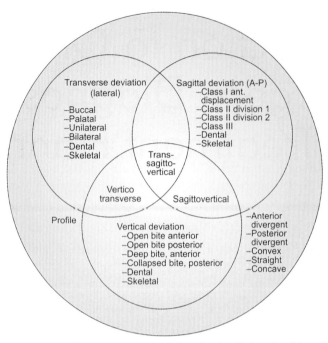

Fig. 24.1: Ackerman and Proffit's representation of five major characteristics of malocclusion via a Venn diagram. This is a convenient way of organizing the diagnostic information to be sure that no important criteria are overlooked

Table 24.1: Mandibular excess: prognathic mandible (prognathism) (Figs 24.2A to D)	
Facial features	*Dental features*
1. Prominent chin is the dominant feature (prominent lower third of the face)	1. Angle's class III molar malocclusion will be seen
2. A concave profile	2. Reverse horizontal overjet in the incisor area
3. Severe cases show lip incompetence	3. Posterior cross bite
4. Steep mandibular plane which may be parallel to high palatal plane (angle over 35°,– Normal 25°)	4. Mandibular anterior teeth may be inclined lingually (Nature's dental compensation) or they may be upright
5. Obtuse gonial angle	5. Maxillary teeth may be protrusive (Nature's dental compensation)
6. Middle third of the face appears relatively deficient	
7. Labiomental fold may be diminished or absent	6. An anterior open bite may be seen
8. Nasolabial angle may be acute	
9. Anterior facial height may be increased	

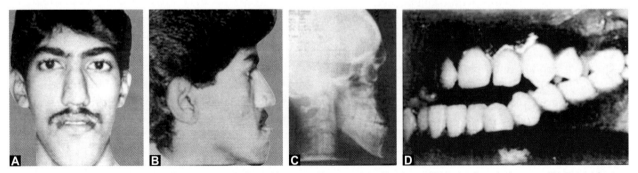

Figs 24.2A to D: Mandibular prognathism: (A and B) Facial features. Front and profile views, (C) Lateral cephalogram, (D) Dental features

Table 24.2: Mandibular deficiency/mandibular retrognathism/micrognathism (Figs 24.3A to C)	
Facial features	*Dental features*
1. A convex profile	1. Angle's Class II molar malocclusion
2. Retruded 'weak' chin. 'Bird face deformity'—in extreme severe cases	2. Increased overjet
3. Short upper lip, curled and protrusive at rest	3. Accentuated curve of spee of lower anteriors
4. An everted lower lip, curled under the protrusive upper incisors with deep mentolabial fold	4. Lower anterior teeth may be tipped forward (fanning) or crowded
5. Acute gonial angle	5. Skeletal deep bite may be present
6. The lip strain will be evident if closure of the mouth is attempted	

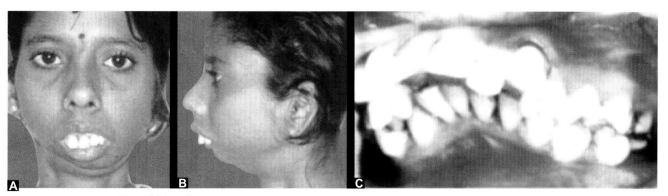

Figs 24.3A to C: Mandibular deficiency: (A and B) Front and profile view; (C) Dental occlusion

Table 24.3: Maxillary excess (long face syndrome): vertical maxillary excess (VME) (Figs 24.4 and 24.5)	
Facial features	*Dental features*
1. Increased height of lower third of the face	1. An angle's class II molar occlusion
2. Recessive paranasal areas	2. A high arched palate
3. Narrow alar base	3. V shaped maxillary dental arch
4. Prominence of infraorbital rims, cheek bones, prominent nose	4. Accentuated curve of spee
5. Large interlabial gap (more than 4 mm) with the lips in repose (incompetent lips)	5. Two variants: (Figs 24.4 and 24.5)
6. Excessive incisor display—Typical 'gummy smile'.	A. With anterior open bite—Excessive posterior maxillary vertical growth. A short or normal ramus. Two thirds of the patients have anterior open bite.
7. Retropositioned or recessive chin	B. Without anterior open bite—Dental compensation with over eruption of incisors (an increased ramus height).
8. Steep mandibular plane	

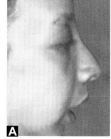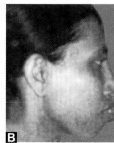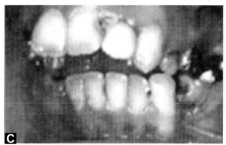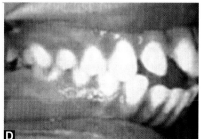

Figs 24.4A to D: VME with anterior open bite: (A and B) Profile view of VME patients, (C and D) dental features of the same patients respectively

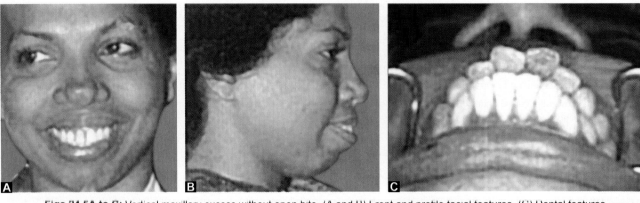

Figs 24.5A to C: Vertical maxillary excess without open bite. (A and B) Front and profile facial features, (C) Dental features

Table 24.4: Maxillary deficiency/vertical maxillary deficiency (VMD) (Figs 24.6A and B)	
Facial features	*Dental features*
1. A short square-shaped face with edentulous appearance	1. Angle's class I or class II molar occlusion
2. Decreased lower facial height	2. Deep overbite
3. The mandible appears square and prominent due to overclosure	3. Mandibular incisors frequently occlude with the palatal gingiva
4. Deep mentolabial fold 'Knobby' appearance of the chin (prominent chin button)	4. Severe attrition of the teeth may be seen
5. Over closure of the lips	

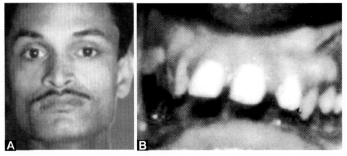

Figs 24.6A and B: Vertical maxillary deficiency (VMD) facial and dental features

Table 24.5: Skeletal bimaxillary protrusion with or without anterior open bite (Figs 24.7 and 24.8)	
Facial features	*Dental features*
1. Convex profile	1. Anterior open bite or edge to edge bite may be present
2. Extreme protrusion of maxillary and mandibular incisors	2. Mild to severe crowding or spaces may be seen
3. Anterior teeth prominent and visible in the frontal and profile views	3. May be associated with a severe tongue thrusting habit
4. Lip strain is evident, if the mouth is closed	4. When severe protrusion of maxillary incisors is seen, accentuated curve of spee with mandibular incisors crowding and deep bite may be seen
5. Lip incompetence	
6. Thick looking lips, with an everted vermilion border and a rolled appearance	
7. Apparent chin deficiency	

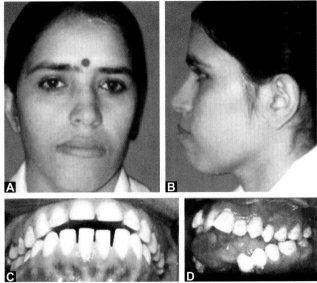

Figs 24.7A to D: Bimaxillary protrusion with anterior open bite (A) Frontal view, (B) Profile view, (C) Dental features, (D) Another bimaxillary protrusion patient's dental occlusion. Note the severe tongue thrust habit

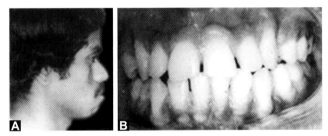

Figs 24.8A and B: Bimaxillary protrusion without anterior open bite: (A) Profile view, (B) Dental features

Table 24.6: Nasomaxillary hypoplasia associated with a prognathic mandible (Figs 24.9A to C)	
Facial features	*Dental features*
1. Flattening of the face	1. Anterior and posterior cross bites
2. Sunken appearance of the face	2. Maxillary incisors tend to be protrusive in relation to the hypoplastic maxilla
3. Prognathic mandible	3. Mandibular incisors upright to the mandibular basal bone
4. Upper lip is flat and relatively short	4. Mandibular posterior teeth have an exaggerated lingual inclination
5. No display of upper incisors	5. Maxillary posterior teeth tend to lean outwards
6. Deepened nasolabial fold	

Table 24.7: Nasomaxillary hypoplasia associated with cleft lip-palate deformities (Figs 24.10A to E)	
Facial features	*Dental features*
• Severe mid-face hypoplasia	• Angle's class III molar malocclusion
• Short, distorted upper lip	
• Asymmetry of the nose (Typical speech 'Nasal Twang')	• Constricted maxillary arch
• Mandible appears relatively prognathic (pseudoprognathism)	• Anterior cross bite
	• Crowding of maxillary teeth

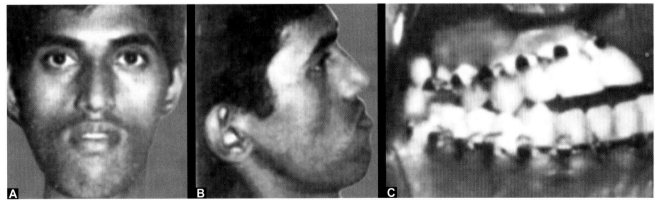

Figs 24.9A to C: Nasomaxillary hypoplasia associated with a prognathic mandible: (A and B) Frontal and profile view, (C) Dental occlusion

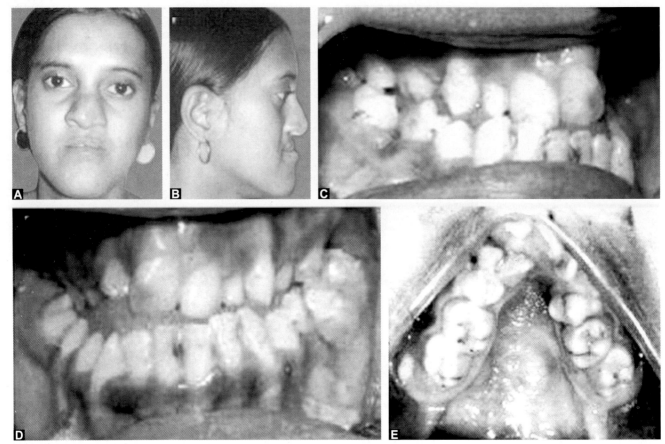

Figs 24.10A to E: Nasomaxillary hypoplasia associated with cleft lip and palate deformities: (A) Frontal view, (B) Profile view, (C) Anterior and posterior cross bite, (D) Dental occlusion, (E) Constricted maxillary arch

Table 24.8: Conditions with facial asymmetry (Figs 24.11 to 24.14)

1. Asymmetrical mandibular prognathism
    a. With anterior open bite
    b. Without anterior open bite
2. Unilateral condylar hyperplasia:
    a. Hemimandibular elongation
    b. Hemimandibular hyperplasia
3. Hemifacial hypertrophy (rare)

Asymmetrical Mandibular Prognathism

With Anterior Open Bite (Figs 24.11A to C)

Clinical features
a. Severe facial asymmetry
b. Eccentric bilateral mandibular protrusion
c. Deviation of the chin
d. High gonial angle
e. Anterior open bite (anterior and posterior cross bite seen unilaterally)
f. Midline of the mandibular arch is shifted

Without Anterior Open Bite (Figs 24.12A to C)

a. Eccentric bilateral mandibular protrusion
b. Deviation of the chin
c. Class III dental malocclusion
d. Associated maxillary hypoplasia
e. No anterior open bite

Unilateral Condylar Hyperplasia

Further divided into 2 types (Table 24.8).

Hemimandibular Elongation (Figs 24.13A to C)

Clinical features
    i. Horizontal displacement of the mandible and chin towards the unaffected side.

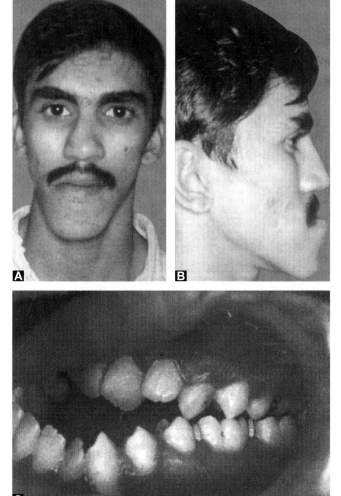

Figs 24.11A to C: Asymmetrical mandibular prognathism with anterior open bite

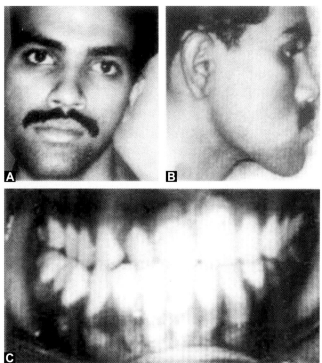

Figs 24.12A to C: Asymmetrical mandibular prognathism without anterior open bite

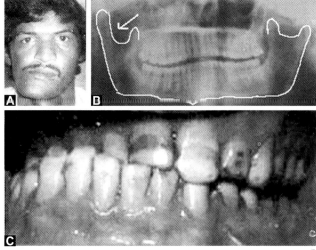

Figs 24.13A to C: Unilateral condylar hyperplasia. Hemimandibular elongation: (A) Marked facial asymmetry in front view of a patient, (B) OPG showing elongation of the neck of the condyle on the affected side, (C) Occlusal plane discrepancy

ii. Usually there is a mild protrusion and lip line slopes down, towards the affected side.

iii. On the unaffected side there may be a lateral cross bite.

iv. The occlusal plane sometimes slopes upward to the unaffected side.

v. Secondary over eruption of the maxillary teeth on the affected side to maintain the functional occlusion.

vi. In severe cases lateral open bite may be present on the affected side.

vii. In the radiographs OPG and PA view elongation of the neck of the condyle with increased ramal height on the affected side will be seen. Condylar head also may show enlargement.

Hemimandibular Hyperplasia (Figs 24.14A to J)

Hemimandibular hyperplasia condition is characterized by a three dimensional enlargement of one side of the mandible, thus, there is enlargement of the condyle,

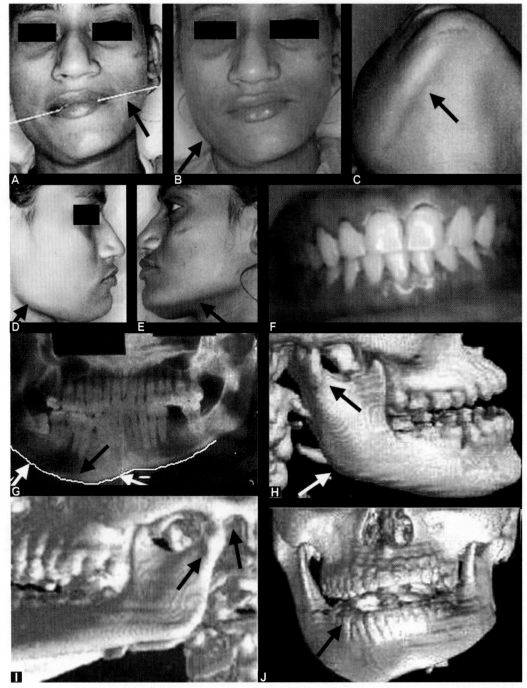

Figs 24.14A to J: Unilateral condylar hyperplasia. Hemimandibular hyperplasia: (A) Occlusal cant, (B) Facial asymmetry, (C) Bowing of (R) inferior border of the mandible, (D) (R) Profile, (E) (L) Profile. On the (R) side, lower level of the inferior border can be appreciated, (F) Occlusion, (G) OPG showing 'Bowing' of the inferior border of the mandible, (H to J) 3D CT scan, (H) Unilateral elongation of ascending ramus and condyle. Enlargement of condyle is seen, (I) Shift of (L) condyle out of fossa, (J) Asymmetry of the lower jaw, unilateral rounding off of the angle and typical bowing of the inferior border of the mandible. Increased height of the body of the mandible is also seen unilaterally

the condylar neck and the ascending ramus and the body. The abnormal growth terminates precisely at the symphysis, giving rise to a sharp 'step' in the mandible at that site and justifying the term hemimandibular hyperplasia.

1. One side of the face appears to be enlarged.
2. Unilateral 'bowing' of the inferior border of the mandible is seen on the affected side.
3. The lip line slopes downward on the affected side.
4. Gross occlusal discrepancies like lateral open bite on the affected side, overeruption of posterior teeth in the maxilla with occlusal cant and increased vertical maxillary height on the affected side may be seen.
5. Associated TMJ pain symptoms may be present.
   Radiographically—the entire hemimandible on the affected side is enlarged and the inferior dental canal is displaced towards the lower border. The OPG demonstrates a pathognomonic appearance.
1. The elongation of ascending ramus (unilateral).
2. Elongation and thickening of the condylar neck (unilateral).
3. An irregular and deforming enlargement of the condyle (unilateral).
4. The angle is characteristically rounded off (unilateral).
5. Typical 'bowing' of the inferior border of the mandibular body—(unilateral).
6. Increased height of the body of the mandible (unilateral).

During active growth phase of hemimandibular elongation and hemimandibular hyperplasia, scintigraphy carried out demonstrates increased uptake in the condyle of the affected side.

TYPES OF SEVERE SKELETAL DENTOFACIAL DEFORMITIES AND ASSOCIATED PROBLEM LIST

1. Esthetic problems
2. Functional problems
3. Psychological problems (Tarnishing self image)
4. Impairment of mastication
5. Impact on digestion—general health
6. Associated speech problems
7. Difficulty in maintaining oral hygiene
8. Susceptibility to caries and periodontal problems
9. Possible TM joint pain dysfunction.

TREATMENT OPTIONS

When a patient has got mild dentofacial deformities, it can be treated with orthodontic tooth movement alone. But, whenever there is severe skeletal dentofacial deformity exists, there are three broad options for treating these deformities.

1. Growth modification
2. Orthodontic camouflage
3. Orthognathic surgery.

Growth Modification

Growth modification or dentofacial orthopedics can be useful in children, where there is growth potential present and modification of the growth can be achieved in some of these patients.

Growth modification can be achieved by using the following:

1. High pull headgear to a complete or partial maxillary fixed appliance.
2. Myofunctional appliances—used for 14 to 16 hours a day.

But this modality has got limitations and only few millimeter changes can be brought about. Myofunctional appliances need to be worn for a long time by the patient and if patient is not co-operative, the desired results cannot be achieved.

Orthodontic Camouflage

Orthodontic camouflage is a biologically acceptable dental compensations, that has been built in, to mask the skeletal malocclusion, brought about by means of orthodontic treatment, in borderline skeletal deformities. Orthodontic camouflage should be carried out, if:

a. Orthodontist is able to carry out biologically acceptable dental compensations
b. With desired soft tissue results
c. Willingness of the patient to co-operate (treatment modality, tolerate prolonged treatment)
d. Growth potential study is done. When quantity, direction or timing of orthodontic treatment is poor, it can bring about disastrous results.

Orthodontic camouflage should be undertaken after careful patient selection/examination for ultimate facial esthetics and occlusal stability. Treatment planning for satisfactory dental occlusion, at the expense of undesirable facial esthetics, is of little value to the patient and should not be attempted.

Orthognathic Surgery

Orthognathic surgery includes surgical repositioning of the jaw and/or dentoalveolar segments. This option is used for the correction of a severe skeletal discrepancy after growth has ceased.

Orthognathic surgery is the art and science of diagnosis, treatment planning and execution of treatment by combining orthodontics and oral and maxillofacial surgery to correct musculoskeletal, dento-osseous, and soft tissue deformities of the jaws and associated structures. In the severe skeletal deformities, orthodontics alone may compromise esthetics and stability and surgery alone, may compromise function and stability.

The objective of orthognathic surgery is to achieve best function, best esthetics and best stability, thereby enhance the personality and lifestyle and channel the patient into self esteem. For the successful outcome of the orthognathic surgery, both orthodontist as well as oral and maxillofacial surgeons are equal partners. Since this treatment modality targets at adult population, time factor is also equally important. The combined surgical orthodontics (orthognathic surgery) also should be aimed at minimizing the total treatment time.

Timing for surgery: In skeletal dentofacial deformities, if patient is having severe psychosocial problems, then only surgery can be undertaken in actively growing patient. But, with the warning, that resurgery may be required later on. Otherwise, the best timing for orthognathic surgery is after the growth potential for the patient is over.

Combined surgical orthodontics demands interdisciplinary team approach of orthodontist and oral and maxillofacial surgeon. The team conference should have proper communication to avoid frustration and disappointing results.

Diagnosis and treatment planning: When the diagnosis and treatment planning for the particular patient is being done, both orthodontist and oral and maxillofacial surgeon should take equal interest. Good communication and proper interaction of the team members are absolutely mandatory, ideally both the members should interview the patient together. Patient's expectations and chief complaint should be taken into consideration and after the detailed treatment plan is decided, patient conference should be held with both the members of the

Table 24.9: Diagnosis and treatment planning	
Phase I	• Assemble the database
	• Synthesize the problem list
	• Diagnosis
	• Team conference
Phase II	• Interdisciplinary problem list
	• Dentofacial problems in order of priority
	• Possible solutions
	• Tentative treatment plan
	• Patient/team conference
	• Definitive plan
Phase III	• Preparatory therapy—endodontic, periodontics, prosthetics, etc.
	• Definitive orthodontic—surgical treatment
	• Continuous team monitoring, re-evaluation interaction, modifying the therapy
Phase IV	• Maintenance

team. All the details of the entire treatment plan and the time and cost factor for the entire treatment should be discussed in detail with the patient. Any questions, doubts on patient's/relative's part should be sorted out at the onset (Table 24.9).

Goal of the diagnostic process is to

1. Produce a concise list of patient's problems
2. Synthesize the various treatment possibilities into a rational plan that gives maximum benefit to the patient.

Collecting Patient's Data

1. Patient's personal data—name, age, sex, race, body type, occupation, hair, habits, physical fitness, any allergies, systemic diseases, airway obstruction problems, previous surgeries, etc.
2. Facial esthetic analysis—frontal, profile
3. Lateral cephalometric analysis—soft tissue, dental, skeletal
4. Occlusal analysis and model analysis:
   • Dental arch form/length,
   • Dental alignment/symmetry,
   • Dental occlusion,
   • Tooth mass relation
5. Final treatment plan:
   • Presurgical orthodontics
   • Surgery plan
   • Postsurgical orthodontics
   • Maintenance.

FACIAL ESTHETIC ANALYSIS

We have to be familiar with the normal facial proportions, before we carry out face to face evaluation of an individual. The entire face is divided into three equal parts—upper, middle and lower thirds. Any change in these proportions can be noted easily in frontal and profile view of the face.

1. Patient is asked to sit upright at the eye level of the clinician. Patient's head should be adjusted in such a way that:
   i. The pupillary plane should be parallel to the floor.
   ii. The plane of the ears also should be parallel to the floor.
   iii. Clinical Frankfort Horizontal Plane (CFHP), i.e. a line from the tragus of the ear to the bony infraorbital rim should be parallel to the floor (this is a natural head position, helpful for standardization of the measurements throughout the treatment sequence).
2. Patient should be examined with the teeth in centric position (tip of the patient's tongue is touched to the most posterior aspect of the palate and teeth are closed together).
3. Patient's lips should be relaxed. (Evaluation of tooth to lip measurement, tooth display, gum display, lip incompetence, chin position, etc.).
4. Patient is asked to look straight and remain steady throughout the evaluation.

   The clinical photographs in frontal and profile view can be taken in this position for records and photographic analysis.

   As mentioned earlier, the face is divided into equal thirds. The upper third is from the hair line to glabella. The middle third is from glabella to subnasale. The lower third is from subnasale to soft tissue menton. The lower third can be further divided from subnasale to upper lip stomion as one third and lower lip stomion to soft tissue menton equaling two thirds. This division can be done both for frontal as well as profile view of the patient. The normal facial proportions are equal thirds. Most of the orthognathic surgery brings about changes in the lower third of the face, therefore preoperative measurements can be taken both in frontal and profile views (Figs 24.15A and B).

Frontal View Analysis (Fig. 24.16)

Larry Wolford and Fields have recommended the evaluation of 14 anatomic relationships in front view analysis which are as follows:

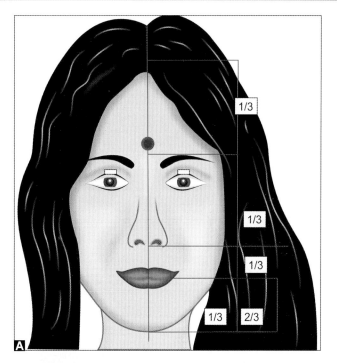

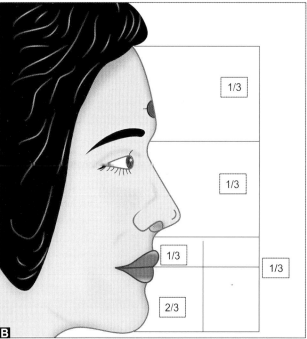

Figs 24.15A and B: Normal facial proportions in: (A) Front view, (B) Profile view

1. The forehead, eyes, orbits and nose are evaluated for symmetry, size and deformity
2. Normal intercanthal distance is 32 ± 3 mm.
3. Normal interpupillary distance is 65 ± 3 mm.
4. The intercanthal distance, alar base width, and palpebral fissure width should all be equal.

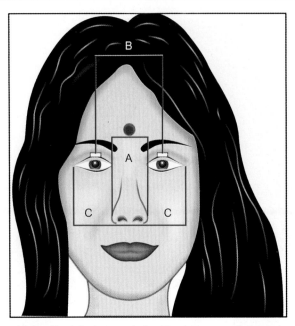

Fig. 24.16: Frontal view analysis. The transverse facial balance. (A) Normal intercanthus distance—32 mm ± 3 mm, (B) Normal interpupillary distance—65 mm ± 3 mm, (C) The width of the palpebral fissures should be equal to the intercanthal distance

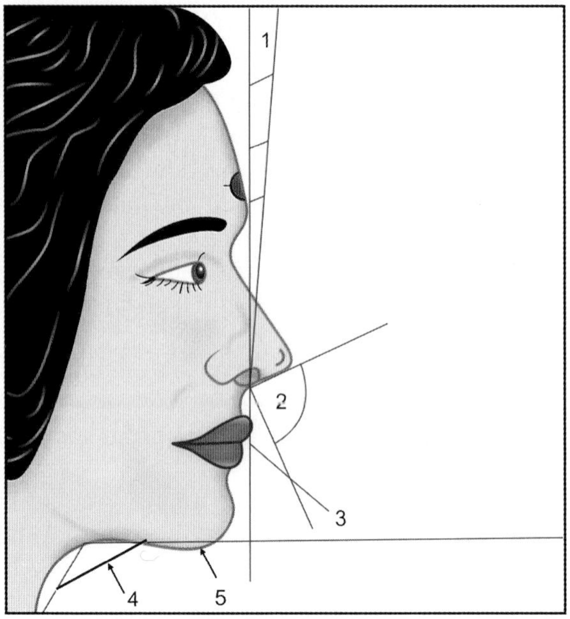

Fig. 24.17: Profile view analysis

5. The width of the nasal dorsum should be one-half the intercanthal distance and width of the nasal lobule should be two-thirds the intercanthal distance.

6. A vertical line through the medial canthus and perpendicular to the pupillary plane should fall on the alar bases ± 2 mm.

7. The upper lip length is measured from subnasale to upper lip stomion. The normal upper lip length is 22 ± 2 mm for males and 20 ± 2 mm for females.

8. A normal upper tooth to lip relationship exposes 2.5 ± 1.5 mm of incisal edge with lips in repose.

9. The facial midline, nasal midline, lip midline, dental midline and chin midline all should be congruent and face should be reasonably symmetric, vertically and transversely.

10. Lip incompetence if present should be measured from upper lip stomion to lower lip stomion with lips in repose and teeth in centric occlusion (0-3 mm).

11. Smile line—during smiling, the vermilion of the upper lip should fall at the cervicogingival margin with no more than 1 to 2 mm of exposed gingiva. Patient should be asked to give full smile to detect 'gummy smile'.

12. The distance from the glabella to subnasale and subnasale to menton should be in 1:1 ratio, providing upper lip length is normal.

13. The length of the upper lip should be one-third the length of the lower facial third.

14. The lower eyelid should be in level with or slightly above the most inferior aspect of the iris.

Profile or Lateral View Analysis (Fig. 24.17)

This is helpful for determining vertical and antero-posterior plane problems of the jaws. The facial profile can be classified into three types: straight, convex and concave.

1. *The facial contour angle:* It is a measure of the relative concavity or convexity of the facial profile. The reference norm ranges between –8 and –11 degrees. This angle is formed between the upper facial contour plane and the upward extension of the lower facial contour plane. If the angle is anterior to the upper facial contour plane, the measurement is quoted as negative.

2. *Nasolabial angle:* The angle formed at subnasale by a line drawn tangent to the base of the nose with a line

drawn from the upper lip to subnasale. The normal range is 100 to 110° in males and 110 to 120° in females. A large angulation is indicative of a convex face, generally associated with a recessive chin.

3.   *Lip position:* The upper lip should protrude ahead of the lower facial contour plane by 3.5 mm. The lower lip should protrude by 2.2 mm.

4.   *Lower lip, chin-throat angle:* The angle between a line drawn from the lower lip to the soft tissue pogonion and a line drawn tangent to the soft tissue contour below the body of the mandible. The normal angulation is 110° ± 8°. A large angulation is indicative of a recessive chin while low angulation suggests an excessive chin.

5.   *The chin to throat length:* The distance between the angle of the throat and soft tissue menton. The norm is 51 mm ± 6 mm. An increased value indicates mandibular prognathism and will be associated with a concave face and an acute lower lip, chin throat angle.

Rest of the vertical proportions are same as frontal analysis (Table 24.10).

Table 24.10: Evaluation of 5 major esthetic masses of the face (Figs 24.16 and 24.17)		
1.	Forehead	:	Nasofrontal angle
2.	Eyes	:	Interpupillary distance (6.5 mm normal)
			Intercanthal distance (3.5 mm normal)
			Outercanthal distance (9.8 mm normal)
3.	Nose	:	Length, width, projection nasolabial angle (90°–120° normal)
4.	Lips	:	Length, width, procumbency, recumbency, interlabial gap (3 mm normal)
5.	Chin	:	Mentolabial sulcus
			Lip chin complex contour
			Prominence, deficiency

Table 24.11: Presurgical data		
Patient's personal data	*Frontal and profile view*	*Dental data*
Name, age	Symmetry and	Dental arch form
Sex	proportion	alignment,
Race	Evaluate 5 major	symmetry, tooth
Body type	esthetic masses	mass relation,
Hair	of the face—	crowding, spaces,
Occupation	Forehead, eyes,	overjet, overbite
Habits	nose, lips, chin	anterior, posterior
		cross bite, edge to
		edge bite, open bite

Oral Examination

1.   Basic occlusal relationship (class I, II, III)
2.   Anterior overbite or open bite
3.   Anterior overjet and any cross bites
4.   Health of the dentition
5.   Tooth size discrepancies
6.   Curve of Wilson
7.   Curve of Spee
8.   Dental crowding or spacing
9.   Missing, carious, nonsalvagable teeth
10. Periodontal evaluation
11. Transverse, vertical or anteroposterior discrepancies
12. Anatomical functional tongue abnormalities
13. Attrition, etc. (loss of vertical dimension).
       TMJ function should be recorded (Table 24.11).

Dental Model Analysis

Dental model analysis can be carried out as routinely done in orthodontics. Arch length measurement, tooth size analysis, tooth position, arch width analysis. Curve of occlusion, cuspid molar relationship, tooth arch symmetry, etc. should be noted.

Clinical assessment, dental model evaluation and cephalometric analysis must be used to establish an accurate diagnosis of a dentofacial deformity.

Cephalometric Analysis

Cephalometric analysis of the lateral radiograph is a two-dimensional diagnostic aid.

Salzman (1964) has proved that cephalometrics can provide valuable information from both a clinical and research basis by the following:

1.   Establishing two-dimensional relationships of craniofacial components.

2.   Classifying skeletal and dental abnormalities with respect to cranial base, skeletal pattern, inter and intra-arch dental relationships and soft tissue profile.

3.   Analyzing growth and development responsible for dentofacial pattern, whether for cranial base configuration, congenital abnormalities, pathologic conditions, or facial asymmetry.

4.   Planning treatment for orthodontic and/or surgical procedures.

5.   Analyzing changes after treatment effectiveness of different treatment modalities and effectiveness of retention.

6.   Determining dentofacial growth changes after treatment.

7. Predicting hard and soft tissue contours before initiation of treatment.

Diagnostic cephalometric radiographs should be taken after patient is placed in cephalometer with head adjusted in natural head position, sagittal plane of the patient's head should be parallel with film (Fig. 24.18).

Lips should be in repose and teeth should be placed in centric occlusion. Soft tissues must be reproduced on the cephalometric film without sacrificing details of osseous structures (Fig. 24.19).

Soft Tissue Landmarks (Fig. 24.20)

Glabella: The most prominent point of the forehead.

Soft tissue nasion: The deepest point of the bridge of the nose.

Subnasale: The point at which the base of the nose merges with the upper cutaneous lip.

Labiale superius: The median point of the upper margin of the upper membranous lip.

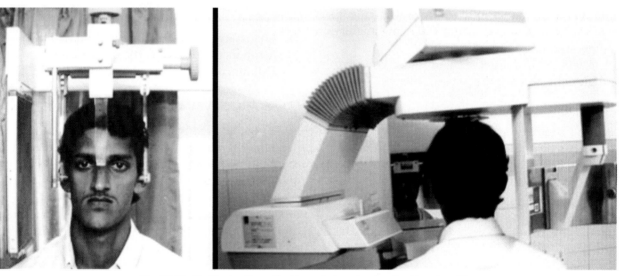

Fig. 24.18: Positioning the patient in cephalometer. A natural head position

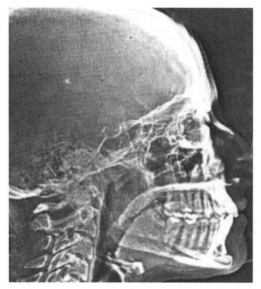

Fig. 24.19: Lateral cephalograph showing hard and soft tissue contours

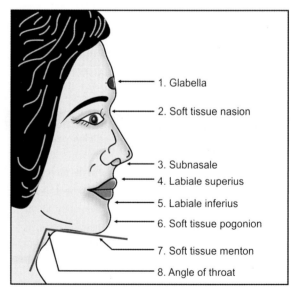

1. Glabella
2. Soft tissue nasion
3. Subnasale
4. Labiale superius
5. Labiale inferius
6. Soft tissue pogonion
7. Soft tissue menton
8. Angle of throat

Fig. 24.20: Soft tissue landmarks

Labiale inferius: The median point of the lower margin of the lower membranous lip.

Soft tissue pogonion: The foremost point on the soft tissue chin in the mid-sagittal plane.

Soft tissue menton: The lowermost point on the soft tissue chin in the sagittal plane.

Angle of throat: The intersection of the horizontal and vertical tangents to the profile of the soft tissue throat.

The upper facial contour plane: It extends between glabella and subnasale.

The lower facial contour plane extends between subnasale and soft tissue pogonion.

Cephalometric Prediction Tracing (Figs 24.21A to C)

The importance of accurately estimating facial growth, based on facial pattern, was recognized as a result of work by Ricketts (1957), that stressed the necessity of predicting facial profile. Fish and Epker in 1980, put forward a method to predict facial profile as a result of surgical orthodontic correction of dentofacial deformities. They advocated surgical movement of skeletal parts (maxilla and/or mandible) with a single acetate sheet overlying the original pretreatment cephalometric tracings.

Bell, Profitt and White (1980), advocated use of the cephalometric prediction with templates to double check the model surgery changes, to predict changes in bony relationships not seen on the dental casts, and to predict soft tissue changes.

a. Prediction analysis presents a simple and accurate method of predicting results of surgical orthodontic treatment.

b. Quantification of the surgical movements necessary to correct the deformity is also possible.

c. It can also accurately predict the resultant facial profile.

d. Provides a visual aid with a single overlay.

e. It can be also used for comparing with actual postsurgical cephalometric tracings for re-evaluating the surgical results.

Posteroanterior Cephalometric Analysis (Fig. 24.22)

Posteroanterior (PA) cephalometric analysis is mainly used for assessing asymmetry of the facial skeleton.

1. First vertical line is drawn joining the midline of the nose and chin and the dental arch—midsagittal line.

2. Second vertical line is drawn passing through the zygomatic arch on either side of midsagittal line.

3. Third vertical line is drawn on either side of midsagittal line passing through the angle of the mandible.

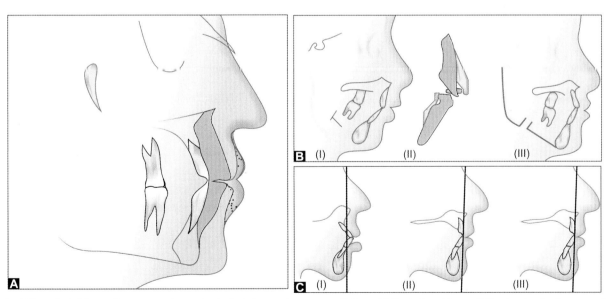

Figs 24.21A to C: (A) Bimaxillary protrusion setback. Soft tissue changes prediction, (B) Cephalometric prediction tracing for the correction of mandibular hypoplasia with class II malocclusion: (I) Preoperative cephalogram, (II) Desired tooth movement prior to surgery, with presurgical orthodontics, (III) Prediction tracing considering the mandibular surgical advancement. Note the changes in soft tissue profile, (C) Comparison of preoperative, prediction and postoperative cephalometric tracings for bimaxillary protrusion case (I) Preoperative cephalogram with soft tissue profile (II) Prediction tracing considering bimaxillary setback surgery (III) Postoperative cephalogram with soft tissue profile

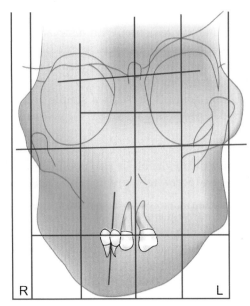

Fig. 24.22: Posteroanterior (PA) cephalometric analysis for assessment of facial asymmetry

These lines will help to evaluate deviation, asymmetry or disproportions of facial skeleton and comparison can be made with the normal side measurements. Horizontal lines are drawn along zygomatic plane, occlusal plane, infraorbital plane, plane of the lower border of the mandible, etc. to assess the deviation in relation to horizontal plane.

A "QUICK CEPH" DENTOFACIAL PLANNER FOR ORTHOGNATHIC SURGERY

Cephalometrics is still imperfectly understood as a clinical tool. Since proper pretreatment assessment can mean the difference between successful and unsuccessful treatment. The purpose of this article is to present clinically useful information which is simple and not so lengthy, so that clinicians are encouraged to use it routinely.

This 'Quick Ceph' '10' measurement analysis will give the most valuable diagnostic, treatment and follow up information in a matter of minutes for evaluating a orthognathic case. A full generation of orthognathic, oral and maxillofacial surgeons, plastic surgeons have been fed on a 'surplus' of cephalometrics, right from its invention by Broadbent. Many a times a clinically useful information may be 'hidden' in a maze of cephalometric analysis like Down's, Steiner's, Tweed's, Jarabak's, Ricketts' and so many others.

The proposed '10' measurement analysis for ortho–gnathic surgery will give a 'quick' assessment as the points and measurements are also simple to locate, identify and trace. When the measurements are color enhanced by using different color pens and pencils, it can also be easily understood by 'Patients' (Tables 24.12 to 24.14).

	Table 24.12: The cephalometric points and planes used in this analysis (Figs 24.23A to D)		
1.	Nasion (N)	:	The anterior most point on the nasofrontal suture.
2.	Anterior nasal spine (ANS)	:	The anterior tip of the sharp bony process of the maxilla near the nasal opening.
3.	Sella (S)	:	The center of the pituitary fossa.
4.	Gonion (Go)	:	A point on the curvature of the mandible derived by bisecting the angle formed by the lines joining tangents to the posterior border of the ramus and the lower border of the mandible.
5.	Menton (Me)	:	The lowest point on the mandibular symphysis.
6.	Pogonion (Pg)	:	The most anterior point on the mandibular protruberance or the symphysis.
7.	Posterior nasal spine (PNS)	:	The most posterior projection of the palatine bones.
8.	Point A (A)	:	The deepest point in the concavity of the maxilla between the ANS and the maxillary alveolar process.
9.	Point B (B)	:	The deepest point in the concavity of the mandible between the pogonion and the mandibular alveolar process.
10.	Subnasale (Sn)	:	The point at which the base of the nose (columella) meets the upper-lip tangent.
	• Mandibular plane (MP)	:	A line drawn tangent to the lower border of the mandible.
	• Sella-nasion plane (SN plane)	:	It is the plane formed by the line joining the center of the sella with the nasion.
	• True vertical line (TV line)	:	It is the line drawn and dropped vertically through the nasion.
	• True horizontal line (TH line)	:	It is the line drawn perpendicular to the true vertical line.
	• Occlusal plane (OP)	:	A line drawn through the region of the overlapping 'CUSPS' of the premolars and the molars.

Table 24.13: The '10' measurement analysis		
Skeletal assessment	Norm (Indian)	Norm (Caucasian)
1. SNA	81.5°	82°
2. SNB	79°	80°
3. ANB	2.5°	2°
4. Post. face Ht./Ant.face Ht. (Jarabak ratio)	65%	65%
5. SN/MP	31.3°	32°
6. Wit's	0 mm in females −1 mm in males	0 mm in females −1 mm in males
7. Chin angle	87.5°	87.5°
Soft-tissue assessment		
8. Nasolabial angle	103°	110°
Dental assessment		
9. IMPA and ⊥ to SN	100,108°	95,104°
10. ⊥ to T	122°	131°

The cephalometric 'norms' used are the established 'norms' for both the Caucasian and the Indian races.

The 'Indian cephalometric norms' have been published by the 'Indian Orthodontic Society' in a ready reckoner form in the year 1990.

Natural Head Position (NHP) (Fig. 24.18)

The 'Natural head position' has been found to be reliable in both Caucasian and non-Caucasian races. Analysis based on NHP have greater clinical application than the traditional method adopted earlier.

It is proven fact that a NHP cephalogram of a patient with dentofacial deformities will differ by at least one or two degrees from the traditional method of a Frankfort head positioning. Hence for patients needing surgical orthodontic treatment, the difference can be very significant diagnostically.

A natural head position cephalogram is taken with the patient looking straight ahead in a mirror. The head should be in its natural position and the patient should be relaxed. The ear-rods and the orbital pointer are then 'lightly contacted' to the skin, this secures the patient in the NHP. Check that the patient's pupil is in the middle of the eye and that he/she is looking straight ahead in the mirror with his/her teeth in occlusion and lips in repose.

The 'X-ray' is then taken. The entire procedure should not take more than 5 minutes.

Case Evaluation (Table 24.15)

The following 'case evaluation' demonstrates the thinking process used with '10' measurements to evaluate an orthognathic problem.

A 30-year-old Indian male patient came for a consultation with the chief complaint of a 'protrusive lower jaw' and that his teeth and jaws bite in 'reverse way' as compared with his family members.
- A lateral cephalogram was taken in the natural head position.
- According to the '10' measurement cephalometric analysis and considering Indian cephalometric norms, the following data was obtained.
- Maxillary/mandibular antero/posterior skeletal relationship as indicated by the angle ANB is −5°. This being a negative value on the higher side confirm a true mandibular prognathism, requiring surgical correction.
- The second skeletal measurement N-ANS is 55 mm (norm is 40 mm) indicates an excessive anterior upper facial height.
- ANS-Me is 68 mm (Norm is 62 mm) also points out that there is an increased anterior lower facial height. The total anterior facial height (N-ANS + ANS–Me) is 123 (norm is 102 ± 5) shows that the total anterior facial height is also excessive.
- The posterior facial height components S-PNS is 55 mm (norm is 32 ± 5 mm) and PNS-MP is 33 mm (norm is 55 mm) reveals that total posterior facial height is within its normal range (of 87 mm) after adding up S-PNS + PNS-MP, i.e. 55 mm + 33 mm = 88 mm. Here the posterior lower facial height could be increased and the posterior upper height decreased in balance by a surgical procedure of LeFort I osteotomy carried out together with a mandibular push-back and clockwise rotation of the mandible.
- The ratio (Jarabak) post. face –Ht/ant. face-Ht works out to be 71.5 percent signifying that the mandible has rotated anticlockwise with a resultant deep bite. This is again provided by the angle SN/MP which for the patient is 28°, implying a skeletal deep bite needing surgical intervention.
- The Wit's reading of −10 mm for the patient, reflects the severity of the anteroposterior jaw discrepancy pointing to the fact that since the patient is a male and the norm for males is −1 mm, he will require a

Table 24.14: The '10' measurement analysis

Skeletal assessment (Figs 24.23A and B)

1.	SNA (norm-82°)	:	Will tell us whether the maxilla is protrusive/restrusive and also in a good vertical position
2.	SNB (norm-80°)	:	Will tell us whether the mandible is protrusive/retrusive. A smaller angle (less than 80°) indicates that the mandible is restrusive. A larger angle (more than 80°) indicates that the mandible is protrusive.
3.	ANB (norm-2°)	:	Will tell us the max./mand. discrepancy of the two skeletal bases. A large value (e.g. 8°) will indicate maxillary skeletal protrusion. A small value (e.g. 0°) will indicate mild mandibular prognathism. A large negative value (e.g. –5°) will indicate true mandibular prognathism.
4.	Post. face HT/Ant. Face HT.(Jarabak ratio-norm-65%) Norms for vertical N-ANS-40 mm ANS-Me-2 mm S-PNS-32 mm PNS-MP-55 mm	:	The vertical components N-ANS and ANS-Me help to diagnose anterior upper and lower facial height problems respectively. S-PNS and PNS-MP help to diagnose posterior upper and lower facial height problems respectively. Any deviations from the normal values quickly suggest of a vertical maxillary excess (VME) or a vertical maxillary deficiency (VMD). Further the Jarabak ratio obtained by the formula will mean as follows: A ratio between 55 and 65 percent indicate backward or clockwise rotation of the mandible with a resultant increase in anterior facial height and a skeletal open bite. A ratio between 65 and 80 percent indicate a forward or a anticlockwise rotation of the mandible with a resultant increase in posterior facial height and a skeletal deep bite.
5.	Anterior face HT SN/MP (norm 31.3°)	:	This angle, if it is more than 32°, confirms a skeletal open bite and if it is less than 32°, confirms a skeletal deep bite, both warranting surgical intervention.
6.	Wit's appraisal Norm is –0 mm in females –1 mm in males	:	Perpendiculars are dropped from points A and B on the occlusal plane. The points of contact on the occlusal plane are labeled as AO and BO. In females AO and BO coincide and hence the reading is 0 mm. In males BO is –1 mm ahead of AO. This measurement is more reliable than SNA and SNB. It is a measure of the antero/posterior discrepancy of the maxillary, mandibular skeletal bases. The severity of an antero/posterior jaw discrepancy will get reflected in a huge Wit's reading in a positive or a negative way. Skeletal class II cases may have a reading of +8 mm or more and True Class III cases may have a reading of –12 mm or more.
7.	Chin angle (norm-87.5°)		The angle formed between the nasion-pogonion line (NPg) to the true horizontal line (TH). It is a very reliable measure of chin *prominence or its restrusiveness or deficiency.*

Soft tissue assessment (Fig. 24.23C)

8.	Nasolabial angle (norm –103 + 5)		The angle formed by a tangent to the columella of the nose (base of the nose) and the upper lip tangent. This angle is a further aid in planning maxillary surgery. Maxilla is to be repositioned posteriorly in case the angle is acute (values of 96° and less) as in class II cases. Maxilla is to be repositioned anteriorly in case the angle is obtuse value of 114° and more as in class III cases. A corrected nasolabial angle within the range of 90°-110° creates a very stable lip support for the patient.

Dental assessment (Fig. 24.23D) :

9.	IMPA and ⊥ to SN IMPA (norm is 90 + 5) ⊥ to SN (norm is 104 + 5)		IMPA is the angle formed by a line passing through the axis of the lower incisor to the mandibular plane (MP). Values of less than 90° indicate mandibular incisor protrusion ⊥ to SN is the angle formed by a line passing through the tip of upper incisor to Sella-Nasion plane (SN-plane). Values of 110° and more indicate upper incisor protrusion and values of less than 95° indicate lesser than 110° indicate upper incisor retrusion. These dental measurements are brought within normal limits by postsurgical orthodontic finish, which will enhances incisal function and stability.
10.	⊥ to —1 (norm is 131°) (Interincisal angle)	:	This angle is formed by a line passing (interincisal angle) through the incisal edge and apex of the root of the maxillary and mandibular central incisors. If the value is less than 115°, it indicates upper and lower incisor protrusion. If the value is more than 150°, it indicates upper and lower incisor retrusion. A corrected interincisal angle within the normal range will lock the occlusion and add to the stability of a surgically corrected case.

surgical correction by 9 mm in the anteroposterior direction.

• The chin angle measures 88.5° (Norm is 87.5°) for the patient. This means that the chin is within its normal skeletal limit with no need for any additional surgical procedures to be performed on the chin.

• The soft-tissue measurement of the nasolabial angle (Norm is 110°) reveals a high obtuse angle of 135° for the patient. Since this angle is more than 114°, it again points to the fact that the maxilla has to be repositioned superiorly and anteriorly to gain lip support.

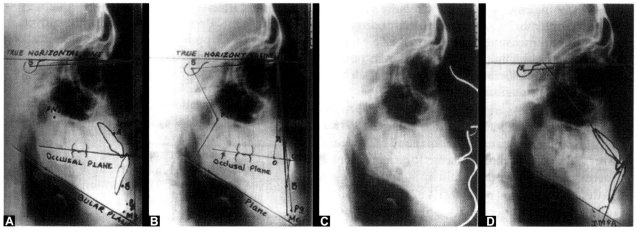

Figs 24.23A to D: The '10' measurement analysis

Ceph Measurements	Norms	Patients Values	Conclusions	Interpretations
Table 24.15: Case evaluation				
1. SNA	81.5°	88°		
2. SNB	79°	93°	Maxillary and mandibular	
3. ANB (SNA-SNB)	2.5°	–5°	Skeletal relationship in A/P plane is a large –ve value than the Norm	Confirms true mandibular prognathism
4. ANT, Facial Ht			Excessive ANT. Upper facial Ht	
N-ANS	40 mm	55 mm	(AUFH)	
ANS-Me	62 mm	68 mm	Excessive ANT. Lower facial Ht (ALFH)	
Total ANT. Facial Ht (N-ANS + ANS—Me)	102 ± 5 mm	123 mm	Total ANT. Facial Ht is excessive	Superior and forward positioning of the maxilla by 10 mm is necessary
Post facial Ht				along with auto rotation and push-back
S-PNS	32 ± 5 mm	55 mm	Excessive post upper facial Ht (PUFH)	of the mandible to balance the profile
PNS-MP	55 mm	33 mm	Post lower facial Ht (PLFH) is reduced	
Total post Facial Ht (S-PNS + PNS—MP)	87 ± 5	88 mm	The total post facial Ht is within normal range	
Jarabak ratio	65%	71.5%	A forward or anti-clockwise rotation of the mandible	Autorotation of the mandible is indicated
5. SN/MP	31.3°	28°	A skeletal deep bite	Surgical correction of the deep bite is warranted
6. Wit's appraisal in male	–1 m	–10 m	Reflects severity of mandibular prognathism	Confirms true mandibular prognathism which requires surgical push-back by 9 mm
7. Chin angle	87.5°	88.5°	The chin or the bony protuberance is within normal limits	No additional genioplasty procedures are indicated
8. Naso-labial angle	110 ± 5	135°	Maxilla will have to be repositioned anteriorly	Maxillary superior and forward repositioning is necessary to gain better lip support
9. IMPA, ⊥ to SN	90°, 104°	87°, 124°	The lower incisors are retrusive while the upper incisors are protrusive	Needs presurgical orthodontics to bring them within the range of 90° and 110°
10. T to ⊥	131°	123°	Indicates maxillary/mandibular incisor procumbency	Needs presurgical orthodontics to get an interincisal angle of 131°

- The dental measurements of IMPA 87° (norm is 90° ± 5) and ⊥ to SN 124° (Norm is 104 ± 5) shows that lower and upper incisors need to be corrected orthodontically to the normal range of IMPA of 95° and ⊥ to SN of 104 ± 5.
- The interincisal angle of 123° for the patient (norm is 131°) also needs orthodontic correction to get a postsurgical, good interdigitated and a stable occlusion, to minimize the chances of a 'relapse'.

FINAL TREATMENT PLAN

Phase I   : Presurgical orthodontic correction of upper and lower incisor inclinations to their skeletal bases.

Phase II   : Superior and forward repositioning of the maxilla by a LeFort I osteotomy with simultaneous mandibular push-back by a sagittal split osteotomy and clockwise rotation of the mandible. The maxillary superior repositioning will be by 8 to 10 mm and maxillary anterior repositioning by 4 mm. The mandibular push back will be by about 5 mm.

Phase III : Postsurgical orthodontic detailing of the occlusion followed by retention.

CONCLUSION

This analysis, hence, has a potential to assess and diagnose orthognathic problems when combined with good clinical judgement to strengthen the surgeon's first impressions on clinical examination.

25 Presurgical Orthodontic Phase

Severe dentofacial skeletal deformity has been described by Proffit and White as "severe problems of jaw function and facial esthetics that require combined orthodontics and surgical treatment."

Normally orthodontic camouflage technique is used for a nongrowing patient with dentofacial deformities. Here, the malocclusion is corrected by conventional orthodontics to position the teeth in the correct relationship to their respective bases of the upper and lower jaws and co-ordinating the relationship of the upper dental arch to lower dental arch and thus camouflaging the skeletal discrepancy.

In combined surgical orthodontics treatment plan, the orthodontic treatment should be aimed at creating a temporary or intermediate malocclusion after removing the nature's dental compensations. **This amounts to relocating the dentition to their respective skeletal bases and unmasking the nature's dental compensations. This will result in worsening the malocclusion temporarily, so that the exact nature of dentofacial skeletal deformity is highlighted.** This will definitely help the surgeon to carry out various osteotomy procedures on the jaw bones with maximum set back or advancement. The results of this fully revealing or maximizing the skeletal deformity and then subjecting it to surgery, will be definitely much stable and esthetically pleasing.

Careful presurgical planning is prerequisite to assure predictable results: Twenty years back, most of the orthodontists used to complete all orthodontic teeth movements before surgery. In combined surgical orthodontic treatment planning, it is a waste of time and undesirable:

1. Unplanned orthodontic treatment for severe skeletal problems results into unsuccessful functional or esthetic results.
2. Referral for surgery thereafter, ends in compromised results.
3. Only desired presurgical orthodontic preparation prior to surgery should be undertaken.
4. Extensive presurgical conventional orthodontics is unnecessary and contraindicated.
5. Orthodontics should be planned to co-ordinate with specific surgical procedures. This practice (a) minimizes total treatment time, and (b) prevents relapse.
6. Inadequate presurgical orthodontics jeopardizes the quality of postsurgical results.

The mechanotherapy and treatment objectives are the opposite of normal orthodontic treatment plan in presurgical orthodontics *(Reversed orthodontics)*.

In orthognathic cases, the 'old cook book' plan of orthodontics is inappropriate.

- Treatment objectives ⎫ Reverse than
- Extraction patterns   ⎬ the conventional
- Type of mechanics   ⎭ orthodontics

Deliberately worsen the occlusion: This enables the surgeon to achieve perfect occlusion and precise jaw positioning. Inappropriate presurgical orthodontics will lead to following problems:

1. The skeletal dento-osseous segments cannot be placed in a satisfactory relationship, because of gross occlusal interferences or gross malposition of the teeth in respect to their supporting bone.
2. Postsurgical orthodontic mechanics could accentuate relapse tendencies.
3. Projected osteotomy cuts would be impossible, because of the proximity to the roots of the adjacent teeth.

The sequence of the entire treatment can be divided into three distinct phases, each with specific objectives, that need to be met for the optimal attainment of the next stage:

1. Presurgical orthodontics
2. Surgery
3. Postsurgical orthodontic detailing.

Meticulous Presurgical Orthodontics

- Lessens the total treatment time
- Controls the relapse tendencies
- Removes the gross occlusal interferences
- Positions the teeth in an ideal relationship to their respective dental bases
- The dental restrictions imposed for the surgical correction of the jaw discrepancy are eliminated
- Allows maximum surgical correction
- Allows proper intraoperative interdigitation
- Significantly reduces operating time and surgical morbidity
- Allows quick and easy postsurgical efficient orthodontic detailing.

The goal, therefore, is to locate the teeth in an optimal and decompensated position, so that the surgical correction is not hindered by the dentoalveolar component and an optimal skeletal and occlusal change can be produced.

▌PRESURGICAL ORTHODONTICS OBJECTIVES

Treat upper and lower dental arches separately/independently. Align the teeth, with inclination and angulation correction:

a. To relieve arch crowding (correct the arch length deficiency).
b. To close the spaces (eliminate tooth size discrepancies).
c. To correct derotations.
d. To eliminate gross dental interferences.

Presurgical Intra-arch Objectives

- Alignment of the incisors in 'ideal' position
- Establishment of correct torque
- Removal of dental compensations
- Increase the severity of vertical and/or horizontal aspects of malocclusion
- Establishment of desired anteroposterior and vertical position of the incisors
- Achievement of arch compatibility on models
- Establishment of class I canine and molar relationships on models
- Create space for segmental osteotomy by root paralleling.

Time Estimation

1. Presurgical orthodontics : 3 to 12 months, (varies with the difficulty in alignment)
2. Surgery—hospitalization : 3-8 days
3. Under surgeon's care : 3-8 weeks
4. Postsurgical orthodontics : 3-6 months (over 6 months due to inadequate preparation)

As orthognathic surgery brings about three-dimensional change/improvement, whenever combined surgical orthodontics is planned, the deformity should be considered in three planes of space. Hence, presurgical orthodontic treatment plan also should be drawn keeping all three planes in the mind.

Presurgical Orthodontic Objectives for Antero-Posterior—Sagittal Plane (AP)

Removal of dental compensations or decompensation phase.

Presurgical Orthodontic Objectives for Transverse Plane

- Differentiation of skeletal from dental problems
- Identification of relative and absolute discrepancies
- Achieve reasonable arch compatibility on the models
- If not, plan for segmental osteotomy procedures.

Presurgical Orthodontic Objectives for Vertical Plane

- Maximizing presurgical orthodontics in open bite cases
- Minimizing the presurgical mechanics in deep bite cases.

  This is essential for the following:

  a. Avoidance of adverse dental relapse potential
  b. Maximizing the speed and efficiency of the treatment.

To Relieve Arch Crowding by Presurgical Orthodontics

- If arch length deficiency is greater than 6 mm, then carry out extractions of teeth
- First premolar extraction gives 7 mm of space
- Whenever the basal bone limit permits, relieve the crowding by multiloop wires, either 014 or 016 Australian Wilcock premium + grade wire (4 to 5 mm space gain) (Table 25.1).
- Additional 3 mm space can be gained by interproximal stripping of 0.25 mm from the mesial and distal surfaces of six anterior teeth.

Extraction Pattern for Presurgical Orthodontics

There is definite difference in extraction patterns chosen for conventional camouflage orthodontics and presurgical orthodontics.

For skeletal class II malocclusion (Figs 25.1A and B), no maxillary tooth extraction or extraction of upper second premolar should be done (This is to prevent over

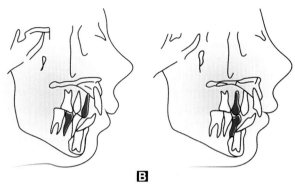

Figs 25.1A and B: Extraction pattern for class II malocclusion. (A) For routine orthodontics, (B) For surgical orthodontics. No maxillary extraction is done, or upper second premolar extraction is done

retraction of the maxillary anterior teeth which would compromise the mandibular advancement) and lower first premolar extraction should be planned to allow leveling of the arch and to correct the lower anterior proclination.

In skeletal class III malocclusion, the extraction pattern chosen will be reverse. In these cases extract upper first and lower second premolars (Figs 25.2A and B).

Extraction of upper first premolar in these cases is done to correct the proclination of the upper anteriors. If the space is needed in the lower arch, then second premolar extraction is done to prevent over retraction of the lower anteriors.

Selection of Orthodontic Appliance

Fixed Orthodontic Appliance System

Fixed orthodontic appliance system is chosen. This appliance is used not only to move the teeth, but also

Table 25.1: Presurgical arch wires used for alignment	
Wire size	*Use*
• .008",.009",.010" supreme grade Australian Wilcock wires	• Excellent properties for alignment without fabrication of loops
• .012",.014",.016" Australian Wilcock wires of premium + grade	• Ideal for correction of rotations, alignment and leveling when used in loop form (traps food)
• Coaxial wires in sizes of 016",.018", .0175",.0195"	• Good properties for correction of rotations and alignment of crowded anteriors at a low cost
• Nickel titanium wires –.014",.016",.018" .016" × .016",.017" ×.025", .016" ×.022"	• Outstanding initial wire for leveling and unraveling crowding gently. Costly wires

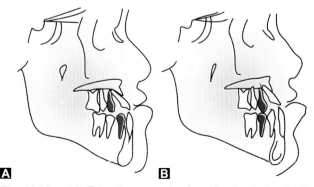

Figs 25.2A and B: Extraction pattern for class III malocclusion. (A) For routine orthodontics, (B) For surgical orthodontics. Extraction of upper first and lower second premolars is carried out

to stabilize them against the stresses encountered at surgery and during maxillomandibular fixation.

Modern preadjusted edge wise .022″ slot appliance with its myriad of variations can be used. In this appliance round or rectangular wire is tied into a bracket slot. It is well-adapted for tooth movement as well as for stabilization of teeth.

Conventional Begg appliance is not suitable for stabilization. Clear or tooth colored plastic brackets or ceramic brackets are not suitable for surgical orthodontics. They are susceptible for breakage and tend to discolor. Bracket placement on the teeth is typical for the usual orthodontic patient, except in the area of a planned osteotomy site, it is advisable to tip the brackets on two adjacent teeth, so that a straight wire will cause root divergence during the presurgical orthodontic phase or to use arch wire bends to produce the desired tooth movements. Sometimes to make the roots divergent at osteotomy site, the right and left canine and premolar brackets are deliberately switched during presurgical treatment phase, it is recommended that all the molars be banded.

Integral hooks—built in hooks in the bracket of molar teeth can be helpful, (or crimpable hooks on the wires) for surgical stabilization and postsurgical finishing, for intra-arch elastic attachments.

Anteroposterior Sagittal (AP-Sagittal) Plane Presurgical Orthodontic Objectives

To remove nature's compensation by correcting the axial inclination of the incisors (achieve ideal axial relationship) (Figs 25.3A and B).

In skeletal class II malocclusion, the maxillary teeth are often retroclined and the mandibular incisors are proclined to compensate for the skeletal discrepancy and to reduce the incisor overjet and to have functional occlusion (nature's compensation).

In these cases, orthodontic decompensation is achieved by uprighting the proclined mandibular incisors and proclining of the maxillary incisors and thereby increasing the amount of overjet to maximum. This will allow surgeon to carry out maximum mandibular advancement (Fig. 25.4).

In skeletal class III malocclusion, the maxillary incisors are often proclined and the mandibular incisors retroclined to minimize the reverse overjet of the incisors and to have functional occlusion (nature's compensation).

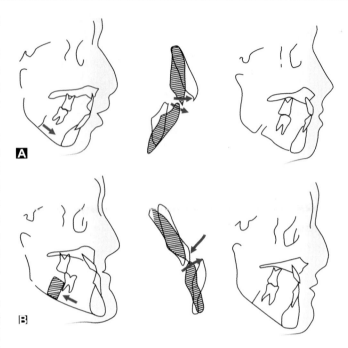

Figs 25.3A and B: Anteroposterior plane presurgical orthodontic objectives. Orthodontic presurgical decompensation to alter the existing overjet. (A) Class II case, (B) Class III case

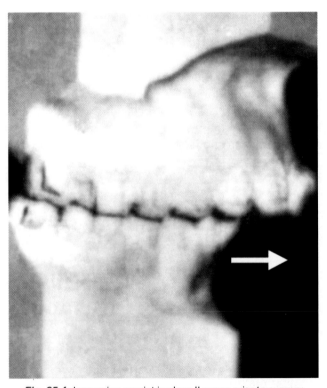

Fig. 25.4: Increasing overjet in class II cases prior to surgery

In these cases, orthodontic decompensation is achieved by making the maxillary and mandibular incisors upright on their respective dental bases and thereby increasing the reverse overjet to maximum. This will allow the surgeon to achieve maximum set back of the mandible with stable occlusion and pleasing esthetics (Fig. 25.3B).

The ultimate goal in AP plane, orthodontic decompensation is to produce sufficient overjet/reverse overjet to allow for the establishment of class I canine relationship on model prior to surgery as well as in the patient intraoperatively. An ideal incisor overjet/overbite produces better chin-lip balance (Use of class III elastics in class II patients to upright or retract the mandibular incisors and help to procline the maxillary incisors or left in their original position Reverse is done in class III cases with class II elastics).

Presurgical Orthodontics Objectives for Transverse Plane

The dentofacial deformities in this plane have commonly defects in the arch width, usually of the maxilla, i.e. posterior cross bites—unilateral or bilateral. They are often combined with AP and vertical problems and also can be associated with deviation of the mandible in centric occlusion.

Transverse plane discrepancies are usually treated either by buccal tipping or bodily movement of posterior teeth. In surgical orthodontics it is important to know (i) whether the problem is skeletal or dental and (ii) whether the problem is relative or absolute.

This is determined by taking upper and lower impressions and making study cast (Figs 25.5A and B). The hand held models are brought into class I canine occlusion to know whether the problem is relative or absolute. A relative problem can be tackled by presurgical orthodontics, but absolute skeletal problem should be solved by planning segmental osteotomies of the maxilla to correct the arch width and arch form. As a rule, orthodontic expansion should be limited to 2 to 3 mm per side (4 to 6 mm total), i.e. not more than half-cusp cross bite. Excessive buccal tipping will cause elongation of lingual cusp, which will interfere with the postoperative result, plus there will be great relapse tendency.

In an isolated skeletal transverse discrepancy, where no other maxillary surgery is anticipated, surgically assisted rapid palatal expansion is a procedure of choice. Where a skeletal maxillary discrepancy is

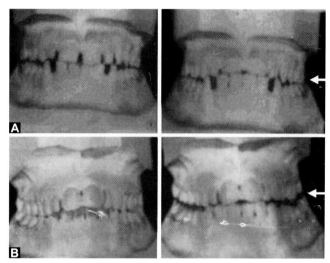

Figs 25.5A and B: (A) Relative transverse discrepancy, (B) Absolute transverse discrepancy

combined with other maxillary problems, multiple segment maxillary osteotomy is indicated (Surgical movement of 5 to 8 mm laterally is possible). Cases with minor dental discrepancies are dealt as routinely. Many times orthodontic minor expansion can be done in the postoperative orthodontic phase, as there will be no more occlusal interferences present.

Presurgical Orthodontics Consideration for Vertical Plane

Vertical maxillary excess (VME) or vertical maxillary deficiency (VMD), i.e. long face and short face cases demand consideration for presurgical orthodontics in vertical plane.

VME with anterior open bite will exhibit typical step behind maxillary canine (a rainbow curve). The level of anterior teeth occlusal plane will be higher than the posterior teeth occlusal plane in the maxilla (Fig. 25.6).

 i. No attempt should be done to close the anterior open bite presurgically.
 ii. Avoid intrusive mechanics in the posterior teeth and concurrently avoid any extrusive mechanics in the anterior region (potential adverse relapse tendencies).
iii. Severe accentuated or reversed curve of Spee should be treated with segmental orthodontics.
 iv. Only dental alignment should be carried out separately in the anterior segment and two posterior segments (level each segment separately).

Skeletal open bites are best treated by segmental maxillary osteotomies, which allow differential vertical

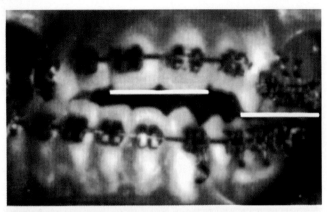

Fig. 25.6: White lines showing anterior and posterior occlusal plane discrepancy in anterior open bite cases. Each segment should be leveled separately by presurgical orthodontics

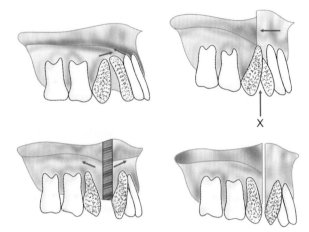

Fig. 25.7: Root paralleling in presurgical orthodontic phase to create a space for segmental osteotomy

movement of anterior and posterior segments. VME without anterior open bite will exhibit nature's dental compensation, i.e. overerupted extruded anterior teeth. In these cases presurgical decompensation with alignment as well as orthodontic intrusion of the anterior teeth will be needed.

Skeletal Deep Anterior Overbite Pattern

Skeletal deep anterior overbite pattern will have three types:
  i. Short face
 ii. Average face
iii. Long face.

In short face or VMD with skeletal deep anterior overbite, there is a need to increase the lower facial height for better esthetic results. No leveling of curve of Spee in the mandibular arch should be done presurgically. Level only the maxillary arch. After surgical advancement of mandible is carried out, lateral open bites will be created in the posterior region. This can be corrected in postsurgical orthodontic phase by tripoding and extrusion of posterior teeth.

In average face and long face with skeletal deep anterior overbite, to prevent increase in the lower facial height, the curve of Spee is leveled by intrusion of anterior teeth prior to surgery.

Root Positioning at the Planned Osteotomy Sites and Retaining the Extraction Spaces

Whenever premolar extractions are carried out for relieving the crowding, the total extraction space should

not be utilized. At least 3 to 4 mm space should be left for making the segmental osteotomy cuts, without jeopardizing the periodontal status of the adjacent teeth. Judicious interproximal stripping can be carried out wherever possible, so that the entire premolar space can be utilized for set back of the anterior segment.

Periapical X-rays of the planned osteotomy region should be taken and if roots are convergent, they are made divergent. The equal amount of space should be created between the crowns as well as roots of the teeth adjacent to the osteotomy sites (Fig. 25.7).

Completion of Presurgical Orthodontic Phase

Fresh records should be taken at the completion of presurgical orthodontic phase. The models should be duplicated. One set is kept for the record and another one handed over to the surgeon for mock surgery or model surgery and preparation of the occlusal wafer splint.

Impressions for models should be taken before fixing the stabilizing arch wire. Interocclusal wafer splints should not be more than 2 to 3 mm thick. (Prior to splint making, the models should be checked whether class I canine and molar relationship can be achieved postsurgically) (Figs 25.8 and 25.9).

Before handing over the patient to the oral and maxillofacial surgeon, a stabilizing passive rectangular wire with multiple lugs soldered or incorporated onto the arch wire (a lug between every two teeth). These should be placed at least three weeks prior to surgery. This will ensure that no further teeth movement will occur and occlusal splint fit will not change at the time of surgery (Fig. 25.10).

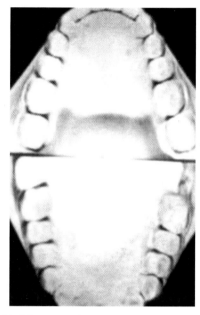

Fig. 25.8: Models prepared at the end of presurgical orthodontic phase

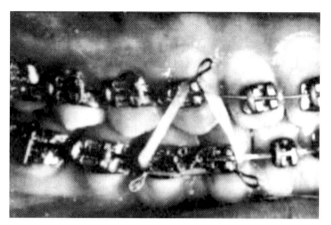

Fig. 25.10: Multiple lugs are helpful in postoperative period for intermaxillary elastic ligation

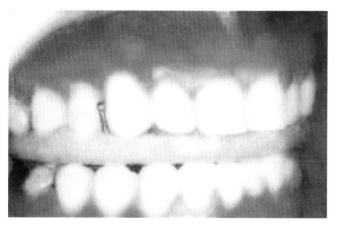

Fig. 25.9: Interocclusal wafer splint

POSTSURGICAL ORTHODONTICS OBJECTIVES

After surgery, 4 to 6 weeks rest is advised for the patient to allow healing and consolidation of osteotomy sites. After the surgeon confirms the satisfactory healing, the interocclusal splint and stabilizing arch wires are removed and replaced by light arch wires to allow the settling of the occlusion. A box or rectangular patterns of light interdental elastics are used including the canines and premolars for desired interdigitation. In deep bite cases where lateral open bites are created, vertical elastic traction should be given in posterior molar region.

Objectives

   i. Closure of all residual spaces.
  ii. Root paralleling at the extraction sites.
 iii. Correcting the incisor torque.
 iv. Correction of residual deep or open bite (extrusion for levelling and settling).
  v. Finer tooth alignment.
 vi. Maximum interdigitation (detailing of occlusion).
vii. Retention phase to readapt and reorient oral musculature to prevent relapse.

Model Surgery (Mock Surgery)

All these years, the oral and maxillofacial surgeons used to 'eyeball' the deformity and decide the surgical plan after model sectioning and aligning them. Now, the total treatment plan is made after using sophisticated tools like cephalometric analysis, photoanalysis, prediction tracings, computer assisted analysis, etc. But, with the present state of the art of the orthognathic procedures, model or mock surgery still holds important key position in the treatment planning and the occlusal wafer splints which are constructed after final mock-up, are still being used as an intraoperative navigator (guide). Cephalometric prediction tracings cannot reproduce three-dimensional view of the patient's dental arch status. Hence, tridimensional models are always helpful for the treatment planning.

Aims of Model Surgery

   i. To locate the problem areas preoperatively.
  ii. To determine the feasible surgical plan.
 iii. To determine the direction of movement of dento-osseous segments.

   iv. To view the osteotomy sites directly.

   v. To obtain the measurements of osteotomies.

   vi. To reduce the operating time.

   vii. To improve the accuracy of overall results.

Hand Articulation

The plaster models should be held manually, in the hand, to carry out analysis of the plaster casts in various occlusal positions. Hand articulation is done:

   i. To plan the presurgical orthodontics.

   ii. To find the existence of a possible tooth mass problem.

   iii. To ascertain the presence of transverse discrepancies.

   iv. To find the ideal site for interdental osteotomy.

   v. To determine the number of segments required to achieve the desired occlusal results.

Prior to model surgery, a thorough clinical examination, cephalometric analysis, dental model evaluation should be carried out. Diagnosis of the patient's problem, considering occlusal and esthetic requirements is done. A tentative surgical treatment plan should be devised.

After the presurgical orthodontic phase is completed, then before fixing the stabilizing wire the fresh impressions are taken and casts prepared. The models are checked with hand-articulation for estimation of the success of the presurgical orthodontics. Model simulation should be done of the anticipated surgical movement. Prediction tracing and model surgery measurements should coincide. Simulate the presurgical orthodontics on the diagnostic models. To meet the patient's esthetic and occlusal requirements the models are hand-articulated in a new position to: (i) align the dental midline, (ii) to achieve maximum interdigitation anteriorly, (iii) to bring canines in an Angle's class I occlusion, (iv) to achieve Angle's class I molar relationships.

Protocol for Mock Surgery

- Cut the model exactly similar to surgery
- Avoid apices or root surfaces of teeth during cutting
- Detect the problem areas—proximity of roots, bony interferences, etc.
- Observe and note the movement of dento-osseous segments—rotations-expansion, etc.
- Reposition the anterior maxillary segment first.

Consider (a) best esthetics and functional requirement (b) axial inclination (c) lip coverage, (d) vertical relationship:

- Achieve maximum interdigitation
- Keep the mandibular model fixed in two-jaw surgery
- Measure and record the AP, transverse and interdental changes
- Re-evaluate and compare with prediction tracing measurements
- Ascertain the difference in intrusion of one side to the other side in facial asymmetry cases in superior positioning of maxilla.

Marking Procedure for Models

To determine the magnitude and direction of the surgical movements in all the three planes, markings on the models should be made and the measurements should be taken using these markings as reference lines.

1. *Base line:* It is drawn 35 mm above the maxillary canine tips and 25 mm above the maxillary first molar cusps tips.

2. *Vertical reference lines (maxillary model):* Parallel to the long axis of the teeth in first molar, canine and between central incisors only. These lines are drawn perpendicular to the base line of the cast. Additional vertical lines can be drawn for segmental surgery.

3. *Transverse markings (expansion or contraction):* Marks on the cusp tips of (R) and (L) canines and on the central fossa of the maxillary first molar. Measure intercanine and intermolar distance.

4. *Anteroposterior marking:* Hold the models in centric relation. Vertical maxillary markings in first molar and canine teeth region are extended till the mandibular teeth.

5. *For interdental osteotomies:* Horizontal lines at the level of tooth apices and at the alveolar crest. Intersecting the previous vertical lines on either side of the osteotomy site.

After the desired mock surgery is done and measurements are recorded, then the models are mounted on the articulator (Mechanical or Hinge articulator) in class I canine and molar occlusion and acrylic wafer splint is constructed (2-3 mm width). This acrylic wafer splint will be used as a guide intraoperatively. Intraoperatively, the osteotomy cuts are modified after checking the fit of the splint.

Orthognathic Surgery: Osteotomy Procedures

HISTORICAL DEVELOPMENT OF ORTHOGNATHIC SURGERY

In 1849, in the United State of America, Hullihen performed first anterior mandibular osteotomy for the patient of distortion of face due to severe burns. The beginning of the early orthognathic surgery was in St Louis, where the orthodontist Edward Angle and the surgeon Blair worked together. In 1897, Blair performed osteotomy of the mandibular body —'St Louis operation'. Thereafter in 1907, he was the first one to describe several operative techniques, for the correction of maxillofacial deformities. Blair was the first surgeon to realize the benefits of the co-operation between orthodontists and surgeons. He wrote in his article "Treating the skeletal deformities is really surgical work, but the earlier a competent, congenial orthodontist is associated with the case, the better it will be for both the surgeon and the patient." Several renowned maxillofacial surgeons invented new methods thereafter, for the correction of skeletal mandibular deformities. In 1955, in central Europe (Vienna), Trauner described inverted L osteotomy of the ramus for the correction of mandibular prognathism. Trauner trained Kole and Hugo Obwegeser, who gave the decisive boost to orthognathic surgery (Table 26.1).

Biological Basis for Orthognathic Surgery

Simple splitting of the bone is known as osteotomy and removal of part of the bone is known as osteectomy. In orthognathic surgery, the jaw bones are intentionally sectioned at various sites to correct the dentofacial deformities and then repositioned at desired position.

The maxillary osteotomies became popular after Bell's extensive research studies on rhesus monkeys in 1969 to 1975. He experimented and studied revascularization and bone healing after various osteotomy procedures. *He provided biological basis for orthognathic surgery and proved that the blood supply to the osteotomized segment will be maintained adequately, if at least one soft tissue pedicle is preserved intact. These studies also demonstrated that as long as the maxilla is pedicled to palatal mucosa and the labial gingiva and mucosa, downfracture of the maxilla with complete mobilization can be accomplished with adequate vascular supply (Figs 26.1A and B).*

Table 26.1: Historical development of orthognathic surgery		
1921	: Cohn-Stock	• Anterior maxillary osteotomies (two stage)
1935	: Wassmund	• One stage anterior maxillary osteotomy
1952	: Converse	• Step osteotomy of the mandibular body for the correction of mandibular prognathism
1954	: Caldwell-Letterman	• Vertical subsigmoid osteotomy of ramus
1955	: Schuchardt	• Developed posterior maxillary osteotomy
1955	: Obwegeser	• Published the famous 'intraoral sagittal split of the mandible'
1958	: Dal Pont	• Modified intraoral sagittal split technique
1959	: Kole	• First to describe bimaxillary surgery for the correction of bimaxillary protrusion. Proposed surgeries for open bite closure and for genioplasty procedures.
1968	: Hunsuck	• Further modified sagittal split osteotomy
1969	: Obwegeser	• Presented a large series of Lefort I osteotomies.
1970	: Obwegeser	• Two-jaw surgery
1974	: Spiessel	• First to apply rigid fixation in orthognathic surgery
1979	: Luhr	• Introduced the miniplate fixation in orthognathic surgery

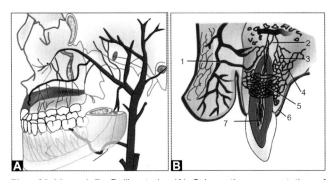

Figs 26.1A and B: Bell's study: (A) Schematic representation of blood supply to maxilla and mandible, (B) Blood supply to anterior maxillary region, showing anastomosing vessels: (1) Labial artery, (2) Apical vessels, (3) Intra-alveolar vessels, (4) Palatal plexus, (5) Periodontal plexus (6) Gingival plexus, (7) Pulp vessels

Various surgical procedures can be performed either in the maxilla or mandible or both together for the correction of dentofacial deformities.

PROTOCOL FOR OSTEOTOMIES

i. Design soft tissue incision to maintain adequate collateral blood supply to the osteotomized segment and to avoid injury to vital structures in the vicinity.
ii. Provide optimum exposure to the site of osteotomy.
iii. Minimum or judicious periosteal stripping.
iv. Gentle soft tissue handling.
v. Design osteotomy cuts without damaging the neurovascular bundle. Determine precise amount of bone cutting required by mock surgery and prepare a occlusal guide splint.

vi. Make osteotomy cuts under constant irrigation with normal saline.
vii. Plan interdental osteotomy cuts without damaging the periodontal status of adjoining teeth.
viii. Design subapical osteotomy cuts at least 4 to 5 mm away from the apices of the teeth.
ix. Remove all the bony interferences while approximating the osteotomized segments.
x. Proper approximation with broad contact of osteotomized segments and stable fixation.
xi. Approximation of the osteotomized fragments in class I canine and molar occlusion (ideal)
xii. Adequate soft tissue coverage to prevent wound dehiscence.
xiii. Proper follow up.

OSTEOTOMY PROCEDURES

Various osteotomy procedures for the correction of dentofacial deformities are given in Table 26.2.

Mandibular Osteotomies can be Divided Into

1. Mandibular body osteotomies.
2. Mandibular ramus osteotomies.

Soft Tissue Incisions for Osteotomies (Figs 26.2 to 26.6)

1. All mandibular body osteotomies, including genioplasties can be performed through 'degloving' vestibular incision taken intraorally. The extension

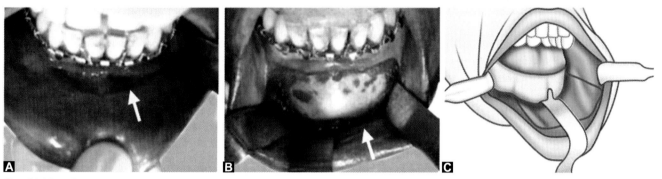

Figs 26.2A to C: (A and B) Intraoral degloving incision and reflection of mucoperiosteal flap till inferior border (C) Diagrammatic representation of degloving technique

Table 26.2: Various osteotomy procedures for the correction of dentofacial deformities

1. **Mandibular body osteotomies**
   i. *Mandibular body osteotomies*—Intraoral procedures
      a. Anterior body osteotomy
      b. Posterior body osteotomy
      c. Midsymphysis osteotomy
   ii. *Segmental subapical mandibular surgeries*
      a. Anterior subapical mandibular osteotomy
      b. Posterior subapical mandibular osteotomy
      c. Total subapical mandibular osteotomy
   iii. *Genioplasties*—Horizontal osteotomy in the chin region
      a. Augmentation genioplasty
      b. Reduction genioplasty
      c. Straightening genioplasty
      d. Lengthening genioplasty

2. **Mandibular ramus osteotomies**
   i. *Subcondylar ramus osteotomy*
      a. Extraoral subcondylar ramus osteotomy (subsigmoid)
      b. Intraoral subcondylar ramus osteotomy (subsigmoid)
      c. Arching ramus osteotomy (extraoral)
   ii. *Intraoral modified sagittal split osteotomy*

3. **Maxillary osteotomy procedures**—Intraoral procedures
   i. *Segmental maxillary osteotomy procedures*
      a. Single tooth dento-osseous osteotomy
      b. Interdental osteotomies
      c. Anterior maxillary osteotomy
      d. Posterior maxillary osteotomy
   ii. *Total maxillary surgery—Lefort I osteotomy*
      a. Superior repositioning of the maxilla
      b. Superior repositioning of the maxilla leaving nasal floor intact—Horseshoe-shaped osteotomy
      c. Advancement of maxilla
         • Simultaneous expansion of maxilla
         • Simultaneous narrowing of maxilla
      d. Inferior repositioning of maxilla
      e. Leveling of maxilla

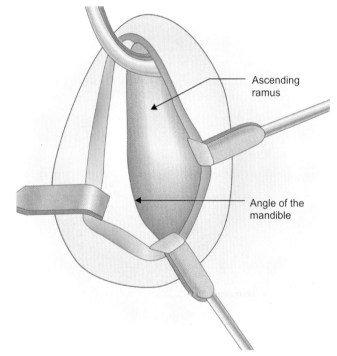

Fig. 26.3: Postramal Hind's or Irby's incision

of the incision will differ depending on the site of osteotomy (Figs 26.2A to C).

2. Intraoral ramus osteotomies can be performed through the incision similar to the incision used for removal of impacted lower third molar.

3. Extraoral ramus osteotomies are carried out either through submandibular Risdon's incision or through postramal Hind's incision (more cosmetic results) (Fig. 26.3).

4. Anterior maxillary osteotomy can be performed by taking three small horizontal vestibular incisions in the region of canine to second premolar on either side and midline incision over the anterior nasal spine. Tunneling of the mucoperiosteal flap can be done to reach the pyriform nasal aperture and the premolar extraction sites. Palatal pedicle is kept intact for maintaining the blood supply. Interdental osteotomies can be performed using the same type of incision (Fig. 26.4).

5. Posterior maxillary osteotomy can be done through buccal vestibular incision starting from first molar to the tuberosity area.

6. Total maxillary osteotomy can be performed by taking complete vestibular incision starting from one maxillary first molar extending to other side maxillary first molar. Again palatal pedicle is kept intact. Other alternative is planning three small vestibular incisions—one in the midline over anterior nasal spine and two on either side, starting from second premolar going toward third molar region and tunneling the mucoperiosteal flap on either side keeping the palatal pedicle intact (Figs 26.5 and 26.6).

Mandibular Body Osteotomy

Mandibular body osteotomy surgical procedures can be performed:
1. Between adjacent teeth.
2. Through pre-existing edentulous space.
3. Through the extraction sites.

Whenever the osteotomies are performed anterior to the mental foramen, it is termed as anterior body osteotomy and if it is carried out posterior to the mental foramen, then it is termed posterior body osteotomy. Midsymphysis osteotomy can be used to widen or narrow the anterior arch width. Posterior body osteotomy is used to correct the level of the posterior segment or posterior cross bite or lingual inclination.

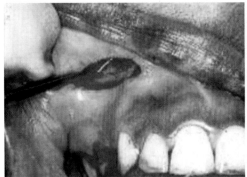 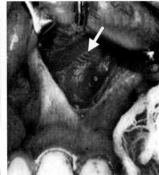 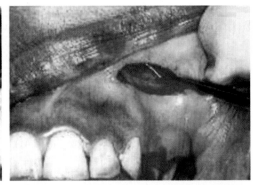

Fig. 26.4: Three small vestibular incisions for anterior maxillary osteotomy procedure. Arrow in the middle picture shows anterior nasal spine is exposed and the horizontal central incision is sutured in a vertical manner for lip lengthening and to prevent scar contraction

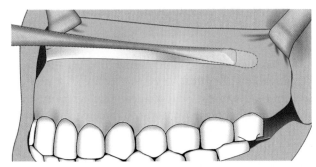

Fig. 26.5: Complete vestibular incision from right first molar to left first molar for LeFort I osteotomy

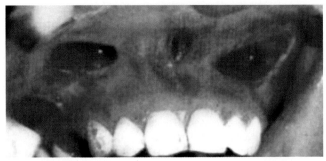

Fig. 26.6: Small incisions in the vestibule for LeFort I osteotomy procedure

Anterior Body Osteotomy (Figs 26.7 and 26.8)

Used in selected cases of:
1. Mandibular prognathism with functional posterior occlusion
2. Class III malocclusion with or without anterior open bite, where the posterior teeth cross bite is dental in nature (can be corrected by orthodontics).

Removal of the first or second premolars is required for the correction of anterior crossbite.

Intraorally, two small vestibular incisions are taken bilaterally, leaving attached gingiva intact into first and second premolar regions, depending on the extraction. Mucoperiosteal tunneling is carried out superiorly till the alveolar crest and inferiorly till the inferior border in the area of extraction. Care is taken not to damage the mental nerve and its branches. A periosteal elevator is inserted lingually through the extraction site subperiosteally to protect the lingual soft tissue during osteotomy cuts. A modified retractor is placed at the inferior border of the body mandible at the proposed osteotomy cut. The vertical osteotomy cut is started in the socket at the alveolar margin involving both buccal and lingual cortices going towards the inferior border. The entire extraction socket should be utilized and the cuts are made parallel to each other or slightly convergent from buccal to lingual for better approximation.

Care should be taken not to remove excessive crestal bone to prevent periodontal defects. The same procedure is repeated on the opposite side. Immediately occlusal splint is tried and osteotomy cuts are modified, if some bony interferences are present. Once the accurate fit of the occlusal splint is achieved, the fragments are stabilized at superior margin by passing figure of eight wires around the necks of the canine and premolar and inferiorly by using miniplate fixation or intraosseous wiring. Wound is closed in single layer. Instead of straight vertical osteotomy, the cut can be modified as step osteotomy to avoid damage to the mental nerve and to have better bony contact.

Posterior Body Osteotomy (Fig. 26.9)

Here, the preservation of neurovascular bundle is of utmost importance. This procedure is not commonly used. It can be used: (i) where there are missing posterior

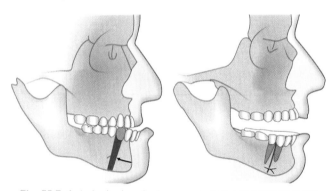

Fig. 26.7: Anterior body osteotomy procedure and setback of the osteotomized segment and fixation with intraosseous wiring

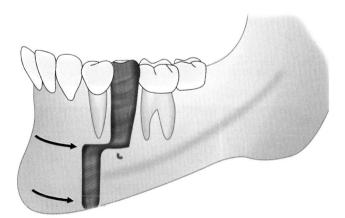

Fig. 26.8: Modified step or Z body osteotomy for anterior body mandible

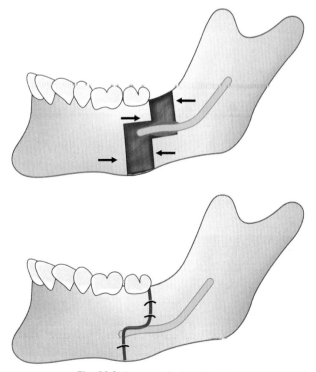

Fig. 26.9: Posterior body osteotomy

teeth, (ii) in selected cases, with class III deformity, and (iii) for correction of crossbite. Vestibular incision, one tooth anteriorly and one tooth distal to the osteotomy site, is taken. This incision can be extended posteriorly up the external oblique ridge for more relaxation. A channel retractor is inserted at the proposed osteotomy site at the inferior border. The cut is started superior to the neurovascular bundle and finished through both the cortices. At the level of neurovascular bundle small window is made by removal of only external cortex and thus exposing the neurovascular bundle. The nerve hook is inserted to pull the bundle toward buccal side and lingual osteotomy cut is completed. Then the neurovascular bundle is retracted gently upward, so that the inferior border cut can be completed. through and through. Same procedure is repeated on the other side and the fragments approximated in such a way that the neurovascular bundle is not damaged. The occlusal splint is fitted properly and the osteotomized segments fixed with either intraosseous wiring or bone plating at the inferior border.

Midsymphysis Osteotomy (Fig. 26.10)

If it is combined with posterior or anterior body osteotomy, then complete vestibular incision can be planned. Thin tapering bur or saw can be used for making the cut in between two mandibular incisors from the alveolar crest to the inferior border. Care is taken to place the osteotomy cuts without damaging the roots of the teeth.

Segmental Subapical Mandibular Surgeries

Segmental subapical mandibular surgeries can be used to reposition the anterior, posterior or entire mandibular dentoalveolar segment.

Anterior Subapical Mandibular Osteotomy (Figs 26.11 to 26.13)

Anterior subapical mandibular osteotomy is very popular technique. It can be used as a single procedure for:
  i. Correcting mandibular dentoalveolar proclina-tion.
 ii. Closing mild anterior open bite.
iii. Leveling an accentuated curve of Spee.
 iv. Correcting mandibular dental arch asymmetry.

It can be used as an adjunctive procedure with other surgical procedures such as:
  i. With anterior maxillary osteotomy to correct bimaxillary protrusion.

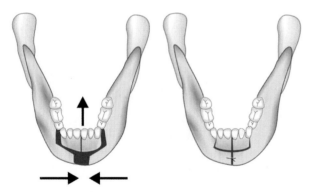

Fig. 26.10: Midsymphysis osteotomy along with anterior subapical mandibular body osteotomy

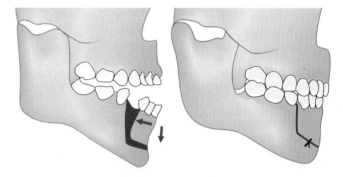

Fig. 26.11: Mandibular anterior subapical osteotomy

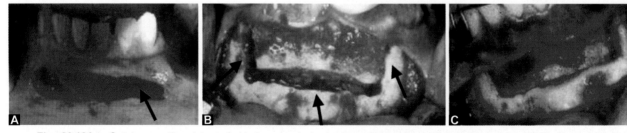

Figs 26.12A to C: Intraoperative picture of anterior subapical osteotomy: (A) Incision, (B) Osteotomy cuts, (C) Final approximation

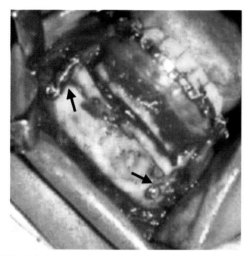

Fig. 26.13: Anterior subapical mandibular osteotomy procedure—an intraoperative picture. Fixation with bone plates is done

ii. With mandibular advancement to level the curve of Spee.
iii. With genioplasty procedure.

Following extraction of premolars on either side, a circumvestibular incision is taken from canine to canine area. The incision is made into the lip and carried tangentially down to the bone. While making the incision the finger is placed on the cutaneous side of the lip to appreciate the depth of the incision, which should limit itself without cutting through the entire lip. Care is taken to locate the mental nerve and protect it. A subperiosteal dissection is carried to the inferior border and the symphysis region is degloved. A periosteal elevator is placed on the lingual side of the extraction socket and vertical cut is made from the alveolar crest till the level of premolar root apex through both the cortices. The same procedure is repeated on the other side. Then both the vertical cuts are connected by the horizontal subapical osteotomy made about 5 mm below the anterior teeth apices.

The segment is mobilized by using an osteotome. An attempt is made to place the teeth into the prefabricated occlusal splint. Bony interferences are removed if necessary and final fitting of the splint is checked and the osteotomized fragment can be stabilized by using miniplate fixation.

The incision is closed in two layers, the muscular and the mucosal layer; and a pressure dressing is given externally.

If anterior subapical mandibular sugery is to be used only for leveling the curve of Spee, then there is no need to extract the teeth. Vertical interdental osteotomies are done between canine and first premolars on either side, using a fine tissue bur and fine osteotome or a saw. Horizontal wedge of bone is removed to depress the anterior fragment.

Posterior Subapical Mandibular Osteotomy Procedure (Fig. 26.14)

Used rarely, as it is technically difficult and there is a high-risk of injury to the inferior alveolar neurovascular bundle. But with the proper skill, it can be used successfully for:
  i. Uprighting the posterior segment which is in extreme linguoversion or buccoversion.
  ii. Closing a premolar or molar space.
  iii. Leveling supraerupted posterior teeth.

A horizontal vestibular incision is taken and the mucoperiosteal flap reflected downwards till the inferior border of the mandible. Here, the anterior vertical cut is taken in the area of missing first premolar or first molar and second vertical cut is placed behind the last existing molar and horizontal cut is taken below the apices of the teeth, protecting the neurovascular bundle. Both the vertical cuts are carried out from the alveolar crest up to the level of neurovascular bundle. The portion of the buccal cortex that overlies the nerve bundle is removed. This window should extend several millimeter posteriorly to the distal vertical cut. The window is made in such a way that the cut extends only in the buccal cortex and the bone is removed with osteotome and saved. After the identification and protection of the nerve bundle, lingual cortex is osteotomized. Both

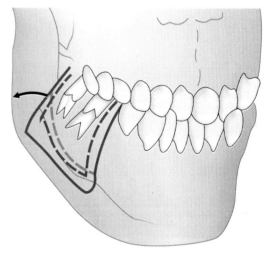

Fig. 26.14: Posterior subapical mandibular osteotomy procedure

vertical cuts are also completed till the horizontal cut level and the entire segment is mobilized with the osteotome in the desired position. The segment can be stabilized by fixing the occlusal splint and by placing a circummandibular wire over the splint. The outer cortical bony plate, which was saved should be fitted back prior to suturing.

Total Subapical Mandibular Osteotomy (Fig. 26.15)

Again not performed routinely, as technically difficult and high-risk of damage to the neurovascular bundle. It can be used to reposition entire mandibular dentoalveolar segment anteriorly, posteriorly or superiorly. For lengthening of lower third of the face or for advancing the mandibular dentoalveolar segment, etc. Here, the location of the horizontal subapical osteotomy is done below the level of the inferior alveolar neurovascular bundle. The level is determined by radiographs and the actual osteotomy location is marked by taking direct measurements from the occlusal plane. The horizontal osteotomy is started initially anteriorly in the symphysis region and proceeds posteriorly. The horizontal

osteotomy cut is completed through the lingual cortex by placing the guiding finger on the lingual side and bur is directed at the angle of 45° from buccal to lingual cortex. The entire horizontal cut is carried just posterior to the last molar. Then a vertical osteotomy is made approximately 5 mm posterior to the last tooth. This cut begins superiorly and carried through and through to the level just above the nerve bundle. The buccal cut is then completed through only the outer cortex and remainder of the lingual cortex adjacent to and below the bundle, is fractured with the osteotome. In advancement cases, care should be taken not to overstretch the nerve. It can tolerate 3 to 6 mm of stretching.

Genioplasties

Genioplasty can be used as a single procedure or it can be used as an adjunctive procedure along with other major osteotomies of the jaw bone (Figs 26.16A to C).

The deformities of the chin should be considered in all three planes—AP, vertical and transverse as the morphology of the symphysis region is highly variable in different individuals, even with the same basic types of dentofacial deformities.

Genioplasties can be used to augment, reduce, straighten or lengthen the chin.

Augmentation Genioplasty (Figs 26.17 to 26.23)

Augmentation genioplasty is used to increase the chin projection. It can be done by:
- Sliding horizontal osteotomy of the symphysis region
- Using autogenous bone graft
- Using alloplastic material—silastic, hydroxyapatite, etc.

Augmentation genioplasty surgical procedure: The entire inferior border of the symphysis is degloved by

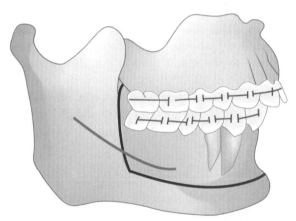

Fig. 26.15: Total subapical mandibular osteotomy

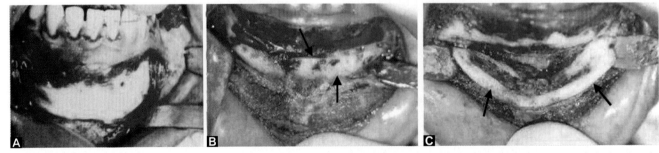

Figs 26.16A to C: Basic genioplasty surgical procedure. (A) Degloving incision, (B) Horizontal osteotomy cut including the inferior border of the chin, (C) Mobilized bony segment ready for genioplasty procedure (Reduction, augmentation, straightening or lengthening procedure)

using vestibular incision. The digastric muscles are separated from the mandible to reduce the tension after advancement. Periosteal releasing incision also should be taken to provide adequate coverage after advancement. Generally, the AP dimension of the symphysis is about 8 to 12 mm. So the same amount of advancement is possible. The horizontal osteotomy cut is made at least 4 to 5 mm below the apices of canines. The cut is completed through both buccal and lingual cortices. The segment is mobilized inferiorly and forward with the help of osteotome. This mobilized segment is pedicled over geniohyoid muscles and some

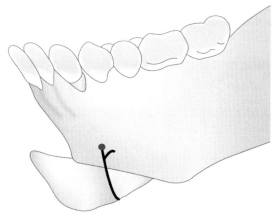

Fig. 26.17: Augmentation genioplasty

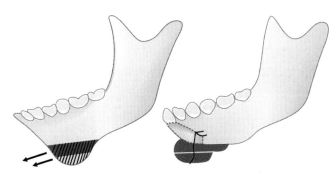

Fig. 26.18: Double sliding augmentation genioplasty

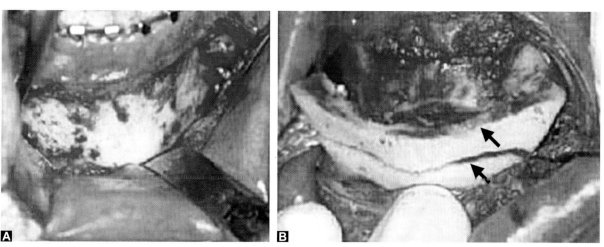

Figs 26.19A and B: Double genioplasty procedure: (A) Surgical exposure through degloving incision, (B) Double horizontal cuts in the anterior chin region to carry out double genioplasty procedure

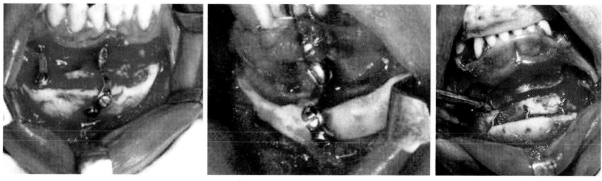

Fig. 26.20: Augmentation genioplasty and fixation

amount of lingual periosteum. Any bony interferences for advancement are removed under direct vision. The mobilized segment should be then advanced into desired position by using towel clips and then external facial contour should be checked and the fragment is positioned to the final desired level. It can be fixed to the superior body with two intraosseous wirings at canine region or two mini bone plates (Figs 26.17 to 26.20).

With major advancement, the periosteal relaxing incision should be made prior to suturing. Suturing is done in two/three layers.

Alloplastic augmentation can be done using the same incision, but which is relatively short in length. On both the sides, little tunneling is done to create a pocket into which the onlay grafting material can be slided for better fixation (Silastic or hydroxyapatite blocks) (Fig. 26.21C).

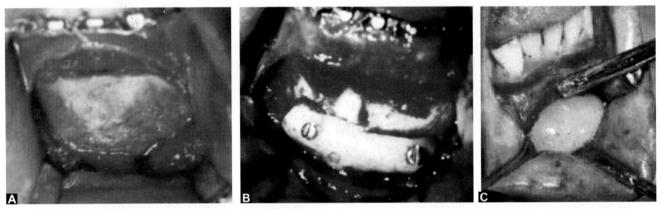

Figs 26.21A to C: (A and B) Augmentation genioplasty with onlay graft, (C) Augmentation with prefabricated silastic graft

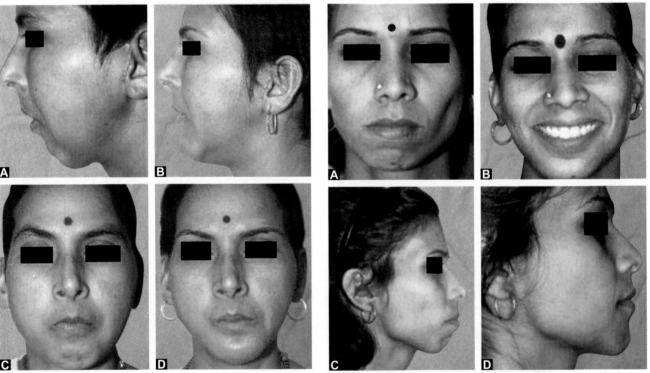

Figs 26.22A to D: Augmentation genioplasty results: (A) Preoperative profile view, (B) Postoperative profile view, (C) Preoperative frontal view, (D) Postoperative frontal view

Figs 26.23A to D: Augmentation genioplasty procedure was carried out to improve the chin contour: (A) Preoperative frontal view, (B) Postoperative frontal view, (C) Preoperative profile view, (D) Postoperative profile view

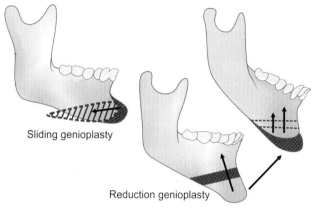

Fig. 26.24: Sliding and reduction genioplasty

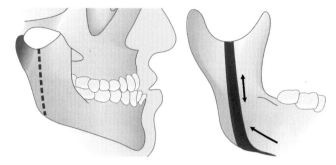

Fig. 26.25: Subsigmoid vertical osteotomy. Caldwell-Letterman osteotomy

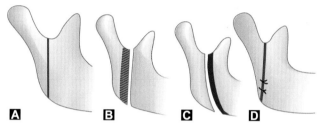

Figs 26.26A to D: Diagram of Caldwell-Letterman osteotomy procedure: (A) Osteotomy cut, (B and C) Decortication of osteotomized segments, (D) Fixation with intraosseous wiring

Reduction Genioplasty (Fig. 26.24)

The reduction of the symphysis region can be achieved both in the anteroposterior and vertical planes or in both planes depending on the need of the patient. This surgical procedure is also used as an adjunctive procedure. Three different types of procedures can be described:

1. Horizontal osteotomy and setback of the fragment. Excess amount of bony wedge, which is left behind is excised and the segment is fixed.
2. Vertical reduction amounts to determining the required vertical movement. Two horizontal osteotomy cuts are made, the lower cut is completed first. Then the superior cut is done and bony wedge is removed. The inferior segment is then pushed upwards and stabilized.
3. Vertical reduction and posterior pushback may be required in some of the cases.

Straightening Genioplasty Procedure

It is indicated in patients with facial asymmetry, where the complete correction of the asymmetry cannot be achieved by appropriate jaw osteotomies, e.g. condylar hyperplasia, TM joint ankylosis, etc. This can be also used in conjunction with anteroposterior (AP), vertical or transverse augmentation or reduction of the chin. The horizontal osteotomy is done and segment is shifted laterally and then contoured to get desired result.

Lengthening Genioplasty

Indicated in patients with short vertical facial height with Cl I and Cl II deep bites. After horizontal osteotomy, the osteotomized segment is pushed inferiorly and bone graft is sandwiched in between to increase the height.

Mandibular Ramus Osteotomies

Subcondylar Vertical Osteotomy

Subcondylar vertical osteotomy was first proposed by Caldwell-Letterman in 1954. The indications for extraoral subsigmoid vertical ramus osteotomy are as follows (Figs 26.25 to 26.28).

i. Major setback of mandible more than 10 mm.
ii. Asymmetric setback of the mandible.
iii. Reoperation of previously operated case.

In this procedure, the ramus is approached through extraoral postramal or submandibular incision and is sectioned from the sigmoid notch to the lower border of the mandible just ahead of the angle (Figs 26.25 to 26.28). The mandibular foramen remains on the distal fragment, thereby avoiding injury to the nerve, and the condyle attached to the proximal segment. After cutting through the pterygomasseteric sling, the angle and inferior border of mandible is exposed. A periosteal elevator is utilized to subperiosteally reflect all the tissues from the lateral aspect of the ascending ramus. The sigmoid notch and coronoid process is also exposed. The hook or curved instrument is engaged at the sigmoid notch and ramus is pulled slightly downwards. A bony prominence corresponding to the lingula and mandibular foramen is located on the lateral

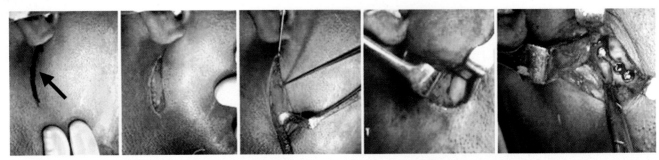

Fig. 26.27: Extraoral postramal incision and different steps of dissection till the exposure of mandibular angle and vertical subsigmoid ramal osteotomy and final bone plate fixation

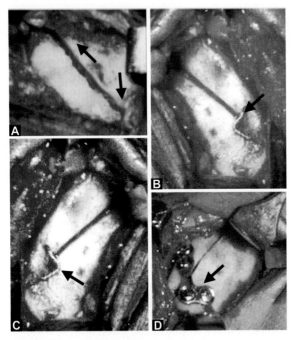

Figs 26.28A to D: Surgical procedure for extraoral subsigmoid ramus osteotomy: (A) Osteotomy cut, (B) Fixation with intraosseous wiring (R) side, (C) (L) Side wire fixation, (D) Fixation with stainless steel L shaped bone plate on (R) side for other patient

surface of the ramus. *This is called as Behrman's bump.* The vertical line going from the sigmoid notch to the inferior border is scratched just posterior to the mandibular foramen with the bur. The cut is started from the sigmoid notch up to the level of mandibular foramen through both the cortices. Care is taken to protect the medial tissues. Then the cut is started from inferior border going up to the level of mandibular foramen. Then both the cuts are joined together. This way if there is any inadvertent injury to neurovascular bundle, which causes hemorrhage, then the two fragments can be quickly separated and the vessel is identified and

ligated. Similar procedure is carried out on the opposite side. After both side osteotomies are completed the proximal fragments are placed over distal fragments and the assistant temporarily locks the mouth in desired occlusion by carrying out temporary inter maxillary fixation (IMF). The decortication of the distal segment is carried out on the lateral aspect of the overlap area and the proximal segment is decorticated on the medial aspect. The proximal segment is then fixed laterally to the distal segment overlapping it with intraosseous wiring or bone plates *(Figs 26.28A to D).* There can be variations of this basic osteotomy procedure. *Subsigmoid oblique subcondylar* osteotomy is advocated *by Robinson and Hinds in* 1955. The cut is extended from the sigmoid notch to the posterior border. *C-shaped or arching osteotomy* can be done by curving the bony cut above the level of mandibular foramen extending it to the anterior border of the mandible, instead of going straight to sigmoid notch. These procedures can be also used for the advancement of mandible along with the use of bone grafts fitted between the distal and proximal segments (Figs 26.29 to 26.31).

Advantages of subsigmoid vertical and oblique osteotomy:

1. Adequate direct access.
2. Adequate control of bony fragments.
3. Good surface contact between the bony fragments.
4. Minimal relapse tendency.
5. Gonial angle contour can be changed.
6. No loss of teeth or arch size.

Disadvantage: It is because of extraoral incision, there is an external scar formation. If the patient has keloid tendency, then this approach is contraindicated. Otherwise careful planning of the postramal incision gives minimum amount of scar, which is hidden behind the shadow of posterior border of the mandible and over the years, scar diminishes.

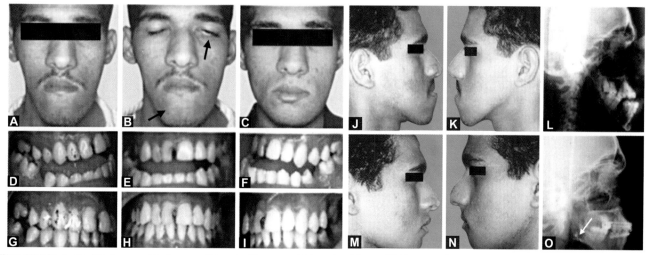

Figs 26.29A to O: (A) Asymmetrical prognathism in 19 years old boy, front face, (B) Preoperative asymmetrical front face showing (L) side Bell's palsy of the eye, (C) Postoperative front face after both sides extraoral subsigmoid osteotomy (surgery) (D to F) Preoperative dental occlusion showing anterior open bite and reverse overjet, (G to I) Postoperative occlusion, (J and K) Preoperative (R) and (L) profile, (M and N) Postoperative (R) and (L) profile, (L) Preoperative lateral cephalogram, (O) Postoperative lateral cephalogram

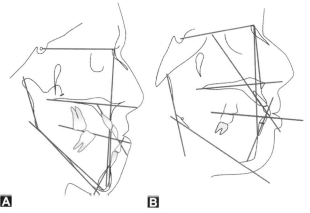

Figs 26.30A and B: (A) Preoperative cephalogram tracing, (B) Post-operative cephalogram tracing for the patient shown in Figures 26.29A to O

Intraoral Vertical Ramus Osteotomy (IVRO) and the Inverted L Osteotomy (Fig. 26.32)

First described by Winstanley in 1968. The indication for IVRO mandibular setback procedure is in mandibular excess patients. This procedure is faster and simpler than the sagittal split ramus osteotomy (SSRO). The rehabilitation time is much shorter and there is lower incidence of inferior alveolar nerve injury. This procedure is also indicated in the patients with TMJ complaints.

For this procedure, the ramus is exposed by taking intraoral incision at the level of mandibular occlusal plane, medial to the external oblique ridge till mandibular first molar. The length of the incision is

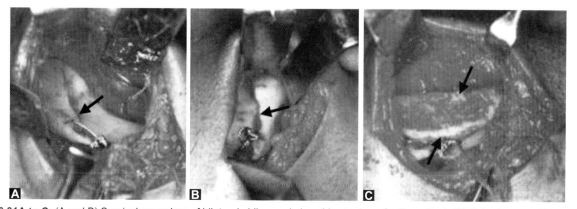

Figs 26.31A to C: (A and B) Surgical procedure of bilateral oblique subsigmoid osteotomy for the patient, (C) Onlay bone grafting on the (R) side ramus after fixation of the osteotomized fragments to correct the flatness on the right side (Arrows)

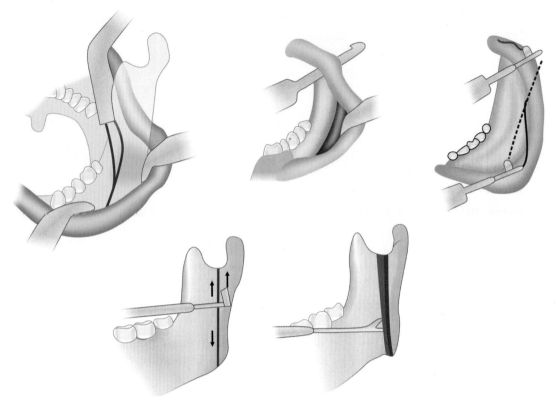

Fig. 26.32: Intraoral vertical ramus osteotomy (IVRO)

about 2 to 3 cm. The mouth is fully opened by inserting a bite block, between the teeth on the opposite side.

The subperiosteal reflection of the entire lateral, posterior and inferior borders of the ascending ramus of the mandible is performed. A J periosteal elevator is used to separate the pterygomasseteric sling. A special curved retractor is used to engage the posterior border of the mandible, thus the ramus can be pulled slightly forward, improving access. The bone cut is made from the sigmoid notch and carried inferiorly to the region of mandibular angle, using a 120° beveled reciprocating saw blade. After completion of the osteotomies on both sides and placement of the mandible into the occlusal splint, IMF is done. The positions of the osteotomized segments is checked. The proximal segment should lie lateral to the distal segment. The approximation of the fragments and fixation is done with intraosseous wiring.

Intraoral Modified Sagittal Split Osteotomy (Figs 26.33 to 26.40)

Bilateral sagittal split osteotomy (BSSO): This is a very popular, most versatile procedure performed on the mandibular ramus and body. First described by

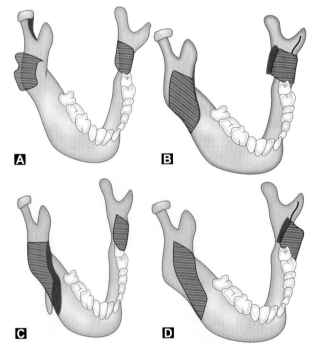

Figs 26.33A to D: Improvements of the sagittal split ramus osteotomy procedures: (A) Obwegeser and Trauner technique 1957, (B) Dal Pont modification 1961, (C) Hunsuck modification 1968, (D) Bell, Schendel and Epker modification 1977-78

Obwegeser and Trauner and later modified by *Dal Pont, Hunsuck and Epker.* This is accomplished through transoral incision, similar to that used for IVRO. The osteotomy splits the ramus and the posterior body of the mandible sagittally, which allows either setback or advancement. This is a highly cosmetic procedure, as it is done intraorally, (no extraoral scar) plus there is broader bony contact of the osteotomised segments ensuring good healing.

For mandibular advancement, there is no need for bone grafts. Thus donor site morbidity and second operative site for the bone graft is totally avoided. BSSO gives excellent results. Only drawback is the technique demands high level of operative skill and experience to minimize the surgical complications.

In 1957, Obwegeser and Trauner first described the sagittal split osteotomy of the ramus region, only by placing buccal and lingual cortical horizontal cuts. The procedure has undergone numerous modifications over the years.

In 1961, Dal Pont changed the lower horizontal cut to a vertical cut on the buccal cortex between the first and the second molars, thereby obtaining broader contact surfaces and requiring minimal muscular displacement with improved access.

In 1968, Hunsuck further modified the technique, advocating a shorter, horizontal medial cut, just posterior to the lingula, (instead of posterior border) to minimize soft tissue dissection. His anterior vertical cut was similar to Dal Pont's (Fig. 26.34).

In 1977, Epker suggested several modifications. These include minimal stripping of the masseter muscle and limited medial dissection. These modifications helped to reduce postoperative swelling, edema, hemorrhage (Fig. 26.33D).

Surgical procedure: A bite block is inserted on the opposite side in between the upper and lower teeth for making easy access and projecting the ramus anteriorly. An incision is made on the lateral aspect of the anterior border of the ramus, overlying the external oblique

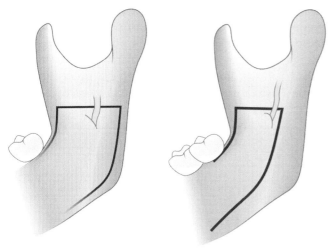

Fig. 26.34: Hunsuck's modification. He advocated a shorter horizontal medial cut just posterior to the lingula instead of extending it till posterior border

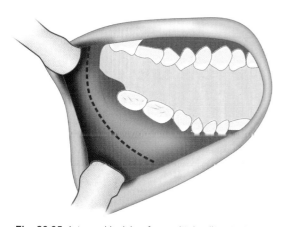

Fig. 26.35: Intraoral incision for sagittal split osteotomy

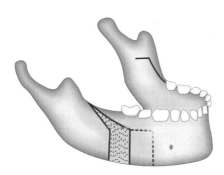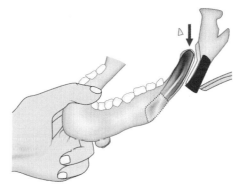

Fig. 26.36: Intraoral sagittal split osteotomy. Arrow—before approximation of osteotomized fragments bony interferences should be removed

ridge, from midway up the ascending ramus (to avoid buccal pad of fat) downward into vestibular depth till mandibular first molar region (Fig. 26.35). The soft tissue dissection is started subperiosteally along the anterior border upwards, towards the coronoid process. Medially the soft tissues are reflected, until the lingula and the inferior alveolar nerve bundle and mandibular foramen is identified. The medial soft tissue dissection is stopped slightly posterior and superior to the lingula. While the medial soft tissues are being retracted, the medial bone cut is made through only the lingual cortex

about 2 mm above the neurovascular bundle and just posterior to the lingula (Fig. 26.36).

Following the completion of horizontal medial osteotomy, cut is then carried down the lateral most aspect of the anterior border of the ascending ramus to the region of the second molar. This osteotomy is made parallel to the lateral cortex. The bite block is removed and the periosteum from the lateral aspect of the mandible is elevated in the molar area till the inferior border of the mandible. For setback procedure, the vertical osteotomy cut is taken lateral to second molar,

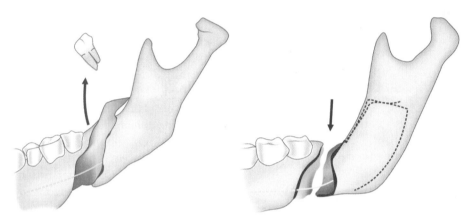

Fig. 26.37: During sagittal split osteotomy, the impacted third molar should be removed with minimum bone loss. Otherwise, inadvertent fracture can occur during the split (arrow)

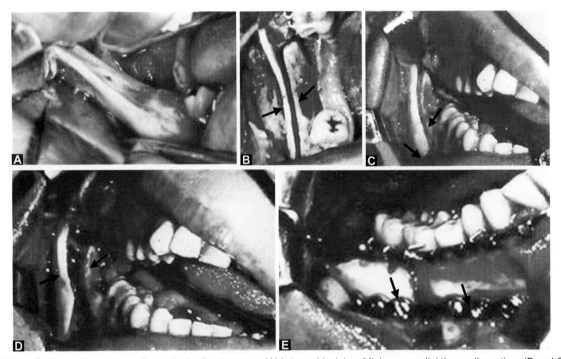

Figs 26.38A to E: Surgical procedures for sagittal split osteotomy: (A) Intraoral incision. Minimum medial tissue dissection, (B and C) Lateral osteotomy cuts, (D) Sagittal split complete. Check for bony interferences, (E) Final fixation with six hole bone plate and screws

however, in major advancement cases, vertical cut is placed forward in the region of the premolar. Vertical cut is completed through the lateral cortex only. *The cut extends through both the cortical plates at the inferior border of the mandible.* With osteotome, all bony cuts are checked for their completeness. Two osteotomes are then inserted and used as levers to separate the segments. Spreader can be used to finally separate the segments. The same procedure is repeated on the other side. In case of advancement, the bony interferences should be checked and the distal fragment is advanced and locked into

desired occlusion. The fixation of the fragments can be done by intraosseous wiring or lag screws or by bone plates (Fig. 26.38).

In case of setback, the distal fragment is pushed back. There will be overlap of the proximal fragment in the molar region. The excess bone on the proximal fragment is cut off by taking another vertical cut, distal to the previous cut, including only proximal fragment. The fragments will be checked now for proper approximation and fixation is carried out. This procedure gives excellent stable results (Figs 26.39 and 26.40).

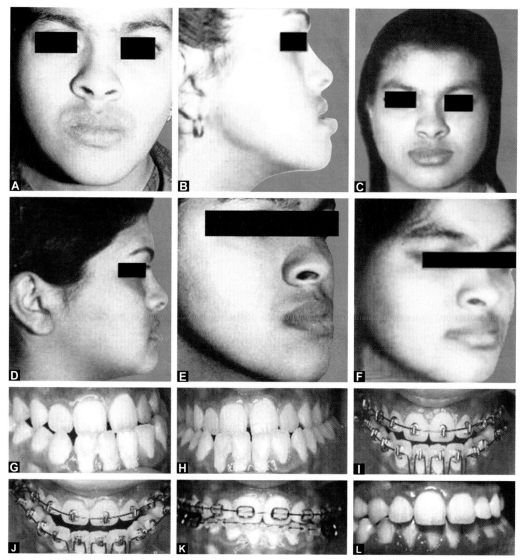

Figs 26.39A to L: A 21-year-old girl with mandibular prognathism: (A) Preoperative front view of face, (B) Preoperative profile, (C and D) Postoperative front face and profile, (E and F) Three-fourth facial view preoperative and postoperative, (G and H) Preoperative dental view. Note the nature's compensation. Upper anteriors are proclined. Lower anteriors lingually inclined, resulting in minimum reverse overjet, (I and J) Presurgical orthodontic phase. Note that the teeth are upright on their dental bases and increased reverse overjet (Decompensation). Bilateral sagittal split osteotomy surgery carried out, (K) Postsurgical orthodontic detailing, (L) Final finished occlusion

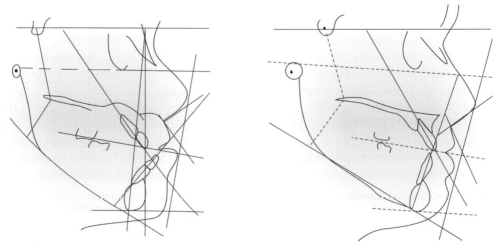

Fig. 26.40: Pre and postoperative cephalometric tracing of the patient shown in Figure 26.39

■ MAXILLARY OSTEOTOMY PROCEDURES

Segmental Maxillary Osteotomy: Surgical Procedures

Segmental maxillary surgery is commonly indicated in the correction of dentofacial deformities, where only a portion of the maxillary dental arch requires repositioning for functional and aesthetic reasons. Single tooth osteotomy is used to correct tooth malposition, dental ankylosis or closure of a diastema. Interdental osteotomy procedure was first advocated by Kole and was used to close diastemas in the maxillary dental arch, much prior to surgical orthodontics came into vogue. Now the diastemas are closed in the presurgical orthodontic phase and the residual spaces are left behind canines, so that the segmental osteotomy can be planned utilizing this available space.

Single tooth dento-osseous osteotomies: The basic criteria for this type of osteotomy is that, there must be sufficient space available between adjacent tooth roots, so that a fine osteotomy cut can be placed without injuring the roots. There should be also adequate space in the dental arch to reposition the osteotomised segment into proper occlusion without interference.

Incision: (a) A horizontal vestibular incision, or (b) multiple vertical incisions can be taken.

Surgery: A horizontal vestibular incision is made one tooth distal to those being mobilized. The mucoperiosteal flap is reflected superiorly exposing anterior nasal spine and piriform apertures of the nose. The nasal mucosa is protected by keeping periosteal elevator at the nasal floor and piriform aperture. The oral mucoperiosteum is reflected only till attached gingiva to maintain blood supply. Vertical interdental osteotomies are then made with a fine fissured bur, through the labial cortex from the nasal floor to the level of attached gingiva (4 mm above the alveolar crest). By keeping the finger on the palatal aspect the cut is completed through palatal cortex. When diastemas are present some amount of bone will have to be removed interdentally to close the spaces and approximate the fragments (Fig. 26.41).

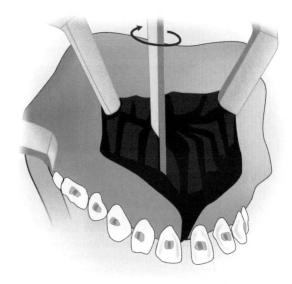

Fig. 26.41: Interdental osteotomies

The alveolar crestal bone is then sectioned with a fine osteotome. Generally, the vertical interdental osteotomy cuts extend into the anterior nasal floor. However, if there is sufficient bone present between the root apex and nasal floor, the separate horizontal cut can be taken, leaving the nasal floor intact. The osteotomized segment is then mobilized into the desired position by using fine osteotome. The occlusal splint is positioned into place and suturing is done.

When multiple, large (4 to 6 mm) diastemas are present, then multiple vertical interdental soft tissue incisions can be taken. The vertical incisions permit the labial mucoperiosteal pedicle to move more freely in addition to having better attachment to the individual segment.

Anterior maxillary osteotomy (Figs 26.42 and 26.43): This is a very frequently used most popular technique for the correction of dentoalveolar protrusion of the anterior maxilla. Correction is accomplished with an anterior maxillary osteotomy with or without a midline split. The anterior segment can be moved superiorly or inferiorly and posteriorly as indicated. It can also be used in conjunction with mandibular subapical osteotomy for the correction of bimaxillary protrusion. The first anterior maxillary setback was performed by Cohn Stock in 1921. *Wassmund in 1935, modified this procedure and advocated that the bony palate be approached by tunneling the palatal mucosa.* He suggested vertical incisions in between the canine and premolar area extending towards the nasal floor. Additional midline

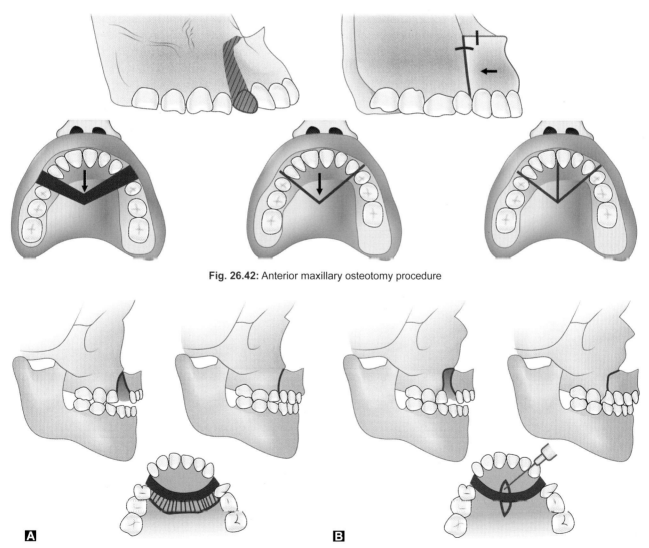

Fig. 26.42: Anterior maxillary osteotomy procedure

Figs 26.43A and B: (A) Wunderer technique, (B) Wassmund technique incision was taken to approach nasal septum and small midpalatal incision, if necessary to complete the palatal cut. *Wunderer* in 1962, further modified the technique by advocating that the palate be approached by an incision taken transversely across the palate, anterior to the planned osteotomy cut. Bony cut is made through the palatal side by reflecting the incision on either side. The anterior segment is pedicled on the labial mucosa (Figs 26.43A and B).

Köle (1959), Heiss (1963) and Steinhauser (1972), described midline splitting of the maxilla. Epker (1980), suggested a horizontal vestibular incision from premolar to premolar region.

Surgical Procedure—(Followed at Our institution) (Figs 26.44A to G)

Normally upper first premolars are extracted on either side. In extreme bimaxillary protrusion both first and second premolars can be extracted to achieve the desired setback of the anterior fragment. In presurgical orthodontic phase, if diastemas are closed after leaving the residual space behind canines, then that space can be used for osteotomy cuts, with or without first premolar extractions, depending on the need. If first molars are carious and unsalvageable, then the vertical cuts can be taken in that available extraction space. Two separate incisions are taken in the buccal vestibule, which allow the preservation of the maximum soft tissue pedicles. One small horizontal incision is taken in the midline to expose the anterior nasal spine (At the end of the surgery, if this incision is sutured length wise, making it vertical, then it will help to increase the upper lip length). Two small horizontal vestibular incisions are taken, one on either side, from canine to first molar region. The mucoperiosteum is elevated superiorly through these incisions to expose the anterior wall of the maxilla and the piriform aperture. Tunneling is done through and through from one side of the incision to another side for achieving proper access and enough mobility for the anterior segment. Careful separation of the nasal mucoperiosteum from the anterior nasal floor and piriform rims is done by using periosteal elevator without tearing the mucosa and without inducing excessive hemorrhage. Inferiorly at the extraction site mucoperiosteum is tunneled till the alveolar crest so that small L-shaped retractor can be placed during osteotomy cuts to prevent damage to the mucoperiosteal flap.

Vertical osteotomies, on the either side using the extraction space are completed through and through the labial and palatal cortices till the level of canine root apices.

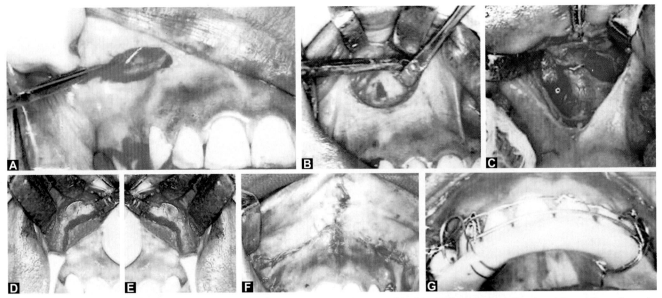

Figs 26.44A to G: Anterior maxillary osteotomy. Intraoperative pictures: (A) Intraoral incision, (B) Periosteal elevator at the piriform fossa to protect nasal mucosa, (C) Midline incision to expose the nasal spine, (D and E) Anterior maxillary osteotomy cuts complete, (F) Inverted Y type suturing for lip lengthening, (G) Prefabricated acrylic splint in position

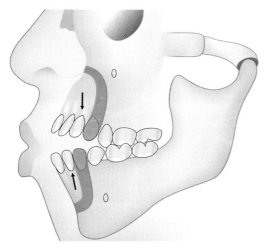

Fig. 26.45: Bimaxillary protrusion can be corrected by anterior maxillary and lower anterior subapical osteotomy procedures

A periosteal elevator is inserted along the lateral nasal wall beneath the nasal mucoperiosteum to protect it during the osteotomy cut. The horizontal osteotomy cut is started from the deepest part of the piriform aperture through the anterior aspect of the lateral nasal wall and 5 mm above the canine root apex and towards the superior end of the vertical cut. During this cut, small retractor is used for proper access and protecting the flap. While carrying out the osteotomy cuts from the labial to palatal side with the bur, a finger is maintained on the palatal mucosa all the while and laceration of the palatal mucosa is prevented by using tactile sense. If a midline split of the anterior maxilla is indicated to expand or narrow the dental arch, then it is completed before final mobilization of the anterior maxilla. It is also important to make the osteotomies through the dentoalveolar

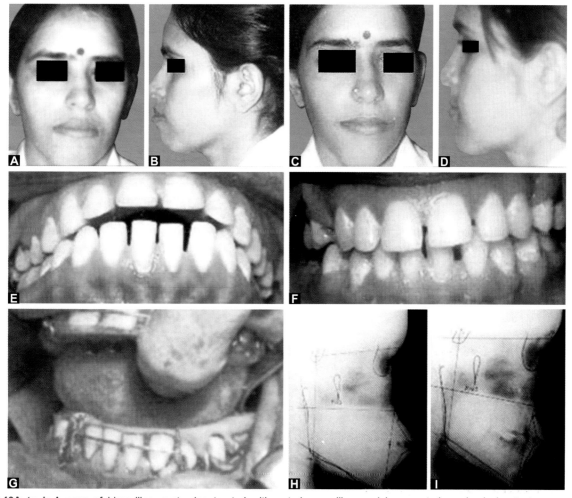

Figs 26.46A to I: A case of bimaxillary protrusion treated with anterior maxillary and lower anterior subapical osteotomy procedures. (A and B) Preoperative front and profile view, (C and D) Postoperative front and profile view, (E and F) Pre and postoperative dental occlusion, (G) Occlusal splints *in situ*, (H and I) Pre and postoperative cephalograms

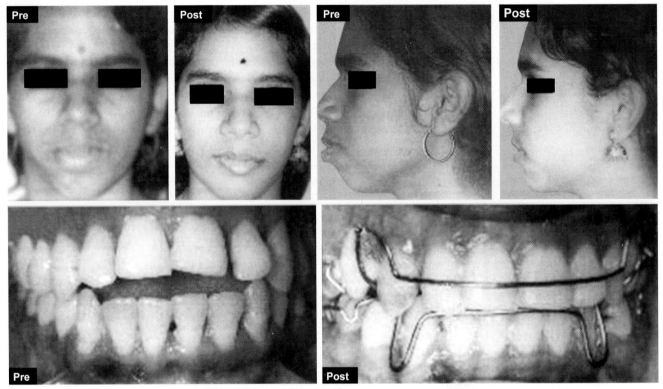

Fig. 26.47: Bimaxillary protrusion treated with surgery

segment towards the osteotomy site on the opposite side. This allows completion of the transpalatal osteotomies easier. Through the small midline incision, the anterior nasal spine is identified and if it is very prominent, then it can be trimmed using ronguer forceps. The nasal septal osteotome is inserted and angled slightly inferiorly to separate the nasal septum. The osteotome is tapped with the hand pressure posteriorly only to the area of the planned transverse palatal osteotomy. The final mobilization of the anterior maxillary segment is done by placing osteotome transpalatally from the vertical cuts going downward and forward. The finger is constantly maintained on the palatal mucosa to avoid laceration. After completion of the transpalatal osteotomy, the anterior maxilla is downfractured with finger pressure. If significant resistance is encountered, then the bony cuts are checked and completed properly.

Following downfracturing, the nasal crest of the maxilla is removed with large round bur, to prevent deviation of the nasal septum, when the segment is repositioned. If the segment is to be placed superiorly, then the midline of the nasal floor can be grooved further.

The occlusal splint is inserted and an attempt is made to place the anterior segment into its predetermined position. If the fragment does not fit properly, then under direct vision the bony interferences are removed selectively. Once the splint is fitted properly, it can be fixed to the maxillary dental arch by interdental wiring. Vertical stability can be achieved by means of intraosseous wiring or bone plates. The two side incisions are closed horizontally with absorbable sutures and midline incision is sutured vertically for lip lengthening. The occlusal splint is kept in place for 3 to 4 weeks.

Advantages of this technique (Figs 26.45 to 26.47):

   i. Simple and versatile procedure.
  ii. Provides direct access to the nasal crest and nasal septum and prevents buckling of the septum.
 iii. Permits removal of the necessary midpalatal bone easily.
 iv. Provides an excellent vascular pedicle.
  v. Complete preservation of palatal pedicle.

Posterior Maxillary Osteotomy (Fig. 26.48)

Originally described by *Schuchardt* in 1959, as a two stage procedure. Now, it is always done as a single stage procedure. The unilateral or bilateral posterior maxillary osteotomy can be used for correction of a wide variety of occlusal and dentofacial discrepancies, which are as follows:

i. To correct crossbite.
ii. To superiorly reposition a supraerupted posterior segment.
iii. To close the posterior open bite by placing it inferiorly, etc.

Access to the osteotomy cuts is taken via a horizontal buccal vestibular incision from the canine to first molar region. The tunneling of the mucoperiosteal flap is done superiorly and inferiorly. By reflecting the mucoperiosteum, lateral maxillary wall and region posterior to the pterygoid plates is exposed.

The level of horizontal osteotomy is marked by scratching with the bur at least 5 mm above the apices of the posterior teeth. The vertical osteotomy cut is done either between the adjoining teeth (interdentally) or by using the extraction site as predetermined. As the horizontal osteotomy extends distal to the second molar, it is tapered inferiorly toward the pterygomaxillary fissure behind the tuberosity region. The horizontal and vertical osteotomy cuts are completed through the palatal cortex by keeping the palpating finger constantly on the palatal mucosa to prevent laceration. Small curved osteotome is used to separate the pterygomaxillary junction and entire posterior segment can be downfractured pedicled on the palatal mucosa. Now the palatal bone can be removed sufficiently under direct vision. After the segment is well mobilized and the planned osteotomies completed, the prefabricated occlusal splint is fitted and wired to the teeth. Direct wire or bone plate fixation can also be done.

LeFort I Osteotomy (Figs 26.49 to 26.61)

The LeFort I osteotomy is another versatile procedure, used frequently to resolve many functional and esthetic problems. This is a very dependable, predictable procedure with low complication rate. Understanding the biological basis of bony osteotomies is very critical. *The revascularization studies* of *Bell* indicate that the maxilla can be mobilized and repositioned and the healing continues, as long as the mobilized maxilla is pedicled on broad soft tissue base. Excellent healing is observed, even if the maxilla is segmented into multiple pieces. The soft tissues of the palate, lateral pharyngeal walls, buccal mucosa provide the vascular channels for healing. There is a rich, anastomosing collateral vasculature present in the facial area which results in excellent repair and healing.

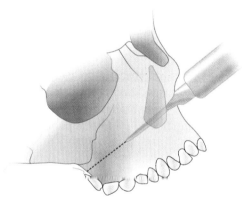

Fig. 26.49: LeFort I osteotomy

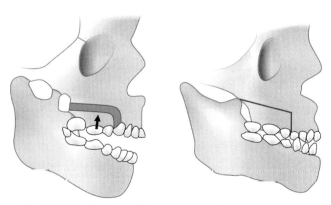

Fig. 26.48: Posterior maxillary osteotomy: Schuchardt technique

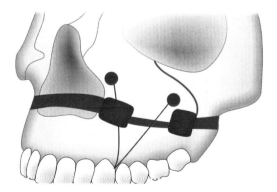

Fig. 26.50: Inferior positioning of maxilla with LeFort I osteotomy, down fracturing and sandwich bone grafts

Indications: The deformities of the maxilla coexist in the multiple planes. Therefore, LeFort I osteotomy can be used to tackle the multifold problems either as a single procedure or in conjunction with mandibular osteotomy procedures.

Whenever required, multiple segmentalization of the maxilla, also can be done.

This procedure is used for surgical repositioning of the entire dentoalveolar segment of the maxilla superiorly, inferiorly, anteriorly and posteriorly, while simultaneously segmentalizing it to widen, narrow, level or improve arch symmetry.

Maxillary Advancement

Indications: Post-trauma patients, cleft lip and palate patients, nasomaxillary hypoplasia, in severe mandibular prognathism to reduce the amount of severe mandibular setback.

This can be done along with simultaneous expansion of the maxilla or narrowing of the maxilla by doing additional midpalatal split of the maxilla.

Inferior Positioning of Maxilla (Fig. 26.50)

Indications: In cases of vertically deficient maxilla, VMD cases, cleft palate cases, bone grafting is necessary after downfracturing of the maxilla. Bone grafts are secured with circumferential wiring or bone plates.

Leveling of Maxilla

Vertical maxillary asymmetry may be idiopathic, but can be also seen associated with hemifacial microsomia, Romberg's disease, unilateral condylar hyperplasia, TMJ ankylosis, etc. The occlusal plane in these conditions is canted transversely, because of either a lack of vertical growth on one side or excessive vertical growth on the opposite side.

The leveling of the maxilla can be done by:
  i. Raising up of one side of the maxilla.
  ii. Lowering one side of the maxilla.
  iii. Simultaneously lowering one side and raising the other side of the maxilla.

The degree of leveling necessary is determined by the clinical evaluation and the posterior, anterior and lateral cephalometric analysis. In adults, it is always necessary to simultaneously reposition the mandible, when the maxilla is being levelled.

Superior Repositioning of the Maxilla (Figs 26.51 to 26.54)

Vertical maxillary excess (VME) cases with typical 'gummy smile' and over-exposure of anterior teeth will require superior repositioning of the maxillary dentoalveolar segment. Vertical maxillary excess (VME) cases are usually presented with coexisting other deformities of the maxilla or mandible or both, including AP (class II malocclusion), transverse (posterior cross, bite) and a vertical (open bite) component. The unique feature of total maxillary surgery or LeFort I osteotomy is that, it permits the simultaneous correction of the vertical, A-P and transverse deformities via appropriate repositioning and segmentalization of the maxilla.

Two basic surgical approaches for superior positioning of maxilla:

Superior Positioning of the Entire Maxilla— LeFort I Osteotomy (Figs 26.51 to 26.56)

Indications:
a. Superior movement less than 5 mm (minor movement).
b. Existing functional nasal septal deviation or excessively large inferior turbinates.
c. Movement of the maxilla as a single unit or minor movement of multiple segments.

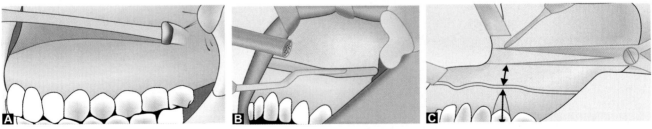

Figs 26.51A to C: LeFort I osteotomy with superior repositioning of maxilla: (A) After vestibular incision subperiosteal tunneling is done, (B) Visualization of the lateral maxillary wall, (C) Reference marks are scored on the bone

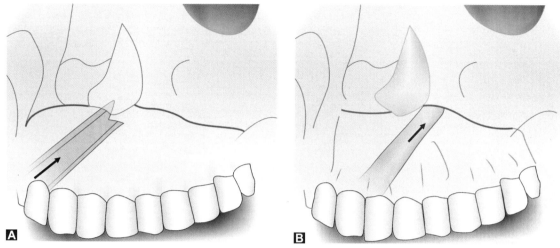

Figs 26.52A and B: Separation of nasal attachments to the maxilla. The septum and vomer are separated from the nasal floor by use of a septal chisel

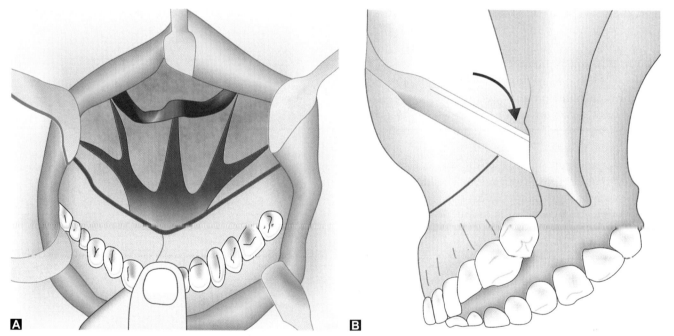

Figs 26.53A and B: (A) Down fracture of the osteotomized maxillary dentoalveolar segment, (B) Osteotome at the pterygomaxillary fissure for disjunction or separation of maxilla from the pterygoid plates

Superior Positioning of the Maxilla Leaving the Nasal Floor Intact (Figs 26.57 to 26.61)

Horseshoe-shaped osteotomy—Modification of LeFort I osteotomy.

Indications:

a. Superior repositioning of 5 to 15 mm (major movement).

b. Pre-existing decreased nasal airway function not related to nasal septum deviation

c. Segmentalization of the maxilla into three to four pieces with considerable movement of the individual segments.

Surgical procedure—LeFort I osteotomy (Figs 26.51 to 26.55): Whenever the vertical changes are planned, it is critical to place an external reference pin and measure to

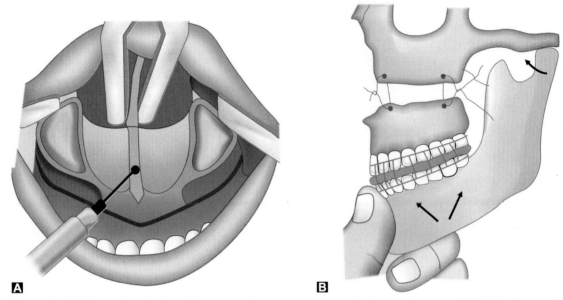

Figs 26.54A and B: (A) LeFort I down fracture. A deep groove is made to accommodate the nasal septum, (B) Guiding the mandible, against the occlusal splint passively and then fixing the fragments with intraosseous wiring

the reproducible point on the maxillary incisors. This is done by placing a Kirschner wire through the skin and into the bone of the nasal bridge.

Intraoral circumvestibular incision is placed high in the buccal vestibule and it extends from the zygomaticomaxillary buttress region anteriorly across the midline. At the midline the incision level is lowered than the posterior region. The incision should be through and through from the mucosa till the periosteum. After completion of the incision bilaterally, the mucoperiosteum is elevated from the anterior aspect of the nasal floor and the anterior aspect of the nasal septum is reflected from the vomerine groove with a periosteal elevator, exposing the anterior floor of the nose. The lateral walls of the maxilla are exposed superiorly and posteriorly, tunneling is carried out till the tuberosity region. No tissue is elevated on the inferior aspect of the circumvestibular incision. The nasal mucoperiosteum is then elevated from the lateral nasal wall beginning at the piriform aperture and extending 10 to 15 mm posteriorly. Once the dissection of the soft tissue is completed, vertical reference points are scratched with the bur at the piriform aperture region, in the canine area and at the zygomaticomaxillary buttress region. Calipers are used to mark a point about 4 mm above the apices of the canine and first molar. These points determine the position of the first osteotomy line.

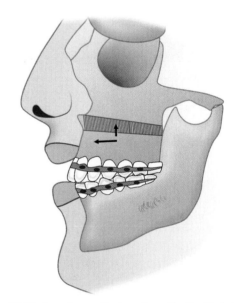

Fig. 26.55: Superior positioning of maxilla. Double LeFort I osteotomy

If superior positioning is to be done then another line is drawn above the first line at a distance equivalent to predetermined superior repositioning.

The periosteal elevator is inserted submucosally at the depth of the piriform aperture and then the osteotomy cut is started from the lateral wall of the

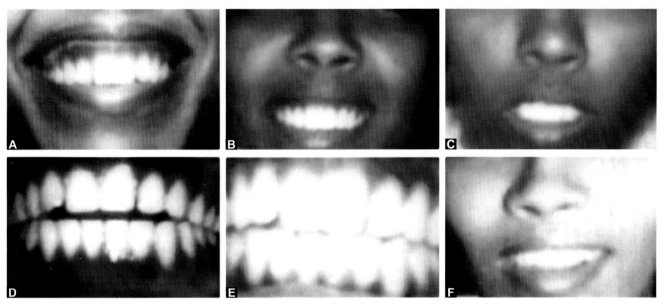

Figs 26.56A to F: LeFort I osteotomy with superior positioning of maxilla for a 22 years old girl with VME, over exposure of gingiva and teeth: (A and B) Gummy smile, (C) Incompetent lips, (D) Preoperative occlusion—anterior open bite, (E) Postoperative occlusion, (F) Postoperative front face. Note the improvement in smile (No gummy smile)

nose, going over the lateral wall of the maxilla, towards zygomaticomaxillary buttress, as the cut extends posteriorly it descends downwards towards the pterygomaxillary fissure. Cut should extend from buccal to palatal bone. After finishing the inferior cut, an identical cut is made superiorly at the predetermined level. The bone in between these two cuts should be removed with the osteotome.

The same procedure is repeated on the opposite side. Finally, pterygomaxillary dysjunction is done by using a curved osteotome, placed behind the tuberosity. The osteotome should be directed downward and inferiorly and light tapping over it will separate the maxillary segment from the ptergygoid plates. Care should be taken that during this procedure the palpating finger is guiding the separation without laceration of the palatal mucosa. The nasal septum osteotome is used to separate nasal septum. A straight osteotome is used to cut the lateral nasal wall posteriorly. The entire maxilla is then downfractured with either manual manipulation or maxillary mobilization forceps. A deep groove is made in the midline with round bur to accommodate nasal septum or alternatively, the inferior portion of the nasal septum is resected to avoid deviation of the nasal septum. Bony interferences at the lateral wall of the nose, posterior tuberosity area should be trimmed

with rongeur and superior positioning of the maxilla is checked. If the maxilla is to be segmentalized, then the vertical interdental osteotomies or osteotomies through the extraction sockets are completed first. The transverse palatal osteotomy can be easily done under direct vision by downfracturing the maxilla inferiorly. After complete mobilization of the maxilla, an occlusal splint is fixed to the osteotomized segment and mandible should be guided passively against the splint, with condyles seated in the fossa. Temporary IMF is done and vertical correction of the maxilla is checked by measuring the calipers. If required, additional bone can be removed by downfracturing the maxilla and pushing it up superiorly after that. The final fixation is done by means of intraosseous wiring or small bone plates at piriform aperture and at zygomaticomaxillary buttress.

Superior Positioning of Maxilla—Leaving the Nasal Floor Intact (Horseshoe-shaped Osteotomy) (Figs 26.57 and 26.59)

Whenever more than 5 to 6 mm of superior positioning of the maxilla is required, the nasal cavity size will be reduced and flaring of the alar bases of the nose will be seen with highly unesthetic results. In order to prevent this undesirable outcome, whenever large amount of

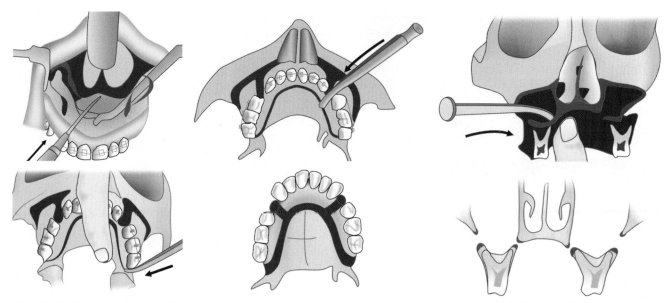

Fig. 26.57: Superior positioning of the maxilla leaving the nasal floor intact. Horseshoe-shaped osteotomy. Modification of LeFort I osteotomy

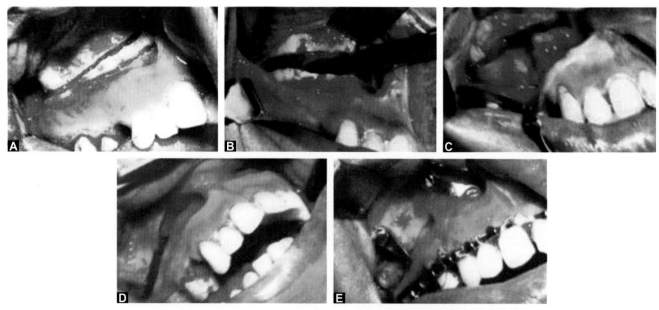

Figs 26.58A to E: A modified LeFort I horseshoe-shaped osteotomy with segmentalization: (A) Double LeFort-I osteotomy cuts only on the buccal cortex, (B) Horse-shoe osteotomy being completed with osteotome after bur cutting, leaving nasal floor intact, (C) After upper first premolars were extracted, anterior segmental osteotomy was carried out, (D) Telescoping of maxillary osteotomized segments and anterior segment pushback, (E) Final fixation with bone plating

superior positioning is required, modified LeFort I osteotomy is carried out.

Horseshoe-shaped osteotomy of the palatal vault, including the dentoalveolar segment and sparing the central palatal vault intact, will allow maximum amount of superior positioning of the maxilla. Here, telescoping of the posterior segments of the maxilla into the maxillary

sinus can be done. The nasal floor is kept intact in spite of maximum superior positioning of the maxilla.

The soft tissue incision and lateral bony wall cuts are same as described earlier. Only after finishing the LeFort I horizontal osteotomy cut through the buccal cortex, vertical interdental or segmental cuts through the extraction sockets are completed. A fissure bur is

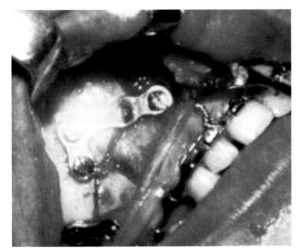

Fig. 26.59: LeFort I osteotomy with segmentalization. Fixation of the fragments is done with L-shaped bone plate and screws

used to begin the transnasal osteotomy through the palate. A finger is kept on the palate to detect the bur as it perforates the palatal cortex. The transpalatal cut is made systematically beginning anterior to the nasal floor and progressing in a lateral and posterior direction into the medial aspect of the antral floor. The transantral cut is usually extended only till the first molar area, thus avoiding injury to the greater palatine neurovascular bundle. Posterior to the first molar, the palatal bone is relatively thin and it can be easily fractured along the palatomaxillary and pterygomaxillary suture areas with curved osteotome with gentle tapping. The maxilla is thus downfractured excluding the nasal floor. This can be achieved by inserting one or two osteotomes into the transnasal portion of the palatal osteotomy between the stable nasal floor and osteotomized

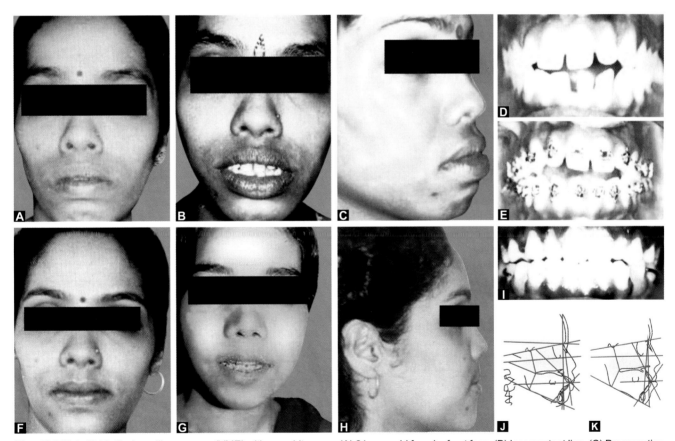

Figs 26.60A to K: Vertical maxillary excess (VME) with open bite case: (A) 21-year-old female, front face, (B) Incompetent lips, (C) Preoperative profile view, (D) Preoperative occlusion with anterior open bite with spaces, (E) Presurgical orthodontics. No attempt was made to treat the open bite. Spaces closed and gathered behind canine teeth, (F and G) Postoperative front face after LeFort I osteotomy with superior positioning with horseshoe-shaped modification and with anterior maxillary osteotomy, (H) Postoperative profile, (I) Postoperative occlusion, (J) Preoperative cephalogram, (K) Postoperative cephalogram

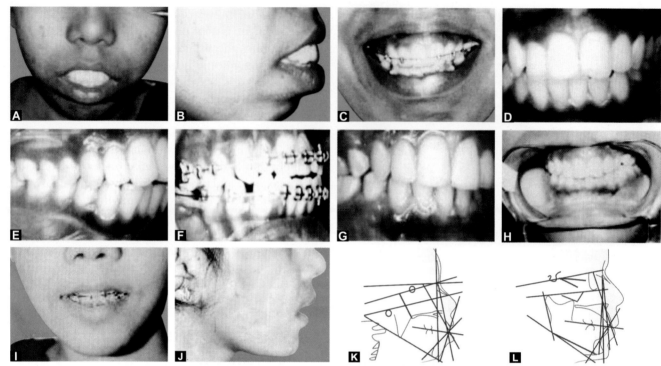

Figs 26.61A to L: Vertical maxillary excess (VME) without open bite case. LeFort I osteotomy—Horseshoe with anterior maxillary osteotomy. (A and B) Preoperative front and profile views, (C) Gummy smile, (D and E) Preoperative occlusion, (F) Presurgical orthodontics, (G and H) Postoperative occlusion, (I and J) Postoperative front and profile views, (K and L) Pre and postoperative cephalograms

dentoalveolar maxillary segment. Whenever excess superior positioning is required, usually large amount of bone is present vertically between the apices of anterior teeth and the nasal floor. After finishing the anterior segmentalization sparing the nasal floor, a horizontal bony wedge can be removed 5 mm above the canine roots. This will allow maximum vertical superior repositioning of the anterior segment without encroaching the nasal cavity. The rest of the procedure will remain the same as described earlier.

Surgical planning for VME cases: Depending on the severity of the deformity, the surgical planning of VME cases needs different procedures to be carried out. They are as follows:

1. a. Superior positioning of the maxilla via total maxillary osteotomy.
    b. Superior positioning of the maxilla via segmental maxillary osteotomy. Autorotation of the mandible brings the chin forward and upward (no need for mandibular surgery).
2. Superior positioning of the maxilla, combined with advancement of the mandible via a ramus osteotomy.
3. Same as (2) plus anterior mandibular subapical osteotomy and segmentalization of maxilla.
4. Additional genioplasty procedure.

S E C T I O N

Maxillofacial Trauma

5

27

Basic Principles for the Management of Maxillofacial Injuries

In view of the large and ever increasing number of facial injuries, it is mandatory for each clinician to have at least some knowledge regarding the primary care and proper referral. Each person subjected to the ordinary risk of everyday life, is a potential candidate for trauma to the face. Various methods for handling maxillofacial trauma have been evolved after the mass casualties which resulted from world wars.

No fixed protocol can govern the treatment of an injured individual, but fundamental principles of treatment with sound surgical basis should be always followed.

  i. Prompt and thorough assessment of injured patient.
 ii. Life threatening situations should be quickly recognized and treated.
iii. Acute trauma care involves many specialities, therefore, proper specialized consultations are asked for.

Treatment of a facial injury should be guided by the functions of the face and its components. *Facial trauma must be considered in a slightly different light than similar trauma elsewhere in the body; where function is the primary concern in a repair. In facial trauma, restoration of a function and esthetics is a must, otherwise a minor facial injury, if not treated properly can become serious problem due to psychological impact.* It is also important to note that

properly executed initial repair of the facial injury often gives better results than multiple secondary procedures. Furthermore, prolonged hospitalization, disability and added expenses can be avoided. Inadequate primary treatment may result in severe deformities, which may be difficult to treat later on without good results. However, even after proper initial primary treatment, there may be need for secondary surgery. This possibility should be discussed with the patient and his/her family.

GENERAL CARE OF THE INJURED PATIENT

General Considerations

When a patient with a severe maxillofacial injury is first seen, an immediate general evaluation must be made to determine if emergency treatment is necessary. Hemorrhage, shock, spinal cord injuries, cardiac arrest, airway obstruction can cause early fatality. Intracranial hemorrhage with associated skull fractures, fractured ribs with pneumothorax or hemothorax, rupture of the spleen or kidney can also pose an immediate danger.

After thorough systemic evaluation and emergency treatment, priorities for treating all injuries can be established. One should not rush into the treatment of an obvious facial injuries prior to complete evaluation. At the same time for some insignificant associated injury, the treatment for facial injury should not be delayed. Soft tissue injuries should be treated within 6 to 8 hours or sooner, whenever feasible. If possible, facial fractures should be treated at the time of the soft tissue repair with the fracture reduction and fixation being done first.

BASIC PRINCIPLES OF TREATMENT OF A SEVERE MAXILLOFACIAL INJURIES

1. Preservation of life.
2. Maintenance of function.
3. Restoration of appearance (esthetics).

In preservation of life, immediate prompt emergency treatment should be instituted by involving various specialities' care.

BASIC ABCs TO BE FOLLOWED FOR PRESERVATION OF LIFE

A: Airway patency maintenance.
B: Bleeding control.
C: Consciousness restoration, circulation maintenance.
Otherwise,
D: Death will follow.

A: Maintenance of Patency of Airway

Maintenance of patency of airway must be given priority consideration, since adequate oxygenation is vital to life (Fig. 27.1).

Maintenance of the airway is dependent on the following:

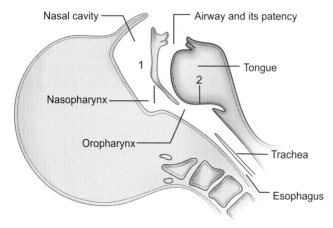

Fig. 27.1: Airway and its patency: (1) Nasopharyngeal airway, (2) Oropharyngeal airway

1. The absence of any anatomical or mechanical barrier.
2. The preservation of the laryngeal reflex.
3. The existence of adequate pulmonary ventilation.
4. The integrity of the respiratory center.

The tissue hypoxia or anoxia is related to the integrity of the respiratory center, the preservation of cough reflex, the efficiency of pulmonary ventilation and the oxygen carrying capacity of the blood. A simple persistent bleeding due to nasal fracture in an unconscious patient, who is lying supine and whose reflexes are depressed by alcohol or drugs, can easily prove to be fatal. Wounds involving tongue, larynx, pharynx with surgical emphysema can bring about airway obstruction. Patient with associated head injury with a deterioration in the level of consciousness may be having depression of the respiratory center. Associated injuries to the lungs may produce 'flail chest' with paradoxical respiration. Pneumothorax, hemothorax, traumatic asphyxia may reduce the pulmonary efficiency.

Clinical Signs and Symptoms of Respiratory Distress (Obstruction)

i. Initially there will be restlessness, apprehension, anxiety.
ii. Tachypnea, tachycardia, pallor.
iii. Rapid, labored breathing (gasping for breath).
iv. Rapid movement or fluttering of the alae of the nose.
v. Crowing sound, stridor, intercostals retraction.
vi. Suprasternal indrawing of the tissues or supra-clavicular retraction.
vii. Decreasing ventilatory excursions, hypercarbia, hypertension.
viii. Progressive cyanosis (may be present with Hb less than 5 gm).

Causes of Respiratory Obstructions Related to Maxillofacial Injuries (Fig. 27.2)

1. Inhalation of blood clot, vomit, saliva, thick mucus or portions of teeth, bone and dentures.
2. Inability to protrude the tongue, because of the posterior displacement of the anterior fragment of the mandible (Bilateral parasymphysis mandibular fractures).
3. Occlusion of the oropharynx by the soft palate after retroposition of the maxilla (fractured maxilla).

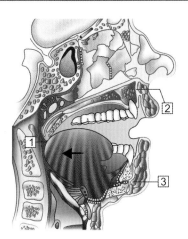

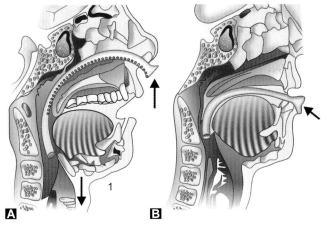

Fig. 27.2: (1) Critical airway obstruction may be seen due to, (2) Retroposition of the maxilla after severe maxillofacial injury, (3) Tongue fall after bilateral parasymphysis mandibular fracture

Figs 27.4A and B: Nonsurgical treatment for airway maintenance after severe maxillofacial trauma: (A) Nasopharyngeal airway tube *in situ*, (B) Oropharyngeal airway tube *in situ*

Treatment for Airway Maintenance (Nonsurgical) (Figs 27.3 and 27.4)

Position of the patient: Supine with neck extended or head turned sideways or patient can be made prone with head down, so that the collection of saliva or blood in the mouth can be thrown out instead of aspiration (Figs 27.3A and B).

Oropharyngeal toilet: All blood clot, saliva, thick mucus or foreign bodies, etc. should be cleared from the oral cavity and throat by digital exploration or by using cotton swabs, if available.

Suction. If the suction machine is available, then catheters should be used to clear the nose, oral cavity and throat.

Anterior traction of the tongue: Control the tongue by the proper positioning of the patient already described or the tongue can be pulled out and it can be maintained in the forward position by using tongue suture or towel clip attached to the patient's shirt collar.

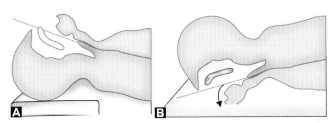

Figs 27.3A and B: Position of the injured patient during transportation: (A) Supine position with head extended, (B) Head turned sideways or downward

Immediate restoration of the position of the soft palate: It can be brought about by doing disimpaction of the maxillary fracture. This is achieved by placing index and middle finger into the mouth hooking behind the soft palate and thumb placed on the alveolus in the incisor region. Head is stabilized by counter pressure with other hand over the forehead. Strong anterior and downward traction will bring the maxilla in the normal position. Immediately one or two well lubricated nasopharyngeal tubes should be inserted to maintain the airway.

  I. Unfavorable mandibular fracture also should be reduced and temporary stabilization with dental wiring should be carried out to prevent the tongue fall.

  II. Mouth to mouth breathing.

  III. Oro or nasopharyngeal airways can be used (Figs 27.4A and B).

  IV. Endotracheal intubation as soon as possible.

Surgical Treatment

A tracheostomy may be indicated in extensive maxillofacial injuries (Figs 27.5A to D).

Indications

a. Lack of tongue control.

b. Gross retroposition of middle third of the facial skeleton.

c. Actual or potential edema of pharynx or glottis.

d. Uncontrollable oro/nasopharyngeal bleeding.

e. Respiratory inadequacy—pulmonary or central nervous system—CNS. In case of dire emergency, a lifesaving oxygen supply can be delivered by puncturing into the tracheal lumen with a 12 or 14 gauge needle for a short time, till adequate airway management is done. In tracheostomized patient, the airway must be monitored carefully. Secretions should be sucked away frequently.

B: Bleeding or Hemorrhage Control

Prompt control of post-traumatic bleeding is a must. Initial digital compression should be given to control the bleeding. Compression dressings also can be used. Major vessels which are cut, should be clamped or ligated. Soft tissue wounds which are deep and extensive should be sutured immediately. Deep wounds also can be packed with gauze till definite measures are taken.

Nasal bleeding can be stopped by using ribbon gauze packing soaked in 1:1000 adrenaline. In some of the cases postnasal packing may be necessary. Anterior nasal packing can be done in addition to postnasal packing (Figs 27.6A to C).

C: Consciousness Restoration/Circulation Maintenance

Initial assessment of the patient will reveal whether the loss of consciousness is due to intracranial injuries or because of hemorrhagic or neurogenic shock.

If the patient is in a state of shock, an immediate venipuncture or a cut down should be performed. A blood sample is sent for cross matching and IV fluids should be started to restore the circulating blood volumes. As soon as possible, blood transfusion can be started. Adjuvant measures like relieving the pain, making the patient comfortable, gentle handling and compression dressings and splinting of fractures can be done simultaneously. Close observation of a patient should be done. All vital parameters like pulse, respiration and blood pressure should be monitored. Control of infection and pain also should be done by administering adequate antibiotics and anti-inflammatory analgesics through IV route. Antitetanus protection also should be thought about. Tetanus antitoxin or toxoid be given immediately. Adequate nutrition also should be planned in order to have speedy recovery. High calorie, high protein diet is helpful. Nasogastric tube feeding may be necessary in severe maxillofacial injuries. Supplementary vitamin therapy should be given.

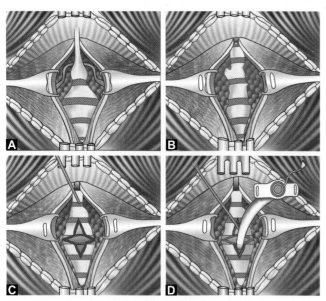

Figs 27.5A to D: Tracheostomy procedure

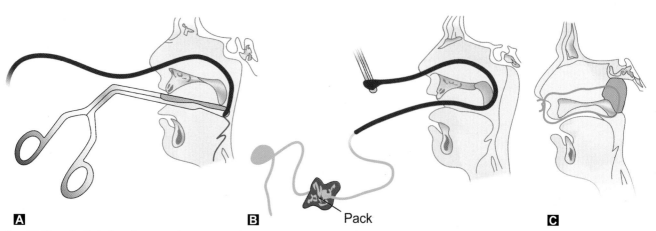

Figs 27.6A to C: Technique for controlling bleeding from the nasal cavity: (A) Catheter passed through the nostril and brought out through oral cavity, (B) Gauze pack tied to the oral end of catheter and nostril end is pulled out to bring the pack upwards, (C) Nasal pack *in situ*

SOFT TISSUE INJURIES

1. Thorough wound cleaning.
2. Gentle tissue handling.
3. Meticulous repair.

} Excellent healing of a facial injury

Facial lacerations should be repaired at the earliest time as soon as patient's general condition allows. Early wound repair lessens edema and prevents the formation of granulation tissue and infection. This will lead toward minimum scar formation. Preferably the facial wounds should be repaired within six to eight hours. Because of excellent blood supply to the facial region, if necessary, safe primary repair can be done even after one or two days.

Wound Management

Prerequisites of wound repair are meticulous wound cleansing and hemostasis. A gauze piece moistened with betadine solution is initially spread over the wound to protect it further from contamination. Surrounding skin of the facial wound should be cleaned gently with liberal application of warm saline, dilute cetavlon or dilute hydrogen peroxide, taking care to swab away from the wound margins. A male patient should be cleanly shaven and female patients should have all cosmetics removed. *The eyebrows should never be shaved*. A careful wound examination including palpation should be carried out to detect foreign bodies (Blood clots, dirt, wooden splinters, broken teeth, denture pieces, glass pieces, tar, hair, bone splinters, etc.). Palpation of these foreign bodies should be done at the depth of the wound, as well as by bimanual palpation. In automobile accidents the dirt or road tar can be embedded in the tissue depth. Solvents, such as ether or benzene, may be needed to remove tar, oil, grease or paint from a wound. Tissue holding forceps or scalpel can be used to remove the embedded foreign matter. To prevent fibrosis or traumatic tattooing of the skin, it is absolutely mandatory to remove these foreign particles.

After the surrounding skin is cleaned and wound palpation and removal of foreign particles is over, then the wound should be irrigated with copious amount of saline solution. Gentle handling of the wound is absolutely necessary. Intraoral wounds also should be thoroughly cleaned with copious saline solution with suction. The eyes also should be carefully irrigated with warm normal saline and inspection should be done for any ocular damage. Laceration of the scalp may be masked due to blood crust, entangled hair, etc. Washing of the area and careful inspection should be done. Conservative approach is chosen as far as debridement of the facial wound is concerned. Hemostasis is also essential for good wound healing. Atraumatic instruments should be used to handle the facial wounds. Fine skin hooks and Adson's tissue holding forceps are very helpful in handling the tissue with a minimum degree of trauma. Gentle sponging of tissues should be done. Approximation of the tissues should be done using finest suture material.

Types of Soft Tissue Wounds and Management (Figs 27.7 and 27.8)

Abrasions

Abrasions caused by the frictional violence, due to friction between an object and surface of the soft tissue. It is presented as raw bleeding areas. The wound is superficial and it denudes the epidermis, occasionally involves deeper layers. Abrasion involves the terminal nerve endings of many nerve fibers and it can be quite painful. Commonly seen as scraps and re-epithelialization occurs without scarring. While deep abrasions may require skin grafting. Abrasions may be contaminated depending on the surroundings. Foreign matter embedding contributes to traumatic tattooing of the skin, foreign body reaction or fibrosis and infection, with delayed wound healing (Figs 27.8A to G).

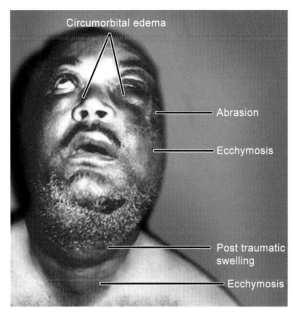

Fig. 27.7A: Clinical picture of a patient, who has sustained a maxillofacial trauma

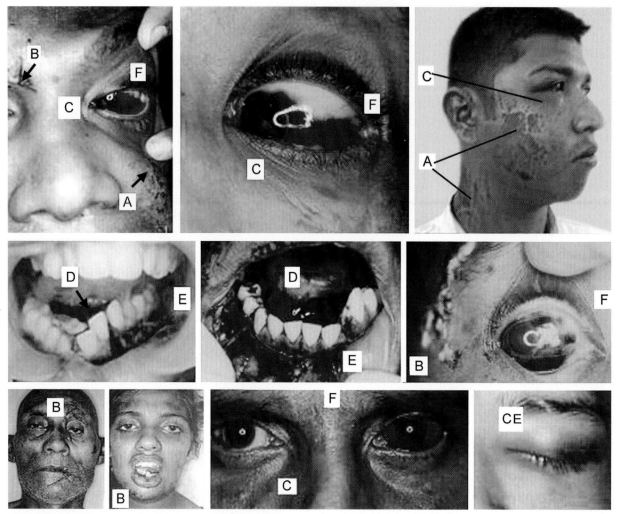

Fig. 27.7B: Different soft tissue wounds in the orofacial region: A—Abrasion, B—CLW sutured, C—Circumorbital ecchymosis, D—Lingual hematoma, E—Intraoral ecchymosis, F—Subconjunctival hemorrhage, CE—Circumorbital edema

Thorough cleaning with profuse saline irrigation, removal of the foreign material, gentle scrubbing with the soft brush to remove sticky material to prevent tattooing, use of surgical soap is required to be done prior to dressing. Topical application of antibiotic ointment with compression dressing promotes good healing. Superficial abrasions can be covered with topical antibiotic application and left open. Slowly the crust of dried blood and serum will form a scab and it will fall off as the healing takes place.

Contusion

Contusion is caused by a blow or fall against a hard or blunt object. Blood extravasates in the subcutaneous or submucous tissue leading to bluish area or bruise. Subcutaneous bleeding is self limiting. This is without

break into the soft tissue surface. Discoloration of the skin or mucosa causes ecchymosis. Important for diagnosis and search for an osseous trauma/fracture is mandatory. Application of ice pack will help to stop further extravasation of blood.

Areas of *ecchymosis* which becomes evident in 48 hours will be seen as bluish black marks and these fade away with change in variety of colors as blue, green, yellow, etc.

Hematomas

Hematomas are localized collection of blood in the subcutaneous or intramuscular or submucosal space. It may be deeply seated or superficial. Contusions and hematomas may be associated with a fracture or rupture of a vessel or vessels. Careful examination may be repeated and

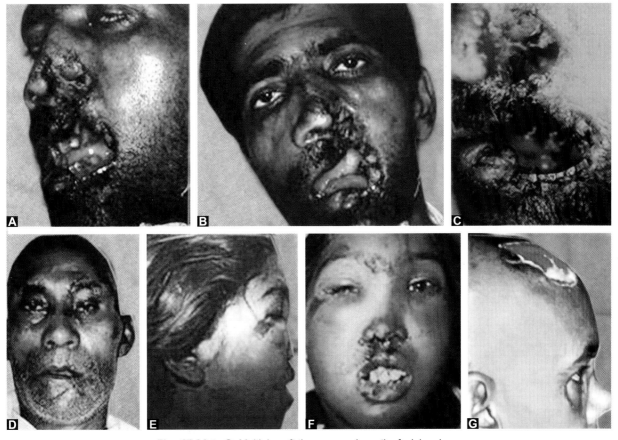

Figs 27.8A to G: Multiple soft tissue wounds on the facial region

X-ray examination is essential for proper diagnosis and treatment. Most hematomas are reabsorbed. Persistent hematoma may require incision and drainage. It cannot be aspirated as blood is partly clotted. Antibiotic cover should be given to prevent hematoma from getting infected.

Lacerated Wounds

Lacerated wounds are most frequent type of soft tissue injuries. Here the tearing of mucosal tissue or skin is seen due to vehicular accidents, low velocity missiles (pistol) or bomb splinters. The margins are contused and lacerated in deep wounds, the muscles are also lacerated and devitalized. There may be associated injury to the underlying vessels, nerves and bone. These wounds are usually highly contaminated with dust, mud, greasy material, tar, glass pieces, bone splinters, etc. *Thorough cleaning, minimum debridement, removal of foreign bodies and proper suturing* (as early as possible) are the steps in the management. Closure should be done in multiple layers (muscle, dermis, epidermis and submucosa and

mucosal closure). These may be superficial or deep. CLW means contused lacerated wounds.

Incised Wounds

Incised wounds are caused by a sharp cutting objects such as knife, dagger, glass piece, tin edge, etc. These are clear cut, gaping, bleeding wounds with minimum contamination. Deep wounds can bring about damage to the vital organs leading towards major complications. The wound should be taken care as early as possible. The wound is cleaned, explored and the bleeding arrested. The wound is closed by primary intention.

Penetrating and Punctured Wounds

Punctured wounds are caused by pointed objects like a knife, bullet, bomb splinter, etc. These wounds are highly deceptive as externally they may appear small, but may be deep penetrating endangering vital organs. Careful clinical examination, X-ray examination and other special investigation may be required.

Crushed Wounds

Crushed wound is caused by road accidents, or a machinery accidents. Crushing of the parts with lacerated skin, devitalization or crushing of the musculature is seen. Damage to blood vessels and nerves with associated profuse bleeding is also observed. The bone/bones are shattered. The wound is highly contaminated. There can be loss of soft/hard tissue.

Gunshot Injuries (High Velocity Missile)

Gunshot injuries are in reality penetrating wounds, but are classified separately, because of the extensiveness of the wounds and the special problems which arise during their management. They are subclassified as: (i) penetrating wounds, when the missile is retained in the wound, (ii) perforating wounds, when the missile produces another wound of exit, (iii) avulsive wounds, when large portion of the soft or osseous structures are destroyed. These wounds are produced by projectiles fired from a gun or fragments of a shell. They may be seen in civilian life or war injuries. Depending upon the speed, shape and striking angle of the projectile, the character of the wound will vary.

High velocity bullets: Small wound of entry and large, ragged wounds of exit. Fragmentation of teeth, bone may serve as secondary missiles, causing extensive internal trauma.

Low velocity projectiles: They become distorted upon meeting resistance and cause comminution and internal damage. Crushing of tissues due to its direct pressure effect around a small area of the track. The necrosed tissues, particularly the devitalized muscles are good nidus for infection.

Multiple metallic foreign bodies are retained in these wounds. The pellets of a gunshot are sterile and they can splinter further, and are seen embedded in the soft and hard tissues at various levels. If usual wound care is not sufficient, then after primary treatment, extensive reconstructive surgery is needed to restore the facial contour.

Treatment of Lacerated Wounds

  i. Cleaning of wound
 ii. Removal of foreign bodies
iii. Debridement
 iv. Hemostasis
  v. Closure in layers—primary closure
 vi. Dressing

 vii. Prevention of infection
viii. Pain control
 ix. Follow-up.

Supportive Therapy

Drains: Superficial wounds do not require drainage. Deeper wounds, particularly, those involving oral cavity, require insertion of penrose or rubber drain. Drains may be placed between the sutures or through dependent stab incision. Drains should be removed after 2 to 4 days.

Dressings: Sofratulle or antibiotic ointment along with dry gauze dressing should be changed in 48 hours. Large wounds need pressure dressing. Sutures can be removed on 5 to 7th day.

Prevention of infection: Strict adherence to sterile technique, wound closure by eliminating all dead spaces and adequate supportive antibiotic therapy and follow up is necessary.

Prophylaxis against tetanus: Whenever there is a inclusion of dirt and debris in the wound, protection against infection by the *Clostridium tetani* organism must be provided. In a person who has been immunized with previous inoculation with the tetanus toxoid, a 'booster' dose of 1 ml of tetanus toxoid should be given as soon as possible. Passive immunity can be produced by administering 1500 units of tetanus antitoxin at weekly intervals, until 3 doses have been given.

Factors Modifying Wound Healing or Leading Towards Failure

  i. Too tight suturing without adequate drainage, may lead towards wound breakdown
 ii. Inadequate pressure dressing—collection of hematoma.
iii. Oral contamination of the wound, with inade-quate closure on the oral mucosa side.
 iv. Secondary hemorrhage.
  v. Inadequate antibiotic therapy.
 vi. Improper asepsis.
vii. Secondary rough handling of the wound.

Inaccurate skin repair, dead tissue, foreign bodies inclusion, compromised vascularity, infection, lack of rest and constant movement and irradiation, delays can hamper the wound healing. General factors like old age, anemia, lack of vitamin C, systemic diseases like diabetes, hepatitis, steroid therapy may delay healing.

Injuries of the Maxillofacial Skeleton

Because of the complex bony structure of the maxillofacial region, any treatment for the extensive injury is quite challenging. Proper attention should be paid towards the restoration of function as well as esthetics.

The facial skeleton is divided into three parts:
  i. Upper third—formed by the frontal bone.
  ii. Middle third—from the frontal bone to the level of upper teeth, or upper alveolus, if patient is edentulous.
  iii. Lower third—the mandible.

Fractures of the middle third of the facial skeleton and/or the mandible are known as 'maxillofacial skeletal injuries' and they can be associated with varying degrees of injuries of the soft tissues. The injuries can vary in severity from simple crack to major fractures of the entire facial skeleton. Incidence of occurrence of maxillofacial injuries is ever increasing due to the fast pace of life and increased violence in addition to the advent of rapid modes of transportations.

ETIOLOGY OF MAXILLOFACIAL INJURIES (TABLE 28.1)

1. Typical causes
   i. Direct violence
   ii. Indirect violence

Table 28.1: Typical causes of maxillofacial injuries
Due to direct violence
a. Altercation, battery, interpersonal fights.
b. Fist fight, blows due to stick, metal rods, bricks, etc.
c. Fall.
d. Road traffic accidents.
e. Occupation hazards (Athletic injury, industrial mishaps).
f. Iatrogenic causes—during dental treatment. Fracture of a tooth, alveolus, maxillary tuberosity, fracture of mandible, etc.
Indirect violence
a. Fall from a height.
b. Counter coup fractures
Due to Excessive Muscle Contraction (Fracture of Coronoid Process).

2. Crush injuries
   i. Automobile accidents/Road traffic accidents (RTA)
   ii. Aeroplane crashes
   iii. Mining accidents
3. High velocity missiles.
4. Predisposing causes:
   a. Local causes: Presence of cysts, osteomyelitis, tumors, presence of third molars, etc.
   b. Systemic causes: Systemic diseases affecting the formation of the structure of the bone.

Most of the severe injuries are caused by road traffic accidents (RTA), when the vehicle driver suddenly puts the break, the head hits the dashboard, steering wheel or the windshield. The various safety measures to be used are seat belts, dashboard padding, telescoping steering wheel, push-away windshield and dashboards with recessed or absent knobs. Now the seat belts are available for all the passengers, whether front seat or back seat. There is a legislation for the compulsory wearing of seat belts in cars, and compulsory wearing of crash helmets for motorcyclists.

Preliminary Examination

After initial steps for preservation of life are taken satisfactorily and patient has been stabilized, then a full examination of the patient is carried out to detect the presence of associated important injuries.

Head injury: To assess the level of consciousness 'Glasgow coma scale' is used. This scale relates clinical observations for motor response, verbal response and eye examination and its responses (Table 28.2). The skull or cranium examination should be carried out for any obvious lacerations or fractures. Level of consciousness also should be assessed:

Table 28.2: Glasgow coma scale
Eye opening—(E)
4—Opens eyes spontaneously
3—Opens eyes to voice
2—Opens eyes to pain
1—No eye opening
Best motor response—(M)
6—Obeys commands
5—Localizes to pain
4—Withdraws to pain
3—Abnormal flexor response
2—Abnormal extensor response
1—No movement
Best verbal response—(V)
5—Appropriate and oriented
4—Confused conversation
3—Inappropriate words
2—Incomprehensible sounds
1—No sounds

i. Fully conscious,
ii. Drowsy patient with disorientation, but responds rationally to spoken questions,
iii. Semiconscious patient, responding irrationally to spoken questions,
iv. Unconscious patient, but responds to painful stimuli (semi coma),
v. Unconscious with no response to painful stimuli (coma). The degree and duration of loss of consciousness is an important indication for the severity of the cerebral damage.

Retrograde amnesia: It is an inability to recall events leading upto the accident.

Anterograde amnesia: It is the failure to remember events immediately following the accident.

Whenever, patient is admitted in an unconscious state with maxillofacial injuries, it may not be due to head injury. Sudden loss of consciousness may be following epileptic fits or cerebral and cardiovascular disasters. The level of consciousness may be also influenced by the action of alcohol or other drugs intake, hypoglycemia or hyperglycemia. Eyes, the spine, the limbs, abdomen and chest should be checked properly. Specialist consultations from neurologist, ophthalmologist, general surgeon should be sought in cases of extensive injuries.

Trauma team: General, cardiothoracic, vascular, orthopedic surgeons, neurosurgeon, anesthesiologist, ophthalmologist, urologists, ENT surgeons, plastic surgeons and maxillofacial surgeons and paramedical staff.

The complete record of the detailed examination for maxillofacial injuries is considered under following steps and it should be preserved for evidence in medicolegal cases.

i. History of the injury to the patient.
ii. General condition on admission.
iii. Extraoral examination.
iv. Intraoral examination.
v. Radiological examination.

History of the Injury to the Patient

A proper history is mandatory for proper diagnosis of facial injuries. A detailed history of the injury should be obtained from the patient, provided he/she is rational and co-operative, otherwise it can be obtained from the relatives, accompanying person or witness at the time of injury.

1. *Who*—The identity of the patient should be ascertained. Name, age, sex, address, phone number, etc. should be recorded.

2. *When*—The date and time of injury should be noted. This will indicate whether it is fresh or old injury. If the patient comes for early treatment, then prognosis is better.

3. *Where*—The surroundings of the injury place is important for knowing the possibility and degree of bacterial or chemical contamination of the wound. Here, the history of tetanus prophylaxis also should be asked and whether patient has received early care elsewhere also should be ascertained.

4. *How*—The mode of injury—the type of violence and direction of the force may give some indication of the nature and extent of the injury. It is also important for medicolegal cases like child abuse, husband or relatives hitting a lady or road traffic accidents.

   If patient gives history of epileptic fit and subsequent fall on the chin or soldier fainting on parade, then midline fracture of the mandible with possible fracture of condylar neck can be suspected.

5. *What* type of treatment was provided earlier (if the patient comes from other center) should be known.

6. *What* is the general health of the patient? Obtaining pertinent medical history may be facilitated by using the AMPLE mnemonic.
   A : Allergies
   M : Medications
   P : Past illness
   L : Last meal
   E : Events related to the injury.
   History of drug allergy, bleeding disorders, pre existing systemic bone diseases, neoplasia with potential metastases, arthritis, related collagen disorders, nutritional and metabolic disorders, endocrine diseases should be asked. Medical and psychiatric problems influencing the management should be ascertained.

7. *Previous history of trauma* also should be recorded for medicolegal purpose.

8. *Length of unconsciousness* also should be recorded for knowing the degree of head injury and proper referral. Prior to subjecting the patient for general anesthesia, neurosurgical clearance should be obtained.

9. *Any history of* pain, vomiting, unconsciousness, amnesia, headache, visual disturbances, confusion after the accident, malocclusion should be noted.

10. *History of amount of bleeding* from various sites—extraoral wound, intraoral wound, nose, ear, etc. should be asked for.

11. *Information about patient's routine medication*—whether patient used to receive insulin, steroids, anticoagulants, etc. prior to accident is also important to know.

12. *Blood group of patient*—whether patient's blood group is known to him?

LOCAL CLINICAL EXAMINATION OF MAXILLOFACIAL INJURIES

Extraoral Examination

Prior to examination, patient's face should be gently washed with warm saline or water and cotton wool swabs should be used to clean dried blood clots or scabs. Oral cavity should be irrigated thoroughly and cleaned with cotton swabs. Mouthwashes can also be used. Evaluation of the facial area should be done in an organized and sequential fashion.

Inspection

Inspection will reveal the presence of edema, ecchymosis and deformity. Associated soft tissue injuries should be noted. Length, breadth and depth of the soft tissue wound should be measured and written. Inspect the nose and ear for the presence of bleeding or cerebrospinal fluid leak. Periorbital edema, ecchymosis, subconjunctival hemorrhage can be noticed (Bruises behind the ear or battle's sign, suggest a skull fracture). A neurological assessment should include careful evaluation of all cranial nerves. Vision, ocular level, extraocular movements, pupillary reaction to light should be carefully evaluated. Visual or pupillary changes may suggest intracranial (cranial nerves II, III, IV and VI) or orbital trauma. Abnormalities of ocular movements may also indicate other central neurologic problems or mechanical obstruction to the movements of the eye muscles resulting from fractures around the orbital area. The eyes, if they are closed due to edema, then the eyelids should be gently separated. If the patient is conscious, the vision is tested in each eye. Then the patient is asked to follow the clinician's finger with his eyes, without moving the head and asked to report if diplopia or double vision is noticed. A note is made of alteration in the size of two pupils and the light reflex is tested. The extent of the subconjunctival ecchymosis and its limits are also confirmed. Motor function of the facial muscles (VII cranial nerve) and muscles of mastication and sensation over the facial area (V cranial nerve) should be evaluated.

Anesthesia, paresthesia or dysesthesia of the lower lip, eyelids, nose, infraorbital areas should be noted.

The nasal complex should be inspected with a speculum and good illumination, for intranasal laceration, septum deviation and hematomas, tip and dorsal contour changes, epistaxis and CSF rhinorrhea.

Palpation (Figs 28.1A to H)

Palpation of the extraoral areas should be started with both the hands, simultaneously on each half of the external face, with gentle but firm pressure. This will help to detect the abnormalities and one can compare the normal side with the abnormal region.

Gentle palpation should start at the back of the head, and the cranium should be explored for wounds and bony injuries. Then the fingers should run over the forehead palpating for any depression. The palpating fingers should be kept in the midline and go sideways over supraorbital rims and infraorbital rims, zygomatic bones and arch. Areas of tenderness, step deformities or abnormal mobility should be noted. The nasal bridge palpation should start from the top till the nasal tip in the center and then sideways. Any crackling if felt, should be noted. Firm digital pressure over these areas, is used to evaluate the bony contours and may be difficult when these areas are grossly edematous. After intranasal cleaning, fresh bleeding or CSF leak should be ascertained.

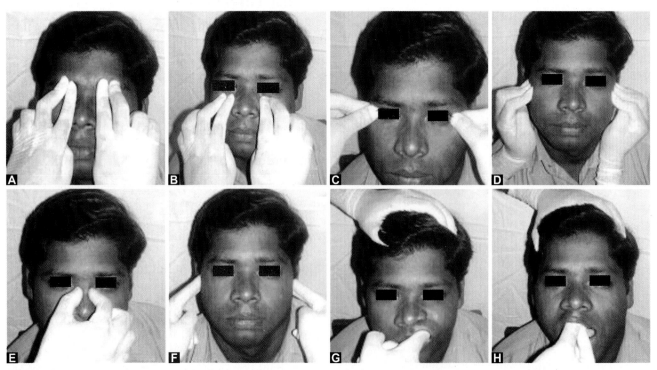

Figs 28.1A to H: Systematic palpation for M/F injuries: Palpation for— (A) Supraorbital ridge, (B) Infraorbital ridge, (C) Lateral margins of orbit, (D) Zygomatic bone and arch, (E) Nasal bones, (F) TM joints, (G) Intraoral palpation in the buccal vestibule for zygomatic buttress, (H) Intraoral palpation for checking the mobility of the maxilla

The cerebrospinal fluid rhinorrhea can be seen in LeFort II and III maxillary fractures (fracture of the ethmoid, sphenoid, frontal bones with dural tear). Here the escape of CSF into the nose is the result of a dural tear associated with the fracture of the cribriform plate of the ethmoid bone. This leak can get arrested in the first few days spontaneously or after the reduction of the fracture. In case of dural tear, there is always a risk of meningitis in early days, after injury or even after some time lapse. Antibiotic cover is important in such cases. Penicillin does not cross the blood-brain barrier. Other group of antibiotics are continued for at least 48 hours after CSF leak has ceased.

Detection of CSF leak may be difficult with associated bleeding in the nose. The mixed blood and CSF leak from the nose produces a classic 'tram line pattern' on the face and a 'halo' effect on the pillow or the bed sheets. This is also known as the ring test. The more viscous CSF forms a central circle rimmed on either side by blood, which diffuses to the edge. CS fluid will not stiffen a handkerchief, while secretions will do so. Characteristic salty taste of CSF in the nasopharynx is experienced by the patient. Patient should be placed in semi-recumbent position and instructed not to strain, sneeze or blow the nose. This is to minimize the risk of increasing intracranial pressure.

Biochemical tests to detect the presence of glucose can be done using Dextrostix, as CSF has a higher glucose content. Determination of the protein content also can be done, if clear fluid (CSF or serum from the blood clot) is seen passing through the nose. CSF contains little protein. Similarly the nasal secretion contains mucin, but no sugar, whereas CSF contains sugar, but no mucin.

The nose should be evaluated for symmetry. Intercanthal distance between the innermost portions of left and right medial canthus is measured. Frequently naso-orbitoethmoid injuries cause spreading of the nasal bones and detachment of the medial canthal ligaments, resulting in traumatic telecanthus (widening of the medial intercanthal distance).

The TMJ function evaluation should be done by placing index fingers on preauricular area or in the external auditory meatus. All the movements should be checked. Then the palpation of the posterior and the inferior border of the mandible should be carried out. Any areas of tenderness and step deformity should be noted.

Intraoral Inspection

Restriction of oral opening, gagging of the occlusion, lacerations, ecchymosis and damage to the teeth and/or alveolus are noted.

There may be presence of blood clots with foetid odor. Buccal and lingual sulci are inspected for wound, ecchymosis or a sublingual hematoma. The loose teeth and gross disturbed alignment of the teeth also should be noted. Occlusion should be checked. Any break or step deformity in the dental arches are found. Palatal mucosa also should be inspected for tear or bleeding areas.

Intraoral Palpation

The buccal and lingual sulci should be palpated for the presence of areas of tenderness, alteration in contour, crepitus, mobility of the teeth, etc. The mandible should be palpated bimanually and the abnormal mobility should be elicited. To assess the maxillary mobility, the patient's head should be stabilized using pressure over the forehead with one hand, and with the thumb and forefinger of the other hand, the maxilla is grasped, firm pressure should be used to elicit maxillary mobility. 'Rock' the maxillary alveolar segments to detect fractures of the alveolus or split in the palate.

Radiological Examination

After a careful clinical examination, patient should be referred for necessary radiological examination. It can be also supplemented by CT scan examinations, whenever the facilities are available.

Minimum X-rays required for the following:
1. *For fractures of middle third of the face*
   - 15° and 30° occipitomental view
   - Submentovertex view
   - Cranial posteroanterior view (skull)
   - Lateral skull view
   - PA view—Water's position
2. *For zygomaticomaxillary complex*
   - Occipitomenton view 15° and 30°
   - PA view—Water's position
   - Submentovertex projection
   - Tomography/CT scan of the orbit
3. *For mandibular fractures*
   - Orthopantomogram—OPG
   - Right and left lateral oblique views of the mandible

- Posteroanterior view of the mandible
- Towne's view for fractured condyles

The occlusal view for mandible or maxilla, intraoral periapical views for individual tooth may be required to be taken.

Fractures of the Jaw Bones

A fracture may be defined as a sudden break in the continuity of bone and it may be complete or incomplete.

Principal factors in fracture are (i) the dynamic factor (blow or impact), and (ii) stationary or static factor (jaw). Dynamic factor is characterized by the intensity of the blow and its direction.

Light blow: Simple fracture or incomplete fracture.

Heavy impact: Compound, comminuted fractures with displacement. Direction will decide the location of the fracture.

Static factor (Physiological age): In younger children, the bone is resilient, the trauma may lead to incomplete fracture. In athletes, the heavily calcified bones resist trauma to some extent. In the static factor physical condition, predisposing causes, anatomical weakness and presence of muscle pull on the fragments are the important considerations.

Classical Clinical Signs and Symptoms of Fracture of the Jaws

1. *A history of injury to the area.*
2. *Pain:* If the patient will complain of pain upon movement either at the site of, or remote from the site of injury, then a fracture should be suspected.
3. *Abnormal mobility:* Presence of abnormal mobility in the dental arches/jaw bones may be detected manually or observed during the movements of the jaws or patient may complain of abnormal mobility at certain site.
4. *Bleeding:* Active hemorrhage may be present or presence of hematoma or ecchymosis may follow a fracture process. In fresh injury, bleeding areas can be inspected by the clinician. Later on, patient should be asked for history of bleeding from oral cavity, nose (epistaxis), and ear, etc.
5. *Crepitus:* Crackling, grating sound can be detected during the palpation of the wound due to the friction of the broken bones over each other.
6. *Deformity:* Obvious facial deformity will be seen depending on degree and direction of the impact. It will also depend on the direction of the fracture line and muscle pull acting on.
7. *Ecchymosis and edema (Swelling):* These signs will be seen within few hours after the trauma. It may be seen extraorally or intraorally depending on the site of fracture and impact.
8. *Loss of function or interference with function:* Mastication of food is interfered. In case of condylar fracture, loss of transmitted movements will be noticed. Speech problems, swallowing difficulty also may arise.
9. *Radiographic evidence:* All cases of suspected fracture must be radiographed. It helps as a diagnostic aid plus provides additional confirmation. It is also important for medicolegal purpose to produce as an evidence.

The general classification of fracture, which is discussed in the mandibular fracture section can be applied to any fracture of the jaw bones.

Basic Principles of Treatment of a Fracture

1. Reduction   ⎫ for re-establishment of form,
2. Fixation   ⎬ function and occlusion with
3. Immobilization ⎭ minimum morbidity.

Aims

i.   Satisfactory facial form.
ii. Satisfactory functional occlusion.
iii. Satisfactory post-treatment range of movements of the jaw.
iv. No second surgery for facial recontouring or malocclusion.
v.   No bone grafting.

1. **Reduction:** Restoration of the fractured fragments to their original anatomical position. The restoration of the fragments to their correct position may be brought about by:
a. *Closed reduction* (Alignment without visualization of the fracture line) (Table 28.3).
   i. Reduction by manipulation.
   ii. Reduction by traction.

No surgical intervention is needed in closed reduction. Alignment of fractured fragments can be done without surgery. Occlusion of the teeth is used as a guiding factor. Fractures in the tooth bearing areas of the jaws are reduced satisfactorily by checking the final occlusion of the teeth.

The closed reduction can be achieved either by manipulation or by traction method.

Table 28.3: Advantages and disadvantages of closed reduction

Advantages

- Inexpensive
- Only stainless steel wires needed (usually arch bars also)
- Easy availability, convenient
- Short procedure, stable
- Gives occlusion some "leeway" to adjust itself
- Generally easy, no great operator skill needed
- Conservative, no need for surgical tissue damage
- No foreign object or material left in the body
- No operating room needed in most cases, outpatient treatment
- Callus formation (secondary bone healing) allows bridging of small bony gaps

Disadvantages

- Cannot obtain absolute stability (contributing to nonunion and infection)
- Noncompliance from patient due to long period of IMF
- Difficult (liquid) nutrition
- Complete oral hygiene impossible
- Possible temporomandibular joint sequelae (MPDS)
- Muscular atrophy and stiffness
- Denervation of muscles; alteration in fiber types
- Myofibrosis
- Changes in temporomandibular joint cartilage
- Weight loss
- Irreversible loss of bite force
- Decrease range of motion of mandible
- Impaired pulmonary function, may be problematic for patient with premorbid pulmonary condition
- Risks of wounds to operators manipulating wires

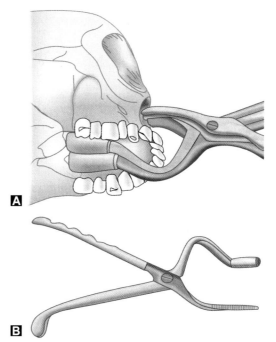

Figs 28.2A and B: (A) Reduction of maxillary fracture using disimpaction forceps, (B) Walsham's disimpaction forceps

i. *Reduction by manipulation*—when the fractured fragments are adequately mobile without much overriding or impaction and the patient comes for treatment immediately after trauma (fresh fractures), then the digital or hand manipulation for reduction can be used. Specially designed instruments for grasping the fragments are available (Disimpaction forceps, bone holding forceps). It can be done under LA with sedation or under GA depending on the need of the patient (Figs 28.2A and B).

ii. *Reduction by traction*
   a. Intraoral traction method.
   b. Extraoral traction method.

In intraoral traction method, prefabricated arch bars are attached to maxillary and mandibular dental arches by means of interdental wiring. Here, the fractured fragments are subjected to gradual elastic traction by placing the elastics, from upper to lower arch bars in a definite manner and direction depending on the fracture line (Figs 28.3A and B). In extraoral traction method, anchorage is taken usually from the intact skull of the patient and different types of head gears are used for various attachments, coming down over the face and connected to the arch bars by elastics and wires. Whenever the traction method is used, patient is encouraged to open and close the mouth slowly, so that the elastic traction starts functioning. Patient should be kept on analgesics for pain control, so that the elastic traction can be smooth. Once the proper occlusion is achieved, then the elastics are replaced by wires to carry out intermaxillary fixation or intermaxillay ligation (IMF or IML). It is also known as maxillomandibular fixation (MMF). After the elastic traction is given, then the patient should be observed for a period of 12 to 24 hours. At the end of 48 hours, if satisfactory occlusion is not achieved, then open reduction is opted for:

b. *Open reduction*—(surgical reduction allows visual identification of fractured fragments) (Table 28.4).

2. **Fixation:** In this phase the fractured fragments (after reduction) are fixed, in their normal anatomical relationship to prevent displacement and achieve

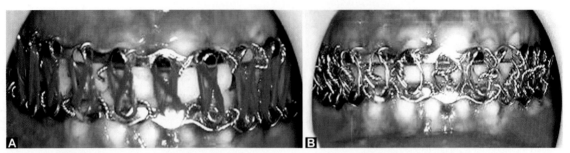

Figs 28.3A and B: (A) Intraoral traction, (B) Intraoral fixation (IMF)/intraoral ligation (IML) with wires

Table 28.4: Advantages and disadvantages of open reduction with rigid internal fixation

Advantages
- Early return to normal jaw function
- Normal nutrition
- Normal oral hygiene after a few days
- Avoidance of airway problem
- Can get absolute stability, promotes primary bone healing
- Bone fragments re-approximated exactly by visualization
- Avoids detrimental effects to muscles of mastication
- Does not require patient's compliance or supervision
- Permits the physical therapy early postsurgically
- Avoids IMF for patient with occupational benefits in avoiding mandible fixation, e.g. lawyers, teachers, sales people, seizure disorders
- Helpful in special nutritional requirements (diabetics, alcoholics, psychiatric disorders, pregnancy)
- Easy oral access (for example in intensive care unit patients)
- Decreased patient discomfort, greater patient satisfaction
- Less myoatrophy
- Decreased hospital time
- Substantial savings in overall cost of treatment
- Lower risk of major complications
- Lower infection rates, improved overall results
- Lower rate of malunion/nonunion

Disadvantages
- Most obvious; need for an open surgical procedure
- Significant operating room time
- Prolonged anesthesia
- Expensive hardware
- Some risk to neuromuscular structures and teeth
- Need for secondary procedure to remove hardware
- "Unforgiving procedure", the rigidity of the plate means no manipulation is permissible
- Needs much operator skill, meticulous technique needed
- Directly compared to maxillomandibular fixation
- Higher frequency of malocclusion
- Higher frequency of facial nerve palsy
- Scarring (extraoral and intraoral)
- Needs sophisticated material
- No bridging of small bone defect (absence of callus)

proper approximation. Fixation devices can be placed internally or externally.

a. *Direct skeletal fixation:* Consists of: (i) *Direct external skeletal fixation,* where the device is outside the tissues, but inserted into the bone percutaneously or (ii) *Direct internal skeletal fixation*—by devices which are totally enclosed within the tissues and uniting the bone ends by direct approximation. In direct external fixation, bone clamps or pin fixation can be used, while direct internal skeletal fixation is carried out with transosseous or intraosseous wiring or using bone plating system.

b. *Indirect skeletal fixation:* Here, the control of bone fragments is done via the denture bearing area. By means of arch bars and IML or Gunning splint, if the patient is edentulous. It can be extraoral or intraoral method.

3. **Immobilization:** During this phase, the fixation device is retained to stabilize the reduced fragments into their normal anatomical position, until clinical bony union takes place. The fixation device is utilized for a particular period to immobilize the fractured fragments. Immobilization period will depend on the type of fracture and the bone involved. For maxillary fractures 3 to 4 weeks of immobilization period is sufficient, while for mandibular fracture it can vary from 4 to 6 weeks. In condylar fracture the recommended immobilization period is 2 to 3 weeks only, for prevention of ankylosis of TMJ.

4. **Next steps** are prevention of infection and gradual rehabilitation of function.

In the teeth bearing region of the jaws, any fracture reduction is guided by checking the occlusion of the teeth. Interdigitation of mandibular teeth against the maxillary teeth is checked and then fixation and immobilization is carried out.

The primary objective in reduction of facial bone fractures is to restore the structures to a normal position of function and contour. This means restoration of normal occlusal relations by proper positioning of the teeth and bony structures. The normal intermaxillary relation is significant as a guide to reposition the bones of the maxillary and zygomatic complex in multiple facial structures. In order to stabilize the reduced facial fractures, some type of anchoring device is applied to maxillary dental arch and mandibular dental arch and intermaxillary fixation is carried out by applying wires or elastic bands between the upper and lower dental arch anchoring devices. The main methods for such fixation are dental wiring, arch bars and splints.

Although reports of teeth being ligated to one another go back as far as 2500 years (Hippocrates), the practicable principle of intermaxillary fixation was formulated after 1887. Gilmer (1887) revived intermaxillary wiring as a method of fracture management. Till today this method can be used very effectively, as it is the simplest method to apply.

There are various methods available for anchoring the dental arches. The type of device to be chosen will depend on the type of fracture, site of fracture, number of teeth present and their periodontal status and availability of the anchoring device.

The anchoring devices can be fitted on the dental arches under local anesthesia with or without sedation, prior to surgical procedure (if at all it is planned) to cut down the total operating time. In case of multiple fractures or extremely unco-operative patient, it can be done under general anesthesia at the time of surgery.

Different Types of Dental Wiring Techniques (Figs 28.4 to 28.8)

   i. Essig's wiring
  ii. Gilmer's wiring
 iii. Risdon's wiring
 iv. Ivy eyelet wiring
  v. Col. Stout's multiloop wiring

Armamentarium for Wiring

1. Presterilized 26 gauge stainless steel wire spool or wires cut into lengths of 20 cm each. Wires are always cut on a bevel, so that the bevel can act as a needle point, to pass through the interdental areas. The wires should be prestretched about 10 percent to prevent loosening after fixing it to the teeth.
2. Two needle holders or wire holders.
3. Wire cutters.

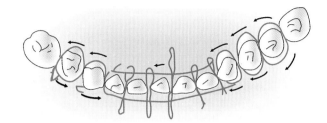

Fig. 28.4: Essig's wiring

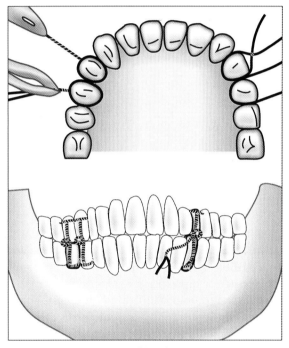

Fig. 28.5: Gilmer's wiring

Essig's Wiring (Fig. 28.4)

Essig's wiring can be used to stabilize the dentoalveolar fractures in individual dental arches, as well as it can be used as anchoring device for IMF. The luxated teeth also can be stabilized using this wiring.

Requirements for this type of wiring is that there should be sufficient number of teeth on either side of the fracture line to take the anchorage.

A 40 cm long, 26 gauge prestretched wire is used. The luxated teeth should be pushed back into their sockets and the stabilization area chosen should be at least 3 teeth away from the fracture line. The wire is passed around the necks of the chosen teeth, one end going from buccal to lingual and other end going lingual to buccal in each interdental space of the teeth (3 teeth away from the fracture line). The buccal end of the wire is stretched to brace the buccal side of the necks of the teeth near the fracture line and on the opposite side of the fracture line again leaving at least 3 teeth on the other side from the fracture line. The same procedure is repeated with the lingual side wire and the ends are then brought out on the buccal side of the last anchoring tooth after lacing the necks of three teeth on the opposite side. Both buccal and lingual wires are brought together and twisted and cut short to be tucked into the interdental space. Now you have two base wires formed, one from buccal side and another from lingual side at the necks of the teeth. The additional small wires are passed interdentally around these base wires to secure them tightly beyond the cingulum. The individual interdental wires are also twisted, cut and adjusted in the interdental spaces, so that the sharp ends do not hurt the patient.

Gilmer's Wiring (Fig. 28.5)

Gilmer's wiring is a direct wiring method of inter-maxillary fixation between the maxillary and mandibular teeth. This is the most common, simple, and practical method, as it secures the teeth and stabilizes the jaw properly. Few firm teeth in the maxilla as well as in the mandible are chosen. At least one tooth anterior and one posterior to the fracture should be available for wiring to assure proper stabilization. It is best, however, to involve multiple teeth, lessening the strain and possible damage to any individual tooth. Wire should not be applied to a tooth directly adjacent to the fracture. A 20 cm long, 26 gauge stainless steel wire is passed around the neck of the chosen tooth. Both the ends are brought out on the buccal surface and manually twisted keeping the twists close to the tooth. Final twisting is completed by grasping both the ends with a wire holder, maintaining lateral traction while twisting, to avoid wire breakage. Couple of teeth are chosen in the individual arches and the twisted wires are left long clamped. After the reduction of the fracture is carried out, then the mandibular wires are twisted tightly together with their corresponding maxillary wires. The finally twisted wires are then cut short and the sharp ends turned into the interdental space. The main disadvantage of this wiring is of requiring complete removal of the wires to open the mouth in emergency situation. Another disadvantage may be the extrusion of the teeth as excess load is subjected, in case very few teeth are chosen for anchorage.

Risdon's Wiring (Fig. 28.6)

Risdon's wiring is a commonly utilized method of horizontal wire fixation. Certain fractures can be treated adequately by this method alone. However, in some cases, additional stabilization may be necessary. In this method usually second molars on either sides are chosen for anchorage. A 26 gauge, 25 cm long wire is passed around the neck of the second molar on each side and both the ends are brought out on the buccal side. Then the ends of both wires twisted together for their entire length, so that the strong base wire is formed on either side, coming toward the midline from each second molar. The two twisted base wires are grasped and crossed at the midline by wire holder and final twisting is carried out adapting these base wires at the neck of the teeth on the buccal side. The excess wire is cut and the ends tucked in the interdental space. The base wire is secured to individual tooth by using additional interdental wires. Here small wires are cut and one

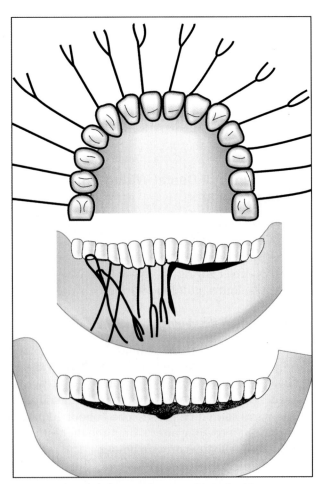

Fig. 28.6: Steps in forming a Risdon's wiring

end of the wire is passed from the distal surface of the tooth below the base wire and brought out towards the lingual side and then brought out on the buccal surface from the mesial interdental space above the base wire. Both these ends are again grasped together and twisted, cut and finished in the interdental space. Each tooth is engaged in the same manner to the base wire, so that the base wire is fully secured to the dental arch. This type of horizontal wiring offers strong fixation.

Ivy Eyelets Wiring (Figs 28.7A to C)

The Ivy loop embraces the two adjacent teeth. A 26 gauge stainless steel wires cut in 20 cm lengths are used. A loop is formed in the center of the wire around the beak of a towel clip or shank of a dental bur and twisted thrice with two tail ends. Such Ivy loops can be preformed and stored in cold sterilizing solution, so that they are available in emergency situation. The two tail ends of the eyelet are passed through the interdental space of the selected two teeth from buccal to lingual side. One end of the wire is passed around the distal tooth lingually and brought out from the distal interdental space over the buccal side and threaded through the previously formed loop. The other wire tail end is carried around the lingual surface of the mesial tooth and brought out on the buccal surface from the mesial interdental space, where it meets the first tail end wire. The two wires are crossed and twisted together with the wire holder and cut short and finished in usual manner. The loop is then adjusted and bent towards the gingiva. The mandibular wire eyelets can be secured to maxillary eyelets by rubber bands or joining wires. One or two Ivy eyelets should be placed in each quadrant.

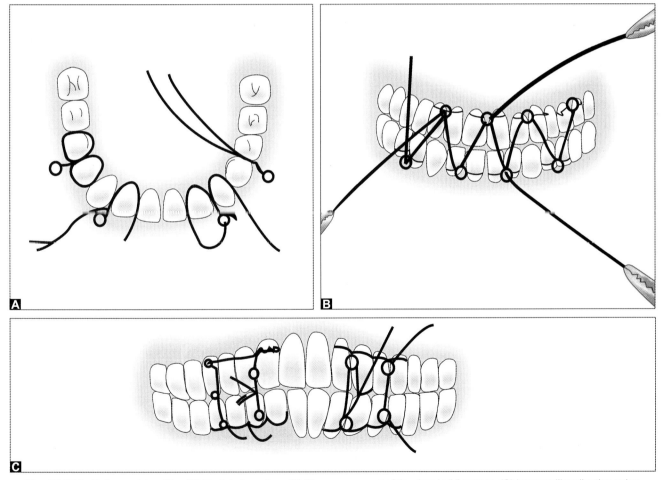

Figs 28.7A to C: Ivy eyelets wiring (A) Eyelets formation, (B) The arrangement of tie wires in 'V' pattern, (C) Intermaxillary ligation using eyelets wiring in a straight pattern

Eyelet wiring is an asset. The rubber bands or bridging wires can be removed, whenever required without disturbing the main wiring and replaced. Even when there is breakage of a wire during fixation, only that eyelet can be removed and replaced.

Col. Stout's Multiloop Wiring (Figs 28.8A to C)

Here, the four posterior quadrants are used for wiring. Four pieces of 26 gauge, 20 cm long wires are required and piece of solder wire or any thick wire is required to make the loops. A piece of solder wire is adapted to the buccal surface of the teeth in the first quadrant, where the wiring is started. The 20 cm long prestretched wire is folded into equal parts, one part is known as stationary wire, will be adapted on the buccal side starting from midline going backward to second molar (or last existing tooth in the arch). The other end of the wire (working end) is then brought distal to the second molar and taken around it on the lingual side. This working end is threaded through the mesial interdental space of the second molar to the buccal side to emerge under the solder wire and the stationary wire. It is then looped around both the wires and back into the interdental space, this time from buccal to lingual side. From the lingual side it goes around the next tooth and the same procedure is repeated for each tooth till midline. The

solder wire can be shifted ahead, once the loop is formed and the loop is twisted three times to form an eyelet. The final finishing is done by grasping both stationary and working ends together and twisting them and cutting short and pressing them in the interdental space. The same procedure is followed in the other three quadrants of the dental arches. If the elastic traction is to be used, then the eyelets should be bent away from the occlusal plane, so that the hooks are formed. If wires are to be used, then the loops are bent toward the occlusal plane. It is desirable to use elastics in the initial recovery period instead of wires. In case of vomiting or emergency airway problem, these elastics can be removed easily.

Arch Bars (Fig. 28.9)

Many types of prefabricated arch bars are available. But the most popular one and commonly used is the *Erich's arch bar.* It is a prefabricated arch bar with hooks incorporated on the outer surface with flat malleable stainless steel metal strip. It provides an effective, quick and inexpensive method of fixation. The bar is available in spool form. The bar should be cut accurately to the length of the dental arch. Accuracy in this regard will prevent injury to the adjacent soft tissues by protruding ends. Each arch bar is to be fixed to the upper and lower dental arches.

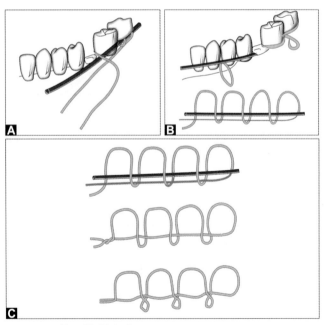

Figs 28.8A to C: Col. Stout's multiloop wiring

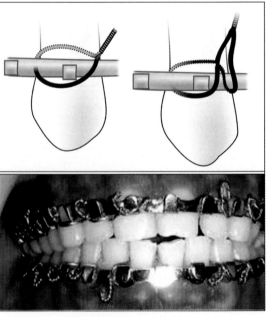

Fig. 28.9: Arch bar fixation

On the upper jaw, the hooks are arranged in an upward direction. The bar is attached to the lower jaw with the hooks in a downward direction. The arch bar should be adapted to the buccal surface of each arch by giving a shape of the arch by bending it. Bending of the arch bar should start at the buccal side of the last tooth progressing past the midline and finishing at the other end. The arch bar is fixed to each tooth, with 26 gauge stainless steel wire, which is passed from the mesial surface of a tooth to the lingual side and back on the buccal side from the distal surface of the tooth. One end of the wire is above the bar and the other below. By twisting the two ends of wire together, the bar is attached securely and firmly to the necks of the teeth on the buccal surface of the arch. The twisting of the wires should be always done in a clockwise manner, so that later on removal of wires can be done in anticlockwise manner. Improper adaptation of the bar, ligation of an insufficient number of teeth and inefficient tightening will result in inadequate stability of the arch bar. Advantages of the arch bar include less trauma because of the thin wire and greater stability in an arch, even if some teeth are missing, because the edentulous gaps can be spanned by this rigid appliance. If some wire is broken in between, the fixation will not suffer and it can be replaced easily. The hooks are flat and do not irritate the tissue. In case of displaced mandibular body fractures, the arch bar can be divided and placed on either side of the fracture line. Elastic traction will reduce the fracture and bring it into normal occlusion. Then the elastics can be replaced by wiring.

The use of Erich arch bar is accepted universally for its obvious advantages.

Custom Made Splints

Custom made appliances are fabricated for individual patient. The splints can be constructed using acrylic material or cast metal.

Indications

1. When the wiring of the teeth will not provide adequate fixation.
2. When horizontal splinting across the fracture zone is required without closing the patient's mouth.
3. When both the jaws are edentulous.
4. In case of growing children, where mixed dentition is present and number of firm teeth for anchorage are not adequate.

5. In case of pregnant women and mentally challenged patients, where IML is not desirable.

Acrylic Splints

  i. Lateral compression splint.
 ii. Gunning splint.

Lateral compression splint (Figs 28.10A to H): It is made for the stabilization of mandibular arch. Mainly used in cases of children, where there is mixed dentition and presence of developing teeth buds (open reduction and direct fixation is contraindicsted). It can be also used in adult mandibular body fracture, where the stability cannot be obtained by means of other type of horizontal wiring methods. The splint can be made up of self curing acrylic, so that the construction is quicker and easy. The first step in the construction is to obtain upper and lower impressions of the dental arches and preparing stone plaster models. On the mandibular plaster cast, the fracture line is marked and the cast is cut at the fracture line. Then the cut cast is assembled by checking the occlusion with maxillary cast and sealed in desired position using sticky wax. Then the 19 gauge wire is adapted to the entire circumference of the mandibular arch at the necks of the teeth, both on the buccal as well as on the lingual side. The bending of this wire should be started on the buccal surface in the midline and taken on the lingual side from distal aspect of last existing molar. On the lingual side, the shape of the wire will be concave adapting to each tooth surface and the end will be brought on the buccal surface going around the last existing molar on the opposite side. The wire will be adapted and brought towards the midline to meet the first end of the wire. This wire will reinforce the acrylic splint, as well as, it will act as a connector to the lingual and buccal flanges of the splint. The acrylic splint is then fabricated from the cast by incorporating the previously bent wire in it. The occlusal surfaces of the teeth should be left open, while constructing buccal and lingual flanges. On the buccal surface of the splint hooks can be incorporated if required. This splint can be fitted to the lower arch by means of interdental wiring or by means of circumferential wiring (circummandibular wiring).

Gunning splint (Figs 28.11A to D): In edentulous jaws, patient's own dentures, suitably modified can be used or specially constructed Gunning splint can be used. Circumferential wiring is used to fix the splint to the mandibular bone and upper denture or splint is fixed to the maxilla by means of peralveolar wiring.

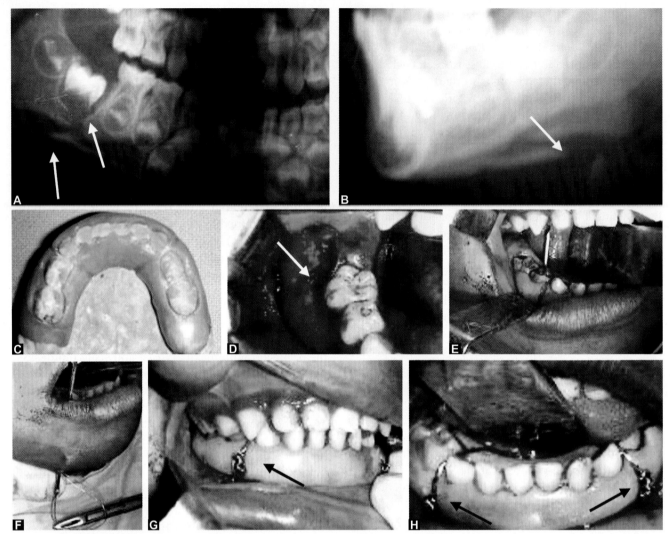

Figs 28.10A to H: (A and B) OPG and lateral X-ray showing fracture in the body mandible in 4 years old child, (C) Lateral compression splint prepared on the cast, (D) Fractured site exposed and reduction done, (E and F) Splint in place and circummandibular wiring is being carried out, (G and H) Final fitting of the splint and occlusion checked

Construction of Gunning Splint

i. Upper and lower impressions taken from the patient's mouth.
ii. Plaster casts made.
iii. Plaster cast cut and assembled (if there is lot of displacement).
iv. Upper and lower base plates adapted.
v. Bite blocks prepared in the posterior region only.
vi. Upper and lower plates with bite blocks constructed using heat cure acrylic leaving the anterior region open for feeding.
vii. Hooks are incorporated on the buccal side of the bite blocks.

viii. Grooves must be made in the both the Gunning splints, in the canine region to prevent the peralveolar and circumferential wires from slipping along the surface of the splint.

Wiring Procedure

Peralveolar Wiring Procedure (Fig. 28.12)

Patient's own upper denture or upper Gunning splint can be fitted to maxillary alveolar ridge by introducing two peralveolar wires in the canine region on either side. The procedure can be done under local anesthesia or general anesthesia if required.

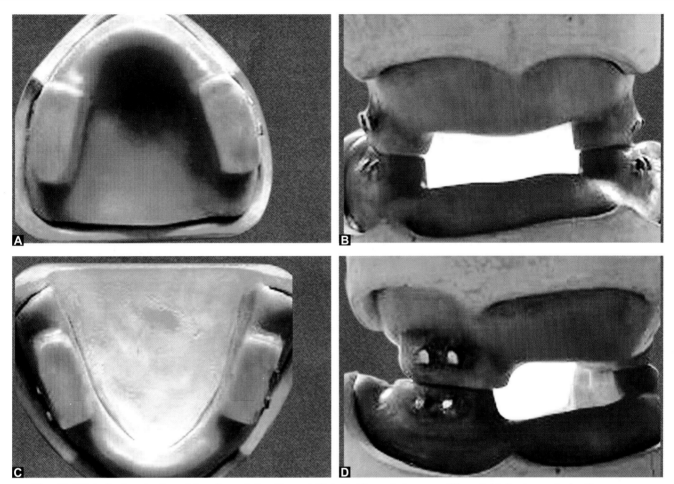

Figs 28.11A to D: Construction of Gunning splint on the cast. Note that the anterior area of the splint is kept open for feeding purpose

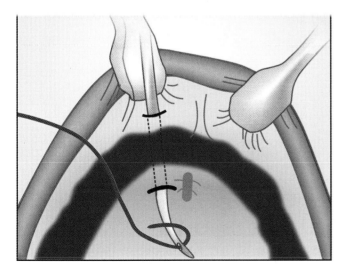

Fig. 28.12: Peralveolar wiring procedure for fitting the Gunning splint to the maxillary edentulous ridge

The splint is firmly placed in the position in the upper jaw and the mucous membrane of the buccal sulcus opposite to the groove in the canine region is pricked by a straight needle dipped in marking ink. This will be corresponding with the entry of the peralveolar wire introducer (Kelsey-Fry bone-awl introducer). A similar mark is made on the palatal aspect at the correct point of emergence of the introducer. With a boring action, the peralveolar introducer is pushed from the buccal to the palatal surface using the marking point as a guide. Once the tip comes on the palatal surface, then 26 gauge wire is threaded through the eye and then the introducer is withdrawn carrying with it the wire on the buccal surface. Both the wire ends are grasped with the wire holder. Same procedure is repeated on the opposite side. The splint is then replaced in the mouth and wires adjusted over it and twisted over the grooves.

The twisted wires are cut and the end should be tucked inward into the grooves.

Circumferential (Circummandibular) Wiring Procedure (Figs 28.13 and 28.14)

Obwegeser's method (Fig. 28.13): This wiring can be utilized (after reduction of the mandibular fracture) for fixation of lateral compression splint or Gunning splint to the mandibular bone. Two wires are passed in the canine region on either side. The procedure is carried

out under general anesthesia after reduction of the fractured fragments.

One can use long, no. 18 hypodermic needle or Kelsey-Fry pattern curved bone awl or specially designed Reverdine needle for passing the wire around the mandibular body.

The lower border of the mandible is palpated in the canine region and the skin is pierced beneath the lower border of the mandible, with the point of introducer, keeping in close contact with the lingual surface of bone, emerges through the floor of the mouth, close to

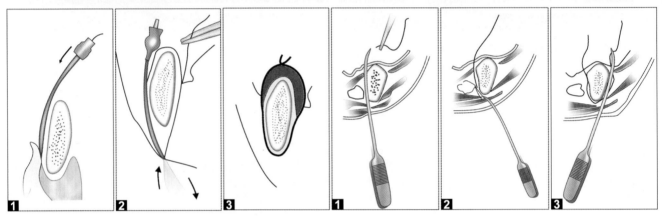

Fig. 28.13: Obwegeser's method of circummandibular wiring

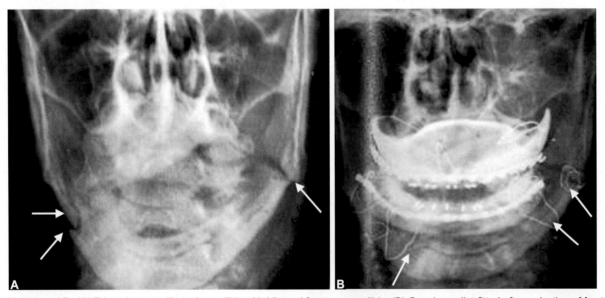

Figs 28.14A and B: (A) Edentulous maxilla and mandible with bilateral fracture mandible; (B) Gunning splint fitted after reduction of fractures with peralveolar and circummandibular wiring. Intraosseous wiring seen at the inferior borders

the alveolar mucoperiosteum. A length of wire 26 or 28 gauge is inserted through the eye of the introducer (or if needle is used through the lumen of the needle) and bent back upon itself. The introducer is then withdrawn along the same pathway, till the lower border is reached. Here, the tip is not withdrawn from the tissues, but is moved around the lower border and directed upwards along the buccal surface of the mandible to emerge through the sulcus. The wire is detached and the introducer withdrawn through the original point of entry. The two ends of the wire are then grasped with wire holder and using the to and fro sawing motion, the wires cut through the intervening tissues and brought in close contact with the lower border of the mandible. Then the splint is adjusted and the lingual and buccal wire ends are twisted together in the region of canine grooves, cut and finished inwards.

Cast metal splints (Fig. 28.15): These splints are fabricated in various metals in the laboratories. It requires impres-sions of both the arches. The lower cast is sawed through the line of fracture. The cast is reassembled in proper occlusion and fixed in position by pouring a base for the cast. The splint is formed till the gingival margins in 28 gauge sheet wax. Occlusal relations are established in the wax-up by checking the centric relation with the opposite cast, while the wax is soft. Then the wax-up is sent for casting procedure and the finished cast splint is obtained. This splint is used in adult patients with few firm teeth available and the splint is cemented to the reduced fractured jaw. These splints

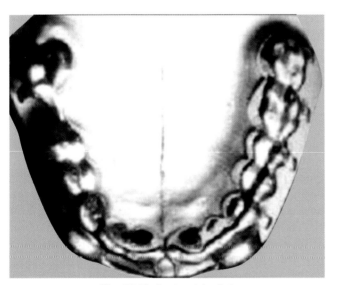

Fig. 28.15: Cast metal splint

are expensive than the acrylic ones plus the construction is time consuming, hence not used routinely.

Methods of Fixation

Fixation is required in the majority of facial fractures.

Treatment without any Form of Fixation

This method is reserved for the following:
  i. Fractures exhibiting minimal displacement and mobility; without occlusal discrepancy or with very minimal occlusal discrepancy.
 ii. Green stick fractures.
iii. Elderly edentulous patients, who are in the high/poor risk category and who have no gross displacement.

Treatment with Intraoral Fixation Alone

This method can be employed for the treatment of the following:
• Dentoalveolar fractures
• Unilateral fracture—maxilla
• Dentulous mandibular body fracture with minimal displacement or no displacement
• Edentulous mandibular body fractures

This fixation can be achieved by the following:
1. The use of an arch bar or suitable type of wiring methods described earlier.
2. Cap splints with locking plates and a connecting bar.
3. Acrylic splints—lateral compression or Gunning type splint.
4. Intermaxillary ligation (IML) or intermaxillary (IMF) fixation—whenever required the jaws are rigidly fixed to each other in centric occlusion. Both the jaws are united as a block, must be fixed to the skull in case of maxillary fractures.

External Fixation (Figs 28.16 to 28.19)

The intact skull serves as a fixation point for the fixation of facial fractures. Usually a plaster of Paris head cap is applied for external skeletal fixation. Rigid connection to the head cap must follow by means of various connecting bars which are attached on both sides to the intraoral arch bars and that lead out of the oral cavity. Small cross-struts on the side bars are used for the application of the elastic traction (Fig. 28.16). Instead of plaster of Paris skull cap, various prefabricated head

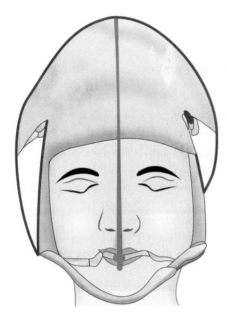

Fig. 28.16: External skeletal fixation with plaster of Paris skull cap

frames can be used. These head frames can be made up of metal or leather straps. These are tiara-shaped head frames directly secured to the head. Head frames provide absolute stability and are more easily applied to an unconscious patient. They can also be used in conjunction with fractures of the frontal bone and cranial vault.

The metallic 'Halo frame' devised by Crewe in 1943 is directly secured to the skull by multiple screw pins inserted into the external cortex of the skull. Vertical rods, bilateral check wires, side bars can be added to the central Halo frame, which is a versatile apparatus of great stability (Figs 28.17 to 28.19).

Different Possibilities for External Skeletal Fixation

1. Plaster of Paris head cap, intraoral arch bars, side bars fixed to the upper arch bar, connection between side bars and plaster head cap by
   a. Bilateral elastic bands.
   b. Bilateral rods and universal joints.
   c. Bilateral transbuccal cheek wires attached to the arch bars.
2. Halo frame (instead of plaster of Paris head cap) with traction and fixation elements and intraoral splints.

The extraoral fixation may be of the following types (Figs 28.19A and B):

1. *Craniomaxillary*—fixation between the skull and maxillary arch is termed as craniomaxillary fixation. This is a rigid direct suspension of the detached middle third of the facial skeleton, which is achieved by connecting the maxillary arch bars to a external head gear. This can be achieved by means of a vertical rod, fixed via universal joints to a projecting bar screwed on the arch bars or splints.
2. *Craniomandibular*—fixation between the mandibular arch and skull is termed as craniomandibular fixation. Here the fractured area of the middle third of the face is sandwiched between intact skull and rigid mandible. This can be achieved by:
   a. Connecting a mandibular splint to a plaster of Paris head cap via an anterior projecting bar and vertical rod, or
   b. Bilateral transbuccal wires from the head caps to a mandibular arch bar.
   c. Halo frame can be used as a fixed anchorage point in both craniomaxillary or craniomandibular fixation method.

Internal Fixation

This type of fixation is achieved entirely or primarily by passing wires within the tissues.

Direct suspension (Figs 28.20 and 28.21): In this method the same principle, as extraoral fixation is used except, the wires are passed subcutaneously from stable skeletal points into the oral cavity and are fixed on both sides to the arch bars under traction (craniofacial suspension). Depending on the type of fracture, the point of fixation may vary. The wires are always passed from a stable point above the fracture line. The various areas for direct suspension of wires can be chosen.
a. Pyriform fossa
b. Zygomatic buttress
c. Zygomatic arch
d. Infraorbital rim
e. Zygomatic process of the frontal bone.

Indirect support: Craniomandibular suspension is brought about by sandwiching the fractured areas between the mandible and some part of the facial skeleton above the fracture line through the medium of suspensory wires connected to a mandibular arch bar. The appropriate sites can be chosen as indicated in direct suspension procedure.

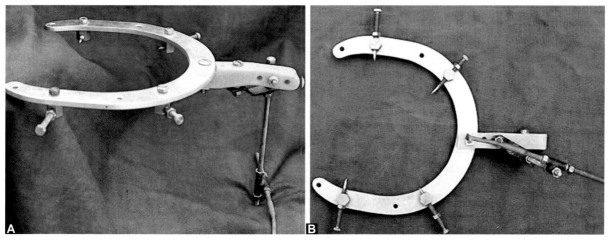

Figs 28.17A and B: The metallic 'Halo frame', devised by Crewe

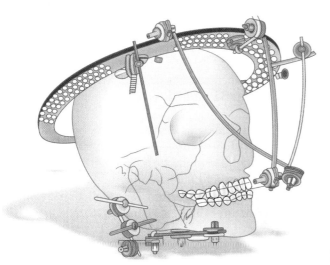

Fig. 28.18: Extraoral fixation device consisting of metallic halo frame, possible combination of rods and universal joints

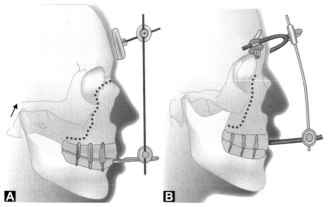

Figs 28.19A and B: (A) Craniomandibular external fixation, (B) Craniomaxillary external fixation

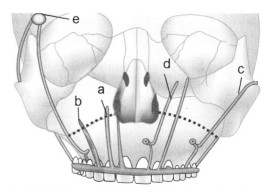

Fig. 28.20: Direct suspension wires at different locations

Transosseous or intraosseous wiring (Fig. 28.22): It can be used at various sites. Open reduction is needed. Here the fractured fragments are approximated in their normal anatomical position after reduction and the holes are drilled on either sides of the fracture line and 26 or 28 gauge stainless steel wire is passed to interconnect the holes and both the ends of the wires are grasped on the outer cortex and twisted, cut and finished. This type of direct internal fixation offers semirigid stability. Most of the times, if occlusal discrepancy exists, then additional IMF is required during immobilization period.

Transosseous or intraosseous wiring can be done at the following sites:

a. Zygomaticofrontal
b. Zygomaticomaxillary
c. Zygomatic bone (comminuted)
d. Palatal processes
e. Frontonasal

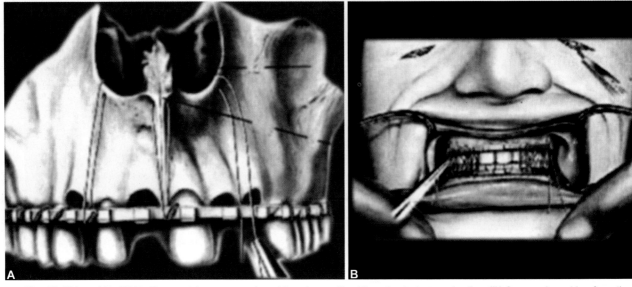

Figs 28.21A and B: (A) Pyriform aperture suspension wiring along with wiring at anterior nasal spine, (B) Suspension wiring from the infraorbital rims on either side to arch bar

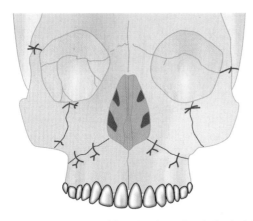

Fig. 28.22: Transosseous wiring at various sites in the facial area

f. Mandibular angle at superior border or inferior border
g. Edentulous mandible at the site of fracture
h. Condylar fractures—subcondylar or high condylar
Wire osteosynthesis is the oldest, simplest and most popular method for internal fixation.

Disadvantages:

• Intermaxillary fixation is always needed
• There is no three-dimensional stability to the fragments
• Interfragmentary pressure cannot be controlled

• Under functional stress, the wire synthesis lacks adequate rigidity, direction control and surface contact
• Delayed healing as compared to bone plate system, because of micromovement at the fracture side.

Direct support: This may be employed in the case of a comminuted orbital floor by utilizing an antral pack or balloon. It can be also used for stabilizing zygomatic complex fractures (Figs 28.27 and 28.28).

Transfixation: Kirschner wires or Steinmann pins may be inserted:

a. From zygoma to zygoma.
b. From zygoma to the maxilla.
c. In mandibular edentulous fractures.
d. In mandibular fractures with extensive loss of bone.

Miniplate osteosynthesis (Figs 28.23A and B): The extraordinarily good results with compression osteosynthesis with plates or lag screws in the mandible have led to the development of similar procedure for the midface. Champy and Michelet introduced miniplate osteosynthesis suitable for facial fracture fixation.

Construction of Plaster of Paris Headcap

Construction of an accurately fitting, firm, comfortable plaster of Paris skull cap is an art, ill fitting, loose headcap will be extremely uncomfortable for the patient and

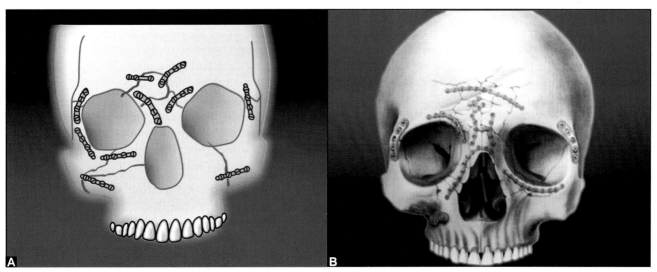

Figs 28.23A and B: Miniplate osteosynthesis

it will not offer desired stability. Patient may develop edema due to friction and complain of dull headache.

Armamentarium

- 12 inches length, 6 inches width of stockinette
- A pair of heavy scissors
- 4 to 5 three inches width plaster of Paris orthopedic bandage
- Various vertical bars, attachments, etc.

Procedure

Male patient's hair should be trimmed, females should have their hair tied up on top of the head with a ribbon. The stockinette sleeve is passed over the patient's head without disturbing the hair. The plaster of Paris bandage is immersed in cold water and first turn is taken round the head just above the supraorbital ridge by putting the bandage tight and shaping it properly. The second bandage is applied rather higher up the forehead than the first bandage and taken well down below the occiput posteriorly. After the first two bandages are in position then the retention ends of the headcap framework is adjusted until they lie accurately against the headcap surface. Then the third bandage is applied over the ends of the framework which are to be embedded in the plaster. The excess stockinette should be trimmed and turned over the wet plaster bandage. Once the plaster sets, then the plaster skull cap with its attachment is firmly secured to the cranium. Various additional attachments/wires are then incorporated and attached indirectly to the dental arch bars; either maxillary or mandibular.

Direct suspension: The principle of internal wire suspension was first described by Adams in 1943. That is the reason why these wires are also called as Adam's suspensory wires. It has got many advantages over external skeletal fixation.

i. No cumbersome apparatus.
ii. Can be used in cases of scalp injuries.
iii. Patients cannot interfere with this type of fixation (mental derangement, cerebral irritation cases).
iv. Simple procedure with minimum armamentarium.
v. Elaborate laboratory facilities are not needed.

Direct suspension of the upper jaw is permissible, when precise articulation of the teeth is not required, e.g. when one or both jaws are edentulous and when immobilization of the mandible is not needed. Fixation of the mandible with maxilla is contraindicated in the presence of severe associated nasal obstruction, unless a tracheostomy is performed.

The internal skeletal fixation of suspensory wires are secured to the arch bars by passing them through holes drilled at the bone by taking small incisions at one of the following sites:

a. Margins of the pyriform fossa of the nasal cavity.
b. Zygomatic buttress.
c. Infraorbital margin—intraoral incision is taken for above three sites.

d. Zygomatic process of the frontal bone (extraoral incision)—after reduction of the fracture has been performed, one end of the wire is passed through the hole drilled in the bone and then returned to the point of origin on the splint or arch bar and the free ends twisted together, thus effecting stable fixation. All the suspensory wires are passed bilaterally on both the halves of the facial skeleton to maintain the balance. The fractured portion of the facial skeleton is in this manner suspended from the intact portion of the skeleton (Figs 28.24A to C).

e. Circumzygomatic wiring—here the wires are passed through the tissues over the zygomatic arches, both ends of the wire being secured to the splint or arch bar.

Procedure for wiring at the zygomatic process of the frontal bone (Figs 28.24 and 28.25): Incision along one of the upper 'Crow's foot' wrinkles overlying the zygomaticofrontal suture or an incision parallel to and within the hair of the outer third of the eyebrow may be employed.

Direct transosseous wiring between the zygomatic process of the frontal bone and the frontal process of the zygomatic bone will have to be carried out as a preliminary measure in the case of fractures of LeFort III type.

A 6 inches long, 26 gauge stainless steel wire is then threaded through the upper hole drilled in the zygomatic process of the frontal bone. The two ends of this wire are passed down the temporoposterior surface of the zygomatic bone to emerge into the buccal vestibule in maxillary second molar region. This passage of wire may be done by using a bone awl or a long, curved hypodermic 18 gauge needle. The attachment of the free ends of the wires is then carried out in the usual manner. Care should be taken that both the wires are not twisted/kinked at any point, so that the subsequent removal is easy.

Circumzygomatic wiring (Figs 28.26A and B): This useful technique was described by Lesney in 1953.

The entire length of the zygomatic arch is palpated and patient's head is turned sideways so the zygomatic arch becomes prominent. An introducer is then entered through small skin stab incision, at the upper border of the anterior aspect of the zygomatic arch, remaining on the medial aspect of it and is inserted within the tissues to emerge in the buccal vestibule in maxillary second molar region. A 26 gauge 10 inches long wire is then threaded in the eye of an introducer and the introducer

is pulled at the upper border of the zygomatic arch. At this point the tip of the introducer is not taken out over the skin surface, but is manipulated back over the lateral surface of the arch and again passed through the tissues toward the buccal vestibule. This way the entire wire encircles around the zygomatic arch. The two loose ends of the wire in the buccal vestibules are pulled to and fro, so that wire cuts through the tissues and comes to lie on the zygomatic arch. Both the ends are then ligated to the dental arch bars as desired.

Direct support: This is mainly used in case of orbital floor fracture or zygomatic complex fracture displacement.

Intraorally the direct support can be given via the maxillary sinus, with the objective of repositioning the fragments and supporting them in position by various means until union has occurred.

Extraorally the orbital floor can be exposed and supported by using bone graft, cartilage graft or some alloplastic material as silastic sheet.

Antral Approach

The mucoperiosteum is reflected from the anterolateral wall of the maxillary antrum following an incision of the Caldwell Luc type. The bone may or may not be fragmented, but an opening is made, just above the canine roots, sufficient to admit the index finger of the operator. The thorough irrigation of the sinus is carried out, loose fragments are removed and entire sinus should be inspected under direct vision. Fractured fragments are reduced digitally.

Antral pack (Fig. 28.27): A long strip of half inch ribbon gauze soaked in betadine or iodoform and lubricated with vaseline is used to pack the antrum. The packing should be started at the back of the floor and laid in layers in an anteroposterior direction. Care is taken not to force the pack tightly at the floor of the orbit, but adjusted in such a way that the ocular level is brought to normalcy. The last end of the pack either may be brought out through the corner of the incision intraorally or through the nose, via a nasal antrostomy.

The pack is not retained for more than two weeks. In case of zygomatic complex fracture, it is reduced first and then the antral pack is inserted.

Balloon catheter (Figs 28.28A and B): Shea and Anthony in 1952, devised a balloon for the purpose of supporting the comminuted orbital floor. Recently the use of Foley's catheter no. 16 or 18 is recommended. The preliminary

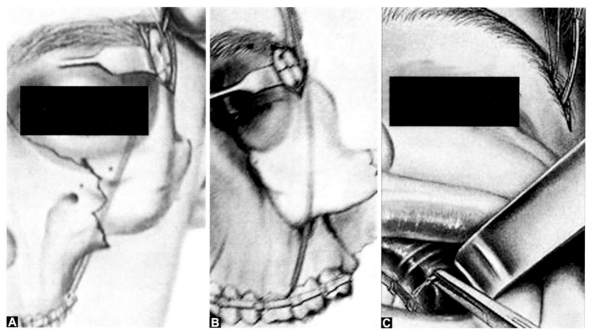

Figs 28.24A to C: Adam's internal suspension wiring at the zygomatic process of the frontal bone. (A) Incision is taken over lateral margin of the eyebrow. Small hole is drilled after exposing the zygomatic process of the frontal bone. Wire threaded through the hole, passing below the zygomatic arch. (B) Other end of the wire is passed over the zygomatic arch. Both the wire ends are brought out in the buccal vestibule. (C) Both the wire ends are tied to the maxillary arch bar for craniomaxillary suspension wiring

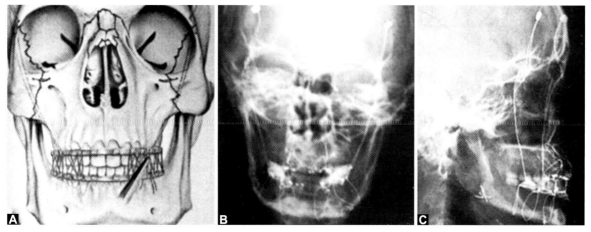

Figs 28.25A to C: (A) Adam's wiring, (B) PA view X-ray showing the Adam's suspensory wiring bilaterally, (C) Lateral view X-ray showing the same with additional circummandibular wiring to secure the splint

procedure is same as described for the insertion of an antral pack. Nasal antrostomy is performed and a curved hemostat is passed from the antrum into the nasal antrostomy. The tips of the hemostat is opened to grasp the tip of the Foley's catheter and the hemostat is pulled into the antrum. The position of the catheter is adjusted in the antral cavity. Then 20 ml of sterile saline is inserted into the rubber stopper of the catheter and the balloon slowly inflated under direct vision, until a satisfactory reduction has been achieved. The balloon is kept for 1 to 2 weeks and then removed, after deflating by emptying the saline, through the nose.

Internal Fixation by Means of Bone Plate Osteosynthesis

The direct internal fixation of the fractured fragments can be carried out by bone plate osteosynthesis method.

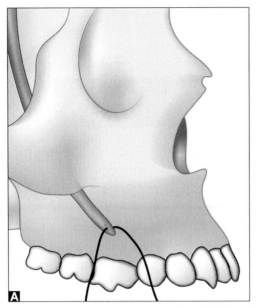
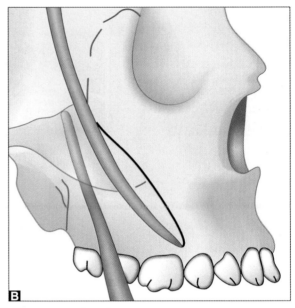

Figs 28.26A and B: Circumzygomatic wiring

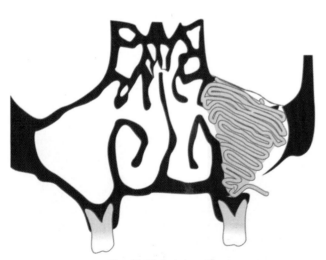

Fig. 28.27: Antral pack

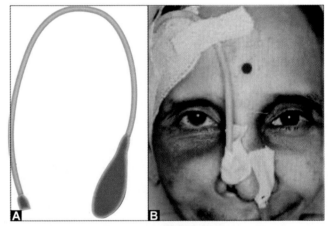

Figs 28.28A and B: Balloon catheter *in situ*

It either totally eliminates the need for IMF or minimizes the period of IMF. Relapse following management of fracture cases was of main concern to all of the treating surgeons in the past. Firm fixation of the fractured fragments is an ideal requirement in order to achieve an uneventful postoperative healing. Rigid internal fixation of these fragments provide three dimensional stability and eliminates the risk of relapse and promotes better osteosynthesis.

Indications

1. Cases where there is absolute contraindications to IMF, i.e. in epileptics, mentally retarded unco-operative patients, asthmatics, alcoholics, drug abusers, pregnant women, etc.
2. When the patient wants to return back to work early.
3. Edentulous patients with loss of bone segments, which need the maintenance of the gap or grafting, if indicated.

4. In subcondylar and angle fractures of the mandible, early mobilization of the joint is required.
5. Atrophic mandible requiring additional reinforcement.

Contraindications

a. In heavily contaminated fractures, where there is active infection and discharge. However, some surgeons advocate the use of compression osteosynthesis in such cases.
b. In badly comminuted fracture, where open reduction may pose risk of compromising vascularity.
c. In children having mixed dentition, where there is a danger of injuring the developing teeth buds.
d. Presence of gross pathological abnormalities in the bone.

Advantages

i. Simple technique.
ii. Decreased intraoperative time.
iii. Most of the time, intraoral approach is sufficient. However, in certain cases extraoral approach may be required.
iv. Direct control of occlusion in intraoral technique.
v. Postoperative intermaxillary fixation is not needed or period of IMF is reduced.
vi. Early return of function.
vii. Reduced hospital stay.
viii. Better esthetics and function, better three dimensional stability.
ix. Minimization of immediate postoperative complications, as mouth is not locked.
x. Better maintenance of oral hygiene.
xi. Nutritional intake does not suffer.
xii. Psychological advantage.
xiii. No weight loss.
xiv. No speech problem.

Precautions: Majority of complications in bone plate osteosynthesis are linked to infections, because of inadequate fixation of the fracture. The following points are important and if neglected lead to compromised results.

a. Strict aseptic procedure is required and precision in the technique is very important.
b. Patient should be kept on preoperative antibiotics and the operation should be undertaken at the earliest.
c. Proper armamentarium should be used and if titanium plates are used, then they should be handled with titanium tipped instruments (Oxidation). Plates and screws also should be made up of the same metal.
d. Plates should be fixed along ideal osteosynthesis lines and minimum 2 screws on each side of the fracture line should be used.
e. The drill bit should be kept perpendicular to the outer cortex.
f. Patient should maintain good oral hygiene.
g. Tension on the flap or infection can lead to wound dehiscence. Careful soft tissue closure (with mobilization of tissue, if required) should be done.

Bone Plate Osteosynthesis (Figs 28.29A to C)

Bone plate osteosynthesis can be carried out using the following:
1. Compression plate with bicortical screw system.
2. Noncompression plate with monocortical screw system.

Experimental and clinical experience has shown that the susceptibility to infection depends on the mobility of the fragments. The bony union can be promoted when the fragments are approximated firmly under pressure against each other. This principle is utilized in the development of compression bone plate system (AO system) by European surgeons. This system offers rigid fixation with intrafragmentary compression. There is no need for IMF postoperatively. Here, there is no intrafragmentary gap or it is less than 0.8 mm. During healing there is no callus formation. But there is primary healing of the bone, characterized by direct restoration of lamellar bone. Osteogenic elements and blood capillaries readily traverse the fracture site, resulting in direct longitudinal bone healing with less remodeling in 3 to 4 weeks. In this technique precision is needed. Occlusal relationship should be checked prior to screw fixation. Otherwise, this highly precise technique, will not allow any occlusal discrepancy correction later on, as it is possible in wire or monocortical bone plate osteosynthesis.

AO System (Figs 28.30 to 28.33)

1. Dynamic compression plate (DCP).
2. Eccentric dynamic compression plate (EDCP).

Plates and screws are made up of stainless steel and need removal later on. These plates are very bulky. Dynamic compression plate system makes compression osteosynthesis possible, because of the screw holes

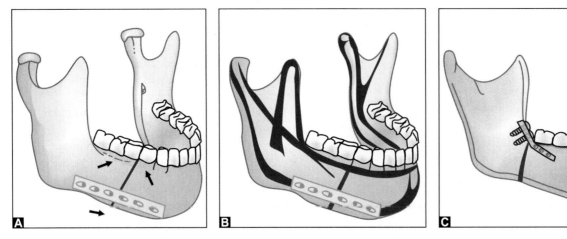

Figs 28.29A to C: Bone plate osteosynthesis (A and B) Rigid fixation. Eccentric dynamic compression plate system (EDCP) (C) Noncompression plating with monocortical screw fixation (Champy's technique)

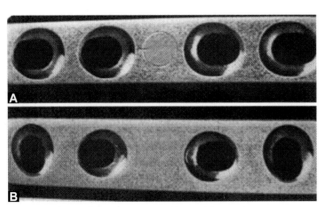

Figs 28.30A and B: AO system plates: (A) Dynamic compression plate, (B) Eccentric dynamic compression plate

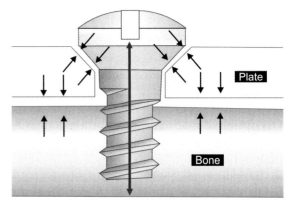

Fig. 28.31: Compressive forces between screw and plate countersink due to the tensile force induced into the screw. Force transmission takes place by the friction between the plate and bone

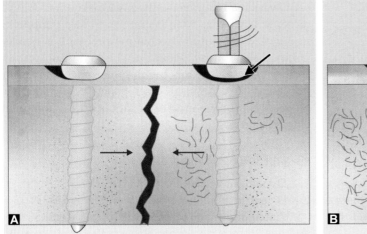

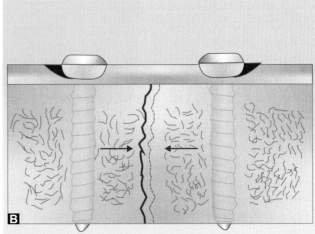

Figs 28.32A and B: Mode of action of DCP (A) Adaptation phase, (B) Compression phase

designed according to the spherical gliding principle for a 2.7 mm screw. In EDCP, the eccentric gliding hole principle is used. In eccentric dynamic compression plate, there are two lateral oblique holes in addition to conventional spherical gliding holes. When the screw with the spherical head is driven into the two inner holes, they provide interfragmentary compression. It is possible by means of two outer holes to produce additional compression at the alveolar margin of the fractured fragment. The two lateral oblique holes take over the function of the tension band in the alveolar margin.

Miniplate Osteosynthesis (Noncompression Monocortical Screw System)

This is a complete different concept than compression bone plate system. This is developed in France by Michelet in 1973 and made clinically popular by Champy in 1975 (Strasbourg Miniplate Osteosynthesis).

Aim: To attain a functionally oriented fracture adaptation. Fixation with miniplate system, which is as small as possible. Application of the plate to the region of the traction side of the bone.

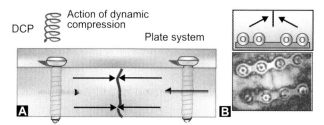

Figs 28.33A and B: Side screw inserted and not tightened. Screw is inserted and tightened first. The screw head moves down the gliding plane of the hole in the plate

Therapeutic Principle: Fixation by Stability

Stability is achieved by a perfect anatomic reduction and intrafragmentary approximation without compression. Champy recognized that in function, it is possible to identify the lines of tension, which when controlled will stabilize the fracture. He also noted that the reciprocal compression force at the lower border, controlled by bone to bone contact across the fracture line. Because these are tensile forces, equivalent to a suspension bridge, small plates will take these loads. Thus, by identifying the lines of tension, miniplate osteosynthesis can be used to obtain immediate jaw function.

The important anatomical issues with monocortical miniplate osteosynthesis are:
1. The location of the dense cortical bone.
2. The location and course of the mandibular canal.
3. Displacing forces acting on the mandible.

Anatomy and Biomechanics of the Mandible

Champy's Ideal Osteosynthesis Lines (Figs 28.34 to 28.37)

Mandible has parabola shaped body. It consists of the outer and inner cortical plates with central spongiosa. The external cortex is strong and thicker in chin region. It is reinforced laterally by the external oblique line—a strong projection. In the chin region, there is a stronger cortex inferiorly at the lower border. By the virtue of its compact bone, it provides good anchorage for osteosynthesis screws. In the tooth bearing areas, alveolar process is of variable thickness. Screw fixation in this area is not possible, due to the anatomy of the roots of the teeth and structure of the bone. The mandibular canal runs from lingula to the mental foramen on a concave course directed upward and forward. Traced

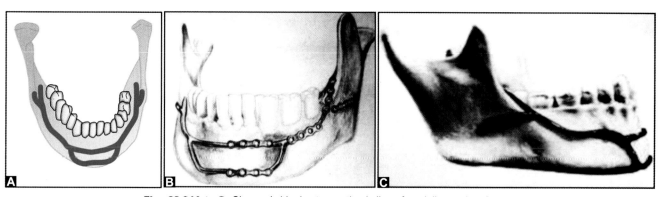

Figs 28.34A to C: Champy's ideal osteosynthesis lines for minibone plate fixation

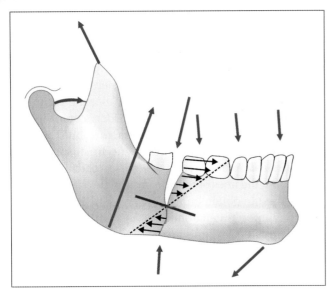

Fig. 28.35: Red line indicates 'the line of zero force' at the mandibular canal level. A fracture is subjected to tensile forces above the line and to compressive forces below the line

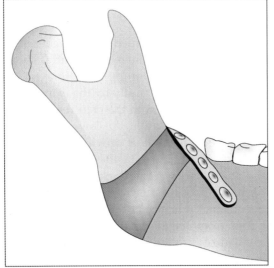

Fig. 28.36: Mini bone plate osteosynthesis at the angle region

from behind forward, the inferior alveolar nerve runs closer to the outer cortex and to the lower border (8 to 10 mm from lower border). Distance between the nerve and the outer cortex ranges between 4 and 6 mm. The mental foramen lies higher than the canine apices (no osteosynthesis).

In every mandibular fracture, the forces of mastication produce tension forces at the upper border and compression forces at the lower border. Therefore, distraction of the fractured fragments will be seen at the alveolar crest region. In the canine region, there are overlapping tensile and compressive loads in both the directions. Besides this torsional forces are also significant.

The experimental exercise on the model and on the fractured mandibles have confirmed the values calculated on the normal mandible is 60 DaN (maximum) in molar region and 100 DaN in the incisor region, allowing for the additional torsional forces. Taking into account these anatomical factors, the determination of these forces allows the establishment of 'ideal osteosynthesis lines' for the mandibular body. It corresponds to the course of a line of tension at the base of the alveolar process. In this region a plate can be fixed with monocortical self-tapping screws. Behind the mental foramen, a plate can be applied immediately below the root apices and above the inferior alveolar nerve. At the angle of the jaw, the plate is most favorably placed on the broad surface of the external oblique line as high as possible. In the anterior region between the mental foramina, in addition to the subapical plate, another plate near the lower border of the mandible is necessary in order to neutralize torsional forces. Second plate is applied parallel to the first plate with a gap of 4.5 mm between them.

Biophysical properties of the osteosynthesis material: It should be bio-inert, biologically well tolerated. It can be miniaturized. It should be strong enough to withstand the bending and tension forces up to 60 to 100 DaN.

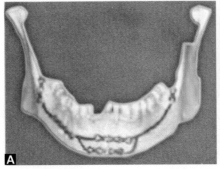
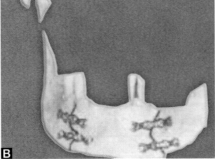
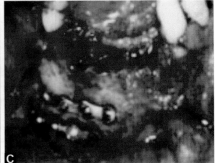

Figs 28.37A to C: Miniplate osteosynthesis at symphysis, parasymphysis, and angle region to neutralize the masticatory forces

Alloy of chrome, nickel and molybdenum with a trace of 0.03 percent carbon ensures good malleability. Screws and plates can be also made up of stainless steel, titanium, etc.

Miniplates: These are available as 2 cm long, 0.9 mm thick and 6 mm wide plates. Screws, plates and instruments should be made up of same material, since variation in material will lead to oxidation reduction phenomena, with detrimental tissue effects. The screws have a thread of 10/10 and in a cortical bone with an average thickness of 3.3 mm, the screws are secured with three turns. This is sufficient for monocortical anchorage.

Points to be Observed
1. The drilling must be precise and must be monoaxial. Otherwise, an unfavorable conical bur hole results.
2. The screws should be self-tapping.
3. The drill must be of the same width as of the screw core.
4. The screw thread must be relatively narrow, so that considerable contact is made in between the turns of the thread, which is 1 mm.

5. Plates must be fixed along the ideal osteosynthesis lines.

Complications: There are few complications directly related to the use of miniplates. The complication rates with respect to infection, delayed union, malunion and malocclusion vary from 5 to 15 percent.

Complications can arise due to:
1. Incorrect diagnosis.
2. Incorrect occlusion.
3. Incorrect osteosynthesis and include:
   • Infection
   • Dehiscence of wound, exposure of plate
   • Malocclusion
   • Fracture mobility
   • Pain at the site of plate
   • Metallic feeling for male patient during shaving.

29 Fractures of the Middle Third of the Facial Skeleton

Fractures of the middle third of the face are seen less frequently than the fractures of the mandible. However, the incidence is increasing due to high speed transportation accidents.

MIDDLE THIRD OF THE FACIAL SKELETON

Middle third of the facial skeleton is defined as an area bounded superiorly by a line drawn across the skull from the zygomaticofrontal suture of one side, across the frontonasal and frontomaxillary sutures to the zygomaticofrontal suture on the opposite side, and inferiorly by the occlusal plane of the upper teeth, or, if the patient is edentulous, by the upper alveolar ridge. Posteriorly, the region is demarcated by the spheno-ethmoidal junction, but includes the free margin of the pterygoid laminae of the sphenoid bone inferiorly.

Bones Constituting the Middle Third of the Face (Fig. 29.1)

These are eight paired bones and two unpaired bones constituting the middle third of the face.

1. The two maxillae.
2. The two palatine bones.
3. The two zygomatic bones and their temporal processes.

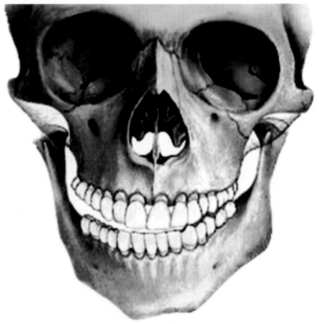

Fig. 29.1: Bones constituting the middle third of the face

4. The two zygomatic processes of temporal bones.
5. The two nasal bones.
6. The two lacrimal bones.
7. The ethmoid bone and its attached conchae-unpaired.

8. The two inferior conchae.
9. The two pterygoid plates of the sphenoid.
10. The vomer—unpaired.

Physical Characteristics of the Midfacial Skeleton

1. The middle third of the facial skeleton is made up of considerable number of bones, which are rarely fractured in isolation.
2. All the bones are comparatively fragile and they articulate in a most complex fashion.
3. The greatest portion of the middle third of the face is made up of the maxilla, which is attached to the cranium and supported by a strong system of buttresses.
   The maxilla is capable of absorbing considerable force by transmission of the force to the adjacent articulating bones. Midface acts as a cushion for the trauma directed towards the cranium from the anterior or anterolateral direction analogous to a 'matchbox' sitting below and in front of a hard shell containing the brain. Violent forces to this region are dissipated or absorbed by fractures of the maxilla and other facial bones, and thus offer protection to the brain and spinal cord (Fig. 29.2).
4. The area of the middle third of the facial skeleton is anatomically complex and complicated, so that fractures of this area are generally comminuted, especially the bones of the nasoethmoidal complex and anterior maxillae. It is this inward crushing causes 'typical dish face deformity.'

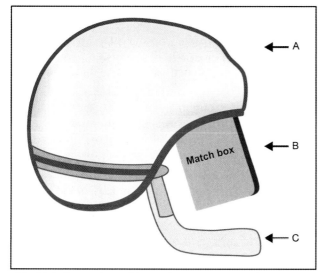

Fig. 29.2: Comparison of the midface to a 'matchbox': A—Skull, B—Midface, C—Mandible

5. The composite structure of this complex bones is so designed that it will withstand the forces of mastication from below and provide protection to the vital structures (e.g. eyes, brain, etc.). The forces of mastication are distributed around the fragile areas of the nose and paranasal sinuses to the base of the skull.
6. This type of structure is able to withstand considerable amount of force applied in a vertical manner from below, but the bones can be easily fractured by relatively small impact, if applied from other directions, i.e. anterior, superior or lateral aspects.
7. The facial bones as a whole, have a very low tolerance to impact forces from the front and sideways. The nasal bones are least resistant, followed by the zygomatic arch, while the maxilla itself is very sensitive to horizontal impacts.
8. If the bones comprising the middle third, are removed from the skull, it will be seen that the frontal bone and body of the sphenoid form an inclined plane, which slopes downward and backward from the frontal bone at an angle of about 45° to the occlusal plane of the upper teeth. The bones of the middle third of the facial skeleton articulate with these strong foundation bones and when fracture occurs, they are crushed or sheared off the cranial base. There is slight amount of backward, but marked downward displacement seen, because of the steep slope of the base of the skull, resulting in the premature gagging of the posterior teeth of the maxilla with the mandibular teeth, causing resultant anterior open bite and lengthening of the face and in extreme cases, the soft palate may be pushed down upon the dorsum of the tongue causing airway obstruction (Fig. 29.3).
9. Any gross disruption of the maxillae will fracture and displace the elements of the nasal septum and nasal bones and expose the paranasal air sinuses to the possibility of infection. In addition, nasal respiration may be impeded by the nasal airway becoming occluded by blood clot (Fig. 29.4).
10. Comminution of the paper thin bone of the orbital floor and medial wall of the orbit readily occurs. Along with backward and downward displacement of the middle third, there is impairment for the support of the eye. Diplopia of a varying degree can occur and is most severe, when there is rupture of the medial or lateral attachments of the suspensory ligament of Lockwood.

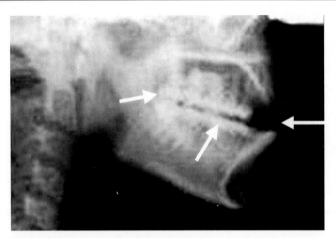

Fig. 29.3: Lateral cephalogram showing the posterior and downward displacement of the middle third of maxilla due to trauma. Note the reverse overjet, anterior open bite, premature gagging of the posterior teeth (Arrows)

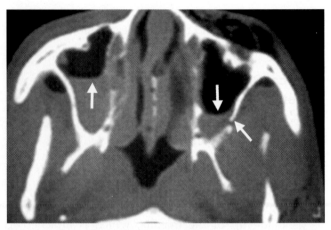

Fig. 29.4: Gross displacement of nasal bones and zygoma will bring about involvement of maxillary sinuses. Bleeding in the maxillary sinuses shows the *fluid collection level* in the CT scan (Arrows)

11. A shearing stress applied to the ethmoidal region results in comminution of the cribriform plate of the ethmoid bone and provides direct access to the anterior cranial fossa. Leakage of cerebrospinal fluid can take place following this injury. It may appear running down the nose mixed with the blood. It is easier to detect when the blood begins to coagulate. If the patient is lying down, then the CSF may pass downward in the nasopharynx and there will be presence of salty taste during swallowing. The flow of CSF will increase, if patient sits up with head inclined forward, coughing, straining or on compression of the jugular veins.

12. The maxillary, palatine, ethmoid, vomer, lacrimal and body of the sphenoid bones are enclosed in mucosa covering large areas of their surfaces, hence the blood supply to any part of the midfacial skeleton is never compromised.

Applied and Surgical Anatomy

The majority of the skeleton of the middle third of the face is composed of wafer thin sheets of the cortical bone with stronger bony reinforcement comprising of the following:

1. The palate and alveolar process.
2. The lateral rim of the pyriform aperture extending upward via the canine fossa to the medial orbital rim and then to the glabella.
3. Zygomatic buttress and the connections to the inferior and lateral orbital margins and the zygomatic arch.

4. The orbital rims.
5. The pterygoid plates.

The bulk of the strength lies in the facial surfaces of the skeleton. Although thin at sites other than those mentioned above, the whole skeleton is strong, because the interconnected laminae provide an excellent cross-braced type of structure.

The maxilla, the composite of the maxillary and palatine bones, forms the largest part of the middle third of the face and contributes to the formation of the orbit, the nasal cavities and the hard palate (roof of the mouth). The body of each maxillary bone is hollowed out by the maxillary sinus.

The body of each maxilla has four processes—frontal, zygomatic, palatine and alveolar. The stability of the maxilla is obtained by bracing against the anterior part of the cranial base. The maxillae are ingeniously designed to resist the forces of mastication, to absorb the shock of the occluding teeth and to distribute the load as evenly as possible over the cranial base.

This load distribution is achieved by the arched shape of the palate, and the abutments of the maxillae against the frontomaxillary, zygomaticomaxillary, and maxillary ethmoidal sutures. Posteriorly a strong buttress is provided by the junction of the pyramidal process of the palatine bone and the pterygoid laminae of the sphenoid bone.

Further support is provided by the vomer and vertical plate of the ethmoid in the nasal cavity. The zygomatic bone redistributes the load to the frontal bone via the zygomaticofrontal suture, and, to a lesser extent, to the temporal bone via the junction of the temporal

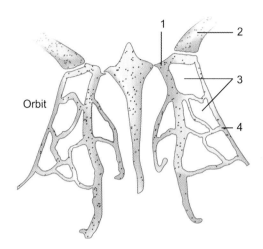

Fig. 29.5: Coronal section of the skull showing delicate laminae framework distributed in a vertical direction. Alignment is along the lines of principle stress: (1) Cribriform plate, (2) Frontal bone, (3) Ethmoid air cells, (4) Lamina papyracea

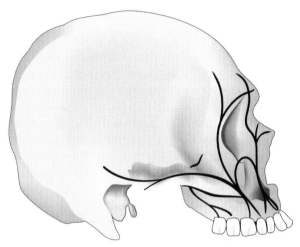

Fig. 29.6: Supporting anterior, middle and posterior vertical pillars of the maxillary skeleton

process of the zygomatic bone and the zygomatic process of the temporal bone. Furthermore, the presence of the maxillary and ethmoidal air sinuses is responsible for the honeycomb type of formation typical of the middle third of the facial skeleton, which is best seen in the coronal section of the skull. The delicate laminae which constitute this lattice framework are principally distributed in a vertical direction, thereby being aligned along the lines of principal stress (Fig. 29.5).

Supporting Vertical and Horizontal Pillars of the Maxillary Skeleton (Figs 29.6 and 29.7)

Vertical pillars: On either side of the facial skeleton, one finds three pillars or buttresses—anterior, middle and posterior.

Anterior or the canine pillar: It starts in the region of the alveolar process of the canine, forms the lateral boundary of the anterior nasal aperture and continues as the frontal process of the maxilla to the frontal bone.

Middle or zygomatic pillar: It starts in the region of the first molar, bends upward and outward as the zygomaticoalveolar crest and the zygomatic process of the maxilla to continue towards the frontal process of the zygoma to end at the zygomatic process of the frontal bone.

Posterior or pterygoid pillar: It is the pterygoid process of the sphenoid bone to which the pyramidal process of the palatine bone is anchored. These vertical pillars are

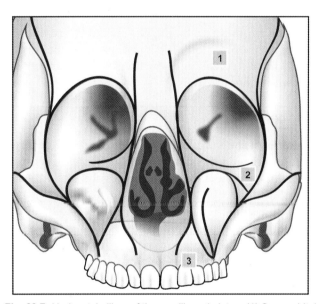

Fig. 29.7: Horizontal pillars of the maxillary skeleton: (1) Supraorbital rim, (2) Infraorbital rim, (3) Alveolar process

braced against each other by the superior and inferior orbital rims and the zygomatic arch.

Horizontal Pillars

1. Supraorbital rims with frontal bone.
2. Infraorbital rims.
3. Alveolar process.

Nerve Supply

The middle third of the face receives its nerve supply from the second division of the fifth nerve. Branches to the teeth pass through the outer cortex of the bone. The infraorbital nerve passes through the infraorbital canal below the floor of the orbit to innervate the soft tissues of the lower lid, the cheek and the lateral aspect of the nose and the upper lip. The palatine branches innervate the mucosa of the palate. The nasopalatine nerve passes anteriorly in the mucosa of the nasal septum bilaterally and through the incisive foramen to innervate the mucosa of the anterior palatine area.

Important Blood Vessels

The third part of the maxillary artery and its terminal branches are closely associated with the fractures of the middle third of the face. Occasionally the artery or its greater palatine branch is torn in the region of the pterygomaxillary fissure or pterygopalatine canal resulting in severe lifethreatening hemorrhage into the nasopharynx. Insertion of postnasal pack will be needed for 24 hours. Adequate reduction of the fracture will prevent further bleeding.

Surgical Anatomy

Fractures of the maxilla are usually the result of direct force and range from simple alveolar fractures to extensive injuries to the bones of the nose, orbit, palate, skull, etc.

Displacement is usually entirely the result of the traumatic force. Muscle contraction plays an unimportant role in the displacement of maxillary fractures, except in those extending into the region of the pterygoid plates, in which displacement of maxilla may be in a downward and posterior direction due to the action of the pterygoid muscles. In complete craniofacial dysjunction associated with fractures of the zygoma, action of the masseter muscle may be a factor in displacement.

1. The lacrimal fossa is formed partially by the maxilla, and injuries to the nasolacrimal duct may be associated with the fractures of the maxilla, which results in epiphora.
2. Damage to the infraorbital and zygomatic nerves can occur unilaterally or bilaterally with zygomatic or maxillary fractures. Here, the anesthesia or paresthesia of the skin of the cheek and upper lip will be present. Full recovery may take up to two years. The anterior, middle, posterior superior alveolar nerves may be damaged, but patient seldom notices the anesthesia of the gum, but if tested with the instrument, areas of anesthesia will be found.
3. Cranial nerves within the orbit may sustain damage. The sixth nerve is most frequently involved, sometimes the contents of the superior orbital fissure are all damaged, in which case ophthalmoplegia, dilation of the pupil and anesthesia within the distribution of the ophthalmic branch of the fifth cranial nerve are noted. Rarely the orbital apex is fractured with resultant damage to the optic nerve and blindness.
4. Optic foramen is a ring of dense compact bone, therefore, invariably fracture line gets deflected away from the foramen protecting the optic nerve. The prominence of the zygomatic bone also protects the orbit from all impinging objects.
5. Fractures involving the orbital walls may give rise to alteration in the position of the globe of the eye (Ocular level). The ocular level is normally maintained by the suspensory ligament of Lockwood, which is attached on the medial side on the lacrimal bone and laterally inserted into Whitnall's tubercle, situated on the inner aspect of the zygomatic bone just below the frontozygomatic suture. Separation at or above this junction will bring about change in ocular level. As the globe of the eye drops, the upper eyelid, follows it downward known as 'hooding of the eye.'
6. If the orbital floor is fractured, there will be herniation of orbital contents into the maxillary sinus. There can be entrapment of tissues resulting in the restriction of the movements of inferior rectus and oblique muscles. There can be temporary or permanent diplopia due to prevention of the upward and outward rotation of the eye.
7. Herniation of the orbital contents into the maxillary sinus or through the thin lamina papyracea of the ethmoid bone on the medial wall of the orbit will lead to enophthalmos.
8. Detachment of the medial canthal attachment of the eye may occur in severe nasoethmoidal complex fractures resulting in traumatic telecanthus.
9. Retrobulbar hemorrhage can cause temporary blindness and exophthalmus.
10. Gross comminution of the antral walls and other fractures involving sinuses can cause bleeding. The sinus will be full of blood and appear hazy in the radiograph. There may be unilateral or bilateral epistaxis depending on the involvement.

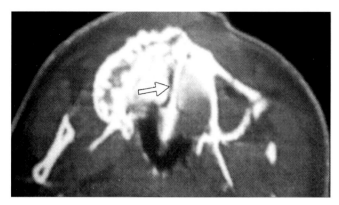

Fig. 29.8: CT scan showing *midpalatal split* of the maxilla along with LeFort II fracture

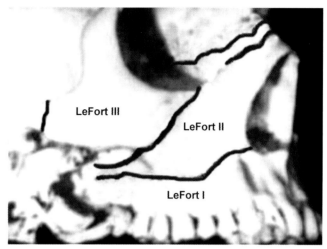

Fig. 29.9: LeFort's classification for middle third of the facial skeleton

11. A depressed fracture of the zygomatic arch or displaced zygoma can cause impingement on the coronoid process of the mandible and it will cause mechanical blockage for the normal movements of mandible. Restricted oral opening will be seen.

12. Midpalatine split of the maxilla is only possible when the injury results from a blow transmitted upward via the mandibular teeth with the jaw open (Fig. 29.8).

CLASSIFICATION OF FRACTURES OF MIDDLE THIRD OF FACIAL SKELETON (FIGS 29.9 TO 29.18)

Classification is mainly helpful for communication purpose. The present precise knowledge of the lines of fracture in the middle third of the facial skeleton, which are produced following injury, is largely due to the experimental studies carried out by a French surgeon, Rene LeFort in 1901 in Paris. Following experimental trauma to the cadaver head and removal of the soft tissues, LeFort discovered that the complex fracture patterns could be broadly subdivided into three groups:

1. LeFort I, LeFort II and LeFort III (Fig. 29.9).
2. Erich's (1942) classified these fractures as per the direction of the fracture line (Figs 29.10 and 29.11).
   i. Horizontal fracture
   ii. Pyramidal fracture
   iii. Transverse fracture
3. Depending on the relationship of the fracture line to the zygomatic bone
   i. Below the zygomatic bone—subzygomatic fractures

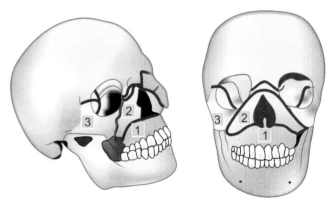

Fig. 29.10: Erich's classification of fractures of the middle third of the facial skeleton: (1) Horizontal fracture, (2) Pyramidal fracture, (3) Transverse fracture

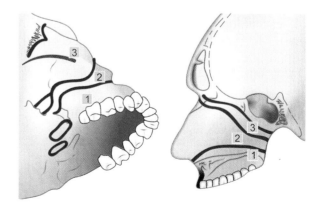

Fig. 29.11: Fractures of the middle third of the face: (1) Horizontal or Guerin or LeFort I fracture, (2) Pyramidal or LeFort II fracture, (3) Craniofacial dysjunction, transverse or LeFort III fracture

ii. Above or including the zygomatic bone—supra-zygomatic fracture

4. Depending on the level of a fracture line
   i. Low level fracture
   ii. Mid level fracture
   iii. High level fracture

5. General classification can be applied to the maxillary fractures (Discussed in mandibular fracture)

6. Rowe and William's classification (1985)
   i. Fractures not involving the teeth and alveolus
      a. Central region
      b. Lateral region
   ii. Fractures involving the teeth and alveolus
      a. Central region
      b. Combined central and lateral region

The most universally used classification is LeFort's classification. Clinically, the identical solitary lines may not be seen, but the direction and description of the lines will help in planning the reduction and fixation. Otherwise, at many places like anterior wall of the maxillary sinus, multiple fragmentation will be seen.

LeFort I Fracture (Low Level, Subzygomatic Fracture) (Fig. 29.12)

It is also called as *horizontal fracture* of the maxilla or *Guerin's* fracture. It is also known as *floating fracture*, as there is a separation of complete dentoalveolar part of the maxilla (pterygomaxillary dysjunction) and the fractured fragment is held only by means of soft tissues. The fractured fragment is freely mobile and the resultant displacement will depend on the direction of the force. Depending on the displacement of a fragment, variety of occlusal disharmony can be seen in this type of fracture (anterior open bite, cross bite, reverse overjet, etc.).

A violent force applied over a more extensive area, above the level of the teeth will result in a LeFort I fracture, which is not confined to smaller section of the alveolar bone. Here, the horizontal fracture line is seen above the apices of the teeth, which detaches the tooth bearing portion of the maxilla from the rest of the facial skeleton. The fracture line commences at the point on the lateral margin of the anterior nasal aperture, passes above the nasal floor, and it passes laterally above the canine fossa and traverses the lateral antral wall, dipping down below the zygomatic buttress and then inclines upward and posteriorly across the pterygomaxillary fissure to fracture the pterygoid laminae at the junction of their lower third and upper two-thirds. At the same time, from the same starting point, the fracture also passes along the lateral wall of the nose and subsequently joins the lateral line of fracture behind the tuberosity. The typical LeFort I fracture is always bilateral, with the fracture of the lower third of the nasal septum. But it can be unilateral also. The displacement will depend on the direction and severity of the force. Posterior, lateral displacement or rotation around its axis can be seen. The LeFort I fracture may occur as a single entity or in association with LeFort II and III fractures.

Clinical Signs and Symptoms of LeFort I Fracture

i. Slight swelling and edema of the lower part of the face along with the upper lip swelling. (Gross edema or facial disfigurement is not present).

ii. Ecchymosis in the labial and buccal vestibule, as well as contusion of the skin of the upper lip may be seen. Laceration of upper lip and intraoral mucosa may be seen.

iii. Bilateral epistaxis or nasal bleeding may be observed.

iv. The most common significant feature is the mobility of the upper dentoalveolar portion of the jaw, which is frequently mobile to digital pressure.

v. Occlusion may be disturbed. Patient will not be able to masticate the food.

vi. Pain while speaking and moving the jaw.

vii. Sometimes there will be upward displacement of the entire fragment, locking it against the superior intact structures, such a fracture will be called as impacted or telescopic fracture. A classical anterior open bite may be seen in this case.

viii. Percussion of the maxillary teeth produces dull 'cracked cup' sound.

LeFort II (Pyramidal or Subzygomatic) Fracture (Fig. 29.13)

Violent force, usually from an anterior direction, sustained by the central region of the middle third of the

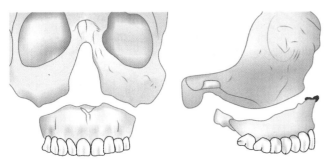

Fig. 29.12: LeFort I fracture lines

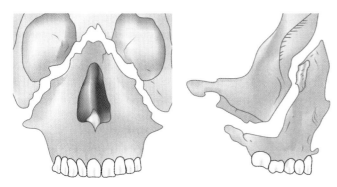

Fig. 29.13: LeFort II fracture lines

facial skeleton over an area extending from the glabella to the alveolar margin results in a fracture of a pyramidal shape. The force may be delivered at the level of the nasal bones.

The fracture line runs below the frontonasal suture from the thin middle area of the nasal bones down on either side, crossing the frontal process of the maxillae and passes anteriorly across the lacrimal bones, immediately anterior to nasolacrimal canal. From this point the fracture line passes downward, forward and laterally crossing the inferior orbital margin, in the region of zygomaticomaxillary suture. It may or may not involve the infraorbital foramen. The fracture line now extends downward and forward and laterally to traverse the lateral wall of the antrum, just medial to the zygomaticomaxillary suture line. As in LeFort I fracture, this fracture line passes beneath the zygomatic buttress, but after that, it inclines rather more abruptly than in the former instance, traversing the pterygomaxillary fissure at a higher level and fracturing the pterygoid laminae approximately midway from its base. Separation of the entire pyramidal block from the base of the skull is completed via the nasal septum.

Clinical Signs and Symptoms of LeFort II Fracture

 i. There is a gross edema of the middle third of the face known as ballooning or moon face. Edema sets in within a short time of injury.
 ii. Presence of bilateral circumorbital edema and ecchymosis (Black eye). Rapid swelling of the eyelids makes examination of the eyes difficult.
 iii. Bilateral subconjunctival hemorrhage confined to medial half of the eye.
 iv. The bridge of the nose will be depressed (flat face). Nasal disfigurement.
 v. If there is impaction of the fragment against the cranial base, then shortening of the face with anterior open bite will be seen.
 vi. If there is gross downward and backward displacement of the fragment, then elongation or lengthening of the face will be seen with posterior gagging of the occlusion with anterior open bite (Dish-shaped face).
 vii. Bilateral epistaxis may be present.
 viii. Difficulty in mastication, and speech.
 ix. Loss of occlusion may be seen.
 x. Airway obstruction may be seen due to posterior and downward displacement of the fragment impinging on the dorsum of the tongue.
 xi. Surgical emphysema—crackling sensation transmitted to the fingers due to escape of air from the paranasal sinuses is seen.
 xii. CSF leak may be present.
 xiii. Step deformity at the infraorbital margins may be seen.
 xiv. Anesthesia and/or paresthesia of the cheek is noted.

LeFort III Fracture (Transverse or Suprazygomatic) Fracture (Fig. 29.14)

It is also known as *high level* fracture. The line of fracture extends above the zygomatic bones on both sides as a result of trauma being inflicted over a wider area, at the orbital level. The force is usually applied from the lateral direction with a severe impact. Here the initial impact is taken by the zygomatic bone resulting in depressed fracture and then because of the severe degree of the impact, the entire middle third will then hinge about the fragile ethmoid bone and the impact will then be transmitted on the contralateral side resulting in laterally displaced zygomatic fracture of the opposite side (craniofacial dysjunction).

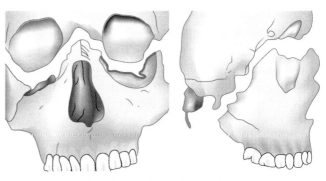

Fig. 29.14: LeFort III fracture lines

In a typically high level LeFort III fracture, the line commences near the frontonasal suture, causes dislocation of the nasal bones and disruption of cribriform plate of the ethmoid bone with tearing of dura mater and consequent CSF rhinorrhea. In such cases, the line of fracture crosses both the nasal bones and the frontal process of the maxilla, near the frontonasal and frontomaxillary sutures and then traverses the upper limit of the lacrimal bones. Continuing posteriorly, the line crosses the thin orbital plate of the ethmoid bone constituting part of the medial wall of the orbits. As the medial orbital wall is very thin, comminution of the fracture line is seen in this region. As the optic foramen is surrounded by a dense ring of bone, the fracture line gets deflected downward and laterally to reach the medial aspect of the posterior limit of the inferior orbital fissure. From this point, the fracture descends across the upper posterior aspect of the maxillae in the region of the sphenopalatine fossa and upper limit of the pterygomaxillary fissures and fractures the roots of the pterygoid laminae at its base.

The inferior orbital fissure constitutes a natural line of weakness and from its anterior and lateral end, on each side a further line of fracture passes across the lateral wall of the orbit, adjacent to the junction of the zygomatic bone with the greater wing of sphenoid. The fracture line separates the zygomatic bone from the frontal bone near the suture and then inclines laterally, running abruptly downward across the infratemporal surface, thus in effect joining the previous line of fracture seen on the medial wall of the orbit. The entire middle third is thus detached from the dense cranial base, the occlusal plane of the maxillary teeth in most instances, being tilted downward and backward so that there is gagging with anterior open bite.

Clinical Signs and Symptoms of LeFort III Fracture

Clinically this fracture appears similar to the LeFort II fracture, but close examination will demonstrate a more serious condition. After stabilizing the head and then gripping of the maxillary teeth with one hand and simple manipulation, will confirm complete movement of the middle third of the face. Mobility of whole skeleton as a single block can be felt.

  i. Gross edema of the face, ballooning.'Panda facies', within 24 to 48 hours.
  ii. Bilateral circumorbital/periorbital ecchymosis and gross edema 'Racoon eyes'. Gross circumorbital edema will prevent eyes from opening.
  iii. Bilateral subconjunctival hemorrhage, where posterior limit will not be seen, when patient is asked to look medially.
  iv. There may be tenderness and separation at the frontozygomatic sutures.This will produce lengthening of the face and lowering of the ocular level. Unilateral or bilateral hooding of the eyes is seen.
  v. Characteristic 'dish face' deformity.
  vi. May be enophthalmos, diplopia or impairment of vision, temporary blindness, etc.
  vii. Flattening and widening, deviation of the nasal bridge.
  viii. Epistaxis, CSF rhinorrhea.

Midline Separation of the Maxilla (Figs 29.8 and 29.15)

A natural line of weakness exists at the sutural interface between the two palatine bones of the maxilla. This is usually associated with high level impact. Any degree of separation of maxillae will result in associated fracture of zygomatic bones as pressure is exerted upon the zygomaticomaxillary suture.

Modification of LeFort's Fracture Classification

At the turn of the century, midface fracture patterns are seem to be far more complex than those produced in LeFort's laboratory in 1901. Fractures involving the cranial base and other midface fracture configurations, including severely comminuted segments of the facial skeleton, are not accurately classifiable using the traditional LeFort scheme. A modified classification system is therefore proposed *by Marciani in 1993* to more precisely define LeFort, NOE (naso-orbital-ethmoidal) and zygomaticomaxillary fracture patterns.

LeFort I   :   Low maxillary fracture
Ia   :   Low maxillary fracture/multiple segments
LeFort II   :   Pyramidal fracture
IIa   :   Pyramidal and nasal fracture
IIb   :   Pyramidal and NOE fracture
LeFort III   :   Craniofacial dysjunction
IIIa   :   Craniofacial dysjunction and nasal fracture
IIIb   :   Craniofacial dysjunction and NOE fracture
LeFort IV   :   LeFort II or III fracture and cranial base fracture
IVa   :   + Supraorbital rim fracture
IVb   :   + Anterior cranial fossa and supraorbital rim fracture
IVc   :   + Anterior cranial fossa and orbital wall fracture

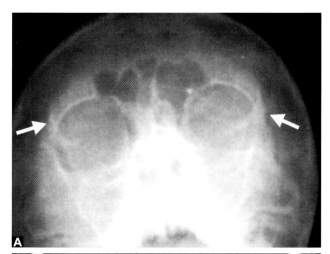

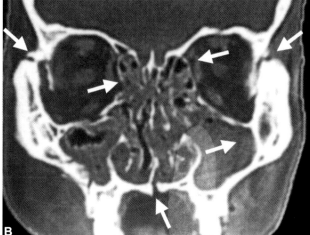

Figs 29.15A and B: High level fracture of middle third of the face with midpalatal split. (A) PA view Water's position; (B) Coronal CT scan showing the break in the continuity at various levels. Note the deviation of nasal septum, haziness of both the maxillary sinuses, bilateral fractures at frontozygomatic sutures, midpalatal split, fractures of nasal bones and maxilla

Rowe and William's (1985) Classification

A. *Fractures not involving the dentoalveolar component*
1. Central region:
   a. Fractures of the nasal bones and/or nasal septum.
      i. Lateral nasal injuries.
      ii. Anterior nasal injuries.
   b. Fractures of the frontal process of the maxilla.
   c. Fractures of type (a) and (b) which extend into the ethmoid bone (nasoethmoid).
   d. Fractures of type (a), (b), and (c) which extend into the frontal bone (fronto-orbitonasal dislocation).

2. Lateral region—fractures involving the zygomatic bone, arch and maxilla (zygomaticomaxillary complex) excluding the dentoalveolar component.

B. *Fractures involving the dentoalveolar component*
1. *Central region*
   i. *Dentoalveolar fractures*—iatrogenic fractures of maxillary tuberosity and floor of the maxillary antrum occur during extraction of maxillary third and second molars. Whenever, the trauma is distributed over a wider area involving the alveolus in addition to the teeth, then a fracture of a block of alveolar bone together with two or more teeth will occur. The complete section is usually palatally driven, but labial or buccal displacement also can be seen. Because of this type of fracture, the occlusion gets disturbed. There will be associated tear of the soft tissues seen. Dentoalveolar fractures should be reduced as early as possible and can be stabilized using horizontal Erich's arch bar fixation or any kind of horizontal dental arch wiring.

   The support of the adjoining firm teeth is taken for stabilization. Before final tightening of the wires, occlusion of the teeth should be checked.

   ii. *Subzygomatic fracture*
      a. LeFort I (low level or Guerin)
      b. LeFort II (pyramidal)

      The above fractures may be unilateral or associated with fracture of zygomatic bone.
2. Combined central and lateral region fractures
   a. High level, suprazygomatic fractures—LeFort III
   b. LeFort III with midline split
   c. LeFort III with midline split + fracture of the roof of the orbit or frontal bone.

■ FRACTURES OF THE ZYGOMATIC COMPLEX

As the zygomatic bone is closely associated with the maxilla, frontal and temporal bones and they are usually involved when a zygomatic bone fracture occurs, therefore these types of fractures are referred to as '*zygomatic complex fractures*' or '*zygomaticomaxillary complex fractures*' or '*tripod fractures*'.

The zygomatic bone usually fractures in the region of the zygomaticofrontal suture, the zygomaticotemporal suture and the zygomaticomaxillary suture. It is unusual for the zygomatic bone itself to be fractured, but in extreme violence, the bone may be comminuted or split across. The isolated zygomatic arch fracture may occur without displacement of the zygomatic bone.

Applied Anatomy

The disarticulated zygomatic bone is a dense, strong structure rather like a four pointed star, slightly curved on flat surface, with the upper point forming the frontal process, the distal point forming the temporal process or anterior section of the arch, the medial point forming the outer half of the inferior orbital rim, and the lower point constituting the buttress, which can be palpated in the upper buccal sulcus. The convexity on the outer surface of the zygomatic body forms the point of greatest prominence of the cheek. Therefore, the zygoma plays a major role in facial contour. The zygoma articulates with four bones—the frontal, sphenoid, maxillary and temporal:

1. The most striking feature is the thickness and strength evident at the zygomaticomaxillary suture area.
2. Medial to this broad sutural interface is an area of extremely thin bone comprising the lateral wall of the antrum.
3. The buttress distributes the masticatory stress to the cranial base and is adapted to withstand a considerable force from below via the broad zygomaticomaxillary suture.
4. A slender temporal process extends posteriorly to form alongwith the zygomatic process of the temporal bone, the zygomatic arch. The coronoid process of the mandible moves between the arch and the infratemporal fossa.
5. The temporalis fascia is attached to the zygomatic bone and arch, whereas, the temporalis muscle is inserted via its tendon into the tip and anteromedial surface of the coronoid process of the mandible. The space between the fascia and the muscle provides a route to approach the posterior surface of the zygomatic bone and the medial aspect of the arch, which is utilized for elevation of the bone during reduction procedure.
6. Rowe has suggested that the displacement of the zygomatic bone can be best understood by reference to rotation about different axes. Here, the *vertical axis* is an imaginary line drawn from the frontozygomatic suture which passes downward

through the center of the body to the buttress. A blow received *in front of* the vertical axis will result in rotation of the horizontal plane, represented by the outer half of the inferior orbital margin and orbital floor. There will be outward movement of the center of the arch. If the blow is received *behind* the vertical axis, then the rotation of the horizontal plane in the opposite direction will be noticed with considerable movement of the arch and outward movement of the rim and floor.

The *longitudinal* or *horizontal axis* is represented by a line at the level of the infraorbital foramen which passes from in front horizontally backward through the center of the body of the bone and the zygomatic arch. An *impact above this level* will result in rotation of the vertical plane with medial movement of the frontal process and a slight outward movement at the buttress. If the impact is received directly on the line then there will be *en bloc* displacement. But with an *impact received from below* the longitudinal axis, then there will be lateral movement of the frontal process and medial displacement of the buttress into the antral cavity.

Classification of the Zygomatic Complex Fracture (Rowe and Killey 1968) (Figs 29.16 and 29.17)

Type I   : No significant displacement
Type II   : Fractures of the zygomatic arch
Type III : Rotation around the vertical axis
      a. Inward displacement of orbital rim
      b. Outward displacement of orbital rim
Type IV   : Rotation around the longitudinal axis
      a. Medial displacement of the frontal process
      b. Lateral displacement of frontal process
Type V   : Displacement of the complex *en bloc*
      a. Medial
      b. Inferior
      c. Lateral (rare)
Type VI   : Displacement of the orbitoantral partition
      a. Inferiorly
      b. Superiorly (rare)
Type VII : Displacement of orbital rim segments
Type VIII : Complex comminuted fractures.

In 1985, Rowe changed his 1968 classification and gave more clinical significance by dividing fractures into stable and unstable varieties. This is similar to the classification created by *Larsen and Thomsen in*

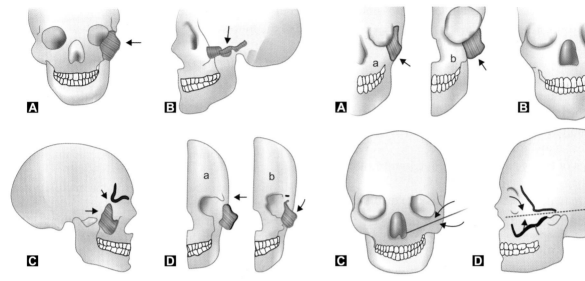

Figs 29.16A to D: Fractures of the zygomatic complex: (A) Group I: No significant displacement, (B) Group II: Zygomatic arch fracture, (C) Group III: Unrotated body fracture, (D) Group IV: Medially rotated body fractures: (a) outward at zygomatic prominence; (b) inward at zygomaticofrontal suture

Figs 29.17A to D: Fractures of the zygomatic complex: (A) Group V: Laterally rotated body fractures (a) upward at infraorbital margin; (b) outward at zygomaticofrontal suture; (B) Complex fractures; (C and D) Directions of force

1968, which is a very simple, yet practical classification for zygomatic fractures.

- Group A: Stable fracture—showing minimal or no displacement and requires no intervention.
- Group B: Unstable fracture—with great displacement and disruption at the frontozygomatic suture and comminuted fractures. Requires reduction as well as fixation.
- Group C: Stable fracture—other types of zygomatic fractures, which require reduction, but no fixation.

Fractures of the zygomatic arch alone not involving the orbit can be classified as follows (Fig. 29.18):

1. Minimum or no displacement
2. V type infracture
3. Comminuted fracture.

Signs and Symptoms

1. *Flattening of the injured cheek* (possibly masked by swelling)—most common displacement of the complex is inward. Immediately following the injury or after the acute phase of the edema is subsided, then an alteration of contour on the affected side is apparent. This is best seen by viewing the patient either from above, by standing behind and above the patient and comparing both the sides of the face or by viewing it from below.

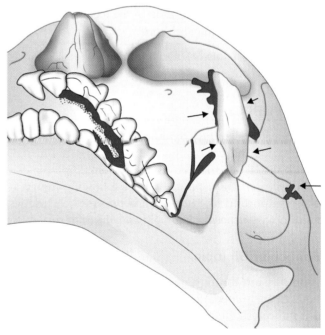

Fig. 29.18: Fracture of the zygomatic arch impinging on the coronoid process of the mandible (Arrows)

2. Unilateral epistaxis may be present.
3. Circumorbital ecchymosis will develop after few hours from effusion of blood into the surrounding tissues. Circumorbital edema can be quite gross.

The examination of the eye may not be possible, till edema subsides.

4. Subconjunctival hemorrhage will be observed at the outer canthus, if the patient is asked to look medially, the posterior limit of the effusion cannot be defined. Such an appearance is indicative of fracture of the lateral orbital wall or floor.
5. Depression of the ocular level/limitation of ocular movement may be seen.
6. Proptosis of the eye may be seen due to retrobulbar hemorrhage.
7. Patient may complain of diplopia and/or blurring of vision.
8. Anesthesia of the cheek, nose and lip may be present.
9. Edema of the cheek and eyelids. Traumatic emphysema can often be detected in the infraorbital region, if air escapes into the tissues from the maxillary sinus.
10. Step deformity of the infraorbital margin.
11. Limitation of mandibular movement.
12. Ecchymosis and tenderness in the upper buccal sulcus, change in sensation of the teeth and gums.
13. Enophthalmos may be seen.

Radiographic examination: Occipitomenton projection is the best projection for the complex.

■ DIPLOPIA

Diplopia is a relatively common complication following fractures of the zygomatic complex. It is a blurred, double vision experienced by the patient. Diplopia can be of *temporary* or *permanent* nature following injury. It is also important to distinguish between two varieties of diplopia—*monocular* diplopia and *binocular* diplopia.

Monocular Diplopia

Double vision through one eye, with the other closed, requires the immediate attention of an ophthalmologist, as it indicates a detached lens or other traumatic injury of the globe.

Binocular Diplopia

When looking through both eyes simultaneously, double vision is experienced by the patient, is common complaint and occurs in approximately in 10 to 40 percent of zygomatic injuries. Diplopia can be caused due to the following:

Physical Interference

1. Intramuscular hematoma or edema of one or more of the extraocular muscles.
2. Disturbance to the attachment of inferior rectus or inferior oblique muscle (change in orbital shape with displacement of the globe causing muscle imbalance).
3. Herniation of periorbital fat into the maxillary sinus (orbital floor fracture).
4. Muscle or periorbital tissue entrapment in the fractured fragments (immediate and temporary diplopia).
5. Development of fibrous adhesions and fat atrophy; (late and permanent diplopia) during post-traumatic healing.

Functional Interference

Orbital floor fracture leads toward displacement of globe due to disturbance to the inferior rectus and inferior oblique muscle.

Enophthalmos and globe ptosis associated with marked displacement of the globe can cause diplopia.

Neurological Causes

i. Paralysis due to neuromuscular injury or edema.
ii. Supranuclear impairments of 3rd, 4th and 6th cranial nerves.
iii. Superior orbital fissure or intraorbital damage.
iv. Intracranial infranuclear injuries may lead to paresis of the nerve or paralysis of a muscle (late serious complication).

Diplopia is a common symptom in the early stages of the injury, which is caused mainly due to edema and effusion (hemorrhage) in and around the region of the extraocular muscles. This type of diplopia is usually temporary, but when there is actual damage to the extraocular muscles or to their nerve supply, recovery is less certain. It can be also caused by enophthalmos, which results when orbital fat herniates through the fractured orbital floor, into the maxillary sinus (a fracture of the orbital floor in isolation is termed as a blow-out fracture). Diplopia due to this reason at the time of injury may not necessarily be a cause for concern, but must be followed closely after reduction of a fracture. Whenever, the level of the eyes is altered, because of injury, there is invariably alteration in the visual axis as well as in the lines of action of the extraocular muscles and results in diplopia.

Alteration of the ocular level depends on the level at which the fracture occurs in the lateral wall of the orbit (Fig. 29.19) (The globe of the eye is supported by Lockwood's suspensory ligament, which is a fascial sling passing from the medial attachment in the region of the lacrimal bone, to be inserted laterally into Whitnall's tubercule, on the lateral wall of the orbit, just below the frontozygomatic suture). If the fracture passes below Whitnall's tubercle, the zygomatic bone can be grossly displaced downward without alteration in the level of the globe of the eye. But if the fracture occurs above Whitnall's tubercle, then alteration of the optical axis results in diplopia.

This is because of the globe getting lowered on one side and thereby the inferior rectus muscle is slightly shortened and the superior rectus is slightly lengthened. Here because of the displacement of the bone and change in ocular level, the upper lid exhibits a typical physical sign known as 'hooding' of the globe.

Diplopia resulting from damage to the extraocular muscles or their nerves is more serious. The extraocular muscles can become trapped within the bony fragments of the floor of the orbit and the inferior oblique muscle is the most commonly affected. Examination of the eye should include testing the fundus for evidence of edema and hemorrhage and testing extraocular muscle function. The result of the examination should be clearly noted so that the progress can be objectively assessed.

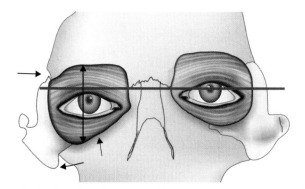

Fig. 29.19: Alteration of ocular level is seen due to the fracture dislocation of the lateral orbital rim. The palpebral ligament is attached to the frontal process of the zygoma. Arrows show the downward displacement of the eye and the palpebral ligament, with displaced bone fragments

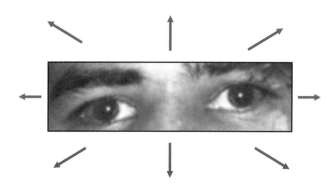

Fig. 29.20: Testing the motions of the eyes in all nine positions of gazes (Arrows). The ninth gaze is the frontal gaze. At the same time diplopia and ocular level is also checked

Testing the Motions of the Eye and Diplopia (Fig. 29.20)

Movement of the eye can be tested by holding a finger or an object at least an arm's length in front of the eyes. The movement of the eye should be examined in all nine positions of the gaze. Simultaneously patient should be asked to report double vision as the finger is moved. The degree of diplopia can most accurately be recorded by means of a Hess chart. The chart shows which of the extraocular muscles is functioning abnormally and by repeating the examination every alternate day, the progress of the diplopia can be monitored. Rapid improvement as shows on the Hess chart indicates that double vision was caused by temporary muscle edema. If, however, the Hess chart remains unchanged in the first week, then the more permanent damage is suspected and future decisions for treatment can be taken.

Differentiating Points for Etiology of Diplopia

Diplopia in the extreme upward and downward gaze is generally due to general edema of the orbit. Diplopia of edema or hemorrhage origin resolves in 5 to 7 days.

Complete lack of eye movement in one direction is due to mechanical interference or neuromuscular injury (Muscle entrapment). If not corrected, it can lead toward permanent persistent diplopia, which is seen in 3 to 15 percent of the patients, due to scar contracture and adhesions either within ocular muscles or between them and other structures.

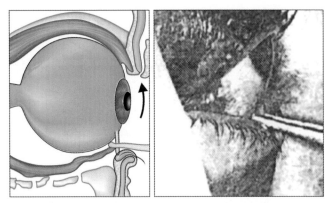

Fig. 29.21: Forced duction test to check the entire range of ocular motion

Neural injuries may cause diplopia only in upward and lateral gaze.

Differentiation between paralysis due to the edema or neuromuscular entrapment can be done by carrying out following test:

Forced duction test: Here a small tissue holding forceps is used to grasp the tendon of the inferior rectus muscle through the conjunctiva of the inferior fornix and the patient is asked for the entire range of motion. An inability to rotate the globe superiorly signifies entrapment of the muscles in the orbital floor (Fig. 29.21).

Hess test: Diplopia can be recorded conveniently by charting the Hess test. The test is based upon the projection of dissimilar images from each eye. The patient sits in front, at a distance of one meter from a screen wearing a red/green goggle. The examiner holds a red test object against the screen and the patient tries to indicate the position of the object by touching it with a green tipped wand. The result of his efforts is charted when his head is held still and he moves his eyes from the primary position to the horizontal right and left extremes of movements. This is repeated when looking above, to the right above and to left above. The equivalent lower positions are also charted.

ENOPHTHALMOS

In simple word Enophthalmos is the inward sinking of the eye. It is a troublesome sequel to the fractures of the zygomatic complex. It occurs following injury due to following:

1. Loss/decrease of volume of orbital contents—herniation of orbital soft tissues in the maxillary sinus or medial wall.

2. Increase in the volume of the bony orbit—due to fractures of its walls. Lateral and inferior displacement of the zygoma or disruption of the inferior and lateral orbital walls or both (can be appreciated by quantitative CT scan).
3. A loss of ligament support.
4. Post traumatic fibrosis, scar contraction and fat atrophy.
5. Combination of all these.

Initially enophthalmos is difficult to diagnose in acute cases, as adjacent soft tissue edema always produces relative enophthalmos.

Clinical Features of Enophthalmos

Clinical features of enophthalmos are accentuation of the upper eyelid hooding, anterior projection of the globe as viewed from above will be reduced on the side of the injury.

Enophthalmos can be corrected by surgical intervention as soon as possible. There is always a difficulty to correct it secondarily because of the fibrosis. Postoperatively, even after restoration of the orbital rims and floor, at the time of surgery, defects occurring posteriorly along the medial or lateral wall or both areas are common and frequently overlooked.

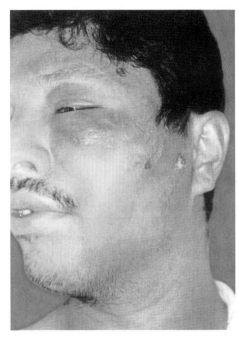

Fig. 29.22: Typical circumorbital ecchymosis and circumorbital edema due to LeFort II fracture

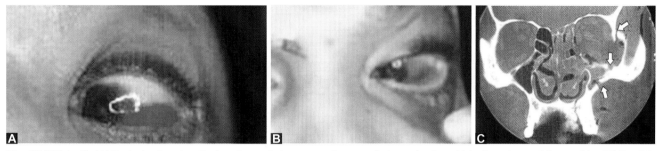

Figs 29.23A to C: (A) Typical subconjunctival ecchymosis in a case of zygomatic bone fracture. Note the edema of the eyelids; (B) Forcible separation of the eyelids and patient is asked to look medially. Subconjunctival hemorrhage is seen at the outer canthus. Note that the posterior limit of the effusion cannot be defined; (C) Coronal CT scan showing the *fracture of the lateral orbital wall and the floor and left zygomatic bone* (Arrows). Note the displacement of the bones and haziness of the left maxillary sinus

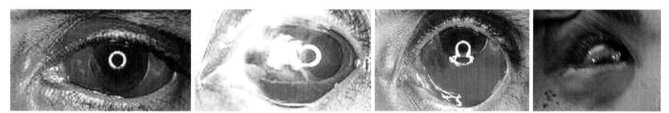

Fig. 29.24: Extensive subconjunctival ecchymosis with pronounced bulging of the conjunctiva in case of fracture of the left zygomatic bone and nasomaxillary process and fracture of the orbital plate of the ethmoid bone. Ocular movements are not affected

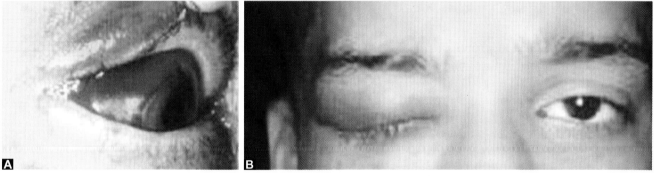

Figs 29.25A and B: (A) Proptosis of the right eye caused by a retrobulbar hemorrhage due to fracture of the zygomatic bone; (B) Swelling and ptosis of the right eyelids due to lymphatic obstruction and injury to the levator muscles

Surgery to reduce the orbital volume is done by placing a space occupying material behind the globe. Glass beads, silicone sheets and sponges, hydroxyapatite, Teflon beads are the nonresorbable materials which can be used to maintain their bulk within the orbit. But there can be problem of extrusion, migration or infection. Cartilage grafts are more popular for rebuilding the orbital volume.

Blindness

Diminished vision or blindness is brought about by retrobulbar hemorrhage or laceration of the optic nerve or hemorrhage into the optic nerve itself. Damage to the retinal artery or injury to optic nerve will lead to permanent blindness.

Retrobulbar hemorrhage will bring about temporary blindness or diminished vision. There will be proptosis, periorbital swelling which will increase in size, retrobulbar pain and dilation of the pupil and ophthalmoplegia (Figs 29.25A and B). Initial conservative treatment will lead to gradual absorption of hemorrhage and full range of motion with gaining the vision will be seen within several weeks. The conservative treatment will consist of ice application, sedative, bed rest, diuretics as IV mannitol and high doses of systemic steroids—3 mg/kg of dexamethasone every 6 hourly (Figs 29.22 to 29.25).

The principles of treatment of midfacial fracture consist of the reduction and fixation of the fractured bones to one another and to the skull. Restoration of the occlusion is a must for the correct reduction of the dentulous jaw segments. The bony framework and buttresses of the midface must also be repositioned or restored and fixed. Restoration of the form will also restore the function. Reduction and fixation can be achieved by either conservative or operative methods. It should be undertaken as early as possible following injury. The sooner the treatment is carried out, the greater the prospects for restoration of normalcy.

After the availability of mini-bone plate system, the conservative methods have largely been replaced by surgical methods. Common to both methods is splinting of both jaws in all cases, in which the alveolar process of the maxilla is involved in the fracture. Fixation of the midface must be maintained by external or internal skeletal fixation until consolidation is achieved. The immobilization to stable skeletal segments of the skull should be maintained for approximately six to eight weeks. IMF is maintained until occlusal disturbances can no longer result, that is, three to four weeks. In case miniplate osteosynthesis has been performed, then there is no need for IMF.

METHODS OF REDUCTION FOR MIDFACE FRACTURES

Manual Reduction

Manual reduction can be carried out in all fresh fractures and where the fragments are not impacted. As a rule, arch bars are first applied to the teeth. The lower jaw serves as a template, so that the occlusion can be checked.

i. *Simple manipulation by hand* is possible in fresh fractures, maxilla is held between the index finger and thumb and brought into normal occlusion. Another method is to fix two double wires encircling the first and second maxillary molars and twisting them individually on either sides. Both the twisted wire ends are held by means of wire holders or hemostats and simultaneously downward movement of the maxilla will help to achieve the normal occlusion.

ii. Dingman and Harding in 1951, suggested the use of dental compound loaded into impression tray for mobilizing the fractured fragment of maxilla. This can be used, where some amount of fibrosis has set in because of delayed treatment. When the impression compound sets, then the firm grip can be taken on the maxillary arch and the handle of the tray is used for rocking the maxilla.

iii. Propescu and Burlibasa in 1966, have described reduction by rubber dam sheets or by means of long ribbon/strip gauze or rubber catheters. Whenever the maxilla is impacted and simple manual mobilization is not possible, then this method can be tried, if sophisticated instruments are not available. The rubber catheter's end is passed from the nostril into the oropharynx and it is grasped with the help of hemostat and brought out of the oral cavity. So, you have one end coming out from nostril and other end through the oral cavity, same procedure is repeated on the other side through the nostril. After grasping all four ends of the catheter and stabilizing the head, maxilla can be rocked into the normal occlusion.

iv. *Reduction by using special instruments*—specially constructed disimpaction forceps can be used to take firm grasp of the maxilla and reduce it into the position.

Rowe's maxillary disimpaction forceps—are available as right and left forceps. Always used in pairs. These are two pronged forceps, where one prong fits into the nasal floor and another one on the hard palate. Anterior traction in the case of a split palate, may be facilitated by the use of the special forceps devised *by Hayton Williams.* These are applied to the buccal aspect of the alveolar process and medial compression exerted until the two halves of the upper jaw are approximated. A screw top is adjusted to prevent crushing of the bone. It is possible to combine the use of these forceps with Rowe's maxillary disimpaction forceps. The stabilized maxillary block may then be disimpacted and drawn forward (Fig. 30.1).

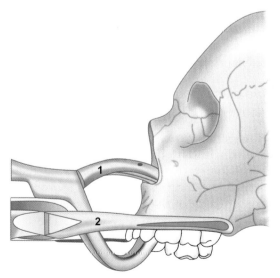

Fig. 30.1: Reduction of maxillary fractures: (1) Rowe's maxillary disimpaction forceps, (2) Hayton William's disimpaction forceps

Reduction by Traction

Repositioning the fractures that are already in a state of partial consolidation or when attempted manual reduction is met with failure, then reduction by elastic traction is tried to interdigitate the fractured fragments. This is mainly used in delayed cases, where the fracture is 10 to 14 days old and no longer sufficiently mobile.

i. Intraoral elastic traction.

ii. Extraoral elastic traction with appropriate extension bars and side bars.

Intraoral intermaxillary elastic traction may be used in an appropriate direction to restore normal occlusion. Once the satisfactory occlusion is achieved, it is replaced by IMF.

Conservative Treatment

Reduction and fixation of the fractured midface is indicated in cases, where surgery is not possible on account of poor general condition of the patient or where there is extensive comminution with tissue loss, making internal skeletal fixation impossible. It may be used also as a supplementary measure with the surgical treatment of midfacial fracture.

Supervised Spontaneous Healing

Fixation may be dispensed with, where mobility at the fractured maxilla is only slight, providing that the occlusion is not disturbed. In such cases the progress of healing is merely supervised. The patient is advised to avoid chewing during the first 2 to 3 weeks and should remain on a liquid or semisolid diet.

Monomaxillary fixation: This method is used when tooth bearing section of the maxilla is not fractured and therefore can serve as fixation point. The arch bar or palatal acrylic plates can be used. This can be used for unilateral fractures of maxilla or higher fractures without occlusal discrepancies. As a rule monomaxillary fixation must be maintained for six weeks.

Intermaxillary fixation (IMF): Intermaxillary fixation is maintained for 3 to 4 weeks and at the end of this period IMF wires and the lower arch bars are removed.

Internal skeletal wire suspension: Many times in addition to IMF, additional support is required for immobilization of the jaws. Craniomaxillary or craniomandibular suspension can be carried out using the stable point above the fracture line. The selection of the site for suspension wire will be dependent on the level of fracture line. The

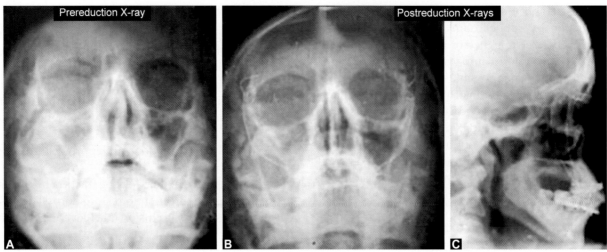

Figs 30.2A to C: Closed reduction with immobilization of fragments using suspensory wirings above the frontozygomatic sutures and IMF

procedure for internal skeletal wire suspension is done through a minor surgery.

- Application of arch bars
- Reduction of fracture by closed method—occlusion is checked
- Fixation of the midface to the base of the skull by means of suspension wires.
- Fixation of the midface by tightening the suspensory wires and intermaxillary fixation
- For edentulous patients, available prosthesis or Gunning splint is used.

LeFort I fracture: IMF fixation by zygomatic arch suspension, if necessary additional suspension at the piriform aperture.

LeFort II: Zygomatic arch suspension or frontal bone suspension. Intraosseous wiring may be done at infraorbital margins.

LeFort III: Intraosseous wiring at zygomaticofrontal sutures and bilateral frontomalar suspension is used after the application of arch bars. Intraosseous wiring may be done at the infraorbital margin, if step deformity exists (Figs 30.2A to C).

Open Reduction (Figs 30.3 to 30.6)

Open reduction is carried out under endotracheal anesthesia with nasal intubation. Intraoral vestibular incision is taken from first molar to first molar region on either side. Mucoperiosteal flap is reflected to expose the fracture line. After identifying the fracture line, in old fractures, an osteotome is inserted to mobilize the

fragment. Disimpaction forceps can be used and the fragment is brought into normal occlusion by manipulation. Temporary IMF is carried out and fracture fragments are fixed under direct vision by intraosseous wiring or mini-bone plates with screws.

For extensive high level fractures of the midface bicoronal incision can be taken. Various skeletal incisions for exposure of midface skeleton are follows (Fig. 30.7):

1. Supraorbital eyebrow incison
2. Subciliary incision
3. Median lower eyelid incision
4. Infraorbital incision
5. Transconjunctival incision
6. Zygomatic arch incision
7. Transverse nasal incision
8. Vertical nasal incision
9. Medial orbital incision.

Fracture of the Floor of the Orbit (Blow-out Fracture)

True blow-out fracture occurs as a result of direct trauma to the orbit with an object larger than the globe size (cricket ball injury) (Fig. 30.8). Here primarily there is an increase in hydraulic pressure within the orbit resulting from compression of the orbital contents. In addition, forces acting on the bone play a part. The fractured orbital floor gives way into the maxillary sinus. At the same time, orbital fatty tissue and sometimes muscles, (inferior rectus and inferior oblique) prolapse into the sinus like a hernia.

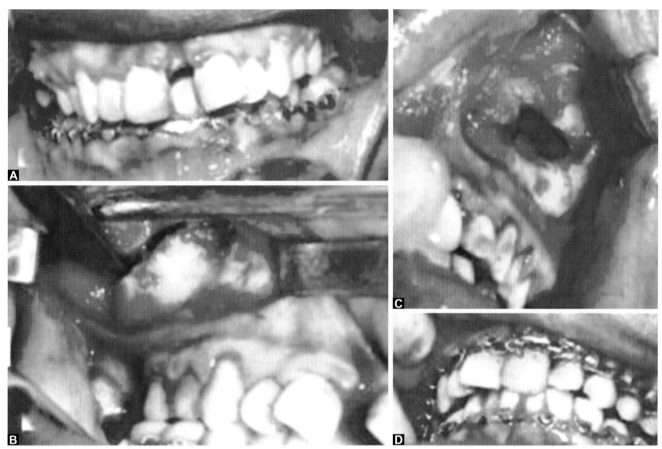

Figs 30.3A to D: (A) LeFort I fracture with midpalatal split-occlusal disharmony, (B) Intraoral buccal vestibular incision to expose the fracture line on right side, (C) Left side surgical exposure to expose the fracture line and bony defect in the anterolateral wall of the maxillary sinus, (D) Fracture reduction done to achieve satisfactory occlusion

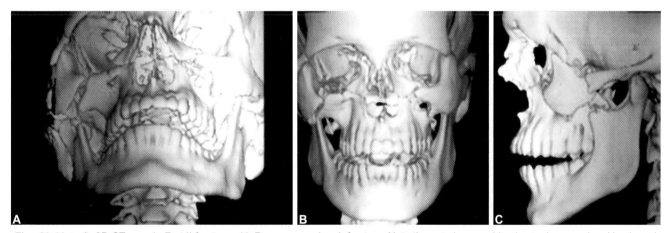

Figs 30.4A to C: 3D CT scan LeFort II fracture with R zygoma and arch fracture. Note the anterior open bite due to downward and backward displacement of maxilla

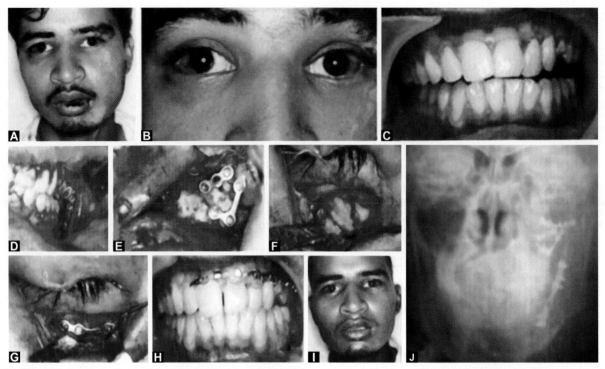

Figs 30.5A to J: (A) Front face after trauma, (B) Subconjunctival hemorrhage with circumorbital ecchymosis, (C) Deranged occlusion, (D) Bone plate fixation after open reduction at L angle, (E) Bone plate fixation at L zygomatic buttress, (F) Infraorbital rim fracture exposed via extraoral infraorbital incision, (G) Bone plate fixation at L-infraorbital rim, (H) Satisfactory occlusion after reduction, (I) Postoperative front face, (J) Postoperative PA view mandible

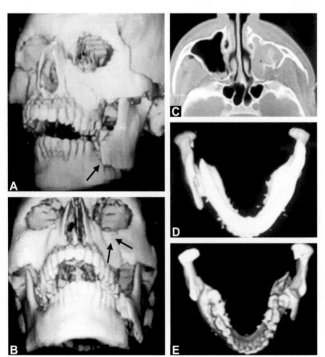

Figs 30.6A to E: CT scan of the patient seen in Figure 30.5 (A and B) 3D CT scan showing LeFort II fracture with L angle mandible fracture (Arrows), (C) Haziness of L maxillary sinus with disruption of sinus walls, (D and E) Gross displacement with overriding of fragments at L angle mandible

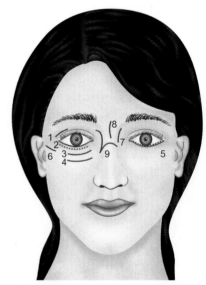

Fig. 30.7: Various facial incisions for exposure of midfacial skeleton

The infraorbital rim remains intact. The fracture may go unnoticed due to the presence of orbital, periorbital edema, hematoma and the clinically intact infraorbital ridge. Enophthalmos with restriction of the extraocular movements and at times diplopia may be

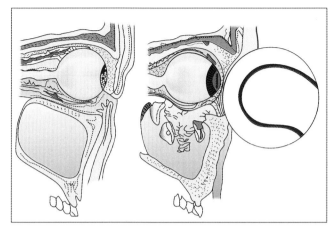

Fig. 30.8: Blow-out fracture of the floor of the orbit. A tennis ball aimed at the globe of the eye forces it posteriorly, compressing the periorbital fat and fracturing the thin orbital floor. Fractured fragments and herniation of periorbital fat will be seen in the maxillary sinus

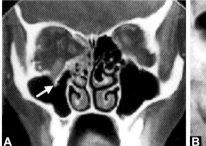
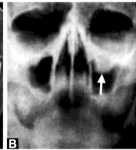

Figs 30.9A and B: (A) Coronal CT scan showing *trapdoor deformity* indicating blow-out fracture of R orbital floor, (B) *Hanging drop appearance in L maxillary sinus* indicating herniation of orbital contents in the sinus due to blow-out fracture

present. Diagnosis can be confirmed by forced duction test and by hanging drop appearance in PA view Water's position radiograph or by CT scan (Figs 30.9 and 30.10).

Treatment consists of surgical exploration of orbital floor and reconstruction of the orbital floor by silastic sheet or bone graft, whenever necessary. Otherwise balloon support or ribbon gauze packing can be used in the maxillary sinus.

TREATMENT OF FRACTURES OF THE ZYGOMATIC BONE

In majority of cases, early operation is advisable, provided that there are no ophthalmic or cranial complications. Whenever there is a gross periorbital edema and ecchymosis, postponement of the operation for 3 to 5 days can be done, but it should not be prolonged more than two weeks.

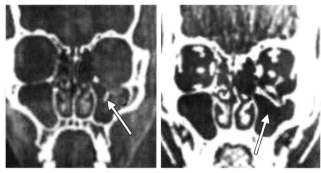

Fig. 30.10: Coronal CT scan showing the blow-out fracture of the floor of the orbit. Herniation is seen in the maxillary sinus

Stable fractures: Simple elevation will be sufficient, because of high degree of stability due to integrity of temporal fascia and the interdigitation of the fracture lines. No additional fixation is required after reduction.
- Type 1   : No treatment
- Type 2   : Unless vertically displaced
- Type 3   : and
- Type 4 (a): Open reduction may be required and transosseous wiring is advisable.

Unstable fractures: Require open reduction and transosseous wiring or bone plating.
- Type 4 (b)
- Types 5, 6, and 7, 8

Operative Technique

The approach of Gillies, Kilner and Stone (1927) is popular for reduction of fractures of zygoma (Figs 30.12, 30.13 and 30.15).

Gillies Temporal Approach (Figs 30.11 to 30.13 and 30.19)

The temporal fascia is attached to the zygomatic arch and the temporal muscle passes downward medial to the fascia to be attached to the coronoid process. Between these two structures a natural anatomical space exists into which an instrument can be inserted and it can be utilized to elevate the displaced zygoma or its arch into position.

Technique: The hair is shaved from the temporal region of the scalp. The external auditory meatus is plugged with cotton to prevent any fluid or blood getting inside. An incision about 2 to 2.5 cm in length is made, inclined forward at an angle of 45 degrees to the zygomatic arch, well in the temporal region. Care is taken to avoid injury to the superficial temporal vessels. The temporal fascia is exposed which can be identified as white glistening

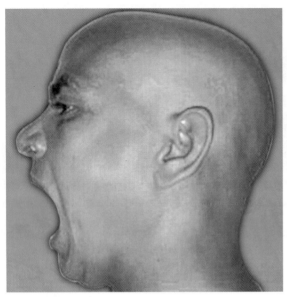

Fig. 30.11: Facial depression seen due to V-shaped fracture of zygomatic arch

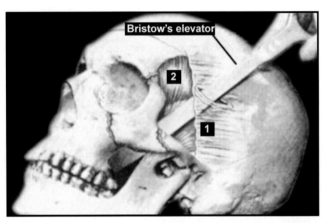

Fig. 30.12: Gillies temporal approach for reduction of zygomatic bone/arch fracture: (1) Temporalis fascia, (2) Temporalis muscle

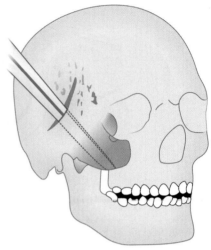

Fig. 30.13: Gillies temporal approach for reduction of zygomatic bone/arch fracture. Diagrammatic representation

elevation procedure care should be taken that pressure is not exerted on the lateral surface of the skull to end up with depressed fracture of the skull). The tip of the elevator is manipulated upward, forward and outward. The snap sound will be heard as soon as reduction procedure is complete. Wound is closed in layers after withdrawing the elevator. Care is taken that after surgery at least for 5 to 7 days, no pressure is exerted on the area till the bone consolidates. Patient is instructed to sleep in supine position or not to sleep on the operated side (Figs 30.14A to G).

Now many operators have modified their own elevators for reducing the fracture of the zygomatic complex, which are available in the market. Any one of these instruments is chosen by the operator and the reduction procedure can be modified changing the direction of the tip of the instrument, depending on the type of fracture. While the tip of the elevator rests on the medial surface of the zygomatic bone, the operator should keep on palpating the external contour with the hand and guide the manipulation till proper positioning of the fragments is achieved.

Intraoral Procedure (Figs 30.15 and 30.16)

Keen's approach (1909): Introral buccal vestibular incision is taken in first and second molar region behind the zygomatic buttress. A pointed curved elevator (Monks' pattern) is passed supraperiosteally up beneath the zygomatic bone. The depressed bone is then elevated with an upward, forward and outward movement.

structure. The incision is taken into the fascia and the fibers of temporalis muscles will be seen. Long Bristow's periosteal elevator is passed below the fascia and above the muscle (Fig. 30.12). Once this correct plane is identified and instrument is inserted through it, downward and forward, the tip of the instrument is adjusted medially to the displaced fragment. A thick gauze pad is kept on the lateral aspect of the skull to protect it from the pressure of elevator while reduction is going on. The operator has to grasp the handle of the elevator with both hands and assistant has to stabilize the head of the patient. (During

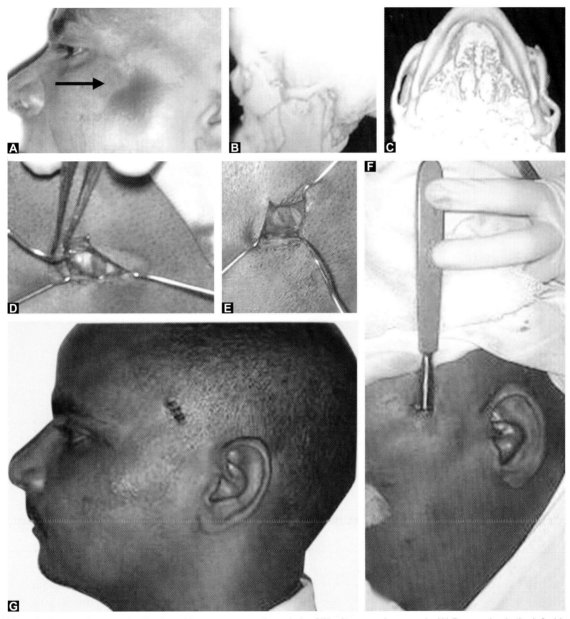

Figs 30.14A to G: Clinical pictures of reduction of fracture zygomatic arch, by Gillies' temporal approach. (A) Depression in the left side of cheek, (B and C) 3 D CT scan showing L zygomatic arch fracture, (D and E) An incision to expose the temporal fascia and muscle, (F) Elevation of depressed fracture with bone elevator, (G) Final suturing after fracture reduction

Alternate methods like intranasal elevation via intranasal antrostomy or oroantral elevations were suggested. Direct extraoral elevation can be done by inserting a sharp curved hook directly through the skin below and above the prominence of the zygomatic bone. Manipulation of the hook reduces the fracture (Figs 30.17 and 30.18).

Gross separation of the zygomaticofrontal suture (Type 4(a), 4(b), 5(a),(b) and (c): Extraoral incision is taken in the wrinkles, one centimeter above the outer canthus or in the line of the outer aspect of the eyebrow. Holes are drilled approximately 0.5 cm away from the fracture ends of the frontal and zygomatic bones. A periosteal elevator is placed on the medial aspect to protect the

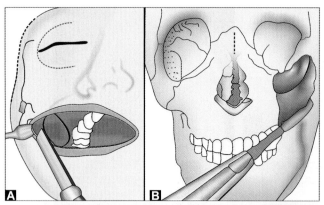

Figs 30.15A and B: Intraoral Keen's approach for reduction of zygomatic bone/arch fracture

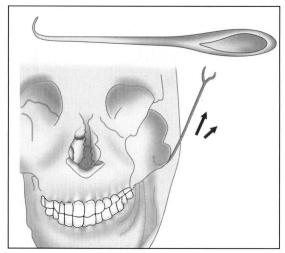

Fig. 30.17: Reduction of zygoma using zygomatic hook

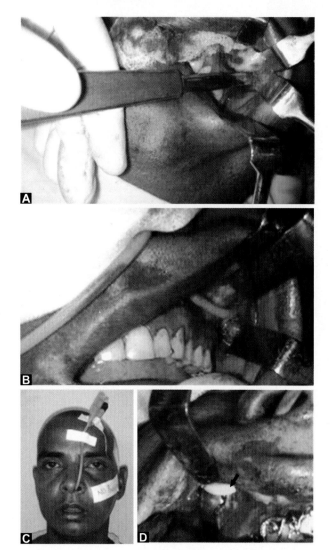

Figs 30.16A to D: (A) Intraoral reduction of zygomatic bone fracture by Keen's approach, (B) Stabilization of reduced fracture by using balloon catheter, (C) Postoperative photograph of the patient, (D) In another patient, support to the fractured zygomatic complex is given by balloon catheter (Arrow)

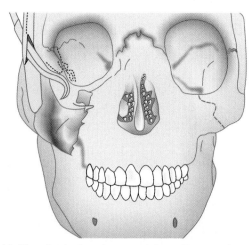

Fig. 30.18: Closed reduction of zygomatic bone fracture using towel clip

eye. The 26 gauge double wire is passed and twisted after passing through both the holes and approximation of the fragments. Instead of wire, 2 hole miniplates can also be used for direct fixation. Wound is closed in layers (Figs 30.20 and 30.21).

Comminution of the orbital floor (Type 6(a)): (Figs 30.22A to G) Use of antral pack or balloon catheter can be done which is previously described.

Comminution and displacement of the orbital rim (Type 7): Direct figure of eight intraosseous wiring can be done through extraoral infraorbital incision or semilunar orbital bone plate can be fixed (Figs 30.23A to E).

Associated coronoid fractures: No separate treatment is indicated. But if coronoid process is completely detached and causing limitation of the oral opening after reduction then it should be excised through intraoral incision.

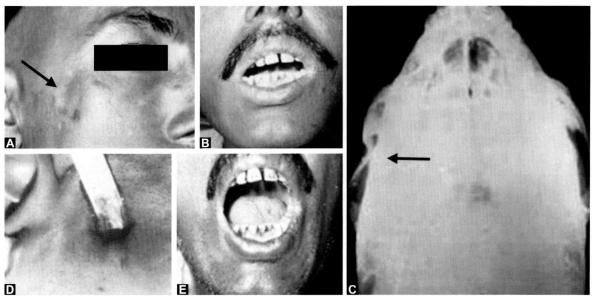

Figs 30.19A to E: Reduction of zygomatic arch fracture by Gillies' method: (A) Typical depression due to depressed V shaped fracture of R zygomatic arch, (B) Limited oral opening due to impingement on the coronoid process by fractured fragments, (C) Jug handle X-ray views *showing fracture of R zygomatic arch*, (D) Reduction by Gillies' method, (E) Improved oral opening after reduction

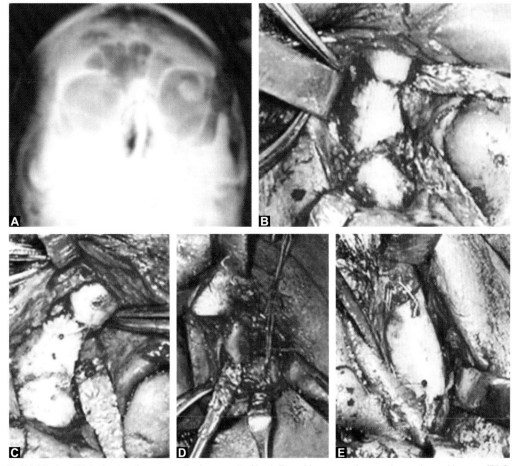

Figs 30.20A to E: (A) PA view Water's showing gross displacement of both R and L zygomatic complex and nasal bones, (B) Surgical exposure of right side fractured frontal process of zygoma, (C) Fixation after reduction with intraosseous wiring on right side, (D) Surgical exposure on the left side frontal process of zygoma showing loss of bone, (E) Autogenous iliac crest bone grafting done

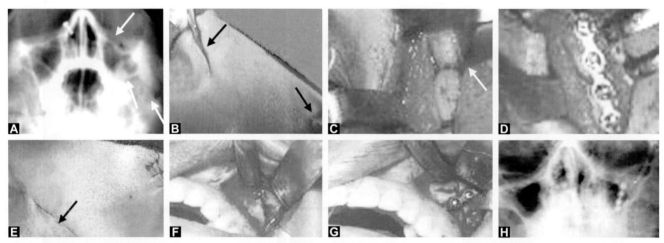

Figs 30.21A to H: Reduction of zygomaticomaxillary complex fracture. (A) Preoperative X-ray (B) Eyebrow incision and Gillies incision (C) Fracture reduction at frontozygomatic suture (D) Bone plate fixation (E) Subcuticular suturing (F) Intraoral vestibular incision to expose the fracture (G) Intraoral bone plate fixation (H) Postoperative X-ray

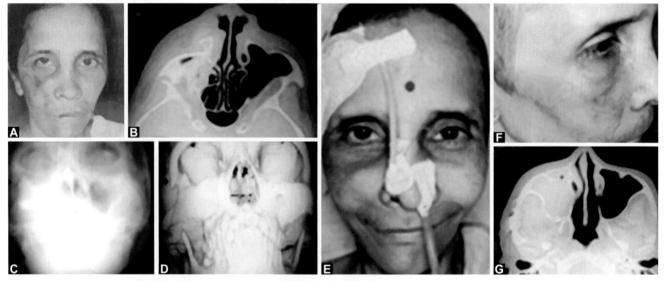

Figs 30.22A to G: Right zygomaticomaxillary complex fracture: (A) Preoperative front face, (B) CT scan (C) PA view Water's X-ray (D) 3D scan showing the displaced R zygomatic bone, (E) Intraoral reduction and stabilization using balloon catheter, (F) Postoperative facial view (G) Postoperative CT scan showing the restoration of fractured anterolateral wall of maxillary sinus

Malunion of the Zygomaticomaxillary Complex

It will show following signs and symptoms:
1. Cosmetic
2. Neurological
3. Antral
4. Masticatory
5. Ophthalmic

Cosmetic: Loss of contour or prominence of cheek will be seen. Correction may be done either by surgical refracturing or camouflaging the deformity by means of onlay bone grafting or alloplastic material like hydroxylapatite blocks.

Neurological: The paresthesia, dysesthesia or anesthesia may be present. Observation for recovery of infraorbital nerve should be done for 6 to 12 months, otherwise surgical exploration of the nerve can be done.

Antral: Persistent sinusitis may be due to the presence of loose necrotic bone pieces or a foreign body, which should be removed via Caldwell-Luc operation.

Masticatory: Depressed zygomatic arch fracture impinges on the coronoid process bringing about limitation of the mandibular movements and opening. In extensive fracture, via coronal incision the arch should be exposed, refractured and stabilized by direct fixation

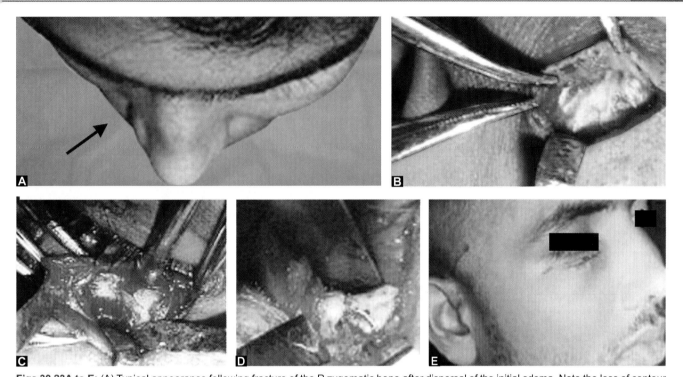

Figs 30.23A to E: (A) Typical appearance following fracture of the R zygomatic bone after dispersal of the initial edema. Note the loss of contour and flattening on right side of the face, (B) Gillies' approach for reduction, (C and D) Open reduction via infraorbital incision for reduction of infraorbital rim fracture and fixation by intraosseous wiring, (E) Postoperative facial appearance

method. Osteotomy and bone grafting can be done if required.

Ophthalmic: Change of the ocular level, diplopia, enophthalmos, occulorotatory restriction are the residual deformities which are difficult to correct secondarily. Exploration and surgical correction can be attempted

FRACTURES OF THE NASAL BONE AND TREATMENT (FIGS 30.24 TO 30.28)

Incidence of nasal fracture is quite high, because of the prominent position of the nose. Nasal fracture is usually the result of direct injury; it can occur as an isolated fracture or it may be combined with other facial fractures. Fractures of the nasal bones and septal cartilage result in not only cosmetic deformity, but also functional disturbance. If early treatment is instituted, reduction and fixation is achieved properly, the disturbance of function can be prevented. If treatment is delayed, then malunion will require more extensive surgical repair. Nasal fractures in children should be generally treated conservatively with closed reduction, because of the growth potential. The nasal fractures are often overlooked in multiple facial injuries. Nasal symmetry,

proper appearance and adequate airway through the nose is important. Careful clinical examination, meticulous reduction and stabilization will give good result and no airway obstruction.

Anterior injuries: Direct, violent, and/or anterior force may result in smash fractures of the nasal bones, the frontal process of the maxilla, the lacrimal bones and the septum. Comminuted fragments may be driven laterally into the orbit or upward into the ethmoid region. Splayed nasal fractures may be associated with damage to the nasolacrimal ducts, the perpendicular plate of the ethmoid, the ethmoid sinuses, the cribriform plate and the orbital parts of the frontal bone. Widening of the intercanthal distance is known as traumatic telecanthus. Buckling of the nasal septum may be seen.

Lateral injuries: Force applied from the side, may involve only one nasal bone with medial displacement, but most commonly in adults, a violent blow from the side results in fractures of both nasal bones and fracture of nasal septum with lateral shifting of the entire bony framework. This is known as 'open book' fracture. In most severe injuries, the septum may be fractured or displaced from the maxillary crest, from the vomerine groove or from

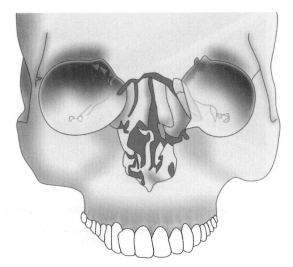

Fig. 30.24: Fractures of the nasal bone

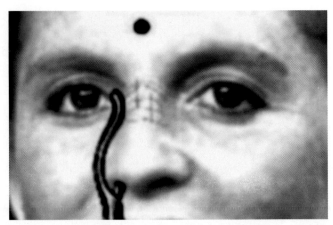

Fig. 30.26: Reduction of nasal fractures

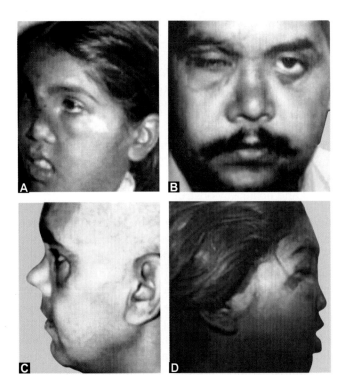

Figs 30.25A to D: Clinical picture of nasal fractures

its attachment at the anterior nasal spine of the maxilla, with displacement into the adjacent airway. Fractures of the septum occur in the vertical plane. There may be telescoping or overlapping seen (Fig. 30.24).

Diagnosis of Fractures of Nasal Bones

A good history and careful clinical examination assisted by proper radiographic evaluation is mandatory and helpful from a medicolegal standpoint. History of previous nasal deformity, trauma, surgery or breathing difficulty should be asked for. Nature and direction of the trauma also should be asked. Patient's chief complaints are usually nasal bleeding, pain, swelling and difficulty in breathing through the nose. Sense of smell also may be lost or diminished. On clinical evaluation, obvious nasal deformities like depressed bridge of the nose, flattening or deviation of the nasal bone may be evident (Figs 30.25A to D). In the fresh fractures, edema, hematoma, lacerations, subconjunctival hemorrhage may be seen. Nasal obstruction may be the result of edema, blood clots, swelling of the nasal mucosa, dislocated bone, cartilage, etc. Subcutaneous emphysema may be present, because of the patient's repeated attempts to blow the nose. Circumorbital ecchymosis will be present. CSF rhinorrhoea may be present. On palpation, crepitation and tenderness will be there. Active bleeding or epistaxis should be taken care immediately.

Radiographic Evaluation

Lateral views of the nasal bones, 15° or 30° occipitomental projections can be taken. A lateral view taken with a small dental film against the side of the nose also provides an excellent detailed study. CT scan is helpful for higher level fractures of the nose.

Management

Closed reduction is the treatment of choice for most nasal bone and/or septal fractures. These fractures should be repaired within 7 to 10 days.

Closed reduction can be done under LA with or without sedation or general anesthesia. It should never

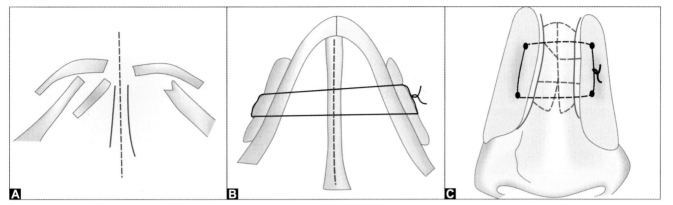

Figs 30.27A to C: (A) Gross displacement of nasal bones, (B and C) Following disimpaction, reduction of fragments, they are stabilized by a horizontal mattress suture of 0.5 mm diameter of stainless steel wire tied over lead plate. Soft tissues are protected by cotton wool rolls

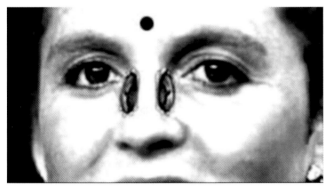

Fig. 30.28: Nasal splint in position

be conducted under intravenous sedation alone. As reduction procedure will provoke bleeding, the trickling of the blood near glottis may provoke a dangerous laryngeal spasm.

If the local anesthesia and sedation are used, it is important to protect the airway by packing ribbon or strip gauze soaked with local anesthetic agent plus vasoconstrictor for hemostasis. The pack is placed in the posterior aspect of the nose with suture attached to it for retrieval. Local anesthetic agent is then injected with vasoconstrictor intranasally.

The two specially designed instruments that are used for repositioning the nasal bones are Asche's and Walsham's forceps. In general, bony fractures should be reduced first, followed by reduction of septal fractures or its dislocation from the maxillary groove. The reduction can be done by using a long, flat, narrow instrument such as Howarth's periosteal elevator. Inferiorly or medially displaced nasal bones are lifted upward and laterally, by using Howarth's elevator into

normal position. The laterally displaced nasal bones are brought into normal position by using Walsham's forceps or digital pressure. Walsham's forceps are used with unpadded blade inside the nasal cavity deep to the nasal bones and the other padded blade externally on the skin over the fractured nasal bones. The bones are manipulated between the blades until adequate mobility is achieved. Anterior traction and medial rotation followed by lateral rotation to reposition the fragments is done (Fig. 30.26). Operator will constantly check the external nasal contour with his palpating fingers. Asche's septal forceps are then introduced on either side of the septum along the floor of the nose and used to realign the septal cartilage in the groove in the vomer and having ironed out any deflection in the perpendicular plate of ethmoid or the vomer are slowly brought upward and forward to elevate the nasal bridge anteriorly. At the end of the reduction, previous nasal pack with the suture is removed. Following complete reduction, internal stabilization is done with nasal packing using half inch ribbon gauze saturated with antibiotic ointment. The pack is placed under direct vision in the superior nasal vault first and then packed inferiorly. Both the nostrils should be packed to support the nasal septum. The pack is removed after 3 to 4 days.

The external dressing consists of padding the area with cotton wool or gauze pieces and stabilizing it with adhesive tape in a 'butterfly' manner secured to the forehead and crossing over the nasal bridge on either side. External splints that may be used include dental impression compound mould, plaster of Paris, metal splints, lead plates or acrylic or prefabricated splints such as Denver splint (Figs 30.27 and 30.28). The external splints are usually left in place for 5 to 7 days after reduction. The splint provides support for the nasal bones as well prevents hematoma and edema of the nasal structures. Nasal fractures associated with maxillofacial injuries should be treated after stabilizing other fractures with miniplate system, so that IMF is not required and airway can be maintained through the oral route as the nostrils will be packed for 3 to 4 days postoperatively.

In extensive unstable fractures open reduction can be opted for. Open sky or bicoronal approach can be used and bone grafting, direct fixation of the fragments can be planned.

31 Applied Surgical Anatomy of the Mandible and Classification of Mandibular Fractures

■ ANATOMY OF THE MANDIBLE

The mandible is the largest, heaviest and strongest bone of the face. The normal mandible provides a normal airway and proper facial contour. A solid movable mandible allows normal chewing, swallowing and speech. Even though, it is a very strong structure, it is prone to injury, because of its prominent position in the facial skeleton. It is a common site of election for receiving intentional or unintentional violence.

The body of the mandible has got horseshoe or parabola shape. Two rami project upward from the posterior aspect of the body. The condylar processes of these rami articulate with the temporal bone to form the TM joints. The mandible has been compared to an archery bow, which is strongest at its center and weakest at its ends, where it often breaks (Fig. 31.1).

The lower jaw is a movable body, which carries the alveolar process and the teeth. The adult mandible is composed of a compact outer and inner plate of cortical bone and a central portion of medullary bone (spongiosa), whose trabeculae are distributed along the lines of maximum stress.

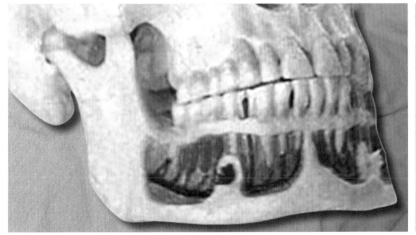
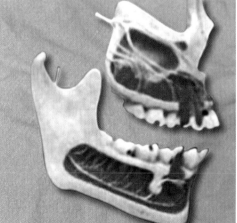

Fig. 31.1: The mandible

The lower portion of the body is heavy and thick and consists of dense cortical bone with little spongiosa and changes very little during adult life. The alveolar process has got lingual and buccal plate of compact but thin bone. The alveolar bone changes throughout the life of a person and becomes adapted to the movements of the teeth or to the loss of teeth. After extraction of teeth, the alveolar process undergoes marked atrophy. After total extractions, due to extreme atrophy, the mental foramen almost comes at the margin of the crest of the ridge. The body of the mandible is naturally strengthened by a strong system of buttresses which extend into the region of the rami.

On the lateral surface, the strong external oblique ridge extends from the body obliquely upward to the anterior border of the ramus. Medial surface is thinner than the lateral surface. But, it is also composed of dense, thick compact cortex. Here, the mylohyoid line extends from the area of the socket of the third molar diagonally downward and forward towards the genial tubercles at the midline. Bony chin is the most vulnerable endangered targeted area, but it is naturally strengthened by the mental protuberances. In childhood, the body of the mandible is weakened by the presence of developing buds of permanent teeth, but naturally protected due to the resilience of the bone.

The ramus consists essentially of two thin plates of compact bone, separated by a narrow portion of cancellous bone. The posterior border of the ramus is strong and rounded.

The bony trajectories transmit and disperse the forces of mastication towards the condyles from the body, thus preventing injury to middle cranial fossa (Fig. 31.2).

Areas of Weakness (Vulnerable for Fracture)

1. The junction of the alveolar bone and basal mandibular bone creates a line of weakness. Dentoalveolar fractures can be seen independently with or without the fracture of basal bone.
2. Symphysis region is formed by the bony union of two halves in the center at first year of life. Symphysis fracture is seen at this line of weakness.
3. Parasymphysis region lateral to the mental prominence is a naturally weak area susceptible for parasymphyseal fracture. This is because of the presence of the incisive fossa and mental foramen.
4. The body of the mandible is considerably thicker than the ramus and the junction of these two portions constitutes a line of structural weakness.

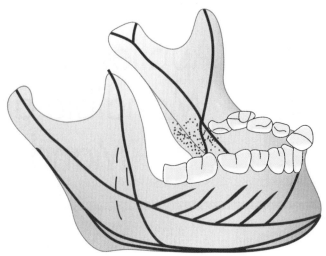

Fig. 31.2: The trajectories of the mandible. The mandible is strengthened by the development of massive compacta, as well as by the trajectories of the spongiosa, in response to the forces of the muscles of mastication

Angle fractures are commonly seen due to the curvature of trajectories in this region.

5. Strength of the lower jaw also varies with the presence or absence of teeth. The presence of impacted lower third molars or excessive long roots of canines make the area more vulnerable for fracture. With the advancing age, the loss of teeth and resorption of alveolar bone leads to a decrease in the vertical height of the mandible, making it prone to fracture.
6. The slender neck of the mandibular condyle renders it particularly liable to fracture as a result of direct violence applied to the chin. This anatomical weakness actually acts as a safety mechanism, as a fracture of the neck of the condyle prevents injury to the middle cranial fossa. Direct blow to the chin region can lead towards fracture of one or both condyles. Sideways blow can bring about fracture of the opposite condylar neck along with parasymphysis fracture at the same side of the blow.
7. As the curve of the mandible becomes progressively more distorted by trauma, the outer and inner compact plates tend to fracture independently. When the fracture passes through the outer plate and reaches the lamina dura of the tooth root, it fractures the root and passes around the root, stripping the periodontal membrane. When the force arrives at the lingual plate, the fracture occurs obliquely at different level than the buccal plate.

This deflection of the fracture line may cause an appearance of double fracture on the lateral oblique view radiograph.

8. Fractures in the tooth bearing area have communication through the periodontal membrane. Therefore, the infection from the oral cavity can travel in the bone through the break. The tooth, denuded of periodontal membrane on some aspect of its root also constitutes a portal of entry of infection into the bone at the site of fracture, plus teeth can become nonvital due to trauma and are also susceptible for infection.

Blood Supply

1. Central blood supply through the inferior alveolar artery.
2. Peripheral blood supply through the periosteum. When a fracture of the mandible occurs, blood vessels involved in the line of fracture are torn. The resultant effusion of blood into surrounding tissues produces ecchymosis and hematoma. If the periosteum on the lingual side is torn, it can lead to sublingual hematoma. The intact periosteum maintains the collateral blood supply. Before the antibiotic era, the teeth in the fracture line were extracted prophylactically to prevent infection (which is no more required).

In the severely atrophic mandible, there is greater dependence on periosteal blood supply than the central supply. Therefore, if open reduction is planned, stripping of the periosteum in such cases should be kept to a minimum.

Nerve Supply

Damage to the inferior alveolar nerve after fracture, results in the paresthesia or anesthesia of the lower lip on the affected side. If the nerve is completely severed, then recovery by regeneration takes 3 to 12 months, usually preceded by 'tingling' sensation, paresthesia and hyperesthesia of the area. The rate of recovery will depend upon the following:

i. Accurate approximation of the nerve ends (proper reduction of fragments).
ii. Elimination of infection
iii. Proper fixation (prevents undue mobility)
iv. Absence of any intervening hard or soft tissue in the inferior dental canal (muscle entrapment in the fracture line or foreign body or bone fragment).

Muscle Action

1. The muscles of facial expression, which are attached on the outer aspect of the anterior part of the mandible and which are inserted into the skin, exert no effect on the displacement of the fragments following mandibular fracture.
2. The muscles originating from the inner aspect of the mandible, the mylohyoid, geniohyoid, genioglossus and anterior belly of digastric exert their effect in centripetal manner. The fractured fragments, therefore, tend to collapse posteriorly or medially.
3. The lateral pterygoid muscle is inserted into the medial fossa on the anterior aspect of the condyle. Therefore, in condylar fractures, the head is displaced anteriorly and medially and may also undergo lateral rotation due to the spasm of the muscle.
4. The mandible anterior to a line passing through the anterior margin of the masseter muscle, is influenced by the depressor group of muscles, while the ramus is influenced by the elevator group.

Factors Influencing Displacement of a Mandibular Fracture

1. Direction and intensity of the traumatic force.
2. Site of fracture.
3. Direction of the fracture line.
4. Muscle pull exerted on the fractured fragments.
5. Presence or absence of teeth.
6. Extent of soft tissue wounds.
   i. If the strong force is directed at particular site, it can result first into direct fracture and also into another indirect fracture on the opposite side. Depending on the direction of the fracture line and muscle pull exerting on the fragments, the resultant displacement will be brought about due to extensive tear of the ligaments as well as supporting soft tissues.
   ii. The body of the mandible is only lightly covered by the muscles which offer very little protection. The ramus, however, is well-splinted by the masseter and medial pterygoid muscles. Therefore, an extensive comminuted fracture in this region shows minimum displacement.
   iii. Presence or absence of teeth on the proximal segment of a fracture line can have influence on the total amount of displacement of proximal segment. Teeth which are present on the

proximal segment may prevent displacement by occlusal contact with the maxillary teeth.

iv Extent of supporting soft tissue wound is also an important factor. Severe tear of the musculature and overlying soft tissues permit wider displacement.

Symphysis Fracture

If the fracture line passes from the labial to the lingual surface in a straight line (rare), the fracture is fairly stable to the influence of the muscles which are attached to the genial tubercle.

If the fracture line runs obliquely, then varying degree of displacement or overlap will be seen. Medial displacement will be due to the action of the mylohyoid muscle and also due to imbalance of the muscles attached to the genial tubercles on either side.

Canine Region Fracture

Common site of fracture, partly due to the length of the canine root weakening the bone and also due to the maximum convexity of the curvature at this site. If the fracture is bilateral, then the total displacement will be much more and can be hazardous, because of the tongue fall and obstruction of the airway.

If the bilateral fracture line in this region runs obliquely forward and medially from the inner to outer cortical plate, then due to the pull of geniohyoid and genioglossus and anterior belly of the digastric muscles, the entire anterior section of the mandible is displaced posteriorly and this leads to tongue fall and airway obstruction.

Body Fracture of the Mandible

Here, if the fracture line is unfavorable, i.e. running from the alveolar margin downward and backward toward the inferior border, then the vertical displacement of the posterior fragment is not so pronounced due to the action of the elevator group of muscles, being counteracted to some extent, by the suprahyoid group of muscles. But, the medial or lingual displacement tends to increase.

Fractures of the Edentulous Mandible

Following extreme alveolar atrophy in the molar regions of the edentulous mandible, these areas are prone to fracture. The bilateral fractures of the body of the edentulous mandible can occur near the posterior attachment of the mylohyoid diaphragm. The mylohyoid muscle level appears to be higher up in this situation, because of extreme atrophy and loss of vertical height of the body of mandible. There is a downward and backward angulation of the anterior part of the mandible seen due to the influence of the digastric and the mylohyoid muscles. This extreme 'bucket handle' displacement may bring about respiratory distress in an elderly patient. Early stabilization of this type of fracture is a must (Refer to Fig. 32.25 in the next chapter).

■ MANDIBULAR FRACTURES

Fractures of the mandible are common in patients, who sustain facial trauma.

A study conducted by Hang et al in 1983, showed the incidence in the ratio of 6:2:1 of mandibular, zygomatic, maxillary fractures respectively. Approximately two-thirds of all facial fractures are the mandibular fractures (nearly 70%) (Tables 31.1 and 31.2).

Sex: Most mandibular fractures are seen in male patients. The ratio is approximately 3:1.

Age: Thirty-five percent of mandibular fractures occur between the ages of 20 to 30 years.

Number of Fractures Per Mandible

i. Unilateral, single   :   53 percent
ii. Bilateral, double   :   37 percent
iii. Multiple fractures :   10 percent

Fifty percent have more than one fracture.

Classification

There are several ways to classify the mandibular fractures:

Table 31.1: Location: As per Olson's study in 1982			
Body fractures	38%	Symphysis	16%
Condyle fractures	29%	Rest of the body	22%
Angle fractures	25%	Ramus fracture	4%
Dentoalveolar fractures	3%	Coronoid fractures	1%

Table 31.2: Etiology of mandibular fractures	
Vehicular accidents	43%
Altercation, assaults, battery, interpersonal violence	34%
Fall	7%
Sports injuries	4%
Industrial mishaps or work accidents	10%
Pathological fractures or miscellaneous	2%

i. General classification.
ii. Anatomical classification.
iii. Relation of the fracture to the site of injury.
iv. Completeness.
v. Depending on the mechanism.
vi. Number of fragments.
vii. Involvement of the integument.
viii. Shape or area of the fracture.
ix. Direction of fracture and favorability for the treatment.
x. Presence or absence of teeth.
xi. AO classification—relevant to internal fixation.

1. Kruger's General Classification (Figs 31.3A to E)

Simple or closed: The linear fracture, which does not have communication with the exterior or the interior. Such a fracture does not produce a wound open to the external environment either through the skin, mucosa or periodontal membrane. It may or may not be displaced.

Examples: Fractures in the region of the condyle, coronoid process, ascending ramus, etc.

Compound or open: This fracture has communication with the external environment through skin or with the internal environment through mucosa or periodontal membrane. All the fractures involving the tooth bearing area of the mandible or where an external or intraoral wound is present involving the fracture line.

Comminuted: A fracture in which the bone is splintered or crushed into multiple pieces. These types are generally

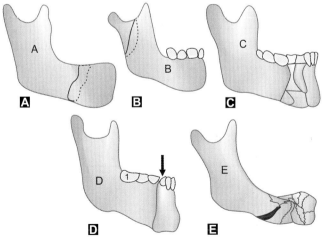

Figs 31.3A to E: (A) Simple fracture, (B) Greenstick fracture. Straight line fractured cortex. Dotted line bent cortex, (C) Compound comminuted fracture, (D) Compound fracture. Arrow-exposed bone, (E) Simple comminuted fracture

due to a greater degree of violence or high velocity impact. Gunshot wounds, where missiles are traveling at a high velocity can produce these fractures.

Complicated or complex: Fractures associated with the damage to the important vital structures complicating the treatment as well as prognosis.

Example: Fractures with injury to the inferior alveolar vessels or nerve, facial nerve or its branches, facial vessels, condylar fractures with associated injuries to middle cranial fossa, etc.

Impacted: Rarely seen in mandibular fractures. More commonly seen in maxilla. This is a fracture in which one fragment is firmly driven into the other fragment and clinical movement is not appreciable.

Greenstick: A fracture in which one cortex of the bone is broken with the other cortex being bent. It is an incomplete fracture seen in young children because of inherent resilience of the growing bone.

Pathological: Spontaneous fracture of the mandible occurring from mild injury or as a result of a normal degree of muscular contraction. This is because of weakness caused due to the pre existing bone pathological processes.

Areas of structural weakness may result from the following:
a. *Generalized skeletal disease*
  i. Endocrinal disorders—hyperparathyroidism or postmenopausal osteoporosis.
  ii. Developmental disorders—osteopetrosis, osteogenesis imperfecta, etc.
  iii. Systemic disorders—reticuloendothelial diseases, Paget's disease, osteomalacia and severe anemia.
b. *Localized skeletal disease:* Various cysts, odontomes, tumours, osteomyelitis, osteoradionecrosis in the local region, presence of impacted third molar, etc.

2. Anatomical Location

Rowe and Killey's classification
A. Fractures not involving the basal bone—are termed as dentoalveolar fractures.
B. Fractures involving the basal bone of the mandible. Subdivided into following:
  i. Single unilateral
  ii. Double unilateral
  iii. Bilateral
  iv. Multiple

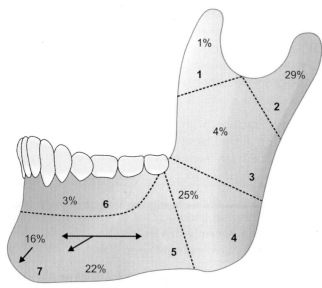

Fig. 31.4: Dingman and Natvig classification of mandibular fractures by anatomic region: (1) Coronoid process, (2) Condylar process, (3) Ramus region, (4) Angle region, (5) Body region, (6) Alveolar process, (7) Symphysis region

Dingman and Natvig classification by anatomic region (Fig. 31.4)

A. Symphysis fracture (midline fracture).
B. Canine region fracture.
C. Body of the mandible between canine and angle.
D. Angle region—triangular region bounded by the anterior border of the masseter to the posterosuperior attachment of the masseter.
E. Ramus region—bounded by the superior aspect of the angle to two lines forming an apex at the sigmoid notch.
F. Coronoid region.
G. Condylar fractures.
H. Dentoalveolar region.

3. Relation of the Fracture to the Site of Injury

 i. Direct fractures.
ii. Indirect (countrecoup) fractures.

4. Completeness

Complete and incomplete fractures.

5. Depending on the Mechanism

  i. Avulsion fracture
 ii. Bending fracture
iii. Burst fracture

 iv. Countrecoup fracture
  v. Torsional fracture.

6. Number of Fragments

Single, multiple, comminuted, etc.

7. Involvement of the Integument

 i. Closed or open fractures.
ii. Grades of severity I to V.

8. Shape or Area of the Fracture

Transverse, oblique, butterfly, oblique surfaced.

9. According to the Direction of Fracture and Favorability for Treatment

a. Horizontally favorable fracture.
b. Horizontally unfavorable fracture.
c. Vertically favorable fracture.
d. Vertically unfavorable fracture.

This classification is aimed towards the angle fractures. Here, the direction of fracture line is important for resisting the muscle pull. When the muscle pull resists the displacement of the fragments, then the fracture line is considered as *favorable*. If the muscle pull distracts the fragments away from each other, resulting in displacement, then the fracture line is considered as *unfavorable (Figs 31.5 and 31.6)*.

The elevator group of muscles exert an upward, forward and medial pull, while depressor group of muscles exert a downward and backward pull in an intact mandible. Whenever there is a break in the continuity at the angle region, then these two muscle groups loose their co-ordinated movements and have

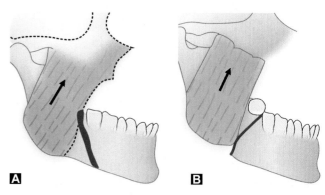

Figs 31.5A and B: (A) Horizontally favorable line of fracture at the angle of the mandible, (B) Horizontally unfavorable line of fracture at the angle of the mandible

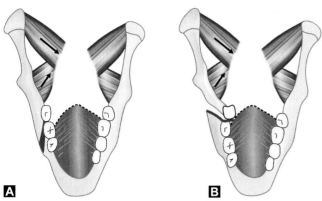

Figs 31.6A and B: (A) Vertically favorable line of fracture through the right angle of the mandible, (B) Vertically unfavorable line of fracture through the right angle of the mandible

independent action. In unilateral angle fracture, posterior ramus fragment is the lesser fragment, while the body of the mandible bearing the teeth becomes the greater fragment. The greater fragment's position is stabilized to certain extent by the occlusion of the teeth, while posterior ramal fragment can show displacement independently.

Here, the direction of the fracture line is responsible for resisting the muscle pull. When the mandible is viewed from the horizontal plane or studied by taking oblique lateral view mandible radiograph, then whether it is *horizontally favorable or unfavorable* line is decided.

a. When the fracture line passes from the alveolar margin, downward and forward, then upward displacement of the posterior fragment is prevented by physical obstruction caused by the body of the mandible. Hence, such a fracture line is termed horizontally favorable.

b. On the other hand, if the line of fracture passes downward and backward, then the upward movement of the posterior fragment is unopposed. This type of fracture is termed horizontally unfavorable. Sometimes the upward displacement can be prevented by the presence of a tooth on the posterior fragment, which comes into contact with maxillary tooth.

c. When the angle fracture is viewed from above, or from the occlusal surface (in the vertical plane), then the buccolingual direction of the fracture line can be studied. Here, the displacement of the posterior fragment can be noticed in the medial direction due to the spasm of medial pterygoid and mylohyoid

muscle. Here, the fracture line which passes from the outer or buccal plate obliquely backward and lingually, will tend to resist the muscle pull mentioned above and is thus termed a vertically favorable type of fracture.

d. When the fracture line passes from the inner or lingual plate obliquely backward and buccally, inward movement of the posterior fragment will take place as a result of the medial pterygoid muscle pull. This type of fracture is termed vertically unfavorable.

This classification is of clinical importance for the treatment planning and fixation, the amount of displacement can be judged and the type of fixation device can be chosen.

10. According to Presence or Absence of Teeth in Relation to the Fracture Line

It is very essential to note the presence or absence of teeth in relation to the fracture line, also the periodontal status, as well as teeth size for planning fixation method. Dentition can be used as the guide for reduction procedure and also can be used for fixation and immobilization. In edentulous patients occlusal guidance is lost. Similarly in deciduous dentition, or mixed dentition, special splints need to be constructed as a 'fixation or immobilization' device.

Kazanjian and Converse classification:

Class I: When the teeth are present on both sides of the fracture line.

a. An adequate number of teeth of suitable shape and stability. Wiring—direct, continuous or multiple loop or interdental eyelet type, use of prefabricated arch bars.

b. An inadequate number of teeth, whose shape or stability is unsuitable.
    Lateral compression splint, arch bars, or cast metal cap splints.

Class II: When the teeth are present only on one side of the fracture line.

a. Short edentulous posterior fragment
    i. If favorable, immobilization of main fragment by interdental wiring or arch bars. Minor displacement can be accepted.
    ii. If unfavorable open reduction with direct fixation is a must.

b. *Long edentulous posterior fragment*
  i. Without displacement—requires conservative treatment
  ii. With vertical and medial displacement—requires open reduction and fixation.

Class III: When both the fragments on each side of the fracture line are edentulous.
  i. Simple or compound fracture without much displacement in the body region—Simple Gunning type splints.
  ii. Simple fractures which are unfavorable. Open reduction and fixation.
  iii. Compound fractures—Surgical intervention.

11. AO Classification (Relevant to Internal Fixation)

1. F: Number of fracture or fragments
2. L: Location (site) of the fracture
3. O: Status of occlusion
4. S: Soft tissue involvement
5. A: Associated fractures of the facial skeleton

Such a classification is helpful in terms of:
  • Patient selection and treatment planning
  • Evaluation of therapeutic results
  • Comparison of different treatment methods
  • Information and communication.

These criteria can be objectified clinically and radiographically:
1. F : Number of fracture
   F0 : Incomplete fracture
   F1 : Single fracture
   F2 : Multiple fracture
   F3 : Comminuted fracture
   F4 : Fracture with a bone defect

2. Categories of localization (site) L1-L8
   L1 : Precanine
   L2 : Canine
   L3 : Postcanine
   L4 : Angle
   L5 : Supra-angular
   L6 : Condyle
   L7 : Coronoid
   L8 : Alveolar process
3. Category of occlusion—O0-O2
   O0 : No malocclusion
   O1 : Malocclusion
   O2 : Nonexistent occlusion—edentulous mandible
4. Categories of soft tissue involvement—S0–S4

The risk of infection and healing depends on the condition of the soft tissues surrounding the fracture.
   S0 : Closed
   S1 : Open intraorally
   S2 : Open extraorally
   S3 : Open intra- and extraorally
   S4 : Soft tissue defect
5. Categories of associated fractures A0-A6
   A0 : None
   A1 : Fracture and/or loss of tooth
   A2 : Nasal bone
   A3 : Zygoma
   A4 : LeFort I
   A5 : LeFort II
   A6 : LeFort III

Grades of severity—I-V

Grade I and II are closed fractures
Grade III and IV are open fractures
Grade V open fracture with a bony defect (gunshot).

Fracture Formula

Right hemimandible	Left hemimandible			
FLO Example	FLO			
Fracture Category	Localization	Occlusion	Soft tissue	Associated fractures
F0	L1	O0	S0	A0
Incomplete fracture	Precanine	Normal occlusion	closed	None

Management of Mandibular Fractures

▐ MANDIBULAR FRACTURES IN CHILDREN

Incidence of facial fracture is less than two percent prior to 5th year of life. However, mandibular fractures in children are most common. Total percentage of facial fractures is less in children, because of the following:

1. Sheltered atmosphere, protection given to children.
2. Decreased facial mass and proportion.
3. Soft consistency of bone.
4. Pliable cancellous bone has got greater proportion with thin buccal and lingual plates.
5. Taut periosteum offers protective mechanism against fracture and its displacement.
    The factors to the child's advantage are as follows:
    a. Faster healing and early bony union. Excellent osteogenic and remodeling capacity.
    b. The ability for adaptation as the deciduous teeth are shed and permanent teeth erupt. Clinical symptoms are same as those of fractures of the lower jaw in the adult. Pain, swelling, malocclusion are the leading symptoms. Abnormal mobility, step deformity in the dental arch will be seen.

The radiographic examination is usually difficult in unco-operative child.

Conservative Therapy

Conservative therapy: Supervised spontaneous healing:

Greenstick fractures are self retentive. In crack fractures or greenstick fractures with no malocclusion, there is no need for fixation. Closed reduction is simple and an attractive solution for them. Patient is advised to take lot of fluids and soft food for 10 to 14 days.

Conservative Treatment with Splints

Lateral compression splints: These are prepared and fixed to the mandibular body with circummandibular wiring (for the children with complete deciduous dentition or with mixed dentition).

Open Reduction

Open reduction is not usually necessary. But, in multiple displaced fractures especially, at the angle and parasymphysis region, open reduction may be needed. Intraosseous wiring or bone plating should be done at the lower border of the mandible without damaging the developing teeth buds (Fig. 32.1).

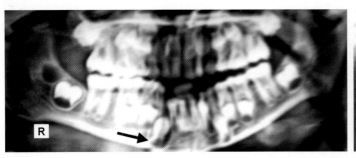 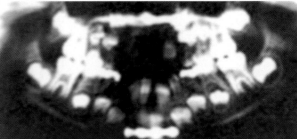

Fig. 32.1: Minibone plating for a symphysis fracture in a child patient

MANAGEMENT OF MANDIBULAR FRACTURES IN ADULTS (TABLE 32.1)

Closed Reduction

Most of the mandibular fractures can be treated by closed reduction. It is often advocated, because of its relative simplicity, low cost and noninvasive nature of treatment. A significant degree of displacement does not preclude the use of a closed reduction to repair a mandibular fracture. The presence of teeth provides an accurate guide for reduction. Teeth may on occasion be brought into contact during reduction, yet be occluding incorrectly owing to lingual inclination of the fractured fragments. Whenever the occlusion is used as an index of accurate reduction, it is important to recognize any pre existing occlusal abnormalities, such as anterior open bite, etc. Wear facets on the teeth, can provide valuable clues to previous contact areas (Figs 32.2A and B).

Indications

1. Nondisplaced favorable fracture.
2. Grossly comminuted fractures.
3. Severely atrophic edentulous mandible.

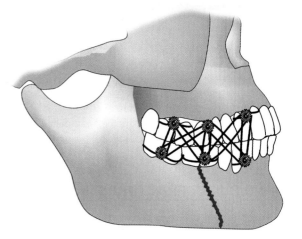

Fig. 32.2A: Closed reduction for mandibular body fracture

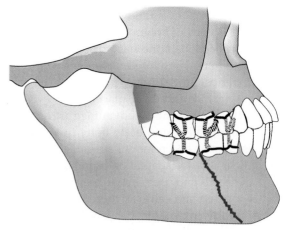

Fig. 32.2B: IMF with Gilmer's wiring after closed reduction of the body mandibular fracture

Table 32.1: Management of mandibular fractures		
1844	Erich and Austin	Preantibiotic era, closed reduction
1847	Buck	Transosseous silver wiring
1943	Gordon	Wire suturing, stainless steel intraosseous wiring plus MMF
1970	Spiessel	AO/ASIF—compression plate
1973	Michelet	Noncompression monocortical screws with miniplate system
1978	Champy	Ideal osteosynthesis lines

4. Lack of soft tissue overlying the fracture site.
5. Fractures in children with developing teeth buds.
6. Coronoid process fractures.

In closed reduction procedure, either dental wiring or arch bars are applied to individual dental arches and satisfactory occlusion is gained after reduction and IMF is carried out. The recommended immobilization period for mandibular fractures correlates with the bony callus stage of secondary bone healing. The average recommended immobilization period for mandibular fractures is 6 weeks. In old age in edentulous mandibular fractures, a longer period of IMF is required.

In edentulous patients, Gunning type of splint can be used. Many times in mandibular body fractures, there is no need for IMF, only horizontal type of fixation will be sufficient. Risdon's horizontal wiring, Erich's arch bar fixation with additional figure of eight wiring for adjoining teeth at the fracture site will give adequate fixation. Cap splints can be constructed whenever possible. Lateral compression splint also is of help in some of the cases, where enough number of teeth are not present for adequate fixation. This type of conservative closed reduction without closing the patient's mouth is very rewarding for the patient.

Advantages of Open Reduction and Direct Fixation

1. Reduction and fixation is done under direct vision.
2. Stable fixation is achieved by better approximation of fractured fragments.

Indications for Open Reduction

Open reduction of mandibular fractures previously was reserved for displaced fractures in the angle and nontooth bearing regions of horizontal mandible. But with the advent of antibiotic era and improved fixation methods, a new paradigm has emerged. Open reduction and rigid or stable fixation may be indicated as the procedure of first choice, when one or all of the following conditions are present:

1. Displaced unfavorable fractures.
2. Multiple fractures.
3. Associated midface fractures.
4. Associated condylar fractures.
5. When IMF is contraindicated or not possible.
6. To preclude the need for IMF for patient comfort.
7. To facilitate the patient's early return to work.

Contraindications for Open Reduction

Open reduction may be contraindicated, when:

1. GA or a more prolonged procedure is not advisable.
2. Severe comminution with loss of soft tissue.
3. Gross infection at the fracture site.
4. Patient refusing open reduction.

SURGICAL APPROACHES TO THE MANDIBLE (FIGS 32.3 TO 32.13)

Adequate exposure of a fracture site allows anatomic reduction of the fragments and proper placement of the hardware. Proper incision design allows adequate access to the fractured mandible with minimum morbidity. In some instances, lacerations provide direct access to the fractured mandible.

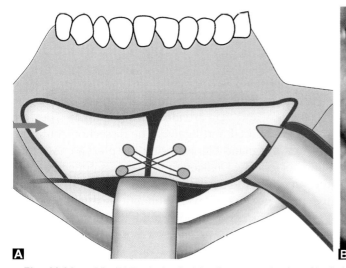
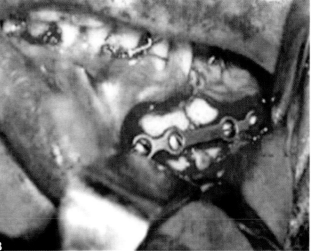

Figs 32.3A and B: (A) Degloving incision for open reduction of body fractures of the mandible, (B) Minibone plating for L parasymphysis fracture fixation via intraoral degloving incision

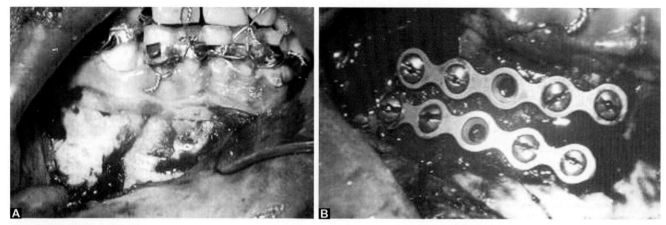

Figs 32.4A and B: (A) Right parasymphysis fracture reduction via intraoral degloving incision. Temporary IMF is done to hold the fragments in position, (B) Double bone plating done to withstand the torsional forces in symphysis region. IMF is released after bone plate fixation

Intraoral Approach—Symphysis and Parasymphysis Region (Figs 32.4A and B)

Termed as anterior, vestibular approach or 'degloving incision'. The lower lip is everted and an incision is created at the depth of the vestibule in the mucosa with a scalpel or electrocautery. Incision is curvilinear and extends anteriorly into the lip. The mentalis muscle will be visible and the fibers are divided in an oblique fashion, leaving a margin of the muscle attached to the bone for closure. The periosteum is divided and a subperiosteal dissection is done to identify the mental nerves. Reduction and bone plate fixation is done. Closure is completed in layers. A pressure dressing is secured to the area to prevent hematoma formation and maintain the position of the mentalis muscle.

Intraoral (Body, Angle, Ramus Region): Transbuccal Incision (Figs 32.5A to D)

Dissection in this region begins with a mucosal incision, that is started with a scalpel or electrocautery, 3 to 5 mm below the mucogingival junction. The incision is created perpendicular to the bone to avoid the mental nerve and it extends over the external oblique ridge. The level of the incision at the external oblique ridge should not be carried superior to the mandibular occlusal plane to avoid herniation of the buccal fat pad. The incision is carried through the periosteum and a subperiosteal dissection is performed. Periosteal elevator is used to expose the lateral border of the ramus. L-shaped retractors can be used during the procedure. To protect the facial nerve, facial artery and vein, the dissection

should not violate the periosteal envelope. Reduction and fixation is done. Closure is completed in one layer.

Extraoral Submandibular Risdon's Incision (Fig. 32.6)

This incision is used to access the mandibular ramus, angle and posterior body. Patient is prepared and draped in routine surgical manner. Important landmarks—the corner of the mouth and the eyeglobe must be visible. Head of the patient is turned sideways. The incision is marked 2 cm below the inferior border of the mandible to avoid damage to the marginal mandibular branch of the facial nerve. Ideally the incision is placed in a relaxed skin tension line (the Langer's lines) (Fig. 32.7). The skin and subcutaneous tissues are incised with a scalpel down to the level of the platysma, and undermining of the skin to allow improved retraction is accomplished with scissors. The platysma is then sharply divided exposing the superficial layer of the deep cervical fascia. The plane of the dissection is carried out through this layer over the superior surface of the submandibular gland. The facial artery and vein are identified (Fig. 32.8). They are clamped, divided and ligated. The dissection continues towards the mandible, exposing the pterygomasseteric sling posteriorly. Division of this layer is done to expose the inferior border of the mandible after cutting through the final periosteal layer. Subperiosteal dissection is performed anteroposteriorly and the desired area of the mandibular body, angle or ramus is accessed. The desired procedure is carried out. Closure is done in layers (Figs 32.9A to C).

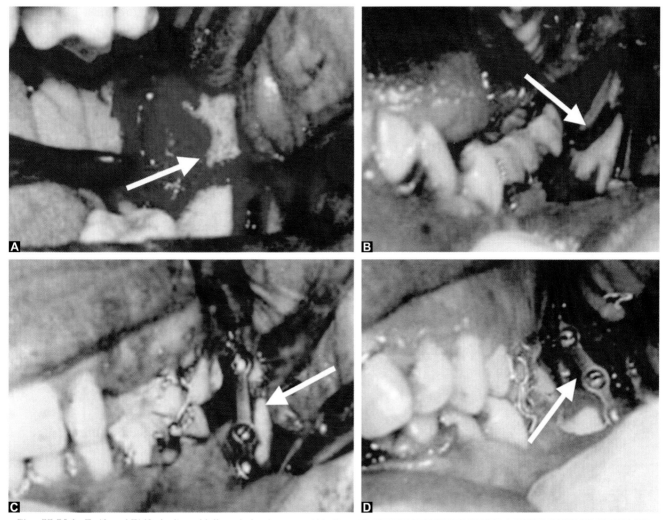

Figs 32.5A to D: (A and B) Reduction of left angle fracture mandible through intraoral transbuccal incision. Fracture fragments brought into approximation and temporary IMF done, (C and D) Bone plate fixation done

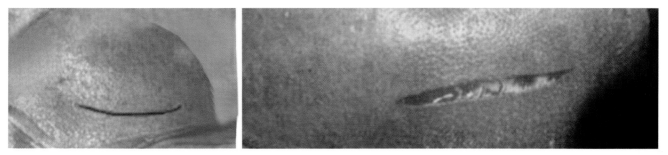

Fig. 32.6: Submandibular Risdon's incision

Transosseous Wiring (Intraosseous Wiring)

Direct wiring across the fracture line is an age old and effective method of fixation of jaw bone fractures. Transosseous wiring can be done through intraoral or extraoral approach. In principle, holes are drilled in the bony fragments on either side of the fracture line, after which a length of 26 gauge stainless steel wire is passed through the holes and across the fracture. After

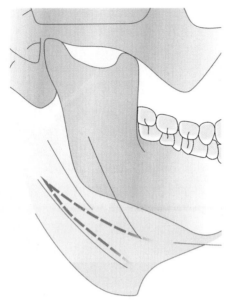

Fig. 32.7: Extraoral incisions are planned following Langer's lines to give cosmetic scar

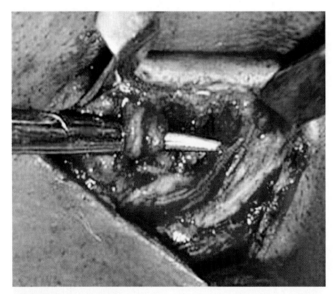

Fig. 32.8: Submandibular incision. Facial artery and vein exposed during dissection, which will be cut and ligated

this initial preparation, the fracture must be reduced independently with the teeth in occlusion before the free ends of the wire are lightened and twisted. The twisted ends are cut short and tucked into the nearest drill hole. The single strand wire fixation in this horizontal manner is the simplest form of fixation with intraosseous wiring. But this can be modified in various ways depending on the need. The variations of the basic technique will depend on the following:

a. Position of fracture.
b. Muscle forces acting on the fragments.
c. Degree of comminution.
d. Number of fragments to be fixed.
e. Nature of the fracture line—oblique, straight, etc.

The variations can be two-hole, four-hole, three-hole technique. Obwegeser's figure of eight wiring, Hayton-William's modification of figure of eight wiring, etc (Fig. 32.10). These variations are mainly used at the inferior border of the mandible through extraoral incision (Fig. 32.11). The intraoral incision for fixation of transosseous wiring at the upper border is chosen for the fractures at the angle with minimum displacement or for the edentulous areas of the body fracture.

Indications for extraoral incision with transosseous wiring at the inferior border:

1. Unfavorable, grossly displaced fracture at the angle of the mandible.
2. Severe overriding of the fragments.
3. Triangular comminuted fracture at the inferior border associated with angle fracture.
4. Fracture of edentulous mandible.
5. Malunited fractures.
6. Nonunion of the fracture.
7. Fractures with large extraoral lacerations.

Intraoral Transalveolar or Upper Border (Superior Border) Wiring (Figs 32.12A and B)

It was first advocated by Sir William Kelsey Fry to control the posterior fragment by drilling a hole through

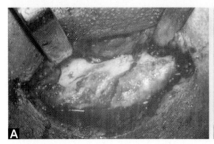
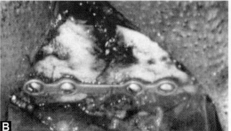
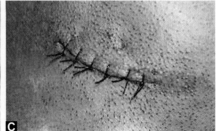

Figs 32.9A to C: (A) Right angle fracture opened via extraoral submandibular incision, (B) Bone plate fixation done, (C) Interrupted suturing done

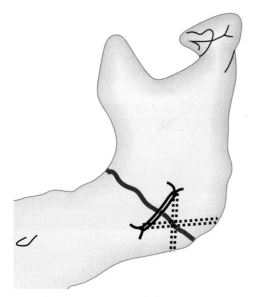

Fig. 32.10: Hayton-William's figure of eight wiring

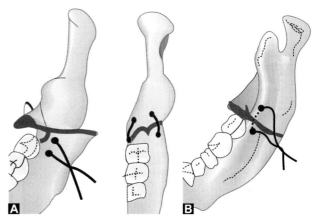

Figs 32.12A and B: Superior border transosseous wiring (intraoral), (A) Superior border wiring engaging both buccal and lingual cortices, (B) Superior border wiring engaging only buccal cortex

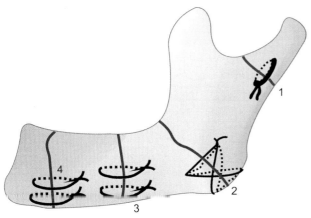

Fig. 32.11: Intraosseous or transosseous wiring (1) For fixation of subcondylar fracture (2) For fixation of angle fracture (3 and 4) For fixation of parasymphysis fractures

the alveolar process of each fragment. Here, the wire is passed through the extraction socket of the third molar tooth, which is invariably involved in the fracture line. Many times, simple loop through only the buccal plate may be adequate. But for better fixation both buccal as well as lingual plates of the alveolar process should be involved and the horizontal mattress type of wiring provides optimum stability. While drilling the holes on either side of the fractured fragments at the alveolar crest, one has to select the site for drilling the holes carefully, so that during final twisting, the thin alveolar bone should not get crumbled down. While drilling the hole on the lingual plate, protection of the lingual nerve

should be done by placing periosteal elevator. This type of wiring is always combined with some form of intermaxillary fixation (IMF).

Extraoral Lower Border (Inferior Border) Transosseous Wiring (Figs 32.10, 32.11 and 32.13)

Fractured fragments are exposed under direct vision through Risdon's incision. After cutting through the pterygomasseteric sling and periosteal layer, the bony fragments are located. The periosteum and tissues on the medial surface are also stripped from the bone for a distance of one centimeter. The end of each fragment is secured with bone holding forceps (Crocodile bone holding forceps, or Kocher's forceps, or Rowe's modified forceps, or Harrison's bone holding forceps) and fractured fragments are brought into approximation by manipulating the bone holding forceps (Figs 32.13A and B). If some soft tissue is entrapped between the fragments or any other debris should be separated or removed. A flat ribbon retractor or tongue depressor is placed under the medial side at the inferior border to protect the underlying soft tissue structures. The entire area should be well exposed by using L-shaped retractors at the upper edge of the incision. The holes should be drilled using small round bur with electrical engine and handpiece with constant irrigation of saline solution (Fig. 32.13C). The first hole should be drilled in the anterior fragment slightly away from the inferior border (No. 1) and at least 0.5 cm from the fracture site.

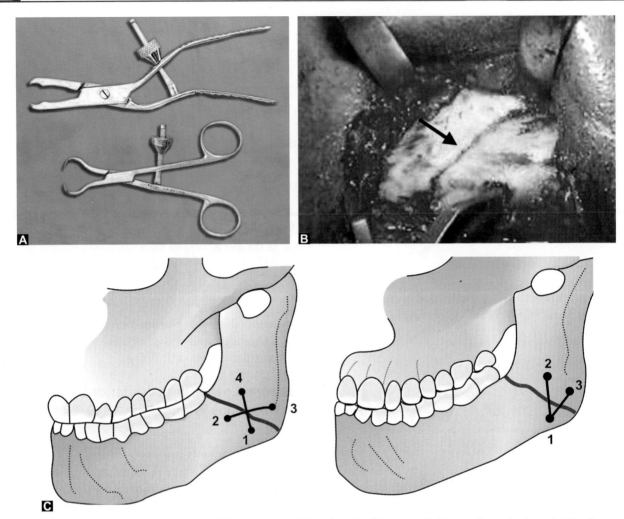

Figs 32.13A to C: (A) Bone holding forceps, (B) Fracture mandible reduced and fragments held in position using bone holding forceps, (C) Transosseous wiring procedure with its variations

The bur hole should be through and through the buccal and lingual cortex. Care should be taken that the hole should be drilled away from inferior alveolar nerve. If four hole technique is to be used, then another hole (No. 2) is drilled above the first hole in the anterior fragment. The ribbon retractor is then repositioned under the posterior fragment. One hole is placed near the inferior border (No. 3) 0.5 cm from the fracture site. Another hole (No. 4) is placed as high as possible above the first one and just below the inferior alveolar canal. Two separate double wires of 26 gauge are cut and one wire is passed from No. 1 hole from buccal cortex to lingual cortex and passed at the posterior fragment to lingual cortex and brought out over buccal cortex from hole No. 4. Then another wire is passed from hole No. 2 and brought out from hole No. 3. Both these wire's ends are twisted individually in criss cross manner after approximating the fragments and ends cut and finished.

Before final tightening of the wires, the assistant should check the occlusion or temporary IML should be carried out. The wires are checked for their tightness and bone holding forceps removed and fracture reduction is inspected. Wound closure is done in layers.

Temporary IML should be removed prior to extubation, if the procedure is done under GA. In the immediate postoperative period, no IML should be given. Next day IML can be done. The sutures should be removed on 5th-7th day. The stainless steel wires remain within the bone permanently and their removal is not necessary, since it is an inert substance and does not give rise to inflammation or irritation of the tissues, unless sepsis has been introduced.

Detached fragments of bone: During surgical procedure, detached portions of the cortical bone may be occasionally encountered, which was not obvious clinically as well as radiologically. Provided that they are attached to periosteum or muscle, they may be wired back into position.

On the other hand, small portions of bone devoid of such attachments with loss of blood supply should not be retained, because they may lead to sequestration at a later date. Such pieces should be therefore removed. However, if a segment of bone removal will lead to a big defect between the bone ends which would lead to nonunion, then in such cases the bone should be replaced back and wired in position as a free graft.

Teeth in the fracture line (Figs 32.14 to 32.17): As per the old concepts teeth in the line of fracture, were considered as a potential impediment to healing for the following reasons:

1. The fractures in the tooth bearing areas are always compounded via periodontal membrane.
2. Due to trauma the tooth can become nonvital.
3. The previous periapical pathology may be present.

The infection can reach the fracture line as a result of any of the above. This will complicate the healing or even lead to a nonunion. In preantibiotic era, therefore, all teeth in the line of fracture were extracted.

Presently, the protocol which is followed is—a tooth in the line of fracture which is structurally not damaged, not subluxated and in functional position in the dental arch should be retained and antibiotics administered.

Controversy also exists with regards to functionless third molars involved in mandibular fractures. If such a tooth helps in stabilizing the fracture, it should be retained (Figs 32.14 to 32.17).

Management of teeth retained in fracture line:

1. Good quality intraoral periapical radiograph to assess the status and plan the treatment, is needed.
2. Proper use of antibiotic therapy should be started.
3. Splinting of tooth, if luxated or mobile should be carried out.
4. Endodontic therapy is carried out, if necessary.
5. Immediate extraction, if fracture becomes infected.

Absolute indications for removal of a tooth in the fracture line:

1. Longitudinal fracture involving the crown and the root, splitting the tooth.
2. Complete subluxation of the tooth from its socket.
3. Pre existing large periapical pathology.
4. Grossly infected fracture line.
5. Bad periodontal status of the tooth and third degree mobility due to periodontitis.
6. Functionless teeth.
7. Advanced caries.
8. Root stumps.

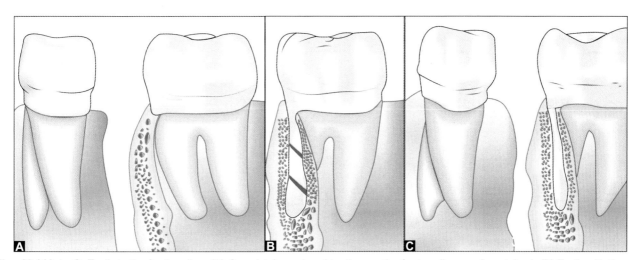

Figs 32.14A to C: Teeth in the fracture line: (A) Completely enclosed teeth near the fracture line can be retained, (B) Teeth with the root fractures, which are exposed in the fracture line are extracted, (C) Teeth with the exposed roots, devoid of bone encasement are extracted or preserved after root canal treatment

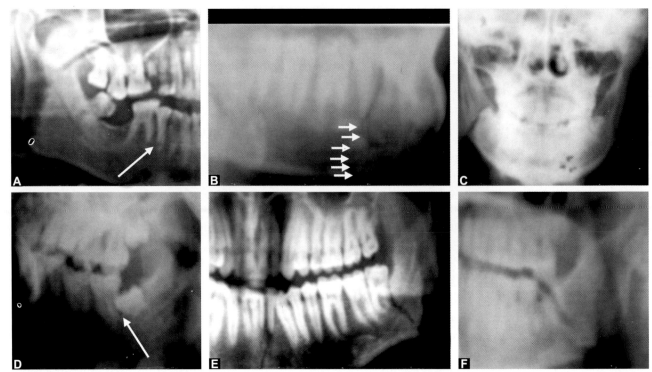

Figs 32.15A to F: Teeth in the fracture line: (A) OPG showing R parasymphysis fracture with broken roots of second mandibular premolar and first molar. Extraction of both the teeth is indicated while fracture reduction and plate fixation, (B) Lateral X-ray showing parasymphysis fracture line passing between two mandibular premolars, (C) PA view showing R angle fracture involving impacted lower third molar, which should be removed at the time of reduction, (D) Lateral X-ray showing L angle fracture, involving impacted third molar, (E) OPG showing L symphysis and angle fracture, involving L lateral incisor and L third molar, (F) OPG showing L side fracture mandible and root fracture of lower third molar

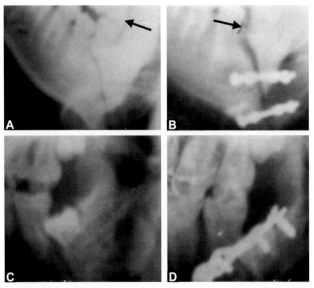

Figs 32.16A to D: (A) Lower left third molar in the fracture line is luxated. Note the premature contact with upper left third molar. Retaining such a tooth will interfere with the occlusion and proper reduction, (B) Postoperative X-ray shows the improper reduction of the fracture and extrusion of the lower left third molar, (C) Fracture line passing between second and third molar, (D) Extraction of third molar, reduction and intraoral plate fixation

BONE PLATING IN MANDIBULAR FRACTURES

Advantages

 i. Rigid or stable fixation.
 ii. Obviates the need for immobilization of the mandible.
 iii. Early return to home and work.
 iv. Soft diet can be taken.
 v. Maintenance of oral hygiene.
 vi. Useful in mentally challenged, physically handicapped patients.
 vii. Maintenance of airway in multiple fractures.

Simple Noncompression Bone Plates

Champy's system made up of stainless steel or titanium can be used with monocortical screws which are self-tapping. It is preferable to use screws 2 mm in diameter and 10 mm in length with titanium plates in order to improve the rigidity of the fixation. The plates are available in various sizes and shapes. Suitable selection of the plate should be done depending on the site and type of fracture to be fixed (Fig. 32.18).

Miniplate Osteosynthesis

Instrumentation is shown in Figure 32.19. For the adaptation of the plate to external cortex of the bone,

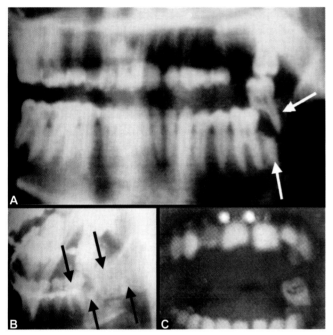

Figs 32.17A to C: (A) OPG showing L side fracture mandible with the displacement of posterior fragment upwards and medially. Root fracture of second L lower molar is seen and the crown is in contact with upper second molar preventing further displacement of posterior fragment, (D) Lateral oblique view L side note the step deformity, (C) Intraoral picture showing the occlusal deformity

a plate bending pliers and a plate bending lever is needed (Fig. 32.20). The bending pliers allow the plate to be adapted over margins and surfaces by virtue of the special indentations in the plate. With the side cutting shears, the plates may be cut to the desired length. The screwdriver incorporates a spring lock device, so that the screws can be easily picked up from the screw rack and screwed into the mandibular bone. The tightening of the screw is finished with another small screwdriver. The screws and plates are made up of the same metal. The mechanical properties of the osteosynthesis material ensure that the induced tension and torsion forces are neutralized. In general, however, physiologic forces acting directly on the bone can be tolerated.

The plates available are—4 hole, 6 hole, 8 to 16 hole plates, in addition to 4 to 6 hole plates with an intermediate bar segment. The plates have a thickness of 0.9 mm. The minimum diameter of the hole is 2.1 mm with a bevel of 30 degree. Self-tapping conical screws are available in lengths of 5 to 15 mm. The screw thread has a diameter of 2 mm, one turn of the screw corresponds to 1 mm penetration into the bone. The diameter of the screw head is 2.8 mm, the counter sinking of the head corresponding to the 30° beveled drill hole in the plate. The drill which is used to prepare hole in the bone has a diameter of 1.6 mm and so is 0.4 mm smaller than the screws used. The difference of 0.4 diameter ensures firm anchorage of the self-tapping screws (Fig. 32.21).

Application of miniplate osteosynthesis (Fig. 32.22): Correct fracture fixation with miniplates is ensured in completely dentulous jaws as well as in edentulous jaws. As a rule, the approach is always intraoral, even in cases in which

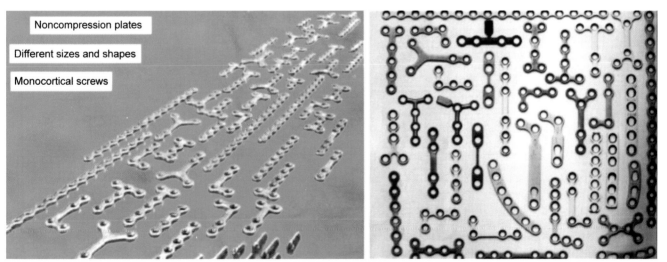

Noncompression plates

Different sizes and shapes

Monocortical screws

Fig. 32.18: Different types of monocortical noncompression plates and screws

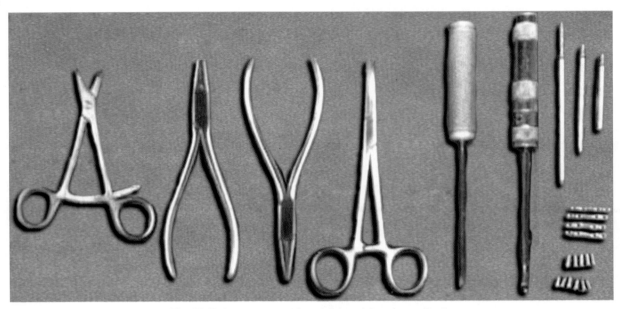

Fig. 32.19: Instruments set for minibone plate osteosynthesis

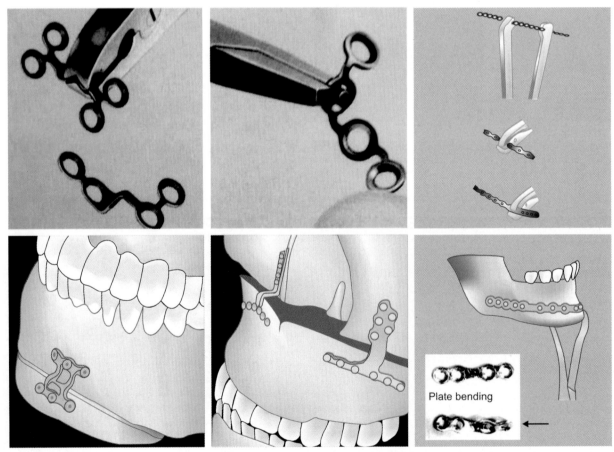

Fig. 32.20: Plate bending—using a plate bending plier and a plate bending lever to adapt to bone contour

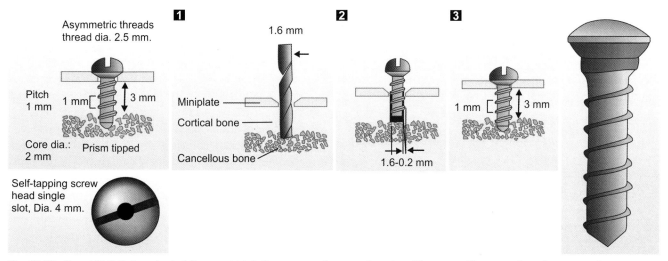

Fig. 32.21: (1 and 2) Drill diameter is 1.6 mm, which is the same as the core diameter of the screw. The screw thread measures 2 mm across. The holes drilled should be monoaxial, (3) All screws are of self-tapping type, with a pitch of 1 mm. For average mandibular cortex thickness of 3 mm, 3 turns of the screw will provide adequate anchorage

jaw injuries are compounded externally. In multiple mandibular fractures, the precise reduction and the establishment of occlusion is more difficult, hence it is advisable to secure the occlusion by interdental wiring, before the osteosynthesis is performed. In the edentulous jaw, manual reduction is generally sufficient. Following reduction, the osteosynthesis lines should be considered. The adaptation of the bone plate should be carried out by using bending pliers (Fig. 32.20). The adapted bone plate should lie passively on the contour of the external cortex, without any gap between the plate and the bone. The plate is adjusted in such a way that minimum two screws can be fixed on either side of the fracture line. The drilling is then performed through the holes in the plate perpendicular to the surface of the bone. The miniplate is fixed in position with the screws. In the case of fractures of the angle of the mandible, the plate should be located on the posterior fragment, medial to the external oblique line, so that it is bent over the surface and the posterior screws are placed in a nearly sagittal direction. In certain cases—with simultaneous fractures of the alveolar process or when impacted wisdom teeth are present, the plate may be fixed to the outer surface of the mandible corresponding in position to the course of the line of tension.

With fractures between the canine and premolars, the mental nerve may be damaged by the application of the plate. It is therefore advantageous to place the concave section of the plate between the screw holes precisely over the exit point of the nerve. In exceptional cases transposition of the nerve to a lower level may be

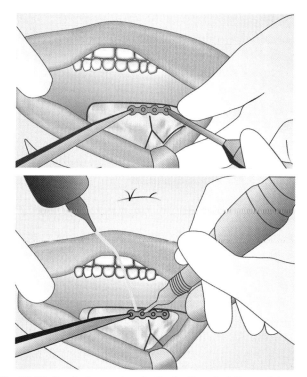

Fig. 32.22: Surgical procedure for the fixation of minibone plates and screws

indicated. To neutralize torsional forces in the symphysis region in between the mental foramina, it is necessary to use two parallel plates. The gap between them should be 4 to 5 mm. It is recommended that the lower plate be fixed first and the subapical plate to be fixed later. In the comminuted fractures or where there are detached triangular pieces of bone, longer plates with six or more screws should be used. In multiple fractures of the body of mandible, after reduction, the fragments are held firmly by temporary IMF. The osteosynthesis is performed first in the teeth bearing section of the jaw, e.g. in midline and angle fracture, the midline fracture is fixed first, this makes it easier to avoid malocclusion.

Complications and management:

Suture dehiscence: It is found if the surgery for osteosynthesis is delayed due to some reasons:

i. Timing of surgery.

ii. Due to inappropriate incision in the region of the attached gingiva, on 4th or 8th postoperative day, the gap will be noticed. In such a case, the sutures are removed and cleaning of the wound with 15 percent hydrogen peroxide is done. Frequent mouthwashes are encouraged. Wound is allowed to heal with secondary intention.

Postoperative infection: This may be due to the following:

i. Inadequate number of screws applied.

ii. Incorrect placement of the bone plates, outside the osteosynthesis lines.

iii. Proximity of the plates to the apical region.

iv. Inadvertent placement of the screws in the teeth bearing area.

v. Lack of maintenance of oral hygiene postoperatively.

Compression Plates

Whenever the plate is applied to the convex surface of the mandible at its lower border, there is a tendency for the upper border and lingual plate to open up with the final tightening of the screws. This leads to distortion of occlusion as well as opening of the fracture line on the other side, in case of bilateral fractures. To overcome this problem and to produce more rigid fixation Spiessel in 1972, Schilli in 1977 devised various designs of compression plates. These compression plates include at least two-pear shaped holes. The widest diameter of the hole lies near the fracture line. The screw is inserted in the narrow part of the hole and at the final movement of tightening, its head comes to rest in the widest diameter of the hole, which is countersunk to receive it. The compression holes in the plate may be positioned one on each side of the fracture line (Spiessel, DCP—Dynamic compression plate).

EDCP—Schilli designed a plate with oblique lateral holes, which direct the compressing force towards the upper border, so that when the plate is screwed firmly into the place, there is no tendency for the fracture line to gape (Figs 32.23A to E).

The entire procedure is too precise and lengthy. Extraoral route is needed. The various complications associated with the use of these bulky plates are metal fatigue, fracture of the plate, necrosis of the bone ends, osteoporotic changes, etc. With the advent of miniplates, the use of original compression osteosynthesis is not done frequently. Though theoretically it offers the most rigid fixation.

Mandibular fractures associated with multiple other facial fractures (Fig. 32.24): The old adage—'inside out and from bottom to top' sequence to be followed, when treating multiple facial fractures. Mandibular fractures should be treated first to restore the lower facial height as well as to achieve the continuity of the lower arch (for guiding the reduction of other fractures).

Edentulous mandibular fractures: With associated medical problems in these patients, there is special challenge in treating these fractures:

i. Alveolar resorption is four times greater in the mandible than in the maxilla.

ii. Inferior alveolar vascular supply to the bone is greatly compromised.

iii. Too little cancellous bone for repair (osteoblastic endosteum).

iv. Normal healing potential is retarded.

v. Open reduction amounts to stripping of periosteum, which impairs osteogenesis, as there is greater dependence on periosteal supply in atrophic mandible.

However, small bone discrepancies (nonanatomic alignment by closed reduction) are usually of no consequences by maturation of the bone.

But, sometimes, due to extreme alveolar resorption, the molar areas may be more prone to fracture. In some cases, it is possible to have bilateral fracture of the body of the edentulous mandible, each occurring near the posterior attachment of the mylohyoid muscle. In the edentulous mandible, the mylohyoid muscle attachment is relatively higher up on the lingual side. Under the influence of the diagastric and mylohyoid muscles pull, there is extreme downward and backward angulation of the anterior fractured fragment. This creates a typical 'bucket handle' type of displacement, which is highly unstable. This type of extreme displacement at times, may cause respiratory distress in an elderly

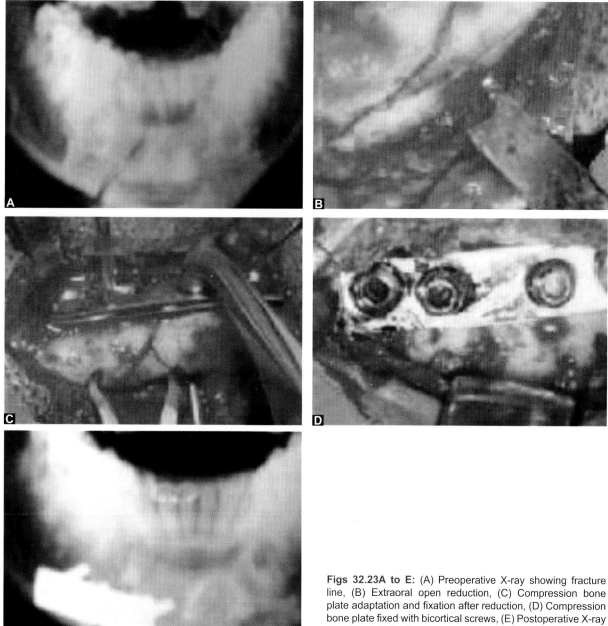

Figs 32.23A to E: (A) Preoperative X-ray showing fracture line, (B) Extraoral open reduction, (C) Compression bone plate adaptation and fixation after reduction, (D) Compression bone plate fixed with bicortical screws, (E) Postoperative X-ray showing rigid fixation

patient. Early stabilization of the fracture is mandatory (Figs 32.25 and 32.26).

Treatment plan for edentulous mandible fractures

  i. Closed reduction with mandibular prosthesis held in place by circummandibular wiring.
 ii. In nonunion or delayed healing, open reduction with titanium mesh.

iii. Severely atrophic edentulous ridge fracture, open reduction with primary bone grafting.

In case of edentulous mandible fractures, many times, nonunion of the fracture is seen due to impaired blood supply or presence of infection, after conservative treatment. During the open reduction procedure, there is typical 'eburnation' of the ends of the fractured

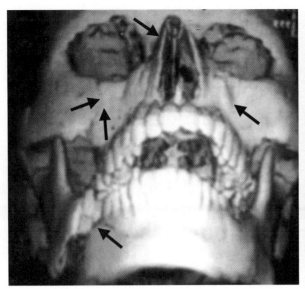
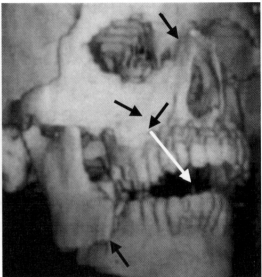

Fig. 32.24: 3D scan showing panfacial fractures. LeFort II, right zygomatic bone, nasal fractures are seen. Right angle mandibular fracture showing gross displacement with overriding of the fragments. Note the loss of occlusion with severe anterior open bite

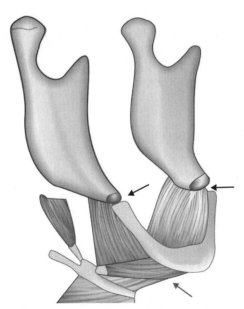

Fig. 32.25: Possible mechanism of producing 'bucket handle' type of fracture of atrophic edentulous mandible. The fracture is seen in the resorbed body of the mandible in front of the posterior attachment of the mylohyoid muscle (red arrow)

fragments is noticed. This is the process, where the outer and inner cortex heals at both the fractured ends of the fragments. Many times soft tissue entrapment is also found between the fracture ends leading to nonunion. In the radiograph, this eburnation is seen as 'elephant foot deformity' in the edentulous mandible fracture (nonunion). In such a situation both the fractured ends should be freshened up, soft tissue entrapment is cleared off and then the fixation should be carried out (Fig. 32.27).

Reconstruction Plates

These are capable of temporary load bearing and therefore useful in comminuted fractures, defect fractures and infected fractures. It is also useful in the case of severely displaced angle fractures. Reconstruction plate absorbs all functional loads to restore the continuity and permits early mobilization, despite extensive fragmentation of the bone. It also spans the comminuted area to preserve the original shape, length and strength of the mandibular arch.

Reconstruction plates must be accurately contoured to avoid fracture displacement and a subsequent malocclusion during tightening of the screws. The use of template simplifies the bending process of the large reconstruction plates. When using a reconstruction plate, the most posterior screw holes to the fracture site, should be placed at least 1 cm away from the fragment end and

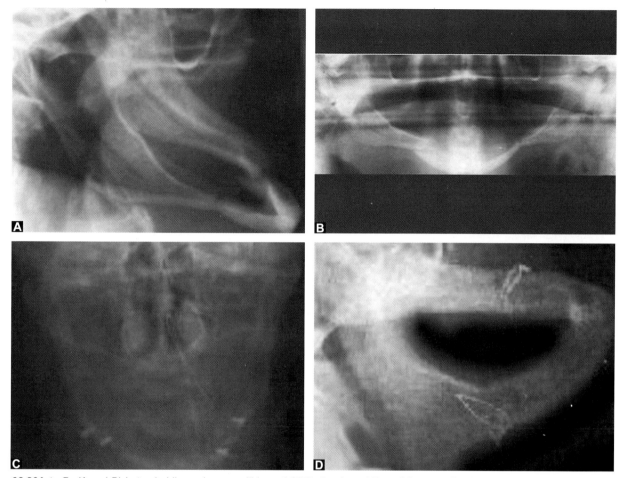

Figs 32.26A to D: (A and B) Lateral oblique view mandible and OPG showing a bilateral fracture of a thin edentulous mandible with typical 'Bucket handle' type of displacement, (C) Open reduction and fixation was done. Postoperative PA view mandible, showing the proper reduction and fixation of the bilateral fractures, (D) Intraosseous wiring fixation in another patient for stabilizing bucket handle fracture

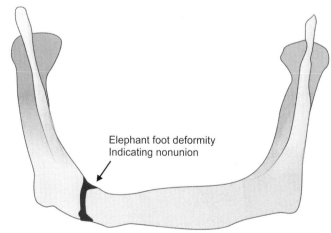

Elephant foot deformity
Indicating nonunion

Fig. 32.27: Elephant foot deformity, indicating nonunion of fracture of the edentulous mandible

four screws in each segment provide the maximum resistance to deformation (Figs 32.28 to 32.30).

Complications of mandibular fracture management: Untoward sequelae such as infection, bleeding, lip numbness, malocclusion, nonunion, malunion, trismus, tooth loss, paresis and cosmetic compromise are reported to range as high as 40 percent or more.

Employment of proper surgical protocols will reduce postoperative complications.

Complications during primary treatment

1. *Infection*—Lowering the patient's local or general resistance will predispose to infection. Pathological fracture, debilitated patients, diabetics, patients on steroid therapy are more prone to infection.

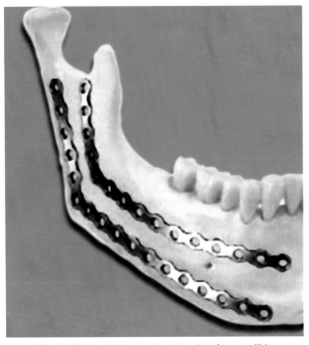

Fig. 32.28: Angled reconstruction plate for mandible

2. *Nerve damage*—Anesthesia of the lower lip due to neuropraxia or neurotemesis of the inferior alveolar nerve is the most common complication. Facial nerve damage may be seen due to penetrating injuries.
3. *Displaced teeth and foreign bodies*—may be swallowed. Chest radiograph should be done and if needed, bronchoscopy should be carried out. Foreign bodies like glass pieces, fragments of teeth can get buried in the soft tissues of the lip. They should be explored and removed.
4. Pulpitis.
5. Gingival and periodontal complications.

Later complications

1. *Malunion*—results due to improper fixation method, early removal of immobilization device, tissue entrapment in the fragments, etc.
2. *Delayed union*—due to local factors such as infection or general factors such as osteoporosis or nutritional deficiency.

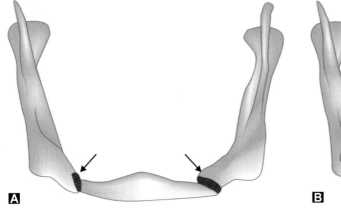
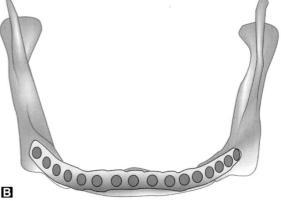

Figs 32.29A and B: (A) Bilateral fracture of edentulous atrophic mandible, (B) Fracture reduction and fixation with reconstruction plate

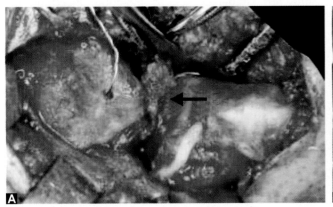
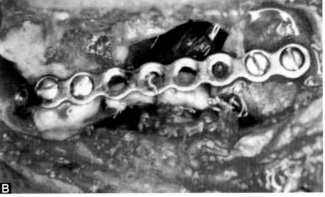

Figs 32.30A and B: (A) Nonunion of the mandibular body fracture. Note the soft tissue entrapment between the fractured fragments, (B) Sliding inferior border bone grafting. Fixation with reconstruction plate

3. *Nonunion*—radiologically, rounding off and sclerosis of the bone ends is seen. This condition is called as 'eburnation'. This is caused by:
   i. Infection at the fracture site.
   ii. Inadequate immobilization.
   iii. Unsatisfactory approximation with tissue entrapment.
   iv. The ultrathin edentulous mandible in an elderly debilitated patient.
   v. Considerable loss of bone and soft tissue.
   vi. Inadequate blood supply after radiotherapy.
   vii. The presence of bone pathology like tumors, etc.
   viii. General diseases, e.g. osteoporosis, nutritional deficiency, disorders of calcium metabolism.
4. Sequestration of bone.
5. Traumatic myositis ossificans—rare.
6. Scars.

33 Fractures of the Condylar Process and Its Management

Incidence of the condylar fracture reported in the literature varies from 5 to 8 percent among all mandibular fractures. The condylar fractures may be a result of direct or indirect impact.

CLASSIFICATION OF CONDYLAR FRACTURES (FIGS 33.1 TO 33.10)

1. Unilateral or bilateral condylar fractures (Figs 33.1A and B)

2. Rowe and Killey's classification
   a. Simple fractures of condyle
   b. Compound fractures of condyle
   c. Comminuted fracture associated with zygomatic arch fractures

3. Rowe and Killey's classification (1968) (Figs 33.2A and B)
   a. Intracapsular fractures or high condylar fractures (Figs 33.3A and B)

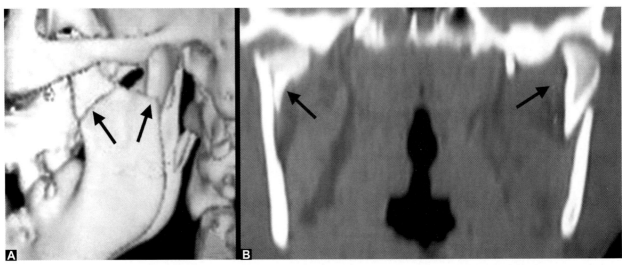

Figs 33.1A and B: Condylar process fracture classification: (A) Unilateral fracture, separate coronoid process fracture is also seen, (B) Bilateral fracture

i. Fractures involving the articular surface (rare).
ii. Fractures above or through the anatomical neck, which do not involve the articular surfaces

b. *Extracapsular or low condylar or subcondylar fractures:* Here the fracture runs from the lowest

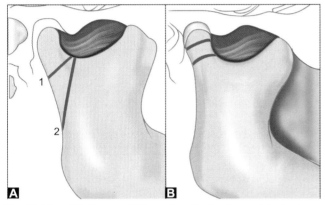

Figs 33.2A and B: Rowe and Killey's classification for condylar fractures: (A) 1—Intracapsular or high condylar fracture, 2—Extracapsular or low or subcondylar fracture, (B) First fracture line is above the attachment of lateral pterygoid muscle. Second fracture line is at or below the attachment of lateral pterygoid muscle, where condylar head is always prone to displacement due to the contraction of the muscle

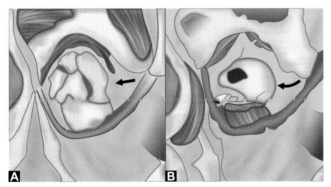

Figs 33.3A and B: Intracapsular fractures. (A) Fracture involving articular surface, (B) Fracture above or through the anatomical neck without, involvement of the articular surface, (Mushroom type)

point of curvature of the sigmoid notch, obliquely downward and backward below the surgical neck of the condyle to the posterior aspect of the upper part of the ramus.

c. Fractures associated with injury to the capsule, ligaments and meniscus.
d. Fractures involving the adjacent bone, e.g. fracture of the roof of the glenoid fossa or the tympanic plate of the external auditory meatus.

4. Clinical classification by MacLennan (1952) (Figs 33.4A to E)
   a. *No displacement:* A crack fracture is seen without alteration of the normal relationship of the condylar head to the glenoid fossa or of the neck of the condyle to the ramus.
   b. *Deviation:* Simple angulation exists between the condylar neck and the ramus.
   c. *Displacement:* Overlap occurs between the condylar process and the ramus. The obliquely fractured condylar fragment lies lateral to the ramus.
   d. *Dislocation:* Disruption takes place between the condylar head and the glenoid fossa. The condylar fragment gets pulled anteriorly and medially by the lateral pterygoid muscle.

5. Wassmund's classification (1934)
   a. *Type I:* Fracture of the neck of the condyle with slight displacement of the head. The angle between the head and the axis of the ramus varies from 10 to 45 degrees. These type of fractures tend to reduce spontaneously.
   b. *Type II:* An angle of 45 to 90 degrees is seen between the head and the ramus. There is tearing of the medial portion of the joint capsule.
   c. *Type III:* The fragments are not in contact. Head is displaced medially and forward due to the pull of lateral pterygoid muscle and spasm. The fragment is generally confined within the area of the glenoid fossa. The capsule is torn and

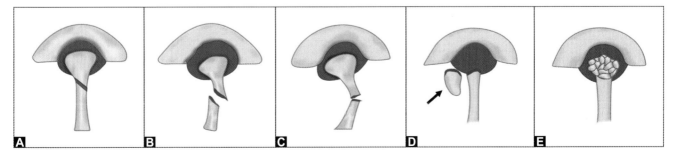

Figs 33.4A to E: MacLennan's classification of condylar fractures: (A) No displacement, (B) Displacement, (C) Deviation, (D) Dislocation, (E) Comminution, (Multiple fragmentation)

head is outside the capsule. Open reduction is advocated.

d. *Type IV:* Fractured head articulates on or forward to the articular eminence.

e. *Type V:* Vertical or oblique fracture through the head of the condyle—rare.

6. Comprehensive classification: Proposed by Lindhal (1977), which required radio-graphs in 2 planes at right angles to each other.

To describe a condylar fracture under this system, the following details must be noted:

a. *Fracture level:* This may be as follows (Fig. 33.5):

i. *Condylar head fracture, intracapsular:* By definition a condylar head fracture is within the capsule and is therefore termed intracapsular.
   - Vertical (anteroposterior sagittal split)
   - Compression (producing a mushroom type of expansion)
   - Comminuted

   A horizontal subdivision would be difficult to differentiate from next category.

ii. *Condylar neck:* The radioconstriction representing the condylar neck corresponds anatomically to region of inferior attachment of joint capsule.

iii. *Subcondylar:* This is the region below the neck, extending down to the most inferior part of the sigmoid notch anteriorly while its posterior limits situated more inferiorly corresponding to the point of maximum curvature of natural concavity of posterior border of the mandible in that region.

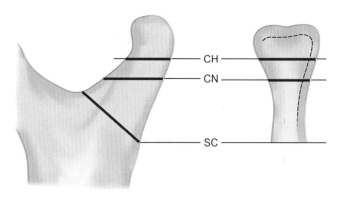

Fig. 33.5: Lindhal's classification: CH—condylar head-intracapsular fracture, CN—condylar neck fracture, SC—subcondylar fracture

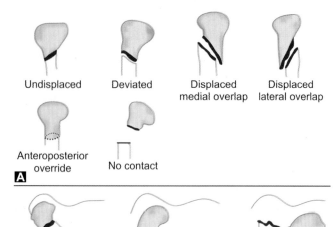

Figs 33.6A and B: Relationship of the condylar fragment: (A) To the mandible ramus stump, (B) To the glenoid fossa

b. *Relationship of condylar fragment to mandible* (Fig. 33.6A):

   This may be as follows:

   i. Undisplaced (or fissure fracture)

   ii. *Deviated:* This is a simple angulation of the condylar process in relation to main mandibular fragment without overlap

   iii. Displaced with medial overlap of the condylar fragment

   iv. Displaced with lateral overlap of the condylar fragment

   v. Anteroposterior overlap is possible, but infrequent

   vi. Without contact between the fragments

c. *Relationship of condylar head to fossa* (Fig. 33.6B)

   The following relationship may be observed:

   i. No displacement—joint space appears normal.

   ii. Displacement—joint space is increased, but condyle is still related to the glenoid fossa. Lindhal subdivided this into slight displacement and moderate displacement, but quantification is difficult.

d. Injury to meniscus: It may be torn, ruptured/herniated in forward/backward direction.

7. Thoma (1945) classified fractures in a simple way taking into consideration the direction of displacement.

A. *Condylar fractures*
  i. Without displacement of condyle
    • Greenstick fracture
    • Intracapsular
    • Extracapsular
  ii. With displacement of condyle
    • Lateral
    • Medial
    • Forward
    • Backward
  iii. With overriding of fragments
  iv. With dislocation in lateral or medial direction
    • Intracapsular
    • Complete fracture dislocation
    • Complete dislodgement of the condyle
    • Dislocation of the fractured part of the head of the condyle
  v. With dislocation in forward direction
    • Anteriorly from the articular eminence
    • Posteriorly from the articular eminence
    • With dislocation and displacement of the meniscus
    • With comminution
    • Old fracture with deformities
      — Pseudoarthrosis
      — Ankylosis
B. *Subcondylar fractures*
  i. Without displacement of fragment
  ii. With displacement of fragment
  Fracture line either extending through head or base of the condyle or neck has been called condylar fracture by Thoma, whereas in subcondylar fracture, the line runs transversely over ascending ramus.
8. Spiessel and Schroll classification (1972) (Figs 33.7A to F)
  i. Nondisplaced fracture
  ii. Low neck fracture with displacement
  iii. High neck fracture with displacement
  iv. Low neck fracture with dislocation
  v. High neck fracture with dislocation
  vi Head fracture

Etiological Factors Leading to Condylar Fractures

Etiological factors leading to condylar fractures may be grouped as:

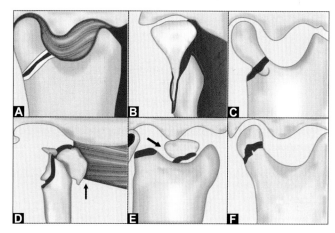

Figs 33.7A to F: Spiessel and Schroll classification: (A) Nondisplaced fracture, (B) Low neck fracture with displacement, (C) High neck fracture with displacement, (D) Low neck fracture with dislocation, (E) High neck fracture with dislocation, (F) Condylar head fracture

1. Intentional trauma—interpersonal violence/fist fight, etc.
2. Unintentional trauma—motor vehicular accidents, fall on the chin, sports injuries, industrial mishaps, etc.

Whenever a blow is received on the lateral side of face, the zygomatic arch protects the condyle and coronoid process. Under these circumstances, the arch may fracture and may be associated with fracture or dislocation of the condyle (Figs 33.8 and 33.9).

When a blow is given on the face resulting in fracture of the mandibular condyle, the position of the fractured condyle in relation to the remainder of the ramal stump will depend on certain factors:
1. The direction and degree of force.
2. The precise point of application of force.
3. Whether the teeth were in occlusion at the time of injury.
4. Whether the patient is partially or fully edentulous (Fig. 33.10).

Fracture with little or no displacement occurs when adequate natural or artifical molar support exists and the teeth are in occlusion at the time of impact.

A variable degree of displacement will take place, if the teeth are separated or the force is received from a lateral direction. Full force of impact will be transmitted to the condyles, resulting in a variable degree of fracture dislocation, if the mouth is widely open or there is inadequate molar support at the time of injury.

If a hard blow is received on the mandible, the force is transmitted on the teeth, which are in occlusion.

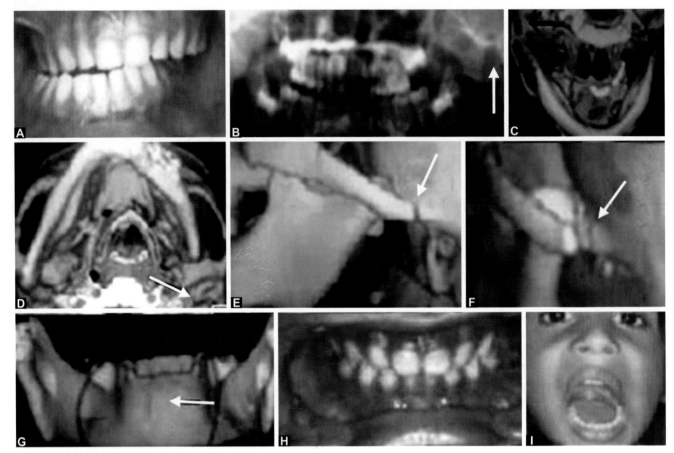

Figs 33.8A to I: Dislocation of condyle with zygomatic arch and parasymphysis fracture: (A) Six years boy came with the history of fall, C/O teeth not occluding and inability to open the mouth wide, (B) OPG showed dislocation of L condyle. Under sedation reduction was tried without success, (C to F) 3D CT scan showing left zygomatic arch fracture at the base, which was not seen in OPG, (G) L parasymphysis fracture seen in 3D CT, mandible with medial rotation and disarticulation, (H) Under GA again intraoral reduction was attempted with failure. E.O preauricular approach was taken to reduce the dislocation of the condylar head back into fossa. Zygomatic arch fracture was reduced and fixed with 2 hole minibone plate. Normal occlusion was achieved, (I) Normal oral opening

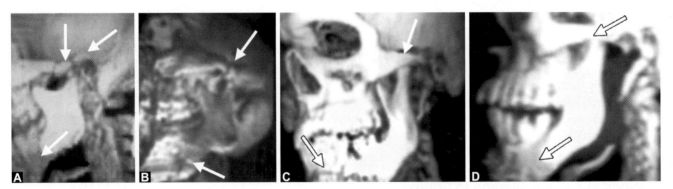

Figs 33.9A to D: (A and B) L zygomatic arch fracture associated with dislocation of condyle and L malunited parasymphysis fracture, (C and D) Another patient with L parasymphysis malunited fracture with dislocation of condyle, which often goes unnoticed

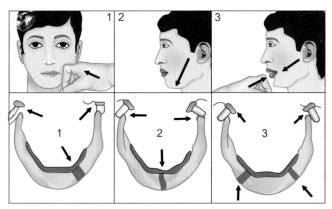

Fig. 33.10: Mechanism of injury to the condyles: (1) Blow, (2) Ground fall, (3) Dashboard RTA injury

When the blow on the face results during posterior or lateral movements, then the indirect stress results in the fracture of the slender neck of the condyle. On the other hand, if the patient receives a blow on the chin, the force of the impact is transmitted upwards and backwards along the length of the mandible. If the blow is delivered with great force, it would force the condylar head through the glenoid fossa, into the middle cranial fossa. This calamity is prevented in majority of the cases, because the slender neck of the condyle fractures due to impact and prevents the condyles from entering into the middle cranial fossa.

When the blow is received in the center of the chin, the distribution of force is equal to both the condyles, resulting in a bilateral indirect fracture through the necks, accompanied by a direct fracture at the symphysis (countercoup type of fractures). This type of injury is more often seen in an epileptic patients or soldiers who fall on the face during parade.

If the patient is wearing a denture or is having the posterior teeth in occlusion at the time of injury, the contact between the upper and lower teeth would minimize the consequences of the impact, but if such protection is not possible, then the patient may sustain a severe fracture dislocation of one or both the condyles.

DIAGNOSTIC FINDINGS OF CONDYLAR FRACTURES

1. Evidence of facial trauma, especially in the area of the mandible and symphysis.
2. Localized pain and swelling in the region of the TMJ.
3. Limitation in mouth opening.

4. Deviation, upon opening, towards the involved side.
5. Posterior open bite on the contralateral side.
6. Shift of occlusion towards the ipsilateral side with possible cross bite.
7. Blood in the external auditory canal.
8. Pain on palpation over the fracture site.
9. Lack of condylar movement upon palpation.
10. Difficulty in lateral excursions as well as protrusion.
11. The occurrence of anterior open bite with bilateral subcondylar fractures. This is associated with posterior gagging of the occlusion.
12. Persistent cerebrospinal fluid leak through the ear is indicative of an associated fracture of the middle cranial fossa (otorrhea).

The diagnosis of fracture of the condyle is usually made on clinical examination and confirmed by radiographic findings.

Clinically, it will be noted that there is asymmetry of the face on the involved side due to, shifting of the mandible posteriorly and laterally towards the affected side (deviation of the mandible). Premature occlusion on the involved side is caused by upward pull of the elevator muscles of the mandible. This results in a class I lever with the fulcrum on the molar teeth on the involved side (Figs 33.11A to C).

An open bite deformity anteriorly and on the opposite side of the mandible is noted. In case of bilateral fracture condyles, the patient will have anterior open bite deformity with premature contact only on the posterior teeth. This is caused by upward displacement of ramus and telescoping of the fractured fragments, due to contractions of the lateral pterygoid muscles. In bilateral condylar fracture, which occurs below the attachment of the lateral pterygoid muscles, the patient is unable to protrude the mandible. In unilateral fractures at the same level, the patient is unable to perform lateral movements to the opposite side, as the lateral pterygoid muscle is out of function on the affected side (Figs 33.12 and 33.13).

Fractures above the level of the lateral pterygoid muscle insertion do not exhibit displacement, as there is absence of contracting muscle attached to the proximal segment. The patient may complain of severe pain in the TM joint and it will be noted that the teeth are separated and do not come into the occlusion on the affected side, because of the hemarthrosis in the joint, which forces the condyles downwards. It may be few weeks before the teeth come into their normal occlusal relationship. In this type of fractures, especially in children, active early

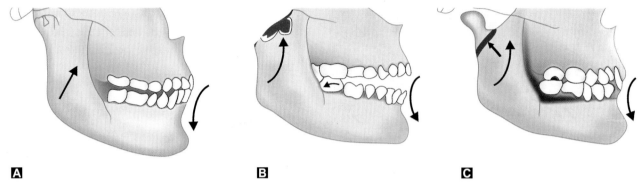

Figs 33.11A to C: Lever principle applied to the mandible

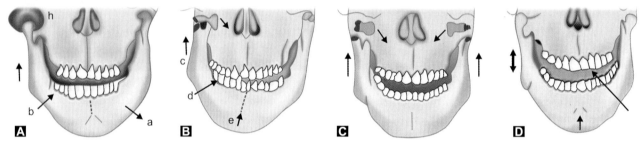

Figs 33.12A to D: Signs of injury to the temporomandibular joint: (A) Effusion, h—hemarthrosis, a—midline shift to contralateral side, b—unilateral posterior open bite, (B) Unilateral fracture dislocation, c—telescoping, d—posterior premature contact, e—midline to ipsilateral side, (C) Bilateral fracture dislocation with anterior open bite, (D) Bilateral dislocation of the condyles without fracture. Note the total inability to occlude

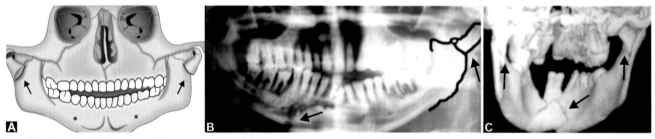

Figs 33.13A to C: (A) Diagram—bilateral condylar fractures with anterior open bite, (B) OPG showing R parasymphysis and L unilateral condylar fracture, (C) 3D CT scan with posterior rotational view, showing bilateral condylar fractures with overriding and symphysis fracture mandible (countercoup fractures)

mobilization of the joint is a must, the parents should be warned about the possibility of the development of ankylosis of the TMJ, if proper treatment is not initiated.

TREATMENT OF CONDYLAR FRACTURES

The management of condylar fractures is divided into: (a) Nonsurgical and (b) Surgical treatment.

Because of the complexity of the functional anatomy of this region, there is a lot of controversy related to

the specific treatment modalities. The decision will vary depending on the age of the patient, the type of fracture, concomitant injuries and associated anatomical findings.

Nonsurgical Management of Condylar Fractures

Most cases of the condylar fractures are best managed through nonsurgical means. The obvious advantage is the avoidance of morbidity and complications associated with surgery.

Conservative method varies from no fixation to employing various fixation devices:

1. Condylar fractures without displacement or with minimum displacement, without much occlusal disturbance and functional range of motion do not require any active treatment. Patient is asked to restrict the movements and semisolid soft diet intake for 10 to 15 days followed by active movements.
2. In case of deviation on mouth opening without much occlusal discrepancy, a simple muscle training in front of a mirror is adequate. On the involved side, class II elastic traction and on the normal side, vertical elastic forces may be beneficial.
3. In cases, where condylar fragment overriding is seen with alteration in ramus height, producing malocclusion, initially elastic traction is given to correct the malocclusion, followed by IMF for 2 to 3 weeks.

Early mobilization is advocated in cases of young children to avoid ankylosis of TMJ.

Surgical Correction of Condylar Fractures

Many a times, ankylosis, malocclusion, continued pain, dysfunction are examples of residual difficulties associated with the conservative management with condylar fractures.

Absolute Indications for Open Surgery

1. Fracture dislocations in the auditory canal or middle cranial fossa (rare)
2. Anterior dislocation with restricted mandibular movements
3. Bilateral condylar fractures associated with a comminuted LeFort III type with craniofacial dysjunction.

Relative Indications (Figs 33.8 to 33.13)

1. Subcondylar fractures with overriding of the fragments with anterior open bite.
2. Anterior and medial displacement of the condylar fragment.
3. In case of delayed treatment, where there is pain and dysfunction associated with malunited fracture.

4. Unilateral or bilateral fractures with loss of the posterior teeth, in either upper jaw or both the jaws.
5. Cases in which position of the condylar fragment interferes with normal function of the jaws.

Surgical Approach to the Condyle

The preauricular approach historically has had a relatively high incidence of facial nerve involvement. Modifications of this approach include an approach to the joint region through a subtemporal fascial-periosteal envelope. Such an approach allows avoidance of the facial nerve branches by staying first posterior and then deep to the nerve. Postramal approach is better for subcondylar fractures.

Methods of Fixation of Condylar Fractures (Figs 33.14 and 33.15)

It can be done by using transosseous wiring or bone plating with miniplating system.

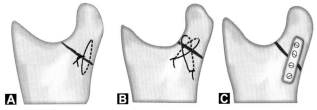

Figs 33.14A to C: Methods of fixation of condylar fracture. (A) Intraosseous wiring, (B) Double intraosseous wiring, (C) Bone plating

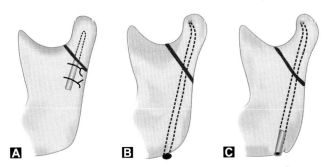

Figs 33.15A to C: Various methods of fixation of condylar fracture. (A) Any long metal tube or hypodermic needle or Steinmann pin is cut and inlaid into the ramus segment and fixed with wires, (B) Long pin or Lag screw is threaded through the ramus into the condylar segment, (C) Petzel introduced a sophisticated technique of fixation. He drilled a hole from the inferior surface through the ramus and then inserted a pin into the condylar segment. After the reduction is done, the pin is cut and a nut is placed at the end of the pin and tightened to offer a compression effect at the fracture site

Various methods using threaded pins have also been described. One of the simplest methods is to use a Kirschner wire or lag screw that is passed from the inferior aspect upwards into the condylar head. Prior to surgery upper and lower arch bars or any other type of wiring to be fixed, so that the actual surgical time is cut down.

Preparation of the patient: The temporal region is shaved preferably the day before surgery. The skin of the preauricular region and the ear are prepared in the usual manner. The patient should be placed on the table so that the sagittal plane of the head is parallel with the table. This often requires that the shoulder be raised with a flat sandbag. Sandbags are also used to maintain the head in the correct position.

Operative procedure: Access to the TMJ is done for high condylar fracture via modified preauricular incision and for subcondylar through postramal approach. Blunt retractors are inserted and the zygomatic arch is located. The depression in the inferior border of the arch denotes the location of the mandibular joint. The mandible at this point may be moved by the assistant, which may produce movement of the fragments and so helps in locating them. As one proceeds, the transverse facial artery and vein may be encountered, cut and tied. Inverted L-shaped incision is taken from the lower border of the zygomatic arch to the outer surface of the ramus.

The procedure from here, depends on whether the condyle is displaced laterally or medially, which is already determined from the radiographs. If the condyle is laterally displaced, then the periosteum of the neck of the condyle is stripped off with a periosteal elevator. The condylar retractor is now inserted from the posterior border going medially to protect the vital structures (Fig. 33.16). The hole is drilled through the outer cortex till the inner cortex. The 26 gauge double wire is passed through the hole and grasped with the hemostat from the medial aspect. The mandibular fragment is located next, since the fragment is under the condyle (if submandibular or postramal approach is taken, then small hole is made at the angle at the inferior border of the mandible, through which double wire is passed and grasped with a hemostat. This wire is pulled downward, so that there is better access for grasping the condylar fragment as well as ramus). By using periosteal elevator and special condylar retractor, another hole is drilled in the ramal fragment. The wire, previously placed in the condylar fragment is now drawn through from the fracture surface by inserting a looped wire in the hole from the outer surface of the ramus. The fracture is then reduced under direct vision and temporary IMF is done intraorally by the assistant. After that the wire ends are twisted together and cut off and the ends are bent over close to the bone. In cases, where condyles are medially displaced, the procedure is reversed. First the mandibular fragment is located by manipulation and same procedure can be repeated as described. After fixation by the wires, the wound is closed in layers and dressing is given. At the end of the operation, temporary IMF should be removed to facilitate extubation and it should be replaced next day. Immobilization is kept for 15 to 20 days.

Minibone plating can also be done instead of intraosseous wiring (Figs 33.17 to 33.20). Here, the fracture should be reduced as described and then the small four hole or two hole bone plate should be adapted

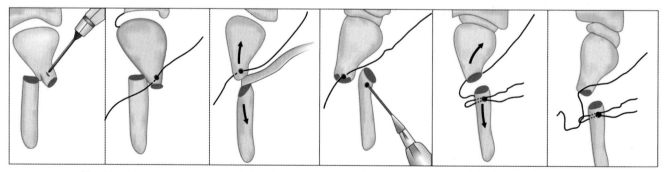

Fig. 33.16: Diagrammatic representation of reduction and fixation with intraosseous wiring for condylar fracture

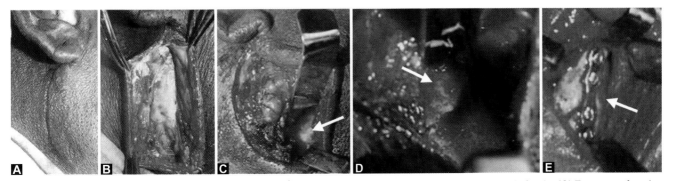

Figs 33.17A to E: Bone plating: (A) Postramal or retromandibular incision, (B) Exposure of parotidomasseteric fascia, (C) Exposure of angle of mandible, (C) Laterally displaced fractured fragment, (E) Reduction and fixation with bone plate

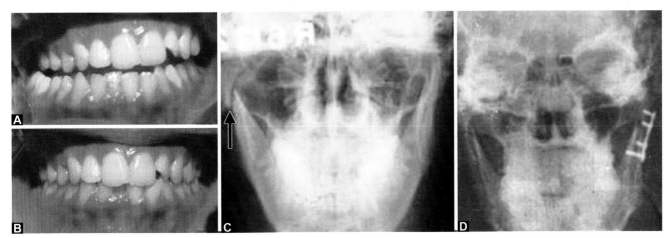

Figs 33.18A to D: A 15-year-old female with history of hit by an autorickshaw: (A) Deranged occlusion with restricted oral opening, deviation of chin towards right side, (B) Postoperative occlusion, (C) X-ray showing unilateral fracture of condylar process, (D) Postoperative X-ray

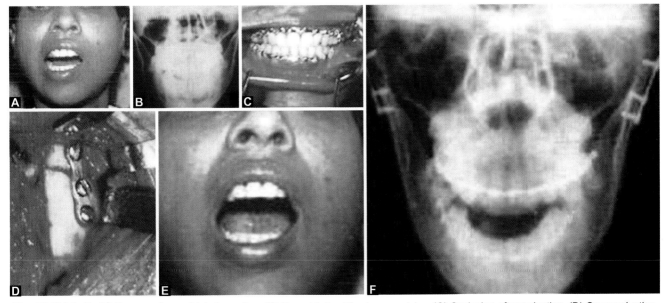

Figs 33.19A to F: (A) Preoperative restricted opening, (B) X-ray-bilateral fracture condyles, (C) Occlusion after reduction, (D) Open reduction, fixation, (E) Postoperative oral opening, (F) Postoperative X-ray

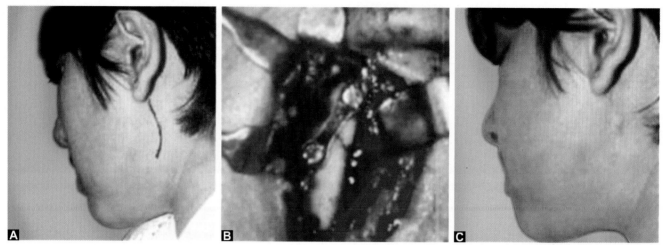

Figs 33.20A to C: (A) Marking for postramal incision, (B) Bone plating for L condylar fracture, (C) Postoperative scar

to the external cortex and fixed with monocortical self-tapping screws. If the high condylar fractured fragment is displaced too anteromedially, then it should be located by depressing the ramal fragment and catching it with the hemostat. Then if it can be fixed back as a free graft to the ramal stump, the attempt should be done (Figs 33.21 and 33.22). But many times condylectomy is recommended, because replantation is not possible.

Malunion (Dysarthrosis or Meta-arthrosis) and Pseudoarthrosis

Dysarthrosis: Here morphological change is seen in unreduced fracture dislocation producing nonarticulating deformed condyle. The malunion results in disturbance in anatomy as well as in function. Patient will

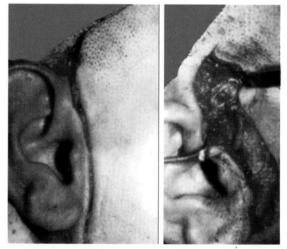

Fig. 33.21: Preauricular incision for exposure of high condylar fracture

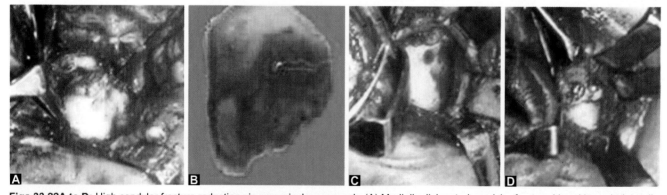

Figs 33.22A to D: High condylar fracture reduction via preauricular approach. (A) Medially dislocated condylar fractured head brought laterally; (B) Condylar head removed in toto, and used as a free graft for replantation, as normal fixation was not possible, (C) Ramal stump is prepared for fixation of condylar head, (D) Replanted head fixed in position with screws

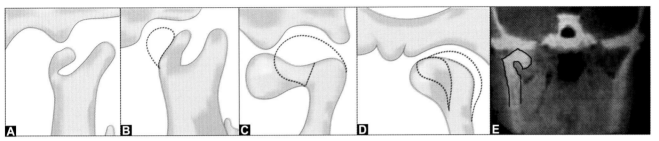

Figs 33.23A to E: Dysarthrosis: (A to D) Diagram of the formation of dysarthrosis, (E) Coronal CT scan showing dysarthrosis of the right TMJ after malunion of medially displaced condylar fragment

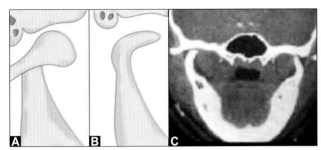

Figs 33.24A to C: Meta-arthrosis of TMJ after malunion of fractured condyle: (A and B) Diagram, (C) CT scan meta-arthrosis of both the temporomandibular joints

have pain and limitation of movements of lower jaw (Figs 33.23A to E).

Meta-arthrosis: It is result of healed fracture in malposition, but it produces no symptoms. These are the type of joints with altered anatomy, but functionally acceptable (anatomically altered, transformed, modified joints) (Figs 33.24A to C).

Pseudoarthrosis: False joint, very painful during normal excursions. Condylectomy may be required.

Preprosthetic Surgery

34　Preprosthetic Surgery

Since the end of World War II, through the development of better materials, the improved accuracy of processing techniques and a better understanding of oral physiology, dental prosthetics has made great strides in increasing the successful use of prosthetic appliances in edentulous patients.

ORAL AND MAXILLOFACIAL PROSTHETICS

By definition oral *prosthetics* is the replacement of missing teeth (lost or congenitally absent) and contiguous oral and maxillofacial tissues, with artificial substitute. The principles of form and function combine to guide the clinical application of prosthodontics towards the most natural cosmetic and functional result.

Nonetheless, there remains a significant number of patients, who can never be made to use dentures effectively, because of bone atrophy, soft tissue hypertrophy or localized soft and hard tissue problems or all of them, which have progressed beyond the point of prosthetic accommodation. It is in these patients, that preprosthetic surgery offers a significant contribution. Many times in the oral cavity pre-existing structures like frenal attachments, exostosis, tori have no significance and there presence do not interference with masticatory

function, when the teeth are present. But, these very nonsignificant structures definitely cause hinderance for denture stability and resultant reduced masticatory function after tooth loss.

Objective of the Preprosthetic Surgery

Objective of the preprosthetic surgery is that to provide a better anatomic environment and to create proper supporting structures for denture construction. Ultimate goal should be rehabilitation of the patient with restoration of the best possible masticatory function, combined with restoration or improvement of dental and facial esthetics. To achieve this goal, maximum preservation of hard and soft tissues of the denture base, is of utmost importance.

Preprosthetic surgery is carried out to reform/redesign soft/hard tissues, by eliminating biological hinderances to receive comfortable and stable prosthesis. (Reform/ redesign denture bearing area to create an oral environment to support a functional prosthetic appliance).

Denture Base Areas of Concern

Maxilla: Maxillary alveolar ridge, labial and buccal vestibular area, palatal vault. Frenal, muscle attachments, tuberosity area, level of floor of the maxillary sinus, nasal floor.

Mandible: Mandibular alveolar ridge, labial, buccal and lingual vestibules, retromolar area, mylohyoid ridge, frenal, muscle attachments, level of genial tubercles, level of mental nerve.

Pathophysiology of Edentulous Bone Loss

Complete denture retention and stability is dependent on the well adapted fit, hydrostatic pressure and physical features of the alveolar process such as contour and height. Over the years, the progressive bone loss, which is seen in the individuals, can negatively impact prosthetic stability, retention and serviceability.

Causes of Bone Loss

- Physiologic
- Environmental
- Pathologic or
- Combination of above causes.

Metabolic factors: Bone loss due to metabolic factors are detailed in Table 34.1.

Aging: Continuous pneumatization of the maxillary sinus, as the age of the patient progresses, in the posterior maxilla. Continuous resorption of the alveolar ridges, after teeth extractions over the years.

Trauma: Bone loss secondary to trauma (during extraction or otherwise) affects the dentoalveolar process and overlying tissue.

Periodontal disease: Generalized bone loss is seen due to extensive periodontal problems. The bone loss will show irregular pattern. Routinely, the alveolar process will show loss in the vertical fashion than the width (width is maintained by the presence of the roots of the teeth).

Combination problems: In case of upper full denture with natural lower dentition, the pressure resorption is seen in the upper alveolar ridge, because of the pressure exerted by the natural dentition. The bone loss is vertical, as well as horizontal especially seen in the anterior maxilla.

Disuse atrophy: It can cause alveolar bone loss. But, it is of less importance, when compared with the bone loss in denture wearers.

Long term denture usage: It is a known fact, that tension forces result in bone opposition and compressive forces result in bone resorption. These forces interact with the edentulous jaw, until a balance is met.

Rate of resorption of residual alveolar ridges depends on:

i. The size, shape, density of the alveolar ridge
ii. The cellular activity of the osteoblasts and osteoclasts
iii. The duration, frequency and direction of any previous occlusal forces to the bone.
iv. Forces generated from the present appliance
v. The patient's resistance to these forces.

Forces applied to the denture bearing areas by the denture are compressive in nature. This results in resorption of the alveolar ridges. Ill-fitting dentures offer excessive compressive forces.

Patterns of Bone Loss

1. Tallgren in 1972, has stated that most of the bone loss occurs in the first year of denture wearing and it is ten times greater, than the loss seen in the following years (probably a period of gaining equilibrium between oppositional and destructive forces).
2. He also demonstrated four times more bone loss in the mandible, than in the maxilla over the years (maxilla distributes the compressive forces over a wider surface area).
3. The direction of resorption in the maxilla differs from the mandibular bone resorption.
4. The usual resorption of the maxilla is on the buccal and inferior portion of the alveolar ridge.

Table 34.1: Metabolic factors of bone loss	
Osteoporosis	*Osteomalacia*
Loss of bone mass, where there is thinning of cortex, with volume loss of cancellous bone	Loss of bone volume
Ratio of organic matrix to mineral matrix is normal	Increase in the ratio of unmineralized organic matrix (osteoid) to mineralized matrix
Due to senile osteoporosis, postmenopausal osteoporosis, hyperparathyroidism, Cushing's syndrome	Due to vitamin D deficiency, renal osteodystrophy, secondary hyperparathyroidism, malnutrition

The pattern of edentulous bone loss (EBL) results in upward and inward loss of structures. In the anterior maxilla, there is less horizontal bone loss and posterior drift of the anterior crest is seen more than in the edentulous mandible. In the posterior maxilla, there is inward drift of the posterior crest. The width of the maxilla is reduced.

5. Because of the progressive resorption over the years, the depth of the palatal vault decreases, and a very thin bone may be present between the floor of the maxillary sinus and the nasal cavity.

6. The mandible resorbs downwards and outwards, causing rapid flattening of the ridge.

7. Tallgren has estimated that the edentulous bone loss (EBL) is upto 1 mm per year, with the greatest loss occurring within 12 to 18 months after extractions.

8. Extractions of teeth done at different times with long-time gaps will exhibit irregular bony ridge pattern.

9. Skeletal morphology has got definite role on the resorption pattern of the edentulous maxilla. People with long faces have more alveolar height than those with short faces. Short face patients have greater biting force, therefore are predisposed to greater bone loss. Pre-existing skeletal deformity will also lead to disturbance in the relationship of the bony ridges.

Mercier in 1995 has described a resorptive pattern of the edentulous ridge (Table 34.2).

Characteristics of Ideal Denture Base Area

The ideal edentulous ridges both maxillary and mandibular should exhibit following features:

Table 34.2: Resorptive pattern of the edentulous ridge (Mercier, 1995)	
1. The ridge is wide enough at its crest to accommodate the recently extracted teeth	Type I—minor ridge modeling
2. The ridge becomes thin and pointed	Type II—sharp atrophic residual ridge
3. The pointed ridge flattens to the level of the basal bone	Type III—basal bone ridge
4. The flattened ridge becomes concave as the basal bone resorbs	Type IV—basal bone resorption

1. Adequate bone support—broad U-shaped alveolar ridge with buccal and lingual/palatal cortices as parallel to each other as possible.

2. Adequate firm soft tissue coverage—the ridge must have adequate coverage of keratinized firm mucosa with uniform thickness. The presence of supple firm tissue, without any irregularities is necessary for maximum peripheral seal.

3. No bony or soft tissue undercuts or prominences.

4. No sharp ridges.

5. No presence of peripheral fibrous tissue bands (scars) to prevent proper seating of a denture.

6. No high muscle or frenal attachments at the crest of the ridge to dislodge the denture.

7. No soft tissue redundancies or hypertrophies on the ridges or in the sulci.

8. No intraoral or extraoral pathology.

9. Proper alveolar ridges relationship in all three planes.

Aims of Preprosthetic Surgery

1. Provide adequate bony tissue support for the placement of RPD/CD—removable partial denture or complete denture (optimum ridge, height and width and contour)

2. Provide adequate soft tissue support. Optimum vestibular depth.

3. Elimination of pre-existing bony deformities, e.g. tori, prominent mylohyoid ridge, genial tubercle.

4. Correction of maxillary and mandibular ridge relationship.

5. Elimination of pre-existing soft tissue deformities, e.g. epulis, flabby ridges, hyperplastic tissues.

6. Relocation of frenal/muscle attachments.

7. Relocation of mental nerve.

8. Establishment of correct vestibular depth.

Treatment Planning and Examination

Preprosthetic surgery is an integral part of the oral and maxillofacial surgery. It comprises of both, basic procedures and the sophisticated techniques of reconstructions and rehabilitation of the oral and maxillofacial region. During treatment planning, there should be co-ordination between the prosthodontist and the oral and maxillofacial surgeon. As the goal of the prosthetic appliance construction is to improve function and esthetics, the requirements to achieve these goals should be discussed by the team members.

The treatment planning will include a thorough medical, surgical and dental history of the patient and medical and dental clinical examination of the patient. This should be supplemented with radiological examination, plus study of the dental casts, whenever indicated. As most of these patients needing preprosthetic surgeries, are in the elderly age group, a thorough medical history should be recorded. Earlier surgical, medical, hospitalization history should be evaluated. Quick assessment of the patient's physical evaluation including vital signs, general functional capacity and psychological status is very important for the treatment planning and its successful outcome. If the patient is on certain long term medications, then their side effects are known to interfere with the surgical plan. Modification/withdrawal (temporary) of these medications may be required prior to planned surgical procedures. Many drugs known to cause xerostomia—caries problems and periodontal problems in partially edentulous patients and may cause burning sensation in the mouth after wearing the full dentures due to loss of salivary lubrication.

Patient's psychological make up is also equally important to receive the prosthetic appliance and to maintain it. Expectations of the patient, willingness and acceptance of the patient to wear the full denture should be known to the clinician. The unwilling, noncooperative patient can be problematic to handle at times. Patient's co-operation, will power and motivation is absolutely mandatory for the success of the treatment.

For the prosthetic appliance, whether it is in the form of partial denture, crown and bridge or full denture or implant based prosthesis, patient's attitude for maintaining oral hygiene should be taken into account. If the patient is unaware, but willing to learn the basic protocols of oral hygiene maintenance, then it will be helpful for treatment planning for type of prosthetic appliance to be offered to the patient. It is also important to know the patient's parafunctional and food/eating habits.

A good clinical examination will include careful assessment of both soft and hard tissues and should include a good facial esthetic examination and radiological examination.

Facial Esthetic Examination

i. Presence of unsupported upper lip
ii. Poor vermilion show

iii. Loss of nasolabial fold or decreased nasolabial fold
iv. Poor/obtuse nasolabial angle with poor projection
v. Excessive lower lip show.

The extent or degree of the above features should be noted.

Intraoral Examination

Examination of the alveolar ridges, both maxillary and mandibular should be carried out along with the soft tissue examination of the entire oral cavity including posterior pharynx. Inspection and palpation should be carried out.

1. Ridge form should be inspected for the amount and contour of the bone.
2. Quality and quantity of the overlying soft tissues of the denture bearing areas to be ascertained (vestibular depth and area).
3. Location of frenal/muscle attachments in relation to the alveolar crest should be noted.
4. Presence or absence of soft tissue and bony pathology should be looked for.
5. Relationship of the maxillary alveolar arch to the mandibular alveolar arch in all three planes.

Systemic evaluation of the alveolar ridge and supporting tissue should be done.

i. Ridge form and contour.
   • Height and width of the ridge.
   • Quality of the ridge—whether flabby, mobile tissue is present over the ridge.
ii. Presence of any gross irregularities in the ridge.
iii. Presence of any exostosis, undercuts, prominences, tori, sharp mylohyoid ridge with severe resorption of external oblique ridge.
iv. Buccal and labial, as well as lingual vestibules evaluation for depth and type of soft tissue.
v. Examination of palatal vault.
vi. Tuberosity area—undercuts, hyperplastic tissue, flabby ridge, etc. Height, width, fibrous or excess bony tuberosity can impair the arch space for fabrication of full or partial denture.
vii. Interarch relationship.
viii. Adequate post tuberosity notching.

Supporting Soft Tissue Examination

1. The amount of keratinized tissue firmly attached to the underlying bone as well as unsupported by the bone should be distinguished from poorly keratinized or freely movable tissue.

2. Inflammatory areas, scars, ulcers, hyperplastic tissues due to ill-fitting dentures should be looked for.
3. Frenal attachments in relation to the alveolar crest—high maxillary labial frenal attachment will need excessive notching in the upper denture to prevent dislodgement. It can be esthetically unpleasing especially in the patients with high smile line. High mandibular lingual frena may affect the design and placement of removable partial denture.
4. Both buccal and lingual vestibular depth should be checked.
5. On the lingual aspect, mylohyoid muscle attachment and genioglossus muscle attachment should be checked.
6. Tongue size and movement is also important for the stability of the denture. Hence needs evaluation.

Radiological evaluation: Radiological assessment should include orthopantograph or panoramic and lateral cephalometric radiographs. In difficult cases, advanced imaging techniques such as computed tomography—dental CT scan can be used. 3D CT scan be used, if cost permits. The radiographs should be studied to detect any presence of bony pathological lesions, presence of impacted teeth, cysts, tumors, root pieces, etc. Bony trabecular pattern, distance of the neurovascular bundle from the alveolar crest, level of mental foramen, the size and pneumatization of the maxillary sinus can be also scrutinized from the X-rays.

Diagnostic models: It should be mounted on an articulator with proper vertical dimension and studied.

PREPROSTHETIC SURGICAL PROCEDURES

Preprosthetic surgical procedures can be classified as (i) *basic procedures* and (ii) *advanced surgery procedures.*

The basic procedures can be carried out under LA on a day-care basis, while advanced procedures will require hospitalization and general anesthesia.

Table 34.3: Bony and soft tissue surgeries	
Bony surgeries	*Soft tissue surgeries*
i. Labial alveolectomy	i. Removal of redundant crestal soft tissue
ii. Primary alveoloplasty	
iii. Secondary alveoloplasty	ii. Frenectomy—labial and lingual
iv. Excision of Tori	
v. Reduction of genial tubercle	iii. Excision of epulis fissurata and palatal papillary hyperplasia
vi. Reduction of mylohyoid ridge	
vii. Maxillary tuberosity reduction and exostosis removal	

The procedures can be carried out for the following:
1. Alveolar ridge correction
2. Alveolar ridge extension
3. Alveolar ridge augmentation.

ALVEOLAR RIDGE CORRECTION (TABLE 34.3)

a. Bony surgeries
b. Soft tissue surgeries

Alveolectomy (Labial) (Figs 34.1A to E)

Surgical removal or trimming of the alveolar process is termed as alveolectomy. Clinically, after extraction, whenever there is a presence of sharp margins at interdental, interseptal or labiobuccal alveolar crest, they should be trimmed with rongeur or round bur and smoothened with bone file. The trimming of the alveolar process should be carried out judiciously. Care is taken that only minimum amount of areas should be trimmed. Too much bone loss will result into poor denture base.

Alveoloplasty (Fig. 34.2)

Alveoloplasty refers to surgical recontouring of the alveolar process. This contouring is done with the purpose to take care of bony projections, sharp crestal

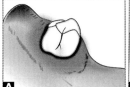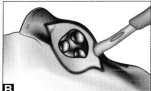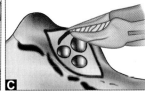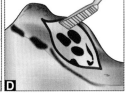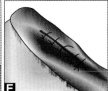

Figs 34.1A to E: Single tooth alveolectomy and alveoloplasty

bone or undercuts. Primary alveoloplasty is always done at the time of multiple extraction or single extraction. Conservation is the key factor in this procedure. Before construction of the prosthetic appliance, maximum efforts should be made to preserve as much of the alveolus as possible. Minimum amount of alveolar bone resorption occurs, if after simple extraction, digital compression of the alveolar cortices is done immediately. This procedure is referred as simple alveoloplasty.

The aim of alveoloplasty is to recontour the alveolar ridge for providing best possible tissue contour for denture support by maintaining as much bone and soft tissue as possible.

Simple Conservative Alveoloplasty with Multiple Extractions (Fig. 34.2)

i. If multiple adjacent teeth are to be extracted in a single sitting, the simple alveoloplasty technique is advocated, if there are no other bony irregularities present. Immediately after extractions, the buccal and lingual plates should be compressed with firm digital pressure and the gingival tissue is repositioned and the entire ridge is palpated for locating sharp bony spicules or undercuts. These should be trimmed with rongeur and the edges smoothened with bone file. In case, if there is any excess redundant tissue is present, then it should

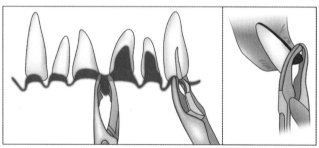

Fig. 34.2: Simple alveoloplasty after multiple extractions

be trimmed with surgical scissors and interrupted suturing should be done.

ii. Elevation of a mucoperiosteal flap and buccal cortex reduction can be done for removal of undercuts with rongeurs or a rotary bur.

Intraseptal Alveoloplasty—Dean's Alveoloplasty with Repositioning of Labial Cortical Bone (Figs 34.3A to D)

- Used in maxilla only (mainly in the anterior region).
- Technique is usually used to reduce gross maxillary overjet.
- To reduce the volume of cancellous bone, maintaining stress bearing cortical bone intact.
- Does not require raising a mucoperiosteal flap.
- Carried out immediately following extractions of anterior teeth.
- Maintenance of periosteal attachment to the labial plate of bone (decreases postoperative bone resorption and helps remodeling).
- It has got ability to reduce a buccal undercut or labial prominence without significantly reducing the height of the alveolar ridge.
- Overall less alveolar bone resorption than with the use of buccal reduction technique. Best long term results.
- Indicated in cases, where adequate bone height exists, but an undercut is present on the buccal aspect of the maxillary ridge.
- Carried out at the time of multiple teeth extractions or early initial postextraction period.
- Two steps—(i) removal of intraseptal bone followed by (ii) repositioning of the labial cortical bone.
- Immediate denture can be planned.

Technique

- Teeth should be extracted without much trauma (atraumatic extractions) to the labial cortex.

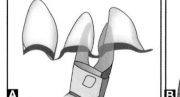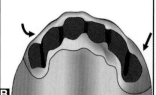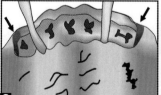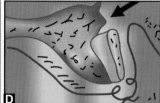

Figs 34.3A to D: Dean's alveoloplasty procedure: (A) Reduction of interdental septal bone, (B) All the septa from canine to canine are reduced, (C) Vertical cuts made at the distal end of the canine sockets, (D) Compression of the fractured buccal plate and suturing

- With straight fissure bur attached to the surgical handpiece or with rongeur, interdental septal bone is cut from canine to canine region.
- With the same bur, vertical cuts are made only in the labial cortex at distal end of the canine extraction sockets bilaterally, without perforation of labial mucosa in the Dean's technique.
- With periosteal elevator/osteotome placed into the base of canine sockets bilaterally, labial cortex is fractured (greenstick fracture attached to labial mucosa).
- Digital pressure is used to compress the fractured labial cortex into the palatal direction.
- Labial plate and palatal plate will come into approximation with each other.
- Any sharp margins at the newly created alveolar crest are filed with bone file.
- Interrupted or continuous suturing is carried out.

Obwegeser's Modification for Intraseptal Alveoloplasty

Repositioning of both labial and palatal cortices (Figs 34.4A to D): It is used when the maxillary overjet is gross and inward compression of only labial cortex is not sufficient to reduce the overjet.
- After cutting the intraseptal bone, an inverted cone vulcanite bur is used to widen the socket at the base
- With small disc or bur, horizontal cuts are made at the base of the extraction sockets in the labial and palatal cortices
- With a straight fissure bur, vertical cuts are then made bilaterally in both labial and palatal cortices in the area distal to canine sockets
- With digital pressure, both labial and palatal cortices are compressed together and sutures given.

If immediate denture delivery is planned, then the denture can be made in clear acrylic, so that it can be used as a template to check for any pressure points. The areas showing blanching should be judiciously trimmed, before suturing. Final fit of the immediate denture should be checked, so that rocking of the denture is not present.

Alveoloplasty after the Postextraction Healing

Many times, multiple extractions are carried out at different times, which results in the irregular ridge. The ridge may be knife edged or multiple areas will show sharp bony spicules, which are very painful to touch. Here, crestal incision is taken and mucoperiosteal flap is reflected judiciously. Care is taken not to tear the flap, as at the sharp points, the separation becomes difficult. The side ways separation with periosteal elevator will help the smooth reflection. Sometimes releasing incisions may be needed. The sharp areas or large undercuts should be trimmed with rongeur or round bur and suturing done.

Elimination of Unfavorable Undercuts

Due to severe atrophy of the mandible (type 3 or type 4) unfavorable prominences may hinder with the proper denture construction. These undercuts are usually seen in the mandibular lingual aspect—genial tubercle prominence, sharp mylohyoid ridge prominence can be noted. Most of the times, the patient will be wearing old dentures and due to resorption over the years, the dentures become unstable and patient may come with the complaint of severe pain on the lingual aspect, at the mylohyoid ridge. Sometimes, ulceration or inflammation at this region is also seen. Patient is asked to discontinue the use of the dentures and surgery should be planned to relieve these undercuts.

Reduction/Resection of the Genial Tubercles

The genial tubercles, the bony attachments of the genioglossus muscle can become an area of interference, due to gross resorption of the mandibular ridge. The level of the genial tubercles in these cases is seen almost at the crestal level on the lingual aspect. A shelf like projection is seen, which will dislodge the lower

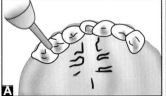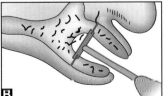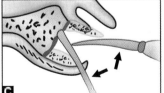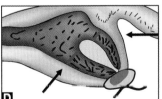

Figs 34.4A to D: Obwegeser's modification for intraseptal alveoloplasty: Repositioning of both labial and palatal cortices

denture with slightest amount of tongue movements, as the peripheral seal on the lingual aspect is not present. Frequently ulceration is also seen over the tubercle area.

- A crestal incision is made from the lower canine to canine region, after infiltration of local anesthetic solution
- No reflection of the flap is done on the labial side
- A full thickness mucoperiosteal flap is reflected to expose the genial tubercle
- The muscle attachment is removed with sharp dissection
- Excision of the tubercle is done by rotary instrumentation or rongeurs
- Smoothening can be done with a bone file
- Copious irrigation of the area prior to suturing is needed.

Reduction of mylohyoid ridge (Figs 34.5A to C): Usually there will be concavity present, immediately below the alveolar crest with prominence of mylohyoid ridge below. This procedure can be performed by using LA pterygomandibular block technique.

- A crestal incision is taken in the posterior ridge region
- Oblique releasing incision is given at the distal end of the incision, going toward buccal cheek area to avoid damage to lingual nerve
- Mucoperiosteal flap reflected on the lingual side to expose the medial surface of the mandible at the mylohyoid ridge region
- The tissue from the floor of the mouth and lingual mucoperiosteum is protected by inserting flat blade of the tongue depressor in between the flap and the bone
- By using osteotome or round bur, the reduction of the mylohyoid ridge is carried out, after dissecting mylohyoid muscle fibers away
- Bone is smoothened with bone file

- Soft tissue flap is returned back and the complete lingual vestibule checked with digital pressure for any sharp areas
- After complete smoothening, the sutures are given.

Excision of Tori

Torus is exostosis/overgrowth of cortical/corticocancellous bone, which is localized to particular area, usually benign and asymptomatic and slow growing. Origin is unknown.

In maxilla: Usually seen in midline of the palate. Incidence—20 percent in females, 10 percent in male patients. Multiple shapes and configurations can be seen. It will vary from single smooth elevation to multiloculated pedunculated bony masses.

In mandible: Found in 8 percent of population, with same incidence in male and females. Usually bilateral tori in the premolar region on the lingual aspect are seen. May be single or multiple or multilobulated. When the teeth are present, tori are of no consequence and usually there are no speech problems associated with them. But after extraction, the upper denture construction or lower partial/full denture construction is not possible, unless tori are excised.

Indications for Reduction/Removal/Excision of Tori

1. An extremely large torus, filling the palatal vault.
2. A large torus, that may extend beyond the post-dam area.
3. Ulceration/traumatization/hyperkeratinization of the overlying mucosa.
4. Deep bony undercuts.
5. Interference with the function—speech-deglutition.
6. Psychological consideration—malignancy/cancer phobia.
7. Food lodgement under the folds and projection of the tori.

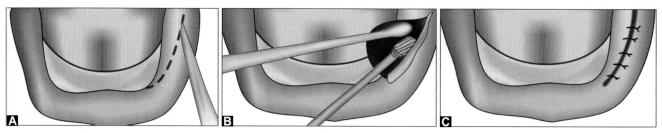

Figs 34.5A to C: Reduction of mylohyoid ridge

Technique for Excision of Palatal Torus
(Figs 34.6 and 34.7)

- LA—bilateral greater palatine and incisive nerve block.
- Anteroposterior linear incision is made in the midline of the palate.
- Y-shaped releasing incisions at one or both the ends of incision.

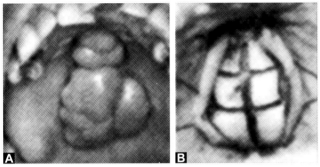

Figs 34.6A and B: (A) Clinical intraoral picture of palatal torus, (B) Reflection of mucoperiosteal flap and retraction sutures and sectioning is seen in this intraoperative picture

- Thin lobulated mucosa should be carefully handled
- Two mucoperiosteal flaps raised with periosteal elevator, from the midline, sideways.
- Retraction sutures can be placed on both the flaps to maximize the exposure.
- The torus should never be excised en mass, because of the proximity to the nasal floor (perforation into the nose—oronasal communication).
- Division of the torus into multiple segments should be done with the bur (vertical and horizontal multiple cuts).
- The small pieces removed with the chisel and mallet.
- Large round bur is used judiciously to final finish.
- Excess soft tissue should be trimmed.
- Continuous 'over and under' type suturing using fine absorbable suture material using atraumatic needle (no trauma to thin mucosa).
- Prefabricated acrylic stent/splint can be given or iodoform tie over pack can be used (to prevent hematoma).

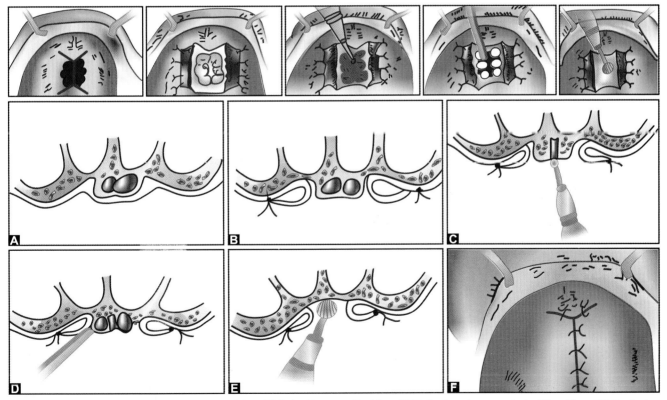

Figs 34.7A to F: Palatal torus and its surgical excision: (A) Palatal torus and incision, (B) Reflection of mucoperiosteal flap, (C and D) Sectioning of torus and removal of multiple small segments, (E) Complete removal of torus and smoothening of palatal vault, (F) Final suturing

Possible Complications

Intraoperative

- Bleeding-injury to greater palatine vessels.
- Fracture of the palatal shelf.
- Oronasal/oroantral perforation.

Postoperative

- Hematoma formation.
- Sloughing/necrosis of the palatal mucosa.
- Gaping/nonhealing wound.
- Oroantral/oronasal fistula.

Mandibular Torus Removal

- LA—pterygomandibular block with local infiltration.
- Incision over alveolar ridge in lower premolar region (edentulous).
- Lingual sulcus incision, without releasing incision in the dentulous patients (prevents damage to the lingual nerve).
- Mucoperiosteal flap is raised, only on the lingual aspect of the mandible, without perforation over the torus area.
- Make a purchase point/groove with the bur, on the medial aspect of the torus, parallel to the medial surface of the mandible from the base to the superior margin.
- Cleavage is taken with the osteotome placed in the purchase groove/trough.
- Gentle tapping to excise the entire torus.

- Smoothening with round bur/bone file.
- Irrigation and suturing.

Possible Complications

Intraoperative

- Injury to submandibular salivary gland duct.
- Excessive bleeding.
- Laceration of the mylohyoid muscle.
- Tearing of the flap.

Postoperative

- Life threatening hemorrhage in the floor of the mouth—infection—airway obstruction.

Maxillary Tuberosity Reduction and Exostosis Removal (Figs 34.8 and 34.9)

- Excess horizontal and vertical bony/soft tissue in the maxillary tuberosity region may interfere with denture construction.
- Excessive bony undercut/mobile or redundant soft tissue/hyperplastic fibrous tissue may be present (or both).
- The excess tissue protrudes into the intermaxillary space to a degree that, there is insufficient space for lower dentures.
  Radiographs are often necessary—OPG or intraoral periapical view:
- To determine the extent of the bone and soft tissue in the enlarged tuberosity region.
- To locate the level of the floor of the maxillary sinus.

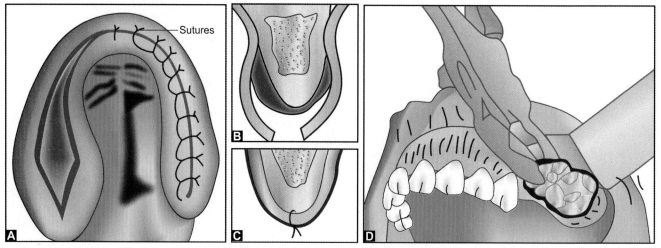

Figs 34.8A to D: Maxillary tuberosity reduction. (A) Incision for tuberosity deformity correction and final suturing (B) Bony reduction and contouring, (C) Suturing, (D) Elimination of buccal exostosis in posterior maxillary area

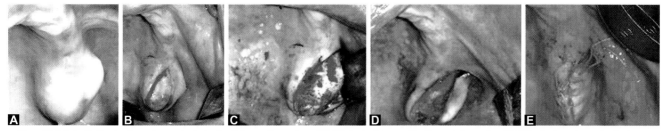

Figs 34.9A to E: Reduction of exostosis in the tuberosity region. (A) Clinical picture of bulbous tuberosity, (B) Elliptical wedge of soft tissue excised, (C) Exostosis exposed, (D) Bony exostosis reduced and contoured, (E) Final suturing

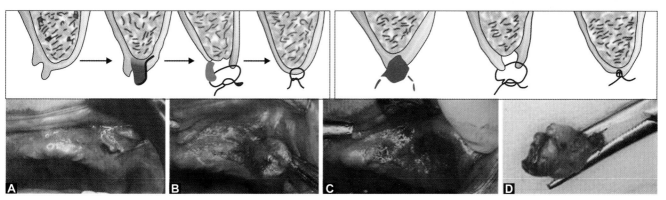

Figs 34.10A to D: Surgical removal of redundant crestal soft tissue

Aims

- To remove the bony/soft tissue irregularities
- To create adequate interarch space for the proper construction of the prosthetic appliance in the posterior area.

Technique

- LA—infiltration or posterior superior alveolar and greater palatine blocks.
- A crestal elliptical incisions from tuberosity to premolar area.
- The mucoperiosteum is undermined and the section of the tissue between the elliptical incisions is removed.
- If the excess soft tissue is fibrous, hyperplastic, then the medial margins of the incisions on both the sides are thinned out tangentially to remove the wedge of excess fibrous tissue till the bony crest.
- If the excess tissue is primarily bone, then rest of the mucoperiosteum is reflected till the vestibular depth.
- Excess bone/buccal exostosis is then removed from the crest of the ridge and from the buccal plate (if excessive undercut exists). This can be accomplished with chisel, mallet or burs.

- After the desired contour is achieved, the excess soft tissue is trimmed along the incision edges to correct the redundancy.
- The flap is sutured and a stent is placed.
- In case of sinus perforation, a collagen matrix can be placed prior to suturing.

Soft Tissue Surgeries for the Correction of Alveolar Ridge

Removal of redundant crestal soft tissue (Figs 34.10A to D): Presence of fibrous, hyperplastic tissue often gives rise to flabby, wobbly ridge form. Dense, fibromatous or the softer and redundant type of tissue results in an unstable base for dentures.
- In maxilla—enlarged tuberosity.
- In mandible—enlarged retromolar pad.

Denture granuloma or hyperplasia: It is seen in the palatal region or at the vestibular depth, obliterating the sulcus or sometimes on lingual aspect of the lower dentures. The tissue is inflamed, fibrous and hyperplastic.

Irrespective of the site, to reduce these hyperplastic tissue, elliptical incisions are taken on either side of the tissue and later on submucosal resection of the excess tissue is carried out, by doing tangential excision or

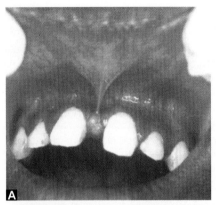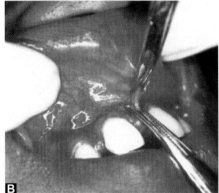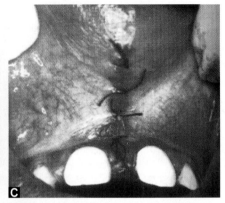

Figs 34.11A to C: Labial frenectomy and suturing procedure

two parallel incisions are taken on the buccal and lingual aspect of the tissues for excision. The patient is instructed to stop using the ill-fitting dentures.

Excision of epulis fissurata: These are the benign, pedunculated lesions present as excessive or redundant tissue of the vestibule, frequently associated with over extension of the denture border or ill-fitting dentures. Sharp excision, electrocauterization, cryosurgery or laser excision can be done.

Palatal papillary hyperplasia: It is due to chronic denture irritation, under an ill-fitting dentures. There can be superimposed *Candida* infection. Denture should be relieved in this area and antifungal agents can be prescribed prior to excision of the lesion. Supraperiosteal excision with a electrocautery can be done.

Frenectomy

Frenal attachment is a thin band of fibrous tissue and a few muscle fibers covered by mucous membrane. Maxillary midline frenum is most commonly seen, lingual frenum is also found in some of the patients. Maxillary and mandibular frena are also found in premolar-molar areas.

Indications: High attachments of labial frena or fibrous bands attached near the alveolar crest in the buccal regions, often displace the dentures during function. Many times ulceration can be seen at the frenal attachments due to impingement of the denture peripheries. One option is to relieve the denture borders at these frenal attachments. But for persistent problem, frenectomy should be considered.

Maxillary midline frenum or labial frenum (Figs 34.11A to C): It usually extends from the upper lip to the crest of the alveolar ridge and it can at times extend toward palate to the incisive papilla. Whenever there is lot of tissue is available, then a cross-diamond excision is used. The base of the frenum at the alveolar crest is grasped with hemostat and incision is taken below and above the hemostat. The surgical defect is created by excision of fibrous band. The closure can be done by interrupted sutures. The small defect at the alveolar crest can be left to granulate.

The Z plasty procedure can be used, when the frenum is broad and the vestibule is short. These type of procedures can be used for eliminating the frenum, as well as for deepening the vestibule (some amount of vertical lengthening can be obtained). It also lessens the tension of the scar band.

V-Y type of incision can be used for lengthening localized area. Broad frena in premolar-molar area can be treated by taking semilunar incision at the mucogingival junction and a supraperiosteal dissection is done. The superior edge of the incision is sutured at the depth of the vestibule to the periosteum and the rest of the raw area below is allowed to heal by secondary epithelialization. Use of prefabricated stent is necessary.

Lingual Frenectomy (Figs 34.12 and 34.13)

Lingual frenum is attached to the crest of the alveolar ridge and it connects to the tongue, below the tip of the tongue in edentulous patient. In dentulous patient, it is attached to the lingual gingiva, behind the mandibular incisors. This condition is also known as tongue tie or ankyloglossia.

Aim of Surgery

- To correct speech
- Prior to denture construction
- To improve the tongue mobility

Technique

- LA—bilateral lingual nerve block with local infiltration.
- Tongue traction suture is taken to improve visibility and control and stabilization of the tongue during procedure.
- One hemostat can be placed at the anterior attachment of the frenum to the tongue and another hemostat be placed at the inferior attachment to the ridge.

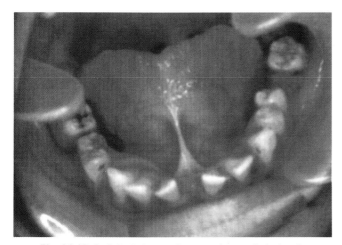

Fig. 34.12: A clinical picture of tongue tie or ankyloglossia

- A cross-diamond incision along the edge of both the hemostats is made.
- Submucosal dissection on either sides to undermine lingual and sublingual mucosa is carried out.
- Dissection of genioglossus muscle fibers is done, if necessary.
- Care is taken to avoid damage to the submandibular duct orifice.
- Suturing done in vertical manner.

Intraoperative Possible Complications

- Injury to superior lingual vessels
- Injury to Wharton's duct/papilla.

Postoperative Complications

- Hematoma in the floor of the mouth
- Pain, restricted tongue movements
- Partial dysphasia.

RIDGE EXTENSION PROCEDURE

Whenever there is an inadequate vestibular depth present, (due to mandibular atrophy and high muscle and soft tissue attachments) to increase the retention and stability of the denture, deepening of the vestibule is considered. To utilize this treatment option, sufficient amount of height of the alveolar bone should be available. In extreme atrophy cases, where resorption of the basal bone has taken place, this option is out of consideration.

Deepening of the vestibule without any addition of the bone is termed as *vestibuloplasty or sulcoplasty or*

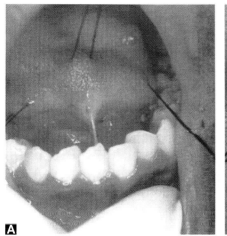
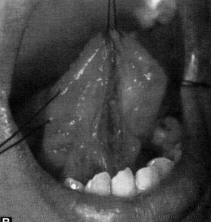
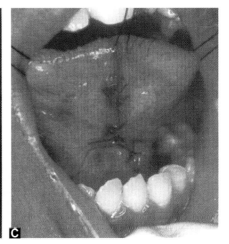

Figs 34.13A to C: Intraoperative pictures of surgical release of lingual frenum

sulcus deepening procedure. Vestibuloplasty can be done in the maxilla or in the mandible or in both the jaws.

Mandibular techniques are further divided into two categories:

1. Those done on the labial side
2. Those done on the lingual side.

Labial Vestibular Procedures

The procedure will be known as transpositional flap vestibuloplasty or lip switch procedure, when the soft tissues from the inner aspect of the lip is shifted to a favorable zone on the alveolar bone, so that the increase in the denture bearing area is achieved.

This method effectively increases the vestibular depth in the mandible, when the patient has a bone height of 15 mm or more in the anterior region. Implants or bone grafts should be considered in the patients having less than 15 mm of bone height in the anterior region. The mucosa must be healthy and exhibit no fibrosis, scarring or hyperplasia.

Kazanjian Technique (1924): Oldest Technique (Figs 34.14 and 34.15)

*   Uses mucosal flap from the inner aspect of the lower lip to increase the depth of the anterior mandibular labial vestibule.

*   Carried out in premolar to premolar region only.
*   Raw area is left on the lip side to heal by secondary intention.
*   Periosteum on the bone is left intact.

Drawback: Severe scarring of the lip mucosa, may decrease the flexibility of the lower lip (Poor long term results).

Procedure (Figs 34.16A to D): A submucosal dissection is done from the inner aspect of the lower lip to the muco-gingival junction, near the alveolar crest on the labial side. A supraperiosteal dissection is directed inferiorly to remove muscle and connective tissue attachments to the desired vestibular depth. The raised mucosal flap is adapted to the depth of the new vestibule and fixed with the sutures or a stent. The raw area on the lip is left alone.

Godwin's Modification (1947)

Mucosal incision on the inner aspect of the lip is designed longer than the proposed vestibular depth to be achieved. The mucosal flap is elevated and pedicled near the crest of the ridge. Near the superior portion of the periosteum attached on the bone, an incision is made and followed by the dissection inferiorly to the desired depth. The periosteum once again is incised at the depth of the previous dissection. The labial periosteal margin is sutured to the incised lip mucosa, then the

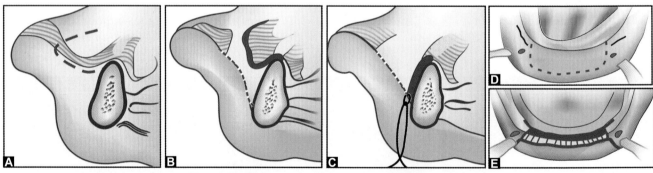

Figs 34.14A to E: Kazanjian labial vestibuloplasty procedure

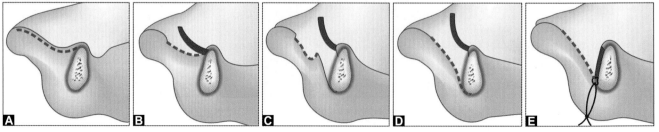

Figs 34.15A to E: Modified Kazanjian technique for mandibular vestibuloplasty

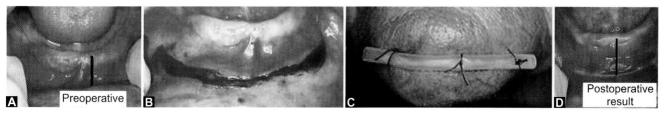

Figs 34.16A to D: Kazanjian vestibuloplasty surgical procedure

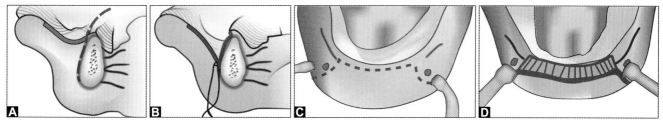

Figs 34.17A to D: Clark's vestibuloplasty procedure

pedicled flap is sutured to the periosteum at the depth of the vestibule. A stent can be used. Postoperatively, extraoral dressing can help the adaptation of the tissue intraorally.

Clark's Technique (Figs 34.17A to D)

- Supraperiosteal flap based on the inner aspect of the lip.
- Leaves raw surface on the bone, covering the inner lip surface, thereby reducing bleeding, postoperative pain and scarring.
- An incision is started slightly labial to the crest along the alveolar ridge.
- Mucosal flap based on the inner aspect of the lip is undermined, till vermilion border, to ensure adequate mobility and overcorrection.
- Supraperiosteal dissection is done, along the labial surface of the alveolar bone till the desired vestibular depth.
- Edge of the mobilized flap is pushed into the new vestibular depth area and held in position by sutures passed through the chin area extraorally and tied around cotton roll or rubber catheter placed below the chin.
- As the alveolar bone is covered by periosteal layer, it heals quickly by granulation.
- Success rate is better than Kazanjian method.

Obwegeser's Modification (1959)

Similar to Clark's method, except the area of the alveolar bone with its periosteal attachment is covered with a split thickness skin graft and held in position by sutures or stent constructed preoperatively. Instead of skin, mucosal graft has also been tried.
- Covers the bone and ensures faster healing
- Reduces chances of postoperative infection
- Less bone loss and scarring.

Lingual Vestibuloplasty

Floor of the mouth extension or floor of the mouth lowering the following:

Soft tissue attachments on the lingual aspect can interfere with prosthetic rehabilitation. Posteriorly the mylohyoid muscle and genioglossus muscle anteriorly, on the lingual surface of the mandible are the two problem areas.
- Technique provides an adequate denture bearing area.
- Eliminates the muscle attachments that dislodge the prosthesis.
- Used in the mandible, when the mylohyoid and genioglossus attachments are close to the alveolar ridge.

Floor of the mouth extension or floor of the mouth lowering can be done by following methods:

Trauner's Technique

- Used for increasing the depth of the floor of the mouth in the mylohyoid region.
- Incision given over lingual side of the alveolar ridge bilaterally, in the posterior region or from second molar to second molar region.
- Supraperiosteal dissection is done to identify mylohyoid muscle.
- Instrument is passed below mylohyoid muscle and muscle separated from the bony attachment.
- Care is taken to avoid lingual nerve damage.
- Fixation of incisal edge of the mylohyoid muscle to a new desired vestibular depth on lingual side by:
  - a. Sutures passed extraorally over the skin at the inferior border of the mandible
  - b. Placement of the skin graft and preformed denture/stent.

Caldwell's Technique

- Entire lingual mucoperiosteal flap is reflected from molar to molar region.
- Mylohyoid ridge is reduced/removed along with the reduction of genial tubercle.
- Mylohyoid muscle and superficial fibers of genioglossus muscles are pushed inferiorly.
- Rubber tubing placed in the lingual vestibule and the flap is held in position at the vestibular depth,

by sutures passed through the skin extraorally, at the inferior border of the mandible.

Obwegeser's Technique (Combination of Buccal and Lingual Vestibuloplasty) (Figs 34.18A to C)

- Incision is given on the alveolar ridge
- Mucosal flap raised buccally and lingually.
- Mylohyoid muscle attachment and only superficial fibers of genioglossus muscle are separated on the lingual side.
- Edges of buccal and lingual flaps attached/sutured to each other, below inferior border of the mandible
- Skin graft is placed over entire alveolar ridge.
- Preformed acrylic stent/denture placed and fixed to the mandible, with circummandibular wiring.

Submucosal Vestibuloplasty Technique (Figs 34.19A to D)

- Useful for maxillary and mandibular labial, buccal vestibules.
- Was first described by MacIntosh and Obwegeser (1967).
- Indicated, when the dentures are unstable, due to shallow vestibular depth and/or high muscle attachments, but with good underlying bone height and contour available.

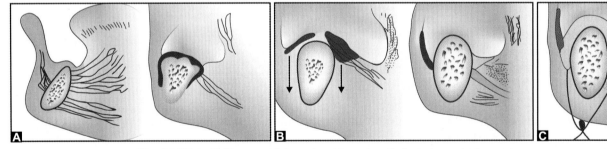

Figs 34.18A to C: Obwegeser's buccal and lingual vestibuloplasty surgical procedure

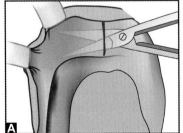
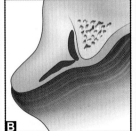
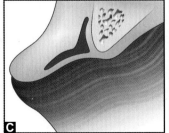
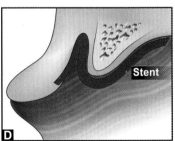

Figs 34.19A to D: Submucosal vestibuloplasty procedure

- The mouth mirror test is used to determine the adequacy of mucosa available.

A mouth mirror is placed in the vestibule and elevated against the bone to the desired vestibular depth. If mobile tissue is present and no abnormal shortening of the lip occurs, then adequate mucosa exists to perform the submucosal vestibuloplasty.

- A vertical midline incision is made in the labial vestibule.
- A supraperiosteal tunnel is made from (R) premolar to (L) premolar area.
- In maxilla, further separate incisions may be given in first molar region for further advancement.
- The intervening submucosal tissue is then excised or repositioned superiorly.
- The new depth is maintained by placement of preformed dentures/stents, which can be fixed to the mandible with circummandibular wiring and to the maxilla by per alveolar wiring.

Maxillary 'Pocket Inlay' Vestibuloplasty (Obwegeser)

The procedure involves surgically creating pockets in the maxillary buttress and the piriform aperture region and denture flange extensions into these pockets improve the total denture retention.

Preoperatively, patient's upper denture is modified with extended labial flanges.

Intraoral incision is taken just above the attached gingiva from one maxillary buttress to the other buttress. Supraperiosteal dissection is performed to create two pockets on either side of the piriform aperture. The dissection is extended superiorly to the level of the attachment of the levator anguli oris muscle. Dissection is also continued in the midline upto the base of the piriform aperture. Perforation of the nasal cavity should be avoided.

The impression of the newly created pouches, is taken using impression compound. The labial flanges of the denture are then covered with the split thickness skin graft. Denture is then inserted into the place. Bilateral circumzygomatic wires and piriform margin wires are used to stabilize the denture, which remains in place for a week.

Advantages

- Patients with only mandibular anterior teeth present, often have pronounced loss of the anterior maxillary alveolus, because of constant occlusal trauma. The above procedure is useful in such cases.

- Increases denture stability and retention by increasing the vestibular area and provides pocket sphincters to grip undercut denture flanges.
- In severe atrophy—tuberoplasty can be combined.
- Deficiency in the nasolabial fold region can be improved.

Mental Nerve Transposition

Many times patients with severe mandibular atrophic ridge, complain of pain after wearing the denture. The cause is the superior position of the mental neurovascular bundle. As the patient starts chewing the food, the pressure causes severe pain. Repositioning of the nerve can relieve the pain. Level of the mental foramen is ascertained with the X-rays. A crestal incision is taken with buccal releasing incisions in the region of premolars. Mucoperiosteal flap is reflected inferiorly to locate the nerve. Dissection below the foramen, till the inferior border of the mandible, should be done and the nerve is freed lightly and held with the hook upward. A bony groove is cut below the mental foramen, only in the buccal cortex. Then the nerve is positioned inferiorly and secured in place with gelfoam and the flap is then sutured.

RIDGE AUGMENTATION PROCEDURES

When the alveolar ridge resorption is so extreme, that the alveolar bone has completely disappeared and in maxilla, the height has been reduced to the point that a nearly flat surface exists between the vestibule and palate and the piriform aperture lies just beneath the gingiva. And in the mandible, the basal bone has shown considerable amount of resorption with the mental nerve positioned almost at the crest and very thin mandibular alveolar ridge exists, which can end up in fracture easily. Vestibuloplasty is out of consideration in such cases, until the replacement of necessary supportive bone is done.

Many techniques have been described in the literature for augmenting the bony architecture of the maxilla and/or the mandible.

Two approaches/options are available: (i) augmentation of alveolar bone (ii) place the implants.

Aims

- Restoration of optimum/near optimum ridge height and width, ridge form, vestibular depth and optimum denture bearing area.
- Protection of neurovascular bundle.

- Establishment of proper interarch relationship.
- Improvement of retention and stability of denture.
- Improve the patient comfort for wearing the denture.

Limitations

- Physical condition of the patient
- Metabolism of the patient (healing capacity)
- Nutritional deficiencies
- Availability of adequate soft tissue coverage
- Compliance of the patient for major surgery

Ridge augmentation procedures can be carried out in the maxilla or in the mandible or both (Table 34.4).

Materials used for Augmentation of Alveolar Ridge

- Autogeneous bone graft—iliac crest, rib grafts.
- Allogenic bone grafts—freeze dried cadaver bone.
- Alloplastic material—hydroxyapatite.
- Metal mesh with autogenous cancellous bone.
- Metal mesh with hydroxyapatite.

Table 34.4: Ridge augmentation procedures

A. *Mandibular augmentation*
   1. Superior border augmentation
      a. Bone grafts
      b. Cartilage grafts
      c. Alloplastic grafts.
   2. Inferior border augmentation
      a. Bone grafts (autogenous or allogenic freeze dried cadaveric mandible)
      b. Cartilage grafts.
   3. Interpositional or Sandwich bone grafts
      a. Bone grafts
      b. Cartilage grafts
      c. Hydroxyapatite blocks.
   4. Visor osteotomy.
   5. Onlay grafting—autogenous, alloplastic, allogenic material.
B. *Maxillary augmentation*
   1. Onlay bone grafting—autogenous/allogenic grafts.
   2. Onlay grafting of alloplastic material.
   3. Interpositional or Sandwich grafts.
   4. Sinus lift procedure.
C. *Augmentation in combination with orthognathic surgery*
   1. Mandibular osteotomy procedure.
   2. Maxillary osteotomy procedure.
   3. Combination procedure.

Mandibular Augmentation

Superior border grafting/augmentation (Fig. 34.20): Davis (1970) has described a technique for ridge augmentation, that uses two 15 cm autogenous rib grafts. One rib is scored at the cortex, followed by contouring the same rib in the shape of the mandible. The rib graft is fixed to the mandible, either with transosseous wiring or circummandibular wiring. The other rib graft is made into corticocancellous particles and moulded around the first rib graft. The surgical flap is then closed. Iliac crest grafting to the superior border also can be used.

Disadvantages

- Donor site morbidity.
- Second surgical site necessary.
- Continued resorption of the grafted sites.
- Soft tissue dehiscence or limitation.

Hydroxyapatite blocks can be used (precarved in a horseshoe-shaped manner blocks are available).

Inferior border grafting (Fig. 34.21): This surgical procedure is indicated, when the alveolar ridge is less than 5 to 8 mm in height and is at risk of pathological fracture.

First described by *Marx and Saunders* (1986), for reconstruction of the mandible following resection.

Modified by *Quinn* (1991)—used for augmentation of atrophic ridge and subsequent placement of implants.

Technique: A supraclavicular incision similar to the incision used in bilateral neck dissection is made, from

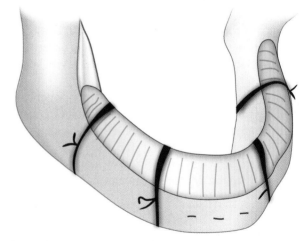

Fig. 34.20: Superior border rib grafting fixed with circummandibular wiring

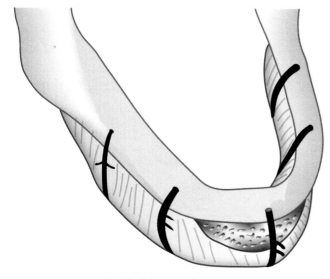

Fig. 34.21: Inferior border grafting

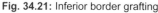

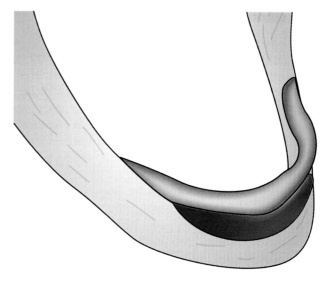

Fig. 34.22: Interpositional graft

mastoid to mastoid region. Subplatysmal dissection, till the inferior border of the mandible is done. Incision through the periosteum is completed from angle to angle. A freeze-dried allogenic cadaver mandible is hollowed out and multiple perforations made into it to allow for revascularization of the packed cancellous bone graft. This allogenic mandible will be used as a tray. The cancellous bone graft is harvested from the iliac crest. The cadaver mandible is then filled with autogenous cancellous graft particles and is fixed to the inferior border with 2-0 vicryl sutures, by circummandibular fixation. The neck flap is closed in tension free manner. Osseointegrated implants can be placed approximately 4 to 6 months following surgery.

Advantages

- Since no surgery is done intraorally, patient's old dentures can be used as transitional dentures
- By using this technique 11 to 17 mm of bone augmentation can be achieved with a resorption rate of only 5 percent over the first several years
- Increased bone height to accommodate implant surgery
- Extraoral flap gives adequate tissue coverage
- Also lower one-third of the facial height is increased. Esthetically better results.

Interpositional Bone Grafts (Sandwich Grafting) (Fig. 34.22)

During this procedure, a horizontal osteotomy is performed, splitting of the residual maxilla or mandible and bone is grafted into this osteotomy gap.

In mandible, sandwich technique is mainly used for augmentation of the anterior mandible, between the mental foramina. The autogenous or allogenic bone or hydroxyapatite grafts can be used successfully. Delivery of the prosthetic appliance is delayed 3 to 5 months for allowing the remodeling of the bone. Secondary vestibuloplasty procedures may be necessary.

Advantages

- Less resorption rate than onlay grafting.
- More predictable long term results.
- Decreased incidence of nerve paresthesia than the visor osteotomy.
- Can be used in conjunction with osseointegrated implants. Implants are placed through the superior free segment of the bone and through the interpositional bone and secured inferiorly within the remaining segment of the mandible. Implant success rate is reported as high as 98 percent with low resorption rate.

Onlay Grafting

When adequate height is present, but width is inadequate for prosthesis in the maxilla or mandible, the option of onlay grafting should be considered. Oldest technique for onlay augmentation with allograft, i.e. hydroxyapatite is advocated by Obwegeser via submucosal vestibuloplasty technique. After creating a tunnel via midline, a putty is formed of hydroxyapatite crystals, mixed with saline/blood, and is injected via syringe into the submucosal tunnel.

Solid or porous blocks of hydroxyapatite have been used as onlay or interpositional grafts to improve the bony defect. The hydroxyapatite powder can be mixed with autogenous bone graft particles.

Osseointegrated implants can be used in conjunction with onlay bone grafting procedure.

A split thickness rib graft/iliac crest bone graft can be used, as an onlay graft in the maxilla or mandible. Rib is more uniform and can be placed in one piece. Iliac crest is placed in blocks or pieces, not uniform.

Advantages

* Improves the height and width of the maxillary alveolar bone
* Can be used both in the anterior and posterior region.

Technique: A high vestibular incision is taken to facilitate good water tight closure and to achieve good undermining of the tissues for relaxation. Mucoperiosteal flap is reflected to expose the defect. Small perforations are made in the external cortex by using small round bur to create bleeding and promotion of clot formation and neovascularization. The grafting material is placed/molded over the external cortex. Placement of barrier membrane helps in regeneration and preservation of the graft. Scoring of the periosteum is done before closure for proper mobilization of the flap.

Visor Osteotomy

The goal of Visor osteotomy is to increase the height of the mandibular ridge for denture support. The Visor osteotomy consists of central splitting of the mandible in buccolingual dimension and the superior positioning of the lingual section of the mandible, which is wired in position. Cancellous bone graft material is placed at the outer cortex over the superior labial junction for improving the contour.

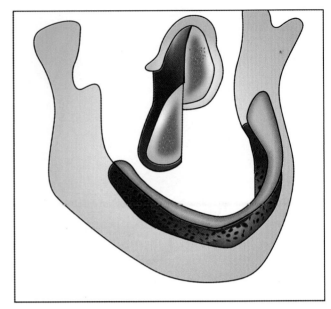

Fig. 34.23: Modified visor osteotomy

Modified Visor Osteotomy (Fig. 34.23)

Consists of splitting of mandible buccolingually by vertical osteotomy only in the posterior regions and a horizontal osteotomy in the anterior region. The posterior lingual segments are then pushed superiorly on both the sides and anterior fragment is also pushed superiorly and fixed with wires to the posterior newly mobilized lingual segments. Corticocancellous bone graft particles with hydroxyapatite granules is placed in the gap between the superior and inferior anterior segments. Rest of the graft material can be molded on the buccal aspect of the posterior segments.

Advantage: Eighty percent of the height is maintained at the end of 3 to 5 years.

Disadvantages

* Nerve paresthesia and dysesthesia.
* Need for hospitalization.
* Donor site morbidity.
* Inability to wear the dentures for 3 to 5 months following surgery.

Sinus Lift Procedure or Sinus Grafting

It is mainly used to assist with the placement of osseointegrated implants in the posterior maxilla. Due

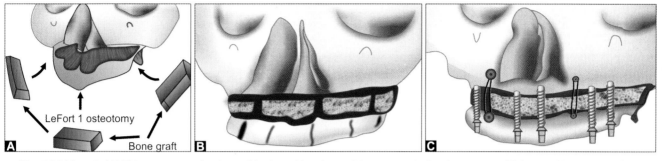

Figs 34.24A to C: (A) Ridge augmentation in combination with orthognathic surgery—LeFort I osteotomy, (B) Interposition bone grafting, (C) Immediate implant fixation

to pneumatization of the maxillary sinus and atrophy of the ridge, the sinus floor is lowered almost to the crest of the alveolar ridge in the posterior region. In order to improve the implant support, the sinus lining at the floor is lifted up surgically and the bone graft is placed between the sinus lining and the inner aspect of the alveolar crest or floor of the maxillary sinus in the posterior maxilla.

Totum (1986) was the first surgeon to perform the sinus grafts. A variety of materials have been used with varying degree of success (autogenous bone, allogenic bone, tricalcium phosphate, hydroxyapatite, calcium phosphate, ceramics and calcium deficient carbonate apatites from bovine bone).

Technique: Intraoral incision is taken on the maxillary crest or slightly on the palatal aspect with vertical releasing incision from canine to tuberosity area. Anterolateral wall of the maxilla is exposed by reflecting the mucoperiosteal flap. A bony window is made with a trap door type osteotomy, just lateral and posterior to the canine fossa.

15 to 20 mm long inferior horizontal osteotomy cut is placed 3 mm above the sinus floor. The anterior vertical osteotomy cut is placed perpendicular to horizontal osteotomy and parallel to the lateral nasal wall, the posterior vertical cut is placed just at the maxillary buttress. The vertical cuts are joined superiorly by placing small bur holes placed at small intervals without completing the superior cut. The trap door type of bony window is then gently lifted up superiorly to expose the schneiderian membrane, which is then lifted up gently from the sinus floor and walls. The gap between the lifted sinus membrane and the floor is filled with the

graft material. For one stage implant a corticocancellous iliac crest bone block can be used. Otherwise a waiting period of 6 to 9 months is advocated before implant placement.

Augmentation in Combination with Orthognathic Surgeries

Many osteotomies have been performed for reconstruction of edentulous atrophied maxilla/mandible.
 i. Anterior maxillary osteotomy.
 ii. Total LeFort I osteotomy, can be used along with interpositioning of the grafts (Figs 34.24A to C). Total maxillary osteotomy with palatal vault osteotomy also can be used for deepening the palatal vault.

Problems Encountered with Augmentation Technique

- Inadequate soft tissue cover.
- Rejection of autografts (failure of union with the host bone).
- Dehiscence of overlying mucosa
- Migration of the graft material
- Resorption of the graft

None of the grafting materials have been considered as ideal or perfect. Each investigator has his own preference and his experience with success rate. Various studies have suggested that autogenous bone grafts either from iliac crest or rib show 28 percent resorption at the end of 6 months, 45 percent at the end of one year, 78 percent at the end of 2 years, 89 percent at the end of 3 to 5 years. But the width of the graft is maintained, though there is vertical bone loss.

Cysts and Tumors of the Orofacial Region

35 Cysts of the Jaws and Oral/Facial Soft Tissues

A cyst is a pathologic cavity or sac within the hard or soft tissues that may contain fluid, semifluid or gas and not always lined by epithelium (It may be lined by epithelium, fibrous tissue or occasionally even by neoplastic tissue) Cyst will be surrounded by a definite connective tissue wall. The cystic fluid either is secreted by the cells lining the cavity or derived from the surrounding tissue fluid. Initially, cysts do not contain pus. It is when the cystic contents become secondarily infected and then the pus develops. Cysts may arise in any of the soft or hard tissues of the orofacial regions.

Originally, since the late 19th century, classifications were based upon clinical and radiologic features, but newer findings and ideas regarding origin and growth have led to some modifications. The classification presented in Flow chart 35.1 is a slight modification of that published by Shear (1983) (Table 35.1). But in 2005, World Health Organization (WHO) reclassified the odontogenic keratocyst as the keratocystic odontogenic tumor. Therefore, we have deleted odontogenic kerato-cyst from the list and it will be discussed in benign tumor section.

CYST FORMATION

Cysts occur more in the jaw bones than any other bones in body, because cysts originate from the numerous rests of odontogenic epithelium, which remains after tooth formation.

Two phases have been recognized in the patho-physiology of cystic lesions:

Cyst initiation—which results in the proliferation of the epithelial lining and the formation of a small cavity.

Flow chart 35.1: Classification of the cysts of jaw, oral and facial soft tissues

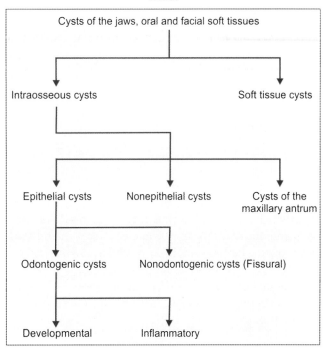

Table 35.1: Intraosseous and soft tissue cysts	
Intraosseous cysts	*Soft tissue cysts*

Epithelial cysts
A. Of odontogenic epithelial origin
  1. Developmental
    a. Primordial cyst
    b. Dentigerous (follicular) cyst
    c. Lateral periodontal cyst—lateral botryoid odontogenic cyst
    d. Calcifying odontogenic (Gorlin) cyst
  2. Inflammatory
    a. Radicular cyst (apical/lateral periodontal)
    b. Residual cyst
B. Of nonodontogenic epithelial origin
  1. Fissural
    a. Median mandibular
    b. Median palatal
    c. Globulomaxillary
  2. Incisive canal (nasopalatine duct or median anterior maxillary) cyst

Nonepithelial cysts (Pseudocysts)
  1. Solitary bone cyst (traumatic)
  2. Stafne's bone cavity
  3. Aneurysmal bone cyst

Cysts of the maxillary antrum
  1. Surgical ciliated cyst of maxilla
  2. Benign mucosal cyst of the maxillary antrum

A. Odontogenic
  Gingival cysts
    a. Adult
    b. Newborn
B. Nonodontogenic
    a. Anterior median lingual cyst
    b. Nasolabial cyst (or nasoalveolar cyst)
C. Retention cysts
Salivary gland cysts
    a. Mucocele
    b. Ranula
D. Developmental/congenital cysts
    a. Dermoid and epidermoid cysts
    b. Lymphoepithelial cyst (cervical/intraoral)
    c. Thyroglossal duct cyst
    d. Cystic hygroma
E. Parasitic cysts
    a. Hydatid cysts
    b. Cysticerocis
F. Heterotropic cysts
    Oral cysts with gastric or intestinal epithelium

Enlargement or expansion—of this cystic cavity, then occurs.

These processes have been clearly defined for epithelium lined cysts, where the initiation is different for each group of cysts, the enlargement process is most likely similar for all epithelium lined cysts, though there may be some variations in the mode of enlargement. Regarding, the bone cysts, little information is available for certain, about their origin and mode of enlargement.

Cyst Initiation

The stimulus for the phenomenon of cyst initiation is not known, other than the inflammatory odontogenic cysts, where clearly it is the infection that is considered as the precipitating factor that results in cystic initiation. In others, it is possible that there is a predisposition in some individuals to form cysts from developing odontogenic epithelium, i.e. from the following:
- Dental lamina and its remnants
- Enamel organ
- Extensions of basal cells from the overlying oral epithelium

- Reduced enamel epithelium,
- Cells rests of Malassez, etc.

Whatever may be the precipitating factor in the initiation of the cystic lesion, it is followed by cyst formation, the factors responsible for which are as follows:
- Proliferation of the epithelial lining
- Fluid accumulation within the cyst cavity
- Bone resorption.

The origin and pathogenesis related to each cystic lesion is discussed in length, later.

Cyst Enlargement

Once cyst formation has been initiated, it continues to grow and enlarge, irrespective of its type and its origin. Following mechanisms have been forwarded, regarding enlargement of cystic lesions:
- Increase in the volume of the contents
- Increase in the surface area of the sac or epithelial proliferation
- Resorption of the surrounding bone and at times
- Displacement of the surrounding soft tissues.

The periosteum is stimulated to form a layer of new bone-subperiosteal deposition.

Increase in the Volume of its Contents

It is generally considered that the volume of the contents of a cyst may increase due to the following factors or their combination, which may bring about cystic enlargement, examples are given below.

Secretions

Mucus secreting cyst, where the lining is mucus secreting, an accumulation of mucus explains the increase in volume.

Transudation and exudation: Inflammatory cysts or the presence of infection—Inflammatory cells, which are commonly present in the capsule, release co-factors, lymphocytes release the lymphokine, osteoclast activating factor (OAF) and monocytes release interleukin -I which stimulates the fibroblasts to release the prostaglandins. These epithelial cells breakdown products produce a *hyperosmolar cyst fluid.*

- *Increased hyperosmolarity*, further draws in the fluid, from the surrounding tissues, as the cyst wall is a semipermeable membrane: thus, the increased hydrostatic pressure, which is much dependent on the type of cystic lining, its permeability and the cystic contents causes cystic enlargement.

- *Increased osmolarity* of the cyst fluid may play a role, in its enlargement, osmotic differences between the serum and cystic fluids is related to the proteins present within the cystic fluid, such as large molecules of globulins, albumin, fibrinogen and fibrin-degradation products, which are responsible for the increase in osmotic pressure of a cyst, which in turn results in cystic expansion.

Epithelial Proliferation

Mural growth in the form of epithelial proliferation, is one of the essential processes by which the surface area of the sac increases, basically by peripheral cell division or by accumulation of cellular contents.

- A multicentric pattern of cyst growth brought about by the proliferation of local groups of epithelial cells as in the keratocysts, results in cystic expansion

- *Collagenase activity* in some cysts such as the primordial and radicular cysts by way of increased collagenolysis could result in cyst expansion

- *Unremitting growth* of certain epithelial linings due to high mitotic values as in keratocysts plays a role in cystic enlargement

- *Presence of low grade infection* stimulates cells such as the cell rests of Malassez to proliferate and form arcades. The number of epithelial layers is then determined by the period of viability of each cell and the rate of maturation and desquamation.

Bone Resorption

As the epithelial cells divide, the cyst is able to enlarge within the rigid bony cavity by the release of bone resorbing factors from the capsule, which stimulate *osteoclast function*, e.g. prostanoids like PGE2 and PGI2 and certain leukotrienes. Differences in the sizes of various cystic lesions could possibly be dependent upon the quantity of release of prostaglandins and other bone resorbing factors.

Cyst Regression

Any process that leads to the involution of the cyst epithelium, e.g. extraction of the necrotic tooth or conversion of the epithelial lining to oral mucosa and reduction of intracystic pressure as with marsupialization may cause the connective tissue capsule to regress and the cavity to be filled by bone or scar tissue.

◼ INTRAOSSEOUS CYSTS

Odontogenic Epithelial Origin

Primordial Cyst

Robinson (1945) first, popularized the term, *primordial cyst* for cysts arising from primordial odontogenic epithelium, i.e. dental lamina or its remnants, odontogenic basal cell hamartias or enamel organ, prior to the formation of calcified structures, thus, this cyst is found in place of a tooth (from the normal series or supernumerary) instead of being associated with one (Fig. 35.1).

Incidence: Primordial cysts comprise approximately about 5 to 10 percent of odontogenic cysts of the jaws and are seen predominantly in the second, third and fourth decades of life, though they can occur in any age group. They have a slight predilection for the males than females.

Site: The primordial cysts have a strong predilection of occurrence in the mandible than the maxilla, about one-half of the former are seen to involve the angle of the

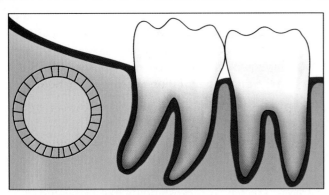

Fig. 35.1: A diagrammatic representation of primordial cyst

mandible with extension for varying distances into the ascending ramus and body mandible. However, they can occur anywhere in the jaws, including the midline, though majority of the cysts are seen posterior to the first bicuspids.

Clinical features: The physical signs and symptoms of a jaw cyst will depend to a certain extent on the dimensions of the lesion. A small cyst is unlikely to be diagnosed on routine examination of the mouth, and is generally detected accidentally on a radiographic examination. In case of the primordial cyst, patients are remarkably free of symptoms until the cysts have reached a large size at times involving the entire ascending ramus. This is because the primordial cyst initially extends in the medullary cavity and clinically observable expansion of the bone occurs late.

The enlarging cyst may lead to displacement of the teeth, percussion of the teeth overlying the cyst may produce a dull or hollow sound. A single missing tooth from the normal series should invite suspicion of the existence of the primordial type cyst. The teeth adjoining the cyst will have vital pulps unless there is coincidental disease of the teeth. Buccal expansion of the bone is commonly seen, lingual and palatal expansion is rare. Large mandibular cysts, invariably deflect the neurovascular bundle into an abnormal position. If acute infection sets in, with accumulation of pus within the sac, neuropraxia of the nerve results with the onset of labial paresthesia or anesthesia. When tension is relieved, with spontaneous discharge of pus via a sinus tract or surgical drainage, sensation returns to normal.

Radiological features: The primordial cyst is usually unilocular, but sometimes have scallped outline, which gives a multilocular appearance. The borders are hyperostotic. The involved tooth is usually missing. The

adjacent teeth may be displaced, diverged or deflected. Primordial cysts in maxilla are smaller than their mandibular counterparts.

When they occur in the periapical region of vital teeth, they can be mistaken for a radicular cyst. They may impede the eruption of related teeth and this results in a dentigerous cyst appearance radiologically.

Pathogenesis: Primordial cyst is generally considered to be a developmental anomaly, which arises from odontogenic epithelium, the main sources being:
- Dental lamina or its remnants
- Basal cells from the overlying oral mucosa
- Enamel organ—by degeneration of the stellate reticulum.

Cyst contents (aspirate): It reveals a thick, granular, yellowish material.

Pathology: The primordial cysts are thin walled and are lined by a regular keratinized stratified squamous epithelium, which is usually 5 to 8 cell layers thick and is devoid of rete pegs. The epithelial cells are arranged in a "Picket Fence" or "Tombstone Pattern". The enucleated lining easily separates from the underlying connective tissue. The capsule is quite thin and normally free of inflammatory cells, and may contain strands of odontogenic epithelium resembling the dental lamina, cell nests and daughter cysts.

Recurrence: Primordial cysts have a pronounced tendency to recur. This aggressive pecularity was first reported by Pindborg and Hansen (1963). The recurrence rate may vary from 5 to 62 percent with most occurring in the first 5 years. Some of the possible reasons reported for this feature are as follows:
- Tendency to multiplicity
- Presence of satellite cysts
- Cystic lining is very thin and fragile, portions of which may be left behind

Treatment: Treatment should always be based on proper clinical assessment, accurate diagnosis and appropriate tests of the cystic aspirate.

Marsupialization is incorrect in principle in the treatment of primordial cysts, owing to their high incidence and tendency to recur.

Bramley (1971, 1974) had very rationally outlined the surgical management of these cysts as follows:
- *Small single cysts with regular spherical outline*, should be enucleated from an intraoral approach, provided the access is good.

- *Larger or less accessible cysts with regular spherical outline*, should be enucleated from an extraoral approach, as an intraoral access would be inadequate and a blind procedure. Care should be taken to ensure that all fragments of the extremely thin lining are removed.
- *Unilocular lesions with scalloped or loculated periphery and small multilocular lesions,* should be treated by marginal excision, i.e. resection of the containing block of bone, while maintaining the continuity of the posterior and inferior borders as in the ascending ramus, angle and body mandible, if there is difficulty of access, extraoral exposure is necessary. If the cystic lining is found to be adherent and in contiguity to the overlying oral mucosa or muscle then it should be excised along with marginal excision. The defect is closed primarily and can be left to heal by secondary intention or can be filled with hydroxyapatite crystals, autogenous bone graft, corticocancellous chips or allogenous bone powder, chips or block
- *Large multilocular lesions with or without cortical perforation*; may require resection of the involved bone followed by primary or secondary reconstruction with a choice of reconstruction plates of stainless steel, vitallium, titanium, use of titanium or stainless steel mesh and bone grafting procedures with iliac crest graft, costochondral graft or allogenous bone grafts.

Clearly, every cyst and every patient should be assessed individually and the treatment planned carefully for each case, whatever form of surgical approach is selected, the patient should be reviewed regularly over a long follow up.

Dentigerous (Follicular) Cyst

A dentigerous cyst is one that results because of the enlargement of the follicular space of the whole or part of the crown of an impacted or unerupted tooth and it encloses the crown of an unerupted/impacted tooth at the cementoenamel junction.

Paget (1863) coined the term dentigerous cyst. They involve teeth of the adult dentition or occasionally supernumerary teeth.

Incidence: The dentigerous cyst is seen more commonly than the primordial cyst, but less common than the apical types. The dentigerous cyst is the most common type of developmental odontogenic cyst, making up about 20 percent of all epithelium lined cysts of the jaws.

The most common age periods for diagnosis are the first, second, third decades, subsequently there is a gradual decline in occurrence. Incidence appears to be equal in both sexes, though some reports, mention a slight predilection for the males and the prevalence is higher for whites than for blacks.

Site: It occurs more frequently in the mandible, than the maxilla. Late erupting teeth are the most frequently involved in descending order are the lower third molars, upper cuspids, upper third molars and the lower bicuspid teeth. Although dentigerous cysts may occur in association with any unerupted tooth, most often they involve mandibular third molars. Other relatively frequent sites include maxillary canines, maxillary third molars, and mandibular second premolars. Dentigerous cysts rarely involve unerupted deciduous teeth. Occasionally, they are associated with supernumerary teeth or odontomas.

Clinical features: Dentigerous cysts have the potential, to attain a large size, often it is the pronounced facial asymmetry or the problem of ill fitting dentures that forces a patient to seek treatment. Pain may be a presenting symptom, if secondary infection supervenes. Clinically, a tooth from the normal series, will be found to be missing, unless the cause is a supernumerary tooth, sometimes, other adjacent teeth may also fail to erupt, may be tilted or otherwise be out of alignment. The lateral expansion causes a smooth, hard, painless, prominence, later as the cyst expands the bone, covering the center of the convexity, becomes thinned and can be indented with pressure on palpation, with further expansion. This fragile outer shell of bone becomes fragmented and the sensation imparted and sound produced on palpation over the area is described aptly as egg-shell crackling, which is also true for other large odontogenic cysts. Still later the cyst lining may come to lie immediately beneath the oral mucosa and fluctuation can be elicited.

Radiological features (*Figs 35.2 to 35.4*): Radiographs will generally reveal a unilocular radiolucency associated with crowns of unerupted impacted teeth; at times a multilocular effect can be seen, when the cyst is of irregular shape due to bony trabeculations. Cysts have a well defined sclerotic margin, unless when they are infected then the margins are poorly defined. With the pressure of an enlarging cyst, the unerupted tooth can be pushed away from its direction of eruption, e.g. the lower third molar may be pushed to the inferior border, or into the ascending ramus, whereas the upper

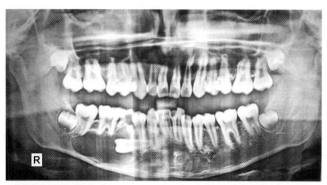

Fig. 35.2: An orthopantomogram (OPG) revealed a single, unilateral, unilocular well-defined corticated radiolucency seen around the crown of horizontally impacted lower mandibular 2nd premolar. It also revealed: grossly carious right mandibular deciduous 2nd molar, over retained right mandibular deciduous 2nd molar and root resorption of right mandibular first and second molar. Circumferential type of dentigerous cyst

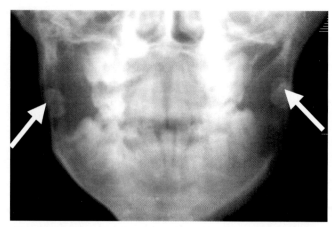

Fig. 35.4: Bilateral dentigerous cysts involving the body and ramus mandible

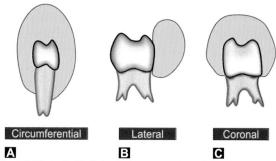

Figs 35.5A to C: Radiological presentation of dentigerous cysts

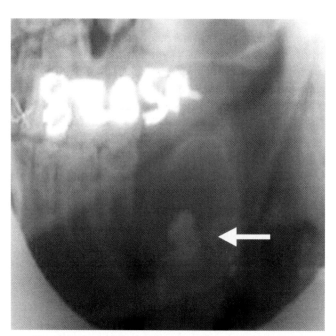

Fig. 35.3: Circumferential type of dentigerous cyst, with mild resorption of second molar

cuspid or incisor may be pushed up into the maxillary sinus or floor of the nose. As compared to the other jaw cysts, dentigerous cysts have a higher tendency to cause root resorption of adjacent teeth. Radiologically, the dental follicle may expand around the unerupted or impacted tooth in three variations, i.e. (a) circumferential (b) lateral (c) central or coronal (Figs 35.5A to C).

Pathogenesis: Dentigerous cysts develop by accumulation of fluid between the reduced enamel epithelium or

within the enamel organ itself of unerupted or impacted teeth. In case of a dilated follicle, a pericoronal width of more than 3 to 4 mm is considered as a cyst. Another possibility suggested for the development of dentigerous cysts is because of degeneration of the stellate reticulum at an early stage of development and is likely to be associated with enamel hypoplasia.

Cystic contents (aspirate): The cyst contents consist of clear yellowish fluid, in which cholesterol crystals may be present, or purulent material, if infection has occurred.

Pathology: The histopathologic features of dentigerous cysts vary, depending on whether the cyst is inflamed or not inflamed. In the noninflamed dentigerous cyst, the fibrous connective tissue wall is loosely arranged and contains considerable glycosaminoglycan ground substance. Small islands or cords of inactive appearing odontogenic epithelial rests may be present in the fibrous wall. Sometimes, macroscopic examination of the cystic lining, may exhibit mural thickenings which on histological examination may exhibit ameloblastic changes. The cystic lining is of reduced enamel epithelium, consists of 2 to 3 cell layers of flat or non-keratinizing cuboidal cells and is attached to the tooth at the cementoenamel junction. The epithelial lining is not keratinized, rarely a dentigerous cyst may form keratin by metaplasia. Because a thin layer of reduced enamel epithelium normally lines the dental follicle surrounding the crown of an unerupted tooth, it can be difficult to distinguish a small dentigerous cyst from simply a normal or enlarged dental follicle based on microscopic features alone. Again, this distinction often represents largely an academic exercise; the most important consideration is assuring that the lesion does not represent a more significant pathologic process (e.g. odontogenic keratocyst or ameloblastoma) (Fig. 35.6).

Presence of sebaceous glands, mucus or ciliated cells in the epithelial lining, is also considered to form as a result of metaplasia. Hyaline bodies may be seen within the epithelium, and clefts from cholesterol crystals may be found in the connective tissue capsule. Epithelial discontinuities may be present, because of intense inflammatory infiltrate in the adjacent capsule or because of partial adherence to enamel.

Treatment: Treatment via an intraoral approach or extraoral is decided by the size of the cyst, adequate access and whether it is desirable to save the involved tooth.

Marsupialization (Partsch surgery): It is indicated in children if the cyst is very large in size and the involved tooth/teeth are to be maintained. The tooth may erupt into occlusion as the defect heals with normal bone, or

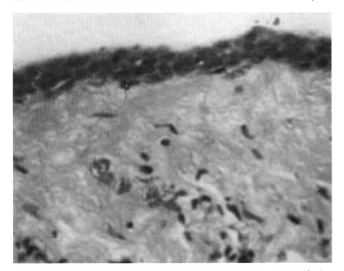

Fig. 35.6: Dentigerous cyst, reveals thin, nonkeratinized stratified squamous epithelium and uninflamed fibrous tissue

orthodontic forces may be used to bring the tooth into occlusion.

Enucleation: Alternatively, the cyst can be enucleated together with the involved tooth in adults, as the possibility of the tooth erupting is low.

In children, an attempt could be made to salvage the tooth, in which case, the lining is separated from the neck of the tooth with a scalpel. This procedure is worth attempting, when root formation is complete, so that the risk of tooth dislodgement is low.

Behavior and prognosis: It is widely believed that ameloblastomas frequently arise in dentigerous cysts, and some have even termed them as preameloblastic lesions. Recurrence is a possibility if some epithelium remains.

Developmental Lateral Periodontal Cysts

Lateral periodontal cysts are found lateral to the roots of vital teeth, and in which an inflammatory etiology or a collateral primordial cyst have been excluded on clinical and histological evidence.

Incidence: This cyst is chiefly found in adults, though it is a recognized entity, it occurs so rarely that no significant conclusions can be drawn regarding specific age or sex predilection.

Site: It occurs more often in the mandible than the maxilla. It is most often related to the mandibular cuspid, bicuspid and third molar roots, followed by the anterior region of the maxilla.

Clinical features: Majority of the cases have number of clinical signs or symptoms and are discovered during routine radiological examination. The associated teeth are vital. At times a gingival swelling may occur on the buccal or lingual aspect, and this must be differentiated from a gingival cyst. The lingual type of cyst involving the mandibular third molar, seems to be more common and if infected can cause a severe spreading infection of the submandibular space.

Radiological features: Radiographs reveal a well defined round or ovoid radiolucency with a sclerotic margin, the lamina dura of the involved tooth is destroyed. Most of the cysts are smaller than 1 cm in size and are seen to be present between the cervical margin and apex of the root. In case of the lower third molar roots, they are seen to be present in the bifurcation, buccally or lingually or against the distal surface of the root.

Pathogenesis: Considering that the lateral periodontal cyst is a distinct entity of developmental odontogenic origin, three possibilities have been suggested regarding its origin, for example:
- Reduced enamel epithelium
- Remnants of dental lamina
- Cell rests of Malassez.

Cystic contents (aspirate): It has a serous caseous content.

Pathology: The cyst is usually lined by a well formed, nonkeratinized, stratified squamous epithelial lining. Localized epithelial proliferations may be seen in the form of plaques. The connective tissue wall, may show inflammatory cell infiltrate.

Treatment: Enucleation is generally, the method of choice, and is easily performed because of the small size and easy access. All attempts should be made to avoid sacrificing the associated tooth.

Botryoid Odontogenic Cyst

The botryoid odontogenic cyst was recognized by Weathers and Waldron (1973), which is thought to arise from odontogenic epithelial rests. It is probable that the botryoid cyst is a *variant of the lateral periodontal cyst.* The gross appearance of the largest lesion was described as resembling a *bunch of grapes,* hence the term *botryoid.* They have been reported to occur within the mandible in the cuspid-premolar region, they give the appearance of a polycystic lesion on the radiograph.

Microscopically, the cysts are divided into multiple compartments, with very thin fibrous connective tissue septae, each cavity is lined by thin, 1 to 2 cells wide, nonkeratinizing sqaumous epithelium, which exhibit 'buds' or 'plaque-like' thickenings of clear cells similar to the lateral periodontal cyst. These thickening could be the source of microcysts in the fibrous wall, giving rise to a polycystic or a multilocular lesion.

Behavior: The lateral periodontal cyst does not have a tendency to recur.

Calcifying Epithelial Odontogenic Cyst (CEOC): Gorlin Cyst (Figs 35.7A to F)

The calcifying odontogenic cyst is a lesion of developmental odontogenic epithelial origin, which is relatively uncommon and bears resemblance to the calcifying epithelioma of Malherbe. It was first described by Gorlin and associates (1962, 1964).

Incidence: Very few cases have been reported, this cyst has no sex predilection. It occurs over a wide age range, but is said to be more common in children and young adults.

Site: They have been described in either jaw, but probably the most common site of occurrence is in the anterior part of the mandible.

Clinical features (Figs 35.7A and B): A large number of cases are symptomless, and are discovered accidently on radiographic examination. Swelling is the most frequent complaint, rarely there is pain. A peripheral or intraosseous lesion may be seen, the latter produce a hard bony expansion and may be fairly extensive. Lingual and palatal expansion may be noted. Some cysts arise close to the periosteum and produce a saucer-shaped depression in the bone, in a few cases displacement of the teeth may be seen.

Radiological features (Figs 35.7C to E): When small, the cyst will be seen between the roots of the teeth. The periphery may be well demarcated or irregular, some lesions are unilocular, whereas others exhibit a multilocular pattern. Cortical perforation may be evident. Calcifications, as irregular radiopaque specks may be seen within the bone cavity, sometimes the calcification can be substantial and occupies a large area of the lesion. The cyst may be associated with a complex odontome or an unerupted tooth. Resorption of the roots of the adjacent teeth may be seen.

Pathogenesis: There is strong evidence that the cyst has an odontogenic origin, the probable sources being:
- Remnants of dental lamina
- Stellate reticulum
- Reduced enamel epithelium.

The epithelial lining appears to have the ability to induce the formation of dental tissues in the adjacent connective wall—therefore, it is quite possible that an odontome, dentinoid alone, or even tumors such as ameloblastoma, odontoameloblastoma, ameloblastic fibroma or ameloblastic fibro-odontoma may be found in the cyst wall, induced by the lining epithelium.

Pathology (Fig. 35.7F): The odontogenic type lining of stratified squamous epithelium is 6 to 8 cells thick and has columnar or cuboidal basal layer of cells, occasionally with nuclei at the ends of the cells, opposite the basement membrane, i.e. they undergo a reversal of polarity reminiscent of the ameloblast. In some areas the lining is thin, in patches, the epithelium proliferates, the cells become swollen and eosinophilic,

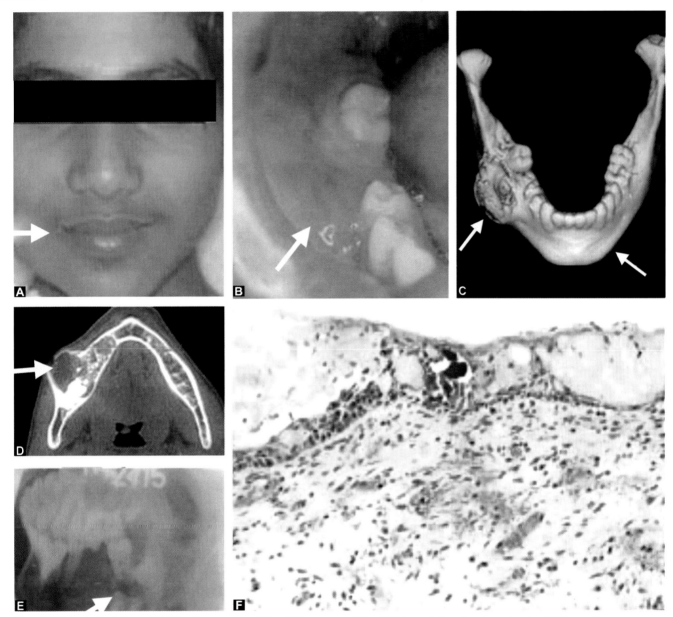

Figs 35.7A to F: Gorlin's cyst: (A) Swelling seen involving right body mandible, (B) Intraoral view showing extensive right buccal expansion due to Gorlin's cyst, (C) 3D CT shows expansion and perforation of buccal cortex due to Gorlin's cyst, (D) Axial CT scan shows radiolucency with speckled calcification and an unerupted, displaced tooth, (E) Radiograph of patient with Gorlin's cyst, (F) Calcifying odontogenic cyst, epithelial lining with ghost cells, foci of calcification and mild inflammation in the cystic wall (Histopathology)

due to a form of keratinization. These are called, *ghost cells*. At first the outline of the cells and their nuclei can still be distinguished, later the outline is lost, the cells fuse and tend to calcify. It is this calcification, which forms the opacities that is seen in the radiographs. The ghost cells are widely separated by intercellular edema. They are enlarged, ballooned, ovoid or elongated, a few contain nuclear remnants, but they are in various stages of degeneration leaving only a faint outline of the nucleus. Irregular amounts of dentin or osteodentin also may be found throughout the lesion. Melanin deposits sometimes may be present in the epithelial linings. The ghost cells, can evoke a foreign body reaction with the formation of multinucleate giant cells in the connective tissue wall of the cyst. In the fibrous wall, strands and islands of odontogenic epithelium may be seen.

Treatment: Simple enucleation is never followed by recurrence. If, however, the cyst is associated with another odontogenic tumor such as an ameloblastic fibroma, then a wider excision will be required. When associated with a complex odontoma, a conservative removal is adequate.

Inflammatory (Periodontal) Radicular Cysts (Fig. 35.8)

The radicular cyst is an inflammatory cyst which results due to infection extending from the pulp into surrounding periapical tissues. It may develop apically, when it is termed as a periapical (periodontal) radicular cyst, or it may develop on the side of the root of a pulpless tooth, when it is termed as a lateral (periodontal) radicular cyst, this cyst should be differentiated from a developmental lateral periodontal cyst which is associated with a vital tooth.

Incidence: As compared to all other jaw cysts, this is the most common of all cysts of odontogenic origin. Males are affected more commonly than females. Very few cases are seen in the first decade, peak incidence is in the third and fourth decades.

Site: The incidence is highest in the anterior maxilla, than the mandible, as the maxillary incisors are most prone to caries, trauma, pulpal death due to development defects and irritating effects of synthetic restorative materials. In the mandible, cysts more commonly involve the mandibular posterior teeth, there may be separate small cysts arising from each apex of a multirooted tooth.

Clinical features: The cyst itself is frequently symptomless and may be discovered, when periapical radiographs are taken of teeth with nonvital pulps. Slowly enlarging swellings are often complained of. Radicular cysts at

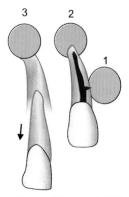

Fig. 35.8: Periodontal cysts: (1) Lateral, (2) Apical, (3) Residual

times attain a large size. Pain may be a significant chief complaint, in the presence of suppuration. Initially, the enlargement is bony hard, as the cyst increases in size, the covering bone becomes thin and exhibits springiness due to fluctuation. In the maxilla, buccal and palatal or only palatal expansion due to the lateral incisor or a palatal root will be noted. In the mandible, lingual expansion is very rare. The mucosa overlying the cystic expansion, as with the other cysts, is at first of normal color; then it may become conspicuous, because of the presence of dilated blood vessels and finally it will take on a profound dark bluish tinge, in case of large cysts. An intraoral sinus tract may be identified with discharging pus or brownish fluid, when the cyst is infected. The involved tooth/teeth will be found to be nonvital, discolored, fractured or with heavy restorations or a failed root canal. They may be sensitive to percussion or hypermobile, or displaced. It may involve deciduous or the permanent dentition. Temporary paresthesia or anesthesia of the regional nerve distribution may be evident as with other cysts when infection is present. Pathologic fracture may be the form of presentation in the mandible, as with other large cysts.

Radiological features: The common description of radicular cysts is a round, pear or ovoid shaped radiolucency, generally outlined by a narrow radio-opaque margin that extends from the lamina dura of the involved tooth/teeth. In case of very large cysts or infected cysts, this peripheral white line is occasionally absent. Root resorption is rare, but may be seen. A lateral radicular cyst may be seen in association with an accessory root canal or lateral perforation during root canal therapy.

Pathogenesis: The epithelial lining is derived from, epithelial cell rests of Malassez in the periodontal ligament, the development of the cyst then occurs in three phases: The exact mechanisms involved in all the phases is debatable.

1. *The phase of initiation:* Chronic low-grade invasion from the pulp leads to the formation of the periapical granuloma. This leads to the activation and proliferation of epithelial rests in the periodontal ligament in the form of strands, arcades or rings.
2. *The phase of cyst formation:* A cystic cavity forms, lined by stratified squamous epithelium due to various possible mechanisms, for example:
    *   Death of the central cells occurs due to increase in the size and reduction of nutrients and oxygen to maintain them

- Central epithelial cells desquamate, others orient towards the periphery, adjacent to the source of nutrition from the connective tissue, or
- Epithelial cells orient towards the periphery to isolate the central necrotic zone.

3. *The phase of enlargement:* Once initiation of cyst has occurred, the continuation of enlargement, may occur due to various different mechanisms, which is true for any cyst, for example:
   - Mural growth
   - Accumulation of fluid
   - Retention of fluid
   - Production of a raised intrastatic pressure.
   - Bone resorption with increase in cystic size (as has been explained in length earlier in the chapter).

Cystic contents (Aspirate): The uninfected cystic fluid is straw coloured or brownish and has cholesterol clefts; a small quantity of keratin flakes may be identified.

In case of a long-standing infection, a dirty-white caseous material may be expressed or frank pus may be present.

Pathology: The cyst is lined by stratified squamous epithelium, the lining may be thin or thick upto 5 mm in size. An inflammatory infiltrate of polymorphonuclear leucocytes will be seen in the lining. Epithelial linings may show the presence of Ruston's hyaline bodies, mucus cells or ciliated cells.

The fibrous capsule is composed of collagen and loose connective tissue. Acute and chronic inflammatory cell infiltrate may be found in the fibrous capsule.

Treatment: Nonvital teeth that are associated with the cyst, can either be extracted (depending on conditions of sufficient bone support and restorative possibilities) or they can be retained, by endodontic treatment and apicoectomy. External sinus tracts should always be excised to prevent epithelial ingrowth. The commonly employed surgical procedure for radicular cysts is enucleation, with primary closure. Very small cysts can be removed through the tooth socket. Large periodontal cysts that encroach upon the maxillary antrum or inferior alveolar neurovascular bundle or the nose, may be treated by marsupialization.

Behavior and prognosis: Some well-documented reports have been published, which contend that squamous cell carcinoma may arise from the epithelial lining of radicular cysts. Browne and other (1972), reported that epithelial dysplasia and keratin metaplasia may precede carcinomatous transformation.

Residual Cyst (Figs 35.9A to F)

A residual cyst is one, that is overlooked after the causative root or tooth is extracted.

Causes: The possible causes are as follows:
- An incompletely removed periapical granuloma or cyst, that potentially enlarges
- An impacted tooth associated with a lateral dentigerous cyst is removed, but the cystic lesion is unrecognized and is left *in situ*, this residual cyst persists and will enlarge
- A cystic lesion develops on either a deciduous tooth or a retained tooth, which either exfoliates or is extracted without knowledge of the underlying pathologic process.

Incidence: It is less commonly seen than in the radicular cysts. It is identified mainly in middle-aged and elderly patients. There is no sex predilection.

Site: The incidence is greater in the maxilla than in the mandible. It is typically seen in edentulous sites (Figs 35.9A and B).

Clinical features: Majority of the cases are asymptomatic and are discovered on radiographic examination (Fig. 35.9B). Occasionally in case of large residual cysts, a pathologic fracture or signs of encroachment on associated structures may be the presenting symptoms.

Pathology: It is similar to the underlying process that was initially present.

Treatment (Figs 35.9C to F): It is similar to that which is employed for a radicular cyst, care should be taken to maintain and preserve the contour of the edentulous ridge.

Multiple Cystic Lesions of the Jaws

Majority of the cases that have been reported of multiple occurrence in the jaw bones, have been of either, primary dentigerous cysts or keratocystic odontogenic tumor or radicular cysts.

Multiple radicular cysts will be associated with several, carious nonvital teeth, generally the maxillary incisors or mandibular posterior teeth. Multiple dentigerous cysts may be present symmetrically in both the

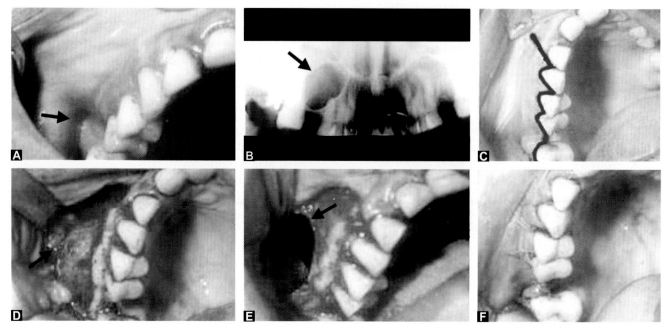

Figs 35.9A to F: Residual cyst: (A) Buccal expansion and missing upper, (R) first molar (extracted earlier), (B) OPG—A residual cystic lesion in 18 regions, (C) Incision, (D) Exposure of cystic lesion, (E) Defect after enucleation, (F) Wound closure

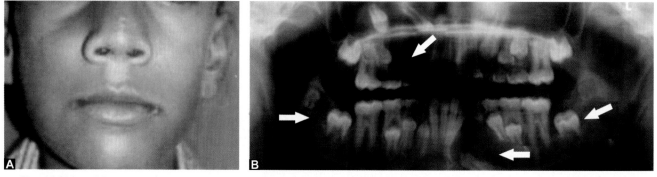

Figs 35.10A and B: Multiple dentigerous cysts: (A) Extraoral view of a 10-year-old child, who had multiple dentigerous cyst, (B) Multiple dentigerous cysts and displaced unerupted permanent teeth (OPG)

upper and lower jaws, involved with unerupted teeth or may be scattered in different quadrants (Figs 35.10A and B).

Intraosseous Cyst of Nonodontogenic Epithelial Origin

Developmental Fissural Cysts (Fig. 35.11)

Fissural cysts are nonodontogenic cysts, that arise owning to epithelial inclusions or entrapments in the lines of closure of the developing facial processes during the embryonic period of life. Each cyst is correlated, with its actual anatomic location.

Median Mandibular Cyst

The mandibular mesenchyme migrates medially from each side and fuses beneath the epithelium to form the mandibular arch, so that median mandibular fissural cysts should not exist. There is no clear cut explanation for these cysts developing in the midline of the mandible, they probably arise from epithelial inclusions in the area of the symphysis.

Incidence: This cyst is less commonly seen than the other fissural cysts. There is no sex predilection.

Site: It is found symmetrically in the midline of the mandible.

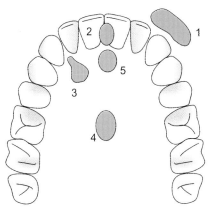

Fig. 35.11: Developmental and soft tissue cysts: (1) Nasolabial, (2) Median alveolar (median mandibular), (3) Globulomaxillary, (4) Median palatal, (5) Nasopalatine

Clinical features: The cyst remains relatively small in size approximately 1 to 3 cm in size. The associated teeth are vital. A labial swelling may be palpable. The teeth may be divergent.

Radiologic features: The cysts are small, generally well-defined, circular or ovoid in shape. The lamina dura of the involved teeth is intact.

Pathology: The cystic lining is of stratified squamous epithelium, the fibrous connective tissue wall may reveal an inflammatory infiltrate.

Treatment: The cyst should be differentiated from primordial cysts or residual radicular cysts. The cyst should be carefully enucleated, without the involvement or damage to the apices of the incisors.

Median Palatal Cyst

Controversy exists on whether the median palatal cyst is a true fissural cyst, that arises because of epithelial inclusion during the fusion of the palatal processes of the maxilla or whether it represents a posterior extension of an incisive canal cyst in case of a *median palatine cyst* and due to an anterior extension in case of *the median alveolar cyst*.

Incidence: It is a rare cyst. There is no sex predilection. It is seen mainly in adults.

Site: It may be seen in the maxillary alveolus, when it is termed as the median alveolar cyst, or in the hard palate, between the incisive fossa and the posterior border of the hard palate, when it is termed as the *median palatal cyst*.

Clinical features: No signs and symptoms exist, unless the cyst becomes large, with expansion of bone and a palpable ovoid swelling in the mid-palatal region or mid-alveolar region.

Radiological features: A maxillary occlusal view will help to identify the ovoid, or irregular radiolucency in the midpalatal region, often it becomes difficult to distinguish the cyst from an extensive incisive canal cyst.

Pathology: The cysts may be lined by stratified squamous epithelium, pseudostratified ciliated columnar or cuboidal epithelium. Chronic inflammatory infiltration may be evidently seen in the subepithelial connective tissue.

Treatment: The cyst should be differentiated from a primordial cyst that may arise from the dental lamina in the midline of the maxilla. Careful enucleation is the line of treatment with primary closure.

Globulomaxillary Cyst

The traditionally described globulomaxillary cyst is also termed as a *lateral fissural cyst*. For years together since Thoma (1937), gave its first description, it has been believed that it arises from nonodontogenic epithelium inclusions at the site of fusion of the globular process of the medial (frontonasal) process and the maxillary process. The globular process is now referred to as the premaxillary process in embryologic terminology.

A critical study of this cyst has led to a lot of controversy, with reports stating that it is improbable for a fissural cyst to develop in this region. It is further reported that, if examined carefully, there were many plausible possibilities of the cyst in this region arising as primordial cysts from supernumerary teeth, developmental periodontal cyst, residual cysts from the primary dentition, lateral periodontal cyst, etc.

Incidence: It is fairly uncommon. It is seen in adults, in either sex.

Site: It is seen between the maxillary lateral incisor and cuspid teeth.

Clinical features: The lateral and maxillary cuspid teeth will be found to be tilted coronally with root divergence. Vitality test will be normal for both the teeth.

Radiological features: If the cyst is small, it is spherical in shape, as it enlarges a typical pear-shaped radiolucency is seen between the maxillary lateral incisor and cuspid with the apex pointing toward the alveolar crest. The lamina dura of both the teeth is preserved. The roots reveal divergence.

Pathology: The epithelial lining is of pseudostratified columnar ciliated epithelium, often derived from the nasal mucosa. The wall which is thick may have concentrations of plasma cells and lymphocytes.

Treatment: Careful enucleation without damage to the adjoining roots of the teeth, followed by primary closure is the definitive line of treatment for true globulomaxillary cysts.

Nasopalatine Duct Cyst

The nasopalatine cyst is a true, nonodontogenic cyst, also referred to as the incisive canal cyst, which occurs because of embryonic epithelial remnants within the nasopalatine canal, that connects the oral and nasal cavities in the embryonic stage.

Incidence: This is the most common type of maxillary developmental, nonodontogenic cyst. It has a slight predilection for the male sex. Majority of the cases are seen in adulthood in the fourth, fifth and sixth decades.

Site: The cyst may arise at any point along the incisive canal, but is seen more commonly in the lower portion of the maxilla, between the apices of the central incisor. Another variant is the cyst of the palatine papilla, which is located solely within the soft tissues in the region of the incisive papilla, at the opening of the canal.

Clinical features: Majority of the cysts remain asymptomatic, as they do not attain a very large size, beyond 1.5 to 2 cm. The notable common symptom is a recurrent swelling, in the anterior region of the midline of the palate, or on the labial aspect between the central incisors, at times the cyst may extend labiopalatally and fluctuation will be positive. Displacement of the teeth is common. The patients most commonly may complain of swelling, pain and discharge. The discharge, often described as a 'salty taste' is seen to originate from a sinus tract at or near the incisive papilla.

At times a burning sensations or numbness is experienced, which is due to pressure exerted by the cyst on the nasopalatine nerves. The central incisors are vital and normal in color, unless they are affected adversely, by trauma or caries.

Radiological features: The nasopalatine duct cyst is seen as a well defined cystic outline, between or above the roots of the maxillary central incisor teeth. It can be round or ovoid, some may appear as heart shaped, because during expansion, they may become notched by the nasal septum or the nasal spine may be superimposed on the radiolucent area or there may be bilateral cysts developing in both Stenson canals. Kay (1972), reported that any radiograph of the fossa, which showed a shadow less than 6 mm wide may be considered within normal limits as a incisive canal fossa in the absence of specific symptoms (Fig. 35.12).

The roots of the central incisors may show divergence and an intact lamina dura around the tooth apices.

Pathology: The type of epithelium found may vary at different levels. It may be stratified squamous at a lower level, more superiorly it may be pseudostratified columnar, cuboidal as well as ciliated. Presence of mucous glands, goblet cells and cilia is highly indicative of their origin within the incisive canal as is the presence of nerves and blood vessels in the fibrous capsule. Hyaline cartilage may be identified in the wall of the cyst.

Cystic contents (aspirate): Aspiration is an important diagnostic aid to rule out a normal incisive canal fossa radiolucency. The viscous fluid content may be mucoid material or even pus if the cyst has been infected.

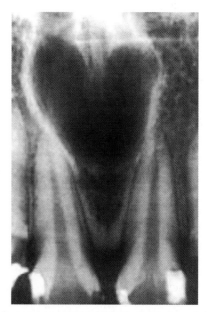

Fig. 35.12: Nasopalatine cyst is typically heart-shaped, between two vital maxillary central incisors

Treatment: Careful surgical enucleation is the line of treatment of nasopalatine duct cysts, by raising a palatal flap after taking an incision along the gingival margins of the teeth, or along the crest of the ridge in the edentulous patient, from canine to canine. The neurovascular bundle is salvaged, the cyst is carefully dissected free, from its bony bed. The flap is returned to its original position and closed by interrupted sutures through the interproximal spaces. Occasionally, an acrylic palatal stent helps in preventing swelling and hematoma formation.

Nonodontogenic Nonepithelial Bone Cysts (Cyst like Conditions)

Solitary Bone Cyst

The term cyst in relation to this lesion is controversial and probably a misnomer, also termed as *traumatic or hemorrhagic bone cyst.* it is not confined to the jaws, as similar lesions are seen elsewhere in the skeleton, commonly at the proximal ends of the humerus and upper and lower portions of the femoral and tibial shafts, where it is known as *unicameral bone cyst.*

Etiology: A number of theories have been forwarded, these include:
- Trauma and hemorrhage with failure of organization
- Spontaneous atrophy of the tissue in a central benign giant cell lesion
- Abnormal calcium metabolism
- Chronic low-grade infection
- Necrosis of fatty marrow secondary to ischemia
- Aberration in the development and growth of the local osseous tissue.

Incidence: The simple bone cyst is not a common lesion, and is seen in the first two decades of life. Lesions occur particularly in children and adolescents between 10 and 20 years of age. Males are affected more often than females, because of the increased exposure of the former to trauma. The relatively infrequent solitary bone cysts in the older age groups might support the theory that the cavities eventually tend to undergo a natural cure.

Site: It is rarely seen in the maxilla. Majority are seen in the subapical region, above the inferior dental canal, in the cuspid and molar region. Occasionally, a lesion may develop in the incisor region (Fig. 35.13(2)).

Clinical features: Usually symptomless and is detected as an incidental finding during a radiographic examina-

tion. The cortex is usually thinned but expansion occurs later on and may first involve the lingual aspect below the mylohyoid ridge where it may be overlooked. The associated teeth are vital, unless involved otherwise. Unerupted teeth usually molars, may be prevented from eruption.

Radiological features: The cyst appears as a unilocular cavity, which when it enlarges pushes up into the interdental bone between the teeth to produce a characteristically scalloped outline to the upper border around the roots of the teeth.

In the anterior region, the outline is usually regular and general shape is round or oval, with no indentations. The roots of related teeth may be displaced, lamina dura is intact; resorption is not seen. Distension of the outer or inner cortical plates is uncommon.

Pathology: When the cyst cavities are opened at operation, they are frequently found to be empty. No visible lining is generally seen, in some cases, a thin membrane, granulation tissue or blood clots may be evident. Loose vascular fibrous tissue membrane with hemosiderin pigment may be seen with small multinucleate cells. The adjacent bone, when included shows osteoclastic resorption on its inner surface.

Cystic contents (aspirate): Aspiration should be done carefully, a deep yellow colored fluid may be obtained. This contains plasma proteins and will clot, if left to stand. From small cysts, a heavily blood stained fluid or fresh blood may be obtained. Some cysts may be

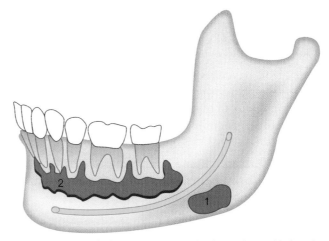

Fig. 35.13: (1) Stafne's idiopathic cavity is always located below the mandibular canal, near the angle of the mandible, (2) Solitary bone cyst is located above the mandibular canal and has a typical scalloped appearance as it often extends between the roots of the teeth

reported empty. It is suggested that they may contain gas such as 'nitrogen', 'oxygen' and 'carbon dioxide.'

Treatment: Surgical exploration is required for diagnosis and usually constitutes the treatment. Gentle curettage stimulates hemorrhage which results in rapid obliteration of the defect and eventual healing by new bone formation.

Stafne's Idiopathic Bone Cavity (Mandibular Salivary Gland Depression)

Although, Stafne's bone cavity is not a cyst, it is included because of their clinical similarity to cysts of the jaw bones and the frequent difficulty in differential diagnosis. It is also known as a *latent bone cyst or static bone cavity.*

Etiology: Various theories have been postulated that include:
- Stafne believed that such cavities are due to failure of the normal deposition of bone during development of the jaws, in an area formerly occupied by cartilage or because of failure of subperiosteal apposition at the lower border
- Developmental defects that are occupied by a lobe of normal submandibular salivary gland
- Close proximity of a lobe of submandibular salivary gland that produces a localized pressure atrophy of the lingual surface of the mandible
- Constricted remains of a solitary bone cyst
- Area of localized necrosis caused by repetitive minor pressure.

Incidence: Relatively uncommon, the largest series have been reported by Stafne (1942). Few defects have been reported in children, though majority have been reported in males over 40 years of age.

Site: They have been reported below the inferior alveolar canal, approximately in line with the position of the third molar tooth toward the inferior border of the mandible, generally unilateral, bilateral defects have been reported (Fig. 35.13(l).

Clinical features: These are symptomless lesions discovered during routine radiological examination, the lesions are nonprogressive.

Radiological features: The depression is rounded or oval, 1 to 3 cm in size and appears as a round or oval defect, below the inferior alveolar canal, posterior to the first mandibular molar. The area of rarefaction is well demarcated by a dense radiopaque line. At times, if the lesion has extended up to the inferior border then cortical bone perforation may be seen.

Pathology: These are idiopathic bone cavities and no diagnostic tissue can be mentioned. These cavities, in fact, are empty. Contrary, they may contain normal salivary gland tissue, lymph node tissue or abnormal glandular tissue.

Treatment: These idiopathic cavities are of no particular concern and once diagnosed as Stafne's cavity, no surgical intervention is warranted. Regular radiological follow up is advised, as they constitute an area of weakness and pathologic fracture can occur.

Aneurysmal Bone Cyst

The aneurysmal bone cyst was first described by Jaffe and Lichtenstein (1942). It is an uncommon hemorrhagic lesion of the bone. *The name is misleading, as it does not contain vascular aneurysm and it is not a true bone cyst.* Though often seen in the long bones and spine, it is rarely seen in the jaws (Figs 35.14 to 35.16). Previously, it has been described as an atypical giant cell tumor, hemorrhagic osteomyelitis, ossifying hematoma or benign bone cyst.

Jaffe and Lichtenstein described this entity with the word 'aneurysmal' to emphasize the 'blown out', distended contour of the affected bone, and the words 'bone cyst' to underscore that when the lesion is entered through a thin shell of bone, it appears largely as a blood filled cavity.

Etiology: Various theories have been postulated, which include the following:
- History of trauma
- Possible relationship with the giant cell lesion
- Variation in the hemodynamics of the area
- Sudden venous occlusion.

Incidence: It is rare, and reports of lesion in the jaws are limited, occurring most commonly in long bones (50 %), the pelvis and vertebrae (20%). In the jaw bones, they account for about 1.9 percent of all ABCs of the skeleton, and about 1.5 percent of all non odontogenic cysts of the jaws. There is no specific sex predilection. It is seen mainly in children, adolescents or young adults.

Site: It is more commonly seen in the mandible than the maxilla, more commonly in the posterior region than the anterior.

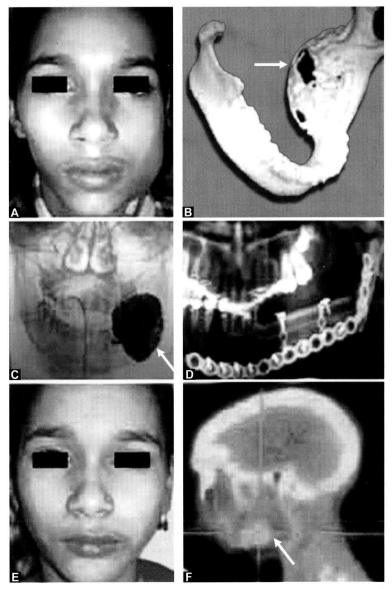

Figs 35.14A to F: Patient with aneurysmal bone cyst: (A) Preoperative frontal photograph, (B) 3D CT scan showing multiple perforations of buccal and lingual cortices, (C) Final glue cast showing glue occupying the lesion, (D) Panoramic radiograph showing fibula flap reconstruction of the mandible, (E) Postoperative frontal photograph, (F) SPECT scan suggesting increased radiotracer uptake at the reconstruction site

Clinical features: The lesions produce firm swellings, the patients may give a history of rapid enlargement, the teeth may show displacement, though they remain vital. Egg-shell crackling may be exhibited. Bruits are not heard and the lesion is not pulsatile.

Radiological features: The lesions are usually unilocular, they may be oval or spherical in shape, causing considerable ballooning of the cortex. They generally show a subperiosteal layer of new bone. At times internal ridges or incomplete septae may give a

multilocular appearance, also described as honey-comb or soap-bubble appearance. Teeth may be displaced and root resorption has been described. The outer cortical plate may be destroyed.

Cystic contents (aspirate): Dark venous blood can be aspirated.

Pathology: The aneurysmal bone cysts (ABCs) are benign, non-neoplastic, expansile, vascular, locally destructive lesions. *WHO classifies ABC as a tumor like lesion and defines it as an expanding osteolytic lesion*

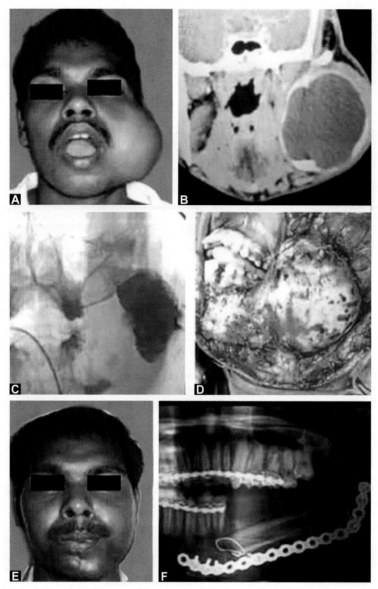

Figs 35.15A to F: Patient no. 2 with aneurysmal bone cyst: (A) Preoperative frontal photograph, (B) CT scan coronal section showing extension of the lesion, ballooning of the condylar and coronoid process, (C) Final glue cast showing glue occupying the lesion, (D) Surgical approach for the resection of the lesion, (E) Postoperative frontal photograph, (F) Panoramic radiograph showing fibula flap reconstruction of the mandible

consisting of blood filled spaces of variable sizes separated by connective tissue septa, containg trabeculae of osteoid tissue and osteoclast giant cells. Other solid areas may have the appearance of fibrous dysplasia, ossifying fibroma or may contain large numbers of multinucleate giant cells, fibroblasts, hemorrhage and hemosiderin.

Treatment: *Various treatment modalities have been reported for ABCs including observation and long term follow up, which may lead to spontaneous regression.*

Surgery is generally hampered by persistent bleeding, but ceases after all the vascular tissue has been removed. Curettage is the choice of treatment, though, incomplete removal in large lesions is liable to result in recurrence in 26 to 53 percent of the cases.

Local excision with bone grafting has been suggested in very large lesions. Radiotherapy is contraindicated as it may result in the occurrence of postradiation sarcoma.

The other methods include (1) curettage along with cryotherapy, (2) percutaneous intralesional calcitonin

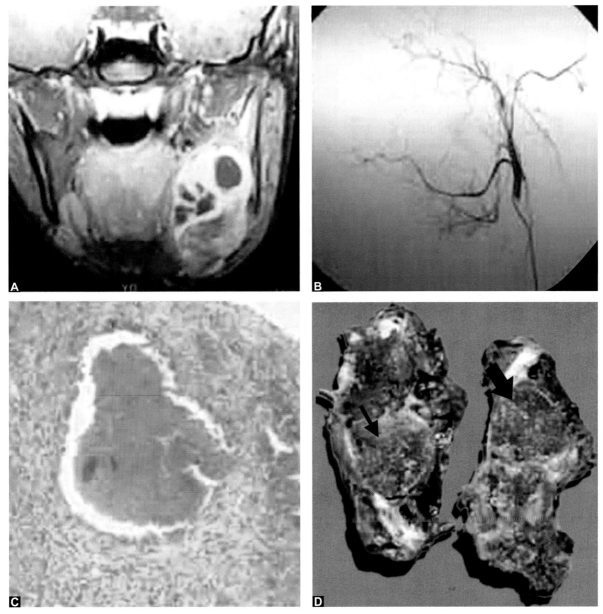

Figs 35.16A to D: Aneurysmal bone cyst: (A) T1-weighted MRI showing hypodense cystic areas separated by septae, (B) External carotid angiography revealing stretching of the facial artery with no vascularity of the lesion, (C) Histopathology showing cavernous spaces separated by septae. Aneurysmal bone cyst, (D) Photograph of the resected specimen showing glue (arrows) in the lesion

injections in combination with methylprednisolone, (3) intralesional injection of a fibrosing agent-Ethibloc-ethicon, (4) arterial embolization followed by en bloc resection.

1. During curettage, massive hemorrage may be encountered, which might require ligation of the external carotid artery as a precautionary measure. Cryosurgery can be supplemented with curettage to decrease the recurrence rate.

2. Intralesional calcitonin injections in combination with methylpredniisolone have been used, but this therapy needs long term repeated multiple injections and the response is unpredictable. The injections are thought to combine the inhibitory antistatic and fibroblastic effects of methylprednisolone with the osteoclastic inhibitory effect and trabecular bone-stimulating properties of calcitonin.

3. Intralesional injections of fibrosing agent may show complete involution or it can be used as an adjunct treatment, wherein the injections may help to limit the blood loss during surgery.

4. Transosseous intralesional embolization followed by en bloc resection. This modality was suggested by Malik and Vinay Kumar (2007) for handling large recurrent lesions to prevent recurrence and to reduce intraoperative massive bleeding. Here, adjunctive intralesional embolization is used preoperatively to decrease the vascularity of the lesion. Initial angiography via transfemoral approach was carried out to assess the feeder vessels and vascularity of the lesion. Percutaneous intralesional embolotherapy under constant fluoroscopic guidance was carried out with diluted n-butyl-cyanoacrylate glue (20 cc). Later on resection of the lesion was done and primary reconstruction using free fibula graft.

It has been reported that embolization occludes vascularity of the lesion, without interfering with the vascularity of the surrounding tissues, which may lead to involution of the soft tissue component. It also brings about sclerosis and ossification. This mineralization becomes apparent 2 to 3 months after embolization.

Cysts Associated with the Maxillary Antrum

Surgical Ciliated Cyst of the Maxilla

These cysts are highly uncommon. They may be labeled as iatrogenic cysts, as the patient will always give a previous history of some surgical procedure that was carried out in the maxilla where in the maxillary sinuses were opened surgically.

Etiology: The cysts develop from the epithelial lining of the maxillary sinus, which was trapped in the surgical incision during closure following a maxillary surgical procedure that involved the sinus lining, e.g. maxillary osteotomies, Caldwell-Luc, or maxillary fractures that had involved the antrum.

Site: The cystic lesion is present in close proximity to the maxillary sinus, but there is no communication between them, as has been proved with radio-opaque dyes.

Clinical features: Patients may complain, of a dull, localized pain in the maxilla; the cystic lesion is otherwise not associated with any tooth.

Radiological features: Radiographs will reveal a well-defined radiolucent expansion of the maxilla, with a radiopaque margin, that is closely related to the maxillary sinus. The cyst may appear to encroach upon the sinus, but in reality, is a separate entity.

Pathology: The cysts are lined by pseudostratified ciliated columnar epithelium.

Treatment: The cysts are best treated by surgical enucleation.

Benign Mucosal Cyst of the Maxillary Antrum

The other terms used for this cystic lesion are *'mucocele'* or *'retention cyst'* of the maxillary antrum.

Etiology: Most of these cysts have been reported to occur due to infection and inflammation of the ducts of the mucous glands.

Incidence: It has been reported commonly, in routine radiographs of the maxilla, with a higher incidence in the third decade.

Site: More commonly seen in the floor of the maxillary sinus, though the other walls also may be involved. Generally unilateral, though bilateral and sometimes multiple cysts may occur.

Clinical features: Majority of the cases are discovered accidentally on radiographs. Though some patients may complain of a dull pain over the antral region, while others may report a sense of fullness or numbness in the maxillary region.

If the lateral wall is involved or the cyst is large in size, then the patient may complain of a nasal obstruction. Others may report, yellowish discharge from the nose or complain of a postnasal drip. Large cysts may produce an obvious swelling in the maxillary region. The cyst is not associated with any teeth.

Radiological features: The cystic lesion is seen as spherical, ovoid, radiopacities within the maxillary antrum, that has a smooth uniform outline. When suspected on an intraoral radiograph, an orthopantomograph must be taken to confirm its existence.

Pathology: The cysts may or may not be lined by epithelium. The secretory type cysts are lined by pseudostratified, ciliated, columnar epithelium and contain mucin. Within the capsule and lumen, a large number of chronic inflammatory cells may be seen.

Treatment: In the symptomatic patient, it is advisable, to remove the cystic lesion via a Caldwell-Luc approach, and enhance drainage via cannulation through intranasal antrostomy, whereas in the asymptomatic patient, it would be best to follow up with periodic radiographs, as most cystic lesions remain static or undergo spontaneous regression with conservative medical treatment with antibiotics, decongestants and antral lavage.

■ SOFT TISSUE CYSTS OF THE ORAL CAVITY

Odontogenic (Developmental) Cysts

Gingival Cysts

The only specific criterion for these lesions is its location in the gingival tissues. There are two types of gingival cysts:

Gingival Cyst of the Adult

Etiology: The cysts possibly arise from:

- Remnants of the dental lamina or cell rests of Serres
- As traumatic implantation cysts
- From enamel organ or epithelial islands of the surface epithelium
- As cystic degeneration of deep projections of surface epithelium or
- Derived from glandular elements.

Incidence: It is relatively rare and has no sex predilection. It is known to occur in adults in the fifth or sixth decades.

Site: They occur more frequently in the mandible than in the maxilla. They appear particularly in the canine and premolar region of the mandible, rarely they may be seen in the anterior part of the jaw.

Clinical features: The cysts are seen in the attached gingiva or the interdental papilla on the labial aspect. The lesions are painless, slow growing swellings that have a smooth surface, may be of normal colour or bluish. They are soft and fluctuant and the adjacent teeth are vital. Occasionally, pressure from larger lesions may cause superficial cortical erosion.

Pathology: The cysts are lined by stratified squamous epithelium and usually contain fluid.

Treatment: Surgical excision is curative and there is no tendency for recurrence.

Gingival Cyst of Infants

Gingival cyst of infants are frequently referred to as *Bohn's nodules or Epstein's pearls.*

Etiology: The cysts arise from epithelial remnants of the dental lamina.

Incidence: Frequency of gingival cysts of neonates is high in newborn infants, but they are rarely seen after 3 months of age.

Site: Bohn's nodules are found on the buccal or lingual aspects of the dental ridges, whereas Epstein's pearls are seen along the midpalatine raphe and are considered to be of nonodontogenic origin.

Clinical features: They appear as discrete white swellings. They may be single or multiple and clinically resemble a mucocele.

Pathology: They have a thin lining of stratified squamous epithelium which may reveal parakeratinization and contain desquamated keratin.

Treatment: No treatment is required as they rupture spontaneously on eruption of the underlying teeth.

Nonodontogenic Fissural Cysts

Anterior Median Lingual Cyst

Incidence: It is a rare lesion, few cases have been reported. It is almost always present since birth.

Site: It is seen to involve the anterior two-thirds of the tongue.

Clinical features: At birth, a fluctuant swelling may be seen involving the anterior two-thirds of the dorsal surface of the tongue.

Pathogenesis: The anterior two-thirds of the tongue develops from paired processes, which develop on the back of the mandibular arch, it is reported that this cyst develops from epithelium entrapped between the lateral tubercles of the developing tongue.

Pathology: The epithelial lining is variable, it may be stratified squamous epithelium, pseudostratified ciliated columnar epithelium or cuboidal epithelium. It may show parakeratinization.

Treatment: Incision and drainage is followed by recurrence. The cyst should be enucleated.

Nasolabial Cyst

Strictly speaking the nasolabial cyst is a true soft tissue fissural cyst that does not occur within bone; therefore the term nasoalveolar is a misnomer, other designations suggested are nasoextra alveolar cyst, nasal vestibule cyst, nasal wing cyst and mucoid cyst of the nose.

Incidence: Nasolabial cysts are uncommon lesions with a wide age distribution. They are seen to occur in the third, fourth and fifth decades of life. They have been seen predominantly in the female sex.

Site: They are seen above the buccal sulcus under the ala of the nose, at the junction of the globular, the lateral nasal and the maxillary processes. They may be unilateral, but bilateral cases have been reported.

Clinical features: Majority of the cases are unilateral though bilateral lesions have been reported. A swelling is seen involving the lip, that lifts up the nasolabial fold and obliterates the labial sulcus. When it bulges into the inferior meatus, it may result in difficult breathing. The cysts are fluctuant and painless unless infected secondarily. Infected cysts may discharge into the nose or mouth.

Pathogenesis: Various hypotheses proposed are as follows:
- Remnants of the nasolacrimal duct
- Lower anterior portion of the mature nasolacrimal duct
- Mucous cysts arising from epithelium lining of the floor of the nose
- Mucous cysts within the mucous glands in the labial sulcus
- Sequestered epithelium from the depths of the groove between the maxillary and lateral nasal process.

Pathology: The epithelium is usually pseudostratified columnar, cuboidal or ciliated. It may be stratified squamous. Goblet cells are present.

Cystic contents (aspirate): The cyst contains straw-colored or whitish mucinous fluid.

Treatment: The cyst should be removed surgically by an intraoral approach. Care should be taken while separating the cystic lining from the nasal mucosa.

Retention (Salivary Glands) Cysts

a. Mucocele
b. Ranula.

Mucocele

Two types of distinct entities described are the *true retention cyst*, which is lined by epithelium and the other is the *mucous extravasation cyst*, which occurs because of the pooling of mucus. It does not have any epithelial lining and is surrounded by compressed connective tissue cells, in some cases only granulation tissue is present.

Etiology: Various reasons that have been forwarded are as follows:
- Obstruction of a salivary duct
- Trauma to a salivary duct which is either pinched or severed
- Trauma to the secretory acini
- Congenital atresia of submandibular duct orifices
- Cystic type of papillary cystadenoma.

Incidence: It is commonly seen in connection with the minor salivary glands. There is no predilection for age or sex. However, it has been reported that retention cysts occurred more frequently in older patients, whereas the extravasation cysts occur more commonly in the younger age group.

Site: Majority of mucoceles are seen to affect the lower lip. With the exception of the anterior half of the hard palate which is devoid of salivary glands. They can occur anywhere in the oral cavity, i.e. cheeks, ventral surface of the tongue, floor of the mouth, retromolar area.

Clinical features: Diagnosis of these cysts is not difficult, generally small in size, they appear as painless, superficial, well circumscribed, swellings on the mucosa. Often approximately, 1 to 2 mm in size. They do not exceed 1 to 2 cm in size. Dilemma in diagnosis may arise when they are deep seated. Fluctuation is positive. Color is variable, it may be translucent or bluish. The mucocele may rupture spontaneously, with the liberation of a viscous fluid. However, in a few days to weeks, additional fluid accumulates and the lesion reappears. This cycle of rupture, collapse and refilling may continue for months.

Pathology: The mucous extravasation cysts, do not have any epithelial lining, and are simply, poorly defined pools containing eosinophilic mucinous material and vacuolated macrophages, granulation tissue and condensed fibrous tissue, may be seen containing lymphocytes, polymorphonuclear leukocytes and eosinophils.

The retention cysts will be partly or completely lined by epithelium which may be of stratified squamous epithelium or of cuboidal cells or pseudostratified columnar epithelium, macrophages may be associated with the epithelium lining.

Treatment: Enucleation of mucoceles is frequently followed by recurrences. They are best treated by surgical excision together with the associated minor salivary gland tissue and surrounding connective tissue. The mucosal margins are then undermined and sutured in apposition.

Ranula

Ranula is a mucocele, that is present on the floor of the mouth, beneath the tongue. Owing to its resemblance to a frog's belly, it has been termed 'ranula'.

Two types have been identified, i.e. *superficial ranula and plunging ranula*.

Etiology: It has been reported that the majority of ranulas occur because of extravasation of mucous due to trauma to the excretory ducts of the sublingual salivary gland.
- *In the plunging type,* this extravasated mucus passes through the mylohyoid muscle and collects in the submandibular region.
- Dilated submandibular ducts could be a causative factor because of *atresia of submandibular duct orifices* is another theory.

Clinical features: A dome-shaped bluish swelling of a superficial ranula may be seen located laterally in the floor of the mouth beneath the tongue. The tongue may be raised or displaced as it enlarges. The swelling may cross the midline. At times, if the swelling is punctured or traumatized, a mucous secretion may be evident. In the 'plunging' type a fluctuant extraoral, submandibular swelling will be seen.

Treatment: Marsupialization results in recurrence. It is advisable to surgically remove the sublingual gland from an intraoral approach for both the superficial or plunging variety. This removes the secreting source and thereby avoids any recurrence.

Nonodontogenic (Developmental) Cysts of the Soft Tissues

Dermoid and Epidermoid Cysts

The *dermoid cyst* is a form of *cystic teratoma*, which is lined by epithelium and in addition reveals the presence of skin appendages, e.g. hair, sebaceous glands or teeth. The *epidermoid* cyst is also lined by epithelium but does not contain any skin appendages.

Incidence: It is uncommonly seen. Age of occurrence is in young adolescents, however, there is no sex predilection.

Pathogenesis: These are nonodontogenic developmental cysts that are thought to arise from epithelial rests persisting in the midline after fusion of the mandible and hyoid branchial arches, it is comprised of a combination of ectoderm, mesoderm and endodermal elements. In 5 percent of the cases, one of the tissue elements can become malignant.

Site: Lateral dermoids are rarely seen, median dermoids are seen in the midline in the floor of the mouth above the geniohyoid muscle or inferior to the geniohyoid muscle, which may be present, superior or inferior to the mylohyoid muscle.

Clinical features: Swellings may be seen as midline swellings or rarely as lateral swellings, in the floor of the mouth and neck. Those above the geniohyoid muscle, elevate the tongue, causing difficulty with mastication and speech. Those present inferior to the geniohyoid muscle, cause a submental swelling, that has been aptly described as a double chin. They are small in infancy but enlarge over the years to several centimeters in diameter. On palpation, a dough-like feel is appreciated (Figs 35.17A and B).

Pathology: Both the epidermoid and dermoid cysts are lined by keratinizing stratified squamous epithelium and contain keratin scales. The dermoid cysts are characterized by the presence of one or more dermal appendages in the wall, such as sebaceous glands, sweat glands, hair follicles, etc.

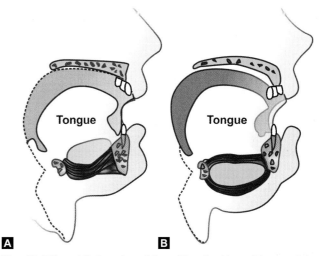

Figs 35.17A and B: Location of dermoid and epidermoid cysts of the oral cavity: (A) Dermoid cyst is visible, in the floor of the mouth, as it elevates the tongue and is present above the mylohyoid muscle, (B) Epidermoid cyst is seen as a submental swelling, as it is located below the mylohyoid muscle

Treatment: Surgical excision is the best line of treatment. For cysts present in the floor of the mouth an intraoral approach, is advisable. For very large cysts present inferior to the mylohyoid musle, an extraoral approach via a horizontal submandibular incision in the midline may be required for better access.

Lymphoepithelial Cysts

Branchial Cleft Cyst (Cervical/Intraoral)

Branchial arch remnants can give rise to cervical cysts, which are more common than intraoral branchial cysts, (Bhaskar, 1966).

Incidence: Overall this is not a common cystic lesion. They may occur at all ages, though they are frequently seen in the young adults between 20 and 40 years of age. There is no sex predilection. They are uncommon in children.

Site: The most common location is at the angle of the mandible anterior to the sternocleidomastoid muscle or the parotid region, less commonly they are seen in the floor of the mouth and the ventral surface of the tongue. Other sites of location are the soft palate, anterior palatine pillar and buccal vestibule.

Clinical features: The lesions vary in size. The neck lesions may reach a size of 10 cm. They are seen as a soft, fluctuant mass at or above cervical sites. Some may develop a fistulous tract and drain externally.

The *intraoral lesions* range in size from 1 to 10 mm. They are submucosal and freely mobile, often they may be confused as mucoceles, lipomas or irritation fibromas, at times, they may drain intraorally via a fistulous tract.

Pathogenesis: It has been postulated that these cysts develop from, either,
- Epithelial remnants of the branchial clefts and pouches
- Residual cervical sinus epithelium
- Salivary gland inclusions in parotid lymph nodes which undergo cystic changes
- Cystic changes within cervical lymph nodes of epithelial inclusions, hence the term benign lymphoepithelial cyst.

Pathology: The cervical cysts are lined by ciliated or nonciliated, pseudostratified columnar epithelium that may contain goblet cells, beneath the epithelium lymphoid tissue may be seen as typical germinal centers or a diffuse, dense infiltrate of lymphocytes. Lumen will contain mucus and desquamated parakeratolic cells.

Intraoral cysts are usually lined by stratified squamous epithelium and lumen will contain a watery fluid. Lymphoid tissue envelops the cystic lining.

Treatment: Aspiration or drainage of these cysts is followed by recurrence. They are best treated by complete surgical excision by a cervical or intraoral approach.

Thyroglossal Duct Cyst

Incidence: Being a relatively rare cystic lesion, there is no significant data regarding age or sex predilection. Although reports reveal highest incidence in infancy and in the second decade.

Site: It can occur anywhere in the midline along the course of the embryonic thyroglossal duct, which extends from the foramen cecum of the tongue into the deep fascia near the thyroid isthmus. Common sites of occurrence are floor of the mouth, area around the hyoid bone and thyroid cartilage region.

Pathogenesis: It is an uncommon developmental cyst. The thyroid gland rudiment develops around the fourth embryonic week, between the derivatives of the first and second branchial arches at the base of the tongue which is recognized later as the foramen cecum. A hollow stalk known as the thyroglossal duct, extends from this foramen cecum through the neck to the thyroid gland. By about the tenth week this duct breaks up and disappears, but cysts may form from residues of this duct at any point along its course.

Clinical features: Classically swellings are seen in the midline, slight lateral positional variations may be seen. On palpation the swellings are soft, tender and movable. Pathognomonic is the movement of the cyst during swallowing and protrusion of the tongue. At times they may cause dysphagia, dysphoria or dyspnea. The size may vary from 1 to 5 cm in diameter.

In 25 percent of cases an associated sinus tract may develop, due to infection. Disfigurement and recurrent infection are common complaints.

Pathology: The epithelial lining is variable, cysts present above the level of the hyoid bone are lined by stratified squamous epithelium while those present below the hyoid bone are lined by ciliated respiratory type or columnar epithelium. However, a single cyst may show different epithelium from one area to another. In the fibrous wall, lymphoid tissue, thyroid tissue or mucous glands may be seen.

Treatment: Complete radical surgical excision of the cyst along with its tract is essential to prevent recurrence. Owing to its proximity to the hyoid bone, a central part of the hyoid bone, approximately 1 to 2 cm may require to be removed during surgery.

Cystic Hygroma

The cystic hygroma, is a type of a lymphangioma, it is a developmental abnormality, in which cavernous lymphatic spaces communicate and form large thin-walled cysts that may grow to an impressive size.

Incidence: Typically they appear in the first few months of life, some may be diagnosed at birth or before the age of 2 years.

Site: Hygromas arise in the sites of primitive lymphatic lakes—on the floor of the mouth, under the jaw, in the neck and in the axillae—but can occur virtually anywhere in the body.

Clinical features: Hygromas that involve the facial tissues and neck produce a swelling that is painless and compressible, the swelling may increase in size over several months to a year, they may remain static or may even regress. The overlying skin may be bluish and transillumination will be positive. Hygromas, may suddenly enlarge when there is an upper respiratory infection presumably because of communication with the lymphatic system. This may cause acute respiratory obstruction and may require an emergency tracheostomy or surgical extirpation.

Pathology: Cystic hygroma consists of dilated cystic spaces lined by endothelial cells.

Treatment: Early excision is recommended, even in the newborn, because although they are not malignant, they tend to infiltrate into the local tissues in and amongst muscle fibers and nerves making them difficult and hazardous to remove at a later date.

There is no satisfactory nonsurgical treatment—a wide variety of sclerosing agents have been tried, unsuccessfully. Surgical extirpation is difficult and tedious. Every effort must be made to remove the cyst wall as completely as possible to avoid a recurrence.

Parasitic Cysts

Rarely parasitic cysts may be seen involving the oral tissues, e.g. hydatid cyst, which occurs in hydatid disease or echinococcosis and is caused by the larvae of *E. granulosus,* i.e. the dog tapeworm.

Cysticercosis of the oral tissues can develop because of the pork tapeworm, *Taenia solium.*

The spread to the oral tissues occurs when the larvae penetrate the intestinal mucosa and then are distributed through the blood vessels and lymphatics when they may get localized in the orofacial tissues.

Heterotopic Cysts

Oral Cysts with Gastric or Intestinal Epithelium

The occurrence of cysts in the oral cavity that may contain gastric or intestinal epithelium is extremely rare, owing to the paucity of reported cases, an analysis is lacking.

Incidence: Most of the cases have been in infants and young children.

Site: Sublingual region, apex and dorsum of the tongue, are the occasional sites of involvement.

Pathogenesis: The origin of these cysts is not defined, it has been hypothesized by Gorlin and Jirasek, that during intrauterine growth, in the 3 to 4 mm embryo the undifferentiated primitive stomach lies in the midneck region not far from the anlage of the tongue, it is quite possible that the ectodermal and endodermal epithelia fuse and mix which explains the cystic lesions in the oral cavity.

Pathology: The cysts are lined partly by stratified squamous epithelium and partly by gastric mucosa. Gastric glands, goblets cells may be seen, occasionally muscularis mucosa may be seen.

Treatment: Surgical excision is the best line of treatment.

General Principles of Treatment of Cysts of the Oral Cavity

Reasons for Treatment of Benign Cysts of the Oral Cavity

- Cysts tend to increase in size and produce facial disfigurement
- Cysts tend to get infected
- Cysts weaken the jaw and can cause pathological fractures
- Some cysts can undergo changes and it is not possible to be certain about a cystic lesion unless the tissue is examined histologically
- Cysts can prevent eruption of teeth—cause disturbance of dentition.

Clinical Presentation (Summary of Signs/Symptoms)

- Before expansion of the jaw is noticeable, most cysts are discovered accidentally on radiographs
- In case of a smooth, rounded expansion of the jaw bones, a cyst should be suspected until proved other-wise
- A change in the fitting of dentures in the presence of a swelling should give rise to the suspicion of a cyst/tumor
- Absence of a tooth from its place in the arch suggests the presence of a dentigerous cyst, particularly in the young
- Presence of a carious, discolored, fractured or heavily filled tooth related to the swelling is suggestive of an apical periodontal cyst
- Tilting of the crowns of the teeth suggests that their roots have been displaced by the expansion of a cyst/tumor
- On extraction of a tooth with a sizeable radicular cyst, cystic fluid may escape from the socket
- Infected cysts may present as painful, tender swellings and may already have discharging sinuses
- Percussion of the teeth overlying a solitary bone cyst produces a dull or hollow sound
- Fissural cysts are generally small in size
- Periodontal cysts, occur anywhere in the dental arch
- Dentigerous cysts are mainly associated with impacted third molars, canines and premolars
- Solitary bone cyst is virtually assigned to the mandible
- Static bone cavity is located beneath the inferior dental canal
- Large cysts usually deflect the neurovascular bundle, paresthesia and anesthesia is rare
- Infected cysts may cause some degree of neuropraxia of the nerve
- As a cyst enlarges a smooth, hard, painless prominence generally on the labial side is seen
- Expansion of the lingual aspect alone can occur with an odontogenic cyst in the ramus or third molar region
- Expansion of both cortical plates is generally indicative of a lesion, other than a cyst
- *Egg-shell crackling* is a term used to describe the fragile outer shell of bone that has thinned out due to the expansion and the sensation and sound produced is like egg-shell crackling
- *Fluctuation* is elicited when the cystic lining lies immediately beneath the mucosa.

Vitality of Teeth

It is essential to perform preoperative and postoperative vitality tests on all teeth related to the cyst regardless of the method of treatment:

- Teeth adjoining primordial cyst, fissural cyst, solitary bone cyst and other nonodontogenic cysts will have vital pulps, unless there is coincidental disease of these teeth
- Apical periodontal cysts are associated with non-vital tooth/teeth
- Lateral periodontal cyst is involved with a vital tooth
- In infected cysts, there may be a temporary absence of a vital response in adjacent teeth, because of pressure interference with sensory transmission from the pulp.

Radiographic Examination

- Periapical radiographs provide a clear and accurate image of small cystic lesions
- Occlusal films of the maxilla, will disclose the amount of palatal bone destruction by a cystic process
- An occlusal view of the mandible, will reveal the expansion of the inner or outer cortical plates
- Extraoral radiographs, provide the full extent of the cystic lesion and help in assessing the damage caused to the adjacent structures, e.g. oblique lateral views, orthopantomographs. PA mandible view helps to reveal both lateral and medial expansion of the ramus. It is also helpful for disclosing a posterior antral cyst
- Anterior cysts of the antrum are best visualized in the Water's projection
- CT scans may be helpful in the assessment of large cystic lesions and multicystic lesions
- In multilocular lesions, differential diagnosis with other multicystic formation such as giant cell lesions, myxomas, hemangiomas and ameloblastomas should be considered.

Radiopaque Dyes

When the size and relations of a cyst are in doubt/its contents may be aspirated and radiopaque dye, e.g. lipiodol, triosil, can be injected prior to further radiography. Injections of radiopaque solution should not be given with great force. Care should be taken to avoid over flow into the soft tissues. After essential radiographs are taken, it is advisable to remove the contrast material by aspiration; remainder of the dye will disperse and be absorbed.

Contrast medium is also useful to follow the progress of regression of a marsupialized lesion.

Aspiration

Aspiration is a valuable diagnostic aid, which may be helpful in distinguishing between a maxillary cyst and the maxillary sinus, between a cystic lesion and a solid tumor mass, between an aneurysmal bone cyst and a central cavernous hemangioma and further it would help in distinguishing various cysts (Table 35.2).

After application of topical anesthesia or after infiltrating a small amount of local anesthetic solution into the overlying mucosa, aspiration is done with a wide bore needle (18 gauge) and a 5 or 10 ml syringe.

A failure to aspirate liquid usually means that a solid tumor is present.

Biopsy

Is a valuable diagnostic aid, in the differential diagnosis of the nature of the cyst or the differentiation in the basic diagnosis between a cyst or tumor. Biopsy is generally performed under local anesthesia or conscious sedation. Care should be taken to place the biopsy incision in such a manner, keeping in mind future surgical exposure, that it will facilitate accurate closure and prevent the setting in of infection, which may delay treatment. The material is then despatched to the pathologist for histopathological examination.

Biopsy prior to surgery is generally advisable for large cystic lesions and when doubt exists.

Assessment: This includes the following:
- Estimation of the size of the cystic lesion
- Extent of bone loss
- Should there be risk of pathological fracture, preparation for suitable splints or IML (intermaxillary ligation) or planning for immediate grafting
- Relationship of the cyst to adjacent structures, i.e. floor of the nose, maxillary sinus, inferior dental nerve, infraorbital nerve, floor of the orbit
- Vital teeth, that have a satisfactory periodontal condition and are functional should be preserved
- Nonvital teeth, which are embedded in sound bone, should be treated by root canal filling and apicoectomy

	Table 35.2: Various aspirates	
Pathology	*Aspirate*	*Other findings of aspirate*
1. Dentigerous cyst	Clear pale, straw colored fluid	Cholesterol crystals
		Total protein in excess of 4.0 g per 100 ml (resembling serum)
2. Keratocystic odontogenic tumor	Dirty, creamy white viscoid suspension	Parakeratinized epithelium
		Total protein less than 5.0 g per 100 ml most of which is albumin
3. Periodontal cysts	Clear, pale yellow straw colored fluid	Varying amounts of cholesterol crystals
		Total protein content is between 5 and 11g per 100 ml
4. Infected cyst	Pus or brownish fluid, seropurulent/ sanguinopurulent fluid, at times paste like or caseous consistency	Polymorphonuclear leukocytes
		Foam cells
		Cholesterol clefts
5. Mucocele, ranula	Mucus	
6. Gingival cysts	Clear fluid	
7. Solitary bone cyst	Serous or sanguineous fluid, blood or empty cavity	Necrotic blood clot
8. Stafne's bone cavity	Empty cavity will yield air	
9. Dermoid cysts	Thick sebaceous material	
10. Fissural cysts	Mucoid fluid	
11. Vascular cyst walls	Fresh blood	
12. Intramedullary cavernous hemangioma	Syringe full of venous blood	
13. Arterial or arteriovenous malformation	Bright red blood Pulsatile, pushes plunger	

- Nonvital teeth which are nonfunctional, mobile and beyond restoration should be extracted
- If bone loss is going to be extensive as in surgical excision, then, consent and preparation for rehabilitation methods such as reconstructive plates, bone grafts and use of other materials, e.g. hydroxyapatite crystals, should be planned
- Acutely infected cysts should be treated with antibacterial drugs, or even drainage prior to surgery should be considered.
- In case of multicystic lesions, efforts should be made to identify a possible syndrome
- Postoperative monitoring of teeth by vitality tests should be done until bone formation is complete.

Operative Procedures

Cysts of the jaws, may be treated by one of the following basic methods:

1. Marsupialization (decompression)
   - Partsch I
   - Partsch II (combined marsupialization and enucleation)
   - Marsupialization by opening into nose or antrum.
2. Enucleation
   - Enucleation and packing
   - Enucleation and primary closure
   - Enucleation and primary closure with reconstruction/bone grafting.

Marsupialization (Decompression)

Principle: *Marsupialization, (Partsch) or decompression, refers to creating a surgical window in the wall of the cyst, and evacuation of the cystic contents.* This process decreases intra-cystic pressure and promotes shrinkage of the cyst and bone fill. The only portion that is removed is the piece removed to produce the window.

Indications

- *Age:* In a young child, with developing tooth germs, or when development of the displaced teeth has not progressed, enucleation would damage the tooth buds.
- In the elderly, debilitated patient, marsupialization, is less stressful and a reasonable alternative.
- *Proximity to vital structures:* When proximity of the cyst to vital structures, could create an oronasal or oroantral fistula, injure neurovascular structures or damage vital teeth, then marsupialization should be considered.

- *Eruption of teeth:* In a young patient with a dentigerous or pseudofollicular keratocyst, marsupialization will permit the eruption of the unerupted tooth or any other developing teeth that have been displaced.
- *Size of cyst:* In very large cysts, where enucleation, could result in a pathological fracture, marsupialization, can be accomplished, through a more limited bony opening.
- *Vitality of teeth:* When the apices of many adjacent erupted teeth, are involved within a large cyst, enucleation could prejudice the vitality of these teeth.

Advantages

- Simple procedure to perform
- Spares vital structures
- Allows eruption of teeth
- Prevents oronasal, oroantral fistulae
- Prevents pathological fractures
- Reduces operating time
- Reduces blood loss
- Helps shrinkage of cystic lining
- Allows for endosteal bone formation to take place.
- Alveolar ridge is preserved.

Disadvantages

- Pathologic tissue is left *in situ*
- Histologic examination of the entire cystic lining is not done
- Prolonged healing time
- Inconvenience to the patient
- Prolonged follow up visits
- Periodic irrigation of cavity
- Regular adjustments of plug
- Periodic changing of pack
- Secondary surgery may be needed
- Formation of slit-like pockets that may harbor foodstuffs
- Risk of invagination and new cyst formation.

Surgical Technique

Partsch I

- *Anesthesia:* The administration of general anesthesia/conscious sedation or simple local anesthesia of the area
- *Aspiration:* Cystic contents are aspirated.
- *Incisions: Types:*
  - A circular, oval or elliptic incision can be taken, 1 cm or larger in size leaving a margin of 0.5 to 1 cm from the gingival margins of the teeth or alveolar crest in the edentulous patient.

– Alternatively, an inverted U-shaped incision can be taken with a broad base toward the buccal sulcus, the mucoperiosteum is then reflected in this case (Figs 35.18A and B).

• *Removal of bone*: Thin bone—When the bone is expanded and thinned out, the initial incision can be extended through the mucoperiosteum, bone and cystic lining into the cystic cavity. The cystic lining and contents are then submitted for histological examination (Fig. 35.18C).

• *Thick bone:* When the overlying bone is thick, bur holes are drilled in a circular shape, which are then connected and the overlying bone is removed carefully with a pair of rongeurs or mosquito forceps.

• *Removal of cystic lining specimen:* The cystic lining is then removed by stabbing a scalpel through the lining against the bone edge, the specimen of lining is then sent for histological examination.

• *Visual examination of residual cystic lining*

• *Irrigation of the cystic cavity*

• *Suturing:* The remaining cystic lining is sutured with the edge of the oral mucosa by continuous sutures or interrupted sutures (Fig. 35.18D).

Alternatively, when a U-shaped incision is taken, then the mucoperiosteal flap which is based on the buccal sulcus can be turned into the cyst cavity covering the margin. The remaining perimeter is sutured to the oral mucosa. It does not matter if the flap overlaps the lining as the cyst epithelium will be destroyed.

• *Packing:* The cavity is then packed with a half or one inch width ribbon gauze, which may be impregnated with an antibiotic ointment, White head's varnish, tincture of benzoin or bismuth iodoform paraffin paste (BIPP). The pack helps to prevent contamination of the cavity with food debris and also provides coverage of the wound margins. With the help of a nontoothed forceps, the ribbon gauze is first laid along the floor of the cavity and is then inserted running from side to side. All packs are generally secured by sutures. The pack is left inside for 7 to 14 days. By the end of 2 weeks, the junction between the lining of the cyst and the oral mucosa around the periphery of the window will have healed (Fig. 35.18E).

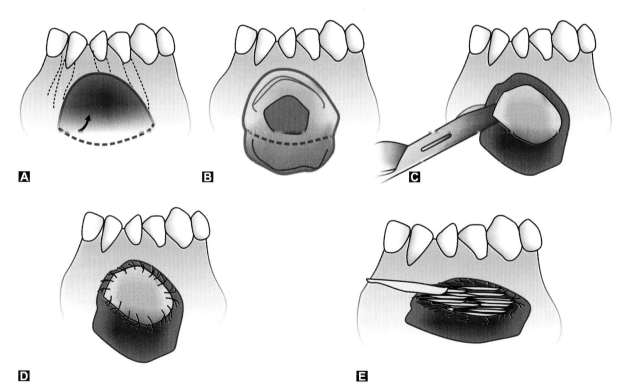

Figs 35.18A to E: Surgical procedure of marsupialization of a cyst in the mandible: (A) U-shaped incision taken on the buccal aspect, (B) Mucoperiosteal flap reflected and bony window created to uncover the cyst, (C) Cystic lining incised with scalpel, portion removed for histopathological examination, (D) Lining sutured to edge of mucosa, U-shaped flap can be tucked into the cavity or excised, (E) Cavity packed with roller gauze

- *Maintenance of cystic cavity:* Careful instructions are given to the patient regarding cleansing and irrigation of the cavity by regular flushing with an oral antiseptic rinse, preferably with a disposable syringe.
- *Use of plug:* A plug may be designed to prevent the contamination of the cystic cavity and preserve the patency of the cyst orifice. The plug should be stable, retentive and of a safe design so that it cannot be inhaled or swallowed. Initially, a plug should be made of a resilient material to avoid irritation to the raw margins, later a well fitting acrylic plug can be made, after taking an impression of the cavity with modelling wax or impression compound. In case of dentures, the plug can be attached to it. The plug may be vented to prevent a pressure build up.
- *Healing:* The cavity may or may not obliterate totally. With time, some degree of a permanent depression remains in the alveolar process.

Modifications of Marsupialization

- ***Waldron's method (1941) or Partsch II:*** This is a two stage technique that combines the two standard procedures, in which, first marsupialization is performed and at a later stage, when the cavity becomes smaller, the procedure of enucleation is performed and the entire tissue is examined histopathologically.

Indications

- Bone has covered the adjacent vital structures
- Adequate bone fill has strengthened the jaw to prevent fracture during enucleation
- Patient finds it difficult to clean the cavity
- For detection of any occult pathologic condition.

Advantages

- Development of a thickened cystic lining, which makes enucleation easier
- Spares adjacent vital structures
- Combined approach reduces morbidity
- Accelerated healing process
- Allows histopathological examination of residual tissue.

Disadvantages

- Patient has to undergo secondary surgery and the possible complications that are involved with any surgical procedure.

Marsupialization by Opening into Nose or Antrum

Advantages

- Primary closure of the oral wound
- Cystic cavity is opened into the maxillary sinus or nasal cavity, thereby reducing intracystic pressure
- Cystic cavity becomes lined with respiratory maxillary sinus or nasal cavity
- Adjacent structures are protected
- Restoration of the normal anatomy of the antral space and nose.

Disadvantages

- Development of an oroantral or oronasal fistula, if there is a breakdown of the wound.

Surgical technique: Cysts that have destroyed a large portion of the maxilla and have encroached on the antrum or nasal cavity, then the cyst is approached from the buccal aspect of the alveolar region.

A gingival curvilinear incision is taken along the involved teeth. Two releasing incisions are made at either end at a 45° angle and extending into the buccal sulcus. Depending upon the status of the teeth, they are either extracted or endodontically treated. A mucoperiosteal flap is raised with a Howarth's periosteal elevator. Generally, in large cysts, an opening already exists in the buccal cortical bone, otherwise, it may need to be enlarged with a pair of rongeurs taking care to avoid damage to adjacent structures such as the infraorbital nerve and the underlying cystic lining.

At this stage, a window is made by removing a portion of the cystic lining as described in the Partsch–I technique, alternatively, it is advocated that the entire cystic lining can be enucleated in one piece.

A second unroofing is then performed by removing the antral lining present between the two cavities. Thus, providing continuity between the cavities. This allows the cyst cavity to become lined with normal ciliated and mucus secreting epithelium regenerating from the respiratory mucosa rather than a squamous epithelium. If the cystic lining has not been removed in toto, then by this technique, it becomes continuous with the lining of the antrum or nasal cavity. Additionally, an intra-nasal antrostomy may be performed. The cavity may be packed with a ribbon gauze soaked with tincture of benzoin or an antibiotic ointment or an antral balloon. This helps to prevent the formation of a postoperative hematoma. The flap is them replaced and a water-tight primary closure is done (Figs 35.19A and B).

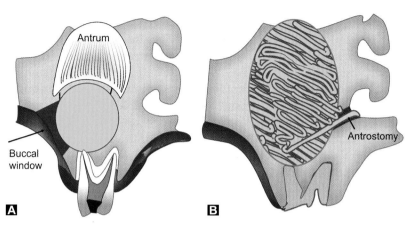

Figs 35.19A and B: Large maxillary cyst extending into the antrum: (A) Cyst approached, buccally a bony window is created, involved tooth is treated endodontically or removed, (B) Portion between cyst and antrum is completely removed. A large nasal antrostomy made, cavity is packed with ribbon gauze

Enucleation

Principle: Enucleation allows for the cystic cavity to be covered by a mucoperiosteal flap and the space fills with blood clot, which will eventually organize and form normal bone.

Indications
- Treatment of odontogenic primordial cysts
- Recurrence of cystic lesions of any cyst type

Advantages
- Primary closure of the wound
- Healing is rapid
- Postoperative care is reduced
- Thorough examination of the entire cystic lining can be done.

Disadvantages
- After primary closure, it is not possible to directly observe the healing of the cavity as with marsupialization
- In young persons, the unerupted teeth in a dentigerous cyst will be removed with the lesion
- Removal of large cysts will weaken the mandible, making it prone to jaw fracture
- Damage to adjacent vital structures
- Pulpal necrosis.

Surgical Technique
- *Enucleation and packing:* This technique if advocated, when it is believed that due to a previous infection or in infected large cysts, a primary closure would be

unsuccessful as it could lead to a breakdown of the wound; or where there is difficulty in approximating the wound edges. In such instances, enucleation is performed and then the cavity is packed as in marsupialization. The wound heals with granulation tissue until epithelialization is complete.
- This method is also used as a secondary measure, when there is a dehiscence after primary closure.

Enucleation with Primary Closure

Surgical Technique

1. *Enucleation of small cystic lesions from an intraoral approach:* Surgery can be performed under local anesthesia, conscious sedation or general anesthesia by an intraoral approach (Figs 35.20A to C).

Incision is carried around the necks of the involved teeth and the adjoining teeth on either side, so that the flap will lie on sound bone. In case of the edentulous patient, incision is placed on the alveolar crest, down to bone. Releasing incisions are given at either ends, which extend into the buccal sulcus, so that the base of the flap is broader. Depending upon the location of the cyst, incision is placed buccally or palatally. A three sided flap also termed as an envelope flap or trapezoidal flap is reflected (Fig. 35.20D). Reflection of the flap is done with a periosteal elevator beginning from under the periosteum of the anterior buccal incision, working parallel to the gingival margin to detach the papillae and push distally (Fig. 35.20E). In certain areas, where a sinus tract may be present or where the cyst has eroded through the cortex and is lying in contiguity with the periosteal layer, reflection may prove to be difficult. Bone is then removed to expose the underlying cystic lesion. In some instances, a window in the bone may already exist, this is expanded with the help of a rongeur. In cases, where the bone is intact, a broad opening is made with the help of a chisel mallet or bone burs. At times, a thin layer of fragmented bone is evident on raising the flap, these tiny pieces are carefully peeled off. The underlying cystic lining is separated with the help of a mosquito forceps and periosteal elevator (Fig. 35.20F).

The underlying cyst lining is now gently eased away from the cavity wall with the help of curved curettes, Mitchell's trimmer or a periosteal elevator. The instrument is applied in such a manner that the concave surface faces the cystic lining (Fig. 35.20G). Care should be taken to prevent rupture of the lining. In areas, where the cystic lining is adherent, a peanut gauze held in the beaks of a hemostat and inserted between the lining and the bony bed, helps to release the cystic lining. Alternately, the cystic contents can be aspirated, so that the size of the sac shrinks and visibility improves. In case of mandibular cysts, separation from the neurovascular bundle is done along the length of the nerve, never across it, or from inside the cyst. The same is applicable for maxillary cysts involving the infraorbital nerve. Difficulty may be encountered when peeling the cyst off the apices of the teeth within the cyst. As far as possible, the cyst should be removed in one piece (Fig. 35.20H).

Teeth that required to be removed are now extracted. In case of endodontically restored teeth, apicoectomy is done and their apices are sealed. Root apices other than planned, if they get exposed during surgery may later require to be filled endodontically. The cyst cavity is then inspected, any residual remnants are removed separately with a mosquito artery forceps. Any tears in the nasal mucosa or antral mucosa are sutured with 3-0 catgut or other absorbable suture materials. Bleeding points are arrested with the help of pressure packs, bone wax, gelfoam, surgical diathermy. Wound is now flushed with normal saline and an antiseptic solution such as povidone-iodine (2%) (Fig. 35.20I).

The cavity may be left to heal or various filling materials have been recommended for packing to obliterate the cavity prior to closure, e.g. resorbable sponge, hydroxylapatite crystals, autogenous bone chips, allogenous bone powder, etc.

The flap is now replaced and interdental sutures are given (Fig. 35.20J).

2. *Enucleation of large, inaccesible mandibular lesions from an extraoral approach:* Large cystic lesions like the pseudofollicular dentigerous cysts that involve the ascending ramus, body and angle mandible are best accessible from an extraoral approach.

Surgery is performed under general anesthesia. Local infiltration is done with normal saline and adrenaline in the concentration of 1:300, 000, this helps in local hemostasis and definition of tissue planes. A submandibular incision, which may at times be required to extend into the postramal region, is taken 1.5 to 2 cm below the inferior border of the mandible. The incision extends through skin and subcutaneous tissues. Blunt and sharp dissection is carried out layerwise through tissue planes, i.e. superficial cervical fascia, platysma and deep cervical fascia. Care is taken to salvage the marginal mandibular nerve, facial artery and vein are clamped and ligated.

Small bleeders are cauterized with a diathermy. The pterygomasseteric sling is divided, the periosteum is incised down to bone and the flap is raised superiorly to expose the underlying bone. Commonly, a bony window already exists, which is then enlarged as described earlier. If not, a suitably sized window is created with a chisel and mallet or bone burs to expose the underlying cystic lining.

Depending upon the extent of the cystic lesion and involvement of surrounding tissues, the surgical procedure of enucleation or marginal excision is performed as advocated by Bramley.

The tissue is sent for histopathological examination. The wound is then inspected. Any remnants of tissue are curretted out as the cystic lining is often thin and easily fragmented. A sharp curette or a bone bur, e.g. a vulcanite round bur with constant sterile irrigation is used to remove a 1 to 2 mm layer of bone around the complete periphery of the cyst cavity.

Stoelinga has advocated the use of Carnoy's solution to reduce the percentage of recurrence of the cysts. The cavity is then cleansed and closed in layers. In very large cysts beyond 4 to 5 cms in size, it is advisable to maintain a vacuum drain in place through the submandibular skin where it is fixed in place. This helps to reduce the dead space and prevents hematoma formation. Deeper layers are sutured with absorbable sutures, skin is approximated with interrupted sutures,

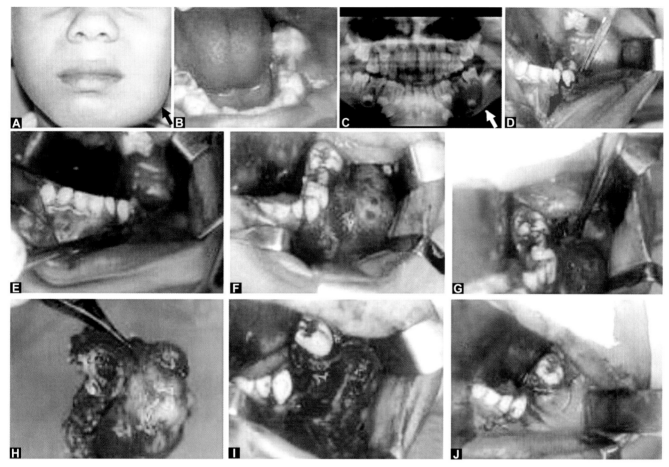

Figs 35.20A to J: Radicular cyst: (A) Extraoral swelling on left side mandible, (B) Intraoral view, buccal expansion and carious 75, (C) Unilocular radiolucency, carious 75, resorption of roots, developing tooth buds, (D) Incision, (E) Mucoperiosteal flap being raised, (F) Cyst exposed, (G) Cyst lining being separated from cavity wall, (H) Entire cyst removed with carious tooth, (I) Wound defect, (J) Wound sutured primarily

vertical mattress sutures or subcuticular sutures for an esthetic scar. The drain is left in place for 48 to 72 hours. Pressure dressing is given.

3. *Enucleation and primay closure with reconstruction/bone grafting:* In large cystic lesions that have perforated and destroyed the cortical plates and inferior border of the mandible that is beyond salvage or is nonexistent. It is advisable to reconstruct primarily with a stainless steel or titanium reconstructive plate. Occasionally, autogenous bone grafts, e.g. iliac crest or costochondral grafts can be used for reconstruction procedures, replacing the lost bone. A water tight closure has to be achieved both intra- and extraorally. Intermaxillary ligation is necessary to help provide immobilization during the healing phase for 4 to 6 weeks.

Complications of cystic lesions
- Fracture (pathological)
- Infection prior to surgery may be acute or chronic
- Postoperative wound dehiscence
- Loss of vitality of teeth
- Neuropraxia in infected cysts
- Postoperative infection
- Recurrence in some cysts
- Dysplastic, neoplastic or even malignant changes.

Suggested follow up
- Long term follow up, at least up to 8 years for primordial cysts for early detection of dealing with any recurrence
- To check postoperative vitality of teeth
- Unerupted teeth that may require orthodontic assistance for eruption

- Orthodontic assistance for alignment of displaced teeth
- Long term follow up of patients with Gorlin's syndrome.

ACKNOWLEDGMENT

For aneurysmal bone cyst cases—Dr Malik and Dr Vinay Kumar would like to acknowledge: *Dr Amresh **S Baliarsing***, Professor and Head, Department of Plastic and Reconstructive Surgery, King Edward Memorial Hospital, Parel, Mumbai, India for carrying out the reconstructive procedures. We would also like to thank Dr *Uday Limaye* and Dr Manish Kumar Srivastava, Department of Interventional Neuroradiology, King Edward Memorial Hospital, Parel, Mumbai, India for carrying out the arteriography and embolization procedures.

36 Benign Tumors of the Jaw Bones

Tumors or neoplasms are new growths of abnormal tissue in the body. They are broadly divided into two groups—benign and malignant, depending upon their behavior pattern and cellular structure. *A benign tumor* grows slowly and is usually encapsulated and it enlarges by peripheral expansion, pushes away the adjoining structures and exhibits no metastasis, however, it may be locally aggressive. *A malignant tumor*, rapidly infiltrates the surrounding tissues, including vital structures and endangers the life of its host. It also shows metastasis in the distant parts of the body usually through lymph and blood streams.

The benign jaw tumors are divided into two broad categories:

i. Odontogenic tumors
ii. Nonodontogenic tumors.

ODONTOGENIC TUMORS

The human odontogenic structures are formed by the inductive interactions between epithelium and mesenchyme. The formation of these structures begin during 5th and 6th week of intrauterine life and continues till about 16th year after birth. During this long period, there is always a possibility of odontogenic lesions developing from these tissues exists; resulting in the development of malformations, hemartomas and neoplasms.

Whenever such lesions are discovered in the oral cavity, clinically or radiologically, the distinctions among these three forms should be made on the basis of clinical and histologic studies.

A *malformation*: It is not neoplastic, but it can cause a functional or esthetic problem, because of its size or anatomical site.

A *hemartoma*: It is a benign lesion composed of a new growth of mature cells on existing blood vessels. (A lesion resulting from faulty development of the embryo).

A *benign odontogenic cyst or self-limiting tumor*: It may show an aggressive or malignant transformation. Therefore, management of such a lesion is always surgical. The surgical modality will vary for individual lesion depending on biological behavior and growth potential of the lesion.

Classification of Benign Odontogenic Tumors

The permutation of different cells of different origin makes the odontogenic tumors a highly complicated group of lesions. Odontogenic tumors are not all neoplasms in the strict sense as some are of a hemartomatous or malformation like nature. In 1946, *Thoma* and *Goldman*, described a classification of odontogenic tumors, based on the tissue cell of origin. It described the induction effects of one tissue (epithelium) on another (mesenchyme) in the pathogenesis of odontogenic tumors. They put these tumors into three broad groups:

i. The lesions primarily derived from epithelium
ii. Those originated predominantly from mesenchyme
iii. A mixed group—both epithelial and mesenchymal tissue shared in the formation of a lesion.

Kramer, Pindborg, Shear in 1992, revised the classification of odontogenic tumors (WHO classification—Table 36.1). This classification is based on embryologic principles, that is, the embryonal inductive influence that the cells of one tissue exert upon the cells of another tissue. In the odontogenic tumors, the tissues are either derived from the ectoderm, namely the enamel organ or the mesenchyme proper (mesoderm). In this classification, the principle of ectomesenchyme was

---

Table 36.1: Classification of benign odontogenic tumors (Kramer, Pindborg, Shear, 1992)

A. *Odontogenic epithelium without odontogenic ectomesenchyme*
   1. Ameloblastoma
   2. Calcifying epithelial odontogenic tumor (CEOT). Pindborg tumor
   3. Clear cell odontogenic tumor
   4. Squamous odontogenic tumor

B. *Odontogenic epithelium with odontogenic ectomesenchyme, with or without dental hard tissue formation*
   1. Ameloblastic fibroma
   2. Ameloblastic fibrodentinoma (dentinoma)
   3. Odontoameloblastoma
   4. Adenomatoid odontogenic tumor (AOT)
   5. Complex odontome
   6. Compound odontome

C. *Odontogenic ectomesenchyme with or without inclusion of odontogenic epithelium*
   1. Odontogenic fibroma
   2. Myxoma (odontogenic myxoma, myxofibroma)
   3. Benign cementoblastoma (true cementoma)

Table 36.2: Histological classification—WHO 2005

Classification of benign odontogenic tumors

A. *Odontogenic epithelium with mature, fibrous stroma without odontogenic ectomesenchyme*
   1. Ameloblastoma, solid/multicystic type
   2. Ameloblastoma, extraosseous/peripheral type
   3. Ameloblastoma, desmoplastic type
   4. Ameloblastoma, unicyclist type
   5. Squamous odontogenic tumor
   6. Calcifying epithelial odontogenic tumor (CEOT)
   7. Adenomatoid odontogenic tumor (AOT)
   8. Keratocystic odontogenic tumor (KCOT)

B. *Odontogenic epithelium with odontogenic ectomesenchyme, with or without hard tissue formation*
   1. Ameloblastic fibroma
   2. Ameloblastic fibrodentinoma
   3. Ameloblastic fibro-odontoma
   4. Odontoma
   5. Odontoma, complex type
   6. Odontoma, compound type
   7. Odonto-ameloblastoma
   8. Calcifying cystic odontogenic tumor
   9. Dentinogenic ghost cell tumor

C. *Mesenchyme and/or odontogenic ectomesenchyme with or without odontogenic epithelium*
   1. Odontogenic fibroma
   2. Odontogenic myxoma/myxofibroma/fibromyxoma
   3. Cementoblastoma

---

introduced. The ectomesenchyme is derived from cells of the neural crest during an early phase in embryogenesis.

In 2005, WHO put forward a new classification, which is known as histological classification (Table 36.2). In this classification, the term odontogenic keratocyst (OKC), which was considered as primordial cystic lesion earlier, is redesignated as keratocystic odontogenic tumor (KCOT) and is newly introduced. This entity will be discussed at the end of this chapter. as a special new reclassified lesion.

Earlier Pindborg and Clausen had proposed a classification (1958) of odontogenic tumors based on embryologic principles, which was modified by Gorlin in 1961 (Table 36.3).

◼ NONODONTOGENIC TUMORS

Nonodontogenic tumors of the jaw include a wide spectrum of different lesions originating from different tissues (Tables 36.4 and 36.5).

Table 36.3: Classification of odontogenic tumors (Gorlin, Chaudhry, Pindborg, 1961)

1. *Epithelial odontogenic tumors*

   A. *Minimal inductive change in connective tissue (Ectodermal origin)*

      1. Ameloblastoma

      2. Adenomatoid odontogenic tumor

      3. Calcifying epithelial odontogenic tumor (CEOT)

   B. *Marked inductive change in connective tissue (Mixed origin)*

      1. Ameloblastic fibroma

      2. Ameloblastic odontoma

      3. Odontoma

      4. Complex odontoma

      5. Compound odontoma

2. *Mesodermal odontogenic tumors*

      1. Odontogenic myxoma

      2. Odontogenic fibroma

      3. Cementoma

         a. Periapical cemental dysplasia (PCD)

         b. Benign cementoblastoma

         c. Cementifying fibroma

         d. Familial multiple (gigantiform) cementoma (Florid osseous dysplasia (FOD)

Table 36.4: Nonodontogenic tumors and fibro-osseous lesions of the jaw bones

A. *Nonodontogenic tumors*

   1. Central fibroma

   2. Myxofibroma

   3. Ossifying fibroma

   4. Osteoma

   5. Osteoid osteoma

   6. Benign osteoblastoma

   7. Chondroma

   8. Giant cell granuloma

   9. Central hemangioma

   10. Benign tumors of nerve tissue

B. *Fibro-osseous lesions*

   1. Fibrous dysplasia of bone

   2. Cherubism (Inherited fibro-osseous bone disease)

   3. Ossifying fibroma

   4. Central giant cell granuloma

Table 36.5: WHO classification of nonodontogenic tumors of the jaws (Kramer, Pindborg, Shear, 1992)

I. *Osteogenic neoplasms*

    Cemento-ossifying fibroma

II. *Nonneoplastic bone lesions*

    1. Fibrous dysplasia of the jaws

    2. Cemento-osseous dysplasias

       a. Periapical cemento-osseous dysplasia

       b. Focal cemento-osseous dysplasia

       c. Florid cemento-osseous dysplasia (gigantiform)

III. *Other cemento-osseous dysplasias*

    a. Cherubism

    b. Central giant cell granuloma

GENERAL PRINCIPLES OF MANAGEMENT OF A JAW LESION

History of the Lesion

Duration: It is very important to know the duration of the lesion.

Prolonged duration → may be congenital

Long duration without pain → benign neoplasm

Short duration, rapid growth → malignant growth

Mode of onset and progress: History of trauma may be obtained in many bone lesions like osteogenic sarcoma. Spontaneous swelling and rapid growing lesion may be malignant, while very slowly growing lesion may be benign growth

Exact site and shape: In a huge swelling it is essential to know the exact site and shape of the swelling for knowing the origin of the lesion.

Progress of the lesion: Whether the swelling has been growing slowly or it has remained stationary for a long time (benign growth). Has it been growing again after a stationary period of months/years (malignant transformation in a benign lesion) or has it been continuously increasing in size (malignant growth)?

Change in character of a lesion: Whether there are ulcerations over the lesions? Fluctuation, softening, etc. are noticed by the patient recently? Whether painless swelling has become painful—secondary infection may have set in the lesion.

Associated symptoms: Pain, abnormal sensations, anesthesia, paresthesia over a region, dysphasia, nasal obstruction—breathing difficulty, tenderness, lymphadenopathy.

Restriction of the oral opening or trismus—due to involvement of pterygoid plates by the lesion it can be noticed.

Similar swelling elsewhere in the body: Multiple involvements due to metastasis.

Loss of body weight: Malignant growth.

Recurrence

Whether the lesion has recurred after the previous surgery?

Habit

Any habits leading to the development of lesion smoking, tobacco chewing, etc.

■ CLINICAL EXAMINATION OF THE LESION

Thorough clinical examination of the lesion, as well as of the entire oral cavity and external facial area including all regional lymph nodes is a must. The quick assessment of general physical examination also should be noted down.

In the oral and maxillofacial region, the examination of the lesion will include inspection and palpation. Percussion is only done for dentition examination and auscultation is reserved for examining suspected vascular lesions. The large lesions should be examined by bimanual palpation to know the intra and extraoral extent of the lesion.

Inspection

i. Number—whether single or multiple
ii. Size
iii. Site or anatomical location of the lesion—palatal swellings may have salivary gland origin, and may not have odontogenic origin
iv. Shape and size of the lesion—whether ovoid, spherical, localized, diffuse, etc.
v. Color of the lesion—whether red or purple (hemangioma), blue (ranula)
vi. Surface—whether smooth, lobulated (benign) or irregular, ulcerated, fungating growth (malignancy)

vii. Whether it is pedunculated or sessile?
viii. Skin over the swelling—red, hot skin will suggest secondary infection.

Palpation

Palpation should be carried out gently and systematically.

Consistency of the lesion: Soft (lipoma), hard or indurated, firm (fibroma), bony hard (osteoma), cystic, etc. It should be also noted whether the consistency is uniform throughout or variable. Whether there is egg shell crackling present? Fluctuation is present?

Presence of pulsations: If the palpation of a lesion reveals a pulsatile quality, a large vascular component is indicated. The 'thrill' can be felt along the lesion. The auscultation with a stethoscope may reveal 'a bruit' or audible murmur.

Fixity: Fixity to the overlying skin/mucosa/underlying structures.

Lymph node examination: Systematic lymph node palpation should be carried out.

Imaging

Imaging modalities like plain radiographs, computed tomography (CT), CT three dimensional reconstruction can be used to know the extent of the lesion. These modalities are mainly used to know the lesion's site, size, shape, presence or absence of intralesional calcifications, any cystic degeneration within the lesion, association or inclusion of the vital anatomic structures, displacement of teeth and root resorption and extent of the lesion, etc. (whether confined to the bone or extended into adjacent soft tissue). In case of malignancy a complete bone scan or scintigraphy can be carried out to find out distant metastasis. Magnetic resonance imaging (MRI) is helpful for knowing the soft tissue extensions and lymphadenopathy. Angiographic studies are carried out for vascular tumors. The actual confirmatory diagnosis of the lesion is made by carrying out histopathological examination following biopsy of a lesion.

Biopsy

Here the tissue is obtained from a living person and sent for histopathological examination for final diagnosis of a lesion.

Selection of a Biopsy Technique

Depending on the nature of lesion, access to the lesion, extent of the lesion and nature of the tissue to be examined, the particular biopsy technique is chosen. Exfoliative cytology, aspiration biopsy, incisional biopsy, excisional biopsy—these are the various biopsy techniques, which can be used for oral lesions. Intraoperative frozen section study also can be used to know the extent of the surgery. Depending on the patient's age, physical health and emotional status, the biopsy procedure can be planned with local anesthesia, sedation or general anesthesia.

Exfoliative cytology: It does not have any role in closed jaw lesion. However, in case of suspected malignancy of the jaw bone, the initial screening can be done by scraping the lesion. The cells obtained from the scrapings are transferred on the glass slide and are stained and examined under the microscope. On many occasions this can give false negative report and hence is not a reliable substitute for biopsy procedure.

Aspiration biopsy: It is done by using a needle and syringe to penetrate the lesion and aspirating the contents of the lesion. It can give valuable information regarding the nature of the tissue. In solid lesions there will be inability to aspirate the fluid or air. In a cystic lesion, a straw colored fluid can be aspirated, while in infected lesion, pus is obtained as an aspirate. Traumatic bone cavity will yield an air aspiration. In vascular lesion, the bright red blood can be aspirated without pulling the piston of the syringe. Bloody aspirate can be obtained from aneurysmal bone cyst or central giant cell granuloma, etc. (Fig. 36.1).

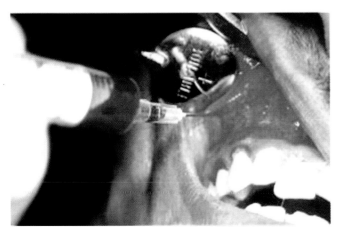

Fig. 36.1: Aspiration biopsy

Aspiration can be carried out for all the lesions, which contain fluid or for any intraosseous lesion prior to surgical intervention. Aspiration can be done by using 18 gauge needle with 5/10 cc syringe. The most fluctuant point of the lesion is selected for the needle penetration. The material obtained from the aspiration biopsy is submitted for (i) pathological examination (ii) chemical analysis or (iii) microbiologic culturing if necessary.

Fine needle aspiration cytology (FNAC): It can be useful for deep seated lesions, e.g. neoplasms of the salivary glands, masses in the neck or soft tissue tumors in the bones. With Silverman needle, it is possible to get a strip of intact tissue 1.5 mm wide and about 1.5 cm long, which can be sectioned and studied like an ordinary surgical biopsy. A negative biopsy is often unreliable. It should be used only as an adjunct to diagnosis.

Excisional biopsy: This is the complete removal of the pathological lesion, which is submitted for histopathological review. Some amount of normal surrounding tissue is also included during total excision of the lesion. It is usually employed for smaller lesions, which can be excised easily without causing much mutilation.

Incisional biopsy: In the larger lesions, the small wedge of tissue is obtained to represent the entire lesion and subjected for histopathological examination. Some rules to be followed during this procedure.

   i. The site of biopsy is chosen carefully after completing the clinical and radiological examination
  ii. The aspiration should be always tried before incisional biopsy.
 iii. The incision should be planned keeping in view, the final surgical procedure.
 iv. Representative areas of the lesion should be incised in a wedge fashion.
  v. Some amount of normal tissue should be included.
 vi. Ulcerated areas, necrotic tissue should be avoided.
vii. Incisional biopsy should be planned without causing injury to the nerves, teeth or blood vessels.
viii. Sufficient amount of tissue should be obtained.
 ix. The specimen tissue should not be crushed.
  x. Deeper biopsies are preferred over superficial one.
 xi. Proper hemostasis is achieved prior to closure.
xii. A nonresorbable tissue barrier may be placed over the bony entrance of the lesion following incisional biopsy to prevent fluid or lesional cell escape into the noninvolved tissue.

xiii. The specimen should be well oriented and marked for proper identification.

xiv. The tissue should be immediately placed in 10 percent formalin solution completely immersed.

PRINCIPLES OF SURGICAL MANAGEMENT OF JAW TUMORS

The goal of treatment is (i) Complete eradication of a lesion (ii) Preservation of the normal tissue as permissible (iii) Excision with least morbidity (iv) Restoration of tissue loss, form and function (v) Long term follow up for recurrence.

Before planning the surgical procedure, the oral and maxillofacial surgeon should discuss the biological behavior, histologic tissue pattern, recurrence rate, etc. with the pathologist and should correlate the clinical, radiological and histopathological findings.

Gold, Upton and Marx in 1991, have presented a standardized surgical terminology for the excision of lesions in the bone. All excisions of the lesions involving the jaw bone can best be described by the following terminologies:

  i. Enucleation
 ii. Curettage
iii. Marsupialization
 iv. Recontouring
  v. Resection without continuity defect (RsCD)
 vi. Resection with continuity defect (RcCD)
vii. Disarticulation

Enucleation with or without curettage, marsupialization are mainly used for the excision of the cystic lesions. Many small benign tumors are nonaggressive and they also can be treated by enucleation, with or without curettage. The surgical procedure is described in the earlier chapter.

Other group of benign tumors, which are locally invasive or aggressive require inclusion of some amount of normal tissue, during excision to lessen the chance of recurrence.

Resection without continuity defect: It is used for such lesions. This is also known as marginal resection (En bloc resection).

Resection with continuity defect: It is carried out for more extensive lesions, which include resection of the inferior border of the mandible.

Partial resection: Here resection of a tumor by removing full thickness portion of the jaw is carried out. In the mandible, this can vary, depending upon the site of tumor, from a small continuity defect to hemi-mandibulectomy.

Disarticulation: Whenever condylar head is included in the resection of the part of the mandible, then the procedure is called as *hemimandibulectomy with disarticulation* and whenever the condylar head is retained for rehabilitation procedure, then the procedure is called as *hemimandibulectomy without disarticulation*.

Total resection: Excision of a tumor by removal of the involved bone is carried out. *Maxillectomy* or *mandibulectomy* procedures can be carried out.

Composite resection: The last group of tumors are the malignant ones. They require much more radical intervention, with wider margins of excision of uninvolved tissue. Surgery may include along with resection of the jaw-neck dissection and dissection of the lymph nodes. Radiotherapy or chemotherapy, either alone or in addition to the surgery, may be used depending on the type of tumor.

Factors to be evaluated before surgery: In order to choose the most appropriate surgical method for individual case, following factors are to be considered:

  i. *Anatomical location of the lesion:* The surgical access to the lesion is an important factor for prognosis. Small benign lesions involving inaccessible areas are more difficult to treat. Example—tumors in infra-temporal region, at the pterygomaxillary fissure, etc. Aggressive tumors in the anterior mandible region will be more accessible and have better prognosis.

 ii. *Aggressiveness of the tumor:* Locally invasive tumors are treated with more wider resection in order to prevent recurrence.

iii. *Size of the tumor and confinement to the bone:* The size of the tumor is important, especially in the mandible. If the inferior border is not involved in the lesion, marginal resection can be carried out without continuity defect. If the tumor is not confined to the bone, that means, if it has perforated the cortices and extended into the soft tissues, then one has to carry out wider resection sacrificing the more amount of normal soft tissue along with the resection of the bone.

iv. *Proximity to adjacent vital structures:* Preservation of the neurovascular structures and teeth is of importance. But, if the tumor is aggressive, then both these important structures have to be sacrificed.

v. *Involvement of maxilla/mandible:* The maxillary tumors have poorer prognosis than those involving the mandible. Proximity to the maxillary sinus, nasal cavity, orbital cavity, cranial fossa, nasopharynx allow these tumors to grow asymptomatically and more extensively to attain a large size with late symptoms.

vi. *Rehabilitation or reconstruction methods:* The rehabilitation or reconstruction is much easier in the mandible than in the maxilla. The continuity of the resected mandible can be maintained by using reconstruction plates. Bone grafting can be done either as a primary reconstruction method or secondary reconstruction method.

The reconstruction of the smaller defects can be done by using bone grafts, alloplastic bone grafts or synthetic material or combination of the above materials.

In the maxilla, after maxillectomy, a denture with obturation can be given to improve speech and mastication.

The microvascular surgery can be considered to reconstruct the lost jaw portion and later dental implants can be given to complete rehabilitation of these patients.

Enucleation with or without Curettage

Indications

1. Surgical excision of the tumors, which tend to grow by expansion, rather than by infiltration of the surrounding tissues.
2. Lesions occurring in the bone with a distinct separation between the lesion and the surrounding bone.
3. Often, there is a cortical margin of bone that delineates the tumor or cyst from the bone.
4. Indicated in following tumors:
   i. *Odontogenic tumors*
      a. Odontoma
      b. Ameloblastic fibroma
      c. Ameloblastic fibrodontoma
      d. Adenomatoid odontogenic tumor
      e. Cementoblastoma
   ii. *Fibro-osseous lesions and nonodontogenic tumors*
      a. Ossifying fibroma
      b. Cherubism
      c. Central giant cell granuloma
      d. Osteoblastoma

   iii. *Other lesions*
      a. Hemangioma
      b. Eosinophilic granuloma
      c. Neurofibroma
      d. Neurilemmoma
      e. Pigmented neuroectodermal tumor

Marginal Resection or Resection without Continuity Defect/Peripheral Osteotomy/En Block Resection

Enucleation of the locally aggressive lesion is not a safe procedure and it makes recurrence almost inevitable. En bloc or marginal resection is indicated in the benign lesions with a known propensity for recurrence, or in those lesions that are incompletely encapsulated or tend to grow beyond their surgically apparent capsule. It is also indicated for recurrent lesion, previously treated by enucleation alone.

Ameloblastoma, calcifying epithelial odontogenic tumor, myxoma, ameloblastic odontoma, squamous odontogenic tumor, benign chondroblastoma, hemangioma are the lesions treated by this method.

This procedure allows complete excision of the tumor, but at the same time a continuity of the jaw bone is retained and thus deformity, disfigurement and the need for secondary cosmetic surgery and prosthetic rehabilitation are avoided.

Intraoral marginal resection: Surgical procedure (Figs 36.2A and B): The circumgingival incision is taken and the releasing incisions can be extended into the buccal mucosa on either side of the lesion leaving at least one or two adjacent teeth on either side. The full thickness mucoperiosteal flap is reflected by using periosteal elevator. Care is taken not to perforate the lesion. If the lesion is perforated, then overlying mucosa should be sacrificed along with the excision of the tumor. The tooth next to the tumor mass should be extracted on either side. The vertical osteotomies are performed through the sockets of the extracted teeth on either side using bur or saw blade.

Both the vertical osteotomy cuts are extended from the buccal to lingual cortex. These cuts are joined with a horizontal cut, placed well beyond the tumor mass including margin of the normal bone. Horizontal cut is also completed through and through the buccal and lingual cortex. The complete excision of the tumor along with some amount of normal bone is carried out

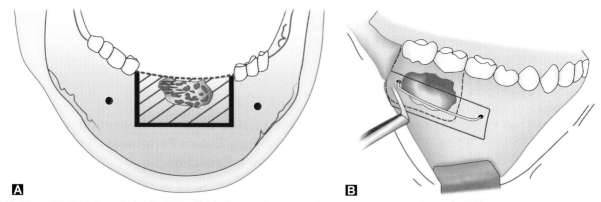

Figs 36.2A and B: (A) Intraoral marginal resection in the anterior region of mandible, (B) Intraoral marginal resection in the posterior region of mandible

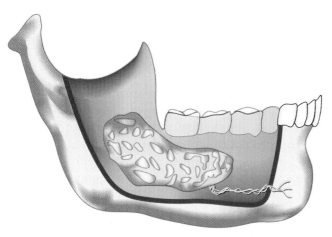

Fig. 36.3: Extraoral peripheral osteotomy

by using osteotome. Teeth involved in the tumor mass are removed with the block in toto. The remaining bony margins should be checked for sharp areas and contoured by using round bur or bone file. The excess mucoperiosteal flap is trimmed off and approximated to suture the wound. This type of excision can be done under local anesthesia with sedation for smaller lesions or it can be planned under general anesthesia.

Extraoral peripheral osteotomy (Fig. 36.3): Since complete resection of large segments involving both the horizontal and the ascending rami or disarticulation of the segment causes considerable amount of disability, this method is useful, which will allow complete removal of the pathology, but is less debilitating than complete resection. The procedure is based on the observation that the cortical inferior border of the horizontal body, the posterior border of the ascending ramus and the

condyle are not generally involved in the benign tumor process. Bone regeneration will start from such areas even though a thin rim of bone is preserved, especially in young patients, result in considerable restoration of the jaw anatomy.

Indications: Large lesions involving posterior mandible.
Operative procedure: In dentulous patients, intraoral crevicular gingival incision is taken around dentulous area, both buccally as well as lingually. Buccinator and mylohyoid muscles are separated after reflecting the mucoperiosteal flap. In edentulous patients there is no need to take intraoral incision.

Extraoral submandibular incision is taken and the inferior border of the mandible is exposed, if required posterior border of the ramus is also exposed. The site of peripheral osteotomy is already decided by studying CT scans or radiographs. The drill holes are made with the electrical dental drill in the healthy bone around the periphery of the lesion. These holes are connected until the tumor mass is separated from the thin span of bone to be retained. The part to be excised is now separated from the attached soft tissue on the external surface. The masseter and buccinator muscles are detached with care, so that not to injure the branches of the facial nerve. Then the mucoperiosteum of the alveolar process is elevated and the specimen is turned outwards to get access to the inner surface to detach the mylohyoid and the internal pterygoid muscles. The temporalis muscle is severed above the coronoid, after which the inferior alveolar nerve and vessels are identified and grasped with a hemostat, ligated and cut off. The remaining bone is now carefully inspected. Intraoral wound is closed with water tight suturing. An immediate bone graft can be inserted through the extraoral wound and fixed with intraosseous wires or bone plates. The wound is closed in layers with a small rubber drain inserted to prevent formation of a hematoma. An external pressure bandage is applied. Careful long term following up is mandatory.

Segmental Resection of the Jaw (Intraoral Approach) (Fig. 36.4)

Indications

1. For treatment of lesions that are infiltrative or have a tendency to recur.
2. Those lesions which extend close to the inferior or posterior border of the mandible, the maxillary sinus or the nasal cavity.
3. It is also used for malignant lesions with high recurrence potential.
4. Recurrent odontogenic tumors with difficulty in examining and gaining an access surgically.
5. Maxillary ameloblastomas with high recurrence rate.
6. Lesions close to the borders of the jaw, with the possibility of postoperative pathologic fracture.

Preoperative assessment: A thorough clinical, radiographic and histologic assessment should be carried out.

Advantages of intraoral approach:

1. Excision of overlying mucosal tissue involved in the lesion is facilitated.
2. Easy access for application of arch bars, extraction of involved teeth, ligation of the inferior alveolar neurovascular bundle, closure of the maxillary sinus and maintaining the forward stability of the tongue, whenever required.
3. An external scar is avoided.

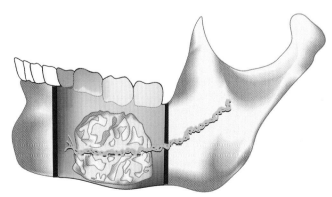

Fig. 36.4: Segmental resection of jaw (Intraoral approach)

4. An extraoral tissues are preserved for a later reconstruction procedure.

Disadvantages of Intraoral Procedure

1. Contamination of the surgical wound by the oral flora.
2. Lack of dependent drainage of the dead space.
3. Difficult access to the most posterior portions of the mandible.
4. The risk of damage to the branches of the internal maxillary artery, deep in the wound.
5. Immediate bone graft reconstruction by oral route has a higher rate of infection and loss of the bone graft (30%).

The patient should be informed of and prepared psychologically for the resulting facial and functional deformity and the reconstruction procedure.

● *Surgical procedure:* For mandibular lesion extending posterior to the mental foramen, ligation of the inferior alveolar neurovascular bundle prior to resection may prevent significant intraoperative hemorrhage. The incision is designed to expose the lesion on both the facial and lingual aspect with or without inclusion of overlying tissues in the specimen. The same incision is extended posteriorly through the buccal mucosa approximately 7 mm lateral and parallel to the anterior border of the ascending ramus and external oblique ridge. Blunt dissection is carried out along the surface of the buccinator muscle to expose the periosteum over the external oblique ridge and anterior border of the ramus. A sharp incision is made through the periosteum and the periosteum is elevated lingually to expose the retromolar area of the mandible, internal oblique ridge and medial surface of the ramus, till the lingula. The inferior alveolar neurovascular bundle is located and a curved aneurysmal needle can be passed around it with a ligature threaded through its eye. The neurovascular bundle is ligated at the higher level above the lingula.

After this, the entire lesion is exposed by reflecting the mucoperiosteal flap on buccal and lingual side till the inferior margin of the mandible. The anterior and posterior bony cuts are then outlined as planned and the cuts are finished by using bur or saw blade from buccal to lingual cortex. In the tooth bearing area, one or two teeth may be removed prior to sectioning the jaw, bony cut can be carried out through an empty socket. Separation of the bony cuts can be completed with an osteotome. The specimen is separated from its bony and soft tissue attachments and inferior alveolar neurovascular bundle is sectioned below the ligature level. Whenever the anterior portion of the mandible is removed, it is mandatory to hold the genioglossus muscles with the hemostat prior to separation from the specimen and then these muscles should be secured with a suture in the forward position to the soft tissues of the chin or to the reconstruction plate to prevent airway obstruction due to tongue fall postoperatively. Primary closure of the wound is done. Intermaxillary fixation or reconstruction plate is necessary to preserve the alignment of the fragments.

Extraoral approach: It may be necessary for difficult approach. The surgical procedure will be same as described earlier for the marginal resection (Fig. 36.5).

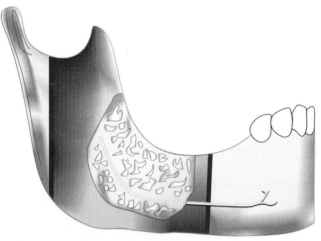

Fig. 36.5: Segmental resection without disarticulation (Extraoral approach)

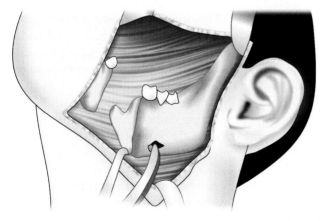

Fig. 36.6: Segmental resection including condyle (Disarticulation)

1. *Segmental resection including the condyle (Disarticulation) (Fig. 36.6):* The surgical approach is through a combined postramal (Hinds) and sub-mandibular (Risdon) incision placed at least 2 cm below and parallel to the inferior and posterior borders of the mandible. After the incision through the skin, subcutaneous tissue and platysma is taken, the dissection plane is made deep to the platysma, along the investing fascia to the inferior border of the mandible. The pterygomasseteric muscle sling and periosteal layer is divided at the inferior border of the mandible. Subperiosteal reflection of the masseter muscle is done along the lateral surface of the mandible to expose the coronoid process, sigmoid notch and condylar neck. The anterior portion of the resection is determined and dissected. Care should be taken to prevent an intraoral communication. (In teeth bearing area the intraoral incision is unavoidable), using the bur or saw blade, the osteotomy is completed. By swinging the specimen laterally, it is freed from its medial attachments subperiosteally. The temporalis muscle is detached from the coronoid process. The condylar head is separated from lateral pterygoid muscle attachment. Care is taken to prevent damage to the maxillary artery and its branches. The specimen is completely removed and the surgical wound is irrigated. The proximal portion of the segment is smoothened to prevent intraoral perforation. Reconstruction plate with condylar prosthesis is placed and fixed on to the proximal stump with screws. The wound is closed in layers after proper hemostasis.

2. *Segmental resection involving the mandibular midline (Figs 36.7 and 36.8):* An incision is made at least 2 cm below the inferior border of the mandible.
   Dissection: Incision is taken through skin, subcutaneous tissue. At the level of platysma muscle, the tissues are undermined. Platysma is cut sharply and dissection is followed to the investing layer of the deep cervical fascia. Incision through this layer is taken till the periosteum at the inferior border of the mandible. The dissection is continued subperiosteally to detach the left and right diagastric as well as the mylohyoid muscle from the medial aspect of the mandible. The genioglossus and geniohyoid muscle attachments are located and a suture is passed around them. Then the muscles are detached from the genial tubercles. The subperiosteal dissection is carried on the buccal surface of the

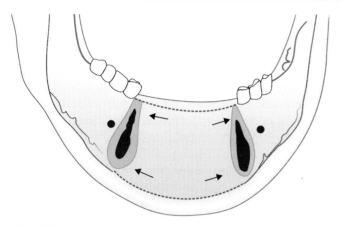

Fig. 36.7: Intraoral segmental resection involving mandibular midline

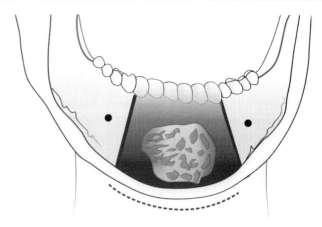

Fig. 36.8: Extraoral segmental resection involving mandibular midline

mandible to expose the planned resection portion. The mental nerves are identified and protected. The lateral extent of the resection is defined in the dentulous jaw by extracting the teeth and placing the bony cuts through the sockets. A mucoperiosteal flap is developed intraorally to free the specimen from the soft tissue attachments. Prior to the removal of the specimen, the remaining segments should be stabilized by carrying out temporary intermaxillay fixation. The reconstruction plate is contoured prior to the excision of the bone and immediately secured it following the resection by means of screws. This prevents the collapse of the segments and allows jaw function during healing and prior to reconstruction and also prevents scar contraction. The oral mucosa Is closed intraorally, using a horizontal mattress suture to obtain as watertight seal as possible. The genioglossus and geniohyoid muscles are pulled forward with suture, which is secured to the reconstruction plate. Extraoral wound is closed in layers.

Maxillectomy

Access to the maxilla is generally obtained by designing the classic Weber-Fergusson incision. The eyelids are closed temporarily by taking tarsorrhaphy sutures. For esthetic good result, it is recommended to tattoo the vermilion border and the other points on both sides of the incision with methylene blue. These points are then matched during closure. The typical incision splits the midline of the upper lip (Fig. 36.9). But better cosmetic results can be obtained by incising along the philtral ridges and then offsetting the incision at the vermilion border (Figs 36.10A and B). The incision is turned

laterally at the base of the columella, then around the alar base and along the side of the nose to within

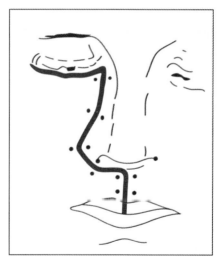

Fig. 36.9: Weber-Fergusson incision

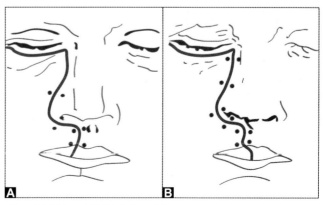

Figs 36.10A and B: Variation of lip split for better cosmetic results

2 mm of the medial canthus. Intraorally the incision is continued down through the gingival margin. It is connected with a horizontal incision at the depth of the labiobuccal vestibule, extending back to the maxillary tuberosity. From here, the incision turns medially across the posterior edge of the hard palate. It then turns 90° anteriorly, several millimeters to the proximal side of the midline, if possible to cross the gingival margin once again (Fig. 36.11).

The incision is carried to the bone, except beneath the lower eye lid, where the orbicularis oculi muscle is preserved. The cheek flap is then reflected back to the tuberosity (Fig. 36.12). The central incisor on the involved side is extracted and the gingival and palatal mucosa are elevated back to the midline. The incision extending around the nose is then deepened into the nasal cavity. The palatal bone is then divided near the midline with a saw blade or bur. The basal bone is then separated from the frontal process of the maxilla with an osteotome. The orbicularis oculi muscle is retracted superiorly, and the bone cut is extended across the maxilla, just below the infraorbital rim, into the zygoma. If the posterior wall of the maxillary sinus has not been invaded by tumor, it is separated from the pterygoid plates with a pterygoid chisel (Fig. 36.13). The entire specimen is removed by severing the remaining attachments with a large curved scissors placed behind the maxilla.

After the removal of the specimen, some amount of brisk bleeding is expected, which is controlled with packing and electrocautery. Branches of the maxillary artery in the pterygomaxillary fissure area may require ligation. While the packing is in place, the specimen should be inspected to make sure that complete tumor has been excised. All sharp bony projections should be trimmed. The flap of the retained palatal mucosa is turned up to cover the medial bony margin. A split thickness skin graft is then sutured to the wound margins to cover the entire defect. Graft is maintained in place by placing softened impression compound ball in the

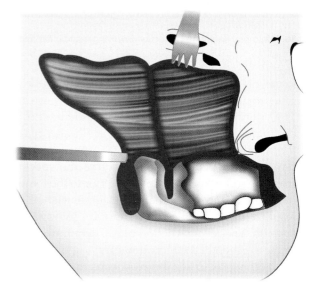

Fig. 36.12: Reflection of cheek flap for maxillectomy

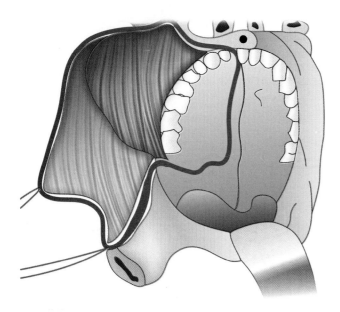

Fig. 36.11: Intraoral incision for exposure of tumor

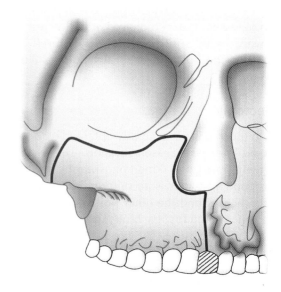

Fig. 36.13: Bony cuts for maxillectomy

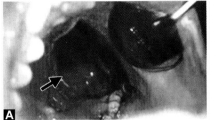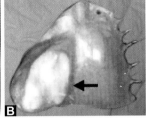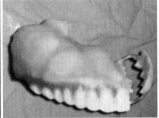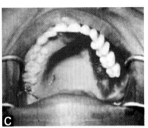

Figs 36.14A to C: Rehabilitation of maxillectomy defect (A) Skin graft in place, (B) Obturator with hollow bulb, (C) Rehabilitation with obturator

defect. The surgical obturator, which is prefabricated, is placed to seal the defect and support the packing. The obturator is fixed to the remaining teeth by means of interdental wiring. The main cheek flap is then turned back and closed in layers (Figs 36.14A to C).

Modifications

1. When the tumor extends up to the roof of the maxillary sinus (but does not invade) the orbital floor should be included in the resection (Fig. 36.15).
2. When the tumor invades the roof of the maxillary sinus, the orbit or the ethmoid sinuses, orbital exenteration is mandatory (Fig. 36.16).
3. The tumors which are confined to the posterior aspect of maxillary sinus may be managed with a more conservative resection that spares the premaxilla (Fig. 36.17).

Postoperative management: Patients are kept in an intensive care unit for the first one or two days for cardiovascular monitoring and necessary maintenance of fluid, electrolyte balance. The patient is kept on liquid diet. Instructions are given for maintenance of oral hygiene. Prophylactic antibiotic therapy is advocated for 5 to 7 days. The surgical obturator is removed after 15 days and the wound is irrigated with warm saline and hydrogen peroxide. Excess skin graft and other debris are removed.

Long term follow up is necessary.

Reconstruction

After surgical resection with continuity defect, there is disfigurement, deviation of the mandible along with resultant altered mandibular movements with facial asymmetry.

Need for Reconstruction

- For the restoration of movements and equilibrium of mandible.

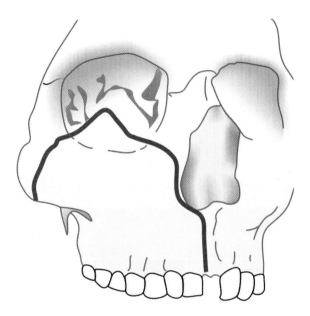

Fig. 36.15: Inclusion of the orbital floor in maxillectomy bony cut

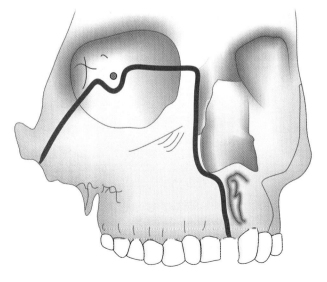

Fig. 36.16: Bony cuts for the orbital exenteration along with maxillectomy

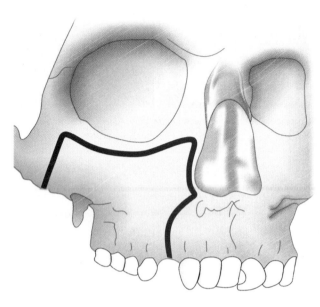

Fig. 36.17: Maxillectomy cut without inclusion of premaxilla

- For maintenance of normal occlusal plane, floor of the mouth and tongue's anatomical position
- For restoration of near normal feeding
- For acceptable esthetics and function
- For more favorable social acceptance.

Timing of Reconstruction

a. **Immediate reconstruction (Figs 36.18 to 36.20)**

Advantages

- Single stage surgery
- Early return of function
- Minimal compromise of esthetics

Disadvantages

- Recurrence in grafted bone
- Loss of graft from infection

Immediate reconstruction can be done by three different ways:

1. Performing surgical excision and grafting, both via intraoral approach.

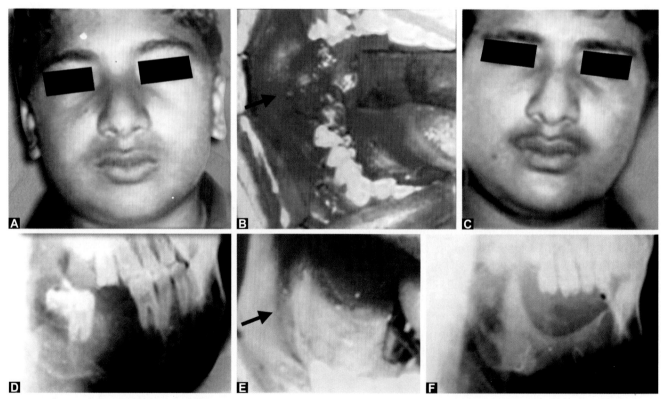

Figs 36.18A to F: (A) A 15-year-old male patient with ameloblastoma in right body mandible, preoperative frontal view, (B) Intraoral lesion view, (C) Postoperative frontal view, (D) Preoperative radiograph showing extent of lesion, (E) Postoperative intraoral view of the healing after segmental resection of the tumor and immediate iliac crest bone graft reconstruction, (F) Postoperative radiograph after six months follow up showing take of the graft

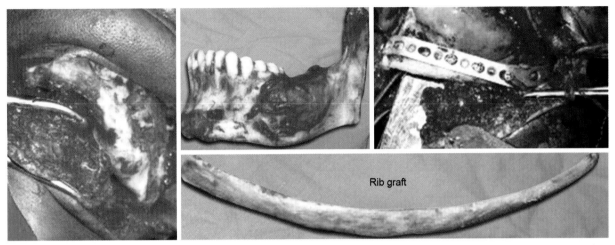

Fig. 36.19: A 30-year-old male patient with ameloblastoma of left ramus and body. Hemimandibulectomy with disarticulation was done, immediate reconstruction with rib graft was carried out

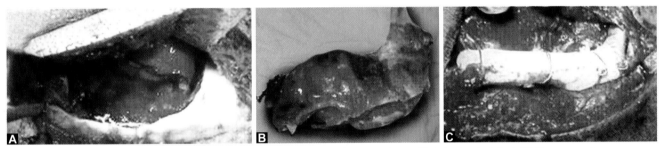

Figs 36.20A to C: (A) Marginal resection of ameloblastoma leaving posterior and inferior border intact, (B) Tumor specimen, (C) Immediate reconstruction with rib graft

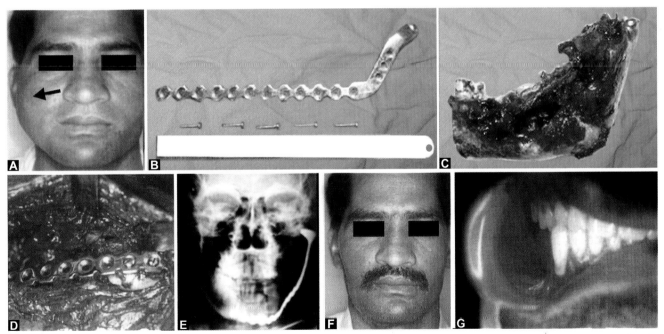

Figs 36.21A to G: Delayed reconstruction (Use of reconstruction plate): (A) Extraoral swelling on right side of the face in a 36-year-old male. Amelobastoma involving (R) body and ascending ramus mandible (B) Reconstruction plate, (C) Tumor specimen after hemimandibulectomy with disarticulation, (D) Reconstruction plate fixation surgery, (E) Postoperative radiograph, (F) Postoperative facial symmetry, (G) Maintenance of occlusion and intraoral postoperative healing

2. Surgial excision utilizing both intraoral and extraoral approach, first obtaining water tight oral closure and grafting done through extraoral approach.
3. Earlier extraction of involved teeth and waiting of 6 to 8 weeks for oral healing and then surgery at second stage, with complete procedure via extraoral approach to avoid oral communication of the graft.

b. *Delayed reconstruction (second stage) (Figs 36.21A to G)*

Here the consideration should be given to maintain the residual mandibular fragments with their normal anatomic relationship with intermaxillary fixation or using a reconstruction plate.

This is to avoid cicatrical and muscular deformation and displacement of segments, which aids in secondary reconstructive efforts at a later date. Usually six months waiting period is observed for recurrence.

ODONTOGENIC TUMORS OF VARIOUS ORIGINS

Tumors Arising from Odontogenic Epithelium without Odontogenic Ectomesenchyme

Ameloblastoma

One of the most significant tumors, which has a long history of recognition and controversy. Opinions differ regarding its terminology, etiology, histological pattern, classification, clinical and biological behavior, diagnosis, treatment aspect and malignant potential, etc.

History: 1st recognized by Cuzack in 1827. Later on Falksson described it in 1879, as follicular cystoid tumor. The term 'Adamantinoma' was used by Malassez in 1885.

Ivy and Churchill coined the term 'ameloblastoma' in 1934.

Robinson has described it as 'usually unicentric, nonfunctional, intermittent in growth, anatomically benign and clinically persistent.

WHO—it is a true neoplasm of enamel organ type tissue, which does not undergo differentiation to a point of enamel formation.

In 1992, WHO classification categorized ameloblastoma as a benign, but locally invasive epithelial odontogenic neoplasm, with strong tendency to recur.

Pathogenesis (origin): According to Thoma, Williams in 1993, the tumor may be derived from various origins.

1. *Late developmental sources:* Cell rests of enamel organ, either remnants of dental lamina or epithelial cell rests of Malassez or remnants of Hertwig's sheath, follicular sacs.
2. *Early embryonic sources:* Disturbances of developing enamel organ, dental lamina, tooth buds.
3. *Basal cells of the surface epithelium of the oral mucosa.*
4. *Secondary developmental sources:* Epithelium of odontogenic cysts, particularly primordial, lateral periodontal cyst, dentigerous cyst and odontomas.
5. *Heterotropic epithelium in other parts of body, especially from the pituitary gland.*

Incidence: It accounts for approximately 1 percent of all oral tumors and 18 percent of all odontogenic tumors.

Age: The age at which the lesion may become clinically evident is as early as the first decade or as late as the seventh decade. Overall average age is 36 years.

No sex predilection: It can occur equally in men and women.

Site: The lesion may occur in either of the jaws. The ratio of ameloblastoma of the mandible to maxilla is 5:1. The sites of predilection are the posterior maxilla and the posterior molar—ramus region of the mandible (60%). In blacks, ameloblastomas occur more frequently in the anterior region of the maxilla.

Classification

a. Central or intraosseous
b. Peripheral or extraosseous. Found in the gingiva and mucosa of the alveolar process.

Clinical features (signs and symptoms): Ameloblastoma is typically asymptomatic and therefore seldom diagnosed in the early stages of development. Remaining undiscovered until the lesional growth produces intraoral and/or extraoral jaw swelling, tooth eruption and dental occlusion disturbances or incidental findings in the radiograph.

Patients complain of slow growing, painless, hard, nontender, ovoid swelling, which is often large in size, as it causes little discomfort in early stage. Other complaints may be mobile teeth, exfoliation of teeth, ill-fitting dentures, malocclusion, ulcerations and nasal obstructions, inability to occlude properly. Later stage with nerve involvement, there will be sensory changes of the lower lip. Pain may be experienced if secondarily infected. Large persistent lesion may exhibit fluctuation, egg-shell crackling.

In the absence of treatment: The ameloblastoma keeps on enlarging and it causes thinning of surrounding bone leading to fluctuation and egg-shell crackling. Since it is not encapsulated tumor, it enlarges and invades into the neighboring tissues by replacing them rather than pushing them as seen in the cysts. Invasion of the medullary space is first feature (bone destruction by direct pressure and distension) when the tumor attains large size with bone erosion, then there is escape into periosteum and mucosa and muscles of the adjoining region.

Root resorption is caused without osteoclastic activity. Locally aggressive invasion in maxillofacial area, may compress vital structures, obstruct airway, impair swallowing, erode major arteries or invade middle cranial fossa. The extensive tumors can cause gross facial deformity.

Size: It may range from lesion as small as 1 cm in diameter and up to disfiguring tumor measuring as large as 16 cm. In maxilla, it may enlarge to involve the maxillary sinus, nasal cavity leading to nasal obstruction and even proptosis of eye (The spread in the maxilla is more extensive, because of cancellous nature of the bone).

Spread: Though it is a benign, locally invasive lesion, in some rare instances or late stages shows spread to distant sites.

The factors contributing to spread include:
1. Duration
2. Extensive local spread
3. Multiple operations/Radiotherapy
4. Proximity to anatomical passage.

Occasional transformation into a malignant form (2–4%) metastasizing to lung and long bones.

Most common sites are lungs and it is considered to be the result of aspiration of tumor cells during extensive manipulation. Metastatic lesions prior to any surgical intervention, give an indication for hematological spread. Other sites, where metastasis is seen include regional lymph nodes, liver, spleen, kidney, long bones, skull, cranium, lumbar vertebrae, ilium, etc.

Radiographic findings

1. The ameloblastoma presents a unilocular (mono-cystic) or multilocular (multicystic) radiolucency in several different forms and shapes.
2. Fifty percent ameloblastomas appear as multilocular radiolucent lesions with sharp borders. Two percent of the ameloblastomas are peripheral. Six percent appear as unicystic lesions.
3. The apparent lesional edge may be distinct or indistinct.
4. Multilocular cyst like radiolucency with compartmentalized appearance due to bony septa. (Honey comb or soap bubble appearance) resembles fibromyxoma, giant cell lesions.
5. Small or large unilocular or multilocular lesion may contain unerupted deciduous or permanent teeth and may resemble a dentigerous cyst.
6. Lesions in dentulous area cause root resorption (30%) and tooth displacement.
7. Buccolingual cortical expansion (80%), this tendency is stronger than a cyst.
8. The displacement of neurovascular bundle at the inferior border is often seen.
9. Maxillary lesions often involve the maxillary sinus and change the normal radiolucency of the sinus to a more opacified appearance.
10. The radiographic image of ameloblastoma is at the most suggestive and not pathognomonic. CT scan—with 3D reconstruction will show the exact extent of the lesion.
11. One of the variants of the ameloblastoma—the desmoplastic ameloblastoma—most often found in the anterior maxilla or mandible appears as a relatively radiopaque lesion, because of its dense connective tissue content (solid type lesion)
12. Differential diagnosis—multilocular lesion—Dentigerous cyst, odontogenic keratocyst, cherubism, giant cell granuloma, odontogenic myxoma, aneurysmal bone cyst.

Histopathology: The ameloblastoma is composed of nests, strands and cords of ameloblastic epithelium, all separated by relatively small amounts of fibrous connective tissue stroma. The characteristic histological features of the ameloblastoma are the orientation of the outer epithelial cell nuclei, which are positioned (polarized) away from the basement membrane.

Two main patterns are seen:

1. *Follicular type (resembles tooth follicle):* It consists of small to large odontogenic epithelial nests (the follicles) and variously shaped and sized ameloblastomatous islands (more common pattern). Cyst formation is commonly seen (Figs 36.22A to D).
2. *The plexiform type:* It consists of interlacing strands of narrow or wide odontogenic epithelial trabeculae resembling the dental lamina. Both these patterns may be observed in the same tumor.

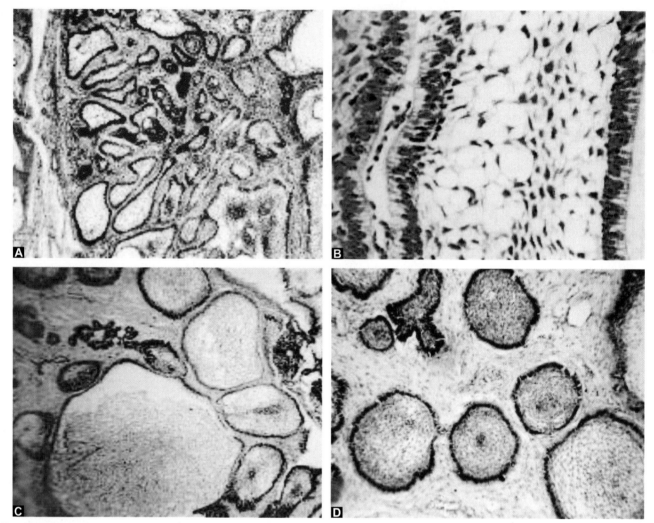

Figs 36.22A to D: Follicular ameloblastoma: (A) Multiple small/large follicles, ameloblastomatous islands in fibrous connective tissue, (B) Peripheral ameloblast like cells with central area resembling stellate reticulum, (C and D) Follicles showing close resemblance to enamel organ

Both these types have a columnar or cuboidal outer epithelial cell layer bordering the connective tissue stroma and enclosing the inner epithelial cells (Fig. 36.23).

Subtypes

1. *Acanthomatous type*—compression of stellate reticulum into a squamoid mass with squamous metaplasia is seen. Sometimes keratin formation in the central portion of the tumor islands is noticed. Occasionally epithelial or keratin pearls may be seen. Usually seen in follicular type of ameloblastoma or peripheral ameloblastoma (Fig. 36.24).

2. *Basal cell type*—bears resemblance to the basal cell carcinoma of the skin. The inner follicular and outer follicular cells may assume a basal cell appearance throughout the lesion.

3. *Desmoplastic type*—variant of solid ameloblastoma. Abundant fibrous tissue stroma can be seen in this variety. Some areas of calcification also can be seen. Marked stromal desmoplasia is noticed. High recurrence rate (Fig. 36.25).

4. *Granular cell type*—stellate reticulum like cells, get transformed into cells with coarse granular, eosinophilic cytoplasm. This type is found to be more aggressive type with high chances of recurrence and metastasis (malignant transformation) (Fig. 36.26).

5. *The mural ameloblastoma*—another name for unicystic lesion, which is found in children and young adults. The ameloblastic epithelium lines the laminal surface and may proliferate into the cyst (mural growth). Often 'budding' aggregates of basal cells, follicular

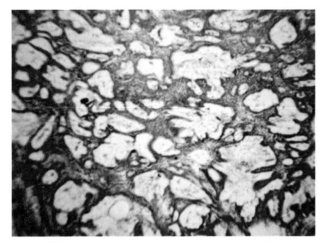

Fig. 36.23: Plexiform ameloblastoma: cord like extensions of odontogenic epithelium resembling the dental lamina, forming a meshwork

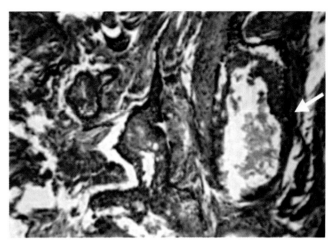

Fig. 36.24: Acanthomatous ameloblastoma: Compression of stellate reticulum into squamoid mass with squamous metaplasia. Arrow—cystic degeneration in the island

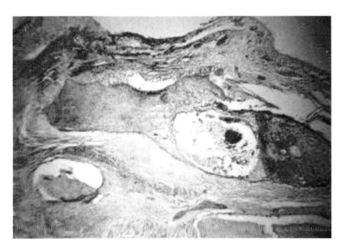

Fig. 36.25: Desmoplastic ameloblastoma: Large islands of odontogenic epithelium surrounded by abundant fibrous tissue stroma. Areas of calcifications noted

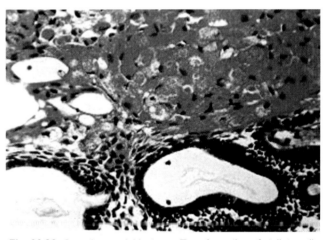

Fig. 36.26: Granular ameloblastoma: Transformation of stellate cells into granular cells seen in the center of the follicle

cells, or plexiform strands extend from the luminal lining into the cystic wall. Further growth of the lesion takes place by creation of microcystic and macrocystic formations in the budding ameloblastic elements that extend and enlarge the primary cystic lumen or the cyst wall by resorption of host bone (Fig. 36.27).

6. *The peripheral ameloblastoma*—origin is from residual or displaced odontogenic tissue in the gingiva or mucosal surface overlying the alveolar process. It may be seen as smooth sessile lesion contained entirely within connective tissue below the epithelial surface or papillomatous type, which infiltrates the surface epithelium. This lesion is not encapsulated like the intrabony ameloblastoma, but is circum-

scribed by stromal connective tissue through which it can infiltrate into the surrounding mucosa as well as penetrate the periosteum and invade the bone (Fig. 36.28).

7. *Malignant subtypes*—the term 'malignant ameloblastoma' is applied, when the metastatic tumor resembles primary tumor with no histological transformation. The term 'ameloblastic carcinoma' is used, when there has been obvious histological transformation towards malignancy of epithelial component and metastatic tumor resembles to a less well differentiated carcinoma, usually an epidermoid carcinoma. These types are rare,

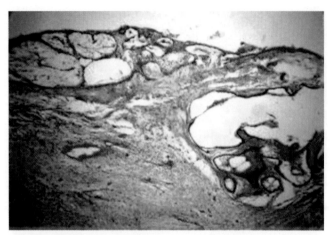

Fig. 36.27: Mural ameloblastoma: Ameloblastic epithelium proliferation into the cystic mural growth

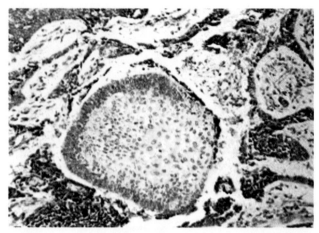

Fig. 36.29: Malignant ameloblastoma: Follicle surrounded by infiltrating cords of tumor

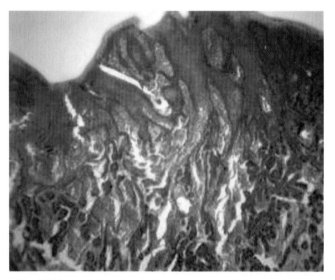

Fig. 36.28: Peripheral ameloblastoma: Streaming of epithelial cells and tumor mass continuity with oral epithelium

aggressive variants with obvious metastasis and poor prognosis, at times inoperable (Fig. 36.29).

Management: Successful treatment is the treatment that renders an acceptable prognosis, causes minimal disfigurement and is based on the behavior and potential of the tumor, the growth patterns of the various physical forms, duration, the anatomic site of occurrence, the clinical extent and size of the tumor and histologic assessment. The treatment modality is also determined considering the age and general health of the patient.

1. Complete eradication of lesion
2. Reconstruction of the resultant defect (Figs 36.30 and 36.31).

Curettage should never be considered as the treatment modality, since intraosseous multicystic lesions' recurrence rate is 55 to 100 percent after curettage, and for intraosseous unicystic lesions—18 to 25 percent.

The characteristic feature of this tumor is that it microscopically infiltrates bone beyond the tumor-bone interface seen in imaging. A safe margin of uninvolved bone is approximately 2 cm for solid and multicystic lesions. This may mean that important structures like inferior alveolar nerve may be resected en bloc with the tumor (Figs 36.32A and B).

For intraosseous, solid/multicystic ameloblastoma:

1. En bloc resection or marginal resection without continuity defect
2. Segmental resection with continuity defect:
   • If cortical bone is resorbed and penetrated, the resection should include periosteal layer.
   • A thin inferior border of the mandible in the first procedure may fracture, if a reconstruction plate is not used to span and support the segment. Retention of less than 1 cm in thickness of an inferior border is not practical and second surgical procedure should be opted.
   • If the complete excision of the tumor is ascertained by clinical and radiographic examination of specimen or intraoperative frozen section, then immediate reconstruction can be undertaken.

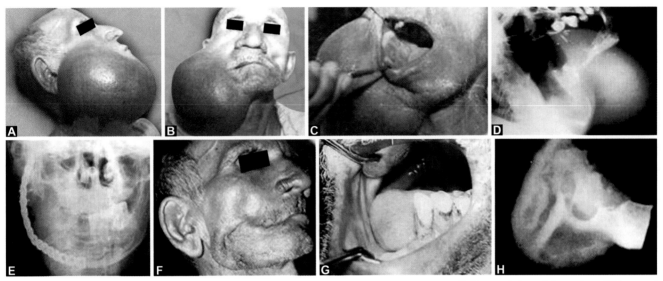

Figs 36.30A to H: Extensive ameloblastoma of right ramus and body in 80 years old male: (A and B) Extraoral view of the patient, (C) Intraoral view of the lesion, (D) Radiograph of the lesion, (E) Postoperative radiograph after hemimandibulectomy with disarticulation and reconstruction plate fixation, (F and G) Postoperative views, extraoral and intraoral respectively, (H) Radiograph of the tumor specimen showing safe margin

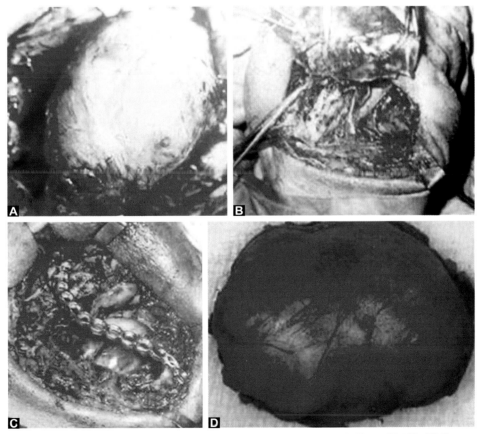

Figs 36.31A to D: Intraoperative pictures of resection of the ameloblastoma in a patient shown in Figure 36.30A: (A) Exposure of the tumor mass through extraoral submandibular incision, (B) Resection of the tumor with hemimandibulectomy with disarticulation of condyle, (C) Reconstruction plate fixation for maintaining the continuity of the mandible, (D) Resected specimen

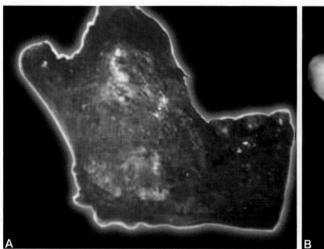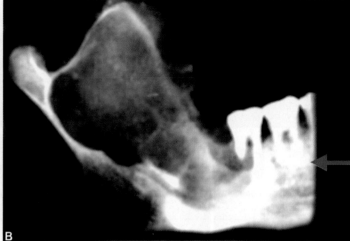

Figs 36.32A and B: Hemimandibulectomy with disarticulation, tumor resection specimen and its radiograph. Note the safe margin of normal bone in resection

- If there is uncertainty about resection margins, reconstruction should be delayed until no recurrence is seen, at least after six months post-operatively.
- Adequate soft tissue coverage should be available, if immediate reconstruction is planned.
- Immediate reconstruction can be done by using an autogenous free bone grafts (iliac or rib graft) or bank allogenic bone crib and autogenous bone marrow with a reconstruction plate.
- Reconstruction plate with or without condylar prosthesis can be used in very old patients, or in cases where secondary reconstruction is planned or where adequate soft tissue coverage is not available.
- If sufficient soft tissue is not available locally, a vascularized composite pedicle graft of bone and myocutaneous tissue can be used.
- In maxilla—aggressive resection is carried out (Figs 36.33A to M).

Jackson and Callon Forte (1996) have given guidelines depending upon anatomical extents:

i. Tumor confined to maxilla without orbital floor involvement—Partial maxillectomy
ii. Tumors involving the orbital floor, but not the periorbital area—Total maxillectomy.
iii. Tumor involving orbital contents—Total maxillectomy with orbital exenteration
iv. Tumor involving the skull bone—Along with skull base resection—Neurosurgical procedure.

Behavior: The multicystic ameloblastoma has a recurrence up to 50 percent during the first 5 years post-operatively. Long term follow up is a must.

Calcifying Epithelial Odontogenic Tumor (CEOT) (Pindborg Tumor)

First described by Pindborg in 1955.

- Origin—epithelial elements of the enamel organ.
- Incidence—uncommon. One percent of all odontogenic tumors.
- No specific sex predilection.
- *Age:* Seen in middle age—30 to 50 years.
- *Site:* Mandible is most commonly involved in the molar region (2/3 of the tumors). One-third of the tumors are found in the maxilla. Marked predilection for the molar region in both the jaws.
- Fifty percent of the tumors are associated with an unerupted or embedded tooth.
- *Signs and symptoms:* Painless, slow growing mass. If encroached on nasal cavity, then produce nasal symptoms like stuffiness, epistaxis, etc.
- *Variety*—(i) Intraosseous, (ii) Extraosseous—nonspecific, sessile gingival masses commonly seen in anterior gingiva.
- *Radiographic features*—depending on the stage of development, CEOT presents variable radiographic picture.

   i. Unilocular or multilocular radiolucency with a well circumscribed border or diffuse lesion.

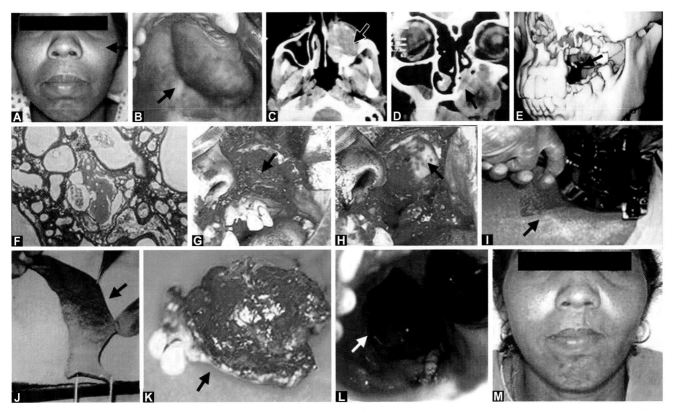

Figs 36.33A to M: A 30-year-old female with recurrent swelling in posterior left maxilla. Patient was operated 5 years back for plexiform ameloblastoma with enucleation: (A and B) Extraoral and intraoral view of the recurrent lesion, (C and D) CT scans—tumor mass involving left maxilla and maxillary sinus and lateral wall of the nose, infraorbital ridge, (E) 3D CT scan—tumor mass involving left maxilla, (F) Biopsy-photomicrography—plexiform ameloblastoma, (G and H) Surgical exposure by modified Weber0Fergusson incision, (I and J) Harvesting of split thickness skin graft to cover maxillectomy defect, (K) Tumor specimen after left maxillectomy and resection of lesion, (L) Postoperative healing of skin graft after 6 months in intraoral view, (M) Postoperative extraoral view 6 months after surgery

ii. Multilocular honey comb appearance—combined pattern of radiolucency and radiopacity with many small, irregular bony trabeculae traversing the radiolucency in multidirection.

iii. Driven snow appearance—scattered flakes of calcification throughout the radiolucency can be seen. Can be seen more concentrated around the crown of the embedded tooth.

iv. Lesion (mainly unilocular) may be associated with embedded tooth.

- *Histopathology:* A locally invasive epithelial tumor characterized by the development of intraepithelial structures, probably of an amyloid like nature, which may become calcified and which may be liberated as the cells breakdown. The areas of calcification form concentric rings termed as *'Liesegang rings'*. These tend to fuse together to form large complex masses.
- CEOT shows some potential for recurrence (15%) and aggressiveness.

- *Management:* Careful excision of the tumor with margin of normal tissue and follow up.

Squamous Odontogenic Tumor

- A rare benign tumor, first reported by Pullon in 1975.
- *Pathogenesis*—presumed to arise from neoplastic transformation of the epithelial cell rests of Malassez within the periodontal ligament of lateral surface of erupted tooth.
- Can be mistaken histologically as an acanthamatous ameloblastoma or a well differentiated epidermoid carcinoma.
- *Age*—ranges from 11 to 67 years.
- No sex predilection.
  Site—maxilla and mandible—equal predilection.
  Maxilla—incisor—canine area
  Mandible—premolar—molar area

Multiple site involvement may be seen. Both jaws may be involved in the same patient.

- Asymptomatic lesions, may experience mild pain, discomfort, tooth mobility.
- Radiographic appearance—nondiagnostic.
    - It may appear as a semicircular or triangular radiolucency with sclerotic/well defined borders.
    - It may be seen associated with cervical portion of the tooth.
- *Histopathology*—varying shaped islands of mature squamous epithelium without a peripheral palisaded or polarized columnar layer.
- Conservative local excision is done for this tumor.

Clear Cell Odontogenic Tumor (CCOT)

- Rare jaw tumor, slow growing lesion, central tumor.
- First described by Waldron in 1984.
- *Age*—above 50 years.
- No sex predilection.
- *Site*—75 percent in the mandible—anterior mandible is the site of predilection, followed by the body and the angle region. 25 percent in the maxilla.
- *Radiographically*—a radiolucent unilocular or multilocular lesion with poorly defined irregular borders. Evidence of bone destruction and root resorption.
- *Histologically*—benign but locally invasive neoplasm, originating from odontogenic epithelium and characterized by sheets and islands of uniform, vacuolated and clear cells.
- Strong potential for local aggressiveness and should be therefore treated radically.

Tumors Arising from Odontogenic Epithelium with Odontogenic Ectomesenchyme with or without Dental Hard Tissue Formation

Ameloblastic Fibroma

- Rare benign neoplasm
- Odontogenic epithelium and odontogenic ectomesenchyme proliferate as a combined soft tissue neoplasm, without the formation of calcified tooth structures.
- *Age*—found in first two decades (20 years)
- *Sex*—both males and females are equally affected.
- *Site*—occurs in both the jaws, but site of predilection is mandible, especially the third molar area.

- *Radiographically*—well defined uni or multilocular radiolucency with sclerotic border. May be associated with unerupted tooth.
    The lesion can be seen from small to large extensive.   Size ranging from 1 to 8 cms.
- *The growth pattern* of ameloblastic fibroma occurs usually by smooth expansion within the jaws, producing cortical bone thinning or resorption. (Finger like projections of the tumor extend into the bone).
- *Histopathology* composed of a cell rich mesenchymal appearing connective tissue in which odontogenic epithelium is predominantly displayed and dispersed throughout the lesion.
- Meticulous surgical enucleation with follow up.

Ameloblastic Fibro-odontoma

- Mixed odontogenic tumor
- Combination of ameloblastic fibroma and forming complex odontoma. The lesion has expansile growth potential of the former and the inductive capability of the latter.
- *Age*—first and second decades (Children)
- *Sex*—more common in males, 3:1 ratio
- *Site*—mandible—premolar—molar region. However, can be found in both jaws.
- Jaw enlargement without symptoms.
- *Radiographically*: Uni or multilocular radiolucency with well defined sclerotic border with radiopacity in the center of the lesion. It may be associated with unerupted teeth or can be seen in place of absent teeth.
- *Histologically*: Cords and strands of odontogenic epithelium dispersed in a cell rich mesenchymal tissue, plus areas of odontogenic epithelium and the mesenchymal tissue form dental papillae and enamel organ. Enamel matrix and dentin are produced in bizarre forms. The tumor is well surrounded by a connective tissue capsule.
- Conservative management with enucleation.

Ameloblastic Fibrodentinoma

- Similar to ameloblastic fibroma, but shows inductive changes that lead to the formation of dentin.
- Rare, benign odontogenic mixed tumor.
- Considered to be a hemartoma rather than a neoplasm.

- *Site*—more common in mandible than maxilla (3:1).
- *Sex*—in males more often than females (2:1).
- *Age*—4 to 60 years of age (mostly below 30 years of age).
- *In children* the lesion may be associated with unerupted or missing deciduous teeth and found in the anterior jaw.
- *In adults*—seen more in posterior region involving permanent teeth.
- Asymptomatic swelling of the jaws.
- *Radiographically*—small or extensive uni or multilocular with well defined borders. Radiopacity may be dispersed throughout the lesion. The associated teeth are often seen to be deeply situated in the lesion.
- *Histologically*—several configurations are seen within a basic lesional format of ameloblastic fibroma. Various stages of induction of dentin may be demonstrated, resulting in lesions that display dentinoid, osteodentin and rarely, tubular dentine. The dentine may be infrequently and poorly mineralized.
- Complete excision of the lesion.

Adenomatoid Odontogenic Tumor (AOT) (Figs 36.34A to P)

- First recognized as separate entity by Stafne.
- The term coined by Philipsen and Birn in 1969.
- It may be considered as hemartoma.
- Incidence—3 to 7 percent of odontogenic tumors.
- *Age*—Younger age group—10 to 20 years (73%) rarely above 30 years.
- *Sex*—Predilection to occur in females—65 percent.
- *Site*—More common in maxilla—65 percent and usually involves the anterior region.
- Associated with impacted permanent teeth (invariably canine tooth in about 74%)
- Painless swelling.
- *Radiologically*—unilocular radiolucency around the crown of an impacted tooth, resembling a dentigerous cyst. Radiolucency may extend apically along the root crossing CE junction. More often the radiolucency show fine calcification (snowflake). The margins are well defined and sclerotic.
- *Differential diagnosis*—Pindborg tumor, CCOT or Gorlin cyst, ameloblastoma.
- *Histopathology.* The lesion is surrounded by a thick, fibrous capsule.
  Shows epithelial cells either polyhedral or even spindle shaped with scanty stroma of connective

tissue. Cells are arranged in sheets, cords or whorled masses, which may form rosette like structure about a central space. Foci of calcification presumed to be abortive enamel formation or dentinoid/cementum like material are seen.
Calcification in several forms may be observed.
  i. Irregular dystrophic bodies.
  ii. Laminated or ring like calcifications
  iii. Large globular masses.
- *Treatment:* Conservative excision or enucleation, because of the capsule is possible. Recurrence is rare with good prognosis.

Odontoma

The term refers to any tumor of odontogenic origin, in true sense. This is the growth in which both epithelial and ectomesenchymal cells exhibit complete or incomplete differentiation of tooth formation. This is considered more as a hemartomatous malformation, also as composite lesion, as it contains more than one tissue.
  Radiographically and histopathologically, it is recognizable in two forms:
1. Compound odontoma
2. Complex odontoma

Compound composite odontoma: It consists of formed calcified toothlike structures or miniature dwarfed teeth (Figs 36.35 and 36.36).

Complex composite odontoma: It is a malformation in which all the dental tissues are represented, with the individual tissues being well formed but occurring in a disorderly pattern. Here the calcified dental tissues are simply found as an irregular mass bearing no morphological similarity to the rudimentary teeth. (Disorderly and haphazard arrangement of calcified dental structure) (Figs 36.37 to 33.40).

- Most common type of odontogenic lesion (< 30%)
- *Age*—first and second decades (10-70 years)
- *Sex*—equal predilection in both sexes.
- *Site*—occurs in both the jaws.

Complex more common in mandible—67 percent.

Compound: More common in maxilla
  Compound odontomas are seen in anterior jaw.
  Complex odontomas are seen in posterior jaw, especially in third molar region.
- Generally asymptomatic
- Radiographically:

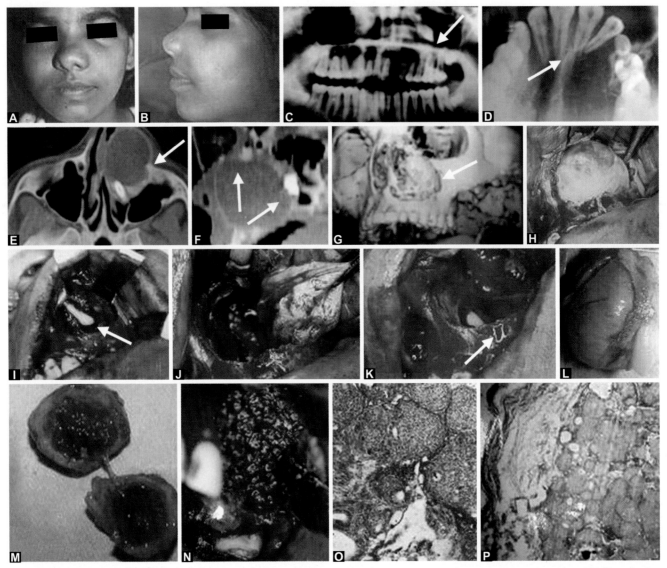

Figs 36.34A to P: Adenomatoid odontogenic tumor in a 14-year-old girl in left maxilla: (A and B) Preoperative extraoral view, (C and D) Preoperative X-rays showing well-defined radiolucency in left maxilla with impacted canine, over retained deciduous lateral incisor and canine, (E and F) Preoperative CT scan—displaced nasal septum and teeth, involvement of maxillary sinus, (G) 3D CT—destruction of anterolateral wall maxilla, orbital floor, deviation of nasal septum, (H) Intraoral exposure of lesion, (I) Upper left lateral incisor on the inferolateral aspect of lesion, (J) Lesion being enucleated, (K) Canine displaced at infraorbital region, (L and M) Excised and cut specimen, (N) Defect filled with hydroxyapatite granules, (O and P) Photomicrograph of AOT—Cuboidal epithelial cells forming rosette like structure. Minimal stromal tissue

– *Compound odontoma*—appears as a radiopaque mass of calcified structures with an anatomic similarity to normal teeth. Seen as a pocket of malformed or dwarfed teeth or toothlike forms surrounded by a narrow radiolucent zone. Sometimes overlying or along side an unerupted tooth or between the roots of a deciduous tooth. It prevents eruption of underlying permanent tooth.

– *Complex odontoma*—may be small, large or occasionally huge, irregular or ovoid smooth, densely radiopaque mass, often surrounded by a thin radiolucent zone. It is frequently overlying a displaced unerupted tooth.

The radiological picture is variable, depending on the stage of formation at the time of incidental discovery. It will range from complete radiolucency in the initial stage to

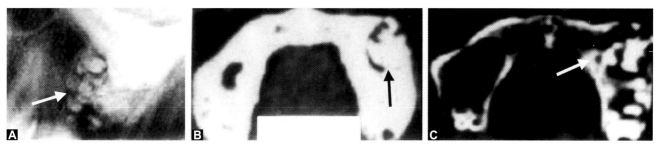

Figs 36.35A to C: Radiograph and CT scan: Compound composite odontoma

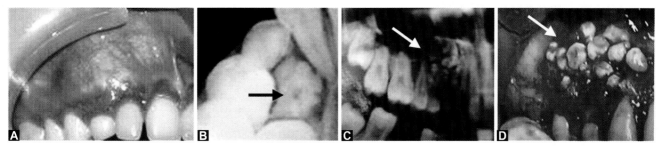

Figs 36.36A to D: Compound composite odontoma: (A) Intraoral buccal expansion, (B) Occlusal view maxilla X-ray showing radiopaque mass on palatal side, (C) OPG showing odontoma (D) Surgical exposure of odontoma

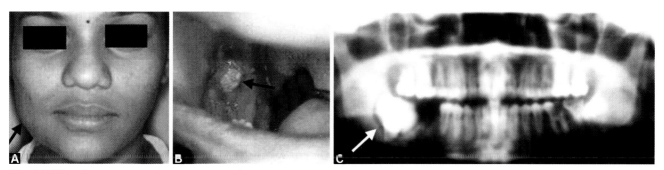

Figs 36.37A to C: Complex odontoma: (A) Extraoral swelling at right angle area, (B) Intraoral swelling in second and third molar area, with small exposed part of complex odontoma, (C) OPG showing dense radiopaque mass with displaced lower third molar, surrounded by thin radiolucent zone. Second molar is missing. First molar was extracted

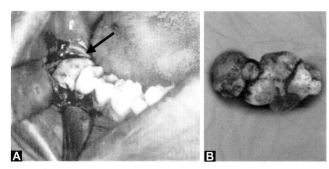

Fig. 36.38A and B: Complex odontoma removed from right third molar region

the stage of 'maturation', i.e. complete calcified structure. Mixed radiolucency and radiopacity can be seen in one lesion also.

- Asymptomatic, shows no expansion of the bone and facial asymmetry.
- Commonly detected on radiographs.
- May show associated unerupted or impacted teeth, associated swelling and infection.
- *Histologically*, the compound odontoma shows a connective tissue capsule. The lesion is composed of anatomically distinct, small, well formed or distorted teeth with enamel, dentine, pulp and

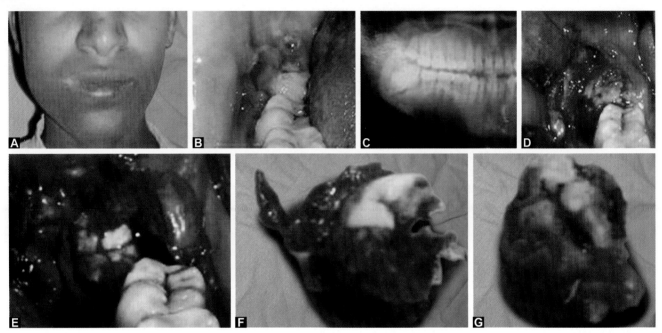

Figs 36.39A to G: Complex composite odontoma: Clinical, radiological, surgical presentation

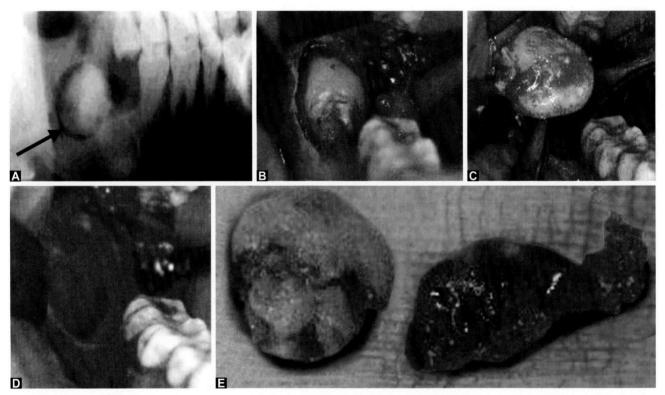

Figs 36.40A to E: Complex odontoma: (A) Lateral oblique view X-ray showing well encapsulated radiopaque mass at angle of the ascending ramus, (B) Surgical exposure of the mass, in a 50-year-old lady, who came with the C/O intraoral pus discharge from right angle region, since 4 months, (C) Surgical removal of the mass, (D) Surgical defect, (E) Complex odontoma and its capsule

cementum. The complex odontoma lacks anatomical organization and consists of calcified dental tissue in a haphazard manner, bound together in a mass of cementum and often surrounded by a thin connective tissue capsule.

- *Management:* Completely calcified complex or compound odontoma is biologically inert and can be left alone.

Reasons for Excision

i. Once detected, patient may be psychologically affected about the diagnosis of the lesion.
ii. To remove the blockade of the favorably placed unerupted tooth underneath or nearby.
iii. To obtain definite diagnosis between the complex odontoma and cementoblastoma or ossifying fibroma or CEOT, etc.
- *Surgical treatment (Intraoral approach):* Adequate amount of overlying bone removal should be done to access the lesion. Compound odontoma is enucleated if the capsule is intact. If the capsule is disrupted, then the individual teeth forms are removed carefully. Small complex odontoma can be enucleated. Large complex odontomas may be fused to the surrounding bone and is very hard. It should be cut into pieces for removal. If excessive force is used to elevate the lesion, the jaw fracture can occur.
- Recurrence is not seen.

TUMORS ARISING FROM ODONTOGENIC ECTOMESENCHYME WITH OR WITHOUT INCLUSION OF ODONTOGENIC EPITHELIUM

Odontogenic Fibroma

- An uncommon, hence poorly understood entity.
- Central benign odontogenic tumor, which contains a moderately cellular fibrous connective tissue stroma with variable amount of inactive odontogenic epithelium.
  The odontogenic fibroma is found:
  i. Intraosseously—central odontogenic fibroma
  ii. Extraosseously—on the gingiva—peripheral odontogenic fibroma.

Central odontogenic fibroma

- Slow, persistant growth and asymptomatic cortical expansion (mainly detected on radiographs)

- *Site*—more commonly seen in mandible. If seen in maxilla—anterior to the first molar.
- *Sex*—males are more affected.
- *Age*—mean age 37 years.
- *Radiologically:* Multiloculated radiolucency with well defined sclerotic margin or an ill-defined nonsclerotic border that merges into surrounding bone. May show extensive root resorption or root divergence. May be associated with unerupted third molars.
- *Histologically:* The connective tissue stroma shows a whorling or interlacing dense collagen matrix with fairly cellular uniform fibroblasts. The odontogenic epithelial component is seen as narrow islands, strands or cords of cuboidal cells. Occasionally some hyalinization or cementum—bone like or dentinoid like calcification can be seen around some of epithelial islands. It is not a capsulated lesion.
- *Differential diagnosis:* Desmoplastic fibroma, myxoma.
- *Management:* Enucleation and curettage.

Peripheral odontogenic fibroma

- *Site*—seen more frequently in the mandible. Most lesions are found anterior to the second premolar. Size—1 to 3 cm.
- The lesions are attached on the gingiva—pedunculated or sessile and have normal gingival color.
- *Sex*—seen equally in males and females.
- *Age*—1st to 8th decade.
- *Treatment*—excision with a margin of uninvolved tissue.

Myxoma (Odontogenic Myxoma or Myxofibroma) (Figs 36.41 and 36.42)

- Central benign, slowly growing, infiltrative tumor of the jaws, which expands the bone and causes destruction of the cortex, with a relatively rare occurrence (9.2 % of all the odontogenic tumors)
- Mostly found in tooth bearing areas of the jaws.
- Occurs both in maxilla and the mandible with a slight predilection for mandible.
- Usually unilateral lesions, but some may cross the midline. Facial asymmetry may be prominent.
- Females are affected more than males—1.5 :1 ratio.
- Wide age range—11 months—70 years.
- The occurrence in children is higher (not below 10 years of age).

- *Pathogenesis:* It is derived from the mesenchymal portion of the tooth germ, either the dental papilla or the follicle, or the periodontal ligament. Apart from its origin being from the mesenchyme or ectomesenchyme of a developing tooth germ. It has also been associated with a myxomatous change of an odontogenic fibroma or residual foci of embryonic tissue.

  A debate still persists whether odontogenic myxoma is truly an odontogenic neoplasm? But its histological similarity to the stellate reticulum of developing tooth, its exclusive occurrence in close proximity and vicinity to the tooth bearing parts of the jaws, occasional association with a missing or unerupted tooth, the presence of odontogenic epithelium, and its rare appearance in any other part of the skeleton establishes its odontogenic origin.

- *Radiologically*—multilocular, small or extensive lesion. May be completely radiolucent or 'soap bubble' or 'honey comb' or 'tennis racket' appearance with irregular, scalloped margins.
- *Differential diagnosis* ameloblastoma, hemangioma, etc.
- *Histologically* characterized by stellate-shaped, angular or rounded mesenchymal cells in a homogenous mucoid stroma, may contain few collagen fibrils. Large and small lesions can resorb cortical bone and penetrate periosteum.

  Based on ultrastructural three principal histological variants of odontogenic myxoma can be distinguished:
  1. Well differentiated fibroblast (30–40%), which appears spindle like on longitudinal section and stellate on cross section.

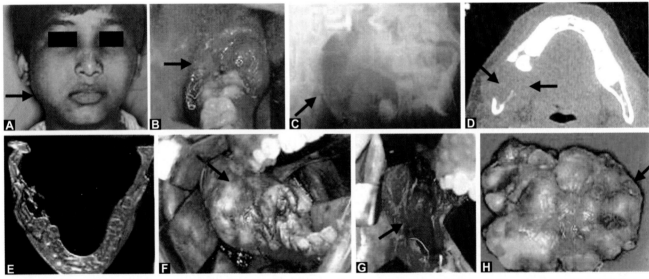

Figs 36.41A to H: Odontogenic myxoma of right mandible in a 10-year-old male patient (A and B) Preoperative extraoral and intraoral view of the lesion, (C) Preoperative X-ray showing the lesion involving ramus and angle region, (D) CT scan showing expansion of buccal and lingual cortices with areas of expansion, (E) 3D CT scan, (F) Exposure of tumor mass by intraoral approach, (G) Surgical defect after excision of tumor mass, (H) Soft gelatinous mass with slimy appearance

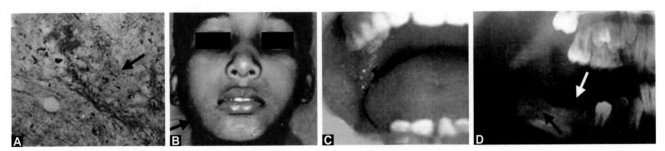

Figs 36.42A to D: (A) Histopathology of odontogenic myxoma (B and C) Postoperative extraoral and intraoral views (D) Six months postoperative OPG showing regeneration of bone

2. Myxoblastic cell (10%), an immature cell with numerous ribosomes, located within an amorphous tumor matrix consisting of acid mucopolysaccharides
3. An intermediate cell having morphological characteristics of both main tumor cell type (40–50%)

- *Macroscopically* gelatinous texture and shiny appearance.
- *Treatment:* As it is infiltrative in nature and absence of encapsulation, recurrence rate is high.
- *Extensive lesions*—excision by resection without continuity defect or resection with continuity defect—including a perimeter margin of tumor free bone. The neurovascular bundle should not be sacrificed routinely. The immediate or delayed reconstruction is dependent upon the clinical and/or histological certainty of complete excision of the tumor.
- Recurrence rate is 33 percent
- Long term follow up.

Benign Cementoblastoma (Cementoblastoma, True Cementoma) (Figs 36.43A to F)

- True neoplasm of cemental origin.
- True cementoma: It is defined by WHO as a neoplasm characterized by the formation of sheets of cementum like tissue containing a large number of reversal lines and being unmineralized at the periphery of the mass or in the more active growth areas.
- It is a rare tumor of connective tissue, forming cementum like calcification, fused to a tooth root.
- *Age*—10 to 20 years.
- No sex predilection.
- Almost equal frequency in mandible and the maxilla. Always in the premolar or molar region.
- Mandibular lesions are found to be attached to a single tooth, while in maxillary lesions they are found to be fused to two or more teeth.
- Slow growing lesion with clinical expansion of the jaw, producing facial asymmetry. Sometimes

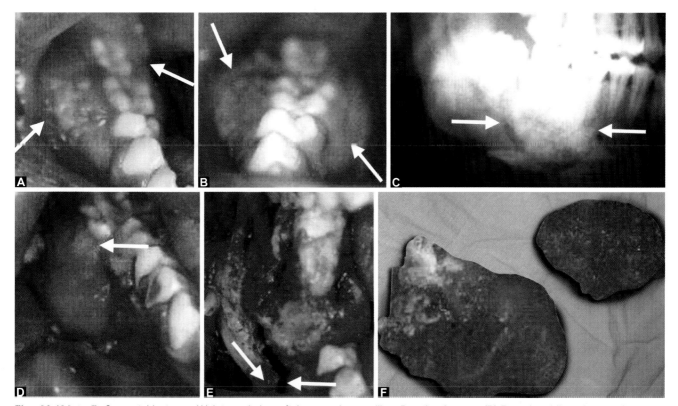

Figs 36.43A to F: Cementoblastoma: (A) Intraoral view of slow growing swelling. Duration 3 years, (B) Buccal and lingual expansion seen, (C) OPG showing well defined, oval radiopaque mass with a radiolucent periphery. The mass is fused to the roots of lower right first and second molars, (D) Surgical exposure of the mass, (E) Thinning out of buccal cortical plate and pathological fracture (arrows) during excision of the mass, (F) Cementoblastoma—excised specimen

resorption of the cortical bone is seen. No discomfort or pain. The affected tooth is frequently vital.

- *Radiographically:* A well defined, round, oval radiopaque mass with a radiolucent periphery, which is fused to a single or multiple roots of a tooth. The affected roots usually show partial resorption.
- *Differential diagnosis:* Condensing osteitis, cementifying fibroma, osteoblastoma, odontoma, etc.
- Histologically
  - Main bulk consists of a dense cementum or osteocemental mass
  - Numerous reversal lines forming a calcified mosaic pattern is seen occupying the central area of the lesion.

At periphery, trabeculae are almost arranged at right angles. Peripheral active fibrous stroma shows unmineralized fine cemental trabeculae bordered by cementoblasts and cementoclasts farther away from it.

- *Management:* As the size of the lesion usually varies between 1 to 3 cm in diameter and the lesion is separated from the surrounding bone by capsular like connective tissue—it can be easily enucleated. Large lesions can be cut into segments for enucleation. Tooth attached to the lesion is extracted with the lesion.

■ NONODONTOGENIC LESIONS OF THE JAWS

Osteogenic Neoplasm

Cemento-ossifying fibroma (COF), Cementifying fibroma.

Ossifying Fibroma (Figs 36.44 to 36.46)

The lesion previously termed as cementifying fibroma was considered as odontogenic tumor. But today it is agreed that these lesions are best classified as osteogenic neoplasms.

- *Origin:* Ossifying fibroma is a benign lesion arising from undifferentiated cells of the periodontal ligament.
- *Age:* Third and fourth decades of life.
- *Sex:* A definite female predominance with female to male ratio—5:1.
- *Site:* Mandible is the most common site—premolar molar area. Maxilla—common site—posterior maxilla.
- *Signs and symptoms:* Small lesions are symptomless and detected on radiological examination. Larger

lesions are painless, slow, but persistently growing swelling of the involved bone, often causing facial asymmetry. Pain and paresthesia are not associated. Gradual expansion and thinning of the buccal and lingual cortical plates is seen.

- *Radiologically:* Well circumscribed lesion with sharply defined border between the lesion and adjacent normal bone. Most often it shows unilocular radiolucency, but varying degrees of radiopacity can be seen. After maturation and mineralization of long standing, the lesion appears as a dense, radiopaque mass surrounded by a thin, well-defined regular radiolucent rim. As the lesion enlarges, it may displace the adjacent teeth and less commonly, cause resorption of the roots. Large ossifying fibroma of the mandible, often may demonstrate a typical downward bowing of the inferior cortex of the mandible.
- *Histopathology:* It may show a fibrous capsule surrounding a tumor or it is well demarcated neoplasm composed of fibrous tissue that contains varying amounts of calcified tissue resembling bone, cementum or both. The tumor consists of a collagenous stroma, containing variable numbers of uniform spindled on stellate cells. The feature which distinguishes ossifying fibroma from fibrous dysplasia is the focal presence of osteoblasts along the surface of the bone deposits. Two types of calcifications are commonly seen—(1) in the form of trabeculae of osteoid and bone (2) basophilic ovoid calcifications that resemble cementum like material.
- *Management:* As the lesion is well demarcated from the surrounding bone, it permits relatively easy separation in one piece or in several large pieces. Intraoral approach by enucleation is the preferred method. Adjacent teeth, neurovascular bundle and bone should be preserved, whenever possible. More extensive lesion may require resection and bone grafting. Recurrence is not seen (Figs 36.44 to 36.46).

Juvenile Aggressive Ossifying Fibroma

This is the uncommon, controversial lesion. It is described in the literature under various terms as *juvenile active ossifying fibroma, aggressive psammomatoid ossifying fibroma.* It is distinguished from the standard ossifying fibroma on the basis of occurrence in a younger age group, tendency to occur in different anatomic sites and aggressive clinical behavior (Fig. 36.47).

- *Age:* Most commonly seen below the age of 15 years in younger children.
- *Site:* Orbital, frontal and ethmoid bones are most frequently involved. The maxilla, paranasal sinuses are more frequently involved than mandible.
- *Signs and symptoms:* Some tumors show rapid progressive growth and enlargement with expansion and thinning of the adjacent cortical bone and invasion of adjacent tissue. Common clinical symptoms include proptosis, exophthalmos, visual disturbances, nasal obstruction and facial asymmetry.
- *Radiographically:* Variable features, depending on the location and the amount of calcified tissue. A destructive, expansile lesion often with well demarcated borders, but it may demonstrate invasion and erosion of the surrounding bone. Varying degrees of radiolucency and opacity may be seen depending on the degree of mineralization.

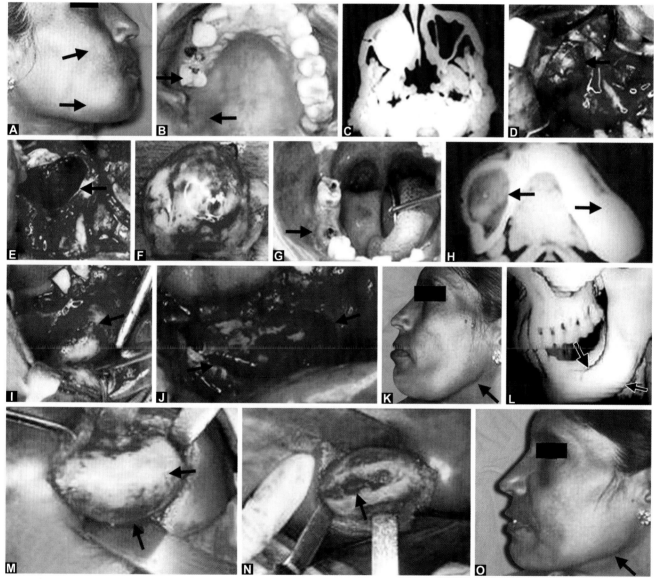

Figs 36.44A to O: Multiple lesions of the jaw bones in a 36-year-old female: (A) (R) maxilla—ossifying fibroma, (R) mandible—radicular cyst, (B) Buccal and palatal expansion, (C) CT scan (R) maxilla, (D) Ossifying fibroma exposed through Weber-Fergusson incision, (E) Tumor mass excision, (F) Tumor specimen, (G) Radicular cyst location, (H) CT scan showing R mandibular radicular cyst and L mandible fibrous dysplasia (I) Radicular cyst—surgical exposure in R mandible (J) Cyst enucleation done, (K) Bowing of inferior border mandible (L) CT scan, (L) mandible-fibrous dysplasia (M and N) shave down recountering surgery for (L) mandible inferior border (O) Postoperative (L) profile after recountouring procedure

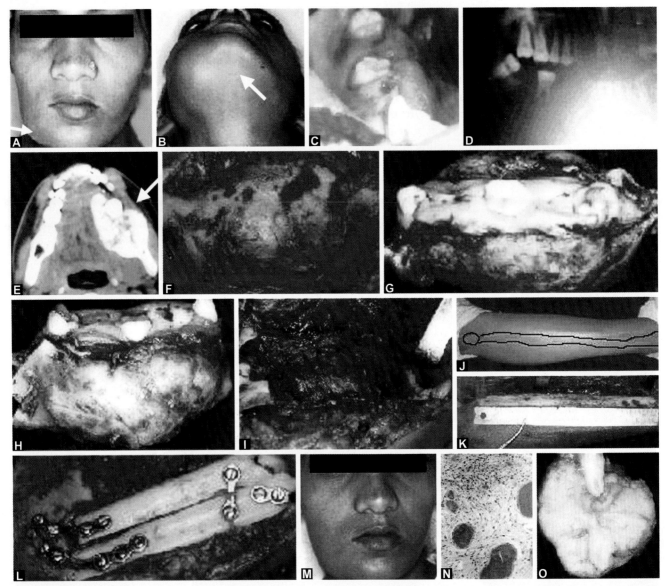

Figs 36.45A to O: Ossifying fibroma, segmental resection, reconstruction with fibular graft: (A and B) Extraoral views of swelling involving (R) ramus and body mandible. Note the bowing and expansion of the inferior border, (C) Intraoral view of the lesion history of exfoliation of 1st, 2nd premolars and 2nd molar. Expansion of the cortices is seen, (D) Radiograph, (E) CT scan showing well circumscribed lesion with sharply defined borders. Mixed radiopaque/radiolucent lesion, (F) Surgical exposure of tumor via submandibular extraoral incision, (G) Occlusal view of the resected specimen showing expansion and fibrous tissue capsule, (H) Segmental resection, (I) Intraoral water tight closure, prior to immediate reconstruction with fibular grafting, (J) Preparation of fibula, (K) Harvesting of fibular graft, (L) Graft fixation with bone plates and screws, (M) Postoperative facial view, (N) Photomicrograph—calcified bodies and cementicles seen in firbous stoma, (O) Cut surface of specimen—pink white gritty surface with fibrous and calcified tissue

- *Histopathology:* The stroma consists of a highly cellular proliferation of spindled to stellate cells with minimum intervening collagen. Small strands of immature cellular osteoid forms within the lesion. Some lesions contain numerous uniform, often laminated structures described as ossicles or psammoma like bodies surrounded by osteoid rims. Some investigators believe that this is the characteristic microscopic feature of this neoplasm.

- *Treatment and prognosis:* Uncertain to state. Recurrence rate is reported as 30 to 58 percent. Complete surgical excision is mandatory. Small accessible lesions are treated with enucleation or peripheral osteotomy. Large lesions require en bloc resection.

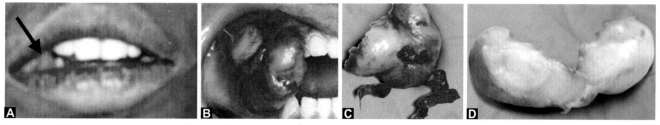

Figs 36.46A to D: Peripheral ossifying fibroma: A 28-year-old female with painless mass of one year duration. Excision of the mass associated with right upper first and second premolars done

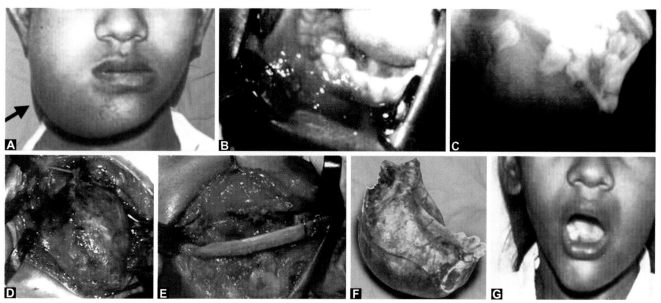

Figs 36.47A to G: Juvenile ossifying fibroma: (A) A 14-year-old girl with large, bony swelling of (R) mandible, (B) Intraoral swelling from (R) canine to retromolar region, (C) X-ray, (D) Surgical exposure of the lesion, (E) Reconstruction with rib graft, (F) Resected specimen, (G) Postoperative facial view and near normal mandibular movement

Osteoma (Figs 36.48 and 36.49)

Osteomas are benign tumors, which consist of mature, compact or cancellous bone. Osteomas are found only in the craniofacial skeleton and rarely found in other bones like clavicles and long bones.

- *Etiology is unclear:* Some appear as true neoplasm of the bone, while other show response to trauma or infection.
- Variety (i) Peripheral osteoma or periosteal osteoma, which arise on the surface of the jaw bone as a polypoid or sessile mass (ii) Endosteal osteoma or enostoses—those which develop centrally within medullary bone.
- *Age:* Detected in young adults. 2nd to 5th decades.
- *Sex:* Predilection not known.

- *Signs and symptoms:* Periosteal osteoma presents as a slow growing, asymptomatic bony hard masses. Asymmetry of the affected bone may be evident, when lesion enlarges to sufficient proportion. The lesion may arise in the maxilla or mandible, especially at the angle of the mandible and lingual aspect of the mandible in premolar/molar area. An osteoma involving the mandibular condyle may cause a slow progressive shift in the patient's occlusion with deviation of the midline of the chin towards the unaffected side.

Small endosteal osteomas are asymptomatic, but large lesions cause progressive enlargement of the affected area. Lesions within the paranasal sinuses may develop symptoms like sinusitis, headaches, ophthalmological problems.

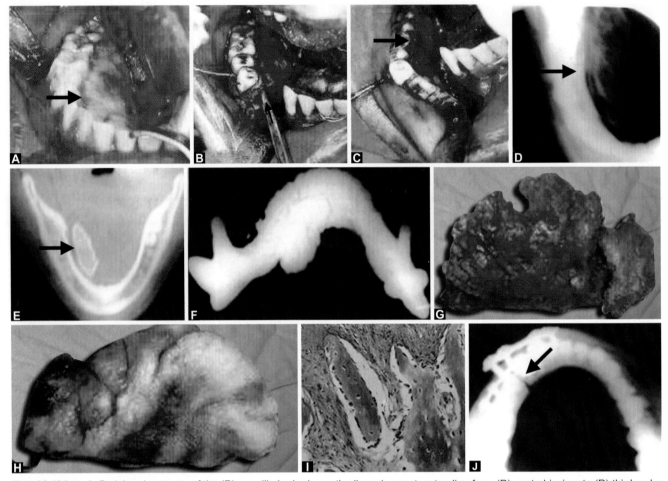

Figs 36.48A to J: Peripheral osteoma of the (R) mandibular body, on the lingual aspect, extending from (R) central incisor to (R) third molar region. (A) Firm, nontender growth in 20 years old male, duration—2 years, (B) Access osteotomy performed in lower (R) canine and premolar region to approach the mass. Excision with the osteotome, (C) Excision complete, (D) Preoperative occlusal X-ray suggestive of osteogenic tumor, (E) CT scan—over hanging lesion on the medial surface of the mandible, (F) 3D scan showing the extension of the mass from (R) central incisor to third molar region. The mass is hanging below the level of the inferior border, (G) Gross specimen—hard tissue mass, (H) Tough, fibrous tissue covering the lesion, (I) Histology of osteoma, (J) Postoperative occlusal view showing fixation of access osteotomy and complete excision of the lesion

- *Radiographically* well circumscribed, densely sclerotic, radiopaque masses. Periosteal osteoma may show a uniform sclerotic pattern at the periphery with a central trabecular pattern.
- *Histopathologically:* Two varieties are seen. (i) Compact osteoma—composed of dense, compact bone with sparse marrow tissue. The bone is mature and lamellar with osteomas and haversian canals (ii) Cancellous osteomas—composed of lamellar trabeculae of cancellous bone and fibro fatty marrow. Osteoblastic activity may be fairly prominent.
- *Treatment:* Conservative surgical excision is done. Osteotome may be used to separate the periosteal osteoma from the attachment of the underlying bone.

Gardner syndrome: It is inherited as an autosomal dominant disorder. The clinical expression of this genetic disorder is variable. But, the most common manifestations are—multiple adenomatous polyps of the colon and rectum, multiple osteomas, dermal and mesenteric fibrous tumors (fibroma), epidermal and trichilemmal cysts of skin. The presence of mutiple osteomas of the facial bones is an important early marker for this syndrome. Such patients and other family members should be evaluated for other clinical manifestations. Some patients may exhibit distinct hyperplastic alterations of retinal pigmented epithelium, which may precede the colonic or osseous lesions. Dental abnormalities such as impacted permanent and

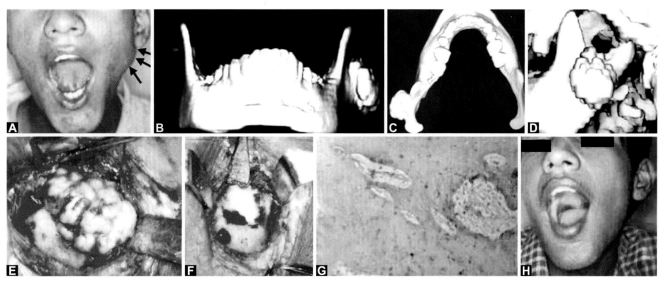

Figs 36.49A to H: Peripheral osteoma on the ascending ramus: (A) In a 16-years-old male, hard, nontender growth below (L) preauricular area. Duration 1 year, (B to D) 3D CT scan revealed a well-defined radiopaque, cauliflower like growth on the external area of ramus, extending till sigmoid notch, (E) Postramal Irby's incision to expose mushroom like bony growth, (F) Excision with osteotome complete, (G) Mature lamellar bone picture, (H) Postoperative view after six months follow up. No recurrence

supernumerary teeth and odontomas may be present in addition to osteomas. Prophylactic colectomy is performed in these patients to prevent transformation of the adenomatous polyps to adenosarcoma or adenocarcinoma.

Benign Osteoblastoma (Figs 36.50A to F)

First described under the name 'Giant osteoid osteoma' by Dahlin and Johnson (1954). Presently accepted term 'Benign osteoblastoma' is suggested by Jaffe and Lichtenstein (1956).

- The lesion is rather uncommon in jaws, seen in long bones and vertebrae.
- *Size*—greater than 2 cm in diameter.
- Vascular osteoid and bone forming benign tumor of bone, characterized cytologically by the abundant presence of actively proliferating osteoblasts and moderate number of multinucleated giant cells in the osteoid tissue.
- It is a central bone tumor.
- Most frequently seen in young patients below 25 years.
- Definite predilection for occurrence in males
- Clinically swelling with or without cortical expansion is noticed, may be of few weeks duration or few years duration. Associated teeth may be mobile.

- Seen in both maxilla and mandible (more) posterior aspect of the jaws.
- It was always misinterpreted as giant cell tumor, but because of ultrastructure histopathological examination demarcation is possible. With few exceptions, tumor osteoblasts resemble normal osteoblasts.
- Radiographic picture—variable. But relatively well defined, mixed radiolucent—radiopaque lesions are seen. When the calcification of the lesion is more, then it appears as a central opacity with a thin radiolucent rim around.
- Intramedullary lesion. A 'sun-ray' appearance of new bone formation may be evident in some lesions misleading to the diagnosis of sarcoma.
- Treatment and prognosis—Complete surgical excision—intraoral approach. Conservative treatment—curettage or local excision also can be done. But follow up should be done for recurrence after conservative treatment.

Osteochondroma (Figs 36.51 to 36.53)

Also known as osteocartilagenous exostosis regarded as the most common benign tumor of bones in the body (1/3 of benign bony tumors). But its occurrence in jaw bone is rare.

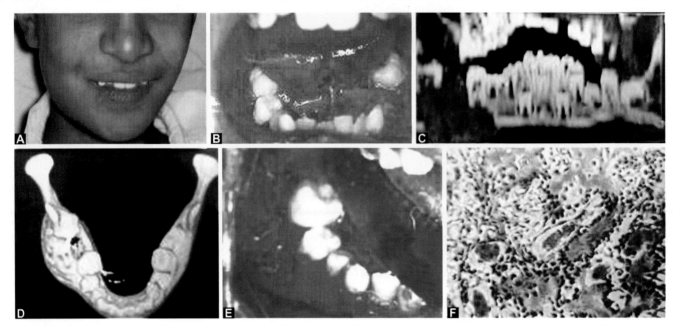

Figs 36.50A to F: Benign osteoblastoma of the right mandibular ramus: (A) Eight-year-old male, with slow growing swelling in (R) side of the lower jaw, since four months, (B) Intraoral bony expansion seen in premolar, molar area with mobility of the teeth, (C and D) OPG and 3D CT scan revealed well-defined radiolucent lesion with buccal and lingual cortical plates expansion in (R) premolar, molar region in the mandible, (E) Intraoral excision of the bluish, grey, firm, gritty mass with multiple lobules was done, (F) Histology: Benign osteoblastoma with moderate number of multinucleated giant cells scattered in osteoid tissue and actively proliferating osteoblasts

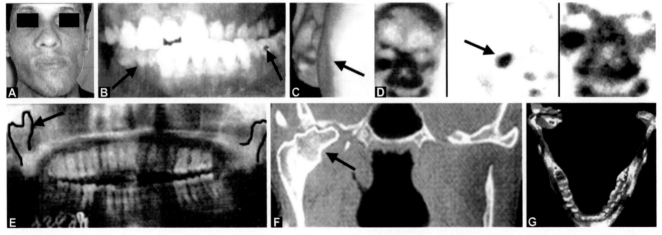

Figs 36.51A to G: Osteochondroma of condyle: (A) A 23-year-old male c/o bony prominence in (R) preauricular area, clicking and inability to carry-out lateral excursion of (R) jaw. Slow growing swelling with deviation of the chin to the left side, causing facial asymmetry, (B) Occlusal derangement with lower midline shift to left side, (C) Visible prominence in (R) preauricular area, (D) Bone scan showing the increased uptake in (R) condylar region, (E to G) OPG, CT scan and 3D scan—well-defined radiopaque/radiolucent mass on the medial aspect of the head of the (R) condyle. Complete excision of the tumor through Al Kayat and Bramley incision was planned

It is not a true neoplasm, but thought to represent a developmental or hemartomatous process of bone. It forms as an exophytic growth from the surface of the affected bone. In the jaw bone mandibular condyle, coronoid process, symphysis, zygomatic arch, posterior maxilla may be involved.

Asymptomatic, bony hard swelling. Involvement of the mandibular condyle may produce unilateral

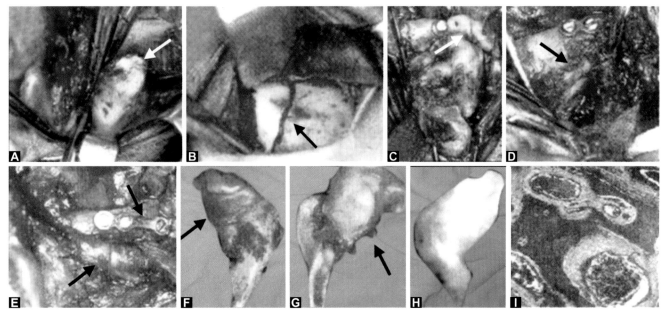

Figs 36.52A to I: Osteochondroma (R) condyle surgery: (A) (R) condyle shifted out of fossa, (B) Risdon's incision condylectomy cut given, (C) Zygomatic arch access osteotomy, (D) Surgical defect after (R) condylectomy along with complete excision of tumor, (E) Temporalis myofacial flap interpositioning, fixation of zygomatic arch by bone plate system, (F and G) Gross specimen—tumor attached to the anteromedial surface of condylar head, (H) Radiograph of specimen—tumor mass is continuous with the parent bone, (I) Photomicrograph of osteochondroma

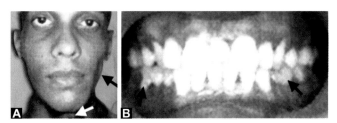

Figs 36.53A and B: Postoperative front face and satisfactory occlusion of the patient seen in Figure 36.51A

posterior open bite, chin deviation away from the affected side with facial asymmetry or bowing of the mandibular ramus.

Radiographs: Show a sessile or pedunculated lesion that is continuous with the adjacent cortex and underlying medullary bone. The bony portion of the lesion shows a central trabecular pattern with well-defined radiopacity. The cartilaginous superficial aspect is less well mineralized.

Histopathology: The surface is composed of a moderately cellular, hyaline cartilage cap covered by a thin, fibrous perichondrium. The deep layer of cartilage exhibits endochondral ossification with deposition of woven bone on mineralized cartilage.

Treatment: Complete conservative surgical excision is done. Recurrence is not reported.

NONNEOPLASTIC BONE LESIONS

Fibro-osseous Lesions of the Jaws

These lesions of the jaw represent a diverse group of lesions that are characterized by replacement of normal bone by a fibrous tissue matrix containing trabeculae of newly formed mineralized bone. This terminology 'fibro-osseous lesion' is not a specific diagnosis, but describes only a process. Fibro-osseous lesions of the jaw include developmental (hemartomatous) lesions, reactive or dysplastic processes. The histopathological picture of these lesions may be remarkably similar. The final diagnosis of these disorders will depend on clinical, radiographic, operative and microscopic features all considered together.

The common fibro-osseous lesions of the jaws are:
1. Fibrous dysplasia of the jaws
2. Cemento-osseous dysplasia
   a. Periapical cemento-osseous dysplasia
   b. Focal cemento-osseous dysplasia
   c. Florid cemento-osseous dysplasia

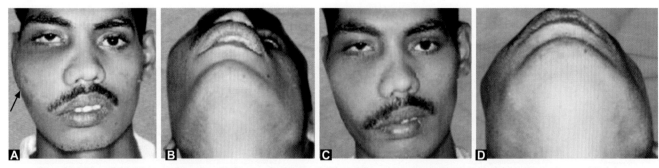

Figs 36.54A to D: A 20-year-old male with fibrous dysplasia of (R) maxilla, zygomatic bone, sphenoid, maxillary sinus, orbital rim: (A and B) Preoperative view showing marked facial asymmetry, (C and D) Postoperative view after debulking

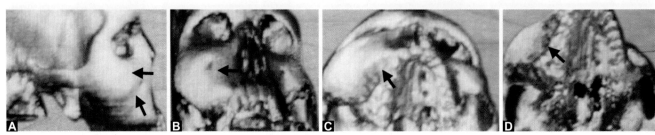

Figs 36.55A to D: 3D CT imaging showing marked expansion of (R) maxilla, zygoma due to fibrous dysplasia. Right orbital volume is reduced, right nasal bones are also involved

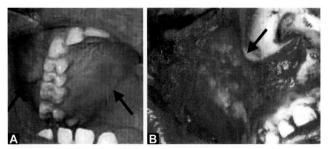

Figs 36.56A to B: (A) Intraoral view showing involvement of right maxilla with buccal and palatal expansion of bone due to fibrous dysplasia, (B) Weber-Fergusson incision to expose the lesion for debulking and recontouring surgical procedure

Fibrous Dysplasia of the Jaws (Figs 36.54 to 36.58)

Fibrous dysplasia was first described by von Recklinghausen in 1891. In 1938, Lichtenstein introduced the term 'fibrous dysplasia'. The pathogenesis is not understood completely, but trauma and endocrine disturbances were labeled as culprits. More recently molecular basis has been identified.

It is a self limiting condition, in which normal medullary bone is gradually replaced by an abnormal fibrous connective tissue proliferation. The mesenchymal tissue contains variable amounts of an osseous matrix that presumably arises through metaplasia and consists only of woven bone.

Types

i. Solitary or Monostotic lesion 80 to 85 percent more common (involving a single bone)
ii. Multifocal or Polyostotic lesion (involving several bones) relatively uncommon.

   a. *In Jaffe type*—three fourths of the entire skeleton may be involved.

   b. *In Lichtenstein syndrome*—the entire skeleton may be involved, along with cutaneous melanotic pigmentation.

   c. *Mazabrand syndrome*—fibrous dysplasia associated with soft tissue myxomas, usually intramuscular (Adjacent to the F.D. lesion).

   d. *McCune-Albright syndrome*—Polyostotic with endocrinopathy—more severe form. Occurs commonly in females. Three percent of the patients with polyostotic fibrous dysplasia have multiple areas of cutaneous melanotic pigmentation (Café au lait macules) and autonomous hyper-function of one or more of the endocrine glands. (Precocious sexual development and onset of puberty).

The skull and jaws are commonly associated in all above forms.

Etiology unknown: Many hypothesis have been proposed.

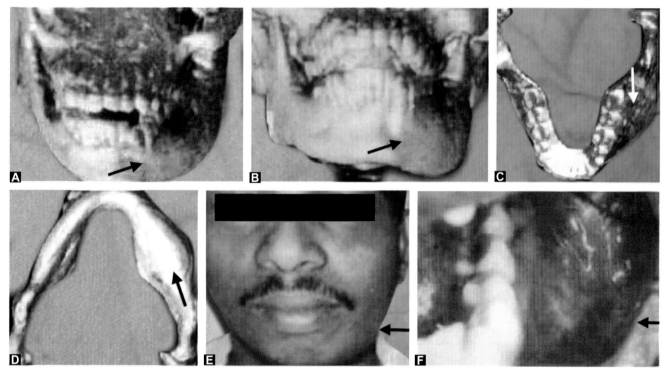

Figs 36.57A to F: A 22-year-old male patient with fibrous dysplasia: (A to D) 3D reconstruction CT scan showing bowing of the inferior border of the mandible and expansion of buccal and lingual cortical plates, (E) Facial asymmetry, (F) Intraoral view showing expansion of buccal cortex and tilting of posterior teeth lingually. Recontouring was carried out

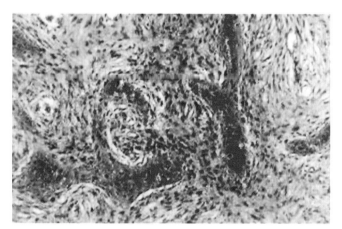

Fig. 36.58: Fibrous dysplasia: Histopathological picture

i. A non-neoplastic, hemartomatous growth resulting from altered mesenchymal cell activity or a defect in the control of bone cell activity.

ii. Focal bone expression of a complicated endocrine disturbance (finding of estrogen receptors in osteogenic cells of a patient)

iii. Inherited basis.

Monostotic fibrous dysplasia of the jaws

- *Onset:* It occurs during the first or second decade of life. Insidious, asymptomatic, painless, slow growing lesion.
- *Sex:* Both males and females are affected equally.
- *Site:* Maxilla is more commonly affected than mandible. Maxillary lesion may extend to include zygoma, sphenoid bone, maxillary sinus and floor of the orbit and are not strictly monostotic. Therefore are termed *craniofacial fibrous dysplasia*. In the mandible, mandibular body is most frequently involved.
- *Swelling* is unilateral, slow growing with progressive enlargement. As the lesion grows, facial asymmetry becomes more evident and it may be the patient's chief complaint.

The fusiform oval (low plateau) firm and smoothly contouring swelling of the affected jaw. Most commonly results from the expansion of the buccal cortical plate. The lingual cortex is rarely involved. In mandible, it may cause a protuberance excrescence of the inferior border. As a rule, the growth of the lesion ceases with skeletal growth.

Teeth involved in the lesion are usually firm, but may be displaced by the bony mass or occlusal level can be changed. The more aggressive clinical form may produce rapid growth, pain, nasal obstruction or exophthalmos.

- *Radiological feature* variable. Ranges from radiolucent to a densely radiopaque mass. Four different pictures can be seen radiologically. (i) The characteristic feature is *'ground glass'* appearance in mature stage, i.e. a homogenous radiopacity with the numerous trabeculae of woven bone or *orange peel appearance*. (ii) In early stage, some lesions may be seen as unilocular or multilocular radiolucencies. (iii) In intermediate stage radiolucent lesion with patchy, irregular opacities similar to Paget's disease can be seen. (iv) A fingerprint bone pattern and superior displacement of mandibular canal can be seen.

In maxilla: There is obliteration of the maxillary sinus by the lesional tissue. Shows increased bone density of base of the skull involving the occipital, sphenoid, roof of the orbit and frontal bones.

The most important characteristic feature of fibrous dysplasia is the poorly defined clinical and radiological demarcating margins of the lesion. The lesion appears to blend into the surrounding normal bone without any evidence of a circumscribed border.

- *Serum chemistry levels* serum calcium, phosphorus and alkaline phosphatase, are within normal ranges because of the slow growth rate.
- *Histologically:* The lesion is essentially a fibrous one, made up of proliferating fibroblasts in a compact stroma of interlacing collagen fibers. Irregular bony trabeculae may be scattered haphazardly or 'c' shaped trabeculae may occur, giving *'Chinese' character appearance*. Bony trabeculae may be coarse woven bone or lamellar. As the lesion matures, spicules of lamellar bone with osteoblastic rimming may be seen.
- *Differential diagnosis* from ossifying fibroma, cementifying fibroma, Paget's disease, osteosarcoma, etc. The usual course of fibrous dysplasia is slow growth for a decade or so, stabilization and slow return to normal. Occlusion and tooth-jaw relation should be carefully monitored during the period of skeletal growth.

Polyostotic fibrous dysplasia (McCune-Albright syndrome)

- The skull and jaws affliction with resultant facial asymmetry

- Simultaneous involvement of both the jaws along with lone bones is seen
- 'Hockey stick' deformity of the femur is seen with leg length discrepancy
- Well defined, generally unilateral tan macules on the trunk, thighs, oral mucosa, known as Café au lait (coffee with milk) pigmentations. The margins of these spots are very irregular in contrast to the spots of neurofibromatosis which have smooth borders.
- Sexual precocity, most commonly seen in females is the common endocrine manifestation.
  (Breast development, pubic hair, menstrual bleeding may be seen to occur within first few years of life in affected girls).

Management: The management of the fibrous dysplasia can be difficult at times. The treatment plan depends on the extent of involvement, functional disability, danger to function, neurologic symptoms and esthetic consideration. Differentiation should be made between monostotic and polyostotic form of the lesion. Complete bone scintigraphy can suggest multiple involvement.

The treatment ranges from observation for minor lesions to radical resection.

Small lesions: Biopsy for confirmation and follow up.

Lesions with functional or esthetic problems: Osseous recontouring via a transoral approach. Resection with bony reconstruction is often not advisable as complete excision is not possible and unnecessary, as the large lesions have poorly defined borders and the disorder is nonneoplastic in nature. The recontouring is done with the contouring round bur or osteotome, while softer lesions can be contoured with a scalpel.

The recontouring is generally undertaken after the active growth stage and during the phase of stabilization. This procedure entails surgical reduction of the lesion to an acceptable contour without any attempts to remove the entire lesion. This is also known as *'surgical shave down procedure'*. 25 to 50 percent of the patients may show variable regrowth of the lesion after recontouring procedure. Radiation therapy is contraindicated, as it carries risk for developing bone sarcoma.

Cemento-osseous Dysplasias

- Most common types of fibro-osseous lesions occurring in the tooth bearing areas of the jaws.
- Precise etiology is not known. May be the result of disorders in the metabolism of cells normally

involved in the production of bone and cementum matrices.

- Microscopically, they consist of fibrous tissue, bone and cementum like calcification.
- On the basis of clinical and radiological features, three disease processes can be seen. (i) Periapical (ii) Focal (iii) Florid cemento-osseous dysplasias. All these forms represent only variants of the same pathological process.

Periapical cemental dysplasia, (periapical cementoma), periapical cemento-osseous dysplasia (Figs 36.59 and 36.60) (Table 36.6)

Differentiation with hypercementosis is done by examining for periodontal ligament space which is present in periapical cemental dysplasia. In multiple radiolucencies, distinction between this condition and

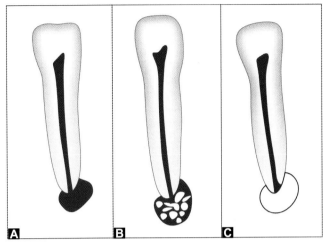

Figs 36.59A to C: Peripheral cementoma: (A) (Stage 1) radiolucent, (B) (Stage 2) mixed, (C) (Stage 3) radiopaque

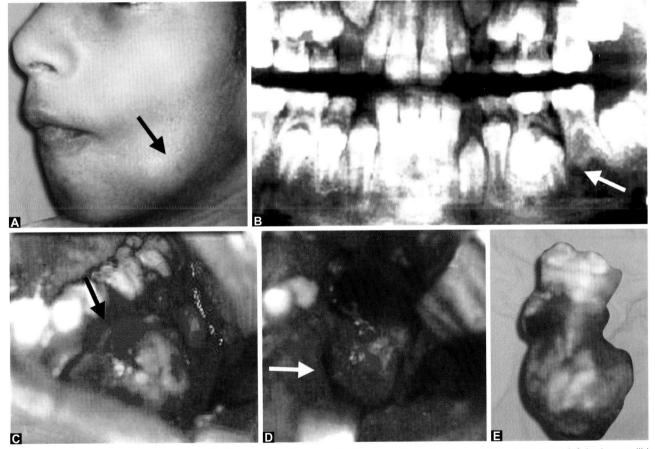

Figs 36.60A to E: Periapical cementoma: (A) Extraoral profile view of a 9-year-old boy showing swelling at the lower left body mandible of 6 months duration, (B) OPG showing well-circumscribed radioopaque mass in relation to lower left deciduous second molar mesial root, (C) Surgical exposure of the mass, (D) Defect after excision of the mass, along with the extraction of lower left deciduous second molar, (E) Specimen-biopsy report-periapical cementoma

Table 36.6: Features of periapical cemental dysplasia

Lesion	Location	Features	Radiographic features
• Stage I Osteolytic stage Radiolucent	• Lower anterior and premolar regions • Involves the periapical bone at the apices of the teeth • Often detected in routine radiographs	• Mainly seen in postmenopausal females, 30–50 years of age. • Common in black females. • Multiple teeth may be involved • Associated with vital non-inflamed pulps. • Asymptomatic self limiting lesions	• Multiple, round to ovoid radiolucent (within 2 cm) lesions at the apices of vital teeth with no sclerotic border. • Differential diagnosis with periapical granuloma difficult.
• Stage II Mixed stage	• Same as above	• Same as above	• Cyst like radiolucency with internal calcific radiopacities. Patchy mottled appearance
• Stage III Radiopaque stage	• Same as above	• Same as above	• Well-defined circular radiopacity bordered by a thin radiolucent band

a radicular cyst can be made on the basis of lack of widening of periodontal ligament space.

Treatment—requires no definitive treatment following diagnosis. Vitality test should be carried out.

Focal cemento-osseous dysplasia

• Seen more in white females.
• 40 to 50 years of age.
• Posterior mandible is more common site.
• Recently described entity that is thought to fall between periapical and florid osseous dysplasia.
• More common than the other forms of fibro-osseous diseases of the jaws.
• Asymptomatic and usually discovered during routine radiographic examination.
• Radiographic appearance may vary from well defined radiolucent lesion to a densely radiopaque mass.
• Many cases involve bone adjacent to the roots of asymptomatic vital teeth or it can be seen in edentulous areas of the jaws.
• Some of these lesions may be associated with the development of idiopathic bone cavities (traumatic bone cyst).
• Differentiation should be made from ossifying fibroma, which tend to separate clearly from bone during surgery in one or many fragments, while focal cemento-osseous dysplasia cannot be separated from the bone easily and is removed by curettage.
• Requires no treatment following the biopsy.

Florid cemento-osseous dysplasia (FOD) gigantiform cementoma:

A rare familial form of disease—also known as familial gigantiform cementoma. WHO in 1992, has used this term as a synonym for florid cemento-osseous dysplasia.

• Shows a striking predilection in adult black women.
• Hereditary, seen only in jaw bones.
• Marked tendency for bilateral, often symmetric involvement. Many times all four posterior quadrants can be involved. Mandible > maxilla.
• Mostly discovered in routine radiographs.
• In some cases, it may be asymptomatic and in others dull pain and an alveolar mucosal fistula may be present.
• Both dentulous and edentulous area may be affected.
• *Radiologially*—typically mottled, mixed radiolucent—radiopaque lesions adjacent to the teeth throughout the affected portions of the jaws can be seen. Cotton-wool appearance similar to Paget's disease. Difference is FOD is limited to jaw bones only.
• Uncomplicated lesions may produce bilateral mild cortical expansion. However, there can be development of osteomyelitis following traumatic episodes like extractions or biopsy or ill-fitting denture trauma, etc. The presence of osteomyelitis with its symptoms like pain, swelling, pus discharge and sequestrum formation can be seen.
• *Histopathology* is similar to the periapical variety. FOD is a reactive type of fibro-osseous bone lesion, originating from the periodontal ligament cells and is characterized by its infiltrative nature into nearby bones resulting in indistinct margins.
• *Treatment*: Florid osseous dysplasia is a non-neoplatic, self limiting process, which requires no treatment following diagnosis. Any form of trauma

or extractions or biopsy should be avoided. Once the lesion becomes complicated and osteomyelitis sets in, then standard treatment like debridement, sequestrectomy, wound care and antibiotics, etc. should be offered.

Familial gigantiform cementoma may show relatively rapid growth resulting in facial deformity. Shave down procedure may not work as the tissue rapidly regrows.

Other Cemento-osseous Dysplasias (Giant Cell Lesions of the Jaw Bones)

A variety of pathological conditions of the jaw bones show the presence of multinucleated giant cells. Of these, the benign, intraosseous, giant cell lesions, though rare in their occurrence in the jaws, have been a source of debate. This group of benign, intraosseous, giant cell lesions comprise of:

1. **Cherubism** is a rare inherited condition affecting the jaws characterized by the replacement of normal bone by a proliferation of fibrovascular tissue containing multinucleated giant cells (Figs 36.61A and B).
2. **The central giant cell granuloma** is, defined by the WHO, as 'an intraosseous lesion' consisting of cellular fibrous tissue that contains multiple foci of hemorrhage, aggregations of multinucleated giant cells, and trabaculae of woven bone (Pindborg 1991).

Cherubism: In 1933, Jones first reported three cases of cherubism in jewish siblings. It was the upward 'looking

towards heaven' upturn of the eyes, combined with the characteristic facial chubbiness of these children that prompted Jones to coin the term 'cherubism' (The term cherubism meaning 'angle face' was coined as such, since the bilaterally swollen mandible creates a resemblance with the cherubs of Renaissance paintings. Cherubs-plump-cheeked little angles) (Figs 36.62A to H).

- It is an inherited autosomal dominant non-neoplastic disorder.
- Pedigrees of families have demonstrated involvement of three or more generations.
- Some cases of cherubism are seen without any family history of disorder. These represent spontaneous mutation.
- It is a rare inherited disorder affecting the jaws and the key feature is replacement of normal bone by

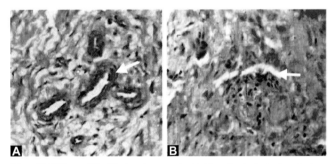

Figs 36.61A and B: Photomicrograph. Multinucleated giant cells in a fibrous stoma. Perivascular cuffing (arrow) with eosinophilic coagulum. Along with clinical picture, suggestive of cherubism

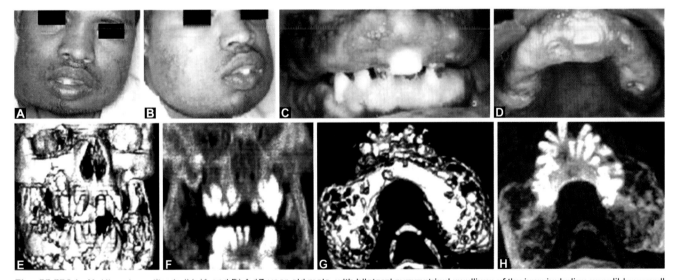

Figs 36.62A to H: Cherubism Grade IV: (A and B) A 17-year-old male, with bilateral symmetrical swellings of the jaws including mandible as well as maxilla. Duration—10 years, (C and D) Intraoral examination showed generalized gingival enlargement, covering almost all the teeth, except anteriors. The gingiva appeared to be firm, hard and leathery, with pebbled surface, (E to H) CT scan—bilateral mandibular, expansile lesions with trabeculated margins associated with enhancing soft tissue within focal areas of erosion are seen in lingual and buccal cortices. Maxilla also shows focal areas of erosion. An osteoid matrix is seen within all these focal areas. Presence of multiple missing and displaced teeth noted

a proliferation of fibrovascular tissue containing multinucleated giant cells.

- It manifests during childhood as early as one year of age. Milder cases may be detected at the age of 7 to 12 years. Age range for most cases—2 to 7 years.
- Sex—male to female ratio—2:1—male predominance.
- Site—most common sites: mandibular angle and ascending rami. The mandible may be first and only bone to be affected. In severe cases, maxilla is also involved.

Clinical presentation—Fordyce in 1976, described the grades of this disorder

Grade I—   Mild, bilateral, symmetrical, posterior mandibular expansion imparting 'chubby' appearance to the face.

Grade II— In addition to mandibular involvement, bilateral maxillary tuberosity involvement will be seen.

Grade III— More extensive, generalized involvement of posterior and anterior regions of the mandible and maxilla. Extensive maxillary involvement causes stretching of the skin of the upper face to expose the sclerae 'eyes upturned to heaven gaze'.

Grade IV— Normally coronoid and condylar processes are spared in cherubism. But in extreme cases of grade IV, there will be involvement of both these processes.

- Bilateral, painless, slow expansion of the affected areas of the jaw (Depending on the grade)
- The facial disfigurement will range from mild to extensive.
- In extensive involvement, there is enlargement and widening of alveolar bone. Developing teeth are often displaced or fail to erupt, malformed or absent.
- The bony expansion is firm and nontender on intraoral palpation.
- The palatal vault may be considerably reduced or obliterated as a result of maxillary expansion.

Extreme tumorous swellings, ultimately cause a grotesque appearance with functional problems involving speech, respiration, deglutition, limited range of jaw motion and mastication. There can be complete obliteration of maxillary sinuses. Visual disturbances can be seen due to unequal globe displacement.

- Regional lymphadenopathy is a common finding in these patients.
- Radiographically—virtually diagnostic picture. Bilateral involvement of the jaws with typically multiloculated, expansile radiolucencies. Expansion

and thinning of the cortices is seen. The coronoid process may be involved with flattening of the sigmoid notch. The condyles are most often spared. Teeth may be displaced, unerupted and appear to be floating in the cyst like spaces. Areas of cortical perforations are commonly seen.

- Computed tomographic scans usually reveal replacement of the affected bone by a soft tissue density. Cortical disruption of the buccal and lingual/palatal sides are easily appreciated as is the superomedial extension of the lesion.

Biologic behavior

- The disorder manifests usually between the age of 2 to 4 years and progresses till the age of seven, where it plateaus or progresses very slowly.
- The earlier the condition manifests, the more aggressive is its course.
- At puberty, the facial deformity remains static and tends to improve during late teens, when the disorder tends to undergo spontaneous involution. The maxillary lesion usually regresses before the mandibular one.
- Facial appearance may return to almost normal by the fourth or fifth decade of life.

Treatment modalities—difficult to standardize. The treatment is usually based on the rate of progression of the lesion, the extent of involvement and the emotional status of the patient.

1. For aggressive lesion with associated functional problems and psychological problems, prompt surgical intervention is needed. Local curettage is the treatment of choice. Packing the defects with allogenic bone powder may aid in rapid osseous healing.
2. Other lesions can be kept under observation.
3. When functional or esthetic problems persist into adult life, surgical intervention, consisting of conservative curettage to debulking of lesions with surgical recontouring is the treatment of choice.

Central giant cell granuloma (giant cell lesion, giant cell tumor) Waldron and Shafer termed it 'central giant cell granuloma' in 1966 (Figs 36.63 and 36.64).

- *Incidence:* Central giant cell granuloma of the jaws is a relatively uncommon lesion.
- *Age:* Occurs predominantly in children, teens and young adults.
- *Sex:* Females are more commonly affected 2:1 ratio to male/female.

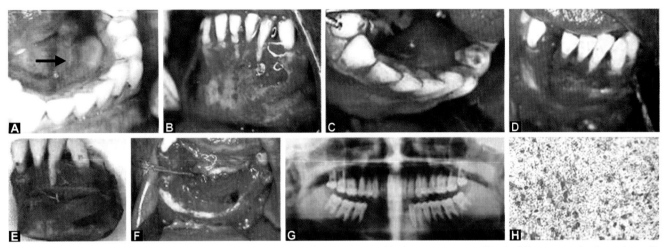

Figs 36.63A to H: Central giant cell granuloma: A 30-year-old female came with the recurrent swelling in (L) parasymphysis region with displacement of associated teeth. History of earlier curettage one year back. (A) Intraorally, a firm, smooth, tender swelling, extending from 31 to 35. Marked buccal and lingual expansion was seen, (B and C) Surgical exposure—note buccal and lingual cortical expansion, (D) Intraoral peripheral osteotomy done, (E) Resected specimen, (F) Resection with continuity, (G) Postoperative, OPG, (H) Giant cells irregularly distributed in a hemorrhagic fibrous stroma

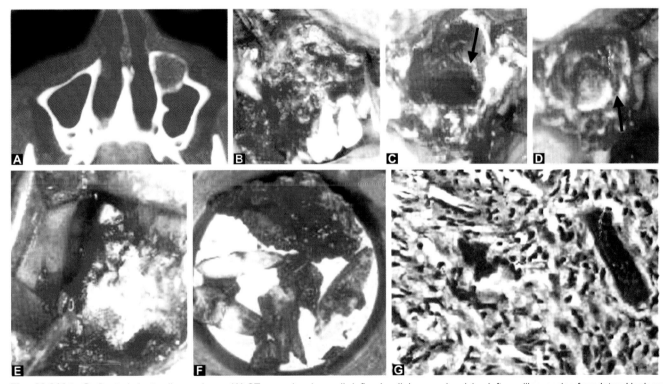

Figs 36.64A to G: Central giant cell granuloma: (A) CT scan showing well-defined radiolucency involving left maxillary region from lateral incisor to second premolar. Expansion of the buccal cortex seen. Anterior involvement of maxillary sinus, (B) Intraoral buccal vestibular incision to expose the tumor, (C) Communication with the max sinus, but no involvement, (D) Use of symphyseal bone graft to seal the communication, (E) Rest of the defect packed with allogenic bone powder, (F) Excised tumor tissue with extraction of teeth, (G) Histopathological picture of central giant cell granuloma—multinucleated giant cells in a spindle cell stroma

- *Site:* 72 percent of the lesions are located in the mandible. Twenty-eight percent in the maxilla. Anterior region is more commonly involved in both the jaws. Multiple giant cell lesions can be seen in one individual involving maxilla and mandible.

Clinical presentation: Giant cell lesions of the maxillofacial skeleton range clinically from slowly growing asymptomatic swellings of the affected jaws, which fail to demonstrate cortical perforation or root resorption to rapidly expanding aggressive tumors characterized by pain, root resorption and a high recurrence rate.

On the basis of the clinical and radiological features they have been divided into two groups:
1. Nonaggressive lesions
2. Aggressive lesions.

Radiologically: Central giant cell lesions present with a range of radiographic features, from incidental findings on routine radiographic examination to large destructive multilocular radiolucencies. The growth pattern of the giant cell granuloma is characterized by out pocketings, with irregular resorption of the cortex. These features are reflected in the radiographs, which gives a impression of septate multilocularity and ill defined border. Honey comb or 'soap bubble' appearances may be seen. Expansion of buccal and lingual cortices may be evident, with occasional cases of cortical perforation.

Histopathology: It is composed of a proliferation of spindled fibroblasts in a variable collagenous stroma. Numerous small vascular channels are evident throughout the lesion.

Multinucleated giant cells are present throughout the connective tissue stroma. The giant cells show variability—small, irregular with 5 to 10 nuclei per cell or large cells with rounded contours and containing more than 20 nuclei. The giant cells are seen around vascular channels aggregated in clusters. In clinically more aggressive lesions, there can be more dense distribution of more nuclear giant cells with less fibrovascular tissue.

Treatment and prognosis: Aggressive curettage of the tumor mass followed by removal of the peripheral bony margins is recommended treatment modality, which results in a low recurrence rate and good prognosis. Aggressive lesions require extensive surgery like resection. Because, the histological features of central giant cell granuloma are similar to those of brown tumor of hyperparathyroidism—investigations like serum calcium, phosphate and parathyroid hormone levels should be done. Recurrence rate is 10 to 50 percent or greater is seen. Long term follow up is necessary.

KERATOCYSTIC ODONTOGENIC TUMOR

Reclassification of the odontogenic keratocyst (OKC) from cyst to tumor.

Historical Background

Mikulicz in 1876, first described the odontogenic keratocyst (OKC) as a part of a familial condition affecting the jaws and as a separate entity. He termed it as a "Dermoid Cyst". In 1926, Hauer introduced the term "cholesteatoma" for it.

Robinson (1945) first, popularized the term, primordial cyst for cysts arising from primordial odontogenic epithelium. He stated that these cysts can arise from dental lamina or its remnants, odontogenic basal cell hamartias or enamel organ, prior to the formation of calcified structures, thus, this cyst is found in place of a tooth (from the normal series or supernumerary) instead of being associated with one. (Tooth is absent in the arch).

Later on, the term "keratocyst" was coined by Philipsen (1956) and was based on the histologic appearance of the cystic lining. This designation, was then widely used and two variants, i.e. orthokeratinized and parakeratinized odontogenic keratocysts were identified.

Pindborg and Hansen in 1963 reported their series of 30 cases of OKC and described the essential features of this type of cyst. It is called keratocyst because the cyst epithelium produces a large amount of keratin which fills the cyst lumen. It also shows distinctive histological features such as flattening of basement membrane, and palisading of the basal epithelial cells, which are characteristics of odontogenic keratocyst.

The odontogenic keratocyst is regarded as a distinctive entity, because of its characteristic histological picture, proliferation kinetics, and aggressive behavior. Therefore, although keratinization may be present in many other types of cysts, the specific histologic pattern of the odontogenic keratocyst separates it from others.

Differences in cytokeratin, epithelial membrane antigen (EMA) and carcinoembryonic antigen (CEA) immunoreactivity between the parakeratinized OKC and the orthokeratinized variety have been demonstrated and the suggestion made that the latter having a considerably less aggressive behavior is different entity and should bear a different name 'orthokeratinized odontogenic cyst (Shear M, 2002).

Keratocystic odontogenic tumor (KCOT) behaves like a tumor in many ways, such as: involvement of large areas of bone, high recurrence rate, distinctive histopathological features, disregulation of PTCH (patched) gene in both nevoid basal cell carcinoma syndrome (NBCCS) and association with other abnormalities (most notably the bifid rib Basal Cell Nevoid Syndrome). Cases of carcinoma arising in KCOT have also been reported. Toller (1967) had suggested that OKCs might be regarded as benign cystic neoplasms.

However, in 2005, The World Health Organization (WHO) reclassified "The Odontogenic Keratocyst (OKC)" as "The Keratocystic Odontogenic Tumor (KCOT)" and added it in its Histological Classification for Benign Odontogenic Tumors Category.

This redesignation of the OKC as the KCOT by WHO is based on the well known aggressive behavior of this lesion,its histology and new information regarding its genetics.

Definition: Benign uni or multicystic intraosseous tumor of odontogenic origin with characteristic lining of parakeratinized stratified squamous epithelium and potential for aggressive infiltrative behavior. WHO recommends KCOT is better term over OKC as it reflects its neoplastic nature.

Etiology and Pathogenesis

Keratocystic odontogenic tumors (KCOTs) are derived from the remnants (rests) of the dental lamina, after this organ has served its purpose. KCOT that occurs in dentate areas of both the maxilla and mandible is probably derived from those remnants. Whether it is developmental or neoplastic in origin is still debated.

Incidence: Keratocystic odontogenic tumor (KCOT) comprise approximately about 5 to 11 percent of odontogenic lesions of the jaws and is seen predominantly in the second, third and fourth decades of life, though they can occur in any age group. It has a slight predilection for the males than females in ratio of 2:1.

In approximately 10 percent, the patients with KCOT, the lesions represent a manifestation of the Basal cell nevus syndrome (BCNS) or nevoid basal cell carcinoma syndrome (NBCCS).

Site: The KCOT have a strong predilection of occurrence in the mandible than the maxilla, about 49 percent of the lesions are seen to involve the angle of the mandible with extension for varying distances into the ascending ramus and body mandible. However, they can occur anywhere in the jaws, including the midline, though majority of the cysts are seen posterior to the first bicuspids. Cases in maxillary anterior, third molar and antrum have also been reported.

Clinical Features

The physical signs and symptoms of a KCOT will depend to a certain extent on the dimensions of the lesion. A small lesion is unlikely to be diagnosed on routine examination of the mouth, and is generally detected accidentally on a radiographic examination. In case of the KCOT, patients are remarkably free of symptoms, until the lesion has reached a large size at times involving the entire ascending ramus. This is because the primordial odontogenic cystic lesion initially extends in the medullary cavity along the path of least resistance, rather than expanding the cortex and clinically observable expansion of the bone occurs late.

The enlarging lesion may lead to displacement of the teeth, percussion of the teeth overlying the lesion may produce a dull or hollow sound, and show perforation of bony cortex. A single missing tooth from the normal series should invite suspicion of the existence of the KCOT. The teeth adjoining the lesion will have vital pulps, unless there is coincidental disease of the teeth. Buccal expansion of the bone is commonly seen, lingual and palatal expansion is rare. Large mandibular lesions, invariably deflect the neurovascular bundle into an abnormal position. If acute infection sets in, with accumulation of pus within the sac, neuropraxia of the nerve results with the onset of labial paresthesia or anesthesia. When tension is relieved, with spontaneous discharge of pus via a sinus tract or surgical drainage, sensation returns to normal. These patients in later stages may present themselves with pain,swelling with discharge and paresthesia of the lower lip and teeth.

Maxillary lesions are more likely to become infected, even if they are small,than mandibular lesions, because of proximity to maxillary antrum and hence are diagnosed at an early age. Enlarging lesions of maxillary antrum may cause displacement and destruction of floor of orbit and proptosis of eye.

Multiple KCOTs are found in children, and are often reflective of multiple KCOTs as a component of Nevoid Basal Cell Carcinoma Syndrome (NBCCS). These multiple cystic lesions, however, may also be independent of the syndrome.

The most characteristic feature is the high rate of recurrence. The lesion showing orthokeratinization or mixed types of keratinization have less recurrence than parakeratinized cysts.

Radiological features: The KCOT can be unilocular or multilocular and is almost always associated with a sclerotic margin. Often, there can be considerable difficulty in distinguishing an ameloblastoma from a multilocular KCOT on radiologic grounds. Majority of the unilocular radiolucencies have a smooth periphery, some may have scalloped margins, which suggest an unequal growth activity (Fig. 36.65). Multilocular cystic lesions can have various radiographic appearances, e.g. one large cyst and some smaller daughter cysts giving the polycystic appearance. It is reported, that later, these cystic lesions fuse with the primary lesion to give the multilocular appearance. Thirty percent of maxillary lesions and 50 percent of mandibular lesions show buccal expansion with resorption of the lower cortical plate of the mandible, as well as perforation of bone. Mandibular lingual expansion may be seen sometimes. When they occur in the periapical region of vital teeth, they can be mistaken for a radicular cyst. They may impede the eruption of related teeth and this results in a dentigerous cyst appearance radiologically, which contain the crown of an unerupted tooth within its cavity (25–40% of cases).

For larger KCOT, with possible cortical perforation, specialized radiographic assessment, such as conventional and specialized films like CT Scan should be undertaken.

Pathogenesis

Mikulicz in 1876, had first described KCOT as a part of a familial condition affecting the jaws.

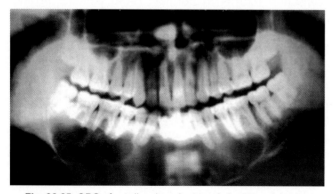

Fig. 36.65: OPG of a unilocular odontogenic keratocyst, having smooth periphery

- KCOT is generally considered to be a developmental anomaly, which arises from odontogenic epithelium, the main sources being:
- Dental lamina or its remnants
- Basal cells from the overlying oral mucosa
- Enamel organ—by degeneration of the stellate reticulum.

KCOT cystic lesion contents (aspirate) KCOT contain a very characteristic thick, creamy, dirty white, viscoid suspension of keratin, which has an appearance of pus, but without an offensive smell (Odorless).
- The smear should be stained and examined for keratin cells
- Electrophoresis, will reveal low protein content, with high albumin to globulin ratio.
- Total protein will be found to be below 4 gm/100 ml, which differentiates the lesion from other cystic lesions. Cholesterol crystals, keratin squames, hyaluronic acid, rushton bodies and heparin and chondroitan sulfate also can be found in the aspirate.

The immunofluorescent studies by Kuusela et al (1982), demonstrated an antigen in the cystic fluid, which is not present in other cystic lesions, nor in plasma or saliva and they named it as *'Keratocyst Antigen'(KCA).*

Histological Features (Tables 36.7 and 36.8)

The KCOT lesions are thin walled and are lined by a regular keratinized stratified squamous epithelium, which is usually 5 to 8 cell layers thick and is devoid of rete pegs. The keratin formed by the epithelium is seen in two variants, parakeratin—in which there is persistence of the nuclei (Fig. 36.66) and orthokeratin—in which the nuclei are absent. Clinically, the parakeratinized variant appears to have a much higher incidence of recurrence. In 80 to 90% of cases). But sometimes, orthokeratinized and both forms are found in different places of the same cyst. Maxillary KCOTs are generally of orthokeratinized variety.

There is well defined often palisaded polarized basal layer, which is of cuboidal or low columnar cells shows budding into connective tissue. It shows increased mitotic activity. The cells superficial to basal layer (stratum spinosum) are polyhedral and exhibit acanthosis. The subepithelial layers show increased collagenolytic activity with paucity of inflammatory cell infiltrate. At intervals there are infoldings of epithelial lining into the fibrous cystic wall (satellite cystic lesion), which along with loss of rete pegs account for increased

Table 36.7: Basic histological features of OKC (Now KCOT)

Pindborg and Hansen in 1963:

1. A thin, uniform thickness, lining epithelium with little or no evidence of rete ridge formation
2. A palisading cuboidal or columnar hyperchromatic basal cell layer
3. A thin, spinous cell layer that often shows a direct transition from basal cell layer
4. A spinous cell layer that frequently exhibits intracellular edema
5. Keratinization that is predominantly parakeratotic, but may be orthokeratotic
6. A keratinized inner cystic surface that is often corrugated, and
7. A thin uninflamed cyst wall

Table 36.8: Histological diagnostic criteria of OKC (now KCOT) by WHO (2001)

The lesion is characterized by a thin fibrous capsule and a lining of keratinized stratified squamous epithelium, usually about 5-8 cells layer in thickness and generally without rete pegs.

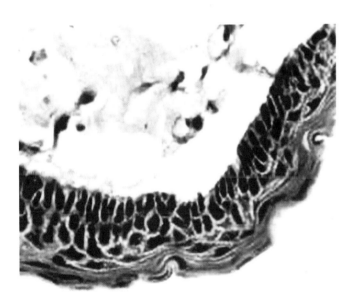

Fig. 36.66: Lining of an KCOT lesion: Parakeratinized epithelium corrugated with tall columnar cells, and devoid of rete pegs

recurrence rates. The histological appearace of the cystic lesion changes in the presence of intense inflammatory process. The adjacent epithelium looses its keratinized surface, may thicken and develop rete pegs or may ulcerate.

The enucleated lining easily separates from the underlying connective tissue. The capsule is quite thin and normally free of inflammatory cells, and may contain strands of odontogenic epithelium resembling the dental lamina, cell nests and daughter cysts. Desquamated keratin may be present in the cystic cavity.

Malignant Transformation

The malignant transformation (MT) of KCOT is a rare, but there is well-documented occurrence to squamous cell carcinoma.

Keratinization alone is a nonspecific finding in KCOT, because other odontogenic cystic lesions also can produce keratin.

Recurrence: KCOT have a pronounced tendency to recur. This aggressive pecularity was first reported by Pindborg and Hansen (1963). The recurrence rate may vary from 2.5 to 62 percent with most occurring in the first 5 to 7 years. Some lesions showed recurrence even after 10 years, hence long term follow up is necessary. When associated with nevoid basal cell carcinoma syndrome or Gorlin Goltz syndrome, the recurrence rate can be as high as 25 to 65 percent.

Some of the possible reasons reported for recurrence are as follows:
- Tendency to multiplicity
- Presence of satellite cysts
- Cystic lining is very thin and fragile, portions of which may be left behind
- Epithelial lining of KCOT have an intrinsic growth potential-clusters of epithelial islands
- Cysts can arise from basal cells of the oral mucosa
- Patients with nevoid basal cell carcinoma syndrome (NBCCS) have a particular tendency to form multiple primordial type lesions.

Brannon in 1976, proposed three mechanisms for recurrence:
1. Incomplete removal of cystic lining
2. Growth of new KCOT from satelite cystic lesions or odontogenic rests left behind during surgery.
3. Development of new KCOT in an adjacent area, that is interpreted as recurrence.

The possible mechanisms of recurrence have also been described by Voorsmit et al. in 1981. They stated that any lining epithelium left behind in the oral cavity may give rise to a new lesion formation. Daughter cysts, microcysts or epithelial islands can be found in the walls of the original lesion. New KCOT may develop from epithelial offshoots of the basal layer of oral epithelium.

Recent factors support emerging molecular evidence that the KCOT is more likely to be a benign cystic neoplasm than a simple odontogenic cyst. Even peripheral KCOTs are known to reoccur.

Genetics

The KCOT behaves like a tumor in many ways, for e.g. involvement of large areas of the bone, high recurrence rate, distinctive histopathological features of the lesion, abnormal function or disregulation of the PTCH (patched) gene—a tumor suppressor gene is noted in both nevoid basal cell carcinoma syndrome associated and sporadic KCOTs, etc. Normally, PTCH forms a receptor complex with the oncogene SMO (Smoothened) for the SHH (sonic hedgehog) ligand. PTCH binding to SMO inhibits growth signal transduction. SHH binding to PTCH releases this inhibition of the signal transduction pathway. If normal functioning of PTCH is lost, the proliferation-stimulating effects of SMO are permitted to predominate (Figs 36.67 and 36.68).

Pathogenesis involves a 2-Hit mechanism with allelic loss at 9q22. The 2 Hit mechanism refers to the process by which tumor suppressor gene is inactivated. The 1st hit is a mutation of one allele which is dominating

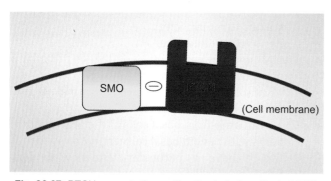

Fig. 36.67: PTCH prevents the proliferation-inducing effect of SMO

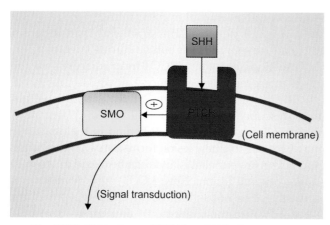

Fig. 36.68: SHH releases PTCH from SMO, allowing signal transduction

inherited has no phenotypic effect. The 2nd hit is the loss of other allele and is known as loss of heterozygosity. In KCOT, this leads to disregulation of oncoproteins cyclin D1 and P53.

Treatment

WHO's reclassification of the OKC as the KCOT, based on behavior, histology and genetics underscores the aggressive nature of the lesion and should motivate clinicians to manage the lesion in a correspondingly aggressive manner.

The KCOT behaves like a tumor in many ways, e.g. involvement of large areas of the bone, high recurrence rate, distinctive histopathological features of the lesion, disregulation of the PTCH (patched) gene in nevoid basal cell carcinoma syndrome, etc. On the other hand, successful treatment by marsupialization denies its tumor characteristics. Truly, cases of carcinoma arising in KCOT has been reported. In fact, the recurrence of the lesion has been reported in a bone graft.

Various treatment modalities have been tried for the successful treatment of the KCOT, ranging from simple curettage, enucleation to resection, but none has been regarded as the ideal treatment and the issue is still a debate in oral and maxillofacial surgery, as to the most effective treatment for this lesion.

According to Ghali GE et al., (2003), as with any odontogenic lesion, initial evaluation must include a through history and physical examination, radiographic studies, and the development of a probable differential diagnosis. Depending on size, location, and behavior, the clinician should decide on an incision versus excisional biopsy. Prior aspiration may be helpful. A careful histological examination and necessity of obtaining biopsy material from various areas to prevent a misdiagnosis of large size lesions, should be always kept in mind in patients with multiple KCOTs, evaluation for the presence of Basal Cell Nevus Syndrome should be undertaken. Large KCOT with possible cortical perforations, deserves specialized radiographic assessment, such as CT scans, in addition to plain X-ray films.

When planning the treatment to minimize/prevent recurrence of the lesion, the following points should be kept in mind.
1. Size and extent of the lesion—surface area measured radiographically of the lesions reported ranged from 2 to 15 cm.
2. Incidence as it relates to patient's age.

3. Location of the lesion in the jaw—association with any vital structure.
4. Presence of perforation or soft tissue involvement.
5. Radiographic appearance—unilocular/multilocular.
6. Primary or recurrent nature of the lesion.
7. Time since the previous treatment, in case of recurrence.

Marsupialization is incorrect in principle, in the treatment of KCOT, owing to their high incidence and tendency to recur. But, in 2002, Nakamura et al. stated that marsupialization, as well as decompression, has the purpose of relieving the pressure within the cystic cavity and allowing the new bone to fill the defect. It consequently, saves the contiguous structures such as tooth roots, the maxillary sinus or the inferior alveolar canal can be saved from surgical damage. It also reduces the size of the KCOT before second surgery. It is more effective in the mandibular body than the ramus region. The characteristics of the KCOT may become less aggressive during the course of marsupialization.

Bramley (1971, 1974) had very rationally outlined the surgical management of these lesions as follows:

- *Small single cystic lesion with regular spherical outline*, should be enucleated from an intraoral approach, provided the access is good.
- *Larger or less accessible lesions with regular spherical outline*, should be enucleated from an extraoral approach, as an intraoral access would be inadequate and a blind procedure. Care should be taken to ensure that all fragments of the extremely thin lining are removed.
- *Unilocular lesions with scalloped or loculated periphery and small multilocular lesions*, should be treated by marginal excision, i.e. resection of the containing block of bone, while maintaining the continuity of the posterior and inferior borders as in the ascending ramus, angle and body mandible, if there is difficulty of access, extraoral exposure is necessary. If the cystic lining is found to be adherent and in contiguity to the overlying oral mucosa or muscle then it should be excised along with marginal excision. The defect is closed primarily and can be left to heal by secondary intention or can be filled with hydroxyapatite crystals, autogenous bone graft, corticocancellous chips or allogenous bone powder, chips or block (Figs 36.69A to E).
- *Large multilocular lesions with or without cortical perforation*; may require resection of the involved bone

followed by primary or secondary reconstruction with a choice of reconstruction plates of stainless steel, vitallium, titanium, use of titanium or stainless steel mesh and bone grafting procedures with iliac crest graft, costochondral graft or allogenous bone grafts.

In the recent studies, Stoelinga and Van Hoelst (1981, 2001, 2003) proposed a more *conservative approach* to large lesions, by treatment with enucleation, excision of the overlying mucosa and/or muscle, if attachment existed to eliminate epithelial rests and/or microcysts and careful cauterization of the bony defect with Carnoy's solution, this they stated prevented recurrence and reported only one case of recurrence in 40 cases over a period of 10 years.

In nutshell, both conservative as well as aggressive approach has been advocated for treatment of KCOT. Conservative method has not gained much popularity, because complete removal of the KCOT can be difficult because of the thin friable lining, limited surgical access, skill and experience of the surgeon,and desire to preserve adjacent vital structures. The goals of treatment should involve eliminating the potential for recurrence while also minimizing the surgical morbidity.

A strict follow-up protocol,which allows for early surgical intervention in case of recurrence, limits the extent of second surgery, thus there is less morbidity. It seems likely that offshoots of the basal layer of the epithelium of the oral mucosa are a major cause for the development of some KCOT and some recurrence.

The most accepted treatment modalities of KCOTs are:
1. Enucleation, followed by cryosurgery
2. Enucleation, followed by adjunctive chemical cauterization using Carnoy's solution along with excision of overlying attached mucosa

Carnoy's Solution

A fixative composed of 60 percent Ethannol, 30 percent chloroform, 10 percent glacial acetic acid.

It is composed of 1 gm of ferric choride, dissolved in 24 ml of absolute alcohol, 12 ml chloroform and 4 ml of glacial acetic acid.

It is applied directly following enucleation. Protein coagulation is thought to limit uptake of these toxic material.

3. Radical excision should be reserved for multiple recurrent lesions

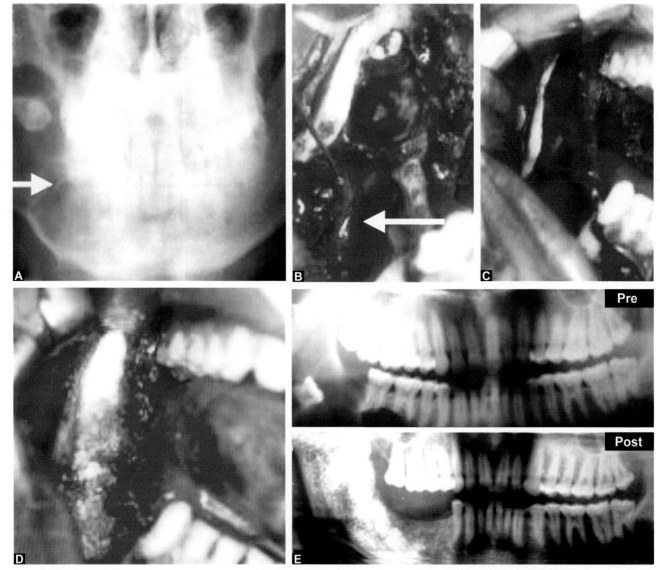

Figs 36.69A to E: KCOT Lesion: (A) Multilocular lesion with a displaced tooth, (B) Enucleation. Multilocularity confirmed at operation. Neurovascular bundle salvaged, (C) Wound defect, (D) Hydroxyapatite crystals packed in defect, (E) Pre and postoperative radiograph showing the lesion and after enucleating, hydroxyapatite crystals within defects

Basal Cell Nevus Syndrome (Gorlin's Syndrome)

Multiple KCOTs may be present solely or may represent *the basal cell nevus syndrome*

Jarisch (1894) first reported this disorder, detailed description was given by Gorlin (1965). It is most likely, a genetic disorder, which is inherited through an autosomal dominant gene. It is seen equally in both sexes. Some of the presenting features are as follows:

Facies
- Frontal and temporoparietal bossing
- Prominent supraorbital ridges in men
- Hypertelorism
- Mandibular prognathism (Figs 36.70A and B)

Skeletal anomalies
- Bifid, fused, rudimentary ribs
- Occult spina bifida
- Bridging of the sella turcica

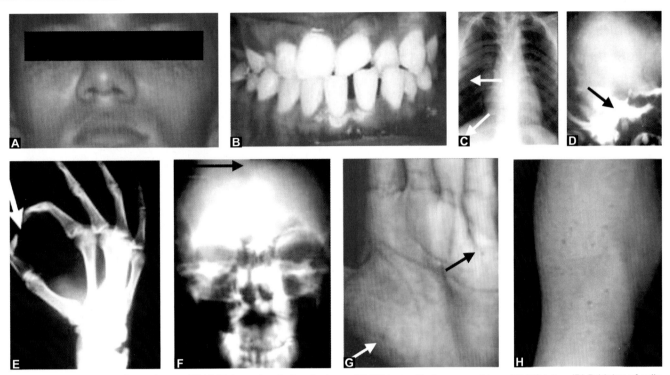

Figs 36.70A to H: Gorlin's syndrome: (A) Multiple nevi and other features, (B) Mild mandibular prognathism, (C) Bifid ribs, (D) Bridging of sella turcica, (E) Shortening of metacarpals, (F) Calcification of falx cerebri, (G) Palmar nevi and dyskeratosis, (H) Multiple nevi on the arm

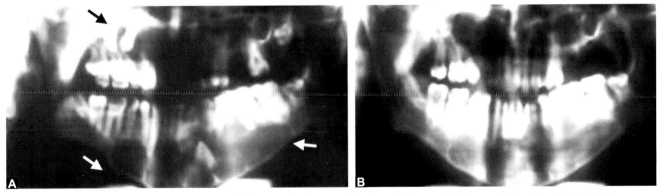

Figs 36.71A and B: Gorlin's syndrome: (A) Preoperative large multilocular radiolucency in the mandible and maxilla bilaterally, (B) Postoperative OPG following enucleation and endodontic treatment

- Shortening of metacarpals
- Calcification of falx cerebri (Figs 36.70C to F).

Skin lesions (Figs 36.70G and H)

- Milia, around eyes
- Dyskeratosis (palms and soles)
- Epidermal cysts (mostly hands)
- Basal cell nevi
- Basal cell carcinomas

Cystic KCOT Lesions

Fifty percent may show multiple KCOTs of the jaw bones (Figs 36.71A and B).

Soft tissue anomalies

- Ovarian fibromata
- Lipomas

Treatment: Shown in Figures 36.72A to F.

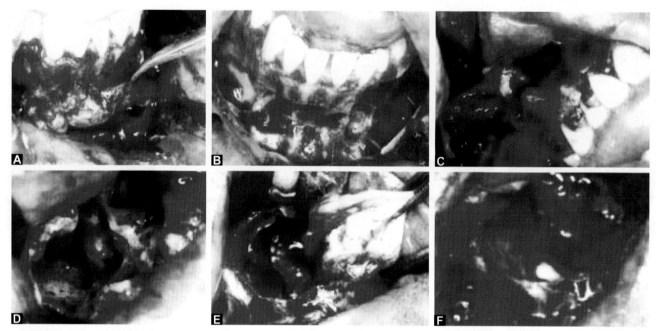

Figs 36.72A to F: Gorlin's syndrome: (A) Enucleation of mandibular lesion, (B) Mandibualr defect, (C) Right side maxillary lesion enucleation, (D) Right side maxillary defect, (E) Maxillary left side lesion enucleation, (F) Maxillary left side defect

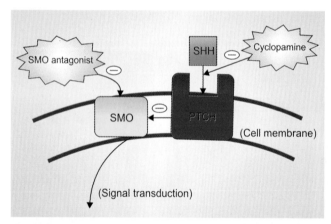

Fig. 36.73: Cyclopamine blocks SHH signal, preventing transduction, SMO antagonist blocks SMO, preventing transduction

Future Trends

Genetic studies have thrown light on new modalities of treatment of the KNOT at a molecular level. These may reduce or eliminate the need for aggressive surgical management.

Taipale et al. in 2000, suggested cyclopamine, a plant-based steroidal alkaloid, inhibit's the cellular response to the Sonic Hedgehog (SHH) signal. It is found that cyclopamine blocks activation of the SHH pathway caused by oncogenic mutation making it a potential 'mechanism-based' therapeutic agent for human tumors, whose pathogenesis involves excess Sonic Hedgehog pathway activity, as it is seen in the KCOT (Fig. 36.73).

Zhang et al. in 2006, postulated that antagonists of SHH signaling factors could effectively treat KCOT. Strategies include the introduction of a wild type form of PTCH inhibiting the SMO molecule by synthetic antagonists and suppressing the downstream transcription factors of the SHH pathway. They suggest intralesional injection of SMO protein antagonist has the greatest potential as a future treatment option.

BIBLIOGRAPHY

1. Blanas N, Freund B, Schwartz M. Systematic review of the treatment and prognosis of the odontogenic keratocyst. Oral Surg Oral Me Oral Pathol Oral Radiol Endod 2000:90;553-8.
2. Nevielle BW, Douglas D. Oral and Maxillofacial Pathology. 2nd edn, 422,594-6.
3. Stoelinga PJW. Long term follow up in keratocyst treated according to a defined protocol. Int J Oral Maxillofacial. Surg. 2001:30;14-25.

Salivary Gland Disorders

37 Diseases of the Salivary Glands

SALIVARY GLANDS: ANATOMY

Oral cavity depicts many pathological processes from the ubiquitous collection of tissues. Proper understanding of these disease processes is a must for a precise diagnosis of these conditions. Several times, the differential diagnosis of the oral lesions includes the diseases of the salivary glands. Thus, a thorough knowledge of their anatomy, physiology, diseases, their etiopathogenesis, differential diagnosis, investigations and treatment is required.

The salivary glands may be classified as major and minor glands. Major glands are paired glands. They are: (i) Parotid, (ii) Submandibular and (iii) Sublingual glands. There are numerous minor salivary glands, which are widely distributed in the oral cavity (Fig. 37.1A).

These glands function to produce saliva, which serves as a lubricant and also has immunologic, digestive and cleansing properties.

Based on the type of secretion, the salivary glands may be grouped as: (i) Serous, (ii) Mucous and (iii) Mixed.

Parotid gland secretion is serous in nature; the minor glands secrete mucous saliva. The sublingual gland secretes both serous and mucous, but predominantly mucous, whereas the submandibular gland secretion is also mixed, but is predominantly serous. Salivary gland secretions contain water, electrolytes, urea, ammonia, glucose, fats, proteins and other substances. Parotid secretions are more concentrated than other salivary glands.

Parotid Gland (Fig. 37.1B)

The parotid gland is the largest salivary gland, the secretion of which is serous in nature. It is pyramidal in shape; the apex is towards the angle of the mandible, the base at the external acoustic meatus. Anteriorly, the gland extends up to the buccal pad of fat and posteriorly encircles the posterior border of the mandible. Parotid gland has two lobes: (i) The superficial and (ii) The deep. They are connected by an isthmus at the posterior part of the gland. The entire gland is covered by a fibrous capsule.

The parotid duct (Stenson's duct) emerges at the anterior part of the gland. It passes horizontally across the masseter muscle, then pierces through the buccinator, to turn at right angles to reach the oral cavity. Stenson's

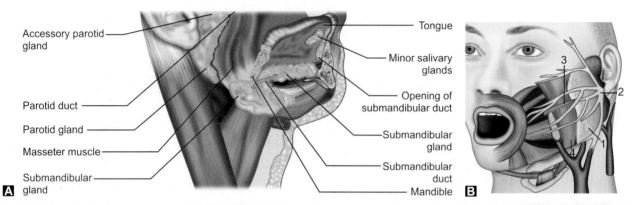

Figs 37.1A and B: (A) Salivary glands of the oral cavity, (B) Parotid gland anatomy: (1) Parotid gland, (2) Facial nerve and its branches, (3) Stenson's duct, (4) Masseter muscle

duct opening is seen as a papilla in the buccal mucosa opposite the maxillary second molar.

Parotid gland has close association with external carotid artery, the retromandibular vein and the facial nerve. The facial nerve emerges from the stylomastoid foramen, branches out from anterior and inferior margins of the gland.

Clinical Considerations

- Because the fibrous fascia is covering the parotid, its inflammatory swelling is tense and hard.
- The parotid duct is wider at some distance before the opening. This leads to the storage of saliva. The epithelial cells and other organic matters can get lodged here causing obstructions, stone formation etc.
- The right angle turn of the parotid duct also leads to stagnation of saliva.
- The close association of the facial nerve with the gland is very important consideration, during the surgical procedures.

Submandibular Gland (Fig. 37.2)

The submandibular gland secretion is both serous and mucous in nature. This gland is located in the submandibular space, extending inferiorly up to the digastric muscle, superiorly the mylohyoid muscle, posteriorly up to the angle of the mandible and anteriorly till the mid portion of the body of the mandible.

The submandibular duct (Wharton's duct) starts from the deep part of the gland, turns sharply at the posterior border of the mylohyoid muscle anteriorly and

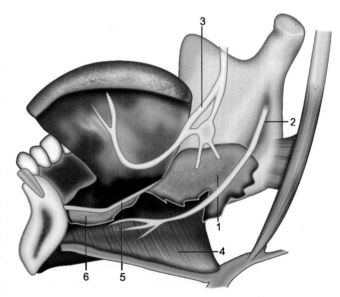

Fig. 37.2: Submandibular gland anatomy: (1) Submandibular salivary gland, (2) Hypoglossal nerve, (3) Lingual nerve, (4) Mylohyoid muscle, (5) Wharton's duct, (6) Sublingual gland

superiorly, crosses the hyoglossus muscle, then reaches the oral cavity. It opens at the sublingual papilla in the floor of the mouth. The submandibular gland is in close association with the facial artery, facial vein, Chorda tympani, branch of the facial nerve and lingual nerve.

Clinical Considerations

- The submandibular gland and duct are placed at a lower level to the oral cavity. It makes the gland prone to retrograde infection by oral flora.

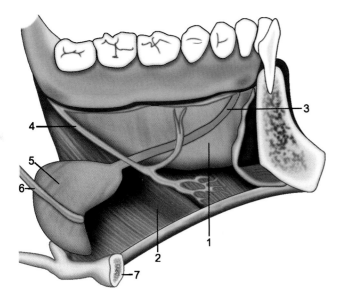

Fig. 37.3: Sublingual salivary gland anatomy: (1) Sublingual gland (2) Mylohyoid muscle, (3) Wharton's duct, (4) Lingual nerve, (5) Submandibular gland, (6) Hypoglossal nerve, (7) Hyoid bone

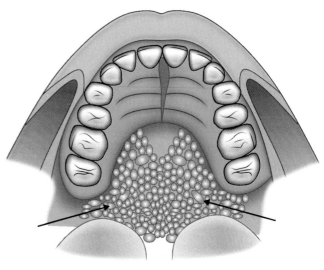

Fig. 37.4: Minor salivary glands in the palate

- Similar to the parotid duct, the Wharton's duct is also wider before reaching the papilla. This can lead to the stagnation of saliva and the organic matter.
- The long and tortuous course of the duct also leads to stagnation of saliva.
- The sharp bend of the Wharton's duct at the posterior border of the mylohyoid muscle allows stasis of the saliva favoring the formation of salivary stones.

Sublingual Gland (Fig. 37.3)

The sublingual glands secrete predominantly mucous saliva. This gland is located in the sublingual space. It is present in association with the sublingual folds below the tongue, and is divided into anterior and posterior parts. It has got many small ducts. In the posterior part, these ducts open through the sublingual folds. The ducts of the anterior part may join to form a large main duct called Bartholin's duct. This either opens though the sublingual papilla or joins with the Wharton's duct.

Minor Salivary Glands (Fig. 37.4)

More than 800 minor salivary glands may be present in the oral cavity. These are in groups scattered all over the mouth. The minor glands secrete mucous secretions. These glands have numerous small ducts.

Clinical Considerations

- The sublingual gland and the minor salivary glands have short ducts, where the chances of stasis are less. Thus, the obstructive lesions don't occur in these glands.
- Since the minor glands are placed superficially on the mucosa, the traumatic lesions such as mucoceles commonly affect these glands.

SALIVARY GLANDS: PHYSIOLOGY

Functions of Saliva

Saliva is a complex fluid, which has several proteins and digestive functions. The protective functions include cleansing, lubrication, maintaining the integrity of the oral mucosa.

The immunoglobulins, lysozymes, lactoferrin, sialoperoxidase, histamine and many other proteins contribute for the antibacterial property of the saliva. There are biologically active peptides, like epithelial growth factor, nerve growth factor and stomatostatin which help in maintaining the integrity of the oral mucosa. They also help in wound healing.

The enzymes such as the salivary amylase, lipase, etc. are important in the digestive action.

Calculus formation: Several proteins in the saliva influence the formation of calculus on the teeth. There are some other proteins like statherin, which will inhibit the formation of calculus. These proteins also inhibit the calculus formation in the salivary glands and the ducts.

CLASSIFICATION OF SALIVARY GLAND DISEASES

Salivary gland diseases may be grouped as follows (Table 37.1).

The following detailed classification also can be considered (Table 37.2).

Table 37.1: Classification of salivary gland diseases

I. *Developmental*
  1. Aplasia—absence of the gland
  2. Atresia—absence of the duct
  3. Aberrancy—ectopic gland

II. *Enlargement of the gland*
  A. *Inflammatory*
    1. *Viral*: Mumps, coxsackie A, CMV, echovirus, parainfluenza virus I and influenza virus
    2. Bacterial
    3. Allergic
    4. Sarcoidosis
    5. Obstructive
  B. *Noninflammatory*
    1. *Autoimmune*: Sjögren's syndrome and Mickulicz's disease
    2. Alcoholic cirrhosis
    3. Diabetes mellitus
    4. Nutritional deficiency
    5. HIV associated

III. *Cysts*
  1. Extravasation cysts
  2. Retention cysts
  3. Ranula

IV. *Tumors of salivary glands*
  A. Benign tumors:
    • Pleomorphic adenoma
    • Warthin's tumor
    • Basal cell adenoma
    • Myoepithelioma
    • Canalicular adenoma
    • Ductal papilloma
  B. Malignant tumors:
    • Mucoepidermoid carcinoma
    • Adenoid cystic carcinoma
    • Malignant pleomorphic adenoma

V. *Necrotizing sialometaplasia*

VI. *Salivary gland dysfunction*
  1. Xerostomia
  2. Sialorrhea

SALIVARY GLAND DYSFUNCTION

Sialorrhea or Ptyalism

It is excessive salivation seen in affected patients. It can be mild, intermittent or continuous profuse drooling. It can cause severe drooling, choking and social embarrassment to the patient. This condition is not so common and can occur due to various causes. Minor sialorrhea can be seen due to local irritation like aphthous ulcers or ill fitting dentures. Idiopathic paroxysmal sialorrhea will have short episodes for 2 to 5 minutes. Profuse salivation is seen in rabies, heavy metal poisoning or after certain medications like lithium and cholinergic agonists. Mentally retarded children also have excessive salivation. Neurologically disabled persons (cerebral palsy) also suffer from this disorder. Drooling of the saliva is also seen after the resection of the mandible, because of poor neuromuscular control. The treatment is conservative. Anticholinergic medication can be tried (atropine). Behavioral modification, physical therapy has been tried.

Suggested Surgical Treatment

• Submandibular gland resection
• Transposition of parotid duct
• Parotid duct ligation.

Xerostomia

This is a subjective sensation of a dry mouth. It affects women more than the men, and seen more commonly in older people, because of decreased glandular secretion due to aging as well as due to some medications which reduce the secretion. Antihistamines, decongestants, antidepressants, antipsychotics, antihypertensives, anticholinergics are known to cause xerostomia.

Other causes of xerostomia are—salivary gland aplasia, aging, excessive smoking, mouth breathing, local radiation therapy, Sjögren's syndrome, HIV infection, etc.

Clinically, dry mouth with foamy, thick, ropy saliva can be noticed. The tongue may have leathery appearance and fissures with atrophy of the filiform papillae. These patients are more prone for oral candidiasis due to reduction in cleansing and antimicrobial action of saliva. Dental decay is rampant with more of cervical and root caries.

Treatment is conservative, maintainance of oral hygiene, use of sialagogues (pilocarpine), modification of medications in elderly patients may help to improve the condition.

Table 37.2: General and etiological classification of salivary gland disorders

A. *General classification*
1. *Developmental anomalies:*
   a. Aplasia/agenesis
   b. Atresia of ducts
   c. Hypoplasia
   d. Congenital fistula
   e. Aberrancy
   f. Accessory ducts and lobes
2. *Inflammatory (sialadenitis):*
   a. *Bacterial:* (i) Acute (ii) Chronic, (iii) Recurrent parotitis of childhood
   b. Specific infections
   c. Allergic
   d. *Viral:* (i) Mumps (ii) Salivary inclusion disease
   e. Post-irradiation
   f. Sialadenitis of minor glands
3. *Obstructive and traumatic:*
   a. Papillary obstruction of duct
   b. Obstruction of duct lumen, e.g. sialolithiasis
   c. Obstruction due to changes in and around duct wall, e.g. strictures
   d. Salivary duct fistula
   e. Frey's syndrome
   f. Mucocele (i) Mucous extravasation cyst (ii) Mucous retention cyst, (iii) Ranula: (a) Superficial, (b) Deep, (c) Plunging
4. *Changes in salivary secretion and composition in disease:*
   a. Functional disorders of salivary glands
   b. Factors influencing salivary flow rate
   c. Xerostomia/dry mouth
5. *Ptyalism (sialorrhea):*
   a. Acute inflammatory conditions, e.g. abscess, herpes infection, aphthae
   b. Tooth eruption
   c. Mental retardation
   d. Parkinsonism
   e. Schizophrenia
   f. Epilepsy
   g. Hg poisoning
   h. Acrodynia
   i. Rabies
   j. Familial dysantonomia
6. *Tumors and tumor-like lesions:* The revised WHO histological classification of salivary gland tumors and tumor-like lesions:
   a. Adenomas: (i) Pleomorphic adenoma, (ii) Myoepithelioma (myoepithelial adenoma), (iii) Basal cell adenoma, (iv) Warthin tumor (adonolymphoma), (v) Oncocytoma (oncocytic adenoma), (vi) Canalicular adenoma, (vii) Sebaceous adenoma, (viii) Ductal papilloma: (a) Inverted ductal papilloma (b) Intraductal papilloma (c) Sialadenoma papilliferum, (ix) Cystadenoma (a) Papillary cyst adenoma (b) Mucinous cystadenoma
   b. *Carcinomas:* (i) Acinic cell carcinoma, (ii) Mucoepidermoid tumor, (iii) Adenocystic carcinoma (cylindroma), (iv) Polymorphous low grade adenocarcinoma (terminal duct adenocarcinoma), (v) Epithelial-myoepithelial carcinoma, (vi) Basal cell carcinoma, (vii) Sebaceous carcinoma, (viii) Papillary cystadenocarcinoma, (ix) Mucinous adenocarcinoma, (x) Oncocytic carcinoma, (xi) Salivary duct carcinoma, (xii) Adenocarcinoma (not otherwise specified), (xiii) Malignant myoepithelioma (myoepithelial carcinoma), (xiv) Carcinoma in pleomorphic adenoma), (xv) Squamous cell carcinoma, (xvi) Small cell carcinoma, (xvii) Undifferentiated carcinoma, (xviii) Other carcinomas
   c. Non-epithelial tumors
   d. Malignant lymphomas
   e. Secondary tumors
   f. Unclassified tumors
   g. *Tumor-like lesions:* (i) Sialoadenosis, (ii) Oncocytosis, (iii) Necrotizing sialometaplasia, (iv) Benign lymphoepithelial lesion, (v) Salivary gland cysts, (vi) Chronic sclerosing sialadenitis of submandibular gland (kuttner tumor), (vii) Cystic lymphoid hyperplasia in AIDS
7. *Autoimmune disorders: (i) Sjögren's syndrome, (ii) Benign Lymphoepithelial lesions: (a) Godwin's (b) Mickulicz disease*
8. *Degenerative disorders:* (a) Hormonal: (i) Diabetes, (ii) Acromegaly, (iii) Gynecomastia, (iv) Pregnancy, (v) Menopause (b) Neurohumoral disorders (i) Cardiac spasm, (ii) Gastric spasm, (iii) Bronchial asthma, (c) Disenzymatic sialosis (Hepatogenic) (d) Sialosis: (i) Metabolic, (ii) Drugs, (iii) Hormonal and, (iv) Hypoglycemic, (v) Malnutrition, (e) Sjögren's syndrome: (i) Primary, (ii) Secondary, (iii) Aggressive, (f) Lymphoepithelial lesions: (Currently, Mickulicz disease: Sjögren's syndrome; and Mickulicz syndrome: Mostly lymphomas)
9. Age changes and oncocytosis

B. *Etiological classification*
   (a) Factors influencing salivary center: (i) Emotions: Fear, excitement, depression, (ii) Neurosis: Endogenous depression (iii) Organic disease: Brain tumor, (iv) Drugs—atropine (b) Factors affecting autonomic outflow pathway: (I) Encephalitis, (ii) Brain tumor, (iii) Accident (trauma to autonomic system), (iv) Neurosurgical operation, (v) Drugs—atropine, (c) Factors affecting salivary gland function: (i) Aplasis (ii) Sjögren's syndrome, (iii) Obstruction, (iv) Infection, (v) Irradiation, (vi) Excision (d) Factors producing changes in fluid and electrolyte balance: (i) Dehydration, (ii) Diabetes insipidus, (iii) Cardiac failure, (iv) Uremia, (v) Edema (e) Ptyalism (Sialorrhea): (i) Acute inflammatory conditions, e.g. Abscess, Herpes infection, Aphthae, (ii) Tooth eruption, (iii) Mental retardation, (iv) Parkinsonism, (v) Schizophrenia, (vi) Epilepsy, (vii) Mercury poisoning, (viii) acrodynia, (ix) rabies, (x) Familial dysantonomia

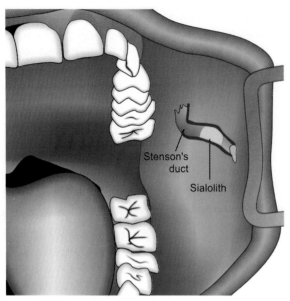

Fig. 37.5: Intraoral view of Stenson's duct and sialolith in the duct

◼ SIALOLITHIASIS (FIG. 37.5)

Sialolithiasis is the formation of sialolith (salivary calculi, salivary stone) in the salivary duct or the gland resulting in the obstruction of the salivary flow. Sialolith is a calcareous substance, which may form in the parenchyma or the duct of the major or minor salivary glands. Though any of the salivary duct may be obstructed by the formation of the sialolith, about 90 percent of the sialoliths form in the submandibular gland. This is because the long, curved Wharton's duct has increased chance of entrapment of organic debris, plus the secretion of this gland is higher in calcium content and thick in consistency and the position of the gland increases the chances for the stagnation of the saliva.

The factors like inflammation; local irritation or drugs can cause stagnation of saliva leading to the build up of an organic nidus, which eventually will calcify. Though the metabolic cause for their formation is suggested, it is not yet established.

Sialolith: The sialolith is a calcified mass with laminated layers of the inorganic material. It results from the crystallization of salivary solutes. The sialolith is yellowish white in color, single or multiple, may be round, ovoid or elongated having the size of 2 cm or more in diameter. The minerals are various forms of calcium phosphate like hydroxyapatite, octacalcium phosphate,

etc. Calcium and phosphorus ions are deposited on the organic nidus, which may be, desquamated epithelial cell, bacteria, foreign particle or product of bacterial decomposition. It is said that the sialoliths grow at the rate of 1 mm/year.

Clinical Features

Sialolithiasis may occur at any age; common in the middle aged persons. When a duct of the major gland is involved, there is pain with the psychic stimulation of the salivary flow. Patients complain of pain and swelling during and after eating the food. The obstruction of the duct by the sialolith causes prevention of salivary flow and increased pressure producing the pain.

On examination, the stone can be palpated, especially, if present at the peripheral aspect of the duct.

Investigations

Radiographs: AP view, lateral, lateral oblique or occlusal view.
Sialography: The radiographs demonstrate the presence of salivary calculi; which can be appropriately located by the sialography.

Complications

- Bacterial infection of the gland may result in the obstruction of long duration.
- *Sialoangiectasis:* Dilatation of the gland and the duct system can happen because of the stasis of the saliva. It may be due to a sialolith, a stricture or chronic infection of the gland.
- The retention of the saliva may result in the formation of mucoceles, especially the mucous retention phenomenon.
- Rarely, the complete obstruction of the duct may result in the atrophy of the gland.

Management

There are several techniques available for the removal of the sialolith. A suitable procedure is selected depending upon the number, size, and site of the stone in the duct or the gland and age of the patient, etc.
- The smaller sialoliths, which are located peripherally near the ductal opening may be removed by manipulation (Called milking the gland).

- Larger sialoliths are surgically removed.
- Sometimes, the stones, which are not impacted, may be extracted through the intubation of the duct with fine soft plastic catheter and application of the suction to the tube.
- Multiple stones or stones in the gland require the removal of the gland.
- Some investigators have successfully used modern techniques like Piezoelectric shockwave lithotripsy to fragment the salivary stones. The fragments pass through the duct, as the salivary flow is stimulated and enhanced by the use of sialogogues.

Transoral sialolithotomy of the submandibular duct (Figs 37.6 to 37.9): Transoral sialolithotomy is the best procedure to surgically remove the submandibular duct stones. This procedure can be carried out under local anesthesia.

The exact site of the stone is located by X-rays and palpation. Following this, a suture may be placed behind the stone to prevent its backward movement. The tongue is lifted and held with the help of a gauze.

Incision is made in the mucosa parallel to the duct taking care not to injure the structures like the lingual nerve and the sublingual glands. After this, blunt dissection is carried out. The tissues are displaced to

locate the duct. Once that part of the duct lodging the stone is identified, a longitudinal incision is made over the stone. The stone is removed using small forceps, in case the stone is large, it is crushed with the help of the forceps. Following this a cannula may be passed to

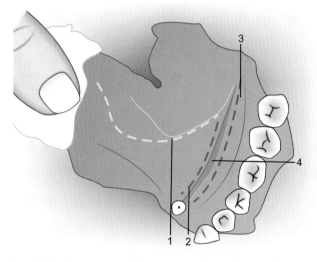

Fig. 37.6: Transoral sialolithotomy of submandibular salivary gland duct: (1) Lingual nerve—superficial course, (2) Incision for anterior stone, (3) Incision for posterior stone, (4) Submandibular duct

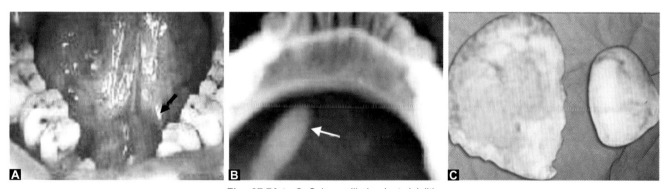

Figs 37.7A to C: Submandibular duct sialoliths

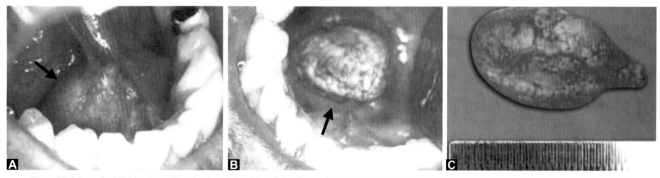

Figs 37.8A to C: (A) Hard swelling in the right side of the floor of the mouth, in an anterior region. Note the inflamed Wharton's duct, (B) Sialolith from (R) Wharton's duct is being explored out, (C) Sialolith after the removal from its bed

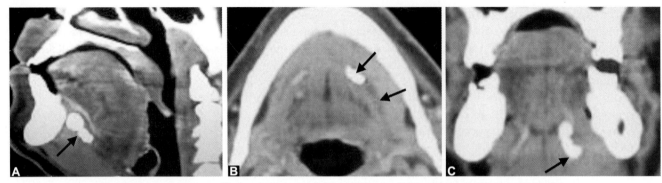

Figs 37.9A to C: Submandibular gland duct sialoliths—CT scan. (A) Sagittal view, (B) Submental view, (C) Coronal view—all showing the presence of sialoliths

aspirate the pieces of stone, mucin, etc. The patency of the duct anterior to the surgical area should be ensured by passing a probe.

Sutures are placed at the level of the mucosa.

Sialadenitis

Inflammation of the salivary glands is known as sialadenitis. Viral infections, bacterial infections, allergic reactions and systemic diseases are the major causes for sialadenitis. It may be acute or chronic.

Viral Infections

Mumps (epidemic parotitis) is the most common viral infection affecting the salivary glands; which is caused by a paramyxovirus. It is an acute, contagious disease, usually affecting the parotid gland. Occasionally, the submandibular or the sublingual glands may also be involved.

This disease is self-limiting one and not dangerous. In these days, the number of cases are reduced, because of the use of the mumps vaccine. It is a disease of the childhood, but when it affects the adults, it leads to greater complications.

Patients suffering from mumps give the history of local epidemic or contact with mumps' patients. This disease has the incubation period of 2-3 weeks.

Clinical features: Initially, the patient may suffer from mild fever, headache, chills, vomiting, etc. followed by pain below the ear and sudden onset of firm, rubbery or elastic swelling of the salivary glands, frequently elevating the ear lobe. In viral parotitis, the glands of both the sides enlarge, which may be simultaneous or one following the other in 24 to 48 hrs. There is excruciating ear pain during mastication. Xerostomia, trismus,

cervical lymphadenitis, tender glands, edema of the overlying skin may also be present. These symptoms usually last for a week. The disease spreads through droplet dissemination as the virus is present in the saliva. Because of the inflammation of the glands, the salivary flow decreases, with the increase in viscosity and turbidity, which increases the chance of ascending infections.

The diagnosis is easy, when the above mentioned features are present. In the absence of secondary infection, there is no suppuration and no pus discharge from Stenson's duct upon pressure on the gland; however, the papilla may be puffy and red.

Complications

- In adults, this viral disease may lead to the inflammation of gonads and central nervous system resulting in meningitis, encephalitis, orchitis, epididymitis, deafness, myocarditis, thyroiditis, pancreatitis, oophoritis, etc.
- In case of secondary infection, it leads to bacterial sialadenitis.

Investigations

- In acute phase, the serum amylase level is increased.
- Demonstration of the antibodies may confirm the disease.

Differential diagnosis: Because the swelling can be near the angle of the mandible, one should not confuse mumps for a infectious swelling from lower molars.

Management: It is self-limiting. Symptomatic relief can be given by antipyretics. Antibiotics can be given to prevent the secondary infection.

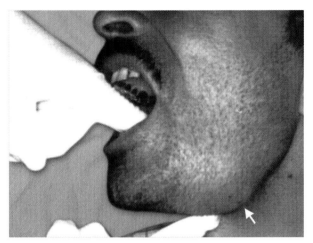
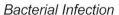

Fig. 37.10: Acute bacterial sialadenitis

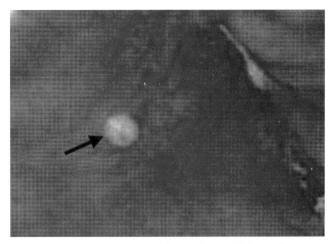

Fig. 37.11: Pus expressed from right parotid duct orifice

Bacterial Infection

Bacterial infection can lead to the inflammation of major salivary glands. Depending on the onset, it may be acute or chronic/recurrent. The bacterial sialadenitis affects the parotid gland more commonly, the submandibular glands are rarely affected.

Acute Bacterial Sialadenitis (Fig. 37.10)

The commensal organisms such as *Staph. aureus, Staph. pyogenes, Strep. viridans, Pnuemococcus, Actinomycetes,* etc. can cause the bacterial sialadenitis. It affects either the neonate and children or debilitated adults with poor oral hygiene. Some drugs like tranquilizers, anti-parkinson drugs, diuretics, anti-histamines, tricyclic antidepressants, etc. decrease the salivary flow, with increased chance of infection of salivary glands.

Clinical features: The disease is characterized by sudden onset of pain at the angle of the jaw, which is unilateral. The affected gland is enlarged and tender and extremely painful. The inflammatory swelling is very tense and doesn't show much fluctuation. The overlying skin is warm and red. There is purulent discharge from Stenson's duct, which can be seen upon pressing the papilla (Fig. 37.11). Patient might present with fever and other symptoms of acute inflammation.

Differential diagnosis: Bacterial sialadenitis can be differentiated from mumps by the discharge of pus at ductal opening.
Investigation: The leukocyte count is high—leukocytosis.

Sialography should not be performed in the presence of suppuration. The pus is collected from Stenson's duct taking care not to contaminate the swab with oral microfloa, for the culture and sensitivity test.

Management

- Antibiotics
- Palliative
  a. Hydrating the patient.
  b. Stimulate the salivation by chewing sialogogues.
  c. Improve the oral hygiene by debridement and irrigation. If there is no improvement.
- Surgical drainage may be done using needle aspiration guided by CT scan or ultrasonography.

Chronic Bacterial Sialadenitis (Figs 37.12 and 37.13)

The chronic or the recurrent type of bacterial sialadenitis may be seen in children and adults. It may be idiopathic or with factors like duct obstruction, congenital stenosis, Sjögrens syndrome and viral infection. All these factors except the duct obstruction by stone are seen commonly in the parotid glands. The microorganisms may be *Strep. viridans, Escherichia coli, Proteus* or Pneumococci. Because these have low virulence, the changes are not sudden.

Clinical features: The disease starts as an unilateral swelling at the angle of the jaw.

The recurrent sialadenitis shows periods of remissions. The gland may undergo atrophy, which results in decreased salivary flow.

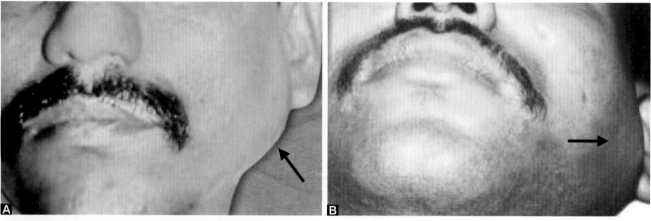

Figs 37.12A and B: Chronic bacterial sialadenitis of (L) parotid gland

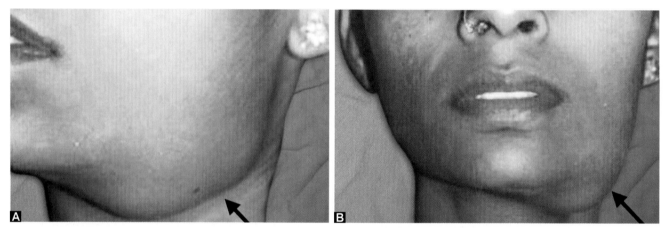

Figs 37.13A and B: Chronic bacterial sialadenitis of left submandibular gland. Note the unilateral swelling at the left angle of the mandible

Management

1. Antibiotics
2. Intraductal infusion of erythromycin or tetracycline
3. Occluding ductal system with a protein solution
4. In intractable cases, excision of the gland.

CYSTS OF THE SALIVARY GLANDS

The cysts of the salivary glands are known as "mucoceles".

Mucocele

This is a swelling due to the accumulation of saliva, as a result of obstruction or trauma to the salivary gland ducts.

Types

There are two types of mucoceles:
1. Extravasation type
2. Retention type.

These two types differ in the pathogenesis. The extravasation type is the common one.

Pathogenesis

Mucous extravasation cyst is caused by trauma leading to the laceration of the duct, commonly of the minor salivary glands, resulting in extravasation of the mucin into the connective tissue. The trauma may be caused by biting of the lip, cheek, pinching of lip by extraction forceps etc. The mucin which extravasates into the connective tissue leads to inflammation drawing the neutrophils and macrophages to the site, which in turn will result in the formation of the granulation tissue, which actually forms the wall of these extravasation cysts (no epithelial lining is seen). Finally scarring results in and around the gland.

Mucous retention cyst: In this case, it is the obstruction of the salivary duct commonly because of a sialolith or may be due to periductal scar, or impinging tumor, resulting in the accumulation of the saliva in the duct. This leads to the dilatation of the duct resulting in a cyst like lesion. These cysts may show the presence of ductal epithelium histologically.

Clinical Features (Figs 37.14A and B)

Mucoceles occur as painless swellings, which may be recurrent (Some patients give the history of increase in size during mealtime).

The common sites of occurrences of mucoceles, especially the extravasation type, are the lower lip and tongue, as they are the common sites for the trauma of the minor salivary glands. The retention type of mucocele is less common and rarely occurs in the lower lip. Instead, it occurs in palate, cheek, floor of the mouth and maxillary sinus.

A well demarcated lesion of the upper lip could be a salivary gland neoplasm than a mucocele.

The extravasation type occurs in 2nd decade and also in children. The retention type occurs in the middle aged persons.

Based on the location clinically, there are two types of mucoceles:
1. Superficial
2. Deep type.

The superficial mucocele resembles a vesicle or a bulla. Since they are placed superficially, the bluish translucency is seen. They are fluctuant. Usually, these cysts are 4 mm to 1 cm in size. The wall is very thin and they rupture easily.

The deep mucoceles are covered by normal appearing mucosa, thus they are different from the superficial ones in the color. They are firm, well-circumscribed lesions and are present for longer period. Some lesions regress and enlarge periodically.

Differential Diagnosis

1. Salivary gland neoplasms
2. Vascular malformation
3. Neurofibroma
4. Lipoma.

Treatment

Mucoceles are treated by surgical excision. It is common to see the recurrence after excision. It can be minimized, if the associated salivary gland acini are also removed.

Ranula (Figs 37.15 and 37.16)

It is a special type of mucocele, which occurs in the floor of the mouth. Since the lesion appears like the belly of a frog, it is called 'ranula'. (Rana-frog) Ranula

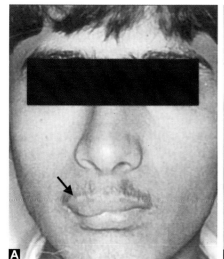
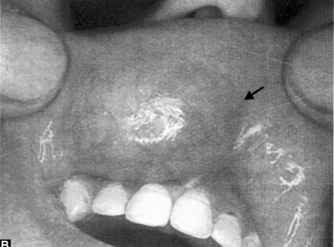

Figs 37.14A and B: Mucocele of the upper lip

is formed because of the trauma to submandibular or sublingual ducts. It starts as a painless swelling on one side of the floor of the mouth. The swelling is fluctuant, and nonpitting on pressure. It may be superficial or deep to the mylohyoid muscle. Superficial ranulas have bluish translucency, the deep ones have the color of the mucosa, soft in consistency and freely movable. When the size of the lesion is significantly large, it may produce the medial deviation and superior elevation of the tongue. A rare variety, which herniates through the mylohyoid muscle resulting as the swelling of the neck is called "plunging ranula". This develops as a result of mucous extravasation.

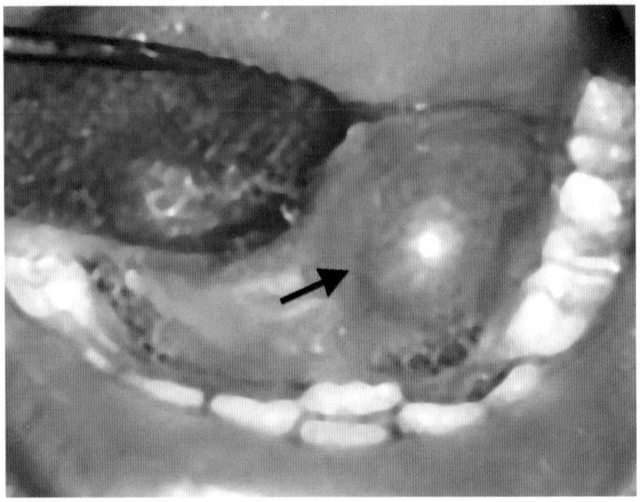

Treatment

Large ranulas may be marsupialized. Due to large size of the ranulas, the mucosa, which is thinned out ultimately, ruptures when injured. The mucoid fluid spills into the connective tissues. As the area heals, the fluid accumulates, thus ranula may show remissions and reappearances.

Differential Diagnosis

1. Angioma (not as firm as ranula)
2. Lipoma (more firm than ranula)
3. Dermoid cyst (in the midline, doughy feeling on pressure).

Fig. 37.15: Ranula in 10-year-old girl

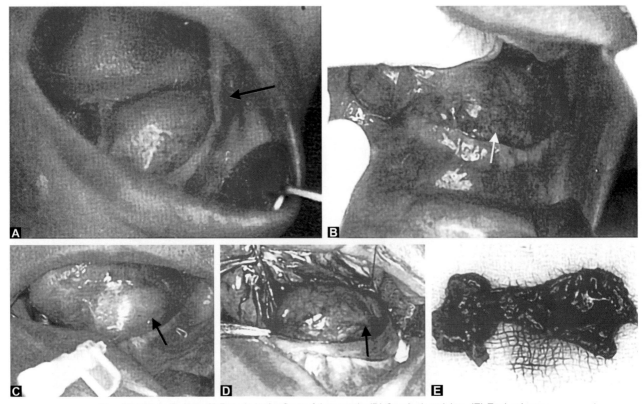

Figs 37.16A to E: (A to C) Ranula in the floor of the mouth, (D) Surgical excision, (E) Excised mass

TUMORS OF THE SALIVARY GLANDS

The tumors of the salivary glands can affect the major and the minor glands. These tumors may be benign or malignant ones.

Benign Tumors

Pleomorphic adenoma, Warthin's tumor, basal cell adenoma, canalicular adenoma, oxyphilic adenoma, myoepithelioma, ductal papilloma, etc. are the benign tumors affecting the salivary glands.

Pleomorphic Adenoma

Pleomorphic adenoma constitutes more than 50 percent of all tumors and 90 percent of all the benign tumors of the salivary glands. It can affect both the major and minor salivary glands; it commonly affects the parotid gland.

This tumor has created lengthy arguments and spirited debate with regards to its histogenesis and management.

Most of the workers believe that the tumor arises from the myoepithelial cell of the salivary gland. The different tissue types of both epithelial and connective tissue elements are seen in the tumor giving the name "mixed tumor".

Clinical features (Figs 37.17A to C): Pleomorphic adenoma most commonly affects the parotid gland, followed by minor salivary glands of the palate, lip, less frequently affects the submandibular gland. Majority of the lesions are seen between 4th to 6th decades, more commonly in females. The tumor starts as a small painless nodule, either at the angle of the mandible or beneath the ear lobe. The nodule slowly increases in size, which may characteristically show intermittent growth. The tumor is well-circumscribed, encapsulated, firm in consistency, and may show areas of cystic degeneration. The tumor is readily movable without fixity to the deeper tissues or to the overlying skin. The tumor can grow to a very large size, but does not ulcerate. Tissue destruction, pain or facial paralysis is not seen.

The intraoral pleomorphic adenomas, which affect the minor salivary glands of the palate, are noticed early, because of the difficulties in mastication, talking, etc. The palatal pleomorphic adenoma may show fixity to the underlying bone, but does not invade the bone.

Pleomorphic adenoma should be differentiated from other benign tumors and hyperplastic lymph nodes. Though the painless nodular, firm growth with no ulceration of the overlying skin, is suggestive of this tumor, it can be confirmed by biopsy. In case of minor salivary gland lesions, which are usually not more than 2 cm in diameter, it is better to perform excisional biopsy.

Differential diagnosis
1. Other adenomas like Warthin's tumor
2. Lipoma
3. Hyperplastic lymph nodes
4. Neurilemmoma of the facial nerve.
   Confirmation of the diagnosis is done by biopsy.

Treatment (Figs 37.18A to F): Pleomorphic adenomas are treated by surgical excision. The parotid tumors are removed with adequate margins, whereas the intraoral lesions can be treated little more conservatively. In case of submandibular tumors, excision of the gland with the tumor is performed.

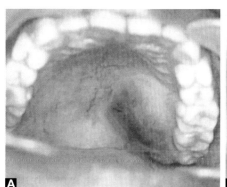 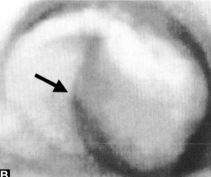 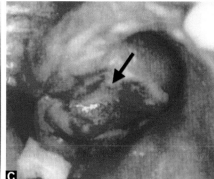

Figs 37.17A to C: (A and B) Pleomorphic adenomas of the palate, (C) Ulceration is seen following biopsy of the lesion

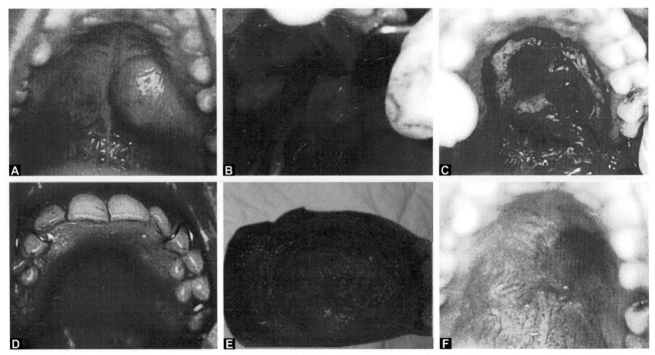

Figs 37.18A to F: Pleomorphic adenoma: (A) Painless growth on the palate of 37-year-old male, (B) Intraoral surgical excision. Hemostat catching the greater palatine artery (C) Denuded bone seen after removal of mass along with mucosa, (D) Raw area is protected by prefabricated splint, (E) Tumor specimen, (F) Satisfactory wound healing with normal mucosal cover

The removal of pleomorphic adenoma should be performed with careful dissection and preserving the facial nerve in case of the parotid tumors. Also, one should take care not to spill any tumor tissue, as they are highly implantable.

Irradiation is contraindicated as the tumor is radio-resistant.

Complications

1. The incomplete excision of the tumor may lead to recurrence.
2. The long standing untreated benign pleomorphic adenomas may undergo malignant transformation. A tumor, which is hard, ulcerates, causes facial paralysis or lymph node involvement could have transformed into a malignant one.

Warthin's Tumor
(Papillary Cystadenoma Lymphomatosum)

This benign tumor affects the parotid glands. Involvement of the submandibular or the minor salivary glands is very rare. Usually, males are affected more commonly in the 5th decade.

Recently, some investigators have highlighted the association of smoking habit in the pathogenesis of this tumor.

The tumor is seen as a firm, nontender, circumscribed mass in the region of angle or ramus of the mandible or beneath the ear lobe. Though both side parotid glands may be affected, the swelling might start on one side following the other.

Sialography: When the tumor attains sufficient size, the sialogram show nonfilling, space occupying, tissue displacing tumor. The diagnosis may be confirmed by biopsy.

Treatment: The tumor is surgically excised.

Malignant Tumors

Mucoepidermoid carcinoma, adenoid cystic carcinoma, malignant mixed tumor, acinic cell carcinoma, are the common malignant tumors occurring in the salivary glands. The malignant tumors can also affect both the major and the minor salivary glands. Usually the malignant tumors occur in elderly people of 50-60 years, i.e. 10 years more than the age group for benign tumors. Some malignant tumors may arise in younger

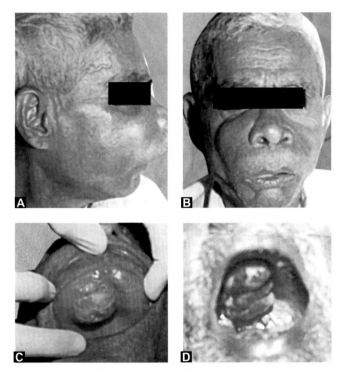

Figs 37.19A to D: (A to C) High grade mucoepidermoid carcinoma, (D) Cylindroma

age group, the most frequent one is mucoepidermoid carcinoma, which can affect the children also.

Mucoepidermoid Carcinoma

This malignant tumor of the salivary glands is famous for it's varied biologic activity, which has created difference of opinion among research workers. The grading of mucoepidermoid carcinoma into low-grade, intermediate grade and high-grade has cleared the doubts about it's behavior. The low-grade tumor behaves almost like a benign tumor with very good prognosis, whereas the high-grade tumor behaves very aggressive. It occurs with an equal distribution between males and females (Figs 37.19A to D).

The clinical features depend upon the grade of the tumor. Thus, it may grow slowly or rapidly; usually as a painless swelling of the parotid or other major salivary gland, or in the minor salivary glands. Intraorally, it may affect the minor glands of the palate, buccal mucosa, tongue and retromolar areas. The high-grade tumor may produce pain, ulceration or facial paralysis, local destruction and metastasis to regional lymph nodes and distant metastasis to the lung, bone and to the brain in later stages.

It is common for intraoral mucoepidermoid carcinoma to undergo cystic degeneration thus mimicking a mucocele clinically. The diagnosis should be confirmed by biopsy.

Intraosseous mucoepidermoid carcinoma: Mucoepidermoid carcinoma can occur intraosseouly within the jawbones; commonly in the mandible. The entrapped mucous glands, the epithelial cells of the odontogenic cysts or aberrant salivary glands present intraosseouly may undergo neoplastic transformation. These tumors are similar in the behavior to the extraosseous variety.

Treatment: The tumor should be surgically excised, the excision should be more radical than for pleomorphic adenoma.

Adenoid Cystic Carcinoma

The adenoid cystic carcinoma is also called as cylindroma, because of its histologic appearance. It may arise as a slow growing swelling, sometimes may mimic a benign tumor clinically and histologically, but has greater potential for local destruction and invasiveness, commonly perineural invasion.

Treatment: Adenoid cystic carcinoma is treated by radical excision. As the tumor is radio resistant, irradiation is not a mode of primary treatment.

Other Malignant Tumors

Basal cell carcinoma, papillary cystadenocarcinoma, serous cell adenocarcinoma, malignant oncocytoma, etc, are some of the other malignant tumors of salivary glands. These tumors are biologically aggressive and should be treated radically followed by irradiation.

◼ NECROTIZING SIALOMETAPLASIA

Necrotizing sialometaplasia is an inflammatory lesion of unknown etiology, which affects the minor salivary glands. Trauma leading to ischemia, acinar necrosis and squamous metaplasia of the ductal epithelium is thought to be the pathogenesis. Since the lesion mimics a malignant lesion, both clinically and histologically, the diagnosis should be carefully done.

Clinical Features

Necrotizing sialometaplasia commonly occurs in men in 5th and 6th decade. Minor salivary glands of the palate; lip or retromolar pad may be affected. The lesion occurs as a large ulcer or ulcerated nodule, which is well demarcated from the normal tissue. The edge of the lesion presents with an inflammatory reaction.

Differential Diagnosis

Necrotizing sialometaplasia resembles the malignant lesions such as mucoepidermoid carcinoma, adenoid cystic carcinoma or squamous cell carcinoma.

Diagnosis should be confirmed by biopsy. One should include adequate amount of tissue in the biopsy, because this lesion can be confused histologically with malignancy.

Management

- Debridement by hydrogen peroxide or saline
- Application of gention violet
- The lesion is self limiting one and heals in 6 to 8 weeks.

◼ SIALADENOSIS (FIGS 37.20A TO C)

There are several conditions which can produce non-inflammatory, non-neoplastic swelling of the salivary gland, which are referred to as sialadenosis (sialoses). The enlargement is painless and usually bilateral, more common in women. Sialadenosis can occur in the following conditions:

- Autoimmune disorders
- Hormonal disorders
- Diabetes mellitus
- Alcoholic cirrhosis
- Diseases of pancreas and kidney
- Anorexia nervosa
- Malnutrition
- HIV–associated salivary gland disorders.

Sjögren's Syndrome

This is a condition originally described as a triad, consisting of dry eyes, xerostomia and rheumatoid arthritis. Now it has been found that patients may present either with dry eyes and xerostomia only (primary Sjögren's syndrome) or with the above two symptoms and accompanying rheumatoid arthritis, systemic lupus erythematosus, polyarteritis nodosa, etc. (secondary Sjögren's syndrome).

Though the etiology is unknown, various causes suggested are genetic, hormonal, infection and immunologic among others. Most authorities support the immunologic mechanism to be the main intrinsic factor in the etiology of this disease.

Clinical Features

Clinically, this disease occurs predominantly in women over 40 years of age, although children or young adults may be affected. The female to male ratio is 10:1.

Typically, patients present with dry eyes and dry mouth due to hypofunction of lacrimal and salivary

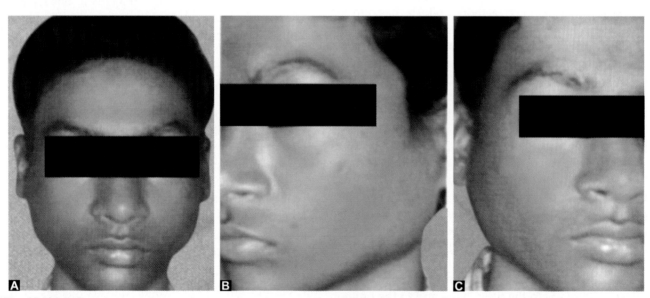

Figs 37.20A to C: Sialadenosis (sialoses)—bilateral, painless, noninflammatory, non-neoplastic swelling of the parotid glands in a 14-year-old male, since six years

glands. This leads to pain, burning sensation and ulcerations on the oral/conjunctival mucosa. Various other glands like nasal, bronchial, vaginal, etc. may also show hyposecretion. Rheumatoid arthritis most frequently accompanies the above symptoms in secondary Sjögren's syndrome. But patients with primary Sjögren's syndrome are seen to manifest parotid gland enlargement, purpura, lymphadenopathy, etc.

Laboratory Findings

The laboratory findings are very important and distinct in the diagnosis of Sjögren's syndrome. Over 75 percent of the patients show a polyclonal hyperglobulinemia and many develop cryoglobulins. Multiple organ or tissue specific antibodies are found, including antisalivary duct antibodies, rheumatoid factor and antinuclear antibodies. Increased sedimentation rate is present in 80 percent of patients.

The Schirmer test consists of placing a strip of filter paper in the lower conjunctival sac. Normal patients will wet 15 mm of filter paper in 5 minutes. Patients with Sjögren's syndrome will wet less than 5 mm of filter paper.

The Rose-Bengal dye test is used to detect the damaged and denuded areas of the cornea. The Break up time (BUT) is performed using a slit lamp and noting the interval between an complete blink and the appearance of dry spot on the cornea.

If two of the above three tests are abnormal, the patient is said to have dry eyes.

Salivary gland function in suspected cases can be measured by using parotid flow rate, biopsy and salivary scintigraphy. Sialochemistry studies have shown elevated levels of IgA, K, Na, etc. in these patients. Sialography demonstrates the cavitary defects which are filled with radiopaque contrast media, producing the "branchless fruit laden tree" or "cherry blossom" appearance.

■ DIAGNOSTIC IMAGING

Diagnostic imaging plays an important role in the evaluation of various disorders of major salivary glands. The modalities used for imaging include:
1. Conventional radiography.
2. Sialography.
3. Ultrasonography.
4. Computerized tomography.
5. Radionuclide imaging.

6. Magnetic resonance imaging (MRI). The abnormalities which can be evaluated by diagnostic imaging can be divided into: (i) Developmental, (ii) Inflammatory, (iii) Autoimmune, (iv) Metabolic, (v) Traumatic, and (vi) Neoplastic.

Conventional Radiography

Radiography of the salivary glands is the widely available technique. It is useful in detecting the calcification within the glands, to know the presence of metastasis to the salivary glands. But radiographs are not useful to know the extent of rapid, destructive, invasive lesions, because the changes can appear in the radiographs only after 30 percent of the mineral content is removed.

The posteroanterior, lateral, lateral oblique and frontal views may be used for the radiography of the salivary glands.

For parotid radiography, patient's head may be turned to 10 degrees to the contralateral side. The intrabuccal view, wherein a periapical film is placed touching the buccal mucosa near the opening of the Stenson's duct is useful to demonstrate the calculi of the Stenson's duct.

Occlusal and lateral oblique views are useful in locating the stones of the submandibular duct.

Sialography (Figs 37.21 and 37.22)

It is a specialized radiographic procedure performed for detection of disorders of the major salivary glands (usually parotid and submandibular glands). The technique was first performed by Carpy in 1902, using mercury as the contrast agent. The technique is employed for examination of both parenchymal (acinar) and ductal abnormalities. It involves cannulation and filling with a radiopaque/contrast agent to make them visible on a radiograph. The procedure indicates the changes in the internal architecture and thus reveals the location and integrity of salivary glands.

Indications

• Detection of calculi or foreign bodies
• Determination of the extent of destruction of salivary gland tissue secondary to obstruction such as calculi or foreign bodies
• Detection of fistulae, diverticuli and strictures
• Detection and diagnosis of recurrent swelling and inflammatory processes

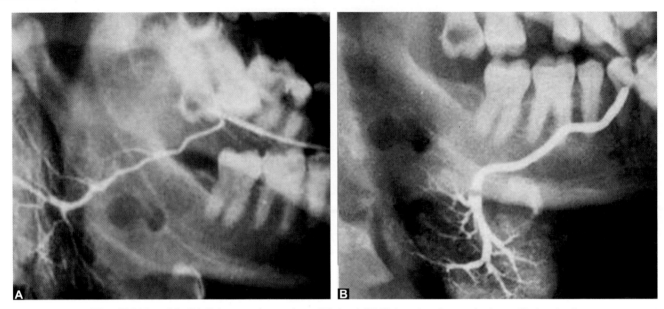

Figs 37.21A and B: (A) Sialogram of normal parotid gland, (B) Sialogram of normal submandibular gland. Note the normal ductal branching pattern in both the sialograms

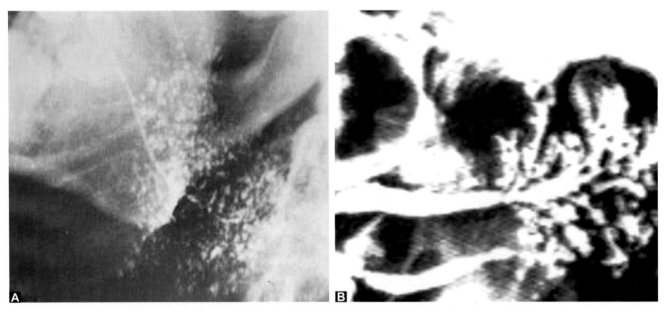

Figs 37.22A and B: (A) Parotid gland sialogram showing sialectasis in Sjögren's syndrome, (B) Lateral view showing sialodochitis changes in parotid gland

- Demonstration of tumor; its size, location and origin
- Selection of the site for biopsy
- Outline the plane of facial nerve as a guide in planning a biopsy or a dissection
- Detection of residual stone(s), residual tumor, fistulae and stenosis or a retention cyst following prior simple lithotomy or other surgical procedures.

Contraindications

a. Patients with a known allergy or hypersensitivity to iodine compounds; and/or other radiographic contrast media. All patients referred for sialography should be asked about possible previous adverse drug reactions to iodine or other radiographic contrast media. These reactions include; marked urticaria, dyspnea, asthmatic attacks, and anaphylaxis.

b. During the period of acute inflammation of the salivary glands (e.g. acute suppurative sialadenitis). In this condition, sialography is contraindicated, because:
   i. The contrast media cause irritation.
   ii. There is increased chance of rupture of duct; and extravasation of contrast media into already inflamed gland.
   iii. There is a potential for retrograde dissemination of pyogenic organisms throughout the gland.

c. Patients scheduled for thyroid function tests in the immediate future. Absorption of iodine present in the contrast material, across the glandular mucosa may interfere with these studies. Sialography should be deferred in patients scheduled for thyroid function tests or such tests should be performed prior to the sialography procedure.

Phases of Sialography

Sialography can be divided into three phases: (a) Ductal phase, (b) Acinar phase and (c) Post-evacuation phase.
Ductal phase of both parotid and submandibular sialogram starts with the retrograde injection of contrast medium and ends when glandular parenchyma starts to become "hazy", reflecting the onset of acinar opacification. The normal opacified parotid ductal system is often described as having a "leafless tree" appearance with a progressive, gradual decrease in ductal caliber, because branching of various ducts occurs throughout the gland.

Visualization of duct(s) draining accessory parotid gland(s) often occur during ductal phase.

The appropriate spot films taken following ductal opacification include: (i) AP, (ii) Puffed AP, views of the cheek, and (iii) Lateral view

Anatomically and sialographically, Wharton's duct can be divided into two distinct segments: (i) Vertical or superficial segment below the level of mylohyoid and (ii) Horizontal or deep segment above mylohyoid muscle. The deep segment unites with the sublingual or Bartholin's duct before entering oral cavity.

The normal opacified ductal system often shows abrupt changes in ductal caliber as branching occurs. This is in marked contrast to orderly arborization seen in intraglandular parotid duct.

The fluoroscopic spot films for opacified submandibular duct obtained during ductal opacification include: (i) Film for horizontal portion of the duct, (ii) AP view, (iii) Lateral oblique of completely opacified ductal system, (iv) Intraoral occlusal view or submental vertex view, using intraoral films are useful in showing pathology involving deep segment of submandibular duct.

Acinar phase: This phase starts with the completion of ductal opacification and ends when there is a generalized increased density to the gland reflecting filling of glandular acini.

The appropriate views for this phase of a sialogram include: AP and lateral views for parotid gland and AP and oblique lateral view for submandibular gland.

Evacuation phase: This phase is useful in assessing the secretory function of gland, as well as, accentuating any ductal pathology not detected in other phases.

This phase can be divided into two distinct subphases: *The first subphase* lasts approximately 60 seconds and assesses the unstimulated, spontaneous clearing of contrast medium from the gland. The second subphase assesses glandular clearing of intraductal and/or intraparenchymal contrast medium following stimulation with a sialogogue, e.g. lemon juice. This phase is performed only if there is incomplete spontaneous clearing of contrast medium during the first phase.

Nonclearing or incomplete clearing of a gland during either phase can be due to: (i) A sialolith and/or stricture, (ii) Extraductal or extravasated contrast medium, (iii) Collection of contrast medium in abscess cavities or (iv) Underlying physiological abnormality.

Contrast Sialography

Contrast sialography can be performed by either:
(a) Lipid soluble or oil-based, or (b) Water soluble agents.

Lipid soluble or oil-based agents: These agents contain 37 percent iodine, e.g. ethiadol. The advantages are: (i) It is not diluted by saliva, (ii) It is not absorbed across glandular mucosa. This results in optimal opacification of both acinar and ductal elements. The disadvantages are: (i) The agents are more viscous, and hence higher injection pressure is required, (ii) The injection is accompanied by greater degree of pain and discomfort, (iii) Any calculus encountered in the duct may be displaced backwards, (iv) When extravasated into glandular parenchyma, it is not readily resorbed; and if present in sufficient quantities, it can cause spray artifacts on subsequent CT studies, (v) Extravasated agents can cause foreign body reaction, and can induce inflammatory reactions and granuloma formation.

Water soluble or water-based agents: These agents contain 28 to 38 percent iodine; e.g. hypaque 50 percent, Hypaque M 75 percent, Renografin 60, 76 percent Sinografin, Isopaque, Triosil, and Dionosil.

The advantages include: (i) They have low viscosity, low surface tension and more miscible with salivary secretion, (ii) The residual contrast medium is absorbed and excreted through kidney, (iii) It is believed that water soluble media coat and outline the calculi more adequately than oil-based. The disadvantages include: (i) The injection is accompanied by little pain and discomfort, (ii) Opacification, generally, is not as good as oil-based media. It is rapidly absorbed across glandular elements, often resulting in overall poor radiographic density and suboptimal demonstration of peripheral ducts and acinar opacification, (iii) It is diluted by saliva.

Technique

Equipment

i.   Polyethylene tubing with a special blunt metallic tip with side-holes for parotid gland injection. A similar tubing for injection into submandibular gland with a end terminal hole.
ii. A 5 to 10 ml syringe
iii. Lacrimal dilator
iv. Contrast medium
v.   Lemon slices or artificial lemon extract in a plastic container.

Procedure

i.   *Identification of the location of duct orifices:* The parotid duct is located at the base of the papilla in the buccal mucosa opposite maxillary 1st and 2nd molar teeth. The area of the mucosa in the vicinity of the orifice is dried with a small sponge. The application of gentle pressure over the area overlying the gland would lead to expression of saliva; in case the gland has some degree of function. The submandibular duct orifice is situated on the summit of a papilla by the side of the lingual frenum.

ii. *Exploration of the duct with a lacrimal probe:* In view of the tortuous course of the parotid duct, patient's cheek must be turned outwards prior to the insertion of the probe into the duct. This eversion of cheek reduces the chances of penetration of the duct at the sharp angles in its course. In case of the submandibular duct, the probe should pass through the considerable length of the floor of the mouth to the level of the posterior border of mylohyoid muscle; approximately 5 cm. In both the ducts, the probe should slide easily back and forth and also rotate freely without dragging.

iii. *Cannulation of the ducts:* The duct orifice is slightly enlarged, and the salivary cannula is inserted into the duct; so that the tissue presses firmly into the orifice to prevent dye reflux. The cannula is held in place by taping the tubing to the face; or by having the patient bite on the tubing wrapped in a sponge.

iv. *Introduction of the radiographic dye:* The dye is slowly introduced into the duct. The amount to be injected for adequate filling of the gland varies from patient to patient; and on the condition of the gland. The amount used is best determined by fluouroscopic observation. The patient is instructed to inform the operator when the gland area feels tight or full. The approximate values of the dye required vary from 0.76 to 1.0 ml for parotid gland, and 0.5 to 0.75 ml for submandibular gland. The injection of the dye should be stopped, if the patient feels mild discomfort, or if the dye is extravasated, and when the gland is full.

Radiographic Projections

• *Lateral oblique projection:* This projection is best to delineate the submandibular gland, as the image is projected below the ramus of the mandible.
• *Lateral projection:* This projection also shows the ductal pattern.
• *Occlusal projection:* This view is useful for sialolith located in the anterior part of Wharton's duct.
• *Anteroposterior (AP) projection:* This projection demonstrates medial and lateral gland structures. In case of parotid, AP projection should be made with mouth open, so that the deeper portion of parotid gland will be visualized. In case of submandibular gland, the chin should be raised in such a way so that inferior border of the mandible and the base of the skull are, approximately at the same horizontal

level, which will prevent superimposition of the gland over either of these two bony structures.

- *Panoramic projection:* This projection is made during the filling phase. It has following advantages: (i) Easier to expose, (ii) Radiation dose is relatively low, (iii) Satisfactory bony details.

At the end of final sialographic views, the cannula should be removed from the duct orifice. The patient is instructed to chew gum; or suck on a lemon; or take other sialogogue, such as 1 percent citric acid solution is given and then asked to rinse the mouth. The purpose of this step is to stimulate glandular function and cause excretion of the dye. The projections; lateral jaw, lateral oblique or AP, should be made again 5 minutes after the removal of the cannula.

Interpretation: Prior to embarking on interpretation of the results of sialography, the normal structures seen on a sialogram should be considered.

1. *Parotid gland:* AP view shows opacification of the parenchyma and ductal system. The two portions, superficial and deep part of the parotid gland, are connected by isthmus in which the ducts are normally stretched which should not be mistaken as pathological finding. Normally, the Stenson's duct is 5 to 6 cm long and 3 mm in width. The distance between the lateral border of mandible and the duct is 2 cm. Lateral displacement of the duct may indicate a possible mass. Accesory parotid gland situated superior to the duct may be present. The ducts in children are finer and delicate than adults.

2. *Submandibular gland:* It is situated in the submandibular triangle in the neck. Wharton's duct is 5 to 6 cm in length and 2 to 4 mm in width. The orifice of the duct is narrower and situated in the floor of the mouth.

The information obtained from a sialogram is the distribution of the ductal pattern, the uniformity of the ductal caliber, the filling or nonfilling of acinar and parenchymal regions. The dye injected into a diseased gland can flow only through an intact duct to areas that are continuous with ductal structures (Tables 37.3 and 37.4).

Table 37.3: Integrity of the glandular architecture in various disease conditions in different phases of sialography

	Calculus	Sialodochitis	Sialoadenitis	Sjögren's syndrome
Filling phase	Feeling defect, segmental strictures, secondary to multiple passage of stones	Segmental constriction, secondary to inflammation and fibrosis	Acinar and terminal ductal ectasia, mildly dilated ducts due to flattening of epithelium	Acinar ectasia and extravasation due to acinar atrophy. Thin and few ductules due to myoepithelial hyperplasia which obliterate the lumen
Emptying phase	Large amount of retained contrast media	Small residue	Small residue	Residue only in acini
Advanced cases	Secondary infection, pseudodiverticulum, abscess, fistula	Combined sialoadenitis and adenitis, abscess, fistula	Irregular cystic formation, sialoadenitis and adenitis, abscess, fistula	Pseudocystic formation, cavitations, superimposed infections

Table 37.4: Glandular architecture in different pathological conditions during the phases of sialography

	Extrinsic tumor	Intrinsic solid encapsulated tumor	Intrinsic encapsulated inflammatory cyst	Intrinsic invasive tumor
Filling phase	Glandular architecture is preserved but displaced acini are compressed and ducts are intact	Glandular architecture remains intact but the intracapsular position of nodular tumor allow it to impinge on ductal system causing localized narrowing surrounding acini may be lacking owing to atrophy	Large cyst stretches the adjacent ducts. No localized narrowing seen, as pressure of cyst is applied uniformly over the length of the duct	Normal ductal architecture is completely destroyed and and replaced by bizarre puddling and a pooling of contrast media
Emptying phase	The ductal system empties normally, since the tumor is extracapsular; glandular parenchyma functions normally	Trapping of contrast medium in the ductal system distal to the site of narrowing is the characteristic of intrinsic tumor	There is no area of localized obstruction of the duct system as in solid tumor, as the contrast medium is almost completely evacuated	Pattern remains essentially unchanged except for further diffusion of contrast medium which occurs as the glandular parenchyma is replaced by invasive tumor which has cost its secretory function

Observations

1. The salivary calculi, stricture or other obstructions appear as radiolucent lesions.
2. In Sjögren's syndrome, sialographs demonstrate many large dye-filled spaces (sialectosis), giving the "Cherry-blossom" or "branchless fruit laiden tree" appearance. The dye could be passing through the weakened salivary gland duct to give this effect.
3. Tumors: Sialography is not useful in case of tumors of the salivary gland. The adenomas of the major glands demonstrate displacement of the glandular structure, which leads to the curving of the collecting ducts giving the "hand holding the ball" appearance.

Radionuclide Salivary Imaging

Radionuclide scanning is a valuable diagnostic tool for major salivary glands. It is useful for evaluation of physiology as well as pathology. It is particularly indicated in patients with suspected obstructive sialadenitis, in whom, the contrast sialography is either contraindicated or cannot be performed due to anatomical or technical reasons. Radionuclide scans differentiate between acute obstructive and nonobstructive sialadenitis. It shows the presence of parenchymal masses greater than 1 cm in diameter; and identifies specific types of tumor.

Procedure

Radionuclide salivary imaging is performed using an oxidized form of technetium 99m (Tc 99m) pertechnetate. Imaging is performed with a gamma camera following IV injection of 10 to 20 µCi of technetium 99m pertechnetate. The activity of the salivary gland is recorded over a given period of time. This information is then used to generate quantitative time-activity curves, as well as, images of salivary glands.

Phases of Radionuclide Salivary Imaging

It represents the physiological process occurring in the glands.

First phase or flow phase: It lasts approximately 15 to 25 seconds and represents the submaximal accumulation of technetium by the gland. It is represented by a line with a positive slope on the time-activity curve. Static images show bolus of activity in major vessels of head and neck.

Second phase or concentration phase: It represents the continued uptake of Tc 99m at a maximal rate. The phase starts 44 to 60 seconds after administration and progresses for next 10 minutes. This phase is represented by a horizontal line on time-activity curve. Static images show an increase in activity in major salivary glands and oral cavity.

Third phase or excretory (washout) phase: This phase is performed following salivary stimulation by a sialogogue, such as lemon juice, applied to the tongue. There is a marked decrease in activity in normal salivary glands within 3 to 5 minutes of stimulation, as well as, a transient increase in activity in oral cavity following stimulation.

Radionuclide salivary imaging does not allow for volumetric quantitation of actual salivary flow.

Gallium Scanning

Gallium-67 citrate, is a radiopharmaceutical useful in evaluation of a number of inflammatory and neoplastic processes involving major salivary glands. Imaging is normally performed 24, 48, and 72 hours following the IV administration of 3-5 µCi of Gallium-67 citrate.

Increased uptake can occur in salivary tumors, lymphoma, acute and chronic inflammation, post-irradiation salivary adenitis, abscess and active sarcoid. Patients with sarcoid often show increased lacrimal uptake reflecting involvement of lacrimal glands.

Computerized Tomography and Magnetic Resonance Imaging

Computerized tomography (CT) and magnetic resonance imaging (MRI) studies provide an excellent soft tissue details. They show (i) lesions and also, (ii) involvement of the adjacent structures. MRI is especially helpful in showing early extension along various neurovascular pathways. CT is especially useful in evaluation of the following:

i. Inflammatory processes involving major salivary glands; as these processes are often associated with sialoliths, which are readily identifiable on CT studies.
ii. CT provides better definition of cyst walls, thereby making it possible to differentiate between various fluid-containing masses, e.g. true cyst, sialoceles, and abscesses.

iii. Contrast-enhanced CT studies; especially useful in evaluation of abscess formation, as hypervascular wall of an abscess will show characteristic enhancement.

iv. Provides better definition of focal osseous erosions or sclerosis.

Computerized tomography (CT) and magnetic resonance imaging (MRI) are important in evaluation of clinically palpable masses involving parotid gland and adjacent structures and their relationship to facial nerve. The relationship of a mass to facial nerve will dictate the surgical approach to be used for its removal. On an axial CT examination the relationship of parotid mass to facial nerve can be inferred by noting the relationship of the mass to retromandibular vein. Lateral displacement of retromandibular vein is indicative of a lesion arising medial to facial nerve, whereas, lack of, or medial displacement of retromandibular vein is indicative of a lesion arising lateral to facial nerve. MRI, by the virtue of its greater soft tissue resolution, is capable of directly visualizing facial nerve, as well as, showing possible early perineural spread in case of a malignancy. MRI also provides better delineation and definition of soft tissue masses.

T2-weighted images provide an insight into the cellularity of salivary gland tumors. Highly cellular masses, e.g. high grade malignancies, tend to have low to intermediate intensities on all images; whereas masses with lesser degrees of cellularity, e.g. benign tumors or low grade malignancies, tend to be bright on T2-weighted sequences.

Techniques of CT Examination (Parotid and Submandibular Glands)

Computed tomography (CT) for parotid and submandibular glands is performed using continuous 5 mm slices through the gland under study. Thinner sections can be used if higher resolution is necessary. It is usually performed in true axial plane. However, semiaxial or direct coronal planes can also be taken.

Salivary CT studies can be done with or without IV contrast. Nonenhanced images show: presence of radiodense sialoliths, glandular enlargement, focal masses, alteration in glandular texture, loss of adjacent tissue planes, focal masses in adjacent structures and adenopathy in adjacent and draining lymph nodes. Enhanced images should be evaluated for; normal glandular enhancement, abnormal enhancing masses (e.g. tumoral enhancement, abscess wall enhancement) and nodal enhancement.

Magnetic resonance imaging (MRI) does not use ionizing radiation to generate images, but relies on a combination of magnetic field and radiofrequency energy. In contrast to CT, in which, it is not possible to obtain direct images in coronal, sagittal planes: with MRI, direct images in axial, sagittal and coronal planes can be obtained. The IV MRI, contrast agents aid in showing and defining: (i) The extent of neoplastic processes involving major salivary glands and (ii) Differentiating between benign and malignant lesions. The widely used MRI contrast agent is gadolinium-DTPA.

Ultrasound Evaluation of Major Salivary Glands

The submandibular gland and larger portion of parotid gland, because of their superficial location, can be readily examined with high resolution ultrasound. The only region that may be difficult to evaluate on ultrasound is the anterior portion of deep lobe of parotid; which is obscured by overlying ramus of mandible. Ultrasound: (i) Differentiates between intraglandular and extra-glandular masses (ii) Demonstrates the presence of solid, cystic, and complex masses and sialoliths.

■ SALIVARY ANALYSIS

The analysis of the composition of saliva though it gives large information, its application in the diagnostic field is not yet known. Both total mixed saliva and secretions collected directly from parotid, submandibular and sublingual glands is useful for the analysis. Cups designed by different investigators are useful in collecting the saliva. Clinical applications are possible in the investigation of the following:

1. Total salivary flow (mixed saliva)
2. Rate of flow
3. Concentration of Na and K in parotid saliva.
4. Salivary phosphate concentration in parotid saliva
5. Sodium and chloride concentration in parotid saliva
6. Salivary IgA concentration
7. Salivary amylase
8. Potassium concentration
9. Calcium concentration
10. Protein content
11. Immunoglobulin content/concentration.

Table 37.5: Salivary analysis		
Investigation	*Observation*	*Condition/diagnosis*
1. Total salivary flow	Decreased Increased	Xerostomia Sialorrhea
2. Rate of flow	Reduced Increased	Sjögren's syndrome Cirrhosis enlargement
3. Na concentration (Parotid)	Increased	Inflammation Sjögren's syndrome
4. K concentration (Parotid)	Increased Increased	Sialadenosis Cirrhosis enlargement
5. Salivary IgA	Increased	Sjögren's syndrome
6. Phosphate conc. (parotid)	Reduced	Sjögren's syndrome
7. Calcium conc. (parotid)	Increased	Cirrhosis enlargement
8. Protein concentration (parotid)	Increased	Cirrhosis enlargement
9. Conc. of amylase	Increased	Cirrhosis enlargement

Table 37.6: Some diagnostic features in salivary gland lesions	
Lesions	*Features*
1. Sialolith	Relationship with food remission and exacerbation
2. Acute sialadenitis	Surrounding area red, erythematous. Warm, tender glands. Pus discharge from ductal opening.
3. Mucocele	Blue, fluctuant, history of recurrence
4. Ranula	Soft, blue, in the floor of the mouth.
5. Associated with AIDS	Multiple bilateral cysts.
6. Pleomorphic adenoma	Slow growing, mobile, painless, nodular, no ulceration, no facial paralysis, periods of inactivity.
7. Warthin's tumor	Elderly male, softer, cystic consistency.
8. Malignant tumor	Rapid growth, surface ulceration, fixation, induration, facial paralysis.

In addition, diagnostic uses of saliva in exfoliative cytology, virus isolation, immunoglobulin concentration, taste dysfunction, etc. are being explored (Table 37.5).

CLINICAL EXAMINATION: DIFFERENTIAL DIAGNOSIS (TABLE 37.6)

Diagnosis of the salivary gland diseases can become a challenge as both the local and systemic diseases can affect these glands. A good correlation of the history, clinical examination, interpretation of radiographic and sialographic images and other laboratory investigations is essential.

History

Duration, Nature and Rate of Growth

The information regarding the duration, nature of onset and rate of growth helps in differentiating the inflammatory and neoplastic lesions.

1. The sudden onset and painful nature suggests an acute inflammatory lesion like mumps.
2. The lesion with long duration and relationship to eating, with episodes of remission and exacerbation suggests obstruction by a sialolith.
3. Slow growing swelling which recurs periodically, suggests cysts of the salivary gland.
4. The benign tumor grows slowly and steadily. Painless swelling of long duration, which is mobile, lobulated suggests pleomorphic adenoma. The true neoplasms can show periods of biologic inactivity, but do not regress on their own.

5. The sudden onset of a painless swelling, which grows rapidly suggests high grade malignant tumor.

Examination

The inspectory findings are important in differentiating lesions. The skin over the inflammatory lesion appears red and edematous. The swellings of the parotid gland appears tense, as it is confined within the fascia.

The changes in the facial musculature should be observed when a malignant tumor is suspected.

Palpation: Bimanual palpation with one finger palpating the lesion, the other finger into the mouth should be carried out. The finger palpation helps in separating the lesions of adjacent structures like branchial cleft cyst, dermoid cyst, inflammation of lymph nodes, etc. The consistency of the uninvolved gland will be normal. Intraoral palpation is helpful for the ductal pathologies. If the intraoral finger can displace the lesion, and it is felt by the extraoral finger, it indicates that it is lateral to the musculature of the mouth.

The gland and ductal opening should be pressed and the secretion should be examined. Purulent discharge indicates bacterial infection. Pain upon palpation indicates inflammation, no pain in case of neoplasms.

Fixation: The mobility of the lesion should be examined. Pleomorphic adenoma, Schwannoma, inflammatory lymph nodes are readily movable. Acute inflammation, abscesses, malignant neoplasms, metastatic lymph nodes are not readily movable.

The indurated hard lesion suggest malignant lesion. Sometimes, the inflammatory lesion of the parotid may also be hard, but it involves the entire gland, whereas the malignant lesion usually involves a portion of it.

Sometimes pathologies of neighboring structures may mimic salivary gland lesions. The lymph nodes situated adjacent to the parotid or submandibular gland may become enlarged due to inflammatory or neoplastic causes.

Osteoma, odontogenic tumors like ameloblastoma, odontogenic keratocyst, lesions occurring at the angle or ramus of mandible, Garre's osteomyelitis, metastatic carcinoma, etc. can be differentiated from salivary gland lesions through radiographs.

◼ SURGICAL MANAGEMENT

Parotid Gland: Superficial Parotidectomy (Figs 37.23A to C)

Indications

a. Tumor: The most common is pleomorphic adenoma,
b. Massive enlargement secondary to: (i) Sjögren's syndrome, or (ii) Calculus in the hilum of gland-calculus is removed without removal of the gland, (iii) Chronic infection.

Approaches

i. Preauricular
ii. Submandibular
iii. Combination of the two approaches.

Preauricular: Incision is taken in the skin. Platysma and superficial fascia dissected. The duct is identified at the anterior border of the gland. The duct is followed backwards through the substance of gland until the calculus; identified and recovered.

Extreme caution should be exercised for the preservation of branches of facial nerve, particularly the lower zygomatic branch, which lies on the surface of the duct just below the accessory parotid. The fascial sheath encasing the gland is closed completely. This prevents saliva leaking into the tissues. A piece of corrugated rubber drain is placed, and the wound is closed over the drain in layers. A pressure dressing is applied over the site of surgery. Superficial parotidectomy surgical procedure is shown in Figures 37.24A to C.

Preventing Injury to the Facial Nerve

Sternocleidomastoid muscle is followed superiorly to find the main trunk. In cases, this route is not successful, a peripheral branch; usually the marginal mandibular, may be found and traced proximally.

Identification of facial nerve may be accomplished by one of the three methods:
i. Direct identification of the main trunk as it exits through the stylomastoid foramen (Lathrop 1949).
ii. Retrograde approach to the trunk from either the mandibular branch, where it passes over the retromandibular vein (Byars 1952), or the peripheral branches alongside the parotid duct (State 1949).
iii. Supravital staining of parotid gland, contrasting the blue normal gland from the unstained tumor and the gleaming white facial nerve fibers.

Complete Excision of Parotid Gland (Figs 37.25 and 37.26)

During complete removal of parotid gland, the prime concern is to conserve the facial nerve and its branches. In malignant lesions, however, this may not be possible and the resultant deformity should be explained to the patient.

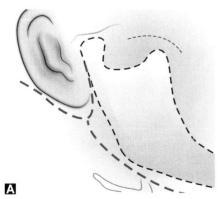
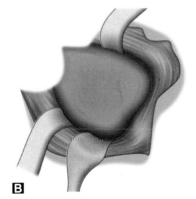
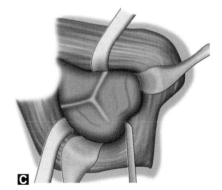

A **B** **C**

Figs 37.23A to C: Surgical exposure for parotid gland excision: (A) Incision for parotid gland excision, (B) Retraction of the ear lobe and anterior flap to expose the superficial portion of the tumor, (C) Superficial portion is freed and elevated from branching facial nerve

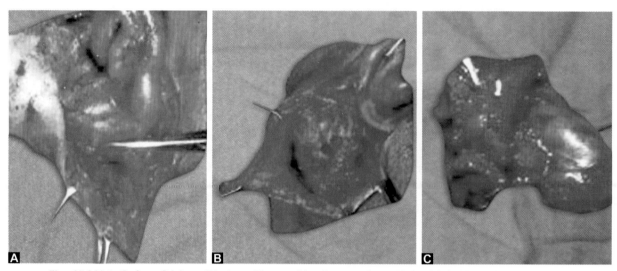

Figs 37.24A to C: Superficial parotidectomy. Pleomorphic adenoma of parotid gland, left side in 42-year-old male
(A) Y-shaped extraoral incision, (B) Tumor mass in superficial lobe of parotid gland is exposed, (C) Superficial parotidectomy, tumor mass

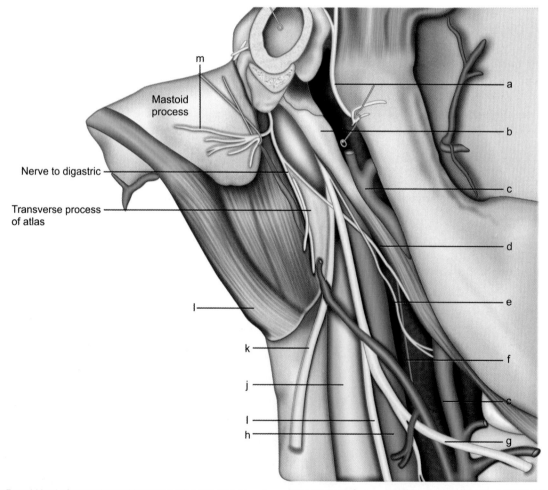

Fig. 37.25: Parotid bed after total parotidectomy: (a) Auriculotemporal nerve (b) Styloid process (c) External carotid artery (d) Stylohyoid muscle (e) Glossopharyngeal nerve (f) Ascending pharyngeal nerve (g) Hypoglossal nerve (h) Internal carotid artery (i) Vagus nerve (j) External jugular vein (k) Accessory nerve (l) Digastric posterior belly (m) Facial nerve. During dissection, it is important to know the anatomy

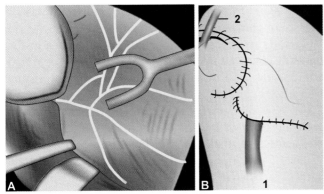

Figs 37.26A and B: (A) Complete excision of parotid gland, (B) Wound closure and placement of soft rubber penrose drains in the upper and lower portion of the closure (1 and 2)

Incision and Dissection (Figs 37.27A to E)

The Y-shaped incision is planned, starting from the superior attachment of the pinna downwards and anteriorly towards the angle of the mandible and anteriorly, forward till the hyoid bone. The second arm of the incision is made posterior to the pinna. The ear lobe is retracted upwards and the skin flap is developed on the cheek side of the incision. An electrical nerve stimulator is used to identify the facial nerve. After the nerve trunk is located, then the course of the nerve is followed and the superficial lobe is freed from its attachments. The Stenson's duct is located, ligated and cut. The deep lobe is approached after this, by further retracting the ear lobe posterosuperiorly. Ligation of external carotid artery and the posterior facial vein is carried out. The facial nerve is then carefully elevated from the deep portion. The retromandibular vein is also divided from its inferior and superior branches and its stumps ligated. The deep portion is gently dissected out of the retromandibular space. This deep portion rests on the styloid process and the stylohyoid, styloglossus and digastric muscles. If the tumor is very bulky, the ascending ramus may be divided and reflected to facilitate the excision of the deep lobe. The mandible is then rewired in position. The wound is closed in layers and a drain is placed.

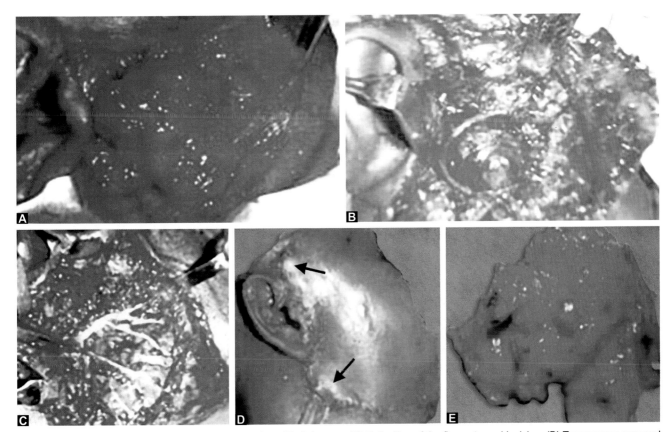

Figs 37.27A to E: Total parotidectomy with preservation of facial nerve: (A) Reflection of the flap-extraoral incision, (B) Tumor mass exposed, (C) Exposure of facial nerve and its branches, (D) Final closure with drain in place, (E) Specimen after total parotidectomy (pleomorphic adenoma)

Submandibular Salivary Gland (Figs 37.28 and 37.29)

Extra-oral Procedures

Procedure for biopsy or excision of the gland: An incision, 4 to 5 cm in length, is taken in the skin in the submandibular region. The incision is placed in, or parallel to the skin creases, about 2 cm below the submandibular border. The wound is deepened through platysma and deep fascia. The branches of facial nerve in the field are identified, mobilized and retracted. The facial vein is identified and ligated. The lower pole of the gland is exposed, grasped with Allis's forceps and turned upwards and forwards. The posterior belly of digastric and stylohyoid muscles are retracted downwards and backwards to expose facial artery lying deeper to the gland. It is ligated and divided. The gland is separated from the lower border of mandible. Here again the facial artery lies lateral to the gland. It is divided and ligated again. With the help of Allis's forceps, the gland is held from the front of lower pole, and the gland is turned backwards, so that the attachment to the posterior border of mylohyoid can be exposed. The gland then can be mobilized and brought down to display the lingual nerve. The nerve is in relation with the upper pole of the gland from the point of emergence of the duct. Extreme caution has to be taken while carrying out the dissection. At times, due to scarring caused by inflammation around an adjoining calculus, the nerve may be adherent. Once the lingual nerve is carefully dissected, and the duct is identified, the mylohyoid muscle is retracted. Then a ligature is passed anterior to ductal pathosis, if it exists. The second ligature is passed posterior to the first one, but still anterior to the ductal pathosis and the duct is sectioned between the ligatures. This prevents the seepage of infected material into the wound. The deep part of the gland, then can be excised. This is preferably ligated and divided. A vacuum drain is kept in the wound, and the wound sutured in layers.

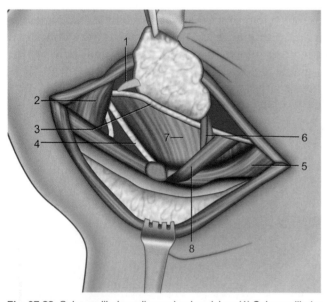

Fig. 37.28: Submandibular salivary gland excision: (1) Submandibular duct, (2) Mylohyoid muscle, (3) Lingual nerve, (4) Hypoglossal nerve, (5) Digastric muscle, (6) Facial artery, (7) Hyoglossus muscle, (8) Stylohyoid muscle

COMPLICATIONS OF SURGERY OF SALIVARY GLANDS

Most of the complications of salivary gland surgery are as a result of damage to nerves. Hence, the complications should be explained to the patient, and informed consent taken, prior to embarking on the surgery.

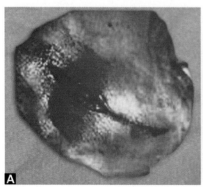 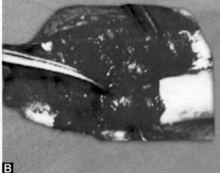 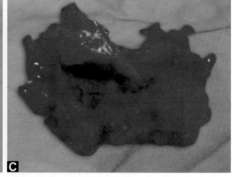

Figs 37.29A to C: Excision of submandibular gland along with the tumor

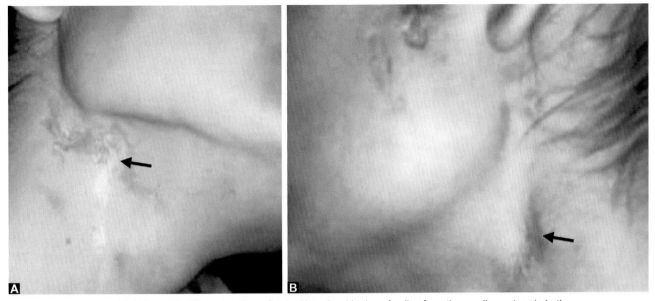

Figs 37.30A and B: Bilateral salivary fistula. Note the dripping of saliva from the small openings in both right and left submandibular salivary gland region. Patient gave history of surgeries for lymphadenitis

Intraoral Approach

i. Anesthesia or paresthesia in the area of distribution of lingual nerve due to damage to lingual nerve, and
ii. Damage to Wharton's duct.

Extraoral Approach

i. Weakness of muscles of facial expression resulting in facial paralysis as a result of damage to the branches of facial nerve. Meticulous dissection should be done in order to minimize the trauma. In case of malignant lesions, however, the resection has to be judicious.
ii. Weakness of muscles of upper eyelid. It is necessary to patch up the concerned eye in order to prevent corneal abrasion.
iii. Auriculotemporal nerve or Frey's syndrome.
iv. Numbness of the ear secondary to severance of greater auricular nerve.

Auriculotemporal Nerve or Frey's Syndrome (see Figs 22.21A and B) Gustatory Sweating

It is a condition wherein sweating and sometimes flushing of the skin in the area of distribution of the auriculotemporal nerve occurs; which is caused by a stimulus to secretion of saliva. It is thought to be the result of damage to auriculotemporal nerve postganglionic parasympathetic fibers from the otic ganglion become united to sympathetic fibers arising from superior cervical ganglion going to supply the sweat glands of the skin.

It rarely occurs and has no treatment. The syndrome can occur in the following circumstances: (i) Surgery of parotid gland, (ii) Surgery of TM Joint, (iii) Injuries to this area of the face, (iv) Injections into this region.

Facial Nerve Paralysis

Commonly, postoperative patients may experience transient facial nerve weakness, primarily involving the marginal mandibular branch, but also occurring in the zygomatic branch. This affects the depressor muscle of the lip and the orbicularis muscle of the eye, respectively. The onset of paresis is usually 1-3 hours postoperatively. Supportive care to prevent corneal irritation may be required during this phase of paresis. Full recovery usually occurs within days to months.

Salivary Fistulae and Sialoceles (Figs 37.30A and B)

Salivary fistulae and sialoceles are uncommon. They consist of a collection of saliva under the skin flap with drainage through the wound. Treatment consists of aspiration of fluid, compression dressings, and removal of salivary stimulants. The problem usually resolves gradually with this simple treatment regimen.

Orofacial Clefts

Cleft Lip and Cleft Palate Management

INTRODUCTION

The dictionary meaning of cleft is a crack, fissure, split or a gap.

The orofacial clefts are congenital deformities, which manifest at birth. Any disturbance during the embryological formation and development and growth of orofacial region will result in the formation of orofacial clefts.

Orofacial clefts are the most frequently occurring craniofacial birth defects.

The zones affected by common orofacial clefts are as follows:
1. Upper lip
2. Alveolar ridge
3. Hard palate
4. Soft palate
5. Nose (not so common)
6. Eyes (not so common).

The old terminology Lagocheilos—harelip is credited to Galen around 120-200 AD.

The commonly accepted terms now used are cleft lip, cleft palate or cleft lip and palate. It is very distressing for the parents, once the child is born with this deformity. The psychological and socioeconomic implications of these congenital deformities can be severe and their management becomes a major issue for health care system. Facial esthetics, speech, mastication, deglutition (swallowing) and dental occlusion, dental set-up can be impaired because of the orofacial clefts (Figs 38.1A to C).

The management of these deformities is challenging and requires multidisciplinary approach, complex long term treatment plan and a rehabilitation programme designed for the individual case. The goals and objectives of the entire treatment plan are aimed at the following:
1. Increased survival rate
2. Improved overall function
3. Improved esthetics
4. Better social acceptance and social integration.

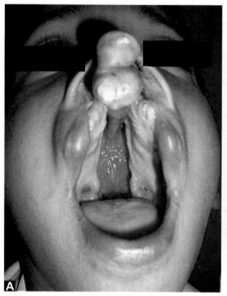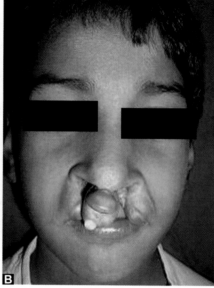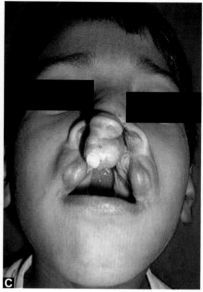

Figs 38.1A to C: Bilateral complete cleft lip and cleft palate deformity. (*Courtesy:* Dr Amresh S Baliar Singh, Head, Department of Plastic Surgery, KEM Hospital, Mumbai, Maharashtra, India)

INCIDENCE

No statistical figures in regard to incidence of cleft lip and palate in India (as a whole) are available. Some International figures are given here.

Fogh-Anderson (1942, Denmark) cited 1:665 as the frequency.

RH Ivy (1963), from the state of Pennsylvania, USA. quoted the incidence of cleft occurrence to be 1:760.M. Oldfield (1959), found the incidence to be 1:600 in UK population.

In India, the survey conducted by Christian Medical College, Vellore, Tamil Nadu, India, reported the incidence of cleft lip and palate in the regional population as 1:639.

Hence, the overall incidence stands out to be 1:700 in live human births.

Fogh-Anderson (1956) from Denmark, while reporting the overall incidence of 1:665 gave the detailed statistics—preponderance of prealveolar cleft in males (65%) than females (35%), and a higher frequency of occurrence of postalveolar clefts in females (66%) than males (35%) (Males are more affected by orofacial clefts, than females by a ratio of 3:2. Cleft lip deformity is more common in males, whereas cleft palates are more common in females). Cleft lip with or without cleft palate is the most common type of facial cleft. Prevalence of cleft lip and palate is 0.77 per 1000 livebirths. Cleft lip is 0.29 per 1000 livebirths and cleft lip with palate is 0.48 per 1000 live births.

Prevalence of isolated cleft palate is 0.31 per 1000 livebirths.

Further giving a break-up of prealveolar clefts in 498 cases, Fogh-Anderson stated that complete clefts were more common than prealveolar clefts. He further stated that in Denmark, of all the cleft lip palate, 25 percent constituted cleft palate alone.

It is now well accepted, that in cases of prealveolar clefts, unilateral clefts (75%) are more common than the bilateral clefts (25%). In cases of unilateral prealveolar clefts, left-sided cleft is more common than the right side.

About 3 to 5 percent of the cleft lip and palates may be associated with congenital deformities of the other parts of the body (Fig. 38.2). Fifty percent of the deformities are combined clefts of the lip and palate. About 25 percent of these are bilateral ones.

ETIOLOGY

Clefts may be caused by hereditary or environmental factors.

Hereditary

Transmission is said to be caused through a male, sex-linked recessive gene. With a family history of cleft lip and palate, preponderance of occurrence is about 40 percent, whereas it is only 18 to 20 percent with cleft palate alone (Fogh-Anderson in 1942). The genetic basis is significant, but not predictable (Fig. 38.3).

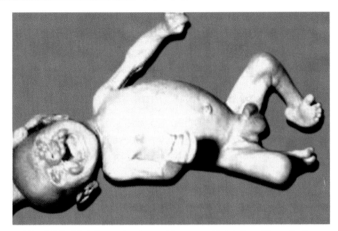

Fig. 38.2: Cleft lip and palate with congenital deformities of other parts of the body

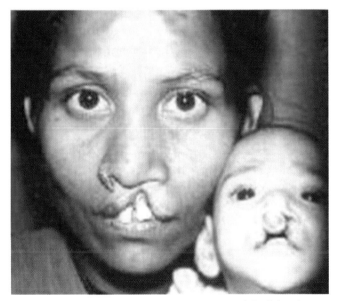

Fig. 38.3: Mother and child with hereditary cleft lip deformity

Environmental Influence

Like in other congenital anomalies various factors, which influence the incidence of cleft lip and palate during pregnancy in the first trimester are as follows:

- Viral infections
- Exposure to radiation
- Influence of drugs—excessive use of antibiotics, steroids, and insulin (it is a potent teratogenic agent) and antiepileptic drugs.
- Deficiency of vitamins A and B
- Anemia
- Anorexia
- Stress
- Excessive consumption of alcohol
- Excessive tobacco chewing and smoking
- Consanguineous marriages are believed to have a significant influence in the occurrence of congenital anomalies (26%).
- Maternal age—older the mother, greater the chance of incidence of congenital anomalies, since there is a greater chance of a defective zygote.

EMBRYOLOGICAL ASPECTS

The embryologic development of the face takes place between 4th and 8th weeks of gestation. The midportion of the face develops immediately anterior to the forebrain by differentiation at broad midline frontonasal prominence. Thickened ectodermal plates, the nasal placodes arise from either side of the frontonasal prominence just above the stomodeum. Progressive elevation of the mesoderm at the margin of the placodes produces a horseshoe-shaped bridge, which is open inferiorly. The limbs of placodes become the median and lateral nasal processes (MNP and LNP) (Figs 38.4A to D).

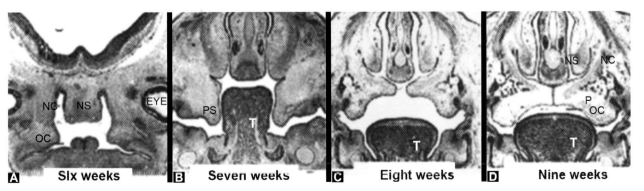

Figs 38.4A to D: Coronal section of the developing palate. NC—Nasal cavity, NS—Nasal septum, P—Palate, OC—Oral cavity, T—Tongue, PS—Palatal shelf

The paired median nasal processes (MNP) merge with frontonasal prominence to form major portion of the frontal process. The median nasal processes coalesce during the 6th week. Their caudal prolongation forms premaxilla and philtrum of the upper lip, columella, nares, lip, cartilaginous portion of the nasal septum and the primary palate. The lateral nasal processes (LNP) form alar region of the nose.

Mandibular arch lies between the stomodeum and the first branchial groove marking the caudal limit of the face. Its paired free ends enlarge and converge ventrally to complete the continuity of the arch during sixth week. The lower lip and the mandible are developed from mandibular arch. Paired lateral elevations of the pharyngeal surface of this arch unite in the midline to form anterior portion of the tongue.

Budding off the mandibular arches are paired postoccular masses of paraxial mesoderm, which constitute maxillary processes (MXP). These masses enlarge toward the ventral surface. The inferior border of the maxilla separates from the mandibular arch. The maxillary processes ultimately coalesce with the mesoderm of the globular process to form upper lip. The cheek, maxilla, zygoma and the secondary palate are derived from the maxillary processes.

The secondary palate is formed by two shelf-like outgrowths from the maxillary processes (MXP). These palatine shelves appear in the 6th week of intrauterine life and are directed on either side of the tongue downward and obliquely. In the seventh week, the palatine shelves ascend to attain a horizontal position above the tongue and fuse together and form the secondary palate.

Anteriorly, the secondary palate fuses with triangular primary palate and the incisive foramen is formed at this junction between 7th and 10th weeks of development. At the same time, the nasal septum grows downward and joins the superior surface of the newly formed palate. The secondary palate makes up 90 per cent of the hard and soft palate, is from the maxillary process.

Formation of the Clefts (Figs 38.5A and B)

In the development of cleft lip and palate, intercontact and fusion between maxillary processes and the median nasal process is normal. The critical problem is failure of LNP to make contact with MNP. The initial MXP-MNP fusion remains intact in early stages of cleft, but in 90 percent of cases, it ruptures later. Clefts of the secondary palate is due to failure of the palatine shelves to fuse together (Figs 38.5 and 38.6).

Medial Nasal Processes (MNP)

Medial nasal processes form the following:
a.   Middle portion of the nose.
b.   The middle portion of the upper lip (Philtrum).
c.   The middle portion of premaxilla, which carries four incisors.
d.   The entire primary palate.

Lateral Nasal Processes (LNP)

Lateral nasal processes forms ala of the nose. Premaxillary segment is continuous with the nasal septum formed by frontal prominence.

Two maxillary processes—MXPs + MNPs complete the upper lip. 2 MNPs + 2 MXPs form the cheek, maxilla, zygoma and the secondary palate.

There are basically two theories forwarded for cleft lip and palate formation.
1.   Theory of Dursy-His (1931, San Francisco) put forward the hypothesis of failure of fusion of the

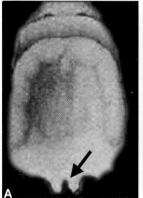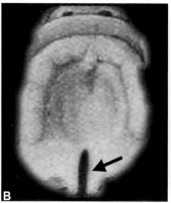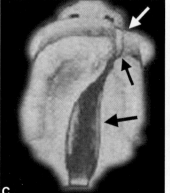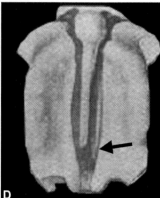

Figs 38.5A to D: Formation of cleft lip and cleft palate: (A) Bifid uvula, (B) Soft palate cleft, (C) The complete cleft-unilateral-involving the lip, alveolar ridge, hard palate, and soft palate, (D) Bilateral complete cleft of the lip and palate

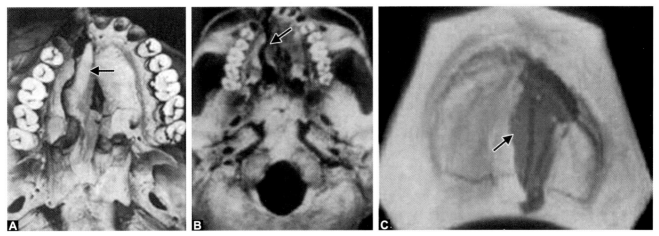

Fig. 38.6A to C: (A and B) Skull with unilateral cleft palate, (C) Model of cleft palate

various facial processes. In fact it sounded a very convincing theory to explain the formation of various degrees of unilateral and bilateral clefts and even the rare midline upper and lower lip clefts. This explained the presence of Simonart's band in an incomplete cleft lip.

The fusion theory is no longer in vogue. The term "process" implies a finger like projection of tissue and "fusion" implies that the projections meet, their epithelial walls disappear and then they grow together. It has now been proved that this is not the case. It is realized that it is not a question of processes, but of localized prominence.

2. Theory of failure of mesodermal migration Fleischmann, a zoology professor (Germany 1910), stated that "cleft palate is the arrest of the disappearance of the epithelial membrane, which remains intact, not penetrated by the adjacent mesoderm." This theory was further endorsed by Victor Veau (1935) and supported by Stark (1954).

Mesodermal migration theory proposes that, as the oral and nasal cavities deepen, there is an increase in the sizes of facial prominences due to the penetration of mesoderm. As more mesoderm enters the area, the bulging increases, so that what used to be a wall of tissue with ectoderm on one side and endoderm on the other side, is transformed into prominence and grooves depending on the amount of mesoderm between the two epithelial layers. Failure of sufficient mesoderm to migrate into a specific area is responsible for the persistence of a groove. With consequent epithelial breakdown, the persistent groove gives way to an established cleft.

It is now accepted that no theory enjoys universal acceptance.

CLASSIFICATION

A. *Davis and Ritchie classification (1922), had anatomical basis:*
   - Group I: Prealveolar clefts (unilateral, bilateral and median)
   - Group II: Postalveolar clefts
   - Group III: Complete alveolar clefts (unilateral, bilateral and median)

B. *Veau (1931) presented a very simple classification*
   - Group I: Cleft of the soft palate only
   - Group II: Cleft of hard and soft palate
   - Group III: Complete unilateral cleft, extending from uvula to incisive foramen and then deviates to one side extending through the alveolus.
   - Group IV: Complete bilateral alveolar cleft.

C. *Internationally approved classification (1967), following Rome Congress based on embryological principle:* This was the basis of the first classification advocated by Fogh-Anderson in 1942, confirmed by Kernahan and Stark (1958) (Fig. 38.7) and later put forward by V Spina (1972) and others. Landmark was the incisive foramen (Table 38.1).

Kernahan has simplified it by representing various clefts in the form of a Y. The anterior portions of the Y depict the lip (1 and 4), the middle alveolus (2 and 5), incisive foramina and the posterior portion (the area of the hard palate from the alveolus back to the incisive foramen (3 and 6), posterior to the incisive foramen,

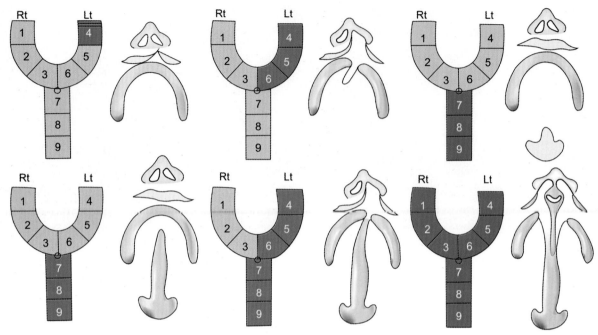

Fig. 38.7: Kernahan's classification

Table 38.1: Internationally approved classification of cleft lip and palate

A. *Group I: Cleft of the anterior (primary) palate*

   a. Lip   Unilateral/Bilateral   Right/Left—total or partial

   b. Alveolus   Unilateral/Bilateral   Right/Left—total or partial

B. *Group II: Cleft of anterior and posterior (primary and secondary) palate*

   a. Lip   Unilateral/Bilateral   Right/Left—total or partial

   b. Alveolus   Unilateral/Bilateral   Right/Left—total or partial

   c. Hard palate   Right/Left—total or partial

C. *Group III: Clefts of posterior (secondary) palate*

   a. Hard palate: Right/Left

   b. Soft palate

D. *Group IV: Rare facial clefts (Figs 38.8A to G)*

the hard (7 and 8) and the soft (9) palate. This facilitates charting of the deformity by residents in a cleft lip and palate clinic.

ASSOCIATED DEFORMITIES AND PROBLEMS

The cleft of the upper lip entails loss of the important orbicularis oris muscle complex. Without the control of this sphincter group of muscles, the developing parts of the cleft maxilla deviate to accentuate the alveolar ridge cleft, when it is seen at the time of birth. In all significant cleft lip cases nostril defect is present, which ranges from mild nostril asymmetry to absence of nasal floor and gross deformity of nasal cartilage and septum. In unilateral cases, the ala on the cleft side is hypoplastic, flared and at lower level than the normal side. The columella will be pulled towards noncleft side. Vertical and horizontal hypoplasia of the maxilla is also noticed on the cleft side. Premaxilla and prolabium are deviated away from the cleft. In bilateral cases, premaxilla and prolabium project anteriorly and the columella is extremely short. There is lack of underlying bony support to the base of the nose. Difference in the dynamics of the growth potential in midline structures as compared to the lateral structures will be evident. Clefts of the palate may be associated with marked underdevelopment of the mandible. In Pierre Robin syndrome along with cleft palate, there is mandibular micrognathia and glossoptosis. The underdeveloped mandible results in tongue fall in the oropharynx, airway obstruction in newborn child.

Structural defects of cleft lip and palate prevent negative oral pressure required for effective sucking. Feeding the child is a major problem in these patients. Palate function is necessary for swallowing and normal speech.

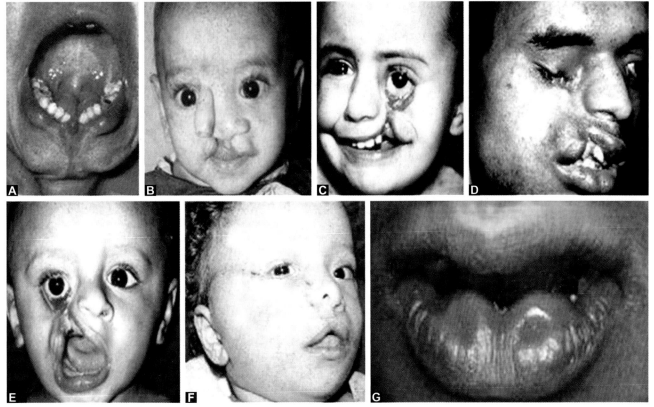

Figs 38.8A to G: Rare facial clefts: (A) Median mandibular cleft, (B) Proboscis nose—double nose with cleft lip-unilateral, (C) Coloboma of the eye with lateral facial cleft, (D) Oro-ocular cleft, (E) Oronaso-ocular cleft, (F) Postoperative view of the same child, (G) Lip pits

The hard palate provides the partition between oral and nasal cavities and soft palate functions with the pharynx in an important valve action referred to as volopharyngeal mechanism. In normal speech, this valve action is intermittent, rapid and variable to effect normal sounds and pressures by deflecting the air stream with its sound waves out of the mouth. Without this valve action, speech is hypernasal and deglutition is impaired. In addition to their actions in the elevation and tension of the soft palate, the levator and tensor muscles affect the opening of the auditory tube (Equalization of pressure by swallowing). When this mechanism of tube opening is impaired, there is greater susceptibility to middle ear infections. There is additional hazard of lymphoid hyperplasia over the auditory tube orifice in the nasopharynx.

Thus, the cleft palate patient will be handicapped with multiple problems of hearing loss from middle ear infection plus defective mechanism of normal speech and deglutition. The growth of the maxilla will be affected in these patients resulting into functional and esthetics impairment and malocclusion.

Dental Problems

Cleft of the alveolus may affect the development of the primary and permanent teeth and the jaw itself. Teeth can be congenitally absent or supernumerary teeth may be seen or crowding or displacement of permanent teeth can be seen. Usually the cleft is seen extending between the lateral incisor and canine areas.

The teeth may be morphologically deformed or hypomineralized and the eruption can be seen at the cleft margin.

The hypoplastic maxilla will have common finding of pseudoprognathism or relative prognathism of the mandible. Early palatal closure will bring about scar contraction and may severely limit the growth and development of maxilla, which will be deficient in all three planes. Constriction of the maxillary dental arch will be seen with narrowing of the palatal vault.

Feeding

The babies can swallow normally, if they are fed directly towards the hypopharynx. But, breast or bottle milk sucking is difficult for babies, as there is no necessary negative pressure in their mouth. The problem can be overcome through the use of specially designed nipples, that have elongated and bigger opening, which extend directly into the hypopharynx. Spoon feeding also helps. During feeding the child will swallow lot of air, therefore the child should not be fed while recumbent and more frequent burping is necessary.

Speech Problems

Retardation of consonant sounds is the most common problem (p, b, t, d, k and g). Speech is affected, hypernasality can remain in these patients, even after the surgical correction. Dental malformation and abnormal tongue position may produce an articulation problem. Hearing impairment aggravates the speech problem further. The speech problem should be treated at earliest, to develop normal articulation skills. Several years of speech therapy may be necessary for acceptable speech level.

◼ AIMS AND OBJECTIVES OF MANAGEMENT OF CLEFT LIP AND PALATE

- To correct the birth defect surgically, so that patient can have acceptable facial esthetics
- To permit intelligible speech
- To correct the dentition to allow normal function and esthetics.

In order to meet medical, surgical, dental, psychological needs of the individual with orofacial cleft birth defect, a multidisciplinary approach is must. Several trained persons like plastic surgeons, oral and maxillofacial surgeons, ENT surgeons, speech therapist, child psychiatrist, trained nursing staff, orthodontist, prosthodontist, pediatricians, etc. are needed to be involved in the overall treatment plan.

◼ GENERAL MANAGEMENT PROTOCOL FOR THE CLEFT PATIENT

1. Immediately after the birth—pediatric consultation, counselling, feeding instructions, evaluation by geneticist to decide whether it is an isolated cleft or if the cleft is part of the syndrome, diagnosis of life expectancy of a child and diagnostic tests.
2. Within first few weeks of life—team evaluation, including hearing testing

3. At 10 to 12 weeks—surgical repair of the lip, 3 to 6 months in India
4. Before age 1 year to 18 months—team evaluation and surgical repair of cleft palate and placement of pressure equalization tubes
5. Three months after palate repair—team evaluation for speech and language assessment
6. Three to six years—team evaluation—Medical, behavioral intervention as needed. Speech therapy, treatment for middle ear infection, fistula repair, soft palate lengthening, psychological evaluation.
7. Five to six years—lip, nose revision if necessary. Pharyngeal surgery.
8. At seven years—Orthodontic treatment phase I
9. Nine to eleven years—Prealveolar bone grafting
10. Twelve years or later—Full orthodontic treatment phase II
11. Fifteen to eighteen years—at the end of orthodontic treatment, placement of implants, fixed bridge, etc. for missing teeth.
12. Eighteen to twenty-one years—when most of growth is completed. Surgical advancement of maxilla, if required.
13. Final nose and lip revision—rhinoplasty, 16 to 18 years.

◼ MANAGEMENT OF CLEFT LIP

Timing of the Lip Surgery

The timing of the lip repair in infancy varies from first 48 hours of life to 6 months of age, depending on the surgeon's judgement. Although, there is always a debate as to when the surgery should be performed, most surgeons follow 'Millard's rule of 10'. Ten weeks of age with 10 gm of Hb and 10 pounds of weight. The trend is shifting toward early repair. In fact few centers like to repair the lip as early as 5 to 7 days post-birth. But in a country like India, where postoperative neonatal care is less than ideal, rule of safety should be applied. It should be safe to anesthetize the child and to look after postoperatively.

Preoperative Evaluation

Total pediatric and ENT checkup should be done for the child, though in a large number of cases, this can be done by the operating surgeon himself. Wherever the need be, help may be sought of other specialists. One should particularly look for the following:

- Upper respiratory tract infection
- Ear infection
- Malnutrition
- Anemia
- Other congenital anomalies particularly cardiac.
- Milestones
- Mental status of the child

Parental counseling is extremely important and its role should never be underestimated.

Feeding

Often the complaint made by parents is about the poor nutritional status of the child due to cleft palate deformity. This is a total fallacy. Though the child is not able to suck like a normal child and tends to take in more air with every sip of the milk, a proper training to the mother can easily overcome this handicap. Spoon feeding is preferred. It is more hygienic. Breast milk can be expressed and fed with a spoon. If desired, the child can be fed with a bottle with teat with a larger hole. In addition the child should be burped frequently to take the air out, which it ingests with the milk (due to large

velopharyngeal port) and feels full without taking in adequate quantity of feed.

Once the date of surgery is decided upon, the child should be weaned off the bottle/breastfeed and should be put on spoon feeding at least a week in advance to let him get adjusted to it.

Operative Procedure (Figs 38.9 to 38.11)

Unilateral Cleft Lip Repair: Millard's Rotation Advancement Principle

The operation is performed under general anesthesia. For endotracheal intubation an oxford tube is preferred. It is then fixed with a stitch to the lower lip in its middle to prevent distortion. Head is placed on a rubber ring. Having draped the patient, the markings are done with pen and ink, usually a sterile toothpick is used dipped in ink (surgical grade). The important landmarks, which are usually present in unilateral cleft lip, are then tattooed with a no. 26 gauge needle.

The lip, ala and the adjoining cheeks are infiltrated with 1:100,000 saline-adrenaline solution, 1 cc or 5 to 10

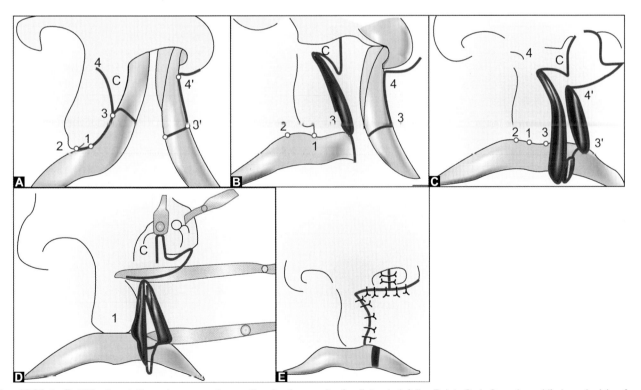

Figs 38.9A to E: Millard's rotation advancement operation for the repair of unilateral cleft lip. Points 2, 1, 3 mark cupid's bow. Incision from 3 to 4 allows for downward rotation of lip. The distance between 3 and 4 should be equal to 3' to 4'. The incision between 3' to 4' creates the advancement flap. The incision from 4' to 5' mobilizes the flap to allow its advancement into the rotation gap. Closure is started by elevating the nostril, permitting small 'C' flap to augment columella

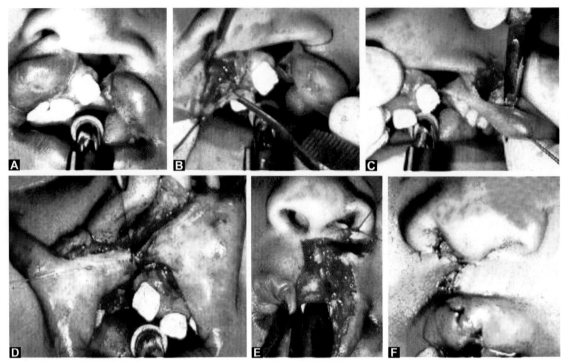

Figs 38.10A to F: Surgical repair of unilateral cleft lip—Millard's procedure: (A) Initial markings, (B) Flap raised on the noncleft side, (C) Skin incision on the cleft side, (D) Intraoral mucosal suturing, (E) Muscular layer and skin suturing, (F) Cleft lip repair complete

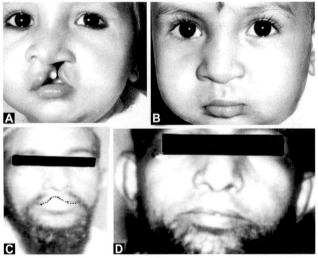

Figs 38.11A to D: Unilateral cleft lip: (A) Preoperative front view in 4-month-old child, (B) Postoperative front view, (C) Preoperative view of 30-year-old male patient, (D) Postoperative view

micrograms per kg body weight can safely be injected. Five minutes wait after injection is desirable. For greater accuracy in incising and suturing and proper alignment of anatomical landmarks, use of magnification loops 1.5 to 2.5 is desirable. Skin incisions are then made with no. 15 blade. Incisions are completed through the

muscle and the mucosa. Simply put, the difference in the height of two peaks of the cupid's bow on the medial element is the exact distance that the higher peak must be lowered into normal position. This is also the exact distance that the interdigitation flap must measure across its widest point, so as to supply a mathematically sufficient amount of tissue to complete the release. The rotation incision provides flap 'C' which is cut free from the lip base attached to the columella. It is freed from the membranous septum to allow columellar advancement. This provides extra length to short columella and also reduces defect at backcut.

The difference in the vertical height of 2 and 3 = amount of release necessary from incision 3-5 + x = width of the point of flap 8-9 = 10, necessary to fill the rotation gap. To achieve requisite rotation, the incision may be carried well past the midbase of the columella. If rotation is still not sufficient, the incision can be carried further across toward the normal side. A "backcut" assures adequate closure without causing obliqueness of the scar or abnormal vertical lengthening of the lip and is a standard feature of all cleft lip repairs. Realignment of vertically attached muscle fibers is very important. Changing their direction from oblique to horizontal enables them to present their ends to the

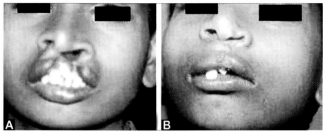

Figs 38.12A and B: (A) Unilateral cleft lip with typical nose deformity, (B) Cleft lip repair without primary nose correction

muscle of the lateral element. Wide undermining of the muscles on the noncleft side should not be encouraged as such action will destroy the natural philtral dimple and philtral column. Freeing the muscle from its skin and mucosa along the edge, offers an advantage in the three-layer suturing.

Primary Nasal Correction

There is great controversy in regards to primary nasal correction at such an early age that it may interfere with the nasal growth. But the release of underdeveloped alar cartilage, correction of the wrongly directed ala and rotating it medially, upward and inward, bringing into its normal anatomical configuration does not interfere with the growth; in fact restoration of normal anatomy allows it to grow in more normal manner (Figs 38.12 to 38.14).

Introduction of flap 'C' into the short side of the columella adds length and contour bringing better symmetry to the central column. Lateral side of flap 'C' still serves as a portion of the nostril sill. The next step is to free the nasal and lip attachments to the maxilla on the cleft side. The extent of freeing depends on the width of the cleft. It must be quite radical in wide complete clefts. An incision along the upper labial sulcus on either side of the cleft with wide undermining and medial advancement of the mucosa depending upon the severity of the cleft, helps to bring the two lip elements (medial and lateral) together and suturing without tension with good buccal sulcus.

Suturing

Flap 'C' is advanced into the columella on the cleft side and fixed with skin sutures of 6/0 ethilon. Then the vermilion pairings are sutured with 4/0 catgut or vicryl to line the sulcus by covering the raw area of the

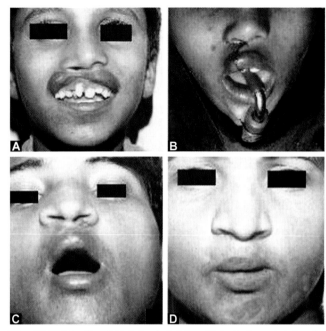

Figs 38.13A to D: (A) Unilateral cleft lip with typical nasal deformity, (B) Repair of the cleft lip along with primary correction of nose, (C) Immediate postoperative results, (D) Nose and lip contour six months postoperatively

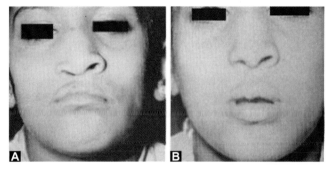

Figs 38.14A and B: Primary correction of the nose: (A) Preoperative view, (B) Postoperative view

alveolus. Simultaneously the lip elements are advanced medially by suturing their upper lining edge to the maxillary mucosa along the labial sulcus on both sides.

Then the key stitch is taken to suture the advancement into the depth of rotation backcut. Muscles on both the sides are then sutured carefully across the cleft. This should be done without tension and in such a manner that skin edges approximate automatically. Skin edges are then trimmed for perfect fit and sutured with 6/0 ethilon. If possible a small 'z' introduced at the mucocutaneous junction helps to prevent peaking, when the scar has healed.

Postoperative

Though the author personally has never used Logan's bow in last 30 years, but surgeons swear by it and if nothing else it protects the lip from external trauma.

Elbow splints are a must for 2 weeks postoperatively.

The child is maintained on spoon feeds for 5 to 7 days and then can use a wati or a glass.

◼ BILATERAL CLEFT LIP

A complete and accurate assessment of the bilateral cleft lip is required before embarking on its surgical correction.
a. Whether the cleft is complete or incomplete.
b. The size and portion of the prolabium and the premaxilla.
c. Presence of anomalies, i.e. lower lip pits, absence of the associated bifid nose, etc.

Principles and Objectives of the Surgical Correction

1. Prolabium should be used to form the full vertical length of the middle of the lip.
2. The vermilion ridge or white line of the inferior border of the prolabium should be preserved.
3. The thin prolabial vermilion is turned down for lining.
4. The thin central prolabial vermilion is immediately built up with the vermilion muscle flaps from the lateral lip segment.
5. Vermilion ridge should come from the lateral lip segments.
6. Upper buccal sulcus should be adequate and at no stage should the central portion of the lip look adherent and tethered to the alveolus.
7. No lateral lip skin should be used below the prolabium.
8. Lengthen the short columella.
9. Premeditated adequate columella planning will avoid the need for later lip re-entry.
10. The creation of continuity of the prolabium with the lateral lip elements joining mucosa for sulcus extension for muscles function. Scar is camouflaged within the philtrum column.
11. Early and permanent alar base positioning.
12. Correct disparity between premaxillary and maxillary segments of the alveolar arch.
13. Repositioning of the severely protruding premaxilla must be done to avoid undue push on the lip.
14. Prevention of collapse of maxillary processes behind the premaxilla.
15. Orthodontia.
16. Bone grafting to stabilize the premaxilla.

Repair Both Sides Simultaneously

Earlier thinking of repairing one side of the lip at one time to convert bilateral lip into a unilateral one is almost outdated today. Simultaneous correction of the lip as well as the nose is done as it obviates the second anesthesia and rehabilitation is faster. Repair in two stages should be reserved only in a small number of cases, where the general health of the child and anesthesia risk overshadows the single stage repair.
1. Freeing of the prolabium from premaxilla.
2. Freeing of lateral lip elements from the maxilla.
3. Forked flaps from the prolabium.
4. Joining of mucosa and muscle to each other behind the prolabium.
5. Lateral vermilion flaps to overlap prolabial vermilion.
6. Banking of forked flaps in subalar incision.

Join alar bases tip to tip. Correction of large defect is achieved by muscle to muscle union in the midline.

Technique of Bilateral Lip Repair (Figs 38.15 to 38.20)

Almost all the methods of lip repair used in a unilateral cleft lip deformity can be used in bilateral lip repair as well.

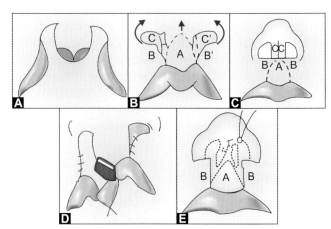

Figs 38.15A to E: Diagram for repair procedure for bilateral cleft lip

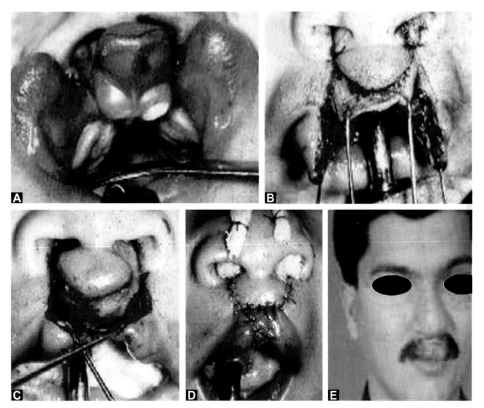

Figs 38.16A to E: Surgical correction of bilateral cleft lip deformity: (A to D) Intraoperative pictures, (E) The same patient 23 years later

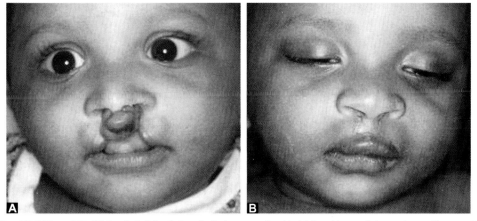

Figs 38.17A and B: Bilateral cleft lip deformity in four-month-old child and immediate postoperative results

The simplest is essentially a straight-line closure and it can produce a satisfactory result. The most popular method for lateral lip repair with older generation surgeons has been the Veau's technique, but the results achieved with Millard's repair have been more pleasing.

While correcting a bilateral cleft lip with Millard's rotation advancement, the only difference, but an important one, is that the flap 'C' is never allowed to cross the midline of the columella. This is to preserve the blood supply to columella. Point 'A' is located medial to lip of the alar base. Point 'C' is placed in the midline of the valley of the cupid's bow on the vermilion ridge. Point 'B' is placed 3 mm lateral to point 'C' on vermilion ridge. If prolabium is wide, forked flaps can be developed and banked in nasal floor to be used later for columellar lengthening. Points A, B are marked on the lateral segments. After marking is completed, saline adrenaline infiltration is used and the operation is proceeded as described for the repair of the unilateral lip.

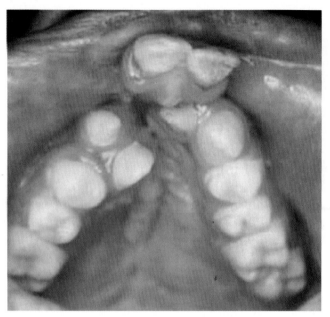

Fig. 38.18: Residual occlusal deformity in 16-year-old male, who underwent surgery for closure of bilateral cleft lip and palate at younger age. Note the premaxilla is unattached to either maxilla and protruding forward unhindered

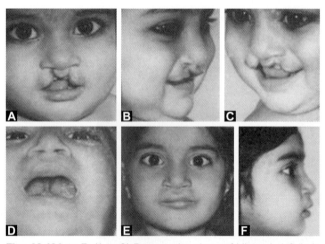

Figs 38.19A to F: (A to C) Preoperative views of bilateral cleft lip in a child of six-month-old (D) Immediate postoperative result, (E and F) Postoperative result three years later

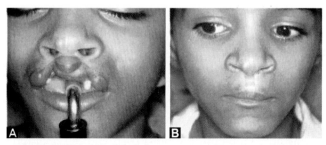

Figs 38.20A and B: (A) Preoperative view of 10-year-old boy, with bilateral cleft lip deformity, (B) Immediate postoperative results

In the complete bilateral cleft, the premaxilla is unattached to either maxilla. Hence there are three components—two maxilla usually equal to each other in size and position and the third central premaxillary element protruding forward unhindered (Fig. 38.18). The complete separation of the central component of prolabium and premaxilla influences the nose, philtrum, musculature, vascularity, nerve supply, growth and the development of all the three elements.

No matter which method of repair is used, certain basic principles remain the same:

a. Observe symmetry of the lip.
b. However small the prolabium, its vermilion must be retained. It should be used to form central part of the lip.
c. Bring muscles into the prolabium. Release muscles in both the segments and try to suture these in the midline, if possible, if not at least bring these into the prolabium, so that the children with repaired bilateral lips can smile normally.
d. Have adequate buccal sulcus. Prolabial lip or the central portion of the lip must be adherent to the alveolus.
e. If for some reason, only one side of the lip is repaired at a time, the second side should be repaired 3 to 4 months later. In such a case one must try to match the previously repaired side.

Columellar Lengthening

In a unilateral cleft lip repair cleft-sided columella is lengthened with the use of the 'C' flap. In a bilateral cleft lip, vertical height of the columella always poses a problem unless the prolabium is quite ample. In such cases if Millard's rotation advancement is used then the banked flaps in the nostril floors are used at second stage at the age of 2 to 3 years to lengthen the columella. If there are no banked flaps, then bilateral forked flaps as described by Millard is used, to lengthen the columella. This improves the lip scars of the previous operation as well.

CLEFT PALATE

Basic Functions of Palate

Sucking

Sucking is effected by an intraoral negative pressure. Lips grasp the object tightly, soft palate moves upward, simultaneously contraction by the buccal muscles and closure of the glottis affects closure of the oral cavity from the nasopharynx.

Swallowing

Swallowing starts as a voluntary movement. Bolus of food is taken to the posterior part of the tongue, then the involuntary movement begins and this helps to take the food into the pharynx. Retroflux of the food into the nasal cavity is prevented by the contraction of palatopharyngeal muscles, which narrow the nasopharyngeal isthmus and the levator palatini muscles draw the soft palate upward and backward to press it against the posterior pharyngeal wall. At the same time tensor palatini muscles open the eustachian tubes to equalize the pressure. Hence the food is not allowed to go back into the oral cavity.

Speech

Speech is produced by the expired air, which is used to vibrate the vocal cords to produce a sound. The sound produced is thus modified by the voluntary changes in the size and shape of the oral and nasal passages. These passages act as a dynamic resonating chamber, e.g. soundbox. The outgoing air may be almost completely stopped in the oral cavity to produce the plosive sounds or may be allowed to go into the nose to produce nasal sounds.

In cleft palate deformity, oral and nasal cavities are not separated from each other, hence the main purpose of repair of the cleft palate is to improve these functions

of sucking, swallowing and speech,which are greatly affected.

Repair of the Cleft Palate (Figs 38.21 and 38.22)

From earlier attempts of stitching together the raw edges to the present day concept of lengthening the palate and repositioning of the palatine muscles, the surgery of palate has attained the more functional concept.

According to Swedish school only soft palate is first closed at 6 to 12 months of age. Hard palate is not repaired till 6 to 8 years of age, lest it may interfere with the growth.

Veau (1931) modified the Langenback's operation of pushback. Wardill (1933-37) evolved four-flap method of repair.

Treatment Guidelines

1. Proper preoperative evaluation is desired.
2. Timing of surgery must be related to the assets and deficits of an individual case.
3. The same surgical procedure can yield different results.
4. The surgeon does not always have complete control of the rehabilitative outcome.
5. Velopharyngeal capability is related to the pharyngeal architecture and to the size and activity of the velum, rather than to the cleft type.

The object of operation is to provide for a mechanism to close the pharyngeal isthmus during speaking and swallowing. Hence the objective of surgery is to obtain a long and mobile palate.

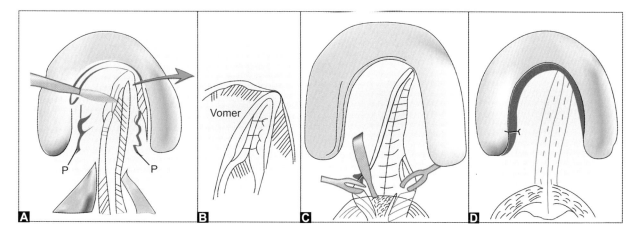

Figs 38.21A to D: Langenback's palatoplasty technique. (A) Bilateral, unipedicled mucoperiosteal flaps based on the greater palatine (P) arteries are elevated, (B) The nasal mucosa is transected and detached from the nasal side of the palatal shelves. Anteriorly, the nasal floor is repaired by suturing the vomerine mucosa to the nasal mucosa on the cleft side, (C) The soft palate is closed in three layers—nasal, muscular, oral. The levator muscles are dissected free from the oral and nasal mucosa and released from the posterior edge of the hard palate. The levator muscles are approximated to each other in the midline, (D) The oral mucosa is reapproximated in the midline with interrupted horizontal mattress sutures

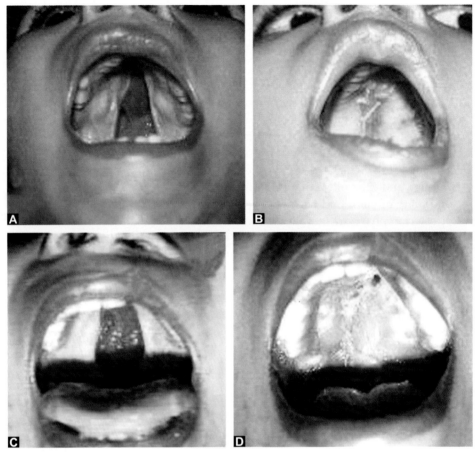

Figs 38.22A to D: Cleft palate repair: (A) Preoperative intraoral view of 12 years girl, (B) Immediate postoperative result, (C) Preoperative intraoral view of 14 years boy and, (D) Immediate postoperative result

Anterior palate is usually closed along with the lip in first stage of the cleft lip repair surgery. A single layer closure of the anterior palate is well accepted. However, a mucosal flap is raised from the cleft side buccal mucosa as described by Muir (1966) can provide buccal layer closure.

Cleft in the alveolar gap is usually closed by a single nasal layer. Buccal side is left with raw area which granulates. Skoog used a mucoperiosteal flap to cover this raw surface and later proved radiologically not only bony fusion of the alveolar cleft is seen, but also the growth of tooth in this segment is observed.

Operative Procedure (Figs 38.23A to D)

Having anesthetized the patient, neck extension is given with the sandbags placed under the shoulders to visualize the palate. A mouth gag – Dott-Kilner or East Grinstead with cheek blades is used to retract the palate. Then saline adrenaline solution 1:1 lac is used to infiltrate proposed lines of incision of the mucoperiosteum and the margins of the cleft. Mucoperiosteal flaps are then raised one from either side. These are island flaps based on greater palatine vessels.

The flaps are elevated to the posterior bony margin. The greater palatine vessels are teased from the foramen and off the palatal flaps for the distance. Next the elevator is passed laterally and posteriorly separating the soft tissues from the medial plate of the pterygoid bone. The palatal muscles are dissected from posterior edge of the hard palate. The free edge of the soft palate is slit open. The amount of posterior displacement of soft palate varies from 1 to 2 cm. Nasal mucosa is separated on the nasal side. Levator muscle aponeurosis and nasal mucosa are carefully separated from the posterior bony margin.

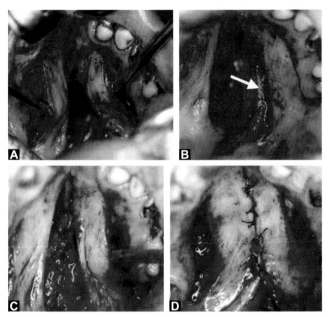

Figs 38.23A to D: Surgical procedure of cleft palate repair: (A) Bilateral unipedicled mucoperiosteal flaps are raised based on the greater palatine arteries, (B) The nasal mucosa is transected, (C) The nasal floor is repaired by suturing the vomerine mucosa to the nasal mucosa on the cleft side, (D) The oral mucosa is reapproximated in the midline

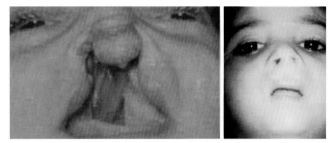

Fig. 38.24: Complete cleft lip and palate deformity and postoperative results

To achieve adequate pushback not only the oral layer, but the nasal layer is also lengthened. It is detached from its attachment to the posterior margin of the hard palate allowing it to move back posteriorly.

Soft palate is sutured using vertical mattress sutures. Suture knots of nasal layer are placed on the nasal side, while that of oral layer, on the oral side. Absorbable suture material (either chromic catgut or vicryl 4/0 in small children and 4/0 in older children and adults, on a Dennis Brown needle) is used. A majority of surgeons still use two layer closure—nasal and oral. But as the functional importance of palate is being recognized more and more, dissection of palatine muscles under magnification and then their suturing in normal anatomical configuration is being preferred. Thus a three-layer closure—first nasal mucosa, second muscle and then the oral mucosa may hold some advantage. Fracture of the hamulus to release tensor palatini is debatable. Often in older children, when the soft palate musculature does not move centrally without tension, hamulus should be fractured and the palatine muscles brought medially and sutured to that from the other side. A cleft uvula must be dissected and muscle uvulae sutured together. Palatine shelves laterally (from where

mucoperiosteal flaps are raised) can be left as such. Their surface granulates quite fast.

In very wide clefts with limited tissue, it may not be possible to achieve full closure. Under these conditions, pushback must never be sacrificed at the cost of complete closure of the cleft. If flaps do not reach till right anterior region, it is quite acceptable to leave a fistula anteriorly for which an obturator can be used.

Postoperative Management

Elbows are splinted in extension. Spoon feeding with only strained liquids (a food particles stick in the oral cavity and become a residue for bacterial growth) is done for 10 days. It is essential that suction with sterile catheters be kept by the bedside at least for first 24 hours. Child should be nursed on his side to avoid the danger of tongue falling back. It is preferable to keep the child following palate surgery in the hospital for 10 days or at least under observation.

COMPLETE CLEFT LIP AND PALATE DEFORMITY

Anterior palate is repaired usually along with the lip. Closure of alveolar cleft provides stability to the maxillary arch. It also helps in closing the oronasal fistula. In infancy this gap can be successfully closed with mucosal or Skoog's mucoperiosteal flap, but in later years a bone graft is required (Fig. 38.24). This provides better periodontal support for teeth bordering the cleft. Most of the centers now favor bone grafting during period of mixed dentition, that is, between ages of 9 and 11 years. Since sagittal and transverse growth of anterior maxilla is completed by 8 years and lateral incisor erupts at 7 to 8 years of age and canine by 11 to 12 years of age. The attached gingiva is used as flaps for alveolar cleft after filling the gap with cancellous bone graft obtained from the iliac crest.

ORTHODONTICS IN CLEFT LIP AND PALATE

One of the major clinical features common to cleft lip and palate is constricted and distorted maxillary arch. The severe the cleft, more severe the arch deformity due to collapse. Following lip surgery due to moulding action, the cleft segment moves medially and arch further collapses. Added to this underdevelopment or severe hypoplasia of the maxilla on the affected side further accentuates the deformity. This leads to malocclusion. Orthodontic treatment is necessary to correct the deformity.

Orthodontic therapy should be started during mixed dentition, and continued through the permanent dentition. Permanent teeth especially, those adjacent to cleft, are malposed, often severely rotated and poorly calcified. They certainly need to be corrected by orthodontia. If necessary, unwanted tooth/teeth can be extracted, specially the supernumerary ones.

Even with complete orthodontic treatment, there is maxillomandibular discrepancy which may need surgical correction in the form of maxillary advancement with or without mandibular pushback, with or without genioplasty.

Maxillary Sinus and its Implications

39 Maxillary Sinus and its Implications

■ GENERAL CONSIDERATIONS

Anatomy

The maxillary sinus was first described in 1651, by Nathaniel Highmore. Therefore, it is also known as *antrum of Highmore*. Maxillary sinuses are two in number, one on either side of the maxilla, and they are the largest of the paranasal air sinuses (Figs 39.1A and B). They communicate with the other paranasal sinuses through the lateral wall of the nose. They may be identical or asymmetrical in size and shape. The average dimensions of the sinus are approximately 3.5 (anteroposterior) x 3.2 (height) x 2.5 (width) cm (Turner 1902). Its volume is 15 to 30 ml. The ostium (3 to 6 mm diameter) opens into middle meatus (Fig. 39.2). It can be described as pyramidal in shape, consisting of a base, an apex and four sides. The base is formed by the lateral wall of the nose. The apex projects laterally into zygomatic process of maxilla; and it may extend into zygomatic bone when the sinus is very large.

The four walls of pyramid are formed by: (i) The roof of antrum or the floor of orbit, (ii) The anterior, and (iii) Intratemporal surfaces of body of maxilla, and (iv) The alveolar process of maxilla which is the floor of sinus.

The roof is formed by thin orbital plate; separating it from orbital contents. The infraorbital canal, containing the vessels and nerves runs down along the roof. The floor is formed by the lateral hard palate; alveolar process of maxilla carrying the roots of premolars and molars. The posterior wall separates the sinus from infratemporal and pterygopalatine fossae. It is pierced by posterior superior alveolar nerves which travel to molar teeth. The anterior wall is the facial surface of maxilla.

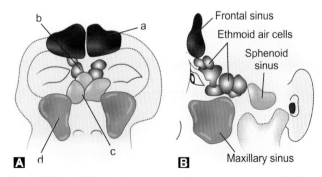

Figs 39.1A and B: (A) Frontal view of paranasal sinuses: (a) frontal sinus, (b) ethmoid air cells, (c) sphenoid sinus, (d) maxillary sinus, (B) Lateral view of paranasal sinuses

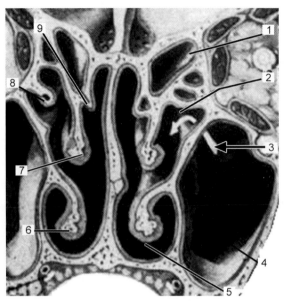

Fig. 39.2: Coronal section through the nasal cavities: (1) Ethmoidal air cells, (2) Middle meatus, (3) Opening of the maxillary sinus, (4) Maxillary sinus, (5) Inferior meatus, (6) Inferior concha, (7) Middle concha, (8) Bulla ethmoidalis, (9) Superior concha

Blood Supply

Blood supply to the mucous membrane is from arteries which pierce the bone; and are derived from facial, maxillary, infraorbital and greater palatine arteries. The veins accompany the arteries, and drain into anterior facial vein and then to pterygoid plexus of veins. The lymphatic drainage of maxillary sinus is through the infraorbital foramen or through the ostium and then to submandibular and deep cervical lymph nodes.

Nerve Supply

Last (1959) described that nerve supply to maxillary sinus is from superior dental nerves (anterior, middle and posterior), and the greater palatine nerve. These are branches of maxillary division of trigeminal nerve. Their pathways are of surgical importance; as there is a possibility of damage to any of these nerves, while doing surgical procedures on anterior and posterior walls of antrum. The anterior superior dental nerve is given off from the infraorbital nerve about 15 mm from infraorbital foramen; and courses down the anterior wall of sinus. The middle superior dental nerve is probably present in more than 50 percent of the cases; and when present it arises from the lateral aspect of infraorbital nerve.

Harrison (1971) described his view, and that it may run in posterior lateral or anterior wall of antrum. The

posterosuperior dental nerve, the same author writes that there are two main offshoots of importance—the superior branch tunnels the lateral wall of the antrum and runs at the level of malar tuberosity; while the larger inferior branch is below, and courses parallel to transverse facial part of anterior nerve.

Embryology (Growth of Maxillary Sinus)

In early stages, maxillary sinus is high in maxilla. Later gradually grows downward, by a process of pneumatization (Table 39.1).

The expansion of the sinuses normally ceases after eruption of permanent teeth. However, occasionally, the sinuses pneumatize further, after removal of one or more of maxillary posterior teeth, and extend into the residual alveolar process. In adults, the apices of the posterior teeth may extend into the sinus cavity.

Physiology

The sinuses are lined by respiratory epithelium; namely, the mucus secreting; pseudostratified, ciliated, columnar epithelium. It is also known as *schneiderian membrane*.

The mucociliary mechanism is useful means for removal of particulate matter, bacteria, etc. The cilia move the mucus and other debris towards the ostium, and subsequently discharged in the middle meatus.

Functions

- Impart resonance to the voice.
- Increase the surface area and lighten the skull.
- Moisten and warm the inspired air.
- Filter the debris from the inspired air.
- Sinuses are located in front of the forebrain, olfactory region, etc. They create "air padding" to provide thermal insulation to the important tissues mentioned above.

Table 39.1: Stages of the growth of maxillary sinus		
Time	*Growth*	*Shape*
3/12 IU	Outpouching in middle meatus	—
Birth	Tubular: 2 cm × 1 cm × 1 cm	
	3 mm per year × 2 mm × 2 mm	Tubular
9 years	60% of adult size	Ovoid
12 years	Antral floor parallels nasal floor	—
18 years	Adult size	Pyramidal

Applied Surgical Anatomy

Relation of the Root Apices with the Floor of the Sinus

In adults, there is a distance of approximately, 1 to 1.25 cm between the floor of the sinus and the root apices of maxillary posterior teeth. Sometimes, the floor of the sinus is in close proximity with the roots of these teeth. The teeth, in close proximity with the sinus vary from study-to-study. Von Bornsdorff (1925) found in his series, that the roots of second molar were closest to the floor. Paatero (1939) also confirmed this finding; with the next in order of frequency were; the first molar, third molar, second premolar, first premolar, and canine (Fig. 39.3).

Low Incidence of Oroantral Fistula in Children Under Fifteen Years

The maxillary sinus reaches its normal adult size by the age of 15 years. Hence, the risk of creating oroantral fistula is less in children and young adults. In adults, the roots are usually in proximity to floor of sinus. The incidence of inadvertent displacement of teeth or roots

into the antrum is also less in young adults (Killey and Kay 1972).

Circumstances with Increased Likelihood of Oroantral Fistula

a. *Large sinuses*:
   i. When sinuses are very large, and the floor gets thinned out, there is a risk of fracture when force is applied during extraction of maxillary posterior teeth. This may result in oroantral fistula.
   ii. Sometimes, the floor of sinus descends down between the adjacent teeth, and also in between the roots of the individual tooth; so that their root apices; especially, the palatal root may cause elevations in antral floor.

b. Unerupted or partially erupted maxillary third molar; such a tooth lies in close proximity to the maxillary sinus. This may lead to its inadvertent displacement into the sinus cavity, especially, if the tooth has conical roots (Fig. 39.4). In such circumstances, attempts to remove the broken root

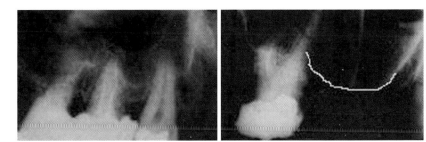
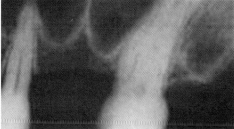

Fig. 39.3: Periapical intraoral X-rays showing close proximity of the roots of upper posterior teeth to the floor of the maxillary sinus

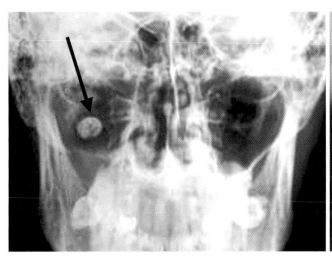
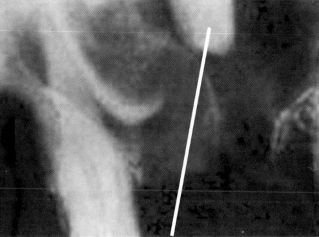

Fig. 39.4: Inadvertent displacement of tooth during extraction into the maxillary sinus

apices, may cause its displacement into maxillary sinus, if extreme care is not taken. The presence of an unerupted third molar in tuberosity constitutes a potential line of weakness. In such cases, if adjacent second molar is extracted, it may result in fracture of the tuberosity.

Lining of Maxillary Sinus

It does not get torn, unless the force of extraction is undue; and the clinician carries out inadvertent postextraction manipulation in the socket. The confirmation of breach in the continuity of maxillary antrum, can be obtained by carrying out routine occipitomental radiographs. These radiographs show radiopacity of maxillary sinus; which persists for ten days to two weeks. Further, in case, there is breach in continuity of lining, there is collection of blood in the maxillary sinus, and which may escape from ostium and may present clinically as unilateral epistaxis.

Cracks and Fractures in the Bony Floor of Maxillary Sinus

These usually heal even if there is accompanying tear in sinus lining. In case, where the clot breaks down, it results in oroantral communication; which, if not noted at the time of extraction either by the patient or by the clinician; evidences itself within ten days, leading to establishment of oroantral fistula and evidences as foul smelling discharge of pus.

Fracture of floor of maxillary sinus, may sometimes occur, following the extraction of upper molars. It is sometimes more easier to extract these teeth in adults than in children aged 7 to 8 years, where the three divergent roots of first molar may be completely embedded in alveolar bone.

Periapical Involvement

Periapical involvement, in the form of acute or chronic abscess in teeth related to floor of sinus, may secondarily involve maxillary sinus. The pus may discharge into sinus producing a fluid level. The extraction of such a tooth, results in blood clot getting infected, and results in creation of oroantral fistula.

Pressure on the Nerves within the Antrum

It may occur in acute sinusitis. The pus formed is unable to escape from ostium into nose; because of its occlusion; caused by inflammation of adjoining mucosal lining.

Tumors Developing in Maxillary Antrum

The anterior and infratemporal walls of maxillary sinus are very thin. The tumors which develop in maxillary sinus may erode these walls and present as swellings of cheek. Tumors may also penetrate floor of maxillary sinus and present as a palatal lump or a swelling in buccal sulcus. The teeth present in the vicinity may get loosened due to bone destruction. The interference with the blood supply to these teeth lead to pulp necrosis which further lead to development of acute apical abscess. In case, the tumor erodes the posterior wall; the posterior superior alveolar nerves may be destroyed; and patient may complain of anesthesia of gingiva or teeth in maxillary molar area.

Involvement of roof of sinus, is as good as involvement of orbital floor. This leads to anesthesia in the distribution of infraorbital nerve; as it lies in a canal in the roof of the sinus and emerges at infraorbital foramen. Further involvement of orbit, the tumor encroaching on the orbit may lead to alteration of pupillary level; the eye is lifted up and proptosis may occur. When the orbital muscles or nerves innervating them are involved, it will lead to strabismus with diplopia. The tumor after occluding the nostril, may protrude through nostril.

Paresthesia in Maxillary Teeth Following Surgical Procedures

The incidence of paresthesia in maxillary teeth following surgical procedures of the lateral wall of the antrum, varies from study to study. In a larger percentage, the sensation gradually returns to normal over a period of time. Very few cases of permanent anesthesia are reported in literature.

Mucous Membrane Lining of Antrum Affected by Infection

If left *in situ*, the normal ciliated columnar epithelium may regenerate, once the infection is taken care of. When the lining is stripped, the nasal mucosa extends through the ostium.

Antral Puncture

Whenever antral puncture is to be carried out; the puncture into the sinus cavity should be made through the middle meatus in children; and in the inferior meatus in adults. The antral puncture or intranasal antrostomy, in the inferior meatus then becomes a point of dependent drainage for maxillary sinus. The floor of maxillary sinus is about 1.25 cm below the floor of the nose.

Canine Fossa

The wall of the sinus is very thin in this area. This area is used for following: (i) Diagnostic aspiration, and (ii) The site for Caldwell-Luc operation; that is, the antral exploration with or without an intraoral antrostomy.

Fractures of the Middle Third of Face

The thin walls of maxillary sinus get easily fractured as a result of trauma. The fractures of middle third of face involve maxillary sinus. Fractures of zygomatic bone show the zygomatic buttress pushed into the sinus; while fractures of middle third of the maxilla—LeFort I, II, and III, show disturbance in the walls of maxillary sinus.

Foreign Bodies in the Sinus

The presence of a foreign body, such as a tooth or root fragment or any other things, it changes its position with movement of head. This change in position can be confirmed by serial radiographs. In case, the foreign body does not move in consecutive radiographs, then it is (i) Either trapped into polyps or thick mucosa; or (ii) Present between the antral lining membrane and the bony wall (Figs 39.5 and 39.6).

Transillumination

It is one of the methods of examination, and can be carried out because of the relative thinness of the walls of the maxillary sinus.

It can be carried out by placing a strong light in the center of mouth of the patient with the lips closed. Upper denture should be removed prior to the commencement

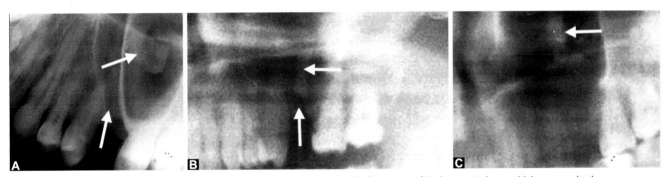

Figs 39.5A to C: Root fragment in the maxillary sinus: (A to C) Presence of broken root piece, which was pushed up in the maxillary sinus. Note the change in the level of the root position in serial radiographs

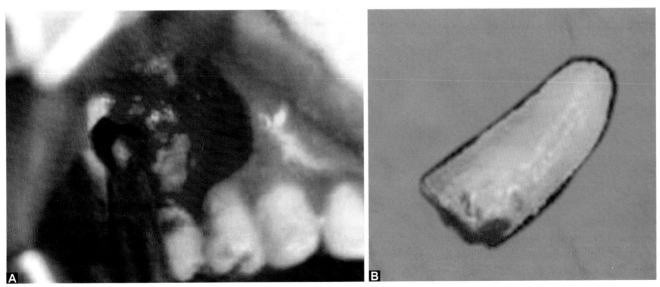

Figs 39.6A and B: (A) Removal of the root piece, which was pushed up in the maxillary sinus, through Caldwell-Luc approach, (B) Root piece recovered

of the investigation. The results of a normal sinus will be a definite infraorbital crescent of light, a brightly lit eye and glowing pupil. In case, the antral cavity contains pus, mucus, polyps, blood and thickened lining membrane, fibro-osseous lesions or a tumor, it will not light up as it was in normal circumstances. The result will also be negative in cases where there is a large abscess overlying maxillary sinus.

Transillumination is certainly, a less accurate method than conventional radiography; but still is a useful method of examination, if the facilities are available.

CLINICAL EXAMINATION OF MAXILLARY SINUS

a. *Extraoral examination:* Pain and tenderness, swelling over the prominence of cheek bones
b. *Intraoral examination:*
   i. Pain and tenderness, swelling over the maxilla between the canine fossa and the zygomatic buttress.
   ii. *Transillumination*: The affected sinus shows decreased transmission of light; due to accumulation of fluid, debris, pus, and thickening of the sinus mucosa.

RADIOLOGY OF MAXILLARY SINUS

The radiological examination is an important aid to clinical examination of maxillary sinus. It provides adequate information to either confirm or rule out various pathological processes involving maxillary sinus. The various radiographs useful are as follows:

1. *Extraoral views:* (i) Occipitomental (OM), (ii) Lateral skull, (iii) Submentovertex (SMV), (iv) Linear tomography, (v) Orthopantomography, and (vi) Computed axial tomography (CAT).
2. *Intraoral views:* (i) Occlusal, (ii) Lateral occlusal, and (iii) Periapical.

Extraoral Views

The knowledge of appearance of a normal radiograph is of a great help in interpretation of radiographs of maxillary sinus. A normal antrum appears as a large air-filled cavity surrounded by various bony structures and dentoalveolar component. The sinus cavity appears radiolucent; and is outlined in all peripheral areas by well demarcated layer of cortical bone. It is always useful to compare the other side in the radiographs. The abnormalities to be looked for include: (i) Evidence of thickening of mucosa on the bony walls (caused by chronic sinus disease), Air-fluid levels (caused by accumulation of mucus, pus, or blood), or foreign bodies.

Occasionally, the apices of the roots of maxillary posterior teeth and impacted third molars are seen projecting into the sinus. In edentulous areas, because of pneumatization of the sinus into the alveolar process, it leads to extension almost to the level of the alveolar crest.

Complete opacification of the sinus can occur by: (i) Mucosal hypertrophy, (ii) Accumulation of fluid, (iii) Filling of the sinus with blood, secondary to trauma, and (iv) Neoplasia.

Disruption of cortical outline may be due to: (i) trauma, (ii) formation of tumors, and (iii) surgical procedures involving the walls of the sinus.

Odontogenic conditions such as granulomas and cysts, may produce radiolucent areas and extend into the sinus cavity. These conditions should be differentiated by their association with the tooth apex, clinical correlation with the dental examination, and the presence of cortical bony margin on the radiograph.

Occipitomental View

The maxillary sinuses can be demonstrated by 15° occipitomental (OM) view radiographs. This view was first described by Water's and Waldron (1915). The presence of pus will produce a horizontal fluid level in this view; provided that there is air above it. As a measure of confirmation of the diagnosis, the view is repeated with the head tilted toward the side of pathology. The fluid level remains horizontal. In case, the fluid is very viscous, the surface may not be completely straight and level (Figs 39.7A and B).

Lateral Skull

This view is helpful in (i) confirming the presence of fluid level and cyst, and (ii) in localizing a foreign body, e.g. root; particularly when the foreign body is located higher up in the sinus.

Submentovertex View

This view is helpful in visualizing the posterior walls of maxillary sinus. The three views together show most of the bony margins of the two antra.

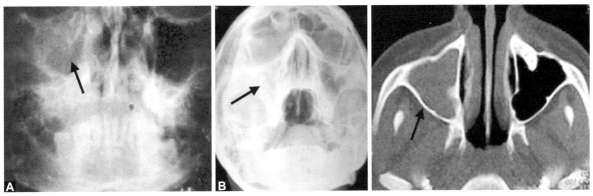

Figs 39.7A and B: (A) PA view of Water's position showing haziness of the (R) maxillary sinus, following extraction of upper right first molar 3 months back. Chronic maxillary sinusitis with oroantral fistula (B) PA view Water's position and CT scan picture of another patient showing complete haziness of (R) maxillary sinus, indicating chronic maxillary sinusitis

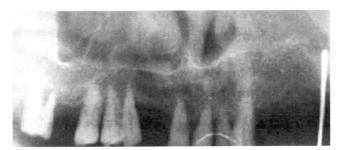

Fig. 39.8: Maxillary panogram showing sinus probe into the maxillary sinus indicating the oroantral communication

Occipitofrontal View

Occipitofrontal view is recommended to detect multi-sinusitis, pansinusitis, if present.

Tomography

This technique provides details of sinus structure; and is indicated for demonstration of following: (i) solid masses within maxillary sinus such as osteoma; and antroliths, and (ii) early erosion of walls of maxillary sinus from malignant diseases.

Orthopantograph

Orthopantograph is helpful in routine detection of lesions such as odontogenic and mucosal cysts of maxillary sinus (Fig. 39.8).

Intraoral Views

The intraoral radiographs are of great value in: (i) locating and retrieving foreign bodies in the sinus such as: teeth, roots, osseous fragments, and also for (ii) careful planning of their surgical removal. These films are useful in demonstration of root fragments in sinus cavity; and also in differentiating the root apices which are intra-antral but extramucosal.

Interpretations

The interpretation of the opacities found in maxillary sinus cannot be specific. In view of the fact that the following structures produce a similar shadow on the radiograph: (i) Transudates, exudates and blood, (ii) Gross mucosal thickening; or blood entirely filled with blood, or pus, or mass of polyp; all produce complete opacity of maxillary sinus. It is impossible to differentiate between them by purely radiological means.

Under normal circumstances, the mucous membrane lining of sinus is about 1 to 2 mm in thickness. The lining in sinusitis, may increase 10 to 15 times. The thickness of antral mucosa also produces a shadow on the walls of maxillary sinus; of a similar density to the substances described earlier.

It is worth noting that thickening of antral mucosa is often seen on routine radiological examination in individuals who are otherwise healthy and asymptomatic. As a matter of fact, 25 to 30 percent of a group of asymptomatic subjects revealed abnormalities ranging from thickening of mucous membrane or polyposis to cyst.

■ INFECTIONS OF MAXILLARY SINUS

Odontogenic Sinusitis

Definition

Odontogenic sinusitis is the inflammation of mucosa of any of the paranasal sinuses. Inflammation of most or all of the paranasal air sinuses simultaneously is known as pansinusitis.

The maxillary sinusitis is usually odontogenic in origin, because of its close proximity with the maxillary teeth. The condition, if not treated, may spread to involve other sinuses.

Etiology

It can be caused by: (i) Infection; periapical abscess spreading into maxillary sinus. Other infections following common cold, upper respiratory tract infection, etc. also can lead to maxillary sinusitis, (ii) Trauma; fracture of antral floor and walls, (iii) Allergy, and (iv) Neoplasms and infected cyst of odontogenic origin (v) Oroantral communication and fistula (vi) Displaced tooth or root.

In case the ostium of maxillary sinus gets blocked, the mucus secreted by secretory cells of the walls gets collected, and the bacterial growth then produces an infection.

Maxillary sinusitis can be classified into: (i) Acute, and (ii) Chronic.

The maxillary sinusitis or inflammation of the antral mucosa is modified due to following factors:
a. Sinus lining is for the air chamber.
b. Ostium is situated in the middle meatus, higher than the sinus floor. Sinusitis is aggravated, whenever the ostium becomes edematous (Because the drainage of the maxillary sinus gets affected).
c. Vascularity of the maxillary sinus is very high.
d. Because of the close relation to the roots of the teeth, there may be referred symptoms to the teeth.

The odontogenic conditions causing sinusitis include: chronic suppuration from granuloma, from an acute abscess; and also from periodontal abscess.

Spread of Infection to Maxillary Sinus, from Apical Abscess

The most common cause of spread of oral infection to maxillary sinus that can be attributed is a periapical abscess (15-20%). The maxillary teeth with roots in close proximity to the floor of antrum, most likely involved in causing such an infection are first molars, second molars, etc. (The teeth vary in different studies). In these areas, antral floor intrudes in between the roots of these teeth.

Clinical Features

Involvement through periapical pathology: The teeth which are involved are first premolars, first molars, and second molars. The presence of abscess causes characteristic signs and symptoms: (i) Severe throbbing pain; when the pus remains confined within bone in apical region. The intensity reduces after 12 to 24 hours as the pus is discharged into antral cavity. (ii) There is only slight swelling of cheek. Patient complains of foul pus running down a nostril; or presence of unpleasant taste or smell. (iii) In case, the tooth is periodontally involved, it may feel loose.

Diagnosis

Appropriate radiographs will reveal, either a totally opaque sinus or a fluid level.

Management

The extraction of the offending teeth carries a risk of perforation and a persistent fistula. In cases of extraction, some authors recommend that the socket be covered with complete soft tissue closure: (i) With antibiotic prophylaxis and taken for at least five days postoperatively; (ii) Decongestants: in the forms of nasal inhalations and drops.

Acute Maxillary Sinusitis

Acute maxillary sinusitis may be suppurative or nonsuppurative (Catarrhal) inflammation of the antral mucosa.

Signs

Extraoral Examination

(i) Tenderness over the cheek, (ii) Anesthesia of the cheek in the area of distribution of infraorbital nerve, (iii) Severe infection may lead to mild swelling of the cheek.

Percussion of maxillary teeth, related to maxillary sinus show tenderness.

Intraoral Examination

(i) Existence of oroantral fistula with or without polypoid mass extruding from the orifice into the socket, (ii) Patient complains of fetor oris, especially when blowing the nose, (iii) Discharge of pus into the mouth from fistula; if opening is obstructed by polyps; the discharge is prevented, (iv) When the middle meatus is the site of drainage, the examination of oropharynx.

Rhinoscopy: Anterior rhinoscopy may reveal pus draining downward (i) Edema and erythema of mucosa and pus discharge flowing onto inferior turbinate bone.

Symptoms

Patient may give history of cold 3 to 4 days prior to the acute attack. There may be nasal blocking following rhinitis. Thick, mucopurulent, foul smelling, discolored nasal discharge may follow. Postnasal discharge with constant irritation requiring clearing of the throat and cough secondary to the nasal discharge may lead to pharyngitis. (i) Heavy feeling in the head. (ii) Constant throbbing pain in upper part of cheek or entire side of the face; which is exacerbated by lowering or bending down. Pain is more severe in the morning and evening. (iii) Maxillary teeth in relation with maxillary sinus on the affected side may be painful. Pain in the teeth often precedes pain in the cheek, (iv) Unilateral foul nasal discharge; which becomes more profuse with lowering down of head, (v) Unilateral nasal obstruction on affected side. There can be occlusion of ostium of maxillary sinus, (vi) The generalized constitutional symptoms are present but in milder form, like chills, fever, sweating, nausea, difficulty in breathing. Anorexia may be due to swallowed pus.

Other Special Examinations

Other special examinations include: (i) Transillumination of maxillary sinus will confirm radiopacity on the affected side. The sinuses when full of pus do not transmit the light through them. (ii) Fiberoptic light probe. This has a source of intense light without production of heat.

Radiography: Water's view (occipitomental 15°) is the most valuable radiograph.
1. *Acute sinusitis:* The affected antrum shows uniform opacity. Sometimes, a fluid level is discernible.
2. *Chronic sinusitis:* The radiograph shows pansinusitis. Fluid level, thickened lining is also seen.

Management

Classical antral regimen includes—bed rest, plenty of fluids, maintenance of oral hygiene. The regimen should be carried out for at least five to seven days.

Antimicrobials: The most suitable against common antral pathogens are: (1) Macrolides: Erythromycin 250-500 mg six hourly for 5 days. (2) Broad-spectrum group: Amoxicillin 250 to 500 mg eight hourly for five days.

Decongestants: These take care of nasal congestion. These drugs reduce the excessive vascularity of lateral nasal wall, thereby improving the opening of the ostium.

i. Nasal drops or sprays, e.g. Ephedrine sulfate—0.5 to 1 percent in normal saline, six hourly.
ii. Xylometazoline hydrochloride 0.1 percent. The decongestant drops not only shrink the swollen and inflamed mucosa, but also help to minimize and eliminate the mucosal discharge. The ostium may now open up and permit free ciliary drainage.

Mucolytic agents: These are used to reduce the viscosity to produce thin mucous secretion. Drugs used—volatile oil preparations are used, Tinc. benzoin, camphor, menthol, chlorbutol, etc. or simple steam inhalation every four hourly can be used. Inhalations of two to three tablespoons full of tincture benzoin co. in a bowl of steaming water for 5 to 10 minutes, 3 to 5 times a day, followed 10 minutes later by 1 to 2 nasal decongestant drops in each nostril. Inhalation is given to maintain or to improve the drainage by the ciliary pathways of the antral lining through the ostium. The steam inhalation tends not only to thin the mucous congestion, and nasal discharges, but also helps to lay down an antiseptic blanket all over the involved antral lining.

Nonsteroidal anti-inflammatory analgesic agents (i) Aspirin (ii) Paracetamol (iii) Ibuprofen.

Chronic Maxillary Sinusitis

Chronic maxillary sinusitis may be due to a persistent dental focus, chronic rhinitis, chronic infection in the frontal or ethmoidal sinuses, allergic conditions, etc.

Pathophysiology

The mucous membrane of the maxillary sinus, due to chronic inflammation may undergo changes like hyperplasia or atrophy. Multiple polyps formation or degeneration of epithelium, where the cilia are lost can be seen. The ostium shows edematous changes causing a complete blocking. The drainage of the sinus will be affected.

The condition sometimes is asymptomatic.
 i. Pain and tenderness in the area of antrum is found usually in acute exacerbations.
 ii. Unilateral foul discharge through posterior nares.
 iii. Cacosmia—a fetid odor with bad taste in the mouth.

Diagnosis

Diagnosis is based on:
a. *History of:* (i) Repeated attacks of acute mucopurulent rhinitis, (ii) Long-standing nasal or postnasal discharge.

b. *Anterior rhinoscopy*: It shows nasal congestion and mucopurulent material in middle meatus.

c. Inspection of oropharynx reveals descending pharyngeal exudates.

d. Presence of an obvious oroantral fistula may be there.

e. Prolapse of polypoidal mass into the mouth forming a lump may be seen.

Transillumination: The sinus reveals radiopacity on the affected side.

Radiography: The findings are: (i) Presence of fluid level, (ii) Thickened lining membrane, (iii) Opaque air space may enclose polyps associated with mucosal thickening, (iv) In case of presence of tooth or root, the characteristic outline is seen within the sinus.

Management

The management requires eradication of related dental complications. If the chronic sinusitis is caused by chronic periapical infection, then affected tooth must be extracted and the socket closed surgically completely as there is a risk of oroantral fistula formation. If there is already a communication with maxillary sinus; if the blood clot fails to organize; and the socket gets infected, then there will be persistent chronic maxillary sinusitis.

There are some factors to be considered in management of chronic maxillary sinusitis, or oroantral fistula:

1. The longer the management is deferred; the greater is the risk of inflammatory changes in lining membrane. The transition to chronic form occurs after a period of two weeks. At this stage, the condition is curable, belated therapeutic intervention adversely affects the prognosis. The lining membrane may get permanently injured and deprived of its capacity for functional recovery. The other irreversible changes, in addition to mucosal thickening and polyposis; include: marked fibrosis, squamous metaplasia and destruction of mucous secreting elements. The ciliary epithelium which normally acts as a scavenger of debris; is destroyed and is no longer capable of its "brushing-up" role. The antrum serves as a factory of massive mucus.

2. There are various grades of chronicity, unless all conservative measures are tried; it is not justified in regarding the case to be irreversible. However, patients with a familial trait for vasomotor or allergic rhinitis are likely to succumb to irreversible disease.

3. In case, the cause is the foreign body, such as tooth or root in the sinus, it is necessary to retrieve these foreign bodies prior to considering any other form of treatment. Concurrent presence of antral polyps, should also be removed. The antral air space is gently irrigated and closure of wound is effected. Routine postoperative treatment with an antibiotic, decongestant and analgesics to be given.

4. The presence of a chronic pyogenic sinusitis subsequent to an oroantral fistula requires surgical closure of fistula. The polyps found at operation should also be removed. Preoperatively, if the antrum is found to be full of pus: (i) It should be irrigated through the fistula, on a daily basis, with a warm normal saline or betadine, or (ii) In certain circumstances, the fistulous orifice needs to be enlarged surgically to enable efficient antral lavage. When the antral washouts appear to be clear, the fistula should be repaired and routine postoperative measures instituted (iii) In cases, where there is no oroantral fistula present, but there is chronic maxillary sinus nonresponsive to other conservative regime, then a surgical drainage should be considered.

Procedure for Surgical Drainage (Fig. 39.9)

A topical anesthesia ointment is applied to the cotton wool, which is inserted along the nasal floor adjacent to the lateral wall of the nose near the inferior turbinate. A sharp trocar and cannula is then introduced along the floor of the nasal cavity inferior to inferior turbinate. The thin medial wall of the antrum is punctured. The trocar is withdrawn and the pus can be drained under pressure through the suction tip. Warm saline irrigation should be carried out daily, till the symptoms settle down.

▌ OROANTRAL COMMUNICATION
▌ AND FISTULA

Definition

a. *An oroantral perforation is an unnatural communication between the oral cavity and maxillary sinus.*

b. *An oroantral fistula is an epithelialized, pathological, unnatural communication between these two cavities.*

The proximity of maxillary second premolar and first molar to maxillary antrum is of great importance. At times, the antral cavity dips down in between the

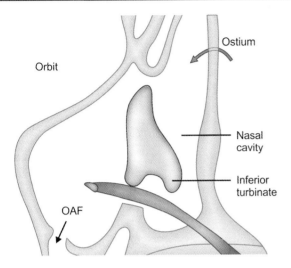

Fig. 39.9: Trocar introduced through nostril into maxillary sinus for surgical drainage and irrigation

roots of maxillary molars resulting in no bone between the roots and the lining of the antrum.

Etiology

Oroantral fistula can result from several causes:
1. Extraction of teeth
2. Destruction of the portion of the floor of the sinus by periapical lesions
3. Perforation of the floor of the sinus and sinus membrane with injudicious use of instruments
4. Forcing a tooth or a root into the sinus during attempted removal
5. Extensive trauma to face
6. Surgery of maxillary sinus; removal of large cystic lesions encroaching on the sinus cavity
7. Chronic infection of maxillary sinus, such as osteomyelitis
8. Teratomatous destruction of maxilla, such as gumma involving palate
9. Infected maxillary implant dentures
10. Malignant diseases such as malignant granuloma.

Extractions

The most common cause of an oroantral fistula is the inadvertent opening of maxillary sinus during extraction of maxillary tooth. The root apices of canines, premolars and molars may be also in close proximity to the floor of sinus. At times, the apices of these teeth intrude into the antral cavity and are separated by the socket from

the sinus lining membrane. Sometimes the root loses its lamina dura due to chronic periapical infection; so that the apex is then in direct contact with the sinus lining. Rarely, the extraction of posterior teeth associated with periapical disease; for example acute periapical abscess, chronic granuloma, or periapical sclerosis is at risk of causing oroantral perforation. But, paradoxically it is the palatal root of the maxillary first molar, which is when broken during extraction, brings about the most frequent creation of an oroantral communication. Also a conical maxillary third molar, which when grasped with the forceps during extraction, slips into the maxillary antrum along with fracture of the tuberosity, and creates an oroantral communication.

A previous history of fistula would necessitate careful radiological assessment of remaining maxillary posterior teeth at the time of removal. Forceps extraction of solitary isolated posterior teeth in an edentulous arch; is also at risk of causing disruption of floor of sinus.

Surgical removal of impacted teeth (e.g. maxillary third molar, supernumerary), submerged, or geminated or hypercementosed, divergent root teeth also carries risk of inadvertent breach in continuity of antrum. Fracture of the maxillary tuberosity during such extraction is the likely possibility.

Apicoectomy on roots of teeth, adjoining the sinus lining.

"Blind" instrumentation, without adequate surgical exposure, in an attempt to retrieve retained apices of posterior teeth is also hazardous; and may result in the root displaced into maxillary sinus through antral perforation.

1. *Facial trauma:* Extensive trauma to middle third of face skeleton, especially if the trauma is due to missiles or sharp objects driven through the mouth into sinus will lead to oroantral fistula. The penetrating injuries, as in gunshot wounds; may result in huge defects of sinus walls.
2. *Surgery:* The various major surgical procedures, that would lead to formation of large fistulae are as follows:
   i. Partial maxillectomy; which is performed for eradication of malignancy or antral neoplasm. This procedure, usually, involves removal of alveolus, part of the palate and antral and medial walls.
   ii. Surgical treatment of large abscess or maxillary cyst may lead to formation of fistula.

iii. *Wrong diagnosis*: Marsupialization done for defects in alveolar antral wall.

iv. Improper planning of incision for Caldwell-Luc operation (The opening in canine fossa will heal if the incision should lie on sound bone).

v. In cases of fractures of zygomatic complex; where the fractures of orbital floor are supported by an antral pack. The pack is kept protruding from the Caldwell-Luc incision and is sutured to buccal sulcus mucosa. At the conclusion of treatment, the pack is pulled out through the opening in buccal sulcus. The orifice, at times, fails to heal and leads to fistula.

3. *Malignant tumors*: Malignant tumors involving maxillary sinus may produce symptoms related to oral cavity, including oroantral communication or fistula in the following ways to produce the symptoms:

    i. By penetration of lateral walls of sinus into mouth.

    ii. By erosion of floor of sinus into mouth.

    In a similar way, neoplasms arising in upper jaw extend into the sinus and lead to fistula formation.

4. *Osteomyelitis*: Osteomyelitis of maxilla is rare; unless, (i) There is underlying systemic disease, such as leukemia, diabetes, uremia, due to kidney disorders, etc. or (ii) Maxillary region has been subjected to irradiation, or (iii) Severe osteitis with bone loss.

5. *Syphilis*: (i) Gummatous lesions of palate may result in an extensive oroantral fistula; as there is the destruction of bone. (ii) Congenital syphilis: The lesions associated with secondary and tertiary forms of syphilis involving nose can arise and extend into mouth.

6. *Implant dentures*: There can be considerable destruction of antral floor in patients with maxillary implant denture. This can be avoided by using sinus lift operation.

Symptoms: Fresh Oroantral Communication: Remember 5 Es

i. *Escape of fluids*: From mouth to the nose on the side of extraction. This happens when the patient rinses or gargles the mouth following extraction of a tooth (Figs 39.10A and B).

ii. *Epistaxis (Unilateral)*: It is due to blood in the sinus escaping through osteum into the nostril. It may or may not be associated with frothing at the nostril on the affected side.

iii. *Escape of air*: From mouth into the nose, on sucking, inhaling or drawing on a cigarette, or puffing the cheeks (Inability to blow cheeks. Passage of air into mouth on sucking).

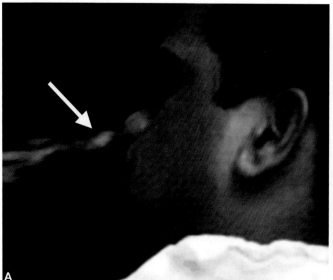
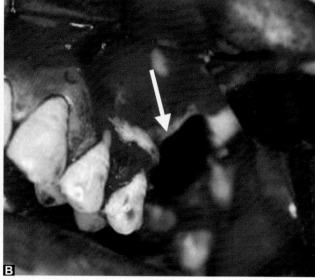

Figs 39.10A and B: (A) Regurgitation of water through nostril. Patient gave history of extraction of upper left first molar 2 months back, (B) Surgical exposure of oroantral communication (Big bony defect)

iv. *Enhanced column of air:* Causes alteration in vocal resonance and subsequently change in the voice.

v. *Excruciating pain:* In and around the region of the affected sinus, as the local anesthesia begins to wear off.

In Late Stage, Symptoms of Established Oroantral Fistula: Remember 5 Ps

1. *Pain*: Previously a dominant feature, is now negligible, as the fistula is established, it allows free escape of fluids.

2. Persistent, purulent or mucopurulent, foul, unilateral nasal discharge from the affected nostril, especially when head is lowered down. Unilateral foul or foetid taste and smell.

3. *Postnasal drip*: The trickling of the nasal discharge from the posterior nares, down the pharynx. The continuous swallowing of the foul mucopurulent discharge may lead to unpleasant taste. This is accompanied by nocturnal cough, hoarseness, ear ache or catarrhal deafness.

4. *Possible sequelae of general systemic toxemic condition*: Fever, malaise, morning anorexia, frontal and parietal headaches and in extreme cases anosmia and cacosmia.

5. *Popping out of an antral polyp*: The persistent infection in the antrum may lead to establishment of chronic long standing oroantral fistula, which may be occluded by an antral polyp. This can be seen as a bluish red lump extruding through the fistula (Figs 39.11A and B).

Fate of Clot

In normal circumstances, penetration of antrum during simple extraction of maxillary teeth, there is formation of a blood clot, which occludes the oral end of the perforation. This usually undergoes organization and the perforation heals uneventfully. Infection of the blood clot from extension from pre-existing periapical infection or as a consequence of maxillary sinusitis, or as a sequel to alveolar osteitis, results in recreation of the fistula.

1. Once infected, the blood clot gets disintegrated and the communication becomes patent.

2. Sometimes, the clot blocking a fistula may be dislodged and blown into mouth as a result of violent nose blowing, or

3. Blood clot may get washed away by vigorous rinsing of mouth.

Persistence of Fistula

Persistence of fistula can result in various problems such as: Inadvertent entry into antrum of food particles, chewing gum, fluids, impression materials, dressings, packs, etc. These substances may result in acute or subacute exacerbation of sinusitis.

Physical signs of oroantral communication can be divided into:

i. Those signs presenting immediately after the formation of communication, and

ii. Those relevant to an established oroantral fistula.

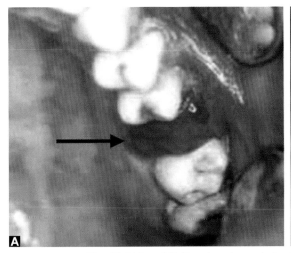 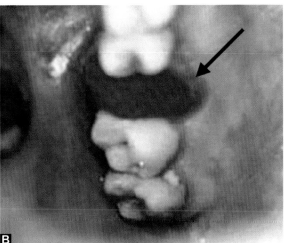

Figs 39.11A and B: Popping of an antral polyp through long-standing oroantral fistula

Recently created communication: Surgery in the immediate vicinity of maxillary sinus; such as extraction of maxillary posterior teeth.

If the extraction demanded more force, however, the extraction was straight forward, and the examination of roots of the tooth revealed that a part of bony floor of antrum is seen adherent to the tooth, then the operator must examine the socket to establish any tear in the lining of sinus.

1. Attempted extraction of maxillary molar root, which disappears as soon as force is applied with an elevator also denotes its inadvertent displacement into maxillary sinus and the presence of coexistent communication.

2. Attempted extraction of a partially erupted upper third molar. The root(s) of such a tooth are adjacent to maxillary sinus, and the application of extraction force results in its displacement into maxillary sinus. This is more likely to occur if the roots of the partially erupted third molar are conical.

Confirmation of the presence of oroantral communication/ fistula: If the fistula is large, it can be assessed from inspection; in case, its patency is not obvious, the nose blowing test is useful. Compression of anterior nares, followed by gentle blowing of nose (with mouth open), causes a rise in intranasal pressure exhibited by the whistling sound as air passes down the open passage. Escape of air bubbles, blood or pus, etc. may appear at the oral orifice. A wisp of cotton-wool held just below the alveolar opening will usually be deflected by the air stream. However, it is important that a suspected antral defect at a site of recent extraction, should not be explored with an instrument. Such a maneuver could lead to breakdown of the blood clot and the seal; and result in a fistula.

Physical Signs of Established Oroantral Fistula

Early signs: The early signs are seen when the blood clot gets disintegrated, so that the breach in the continuity of antral lining remains patent; (and seal is unbroken): (i) As a result of infection, (ii) Forceful nose blowing, (iii) Excessive rinsing of mouth.

Late signs and symptoms: Due to involvement of sinusitis or established oroantral fistula with or without rhinitis: (i) Signs and symptoms of sinusitis and rhinitis, (ii) Escape of air or fluid through nostril, and (iii) Development of a lump (Polyp).

On examination: Inspection (i) Discharge of foul smelling pus from the orifice (occlude patient's nose and ask him to blow). Sometimes, the pus does not descend freely; may be due to occlusion of sinus orifice by polyps.

Careful insertion of an instrument into the antrum, the mass gets pushed to one side and then the flow of pus can be seen with blowing the nose.

Signs of Acute Sinusitis

i. Tenderness over the maxilla, especially in the infraorbital region.

ii. Mild edema of cheek in infraorbital soft tissues.

iii. Rarely, patient gets earache, as a referred pain from antrum. This is attributed to acute otitis media.

iv. Percussion of maxillary premolars and molars related to affected sinus will lead to pain.
Examination of nose with a speculum shows nasal congestion (red, shiny and swollen mucous membrane around ostium).

v. Presence of pus or mucopurulent discharge in middle meatus. This comes from sinus, through ostium, from over inferior conchae onto floor of nose.

vi. *Oropharynx:* Mucopurulent discharge trackling down posterior wall of pharynx.

Signs and symptoms of chronic sinusitis associated with OAF: (i) Impairment of sense of smell, (ii) Foul smelling of mucopurulent discharge seen under middle conchae or in postnasal space, (iii) Mild tenderness over infraorbital region.

Intraoral examination: (i) Descending postnasal flow of mucopurulent discharge, (ii) Herniation of polyp into middle meatus, and (iii) Prolapse of polyp through the fistula.

Sometimes, the oroantral fistula remains asymptomatic; in case, where the oral orifice is large and permits free drainage from antral cavity. The signs and symptoms of acute and chronic sinusitis occur usually, if the fistulous tract is narrow and does not permit free drainage.

Possible Sequelae

1. A newly created fistula, is likely to persist, if one or more of the following contingencies apply:
   a. Interference with normal healing process of the orifice by: (i) Instrument, or probing of orifice, and (ii) Indiscriminate packing, (iii) Exploration of socket, (iv) Vigourous rinsing, (v) Injudicious use of caustic substances, or (vi) Introduction of hemostatic agents

b. Traumatic extraction which resulted in: (i) Soft tissue loss or, (ii) Gross damage to gingival margins peripheral to the gap.
c. Secondary infection of a postextraction or a preexisting sinusitis.
d. When the diameter of the perforation is greater than 4 mm, or the depth of socket is more than 5 mm. Forcible dislodgement of an infected clot through the antral floor.
e. The presence in the wall of the fistula of denuded root of an adjacent tooth.
2. Sometimes, the sinus lining membrane remains intact despite a break in the bony antral floor during an extraction. Under such circumstances, immediate measures should be taken. As a precautionary measure, strenuous noseblowing should be avoided. Such an act may rupture the antral lining and convert the minor defect into a fistula.
3. Extrusion of a dislocated root into nasal passage or nasopharynx and sometimes larynx with pulmonary inhalation. The various factors that play a role in these situations are; posture, effects of gravity; the fragment getting sneezed out; can be ingested. Foreign bodies may get dropped into mouth via the fistula. They either get thrown out or ingested or aspirated.

Management

Purpose

The closure of oroantral fistula should be performed: (i) To protect the sinus from oral microbial flora

(ii) To prevent escape of fluids and other contents across the communication. (iii) To eliminate existing antral pathology (iv) To establish drainage through inferior meatus. A fistulous tract present for more than 14 days should be considered as a chronic fistula.

Treatment of Early Cases

Cases where oroantral communication is recent and formation of fistula is not established.
1. Ideal treatment (i) is immediate surgery repair to achieve primary closure, and (ii) simultaneous antibiotic prophylaxis to prevent sinus infection (Figs 39.12 and 39.13).
The immediate primary closure is done by a simple reduction of the buccal and palatal socket walls, to allow coaptation of buccal and palatal soft tissue flaps to close over the defect. A protective acrylic denture or splint can be used to provide a barrier to the inadvertent entry of food particles.
The result of such a treatment would depend upon: (i) Skill and experience of the clinician, (ii) Surgical facilities available, (iii) Whether the communication is complicated by the presence of a tooth or root in maxillary sinus or not.
2. *Ideal circumstances*: That is where patient is under GA, a surgical procedure can be carried out in operation theater, a tooth or a root can be easily removed from the antrum via the orifice; even if the procedure would entail a slight enlargement of the orifice.
While the similar is to be performed under LA, in a dental chair; regardless of the operator's skill

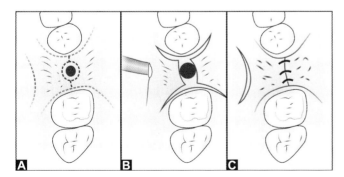

Figs 39.12A to C: Closure of accidental oro-antral communication in the dentulous arch (A) Incisions are made around the teeth and antral opening. A relaxing incision is made on the palate (B) Mucoperiosteal flaps raised and the buccal and palatal alveolar walls are reduced with rongeur, (C) Interrupted suturing done

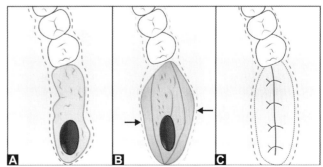

Figs 39.13A to C: Closure after large defect due to tuberosity fracture along with extraction of teeth and oroantral communication: (A) Large defect, (B) Reduction of buccal and lingual walls permits the approximation of flaps, (C) Flaps sutured

and experience; and the facilities available; it is not advisable to explore the antrum for the recovery of the tooth or the root. Moreover, the patient may not give consent for such a procedure.

The various procedures that can be employed are: (i) Complete closure of socket by careful approximation of buccal and palatal gingival margins, (ii) Additional procedures may be required, such as: (a) Reduction in height of underlying alveolar bone, and (b) Relieving incisions in adjacent tissues, and (c) Referral of the patient to an oral and maxillofacial surgeon.

Supportive Measures

1. *Antibiotics:* The prime objective is: (i) Prevention of secondary infection at the site of wound, and (ii) Control of coexisting or pre-existing infection of antrum, if any. The selection of antibiotic should be done on the basis of culture and sensitivity testing:
   i. *Penicillin and its derivatives*: These are used until symptoms begin to subside. It can be started with IV route, and later switched over to oral route. Penicillin V 250 to 500 mg six hourly is adequate.
   ii. In case, the organisms are resistant to penicillin, a broad spectrum antibiotic is prescribed.
2. *Nasal decongestants*: This term applies vasoconstrictor nasal drops and sprays and inhalations. These encourage the drainage of pus and secretions. These do not interfere with ciliary action; however, produce shrinkage of nasoantral mucous membrane and aeration of sinus.
   The available preparations are: (i) Ephedrine nasal drops (0.5%), instilled intranasally every 2 to 3 hours. The correct method of using is the recumbent position with the head inclined to the affected side, (ii) Steam inhalations: when the nose is clear subsequent to the use of decongestant drops or sprays; steam inhalations are helpful in encouraging drainage. It also helps in thinning down the mucous, pus and has a soothing effect, (iii) Benzoin and menthol inhalations: A teaspoonful is added to a pint of hot (not boiling) water and the vapors are inhaled for 10 minutes twice a day, after covering the head.
3. *Analgesics:* Nonsteroidal anti-inflammatory agents: (i) Aspirin 500 mg 1 to 3 tablets 4 times daily. (ii) Paracetamol 500 mg three times daily, (iii) Ibuprofen 400 mg three times daily.

Temporary Therapeutic Measures before Surgical Closure

The ideal treatment is immediate surgical repair combined with supportive measures; because: (i) Success of closure is more likely and (ii) Infection is unlikely and (iii) Easier to recover the displaced tooth or root fragment.

Delay in treatment carries risk of displacement of a root fragment, to a less accessible area of antrum, e.g. tuberosity, recess, lodgment in the inter-radicular areas of molar teeth or even in between the roots of single tooth; which form invaginations of antral floor.

Provisional or temporary measures which effect satisfactory repair include: (i) Whitehead's varnish pack, or (ii) Denture plate.
1. *Pack*: A strip gauze or ribbon gauze is used to pack over the socket and secured with sutures. Superficially, the pack is further supported by a horizontal mattress suture.
2. *Denture plate*: It is indicated when surgical repair of fistula is to be deferred. The purpose of the appliance is to provide a barrier to prevent entry of food particles into the antrum. The orifice in the socket is covered with a piece of gauze or tulle grass; a well-fitting denture plate is constructed to entirely cover the opening.

Whitehead's varnish
- Benzoin 10 parts 44 g.
- Storax 7.5 parts 33 g.
- Balsam of tolu 5 parts 22 g.
- Iodoform 10 parts 44 g.
- Solvent—ether to 1 fl oz or 100 parts.

Treatment of oroantral communication seen within 24 hours of accident: If the case of oroantral communication is seen within 24 hours of its occurrence, and if the edges of the wound are clean; it should be closed immediately. The usual postoperative treatment of antibiotics, nasal drops and inhalations prescribed. In a situation where the case is not complicated by displacement of a tooth or a root into the antrum, it can be closed by a buccal flap and sutured under local anesthesia.

If the situation is complicated by displacement, the case is best treated by immediate surgery in the operation theatre under GA.

Treatment of Delayed Cases

Treatment of cases seen more than 24 hours after accident: When a period of 24 hours has elapsed, the soft tissue margins of fistula often get infected. It is preferable to defer the surgical closure until gingival edges show sound healing, i.e. approximately three weeks.

As a prophylactic measure, antibiotics, analgesics and decongestant should be prescribed. Killey and Kay reported that a large percentage of cases with a small oroantral fistula heal in response to this form of treatment.

In case, (i) there is purulent discharge from fistula; or (ii) the patient develops signs of acute or chronic sinusitis; then the maxillary sinus should be gently irrigated with warm normal saline.

Treatment of oroantral fistula of long duration (more than a month): In these cases, the fistulous tract is usually well epithelialized. Surgical closure is required, (i) Patient presents 2 to 3 weeks after extraction, (ii) Complain of foul taste in the mouth, (iii) Pus discharge from fistula into the mouth, which is increased with nose-blowing.

Management

The drainage of maxillary sinus is established through the fistula by enlarging it surgically, and the sinus should be gently irrigated daily with normal saline until it is clear.

Supportive medical treatment is instituted. When the acute condition subsides, surgical repair is undertaken.

Surgical Procedures Used in Closure of Oroantral Fistula

The surgical procedures can be divided into three groups: depending upon the type of flap used: (i) Buccal, or (ii) Palatal flap, and (iii) Combination of both.

Essential Features of the Procedure

1. The free end of the flap should have an adequate blood supply. The buccal flap is so designed, that the base should be wider than the apex; to ensure adequate vascularization at the apex. The palatal flap should be so designed that the greater palatine vessels are incorporated in the transposed tissues; and should be long enough to swing across the fistulous opening without tension or twisting at the base.
2. Suture line is well-supported by sound bone.
3. Mobilization of either buccal or palatal flap should be done in such a manner that there is no tension on the suture line.

There is a theoretical objection to buccal flap operation. It tends to obliterate the buccal sulcus, and renders the subsequent prosthodontic procedures more difficult. In reality, this does not occur, because of undermining of the flap by releasing incisions.

The palatal mucosa tends to produce some deformity, i.e. ridging, but this tends to regress in due course of time. When the palatal flap is rotated over the fistula, an area of denuded bone is left in the anterior part of palate. This is temporarily covered by gauze pack soaked in Whitehead's varnish. This dressing is secured across the defect with sutures and gets gradually covered with granulation tissue.

Buccal Flap Advancement Operation

It was originally described by Von Rehrmann in 1936. It is the most satisfactory method of closing oroantral fistula. This is according to the principle of periosteal release described by Berger in 1939.

Procedure:

1. *Injection of LA in the mucobuccal fold:* It reduces local capillary bleeding by vasoconstriction at the time of operation, reduces the risk of formation of postoperative hematoma.
2. *Excision of fistulous tract:* An incision is made around the fistulous tract 3 to 4 mm marginal to the orifice. As the soft tissue aperture of the communication is almost always smaller, than the diameter of bony defect. The entire epithelialized tract along with associated antral polyps is dissected out and excised gum margins are freshened with blade no. 11.
3. Two divergent incisions are taken with blade no. 15, from each side of orifice into buccal sulcus for a distance of 2.5 cm. These incisions are made down till the bone. While extending the incisions towards cheek, care must be taken to avoid injury to papillae and duct of parotid salivary gland. Mucoperiosteal flap is reflected carefully. Inspection of bony margins of the alveolar ridge is done. Reduction and smoothening of the same is carried out.
4. *Advancement of buccal flap:* In situations, where the buccal mucoperiosteal flap falls short of covering the fistula; the flap can be advanced. A horizontal incision is made in the periosteum, as high as possible. This will allow advancement of buccal flap. It is advisable only to cut those areas in periosteum which are preventing its advancement. There is no need to cut through the periosteum at the entire base of flap.

5. *Inspection of maxillary sinus:* Maxillary sinus should be carefully inspected for evidence of infection, either through fistula or by illumination, or with a fiberoptic light. Any polypoidal masses or other diseased tissue should be removed. Antrum gently irrigated with warm normal saline.

   In case, if antral pathology is present, Caldwell Luc procedure should be carried out before the final closure of fistula.

6. *Arrest of hemorrhage:* Complete arrest of hemorrhage to avoid formation of hematoma.

7. *Closure of wound:* The mucoperiosteal flap is sutured into position across fistula with interrupted sutures.

8. Postoperative medications: (i) Antibiotics, (ii) Analgesics, and (iii) Nasal decongestants and inhalations.

9. Restriction to soft diet.

10. Instructions to patients: (i) to avoid sneezing, (ii) to explore the wound with tongue, or deliberately sucking air or fluid through it.

11. To avoid nose blowing in early stages: (i) it creates back pressure on sutures before consolidation is complete, and (ii) causes surgical emphysema through mucoperiosteal flap into soft tissue of cheek.

12. Removal of sutures 7 to 10 days postoperatively.

13. *Review:* Patient is reviewed regularly to observe progress, clinically and radiologically.

Modified Rehrmann's Buccal Advancement Flap (Figs 39.14 and 39.15)

Here, after mobilization of the buccal flap and after taking the releasing periosteal incision, the free end of the flap which is to be sutured to the palatal mucosa is modified. A step is created along the entire length of the free end of the buccal flap in the submucosal area, by removal of 1 to 2 mm of mucosal layer, keeping the submucosal layer intact (de-epithelialization). This denuded flap margin is then pulled below the palatal mucosal edge by few vertical mattress sutures. By this procedure, the step in the submucosa will come in approximation with palatal edge, which is closed by means of interrupted sutures. This ensures double layer closure.

Intranasal Antrostomy

It is performed to facilitate the drainage at the conclusion of an operation performed: (i) To close an oro-antral fistula, or (ii) To remove a tooth or a root from sinus.

Drawbacks: It is a controversial surgical procedure for the following reasons: (i) It cannot drain the sinus, satisfactorily; as the point created for drainage is not at the point of dependent drainage; due to the fact that antral floor is about 1.5 cm below nasal floor, (ii) It also

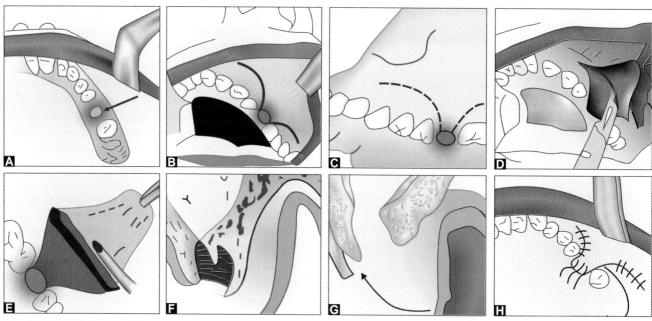

Figs 39.14A to H: Oroantral fistula closure by buccal advancement flap. Modified Rehrmann's procedure: (A) OAF, (B and C) Outline of buccal flap, (D and E) Reflection of buccal mucoperiosteal flap. Relieving incision high up through the periosteum, (F) Sagittal section—Rehrmann buccal flap, (G) Modified Rehrmann flap with de-epithelialization of the margin of the buccal flap, which is tucked under the palatal flap over the periosteum. This ensures double layer closure. Buccal and some palatal alveolar bones are reduced with rongeurs, (H) Initial mattress suturing to pull the margin of the flap and then interrupted suturing is carried out

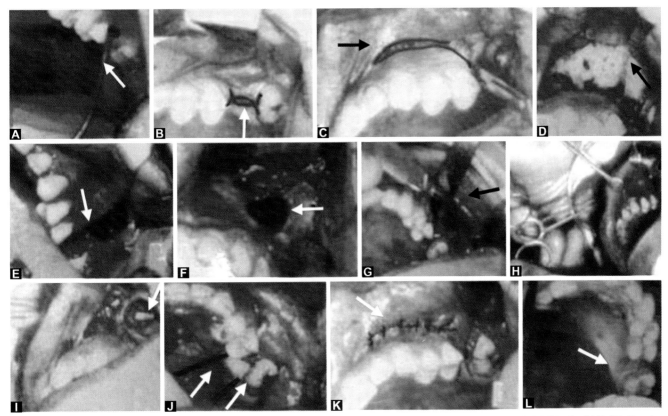

Figs 39.15A to L: Surgical procedure for closure of OAF by modified Rehrmann's buccal advancement flap: (A) Probe in OAF, (B) Circular excision of the margins of OAF, (C) Outline of buccal flap, (D) Reflection of mucoperiosteal flap and exposure of anterolateral wall of the maxillary sinus, (E) Bony defect due to traumatic extraction, seen communicating with the antrum, (F) Window made to access maxillary sinus, (G) Periosteal cut to mobilise the buccal flap, (H and I) Nasal antrostomy procedure, (J) Initial mattress suturing to pull the buccal deepithelialized margin underneath the palatal mucosa, (K) Complete suturing, (L) Satisfactory healing

interferes with ciliary pathways; thus impedes normal physiological drainage of sinus.

Surgical Procedure for Intranasal Antrostomy (Figs. 39.16A to D)

i. A small-sized osteotome or gouge is pushed through the inferior meatus in the nasal cavity, into the maxillary sinus. Then a big curved artery forceps is passed through this opening and a iodoform impregnated ribbon gauze pack's end is grasped into its beak and pulled out into the nostril. Here a single knot, which is put in the ribbon gauze will help to keep it secured in the nostril. The other end of the ribbon gauze is then used to systematically pack the maxillary sinus cavity in multiple folds, after achieving proper hemostasis (after Caldwell-Luc operation).

ii. An antrostomy can be performed by removing approximately 1 cm of the medial wall of the antrum, which bulges into the sinus below the level

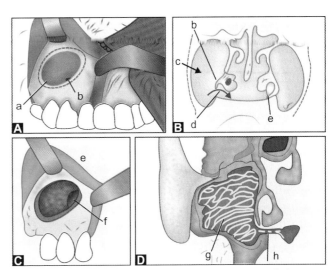

Figs 39.16A to D: Intranasal antrostomy: (a) Posterior wall of antrum, (b) Medial wall of sinus bulges into antrum below interior nasal meatus, (c) Maxillary sinus, (d) Arrow—antrostomy to the level of floor of the nose, (e) Inferior meatus, (f) Antrostomy complete, (g) Antral packing with ribbon iodoform gauze, (h) End of the ribbon gauze brought out through the nasal antrostomy into the nostril

of the inferior turbinate. This antrostomy should be extended to the level of the floor of the nose. The nasal mucosa is then incised from the antral surface on three sides and the nasal mucosal flap thus created is reflected into the antrum.

Palatal Pedicled Flap: Rotational Advancement Flap Operation (Figs 39.17A to C)

Technically slightly more difficult than buccal flap operation. The palate gets its blood supply from greater palatine arteries, which emerge from greater palatine foramen; and run forward in the palate, somewhat midway between gingival margin and the midline of the palate. Ashley (1939) devised the palatal flap operation, where a palatal flap is rotated across fistula, so that the suture line rests on sound bone on buccal side of the orifice. Although palatal tissue is less elastic, it is thicker than the buccal tissue. The abundant blood supply in the palatal tissue promotes satisfactory healing. Procedures involving palatal flaps do not affect the buccal vestibular height. Palatal rotational-advancement flap provides adequate mobility and tissue bulk to the flap. However, it requires the mobilization of large amount of palatal tissue, and it often kinks following the rotation of the flap, which may predispose to venous congestion. Kruger suggested a V-shaped excision of the lesser curvature of the flap to minimize folding.

Ashley's Operation

(i) *Local anesthesia:* It is given to reduce bleeding.
(ii) *Excision of fistulous tract:* The tract is dissected out

by taking an incision around fistula, about 2 mm away from epithelialized edge. (iii) *Marking out of proposed palatal flap:* This is done with Bonney's blue ink before operation, (iv) *Raising a palatal mucoperiosteal flap:* Care is taken not to damage greater palatine artery, (v) Maxillary sinus is inspected and cleared of polyps; and irrigated with normal saline or betadine, (vi) Trimming of buccal mucoperiosteum: This is done in order to give bony support to suture line, (vii) Rotational advancement of the palatal pedicled flap to approximate the buccal margin with interrupted sutures.

Combination of Buccal and Palatal Flaps (Figs 39.18A and B)

An attempt to close larger defects by local flaps often leads to failure. Mobilization of both palatal and buccal flaps helps to have two layered closure. Used only in selected cases or where there is history of earlier repair with failure. The combination of inversion and rotational advancement flaps or hinged and palatal rotational advancement flaps can be used. A double layer closure not only improves the strength of the flaps, but also minimizes contraction and risk of infection.

Caldwell-Luc Operation

George Caldwell in 1893, from New York described a method of gaining entry into the maxillary sinus via canine fossa with nasal antrostomy. Henri Luc in 1897, from Paris also reported the same procedure as his own. Later on the procedure was accepted as Caldwell-Luc operation worldwide.

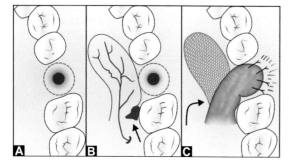

Figs 39.17A to C: Ashley's palatal pedicled rotational advancement flap for closure of oroantral fistula (A) Circular excision of tissue around the fistula, (B) Palatal rotational advancement flap based on the greater palatine vessels. The kinking of the flap may be minimized by excision at the lesser curvature of the flap (dark area) Kruger's modification, (C) Final closure. Raw palatal area can be protected by placing iodoform gauze pack

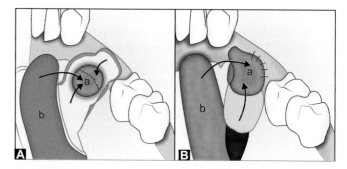

Figs 39.18A and B: Combined local flaps for closure of OAF (A) Hinged buccal and palatal rotational advancement flap—a and b, (B) Inversion flap-A and palatal rotational advancement flap—b. The hatched area is excised to facilitate the rotation of the palatal flap

Indications

1. Open procedure for removal of root fragments, teeth or foreign body or an antrolith (stone) from the maxillary sinus.
2. To treat chronic maxillary sinusitis with hyperplastic lining and polypoid degeneration of the mucosa.
3. Removal of cysts or benign growths from the maxillary sinus.
4. Management of hematoma in the maxillary sinus and to control post traumatic hemorrhage in the sinus.
5. Zygomaticomaxillary complex fractures involving floor of the orbit and anterior wall of the maxillary sinus.
6. Removal of impacted canine or impacted third molar.
7. Along with closure of chronic oroantral fistula, associated with chronic maxillary sinusitis.

Caldwell-Luc Surgical Procedure (Figs 39.19A to D)

i. The surgical procedure can be performed under LA with sedation or under GA—which is the preferred method.
ii. A semilunar incision is planned in the buccal vestibule from canine to second molar area, just above the gingival attachment.
iii. A mucoperiosteal flap is elevated with the help of periosteal elevator till the infraorbital ridge. Care is taken to prevent injury to infraorbital nerve.
iv. An opening or window is created in the anterior wall of the maxillary sinus with the help of chisels, gouges or dental drills. The opening is enlarged carefully in all directions with Rongeur forceps, to permit the inspection of the sinus cavity. The size obtained should be about the size of the index finger. This is to facilitate the palpation of the sinus lining with the introduction of index finger into the sinus cavity. The opening or window created should be well away from the apices of the roots of the maxillary teeth.
v. Pus should be sucked away from the sinus and a thorough irrigation of the maxillary sinus is carried out with copious saline wash.
vi. Inspection of the maxillary sinus is done and removal of root, tooth gauze, cotton or stone or bone wax, etc. can be done at this stage.
vii. The thickened, infected lining of the maxillary sinus can be elevated with Howarth's periosteal elevator and removed and sent for histopathological examination.
viii. If there is profuse bleeding, then the sinus can be packed with ribbon gauze soaked in adrenaline 1:1000 for 1 or 2 minutes.
ix. The antral cavity again is irrigated and can be packed with iodoform ribbon gauze. The end of the same can be removed through the nasal antrostomy or through the small incision in the buccal vestibule.
x. The incision is closed with 3-0 silk.

Postoperative management: Antibiotics, analgesics, anti-inflammatory drugs for 5 days. Pack removal on the 5th day. Tinc. benzoin inhalation three times a day, followed by nasal drops. Patient is instructed not to blow the nose, have soft diet and no vigorous gargling.

FUNCTIONAL ENDOSCOPIC SINUS SURGERY

Purpose

The purpose of functional endoscopic sinus surgery (FESS) is to restore normal paranasal air sinuses mucociliary function.

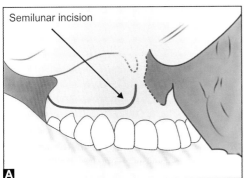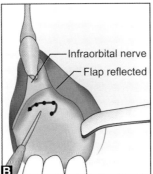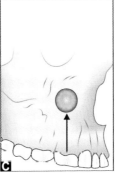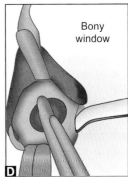

Figs 39.19A to D: (A) Intraoral incision for Caldwell-Luc operation, (B) Creation of bony window with drill, (C) Perforation area for window, (D) Enlarging the bony window at the anterior maxillary wall with rongeur or bur

Historical Background

Hirschmann has been credited as the first surgeon to have attempted nasal and sinus endoscopy with a modified cystoscope in 1901. There are various reports in German literature on endoscopic treatment for sinusitis. The surgical landmarks were initially described in detail by Mosher with his principles of ethmoidal and frontal sinus surgery (1912, 1929). Later, Van Alyea, in 1939, described the anatomy of ethmoidal sinus in great details.

The first description of endoscopically examining nasal cavity and the antrum of Highmore was published by Maxwell and Maltz in 1925. They suggested that sinusscopy should be utilized for diagnosis, and described methods for maxillary endoscopic sinusotomy via the inferior meatal and canine fossa routes.

The functional endoscopic surgical dissections of the ostiomeatal unit of ethmoidal and frontal sinusitis were described in English literature, simultaneously, by Messerklinger and Wigand in 1978, in independent publications. Stamberger and Kennedy, with the help of CT scans and pluridirectional tomograms, improved upon the original description of the technique as described by Messerklinger.

Endoscopic Sinus Surgery

There are four complementary developments which have contributed to the advancement of FESS. (i) *Antibiotics:* Antibiotics are credited as the first significant discovery that opened way for development of limited sinus surgery. (ii) The substantiation that the anterior ethmoid sinus is the underlying key anatomical cause for frequent sinusitis. Infection that begins in the anterior ethmoidal sinus frequently spreads into the maxillary and frontal sinuses. Once ventilation and drainage is established, the sinus can return to normal function. (iii) High-resolution computed tomographic (CT) examination of the paranasal sinuses has allowed for more precise identification and localization of sinus disease. (iv) Advanced endoscopic instrumentation has markedly improved paranasal air sinus visualization and contributed improvement in surgical techniques.

Indications

(i) Recurrent sinusitis with stenosis at the osteomeatal unit which have been refractory to medical treatment. (ii) Chronic hyperplastic sinusitis with obstructive nasal polyps. (iii) Chronic sinusitis with mucocele formation. Patients with frontal sinus mucocele which are laterally placed are not good candidates for this type of surgery. (iv) Fungal sinusitis in patients with diabetes or immunocompromised status are candidates for this type of surgery. (v) Neoplasms. (vi) Orbital cellulitis/abscess unresponsiveness to medical treatment.

Relative Indications

(i) Repair of cerebral spinal fluid leaks. (ii) Selected nasofrontal recess/frontal sinus mucoceles. (iii) Orbital decompression in bilateral exophthalmos. (iv) Sinus-mediated cephalagia.

Diagnosis

The success of FESS depends upon an accurate diagnosis of osteomeatal complex disease; either in the form of mucus, or polypoid changes in the area of hiatus semilunaris or infundibulum.

The various factors employed are:
i. Routine sinus radiographs. They are not of much value in revealing early paranasal sinusitis.
ii. Anterior rhinoscopy with a speculum. It only provides a partial examination of nasal cavity.
iii. *Nasal endoscopy:* It reveals a complete examination of nasal cavity and the osteomeatal complex.
iv. *Computed axial tomography (CAT):* It is used to confirm disease of osteomeatal complex and paranasal sinusitis. However, it is relatively expensive and requires radiation exposure.

Endoscopy of Maxillary Sinus

The topical anesthesia (4% cocaine soaked cotton) is applied to the sublabial area over the canine fossa. Then 1 percent lignocaine with 1,00,000 adrenaline is injected in this area. A small stab incision is made with Bard-Parker blade no. 11 or 15, a 5 mm mucous membrane trocar is used to enter the upper lateral part of canine fossa. The orbital rim should be palpated and the eye protected by keeping a finger on the rim during the puncture of the sinus. The trocar and the cannula are slowly rotated while entering the sinus in a posterior direction. The sinus, then can be examined with a telescope. A biopsy can be taken with an optical biopsy forceps through the cannula. The patient should avoid blowing nose for at least a week postoperatively, to avoid subcutaneous emphysema.

Types of Functional Endoscopic Sinus Surgery

The classification is based on the extent of disease involvement of sinuses prior to surgery, and the underlying medical condition. Anand and Panje's classification is as follows:

Type I: Nasal endoscopy and uncinectomy with or without agger nasi cell exenteration. *Indications:* (i) Isolated osteomeatal thickening of mucous membrane, (ii) Infundibular disease, (iii) Patent maxillary sinus ostia without maxillary sinus membrane thickening and/or cysts, (iv) Unsuccessful prior inferior maxillary sinus antrostomy and/or antrostomy with irrigation, (v) Prior septoplasty/adenoidectomy with continued paranasal sinus symptoms. (vi) Anterior agger nasi cell infection presenting as dacrocystitis or erythema at the medial fornix of the eye.

Type II: Nasal endoscopy, uncinectomy, bulla ethmoidectomy, removal of sinus lateralis mucous membrane and exposure of frontal recess/frontal sinus. *Indications:* (i) Osteomeatal thickening of mucous membrane. (ii) Evidence of anterior ethmoid sinus opacification, including obstruction of infundibulum. (iii) Limited frontal sinus recess disease. (iv) Unsuccesful prior inferior maxillary sinus antrostomy and/or antrostomy with irrigation. (v) Prior septoplasty/adenoidectomy with continued paranasal sinus symptoms.

Type III: Type II plus maxillary sinus antrostomy through the natural sinus ostium. *Indications:* Type II with: (i) Evidence of maxillary sinusitis as evidenced by membrane thickening and/or opacification, (ii) Stenotic or oedematous maxillary sinus ostium.

Type IV: Type III surgical technique with complete posterior ethmoidectomy. *Indications:* As per type III with: (i) Total ethmoid involvement, (ii) Nasal polyposis with extensive ethmoidal and maxillary sinus disease, (iii) Unresponsive to therapy for underlying systemic medical causes, e.g. persistent nasal sinus polyps despite steroid and antibiotic therapy. (iv) Prior type I or type II FESS without response or progression of sinus disease.

Type V: Type IV surgical technique with sphenoidectomy and stripping of mucous membrane. *Indications:* As per type IV with. (i) Evidence of sphenoid sinusitis, and (ii) Pansinusitis and rhinitis.

Surgical Technique

Functional endoscopic sinus surgery (FESS) can be performed under local or general anesthesia. General endotracheal anesthesia is preferred by some otorhinolaryngologist.

The patient is placed in supine position at 15° reverse Trendelenberg. The nose is additionally anesthetized with 4 percent cocaine-soaked cotton pledgets placed in middle meatus and along the entire length of middle turbinate. One percent lignocaine with 1:1000 epinephrine is used for injection of greater palatine foramen. Additional injection in the middle meatus perimeter (uncinate, middle turbinate) are also done.

Endoscopies of maxillary sinus may be performed either via canine fossa or through a maxillary sinus antrostomy. Polyps or cysts may be biopsied or removed through either approach. The middle turbinate is reflected medially as the initial step of the surgery. In case, the nasal septum interferes with adequate visualization of osteomeatal unit, a septoplasty or, submucous resection of septum, should be performed before continuing with endoscopic ethmoidectomy.

An infundibulectomy is then performed using Freer elevator or sickle knife. Palpation of the uncinate process with cutting instruments will determine the limits of the uncinate process before reaching the denser bone of pyriform process. The uncinate process is relatively soft, while the pyriform process is hard. The Freer elevator or sickle knife is inserted immediately anterior and inferior to insertion of middle turbinate. This incision is carried interiorly toward the natural ostium of maxillary sinus (Kennedy, 1985). This exposes the base of infundibulum and anterior wall of bulla ethmoidalis. The uncinate process is then removed with a Blakesley-Wilde forward biting forceps.

The uncinectomy allows entry into anterior ethmoid sinus and makes ethmoidal bulla and natural maxillary sinus ostium to be visible. In case, there is evidence of maxillary sinus disease; or maxillary sinus ostia stenosis, the latter is opened following uncinectomy. The ostium is located at the same level as the anterior inferior edge of middle turbinate.

The bone in anterior region to lacrimal duct is not damaged by overzealous removal of bony tissue. The superior part of ostium should not be opened until the surgeon is certain about the location of bony orbital floor.

If the disease lies in middle or posterior ethmoidal sinus, bulla ethmoidalis is opened. The anatomical landmark encountered posterior to bulla is the lateral attachment of middle turbinate called ground lamella. This relatively dense bone is removed with a pair of upbiting straight Blakesly-Wilde forceps. One ground lamella is removed; entry into the posterior ethmoidal sinus area is gained. The surgeon always works in inferomedial region of sphenoid sinus ostium. The superior and lateral areas are close to optic nerve and carotid artery.

To conclude the surgery, all the diseased mucous membrane is removed. Overzealous removal of septa and normal appearing mucous membrane is not advocated.

Sphenoid Sinus

The surgery for sphenoid sinus needs to be done carefully. The surgeon has to be familiar with the location of sphenoid sinus ostium. The surgeon should have CT scans in view during the procedure. Once sphenoid sinus is identified, a forward biting forceps is used to puncture the sinus. A Kerrison sphenoid punch is used to remove the medial and inferior walls. The optic nerve travels in a lateral to medial direction crossing the superolateral wall of sphenoid sinus.

SECTION 11

Orofacial and Neck Infections

40

Orofacial and Neck Infections and their Management

Infections of orofacial and neck region, particularly those of odontogenic origin, have been one of the most common diseases in human beings. Despite great advances in health care, these infections remain a major problem; quite often faced by oral and maxillofacial surgeons. These infections range from periapical abscess to superficial and deep neck infections. The infections generally spread by following the path of least resistance through connective tissue and along fascial planes. The infections spread to such an extent, distant from the site of origin, causing considerable morbidity and occasional death.

Early recognition of orofacial infection and prompt, appropriate therapy are absolutely essential. A thorough knowledge of anatomy of the face and neck is necessary to predict pathways of spread of these infections and to drain these spaces adequately.

This chapter deals with various types of orofacial and neck infections, with necessary description of numerous fascial spaces; with special reference to their involvement, surgical anatomy, clinical features,

principles of their management with the surgical techniques used for drainage or decompression of the infections by intraoral or extraoral routes, and finally modes of their spread and the complications that would be encountered if these cases are left untreated, are also discussed.

ETIOLOGY

Infections in the orofacial and neck region usually originate from following sources:

A. *General classification*: It is based on the origin of the infection.
1. *Odontogenic*: The majority of infections in orofacial and neck region belong to this group. Odontogenic infections arise within jaw bones, and can be classified as those arising from:
(i) Pulp disease, (ii) Periodontal disease, (iii) Secondarily infected cysts or odontomes, (iv) Remaining root fragment, (v) Residual infection, and (vi) Pericoronal infection.

These manifest in the following forms:
(i) Periapical abscess, (ii) Periodontal abscess, (iii) Infected cyst, (iv) Residual abscess, and (v) Pericoronal abscess.
2. *Traumatic*: Occasionally, trauma from penetrating wounds of soft and hard tissues of the face can lead to orofacial infection.
3. *Implant surgery*
4. *Reconstructive surgery*
5. Infections arising from contaminated needle punctures.
6. *Others*: This group includes instances of orofacial infections arising from other factors such as infected antrum, salivary gland afflictions, etc.
7. Secondary to oral malignancies.
B. *On the basis of causative organisms*: Orofacial infections can be classified as:
1. *Bacterial infections*:
   a. The odontogenic infections encountered in orofacial region are mostly bacterial infections.
   b. Nonodontogenic infections: (i) Tonsillar, and (ii) Nasal infections which are more common in children, and (iii) Furuncle of overlying skin.
2. *Fungal infections*: These infections have slow rate of spread. These are difficult to diagnose in early stages.
3. *Viral infections*: The literature does not show sufficient reports about these conditions of odontogenic origin.

Irrespective of the original source of infection, once it has been established within the soft tissues, its further spread tends to occur in uniform fashion.

PATHWAYS OF ODONTOGENIC INFECTION (FIG. 40.1)

Serious dental infection, spreading beyond the tooth socket, is more common due to the pulpal infection than the periodontal infection.

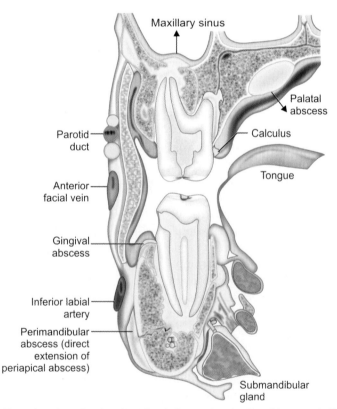

Fig. 40.1: Frontal section of oral cavity at level of second molar. Possible spread of infection starting with simple caries and calculus. Abscess formation at various sites

Invasion of the dental pulp by bacteria after decay of a tooth
↓
Inflammation, edema and lack of collateral blood supply
↓
Venous congestion or avascular necrosis (pulpal tissue death)
↓
Reservoir for bacterial growth (anaerobic)
↓
Periodic egress of bacteria into surrounding alveolar bone

The periapical infection progress can vary according to the:

   i.   The number and virulence of the organism.
   ii.   Host resistance.
   iii.   Anatomy of the involved area.

Odontogenic Infections

Types of infection: (A) Acute, and (B) Chronic.

Acute Stage

In the acute stage, the infection spreading in the soft tissues can take the following forms in the clinical situations. (1) Abscess, (2) Cellulitis, and (3) Fulminating infections.

1.   *Abscess:* It is a circumscribed collection of pus in a pathological tissue space. A true abscess is a thick-walled cavity containing pus. The suppurative infections are characteristic of staphylococci, often with anaerobes, such as bacteroides, and are usually associated with large accumulation of pus, which require immediate drainage. These microorganisms produce coagulase, an enzyme, that may cause fibrin deposition in citrated or oxalated blood.

2.   *Cellulitis:* It is spreading infection of loose connective tissues. It is a diffuse, erythematous, mucosal or cutaneous infection. It is characteristically the result of streptococci infection; and does not normally result in large accumulation of pus (Table 40.1).

   Streptococci produce enzymes such as streptokinase (fibrinolysin), hyaluronidase, and streptodornase. These enzymes break down fibrin and connective tissue ground substance and lyse cellular debris, thus facilitate rapid spread of bacteria along the tissue planes.

   Antibiotics may arrest the spread of infection; and may bring about complete resolution of the condition. However, in cases refractory to antibiotic coverage, pus pockets should be suspected; and in such cases, exploration and drainage should be done.

3.   *Fulminating Infections* of the various spaces in the orofacial region. Here, the infection involves the secondary spaces involving vital structures, along the pathway of least resistance.

Acute Infection (Figs 40.2A to C)

The odontogenic abscesses present in the following forms:

a.   *Acute periapical abscess:* An odontogenic abscess usually arises and remains in the confines of alveolar bone. This is referred to as acute periapical abscess.

b.   *Acute dentoalveolar abscess:* Once the infection has crossed the confines of alveolar bone and comes to lie in the neighbouring soft tissues, and if it gets localized, it is referred to as acute dentoalveolar abscess.

c.   Acute periodontal abscess.

d.   Acute pericoronal abscess.

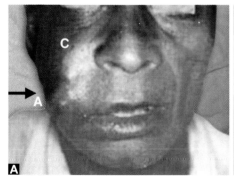 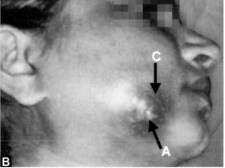 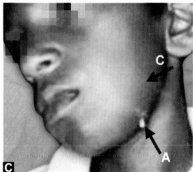

Figs 40.2A to C: Acute odontogenic infection: Clinical extraoral picture of (A) Acute abscess due to periapical pathology. Note the multiple pointing areas, (C) Cellulitis

The infection follows the path of least resistance. The important and the deciding factor, in the involvement of the fascial spaces, is the relationship of root apices of molars with the mylohyoid line. The abscess related to mandibular second and third molars, usually, perforates the lingual cortex and spreads to the submandibular space; as the root apices of these teeth lie below the mylohyoid line. The abscess related to premolars and first molars, involves the sublingual space, as the root apices of these teeth are situated above the mylohyoid line.

Chronic Stage (Figs 40.3A and B)

In the chronic stage, the odontogenic infection can present itself in the following forms:
1. *Chronic fistulous tract or sinus formation:* Abscesses neglected for a long time discharge intraorally or extraorally. When the abscess discharges through the skin; the sinus may appear in a location unfavorable for drainage; and the resulting scar is always thickened, puckered, and depressed and more obvious esthetically prominent.
2. Chronic osteomyelitis
3. Cervicofacial actinomycosis. (2) and (3) are described in next chapter.

General Course of an Odontogenic Abscess

1. *Early stage:* There is intrabony collection of pus. The adjoining soft tissues do not undergo any necrosis.
2. *Intermediate stage:* Perforation of cortex: With perforation of the cortex, the infection progresses; soft tissues become indurated and brawny. Subsequently, a small area of central softening can be

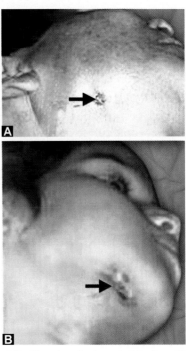

Figs 40.3A and B: Chronic odontogenic infection. Clinical extraoral pictures: (A) Chronic extraoral draining sinus tract, (B) Chronic fistula and exposed bone due to chronic odontogenic osteomyelitis

palpated. This represents the central necrosis due to bacterial propagation and loss of blood supply. At this stage sometimes, it is really difficult to judge whether or not to do an incision and drainage. However, if there is firm, brawny swelling, suppuration usually occurs unless the causative micro-organisms are streptococci.

Some clinicians feel that this is the time to intervene surgically either by, (i) doing incision and drainage; or (ii) extraction of the offending tooth; while the soft tissues are still soft and doughy to touch. In such circumstances, the surgical intervention results in removal of the source of infection; and the soft tissues may not progress to suppuration and may undergo resolution.

If untreated or improperly treated, acute/chronic infection can lead to:
  i.   Focal osteomyelitis.
  ii. Widespread osteomyelitis
  iii. Fistulous tract (intraoral or extraoral) formation.
  iv. Intraoral or cutaneous soft tissue abscess.
  v.   Cellulitis.
  vi. Bacteremia-septicemia.
  vii. Deep facial space infection.
  viii. Ascending facial cerebral infection.

Table 40.1: Differences between cellulitis and abscess		
Characteristics	*Cellulitis*	*Abscess*
Duration	Acute phase	Chronic phase
Pain	Severe and generalized	Localized
Size	Large	Small
Localization	Diffuse borders	Well-circumscribed
Palpation	Doughy to indurated	Fluctuant
Presence of pus	No	Yes
Degree of seriousness	Greater	Less
Bacteria	Aerobic	Anaerobic / mixed

Acute Periapical Abscess

Etiology: The main cause is infective necrosis of pulp. Causes of infective necrosis of pulp include: (i) Carious involvement, (ii) Contamination of traumatic exposure of pulp, (iii) Sterile necrosis, where apical vessels are torn by blow on the teeth, or (iv) following inadvertent chemical or thermal damage to pulp.

Micro-organisms from infected pulp invade periapical tissues. The entry to periapical tissues is gained usually through (i) apical foramina; and in such circumstances, the infection is truly periapical, Occasionally, the entry is through (ii) accessory canals, (iii) an endodontic perforation, (iv) an opening in the floor of the pulp chamber of a primary molar, (v) from an area of surface resorption, or (vi) root fracture. In these circumstances, the abscess develops on the lateral aspect of root or at the root furcation or in the vicinity of root fracture, as the case may be.

Clinical features: Severe throbbing pain in the affected tooth. The offending tooth may show carious involvement, and may be sensitive to percussion. Mobility may or may not be present.

Radiographic presentation: The involved tooth shows carious lesion with periapical pathology, root fracture, erosion or absorption as the case may be. It also shows periapical radiolucency, areas of resorption; and the different types of radiolucencies involving the root fractures.

Treatment: The treatment modalities comprise of the following: (1) Antibiotics, (2) Analgesics, (3) Drainage through the pulp chamber, (4) Extraction of the offending tooth, or (5) Endodontic treatment.

Acute Dentoalveolar Abscess (Table 40.2)

This disease entity is a continuation of periapical abscess.

Clinical features:

1. *Pain:* The severity of pain depends upon the stage of the disease process.
2. Submucosal swelling in the sulcus, usually on the outer aspect of alveolar process. Fluctuation may be elicited after few days. If left untreated, the swelling bursts and produces sinus tract discharging pus.

Radiographic presentation: There is no appreciable difference in the presentation of the two entities radiographically, except that the area of radiolucency may be more marked in dentoalveolar abscess.

Treatment: The same treatment modalities hold true for dentoalveolar abscess. In addition, intra or extraoral incision and drainage may be required.

Acute Periodontal Abscess

Etiology: It arises in periodontal membrane adjacent to a periodontal pocket.

Clinical features: Dull pain, rarely severe, and variable in intensity. Pus discharges via gingival pocket. It may produce a sinus on either inner or outer aspect of alveolar process; and rarely tracks through the skin.

Periodontal abscesses are uncommon in children and an acute swelling close to gingival margin of a primary molar is usually a periapical abscess.

▇ MICROBIOLOGY

The aerobic bacteria found in odontogenic infection are primarily gram positive cocci, most are viridans

	Table 40.2: Differential clinical features between acute periapical and acute periodontal abscesses		
	Features	Acute periapical abscess	Acute periodontal abscess
1.	Pain	Severe and throbbing	Severe and throbbing
2.	Age	Common in adults	Uncommon in children
3.	Pulp	Necrotic and infected	Vital
4.	Swelling	Usually, over the apex	Usually, over the gingival third of the alveolar process
5.	Sinus discharge	May be present	May be present
6.	Tenderness to percussion	Present	Present
7.	Mobility	Later stages	Early stage
8.	Origin	Arises from pulp	Arises in relation to periodontal pocket

streptococci species, include *Strep. milleri, Strep. sanguis, Strep. salivarius, strep. mutans.* These oral streptococci are also known as α-hemolytic streptococci, which account for about 80 percent of aerobic bacteria found in odontogenic infection.

Some anaerobic cocci appear similar, morphologically, to staphylococci. They were named previously as peptococcus. DNA probe investigation has shown that peptococcus and peptostreptococcus are the same bacteria.

There are two main groups of bacteriodes. First is Oropharyngeal group, which is found in the mouth and contributes to odontogenic infections.

The other group found in the gut—the enteric Bacteroides, they include *B. Fragilis, B. Vidgatis, B. Distasonis, B. thetaiotaomicron, B. Ovatis.* They are rarely seen in oral cavity and mostly do not cause odontogenic infections.

Oropharyngeal bacteroides divided into: (a) Porphyromonas, and (b) Prevotella.

a. *Porphyromonas:* It includes *P. asacchrolyticus, P. Gingivalis,* and *P. endodontalis.*
b. *Prevotella:* It includes *P. melaninogenicus, P. buccae, P. intermedius, P. oralis, P. loescheii, P. ruminocola,* and *P. denticola. Prevotella intermedius, Porphyromonas gingivalis,* and *Porphyromonas endodontalis* appears to be most pathogenic among them.

These gram negative anaerobic rods, are usually susceptible to most antibiotic, but they are 25 percent resistant to penicillin V and nearly 50 percent resistant to cephalexin, and other first generation cephalosporin.

The other group of anaerobic gram negative rod is the genus Fusobacterium. Fusobacterium, like bacteroides are pathogenic and have the ability to destroy tissues through production of proteolytic enzymes and endotoxins. Fusobacterium is usually sensitive to penicillin and penicillin like drugs, but are frequently resistant to erythromycin.

Fusobacterium species appears to be the most virulent and when in combination with *Strep. milleri,* commonly seen in aggressive odontogenic infections that have descended into the lateral pharyngeal and retropharyngeal spaces and also into the mediastinum.

Medical Therapy

Consists of supportive care—Hydration, soft or liquid diet, rich with high protein, analgesics and use of antiseptic mouthwashes to maintain the oral hygiene.

Antibiotic Therapy

The antibiotic therapy should be decided after knowing the patient's systemic condition status.

i. *In noncompromised patient with well localized abscess-surgical drainage and dental therapy will resolve the infection without antibiotic cover.* In cases of poorly localized, extensive abscess and diffuse cellulites, antibiotic therapy is a must.
ii. In compromised patients, as well as in patients with systemic signs and symptoms like trismus, airway compromise, fever, etc. antibiotic cover is mandatory.

Patients with diminished host defence, like uncontrolled or insulin dependant diabetics, immunosuppressed patients, chronic alcoholics, intravenous drug abusers, patients on renal dialysis also require antibiotic cover. In these patients, there is always a danger of sudden serious sepsis spreading from even a small septic focus.

Choice of Antibiotic Therapy

Initially always empirical antibiotic selection is done, based on the knowledge of microbiological study of the flora of oral infection. Later on after knowing the laboratory results of culture and sensitivity testing, specific antibiotic is instituted.

Penicillin is an empirical drug of choice, since last many decades. But, now studies have shown that β-lactamase producing organisms such as bacteroids are insensitive to penicillin. Thirty percent of the microorganisms are reported as resistant. As these orofacial infections are a mixed flora of aerobes and anaerobes, the bacterial synergism that enhances growth of these different types of organisms may be disrupted by the use of penicillin and metronidazole can supplement the penicillin.

Oral clindamycin, amoxicillin-clavulanic acid (Augmentin), 1st and 2nd generation cephalosporins are also useful in orofacial infections.

In compromised patient's—Clindamycin alone or in combination with Gentamycin or 1st or 2nd generation cephalosporins can be used parenterally.

Surgical Therapy

Surgical Technique for Incision and Drainage of an Abscess

Incision and drainage helps

i. To get rid of toxic purulent material
ii. To decompress the edematous tissues

iii. To allow better perfusion of blood, containing antibiotic and defensive elements
iv. To increase oxygenation of the infected area.

The abscess is drained surgically and simultaneously dental treatment also should be instituted to achieve quick resolution. It involves the blunt exploration of the entire anatomic space or the abscess cavity; with the opening up of all the tissue planes within the abscess cavity. The abscess cavity is then irrigated with betadine and saline solution. A drain is inserted into the depth of the space. It may simply pass through a single incision and remain in the depth of the space, or it may be a through and through drain. The drain is secured to one of the margins of the incisions with a suture; or to itself, in case of a through and through, intra- to extraoral drains; and left *in situ*, which can again be in the same fascial space or through another fascial space.

Hilton's Method of Incision and Drainage (Figs 40.4A to H)

The method of opening an abscess ensures that no blood vessel or nerve in the viscinity is damaged and is called Hilton's method.

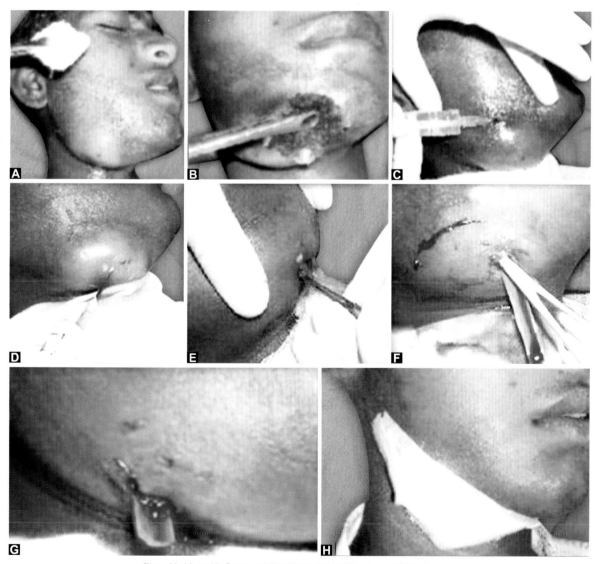

Figs 40.4A to H: Steps in Hilton's method of drainage of an abscess

Steps

1. *Topical anesthesia*: Topical anesthesia is achieved with the help of ethyl chloride spray.
2. *Stab incision*: Made over a point of maximum fluctuation in the most dependent area along the skin creases, through skin and subcutaneous tissue.
3. If pus is not encountered, further deepening of surgical site is achieved with sinus forceps (to avoid damage to vital structures).
4. Closed forceps are pushed through the tough deep fascia and advanced towards the pus collection.
5. Abscess cavity is entered and forceps opened in a direction parallel to vital structures.
6. Pus flows along sides of the beaks.
7. Explore the entire cavity for additional loculi.
8. *Placement of drain*: A soft yeat's or corrugated rubber drain is inserted into the depth of the abscess cavity; and external part is secured to the wound margin with the help of sutures.
9. Drain left for at least 24 hours.
10. *Dressing*: Dressing is applied over the site of incision taken extraorally without pressure.

Purpose of keeping the drain: The purpose of drain is to allow the discharge of tissue fluids and pus from the wound by keeping it patent. The drain allows for debridement of the abscess cavity by irrigation. Tissue fluids flow along the external surface of a latex drain. Hence, it is not always necessary to make perforations in the drain, which could weaken and perhaps cause fragmentation within the tissues.

Removal of drains: Drains should be removed when the drainage has nearly completely ceased. Drains have shown to allow ingress of skin flora along their surfaces. Some form of drains, such as latex drains in particular, are irritating to the surrounding tissues and may stimulate some exudates formation on their own. Thus, drains are usually left in infected wounds for 2 to 7 days (Flynn 2000).

■ SPREAD OF OROFACIAL INFECTION

Routes of Spread

The routes by which the infections can spread are as follows:
a. By direct continuity through the tissues.
b. By lymphatics to the regional lymph nodes and eventually into the blood stream. When the infection gets established in the lymph nodes, secondary abscesses may develop. The spread of infection from the lymph nodes into the tissues results in secondary areas of cellulitis or tissue space abscess.
c. *By the blood stream*: Rarely, local thrombophlebitis may propagate along the veins, entering the cranial cavity via emissary veins to produce cavernous sinus thrombophlebitis. The micro-organisms or infected emboli may get swept away into the bloodstream, leading to bacteremia, septicemia, or pyemia with the development of embolic abscesses (Table to 40.3).

S. No.	Lymph nodes	Areas drained
	Table 40.3: The lymph nodes in the face and neck region and the areas of drainage	
1.	Submental	Tip of the tongue, part of the floor of the mouth in the midline, mandibular incisors, related gingivae, middle alveolar process and basal bone of the mandible, midportion of lower lip and chin.
2.	Submandibular	All maxillary teeth, mandibular teeth except incisors, inferior nasal cavity, palate, body of tongue, upper lip, lateral portion of lower lip, angle of mouth, medial angle of eye, and submental lymph nodes.
3.	Accessory facial • Infraorbital	Skin of the medial angle of eye, skin of anterior face, superficial part of nose.
	• Buccal	Skin of anterior face, mucous membrane of lips and cheeks.
	• Mandibular	Skin over mandible, mucous membrane of lips and cheeks.
4.	Preauricular	Skin inferior to temple, external auditory meatus, lateral part of forehead, lateral part of eyelids, posterior part of cheeks, portion of outer ear, parotid gland
5.	Postauricular	External ear, scalp above and behind the ear.
	• Infra auricular, occipital	Pre and postauricular nodes. Scalp posterior to ear, occipital region.
	• Superficial cervical	Pinna and adjoining skin, pre and postauricular nodes.
	• Deep cervical	Submandibular, submental, inferior auricular, tonsillar and tongue nodes.

Factors Influencing Spread

Some infections progress more rapidly into deep fascial spaces than others. This may be because of: (A) General factors, and (B) Local factors.

General Factors

It includes: (a) Host's resistance; or immunocompetence of the host, and (b) Virulence of micro-organisms; and (c) Combination of both.

a. *Host resistance:* They depends upon: (i) Humoral factors, and (ii) cellular factors.
   i. *Humoral factors* involve immunoglobulins derived from B lymphocytes or plasma cells and complement.
   ii. *Cellular factors* include polymorphonuclear leukocytes, monocytes, lymphocytes, and tissue macrophages.

b. *Virulence of micro-organisms:* It is determined by invasiveness of the causative micro-organisms. These include production of lytic enzymes, potent endotoxins and exotoxins, and interference with or resistance to host humoral and cellular defences.

   Rapid progression of infection occurs in necrotizing fascitis, especially in immunocompromised host, particularly when virulent strains of β-hemolytic streptococci are involved.

c. *Compromised host defences:*
   1. Uncontrolled metabolic diseases, such as, uremia, alcoholism, malnutrition, severe diabetes.
   2. *Suppressing diseases:* **Leukemia**, lymphoma, malignant tumors.
   3. *Suppressing drugs:* Cancer chemotherapeutic drugs, immunosuppressive drugs.

Local Factors

Once the balance between host resistance and bacterial pathogenicity is lost in favor of invading organisms, then the spread of infection progresses. The following are the barriers:

Intact anatomical barriers—(i) *Alveolar bone:* It is the first locally limiting barrier to further spread of a periapical infection. As the infection progresses within the bone, it spreads in the radial manner; and extends to the cortical plates. The site of perforation of the cortex is dependent upon proximity of the root apices to alveolar process. (ii) Periosteum: It is the next local barrier. This structure is better developed in mandible; and hence can delay further spread leading to development of a sub-

periosteal abscess. It does not provide much resistance and the infection spreads into adjacent surrounding soft tissues. (iii) Adjacent muscles and fascia; it is the next site of localization.

The final outcome of spread depends on host's defence mechanisms.

Pathways of Dental Infections (Fig. 40.5)

From a tooth, once the infection crosses the apex, spread of infection depends upon the following factors:
(a) Virulence of micro-organisms, (b) Resistance of the host, and (c) Anatomy of the involved area.

1. *Infection in the periapical area*: Focal osteomyelitis. If the infection remains confined to the periapical area, chronic periapical infection develops. This may sometimes lead to sufficient destruction of bone with well demarcated corticated radiolucency seen on a radiograph. This is known as focal osteomyelitis.
2. Widespread osteomyelitis
3. The infection process may proceed into deeper medullary spaces and lead to widespread osteomyelitis.
4. Formation of fistulous tracts through alveolar bone which exit into the surrounding soft tissue.

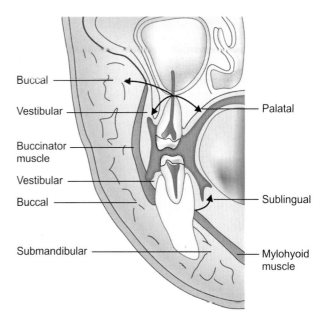

Fig. 40.5: Potential routes of spread of periapical infection. Muscle and fascial attachments determine the direction of spread. Extension beyond these attachments leads to deep space involvement

Anatomical Factors Influencing the Direction of Spread

1. The site of the source of infection such as upper or lower jaw, and the particular segment of the jaw involved.
2. The point at which the pus escapes from the bone and discharges into the soft tissues either labiolingually or buccopalatally.
3. The natural barriers to the spread to pus in the tissues such as layers of fascia or muscle or the jaw bones.

Anatomical Considerations in Dentoalveolar Infections

The fate of a dentoalveolar abscess is dependent upon anatomic position of the apices of the roots from which it originates, especially, the muscle attachments, particularly buccinator and mylohyoid muscles.

It is unusual for an acute dentoalveolar abscess or fistula to appear distant from its site of origin. Infection usually follows the path of least resistance.

Maxilla

A swelling or fistula in the posterior part of hard palate is usually related to the palatal roots of adjacent molars. Infections of upper teeth manifest themselves depending upon the anatomic location of their root apices. Maxillary incisor and cuspid roots lie closer to thin labial plate of bone than to thicker palatal bone. Hence, their infections are usually observed as bulging submucosal (vestibular) abscesses or fistulae in labial sulcus.

The muscles of upper lip arise from alveolar bone, are quite thin, and have little influence on spread of infection.

Infections arising from maxillary bicuspids and molars, may extend buccally and palatally, because of multiple roots. Infection from maxillary bicuspids may extend into connective tissue of buccal vestibule and may spread superiorly, causing cellulitis of the eyelids. The attachments of buccinator muscle are usually well above the root apices of bicuspids, however, extension into buccal space may occur.

The infection from maxillary molars may exit from alveolar bone, either buccally, palatally or posteriorly. The common site for abscess is buccal vestibule, however, buccal space may be involved. The involvement of the palate is uncommon, as the palatal roots are long.

The superior spread of infection into maxillary sinus is not common. The spread of infection posteriorly, may involve the masticator and pharyngeal spaces and spread superiorly into infratemporal space.

Mandible

Infection of mandibular incisors and cuspids, usually presents as a bulging erythematous mass, deep in labial sulcus. If the infection spreads from bone deeper to the origin of mentalis muscle, the submental space gets involved. Infection of mandibular third molars, is frequently pericoronal (pericoronitis); but can be related to root apices, if caries has involved the pulp of the unerupted or erupted tooth. The pathway of infection from the mandibular third molars may be seen to involve buccal vestibule, buccal space, masticator space, and parapharyngeal spaces.

▌ EVALUATION OF THE PATIENT WITH OROFACIAL INFECTION

Patients with an orofacial infection, may present themselves with various signs and symptoms ranging from unimportant to the extremely serious. A quick assessment of the situation is a must.

If the patient
   i. Toxic
   ii. Exhibits central nervous system changes and
   iii. Airway compromise.
Then
   i. Immediate hospitalization
   ii. Aggressive medical treatment
   iii. Aggressive surgical intervention (including intubation and tracheostomy) should be done.

The basic principles of patient evaluation must be followed. These include: complete history, physical examination, clinical features, appropriate laboratory investigations, radiological investigations, and proper interpretation of findings. Adherence to the basic principles helps in arriving at an accurate diagnosis and instituting appropriate treatment.

History Taking

It helps in obtaining information regarding the origin, extent, location and potential seriousness of the problem. The following information may be stressed: (a) History of present illness; especially, onset. (b) History of toothache; or headache, or chills; their nature, location, and duration. (c) Previous hospitalization with infection;

the treatment instituted and it's response. (d) Previous trauma to soft and hard tissues in the region. (e) History of recurrent infections, (f) History of recent rate of increase in extent of swelling, or airway difficulty.

Physical Examination

General Examination

It includes: (i) Examination of thorax, (ii) Abdomen, (iii) Extremities, (iv) Heart and its murmurs, (v) Recording the vital signs: this serves as a useful baseline for noting progression or regression of disease process. Pulse rate is increased, 10 beats/minute for each degree F of rise in temperature.

Regional Examination

It comprises of a comprehensive physical examination and includes the following: (i) Skin of face, head and neck, (ii) Swellings, injuries and areas of tenderness over maxillary and frontal sinuses, (iii) Sinus tracts and fistula formation, (iv) Enlargement of underlying bone, (v) Enlargement of salivary glands, (vi) Enlargement of lymph nodes.

Extraoral examination: A comprehensive regional examination would include:
(1) *Inspection*: (a) Skin of face (redness), head and neck, (b) Swelling, injuries, (c) Fixation of skin, or mucosa to underlying bone, and (d) Sinus or fistula formation.
(2) *Palpation*: (a) Size of swelling, (b) Tenderness, (c) Local temperature, (d) Fluctuation, (e) Enlargement of underlying bone, (f) Salivary glands, (g) Regional lymph nodes (enlargement, tenderness).

Intraoral examination: The examiner should have a good light for the examination of the oropharynx, while slightly depressing the tongue, in order to visualize swelling of tonsillar pillar and deviation of uvula away from the affected side.

(1) Trismus: The interincisal opening should be measured. (2) Teeth: their number, presence of caries, and large restorations, and mobility. (3) Localized swelling and fistulae. (4) Sites of tooth extraction. (5) Percussion: It is useful in determining hypersensitivity. It is performed with a metallic instrument or a tongue blade. (6) Heat and cold testing. (7) Electric pulp testing. (8) Visualization of Stenson's and Wharton's ducts: The flow of saliva from the two ducts on both the sides should be examined. (9) Soft palate, tonsillar fossa, uvula and oropharynx. (10) Displacement of tissues, presence of swelling, and drainage of pus.

Ophthalmologic examination: It includes, assessment of extraocular muscle function, proptosis, or swelling of eyelids, and dorsum of root of the nose.

Clinical Features

a. *Signs of infections:* The cardinal signs of inflammation are usually present to some extent.
   i. *Rubor or redness:* This is usually present, when the infection is close to the tissue surface; especially in individuals with light complexion. It is due to vasodilation.
   ii. *Tumor or swelling:* It is due to the accumulation of inflammatory exudate or pus.
   iii. *Calor or heat:* It is due to pouring of warm blood from deeper tissues at the site of infection, increased velocity of blood flow, and increased rate of metabolism.
   iv. *Dolor or pain:* It is due to (i) The pressure on sensory nerve endings, caused by distension of tissues (edema or spreading of infection), (ii) Increased tissue tension: The action of liberated or activated factors; such as kinins, histamin, or bradykinin like substances, (iii) Loss of tonicity of injured tissues, (iv) Functio laesa: or loss of function of the affected part. It is caused by mechanical factors and reflex inhibition of muscle movements associated with pain. This is reflected in difficulty in chewing and swallowing and respiratory embarrassment.
b. *Fever/Pyrexia:* It is one of the most consistent signs of infection. (97.7°F to 99.5°F—normal oral temp.)
   Other conditions, which may manifest pyrexia include:
   i. Noninfectious inflammatory disorders; such as rheumatoid arthritis
   ii. Excess catabolism as in thyrotoxicosis.
   iii. Neoplastic disease such as lymphoma
   iv. *Postoperative:* Release of endogenous pyrogens, which stimulate the hypothalamic thermoregulation centers.
c. *Repeated chills:* It is common in bacteremia and pyogenic abscesses.
d. *Headache:* It is usually associated with fever, and is thought to be due to stretching of sensitive structures surrounding dilated intracranial arteries.

e. *Lymphadenopathy:* The condition of lymph nodes depends upon whether the condition is acute or chronic. In acute infections, the lymph nodes are soft, tender and enlarged. The surrounding tissues are edematous and overlying skin is erythematous/ reddish. In chronic infection, the lymph nodes are firm nontender and enlarged. The edema of surrounding tissues may not be present. The location of enlarged lymph nodes often indicates the site of infection.

Suppuration of lymph nodes occurs, when the causative organism has overcome the local defence mechanism in the node; resulting in excessive cellular reaction and collection of pus.

f. *Others*:
   i. Presence of draining sinuses or fistulae
   ii. Difficulty in opening mouth
   iii. Difficulty in swallowing
   iv. Increased salivation
   v. Changes in phonation
   vi. Difficulty in breathing
   vii. Bad breath.

Clinical Symptoms of Possible Life Threatening Infections

   i. Respiratory impairment
   ii. Difficulty in swallowing
   iii. Impaired vision or eye movement or both.
   iv. Change in voice quality.
   v. Lethargy.
   vi. Decreased level of consciousness.
   vii. Agitation, restlessness due to hypoxia.

Toxicity—Signs and Symptoms

   i. Pallor
   ii. Rapid respiration, throbbing pulse.
   iii. Fever, shivering
   iv. Appearance of illness.
   v. Lethargy.
   vi. Diaphoresis.

Central Nervous System Changes Associated with Infection

   i. Decreased level of consciousness
   ii. Evidence of meningeal irritation-severe headache, stiff neck, vomiting.
   iii. Edema of eyelids and abnormal eye signs.

Radiological Examination

Conventional Radiography

The radiological examination: The radiological examination is helpful in locating the offending teeth or other underlying causes. The various radiographs useful are: (i) Intraoral periapical radiographs, (ii) Orthopantomographs (OPG), (iii) Lateral oblique view of the mandible, (iv) AP, and lateral view of the neck for soft tissues can be helpful in detecting retropharyngeal space infections.

Other Diagnostic Aids

The other diagnostic imaging aids play a vital role in the management of infection of fascial spaces of face and neck. It helps the surgeon, to know the anatomic extent of the fascial space infections, which aids in surgical drainage of the abscess and inflammatory exudate.

CT guided needle aspiration of fluid collections can be used to obtain material for microbial analysis. The imaging techniques can be broadly classified into following:

(1) Computed tomography (CT scan), (2) Magnetic resonance imaging (MRI), (3) Nuclear medicine, (4) Xeroradiography. These help in diagnosing extension of infection beyond maxillofacial region.

CT scan: It is the "gold-standard", in head and neck imaging. CT and other X-ray images are based on a single factor, i.e. the X-ray beam is attenuated by the tissue present, according to its electron density. CT scan is the most widely used advanced imaging modality in the evaluation of the fascial infections. CT shows the extent of soft tissue involvement, i.e. (a) Showing complete extent of inflammatory process, (b) Epicenter of inflammatory process, (c) Differentiating between myositis-fascitis, and abscess formation. And (d) accurately demonstrating the status of airway and involvement of various group of lymph nodes.

CT shows extent of osseous involvement adjacently, and demonstrates early periosteal reaction associated with osteomyelitis.

CT findings, associated with fascial space involvement include edema and ill-definition of various muscles (myositis) and fascial planes (fascitis), airway displacement or deformity of the soft tissues, air from gas forming pathogens, enhancing the inflammatory masses, fluid collection within involved space, abscess formation evidenced by a hypodense area representing an accumulation of exudates or necrotic tissue surrounded by an enhancing wall and osteomyelitis of involved bone.

Interventional procedures like:

1. Fine needle aspiration of fluid collection: To obtain material for microbial analysis,
2. Abscess drainage and drain placement can be done with CT guidance.

CT View of Various Spaces (Figs 40.6 and 40.7)

Submandibular Space

Normal View: (Axial View)

1. *Submandibular space proper:* The superficial lobe of submandibular gland appears as a well defined soft tissue density, usually surrounded by a flat plane

2. Submandibular group of lymph nodes, are homogenous nonenhancing appearance and never exceed 1.5 cm in diameter.
3. Deep lobe of submandibular salivary gland is not well defined in axial view, since its CT density is close to that of adjacent soft tissues of the floor of the mouth; but it can be identified by coronal section.
4. Mylohyoid muscle appears as a band of soft tissue density, through its origin, adjacent to the medial aspect of mandible. (On coronal section, it appears as a coronal sling extending between the medial aspect of hemimandible).
5. Genioglossus muscle appears as a paramedian muscular band separated by a low density vertical cleft or midline lingual septum. In the inflammatory processes, there is loss of soft tissue plane of submandibular space.

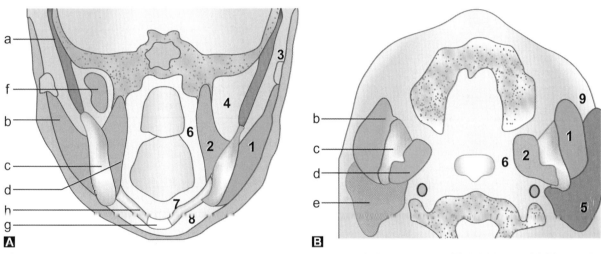

Figs 40.6A and B: CT scan anatomy of fascial spaces—Masticatory space: (A) Coronal image, (B) Axial image. (1) Masseteric region, (2) Medial pterygoid region, (3) Superficial temporal region, (4) Deep temporal region, (5) Parotid space, (6) Parapharyngeal space, (7) Sublingual space, (8) Submandibular space, (9) Adipose tissue lateral to the masseter muscle: (a) Temporalis muscle, (b) Masseter muscle, (c) Mandible, (d) Medial pterygoid muscle, (e) Parotid gland, (f) Lateral pterygoid muscle, (g) Hyoid bone, (h) Mylohyoid muscle

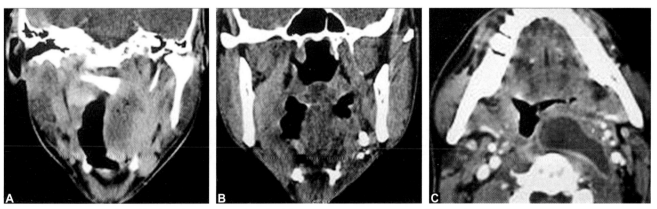

Figs 40.7A to C: (A and B) Coronal CT scan showing involvement of L parapharyngeal space, (C) Axial image also showing the involvement of L parapharyngeal space

Lower axial CT scan, a low density area between the mandible and mylohyoid muscle represents submandibular space.

In coronal view, submandibular space is seen between medial aspect of mandible and mylohyoid muscle.

Sublingual Space

Low density area between the paramidline, genioglossus muscle medially and mylohyoid muscle and medial surface of mandible laterally. Lingual blood vessel, a very important landmark, clearly seen with IV contrast infection. Hyoglossus, styloglossus muscle complex, appears as a thin curvilinear muscle complex medially.

On Axial CT, through inferior mandible, the anterior belly of digastric is seen in digastric fossa in the undersurface of anterior mandible.

Axial CT below the level of mandible, shows paired anterior bellies of digastric below the subcutaneous tissue of neck extending between anterior mandible and greater cornu of hyoid bone.

Masticatory Spaces

It is a distinct deep facial region, bounded by layers of deep cervical fascia. This fascia provides early barrier to spread of infections. Once the fascial boundaries are breached, masticator space infection leads to complex drainage problem.

Patient with masticator space infection are difficult to examine clinically because of accompanying trismus.

CT can be recommended in case of clinically suspected masticator space infection.
CT can demonstrate:
a. The presence of only inflammatory change with no focal pus (cellulitis) precluding surgical drainage.
b. The presence of osteomyelitis, necessitating subperiosteal drainage.
c. Involvement of multiple spaces, besides masticator space, requires more extensive drainage procedure.
d. Presence of pus confined to masticator space, permitting intraoral drainage.

General Principles of Therapy for the Management of Acute Extensive Orofacial Infection

The management of acute odontogenic/orofacial infection comprises of:

1. Immediate hospitalization
2. Aggressive medical treatment (Supportive treatment along with antibiotic therapy)
3. Aggressive surgical intervention (including intubation and tracheostomy) should be done.
   Surgical management: It consists of (i) Extraction of the offending tooth or teeth, (ii) Incision and drainage or a (iii) Combination of both.

Antibiotic Therapy

Recent reports have shown, that on the basis of the recent changes in the antibiotic sensitivity patterns of the most frequent pathogens of orofacial infections, penicillin may no longer be the empiric antibiotic of choice for serious cases requiring hospitalization. Many recent studies, in outpatients, however, have confirmed that there is no difference in ultimate therapeutic success between penicillin and clindamycin, amoxicillin, with or without clavulanic acid; and cephradine.

Indications for use of Antibiotics

(i) Acute onset of infection, (ii) Diffuse infections, (iii) Compromised host defenses, (iv) Involvement of fascial spaces, (v) Severe pericoronitis, and (vi) Osteomyelitis.

Selection of antibiotics: For treating odontogenic infections are as follows:
a. In case, there is no exudates available for culture and antibiotic sensitivity of organism(s) involved before initial therapy, then the initial selection is made on empiric basis.
b. When pus is present, a smear can be Gram stained to provide the basis for a presumptive diagnosis and selection of antibiotic.

In general, bactericidal antibiotics should be preferred to bacteriostatic antibiotics; as these can independently destroy the invading organisms. On the other hand, bacteriostatic antibiotics, only prevent multiplication of bacteria; and depend on host's defence mechanisms for eradication of organisms.

Spectrum: It is preferable to use antibiotic with the narrowest spectrum, which are effective against the organisms involved in the infection. The use of a broad spectrum antibiotic should be avoided; as (i) It increases risk of development of resistant microbial strains; and (ii) Also increases risk of superinfections, by disrupting the normal bacterial flora in various body cavities; and permit nonpathogenic bacteria to proliferate and cause disease.

Supportive therapy: It involves those modalities which aid the patient's own body defences. It consists of the following: (i) Administration of antibiotics, (ii) Hydration of patient through IV route, maintain adequate nutritional status—high protein intake through Ryle's tube feeding (iii) Analgesic, (iv) Bed rest, (v) Application of heat in the form of moist pack and/or mouthrinses. (vi) Opening the tooth for drainage.

Principles of Surgical Management

Determination of severity of infection: It is necessary to do a thorough examination of a patient with severe infection, such as evaluation of the airway in the form of difficulty in breathing, swallowing, speaking, or handling secretions, etc. A change in quality of voice indicates a swelling in or near glottis, such as in parapharyngeal spaces (both lateral and retropharyngeal), or epiglottis. Other findings that may be obscured are as follows: which are usually indicative of parapharyngeal infection:

a. Occasionally, the patient may exhibit an abnormal head posture, or a lateral deviation of head, in an attempt to position upper airway over the deviated trachea, as in a lateral pharyngeal space infection.

b. In case of increased upper airway resistance, the patient may use the accessory muscles of respiration such as platysma and intercostals.

Ability to protrude the tongue past the vermilion border of the upper lip is a fairly reliable sign that the sublingual space is not severely involved.

Determination of the anatomical location of infection: It is necessary to determine the precise location and involvement of different oral, fascial and cervical swelling associated with each of the superficial and deep fascial spaces involved.

Evaluation of the host defenses: The most common diseases that compromise immune system are as follows (Flynn 2000):

a. Diabetes mellitus
b. Steroid therapy within the past two years:
    i. Asthma
    ii. Autoimmune or inflammatory disease
    iii. Organ transplant therapy
c. Cancer chemotherapy within the past year
d. Renal dialysis
e. HIV seropositivity

f. Primary immunodeficiencies
    i. Wiskott-Aldrich syndrome
    ii. Fanconi's syndrome
    iii. Agammaglobulinemia
    iv. Agranulocytosis.

It is important for the surgeon to recognize the situation of immune compromise in patient with orofacial infection and modify the treatment accordingly. Some of the modifications include: (a) Use of bactericidal antibiotics, such as beta-lactams, high doses of clindamycin, metronidazole, vancomycin, and aminoglycosides. The antibiotics to be avoided in immunocompromised patients include: macrolides and tetracyclines.

Decision on the setting of care: The following criteria justify hospital admission of patient with orofacial infection (Flynn 2000): (1) Fever over 101°F, (2) Dehydration, (3) Impending airway compromise, (4) threat to vital structures, (5) Infection of deep cervical space or masticator space, (6) Need for general anesthesia, (7) Need for inpatient control of systemic disease.

Anesthetic implications: The cases of trismus, where the interincisal opening is less than 30 mm, are reported to be associated with a significant increase in likelihood of difficult intubation (Frerk 1991). The surgeon can use this guideline in communicating with anesthesiologist and discuss the hindrance to access to instrumentation of airway. Other studies reported that trismus, because of infection may relax under general anesthesia (Loughman and Allen 1985). The ratchet type mouth prop is very useful to open the mouth during intubation procedures.

Another commonly available method for determining adequacy of respiratory function in infected patient is pulse oximeter. A patient with no pulmonary disease, where the O_2 saturation is below 96 percent in room air, which declines over a period of time and rises again with administration of O_2; is indicative of compromised airway, which requires immediate attention.

Secure the airway: The first step in the management of such a patient is to secure the airway. The commonly used airway management techniques appropriate for the infected patient are listed below (Flynn 2000):

a. Tracheotomy under local anesthesia
b. Cricothyroidotomy under local anesthesia
c. Fiberoptic intubation
d. Blind awake intubation

e. Bullard laryngoscopic intubation
f. Transtracheal jet ventilation
g. Inhalation induction with asleep intubation.

The techniques have their advantages and disadvantages; and should be appropriate for individual infected patient.

Needle decompression (Figs 40.8A to D): A simple useful technique, which is helpful to prevent aspiration of infected material is "Needle decompression" of abscess before intubation. This technique is especially appropriate in cases of pterygomandibular, peritonsillar, or lateral pharyngeal abscess that has thinned the distended overlying mucosa that is likely to rupture during passage of endotracheal tube.

Advantages: (i) It reduces the likelihood of sudden discharge of large amounts of pus into the airway. (ii) It redirects the flow of pus intraorally or extraorally, where it can readily be suctioned. (iii) It also allows immediate submission of an appropriate culture specimen, especially, if the puncture site has previously been prepared with antiseptic solution.

Disadvantages: (i) Discomfort to the patient. (ii) Bleeding from the site of puncture.

Surgical drainage: Some authors advocate that drainage of all spaces involved by cellulitis or abscess caused by odontogenic infection, should be done, as soon as possible after diagnosis.

The rationale for the more aggressive approach includes the following, however, final resolution requires further investigations:
1. It is impossible to diagnose deep space infections either by clinical or radiological examination with 100 percent accuracy.
2. Drainage of cellulitis seems to abort the spread of infection into neighboring deep fascial spaces.

3. Adequate culture specimen can be obtained from cellulitis fluid.
4. Physical debridement and irrigation of infected space may hasten healing by decreasing the size of bacterial inoculum and the amount of necrotic tissue present.
5. Early drainage may prevent later colonization of the site by more highly antibiotic resistant microorganisms.
6. Length of stay in the hospital may be decreased.

Guidelines for placement of incisions in infected cases:
1. Incisions should be placed in the most dependent areas.
2. Incisions should be parallel to the skin creases.
3. Incisions should lie in an esthetically acceptable site as far as possible.
4. Incisions should be supported by healthy underlying dermis and subcutaneous tissue.
    Placing the incision through the thin, often shiny skin directly overlying the abscess, which normally gets undermined by an abscess burrowing its way to the surface; results in a puckered contracted scar which gets collapsed into abscess cavity.
5. Incisions placed intraorally, should not cross frenal attachments, and should be placed parallel to nerve fibers in the region of mental nerve.
6. The removal of the cause; such as an infected tooth, a segment of necrotic bone, a foreign body, if not already done, then should be done at the time of incision and drainage procedure.

CT-guided percutaneous drainage: This technique employs a CT-guided catheter to drain well localized abscess. It is indicated for deep neck abscesses.

It is introduced percutaneously and guided into the abscess cavity. It's advantage is that it helps in precise

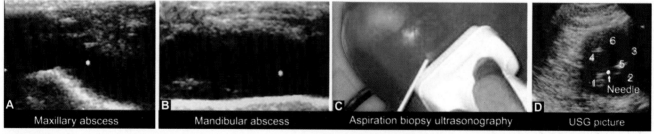

Figs 40.8A to D: Needle decompression of an abscess using USG guided needle aspiration method: (A and B) Confirmation of maxillary and mandibular abscess formation through ultrasonography. Well-defined hypoechoic zones are noted. (C and D) USG guided needle aspiration helps in proper localization of pus, its volume and depth from the skin, 14 to 18 gauge cannula is used to collect the pus and decompress the abscess. Pus is sent for culture and antibiotic sensitivity test

locating the abscess cavity without extensive dissection and minimizes scarring. It is performed in a radiology department.

After performing incision and drainage, a specimen is obtained for Gram staining and culture; and the catheter may be left *in situ*, to serve as a drain.

Extraction of tooth in the presence of acute abscess: This is a controversial subject. One school of thought believes that there is potential spread of infection by manipulation of tooth during extraction. The other school of thought challenges this view and believes that early extraction leads to early resolution of infection by eliminating the source of infection and by providing a portal of drainage.

There are numerous studies reported in this regard; which suggest that immediate extraction of offending teeth does not cause dissemination of infection; and may result in lesser postoperative complications than later extractions. However, these studies are not conclusive. It is worth while considering administration of antibiotics prior to carrying out extraction of offending tooth during acute stage of infection.

Medical supportive therapy: The ultimate success of the surgical and antibiotic therapy for serious orofacial infections depends upon adequate control of systemic diseases that may affect the host's resistance mechanism. The most common serious immunocompromising disease is diabetes mellitus, especially the insulin-dependent type. A good control of blood sugar level has been shown to affect host's resistance favorably.

Presence of fever in a serious infection increases patient's metabolic requirements and fluid needs significantly. The minimal daily fluid requirements are increased by 300 ml per degree of fever per day. Similarly, caloric requirements are increased by 5 to 8 percent per degree of fever per day. In order to meet these fluid requirements, an intravenous infusion of 100 ml per hour should be maintained; to meet the basic fluid needs, and in addition, replacement for the increased fluid losses, because of fever and diarrhea or any other unusual fluid losses. Hypotonic IV solutions, such as one fourth or one half normal saline (NS) with or without dextrose are suggested in order to provide excess free water to replace insensible losses. In case, oral intake has been impaired, by pain, swelling, drains, endotracheal intubation, parenteral nutrition may be required to be given. During prolonged hospital stays, it may be necessary to monitor patient's electrolyte balance,

and provide additional supplements if necessary. This is more important in cases of necrotizing fascitis, where hypocalcemia may be caused by sequestration of calcium ions in necrotic fat molecules.

Review and re-evaluation in the postoperative period: The review of the patient in the postoperative period can be divided into two stages:

a. *Early postoperative phase:* The patient is reviewed for: (i) Maintenance of airway, patency and extubation, and (ii) Monitoring local and systemic signs of recovery

b. *Late postoperative phase:* It includes: (i) Effectiveness of antibiotic therapy. (ii) Care of the surgical wound. In infected patients, it includes frequent wound irrigation and change of dressings, and removal of drain.

The swelling normally decreases by 48 to 72 hours postoperatively, allowing for a temporary rise in swelling because of surgical trauma. Trismus and WBC Count, usually tend to reduce by 24 to 48 hours after surgery. The degree of malaise is supposed to be the earliest and the sensitive systemic indicator. Hence, when the patient feels simply better, it is a good sign.

A review of the case, does not show any improvement by 48 to 72 hours postoperatively, then a re-evaluation should be done for the following: (i) Effectiveness of the wound drainage, (ii) Antibiotic therapy, and (iii) A search for a previously undetected source of infection.

Postoperative CT examination has been very useful in identifying the adequacy of surgical drainage.

The criteria for changing antibiotics in the post-operative period are as follows: (1) Development of allergy or toxicity. (2) Clinical deterioration after 48 hours of antibiotic therapy, if: (a) Repeat surgery has been done, or (b) Postoperative CT demonstrates adequate surgical drainage. (3) Culture and sensitivity or Gram stain indicating resistant micro-organisms, (4) Necrotizing fascitis (use broad spectrum antibiotics).

Rehabilitation: The patient can be discharged from the hospital after having an afebrile period of 24 hours or more, and be able to consume at least adequate amount of liquid diet. Usually all the drains have to be removed prior to the discharge of the patient from the hospital. The outpatient follow up interval should be frequent at first. A deep seated infection, sometimes may resume draining after having stopped before discharge. This may be an indication of resistant organisms. In the absence of worsening signs of infection, this may be treated successfully with a change of antibiotic, especially a broader-spectrum antibiotic. Physiotherapy for trismus should be gentle, to avoid tearing of inflamed masticatory muscles. Encourage the patient to seek immediate and regular preventive and restorative dental care.

▇ POTENTIAL SPACES

Odontogenic infections are frequently encountered in the practice of oral and maxillofacial surgery. Many of these infections can be managed by tooth extraction, endodontic therapy, surgical treatment, including drainage with adequate antibiotic coverage. These infections often respond to surgical and antimicrobial management, however, they have the potential to spread through the fascial planes in the head and neck region to compromise vital structures in the region or involve distant structures. The perusal of literature shows numerous reports of odontogenic infections involving intracranial structures, the orbit, and the mediastinum.

The more commonly involved region is the airway. Airway compromise can occur either at presentation or secondary to postsurgical edema. If prompt treatment is not instituted with immediate recognition of the situation, it can lead to life threatening episode and even death. Fortunately, new antibiotics and diagnostic techniques have reduced the morbidity and mortality of infection in the head and neck dramatically. Whenever, confronted with an acute, life threatening condition due to maxillofacial infection, one must adhere to sound surgical principles, protocols for its management.

Shapiro defined fascial spaces as potential spaces between the layers of fascia. These spaces are normally filled with loose connective tissues and various anatomical structures like veins, arteries, glands, lymph nodes, etc. (space is a misnomer. There are no voids in the tissues in actual reality).

Organization of Cervical Fascia (Fig. 40.9)

1. Superficial fascia
2. Deep fascia:
    a. Superficial layer (anterior)
    b. Pretracheal fascia (middle layer)
    c. Prevertebral fascia (posterior deep layer).
    Pus tends to accumulate in these specific region which are referred to as tissue spaces; none of which are actual spaces until pus is formed. Some of these *potential spaces* are compartments which contain structures such

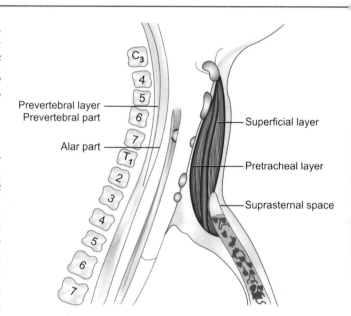

Fig. 40.9: Cervical organization of fascial layers of the deep fascia

as submandibular salivary glands, the buccal pad of fat or groups of lymph nodes. Normally, these structures are surrounded by loose connective tissue, which can easily be stripped by finger pressure to produce a cavity. The pus destroys the loose connective tissue and separates the anatomical boundaries of the compartment as it increases in volume, thus creation of an abscess cavity bounded by muscle, tissues and bone.

The anatomical spaces around the jaws where pus tends to accumulate: The infection in orofacial region, does not spread haphazardly through the loose connective tissue, but tends to accumulate in these potential spaces around the jaws. The detailed knowledge of their surgical anatomy, mainly the boundaries, and the related anatomical structures is important, as it facilitates planning of proper surgical drainage. Many of these spaces communicate with each other.

Pus, once collected, penetrates the fascial and muscle barriers, and eventually reaches the overlying skin.

A muscle is attached to bone by Sharpey's fibers, the attachment is mostly strong and tendinous, but the muscle, may be, in part attached mainly to the periosteum so that it and the periosteum together are readily stripped from the surface of the bone. Here again, a potential space exists deep to the muscle if infection gains access to this plane of cleavage. As pus gets accumulated, it elevates the periosteum from the

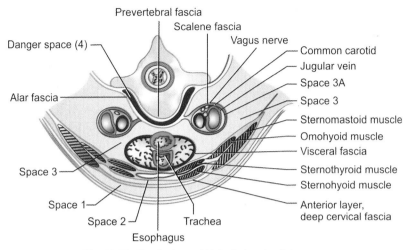

Fig. 40.10: Grodinsky and Holyoke's potential spaces

bone to form an abscess cavity until its spread is limited by the more tendinous part of the muscle.

The narrow interval between muscles also contains a layer of loose connective tissue which permits independent movement of the layers. Here again pus can accumulate to produce an anatomically defined cavity.

Grodinsky and Holyoke in 1938, described these potential spaces as follows (Figs 40.10 and 40.11):

1. *Space 1*: The potential space superficial and deep to the platysma muscle.
2. *Space 2*: The space behind the anterior layer of deep cervical fascia.
3. *Space 3*: Pretracheal space—lies anterior to trachea. Pretracheal space infection leads to mediastinitis. Here, the fascia fuses with the pericardium and the parietal pleura, which explains the occurrence of empyema and pericardial effusion in mediastinitis.
4. *Space 3*: A viscerovascular space (***Lincoln's highway*** as coined by Mosher)—is the carotid sheath from the jugular foramen and carotid canal at the base of the skull to the pericardium or middle mediastinum. Infections in this space are usually associated with internal jugular vein thrombophlebitis or carotid artery erosion.
5. *Space 4*: ***Danger space*** is a potential space between the alar and prevertebral fascia. It extends from the base of the skull to the posterior mediastinum, as far as the diaphragm. Oropharyngeal infections can enter the posterior mediastinum via the retropharyngeal space to the danger space, which is continuous with the posterior mediastinum. The spread of infection

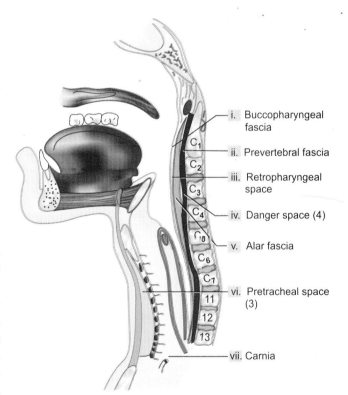

i. Buccopharyngeal fascia

ii. Prevertebral fascia

iii. Retropharyngeal space

iv. Danger space (4)

v. Alar fascia

vi. Pretracheal space (3)

vii. Carnia

Fig. 40.11: Sagittal section of the neck showing spaces 3 and 4 and also the close proximity of retropharyngeal space to the danger space through the alar fascia: (i) Buccopharyngeal fascia, (ii) Prevertebral fascia, (iii) Retropharyngeal space, (iv) Danger space-4 (v) Alar fascia, (vi) Pretracheal space-3 (vii) Carina

from the retropharyngeal space occurs mostly at the fusion of the alar and visceral fascia between C6 and T4 by rupturing through the alar fascia.

Space of Burns: Suprasternal Space (see Fig. 40.9)

The superficial fascia splits below the level of the hyoid bone to form two spaces:

a. It forms the lower part of the roof of the posterior triangle, the fascia splits into two layers, both of which are attached to the clavicle.

b. It forms the lower part of the roof of the anterior triangle and the fascia splits to form the suprasternal space or the space of 'Burns'. The layers pass down to be attached one to the anterior, the other to the posterior border of the manubrium sterni.

Between these layers following structures are present:

i. The sternal head of the sternocleidomastoid muscle.

ii. The communication between the anterior jugular vein.

iii. Lymph glands.

iv. The interclavicular ligament.

■ CLASSIFICATION OF FASCIAL SPACES

Based on the Mode of Involvement

i. Direct involvement: **Primary spaces**—(a) Maxillary spaces (b) Mandibular spaces.

ii. Indirect involvement: **Secondary spaces.**

Spaces involved in odontogenic infections:

a. *Primary maxillary spaces:* Canine, buccal, and infratemporal spaces.

b. *Primary mandibular spaces:* Submental, buccal, submandibular, and sublingual spaces.

c. *Secondary fascial spaces:* Masseteric, pterygomandibular, superficial and deep temporal, lateral pharyngeal, retropharyngeal, and prevertebral spaces, parotid space.

Based on Clinical Significance

i. Face—buccal, canine, masticatory, parotid

ii. Suprahyoid—sublingual, submandibular (submaxillary, submental), pharyngomaxillary (lateral pharyngeal), peritonsillar.

iii. Infrahyoid—Anterovisceral (pretracheal)

iv. Spaces of total neck—retropharyngeal, space of carotid sheath.

Potential Primary Spaces Related to Upper Jaw

Upper lip: An abscess occurring in upper incisors or canine region leads to infection of the base of upper lip.

The abscess is formed on the oral side of orbicularis muscle; and therefore, is a vestibular abscess, and tends to point in the vestibule.

The direction is guided by the origin of orbicularis oris muscle, which is beneath anterior nasal spine. This results in pointing of the abscess towards the apex of lateral incisor. The abscess, rarely points in the floor of nose, where it can be mistaken for a boil of the nose.

Involvement of upper lip on outer surface of orbicularis oris muscle occurs due to skin infections, such as, furuncle.

Infections, in the area of upper lip, incisors and canine, may give rise to orbital cellulitis, or cavernous sinus thrombophlebitis. The path taken by infection is from superior labial venous plexus to anterior facial vein; then in a retrograde direction, via, ophthalmic veins to cavernous sinus. This pathway is facilitated because of absence of valves in these veins.

Treatment: The abscesses in the region of upper lip are treated in the following ways:

1. Antibiotic therapy
2. Incision and drainage
3. Extraction of offending tooth/root canal treatment.

Differential Diagnosis of Swellings of Upper Lip

1. *Trauma to upper lip:* Any trauma to upper lip can produce a considerable size of swelling.

2. *Trauma to upper incisor:* Any trauma to upper incisors can produce swelling of upper lip. It starts to subside after 48 hours.

3. *Hypersensitivity reaction*

   a. Allergic swellings of upper lip may arise with local application of various substances from toothpaste to lipstick. The enlarged lip appears to be soft and non tender; and reduces in size with antihistaminics.

   b. Other edematous swellings: (i) Merkerson-Rosenthal syndrome. This syndrome presents with swollen lip, fissured tongue and facial palsy.

Biopsy of lip will reveal, noncaseating Langhan's giant cell granulomas, which if associated with neuropathy, is likely to be sarcoidosis; and if associated with granulomatous bowel disease, then it is Crohn's disease.

4. *Cysts:* Cysts of jaws produce swelling in vestibule which extend and cause enlargement of upper lip; such as nasopalatine cyst or any odontogenic cyst in upper incisor region.

   Nasolabial cyst: It produces a prominent swelling in the region of nasolabial fold; as it lies against bone between ala of the nose and upper lip.

5. *Neoplasms:* Occasionally, such tumors as pleomorphic adenoma or mucoepidermoid carcinoma may arise in labial tissues. These are usually firm in consistency.

Canine Fossa Involvement (Infraorbital Space)

a. Odontogenic infections
b. Nasal infections; less frequent.

   Periapical abscess of cuspids. Usually presents as labial sulcus swelling; and less commonly as palatal swelling.

   Periapical abscess, which discharges bucally from an upper canine or first premolar; may lead to accumulation of pus in canine fossa, deep to muscles of facial expression moving upper lip.

Involvement: The teeth which frequently give rise to abscess in the area are the maxillary canines and premolars and sometimes the mesiobuccal root of first molars. The periapical abscess discharges buccally superior to the origin of the caninus muscle and pus accumulates in the canine fossa.

Surgical anatomy—Boundaries (Fig. 40.12): Superiorly, levator labii superioris alaque nasi, levator labii superioris, and zygomaticus minor muscles.
- Inferiorly, caninus muscle
- Anteriorly, orbicularis oris,
- Posteriorly, buccinator muscle
- Medially, anterolateral surface of maxilla.

a. *Canine with short root:* Levator anguli oris takes origin from bone below the origin of levator anguli oris, i.e. infraorbital foramen, and levator labii superiors, above foramen and overlaps the anguli oris. The pus from a periapical abscess will emerge and tends to point in upper buccal sulcus, as buccinator muscle has no attachment to bone anterior to first molar.

b. *Canine with a long root:* The root apex in these cases, is above the origin of canine muscle, but below the origin of the quadratus muscle. The pus from periapical abscess may emerge above the origin of levator anguli oris. In such situations, pus escapes to the space between levator labii superioris and levator labii superioris alaque nasi, containing the branches of the infraorbital nerve and blood vessels. The infection may finally spread anteriorly through the gap between the angular and infraorbital heads of the quadratus muscle and emerges under the skin just below the inner corner of the eye, or escape posteriorly between the infraorbital head and zygomatic head of the quadratus muscle, emerging under the skin, just below the outer corner of the eye.

Clinical features (Figs 40.13 and 40.14):
- Swelling of cheek and upper lip (vestibular abscess).
- Obliteration of nasolabial fold (pus accumulates in canine fossa).

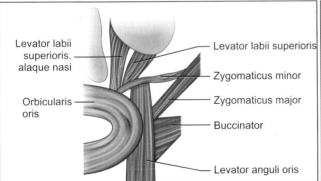
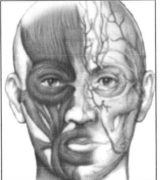
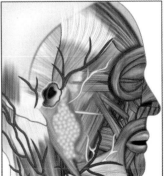

Levator labii superioris. alaque nasi

Levator labii superioris

Zygomaticus minor

Zygomaticus major

Orbicularis oris

Buccinator

Levator anguli oris

Fig. 40.12: Canine fossa space (infraorbital space) and its boundaries, anatomical pictures showing its vital relations

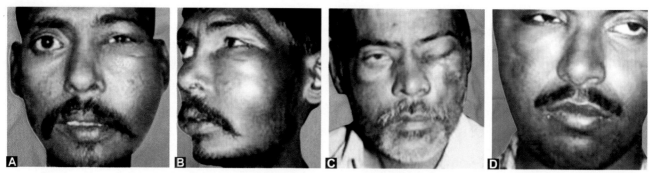

Figs 40.13A to D: Extraoral clinical pictures of canine fossa infection

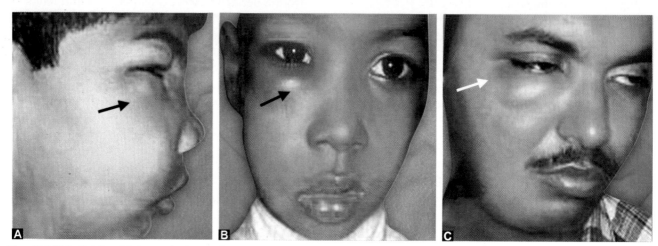

Figs 40.14A to C: Infraorbital or canine fossa infection. Clinical extraoral pictures of three different patients. (A) Note the obliteration of nasolabial fold and infection tracking towards medial canthus of the eye, (B) Infection tracking towards lateral canthus of the eye, (C) Along with canine fossa infection, there is spread of infection in the infratemporal region (arrow)

- Drooping of angle of the mouth.
- Edema of lower eyelid; it indicates pointing of abscess below medial corner
  a. *Extraoral—Early phase:* Usually on the first or second day, there is an inflammatory enlargement of the upper lip, and the angle of the mouth is seen to droop. Obliteration of nasolabial fold. Periorbital edema: *Late phase—* This usually occurs on the second or the third day.
- Marked periorbital edema; forcing the eyelid to close.
- Redness and marked tenderness of the facial tissues.
- When the infection progresses to chronic stage, it may result in production of chronic fistula in the cleft area between the levator labii superioris alaque nasi, and zygomaticus minor muscles near the medial canthus of the eye.
  b. *Intraoral:* The offending tooth is mobile and is tender to percussion.

Incision and drainage: The approach to this area is through the mucosa of buccal vestibule in the region of lateral incisor and canine. A curved mosquito forceps is inserted superior to the attachment of caninus muscle, and the infraorbital space is entered. Pus is evacuated and a drain is inserted and is secured to one of the margins with a suture.

Palatal abscess (Figs 40.15A to D): Involvement: Periodontal abscesses from palatal pockets and apical abscesses from the palatal roots of the posterior teeth are the source of palatal infection. Occasionally the lateral incisor is the frequent cause, as the infection can migrate posteriorly, as far as the soft palate owing to the more palatal orientation of it's roots.

*Surgical anatomy: Boundaries—*The palatal space is bounded by the cortical plate of hard palate inferiorly, and the overlying periosteum and mucosa superiorly; and laterally by the alveolar process of maxilla and the teeth.

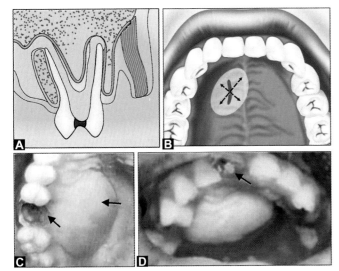

Figs 40.15A to D: Palatal subperiosteal abscess (A) Periapical pathosis pathway to the palate, where the pressure of the accumulated pus elevates the thick mucoperiosteum, (B) Incision for a palatal subperiosteal abscess. The incision should be planned along the medial border of the swelling to avoid damage to the palatine arteries. Hemostat should be inserted along with the dotted arrows to drain the pus completely, (C) Clinical picture of palatal abscess. Note the offending tooth, which should be extracted or treated endodontically, (D) Clinical picture of another palatal abscess due to periapical lesion of right upper central incisor, which is being treated endodontically

Clinical features: Intraorally, a well defined circum-scribed fluctuant swelling is seen, which is confined to one side of the palate, adjacent to the offending tooth. Discoloration may not be present. The offending tooth is tender to percussion.

Incision and drainage. An anteroposterior incision is made through the mucosa, down to the bone, keeping in mind the course of greater palatine nerve and vessels. A curved mosquito forceps is inserted and the pus is evacuated. A small piece of rubber drain is inserted into the abscess cavity and secured with a suture.

Buccal Space Involvement (Figs 40.16 and 40.17)

Buccal space is the potential space between buccinator and masseter muscle.

Boundaries

- *Anteromedially:* Buccinator muscle
- *Posteromedially:* Masseter overlying the anterior border of ramus of mandible
- *Laterally:* By forward extension of deep fascia from the capsule of parotid gland and by platysma muscle.

- *Inferiorly:* Limited by the attachment of the deep fascia to the mandible and by depressor anguli oris.
- *Superiorly:* The zygomatic process of the maxilla and the zygomaticus major and minor muscles.
  Contents: Buccal pad of fat, Stenson's (parotid) duct, facial artery.

Teeth commonly involved: Maxillary and mandibular premolars and molars. The location of the root tip to the level of origin of buccinator muscle determines the spread of infection either intraorally into the vestibule or deep into the buccal space. Pericoronitis in lower third molar—pus can travel forward along the channel formed by the muscle attached to the sloping external oblique ridge and the body of the mandible. In this case, pus pools intraorally opposite 1st or 2nd molars. If pus penetrates the muscle in the retromolar area, then it is directed laterally into the buccal space.

Clinical features (Figs 40.18A to C): When pus accumulates on oral side of the muscle—'Gum boil' is seen in the vestibule.

If pus accumulates lateral to the muscle, prominent extraoral swelling is seen extending from lower border of mandible to the infraorbital margin and from the anterior margin of masseter muscle to the corner of mouth. Sometimes edema of the lower eyelid is seen.

Spread: Continuation with pterygomandibular space to infratemporal space along the fascia, accompanying the Stenson's duct. To submasseteric space—if infection tracks backwards and penetrates the paratidomasseteric fascia.

Incision and drainage: Horizontal incison through the oral mucosa of the cheek in the premolar, molar region. If the pus is lateral to the muscle, then the muscle is penetrated with curved mosquito forceps to enter the buccal space. Drain is placed and secured with suture.

Differential diagnosis:

1. *Cellulitis:* It is caused by *H. influenzae*. It is usually seen in infants and children under 3 years of age. Usually, there is high fever, for at least 24 hours prior to appearance of clinical manifestations.
2. *Erysipelas:* There is rapid onset, dark red swelling, and associated otitis media frequently present.
3. *Crohn's disease:* (Recurrent buccal space abscess) It is a segmental transmural intestinal disease. There is intermittent abdominal pain, fever, weight loss, and diarrhea. It is characterized by inflammatory granulomas present over entire length of GI tract

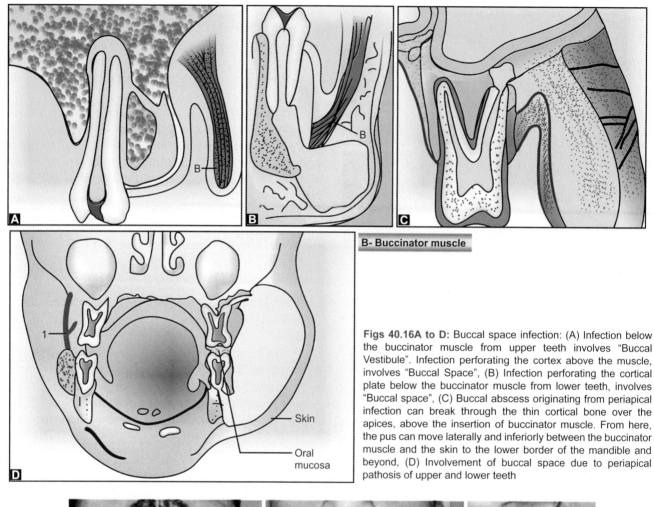

B- Buccinator muscle

Figs 40.16A to D: Buccal space infection: (A) Infection below the buccinator muscle from upper teeth involves "Buccal Vestibule". Infection perforating the cortex above the muscle, involves "Buccal Space", (B) Infection perforating the cortical plate below the buccinator muscle from lower teeth, involves "Buccal space", (C) Buccal abscess originating from periapical infection can break through the thin cortical bone over the apices, above the insertion of buccinator muscle. From here, the pus can move laterally and inferiorly between the buccinator muscle and the skin to the lower border of the mandible and beyond, (D) Involvement of buccal space due to periapical pathosis of upper and lower teeth

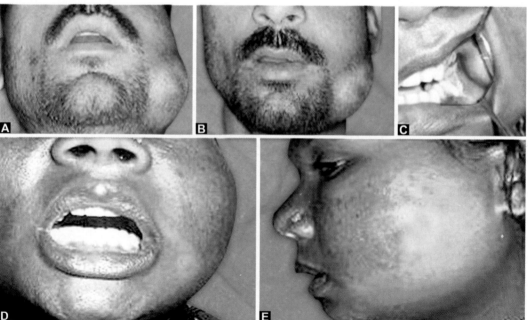

Figs 40.17A to E: Clinical picutre of buccal space involvement

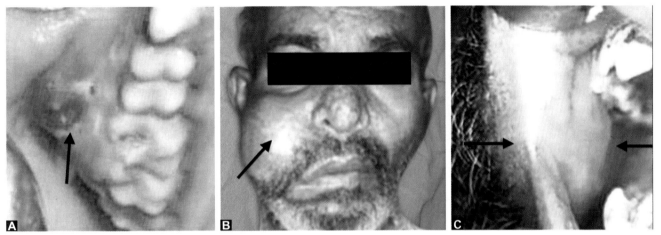

Figs 40.18A to C: (A) Periapical infection moving below the insertion of buccinator muscle, clinically exhibits as vestibular abscess or gum boil, (B) Periapical infection moving above the insertion of buccinator muscle, clinically seen on extraoral picture. Buccal space involvement is seen, (C) Intraoral clinical picture of the buccal space involvement by pus between the buccinator muscle and the skin and the oral mucosa

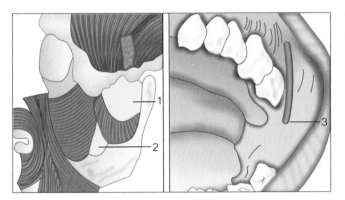

Fig. 40.19: (1) Infratemporal space, (2) Buccal space, (3) Intraoral incision for the drainage of infratemporal space along the anterior border of ramus

from mouth to anus. These granulomatous lesions and ulcerations can progress to the buccal space abscess.

Infratemporal Fossa Space (Fig. 40.19)

It is also called 'retrozygomatic space' by Sicher, as it is partly situated behind the zygomatic bone.

The space is continuous with upper part of pterygomandibular space anteriorly. However, it is separated from it by lateral pterygoid muscle posteriorly. Thus, the infratemporal fossa forms the upper extremity of pterygomandibular space.

Involvement: (i) Infections of the infratemporal space arise from the infection of the buccal roots of the maxillary second and third molars, particularly, from unerupted third molars, and (ii) Local anesthesia injections with contaminated needles in the area of tuberosity, (iii) spread from the other spaces infection.

Surgical anatomy:

i. *Boundaries:*
   - Bounded laterally, by ramus of mandible, temporalis muscle and it's tendon;
   - Medially, medial pterygoid plate, lateral pterygoid muscle, medial pterygoid muscle, lower part of temporal fossa of the skull and lateral wall of pharynx.
   - Superiorly by infratemporal surface of greater wing of sphenoid and by zygomatic arch.
   - Inferiorly, lateral pterygoid muscle, which forms the floor of the fossa, and its lower head is said to mark the border between pterygomandibular and infratemporal spaces.
   - Anteriorly, infratemporal surface of maxilla.
   - Posteriorly, parotid gland.

ii. *Contents:* The fossa contains origins of medial pterygoid and lateral pterygoid muscles. The lower head of lateral pterygoid muscle borders the pterygomandibular and infratemporal spaces. It contains pterygoid venous plexus of veins. It is traversed by maxillary artery, mandibular nerve, and middle meningeal artery.

Clinical features (Figs 40.20A to F):

a. *Extraoral:* The following features are usually seen:
   (i) Trismus: marked limitation of oral opening,
   (ii) Bulging of temporalis muscle, (iii) Marked

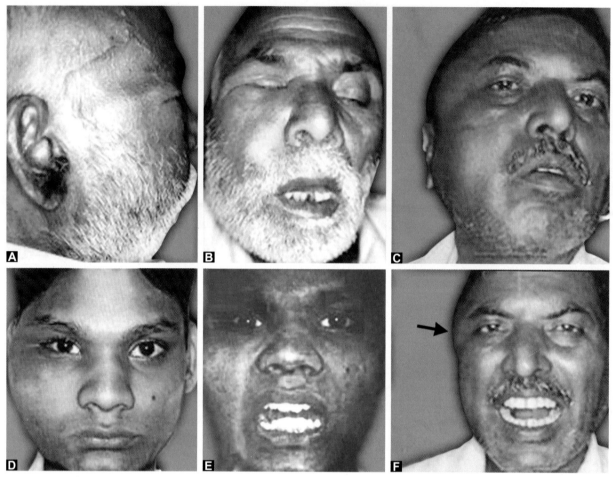

Figs 40.20A to F: Clinical pictures of involvement of infratemporal space due to odontogenic infection

swelling of the face on the affected side in front of the ear, overlying the area of the temporomandibular joint, behind the zygomatic process. (iv) The eye is often closed and is proptosed.

b. *Intraoral:* Swelling in the tuberosity area. Elevation of temperature up to 104°F.

Incision and Drainage

a. *Intraoral approach:* If the trismus is not marked, and fluctuation is detected early, an intraoral incision is given in the buccal vestibule opposite the second and third molars.

The exploration is carried out medial to coronoid process and temporalis muscle upwards and backwards with a sinus forceps, or a curved hemostat. The space is entered, and drained; and a small piece of corrugated rubber drain is kept and secured with a suture.

b. *Extraoral approach:* In severe intractable infection, extraoral incision is the only method of drainage.

Incision is made at the upper and posterior edge of the temporalis muscle, within the hairline. A sinus forceps is then directed upwards and medially. Pus is evacuated; rubber drain is inserted and secured with a suture, and dressing is given.

Despite appropriate and prompt treatment, the condition takes long time to resolve. The restriction of mouth opening persists for long time over a few weeks, and improves in due course of time with active physiotherapy with jaw exercises. In case of failure to improve mouth opening, the following procedures are resorted to; (i) temporalis myotomy and (ii) excision of coronoid process.

Spread: Pus can extend upwards to involve the temporal space, or inferiorly it may perforate the lateral pterygoid muscle, to involve the pterygomandibular space.

Further, infection of infratemporal space should always be regarded as a serious event, because of the proximity of pterygoid plexus of veins, from which infection can track upwards to the cavernous sinus via: (i) The deep facial veins, or (ii) Emissary veins. And via other foramina directly from the infratemporal fossa to the middle cranial fossa. Emissary veins connect these with cavernous sinus through sphenoidal emissary foramen (E of Vesalius), foramen lacerum, foramen spinosum, and foramen ovale.

Thus, rarely, it may involve central nervous system; which is presented as headache, irritability, photophobia, vomiting, and drowsiness.

Potential Primary Spaces Related to Lower Jaw

Submental Space

Involvement: It is involved most frequently by the infections originating from the six anterior mandibular teeth; then perforate the cortical plate below the origin of mentalis muscle labially; and mylohyoid lingually.

The space can be secondarily involved due to infection of submental lymph nodes, following lymphatic spread from lower incisors, lower lip, skin overlying the chin, anterior part of the floor of the mouth, tip of the tongue and sublingual tissues.

Surgical anatomy

i. *Boundaries (Fig. 40.21)*
   • **Lateral:** Lower border of mandible, and anterior bellies of digastric muscle.
   • **Superior:** Mylohyoid muscle.

• *Inferior*: Suprahyoid portion of the investing layer of deep cervical fascia, which is in turn covered by the platysma, superficial fascia and skin.

ii. *Contents*: Submental lymph nodes, and anterior jugular veins. The lymph nodes lie embedded in adipose tissue, and hence, submental abscesses tend to remain well circumscribed.

Clinical Features (Figs 40.22 and 40.23)

a. *Extraoral findings:* Distinct, firm swelling in midline, beneath the chin. Skin overlying the swelling is board like and taut. Fluctuation may be present.

b. *Intraoral findings:* The anterior teeth, are either non-vital, fractured or carious. The offending tooth may exhibit tenderness to percussion and may show mobility. The patient may experience considerable discomfort on swallowing.

Incision and drainage (Figs 40.23A and B): It is performed by making a transverse incision in the skin below the symphysis of the mandible. Blunt dissection is carried out by inserting a Kelly's forceps or sinus forceps through this incision, upward and backward. A small piece of corrugated rubber drain is inserted in the abscess cavity, and is secured to one of the margins of the wound with a suture.

Spread: The infection can spread: (i) Posteriorly, to involve submandibular space, or (ii) It may discharge on the face, in the submental region.

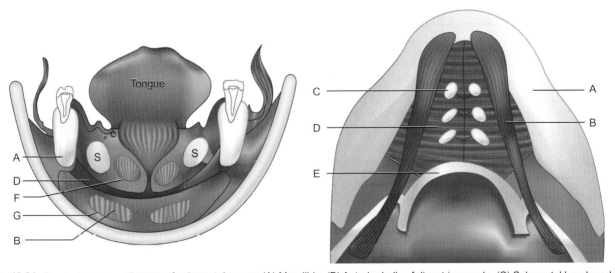

Fig. 40.21: Surgical anatomy diagram of submental space: (A) Mandible, (B) Anterior belly of digastric muscle, (C) Submental lymph nodes, (D) Mylohyoid muscle, (E) Hyoid bone, (F) Geniohyoid muscles, (G) Cervical fascia

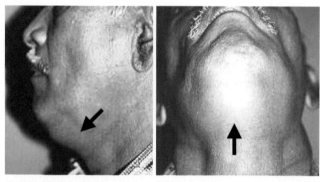

Fig. 40.22: Clinical extraoral picture of submental space involvement due to odontogenic infection

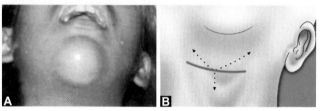

Figs 40.23A and B: (A) Extraoral clinical picture of typical submental space infection due to lower anterior teeth periapical pathology, (B) Incision and drainage for submental space abscess

Submandibular Space

The space lies between the anterior and posterior bellies of the digastric muscles. The upper part lies beneath the inferior border of mandible and the lower part lies deep to the investing layer of deep cervical fascia. The submandibular spaces are considered to be the anterior extensions of parapharyngeal space.

Involvement: (i) It is involved most frequently by infections originating from the mandibular molars. The pus perforates the lingual cortical plate of mandible, inferior to the attachment of mylohyoid muscle, and passes directly into the submandibular space. (ii) The infection from the submandibular salivary gland may pass via lymphatics to the submandibular lymph nodes. (iii) It is also involved, as an extension of infection from submental space; or from the submental lymph nodes via the lymphatics; when the nodes fail to contain the infection within them. (iv) It is also involved by an infection originating from the posterior part of sublingual space. (v) It is also involved from infection originating from middle third of the tongue, posterior part of the floor of the mouth, maxillary teeth, cheek, maxillary sinus and palate.

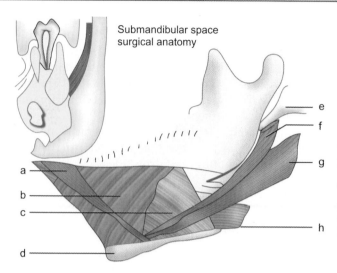

Fig. 40.24: (a) Anterior belly of digastric muscle, (b) Mylohyoid muscle, (c) Hyoglossus muscle, (d) Hyoid bone, (e) Styloid process and stylohyoid ligament, (f) Stylohyoid muscle, (g) Posterior belly of digastric muscle, (h) Middle constrictor muscle

Surgical anatomy: Boundaries (Fig. 40.24):
- Anteromedially, the floor is formed by mylohyoid muscle, which is covered by loose areolar tissue and fat.
- Posteromedially, the floor is formed by hyoglossus muscle.
- Superolaterally, medial surface of mandible below the mylohyoid ridge.
- Anterosuperiorly, anterior belly of digastric.
- Posterosuperiorly posterior belly of digastric, stylohyoid and the stylopharyngeus muscles. Laterally, platysma and skin.

Contents: Superficial lobe of submandibular salivary gland and submandibular lymph nodes, facial artery and vein.

Clinical features (Fig. 40.25):
a. *Extraoral:* (i) Firm swelling in submandibular region, below the inferior border of mandible. (ii) Generalized constitutional symptoms, (iii) Some degree of tenderness, (iv) Redness of overlying skin.
b. *Intraoral:* (i) Teeth are sensitive to percussion. (ii) Teeth are mobile, (iii) Dysphagia, and (iv) Moderate trismus.

Incision and drainage (Figs 40.26A and B): An incision of about 1.5 to 2 cm length is made 2 cm below lower border of mandible, in the skin creases. Skin and subcutaneous tissues are incised. A sinus forceps is

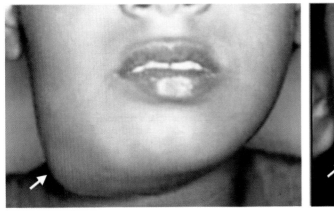
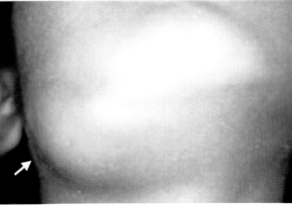

Fig. 40.25: Extraoral clinical picture of right side submandibular space involvement

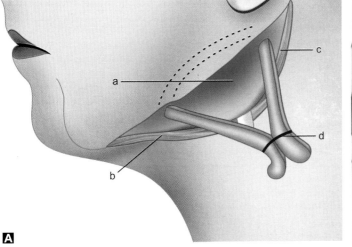

A

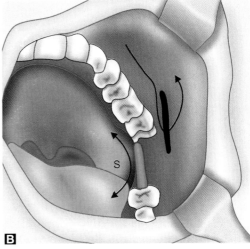

B

Figs 40.26A and B: (A) Submandibular space extraoral drainage. The drains are inserted superiorly and medially to the inferior border of the mandible.(a) Submandibular space swelling, (b) Ant. belly digastric. (c) Post. belly digastric. (d) Rubber drains secured with suture. (D) Intraoral incision for drainage of submandibular space infection (Red). Black incision line is for infratemporal space

inserted through the incision superiorly and posteriorly on the lingual side of the mandible below the mylohyoid to release pus from submandibular space. A corrugated rubber drain is inserted in the abscess cavity and is secured with a suture and dressing is applied.

Spread

i. There are no major anatomic barriers between the two submandibular and submental spaces. Hence, infection can extend into the submental space.

ii. There are no anatomical barriers, hence infection can spread extend easily across the midline, and involve the submandibular space on the contralateral side.

iii. The submandibular space communicates with sublingual space around the posterior border of mylohyoid muscle (Fig. 40.27).

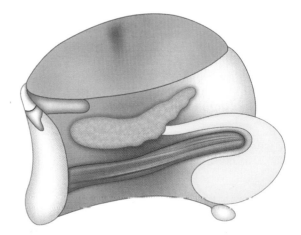

Fig. 40.27: Communication of submandibular space with sublingual space around the posterior border of mylohyoid muscle

iv. Infection can spread backwards to involve para-pharyngeal spaces.

The spread of infection can also be by direct continuity; and is influenced by the attachment of mylohyoid muscle, in relation to the level of root apices of mandibular teeth.

Differential diagnosis:

1. Secondary deposits of a malignant neoplasm or
2. Lymphoma arising in the lymph nodes of upper neck. These may undergo necrosis and present as a fluctuant swelling.
3. TB lymphadenitis.

Infiltration of surrounding tissues by neoplasms will produce swelling and induration resembling cellulitis. However, the redness of the overlying skin will be less marked as well as the degree of tenderness. Incision of the swelling, if carried out, will reveal fragments of the necrotic tissue with the liquefied neoplasm. In such cases biopsy will establish the diagnosis.

Sublingual Space

This space is a V-shaped trough lying lateral to muscles of tongue, including hyoglossus, genioglossus and geniohyoid.

Involvement: The teeth which frequently give rise to involvement of sublingual space are the mandibular incisors, canines, premolars and sometimes first molars. The apices of these teeth are superior to the mylohyoid muscle. The infection perforates lingual plate below the level of the mucosa of the floor of the mouth and passes into the sublingual space.

It is a paired space; but the two sides communicate anteriorly. This space communicates with submandibular space around the posterior border of mylohyoid muscle.

Surgical anatomy (Fig. 40.28)

Boundaries: It is covered superiorly only by the mucosa of floor of the mouth.
- *Inferiorly*: Mylohyoid muscle.
- *Laterally*: Medial side of the mandible, above the mylohyoid muscle.
- *Medially*: Hyoglossus, genioglossus and genio-hyoid muscles.
- *Posteriorly*: Hyoid bone.
- Laterally and inferiorly by mylohyoid muscle and lingual side of mandible.

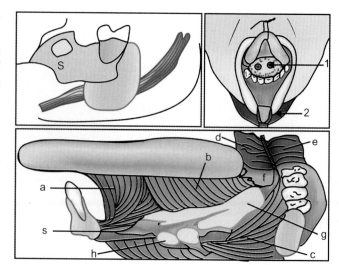

Fig. 40.28: Sublingual space anatomy: (a) genioglossus, (b) hyoglossus, (c) mylohyoid, (d) sup. constrictor, (e) buccinator, (f) styloglossus, (g) Deep part of submandibular gland, (h) Sublingual gland. (S) Sublingual space (1) Sublingual space infection intraoral swelling. (2) Submental swelling

Contents: Major contents include: Geniohyoid and genioglossus muscles, the hyoglossus muscle complex. It also contains (i) Deep part of the submandibular salivary gland and it's duct anteriorly, (ii) Sublingual salivary gland, (iii) Lingual nerve, and (iv) Hypoglossal nerve.

Clinical features (Figs 40.29A to G):

i. *Extraoral:* There is little or no swelling. The lymph nodes may be enlarged and tender. Pain and discomfort on deglutition. Speech may be affected.
ii. *Intraoral:* Firm, painful swelling seen in the floor of the mouth on the affected side. The floor of the mouth is raised. The tongue may be pushed superiorly. This will bring about airway obstruction. The ability to protrude the tongue beyond the vermillion border of upper lip is affected.

Incision and drainage (Fig. 40.30):

i. *Intraorally:* An incision is made close to the lingual cortical plate, lateral to the sublingual plica, as the important structure at this site is the sublingual nerve which is deeply placed and less likely to be damaged by this approach. The other important structures lie medial to the plica and include the Wharton's duct, sublingual artery and veins and the lingual nerve. The sinus forceps is then inserted and opened to evacuate the pus.

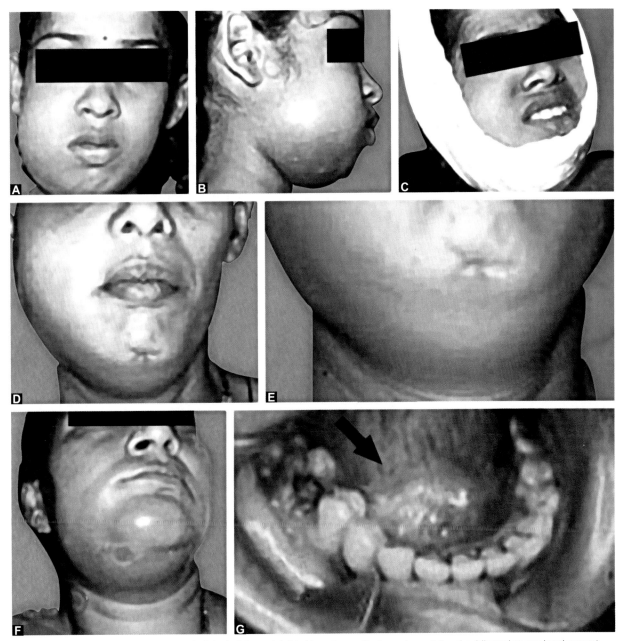

Figs 40.29A to G: (A to F) Extraoral clinical picture of right side submandibular, submental and sublingual space involvement
(G) Intraoral clinical picture of raised floor of the mouth, indicating involvement of sublingual space

ii. *Extraorally:* When both the submental and sublingual spaces contain pus, they can be drained via a skin incision placed in the submental region, pushing a closed sinus forceps through the mylohyoid muscle. Similarly, when the submandibular space is involved, a sublingual space abscess can be approached and drained through an incision in the skin overlying the submandibular space, via the submandibular space.

Spread

i. Infection always crosses the midline, and can affect the space on the opposite side.

ii. Infection from the posteroinferior part of the space, can spread around the submandibular gland into submandibular space, and again can spread posteriorly, via the tunnel under the superior constrictor for the styloglossus into the pterygomandibular and parapharyngeal spaces.

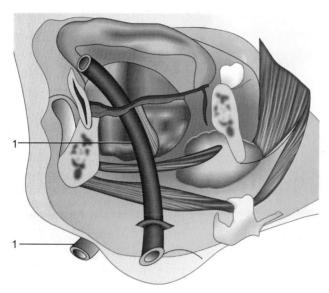

Fig. 40.30: Through and through intra to extraoral drainage of a submental and sublingual space infection. (1) bilateral through and through drains

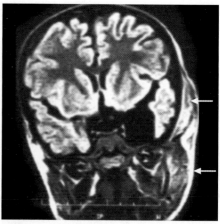

Fig. 40.31: MRI scan of a 6-year-old child suffering from left side temporal abscess due to periapical pathology of lower left 2nd deciduous molar. Ascending infection is seen after involving the masticatory space (Arrows)

iii. Infection can also spread via the lymphatics to the submental or submandibular lymph nodes.

iv. The sublingual space is separated from the sub-mental space by the mylohyoid muscle, which forms a complete diaphragm in the floor of the mouth. The spread to the submental region occurs most often as a result of lymphatic spread to submental lymph nodes. However, there are also, perforating arteries which pass through the mylohyoid to form anastomosis between sublingual and submandibular arteries which accompany the nerves to the mylohyoid. In some patients, infection can spread to the submental space through the apertures formed by these perforating arteries.

Secondary Potential Fascial Spaces

Temporal Space (Fig. 40.31)

Involvement is secondary to the initial involvement of pterygopalatine and infratemporal space.

Surgical anatomy: Temporal pouches are fascial spaces in relation to the temporalis muscle. They are two in number: (1) Superficial temporal space (2) Deep temporal space. The superficial temporal pouch lies between the temporal fascia and temporalis muscle. The deep temporal pouch lies deep to the temporalis muscle and the skull. Below the level of zygomatic arch, superficial and deep temporal pouches communicate directly with the infratemporal and pterygopalatine fossa.

Clinical features: Pain, trismus. Swelling over temporal region may or may not be present.

Incision and drainage (Fig. 40.32): Extraoral incision in temporal region, well above the hairline, 45° to zygomatic arch. The hemostat is inserted above and below the temporalis muscle.

Parotid Space (Figs 40.33 and 40.34)

Involvement: (i) The infections are either blood-borne, or occur as retrograde infections through the Stenson's duct. (ii) The gland is strongly attached to it's fascial covering, i.e parotid fascia, and there is very little intervening loose connective tissue. This makes extension of odontogenic infections into the parotid space usually very difficult. (iii) However, the gland is contiguous to submasseteric, pterygomandibular and lateral pharyngeal spaces; and on rare occasions the parotid space can be involved by an odontogenic infection from one of these spaces.

Surgical anatomy: **Boundaries**—The space is formed by splitting of the superficial layer of deep cervical fascia surrounding the parotid gland, and lies posterior to the masticatory space.

Inferiorly: Stylomandibular ligament, which separates parotid space from the mandibular space.

Contents: Parotid gland and parotid lymph nodes, facial nerve, retromandibular vein, and external carotid artery.

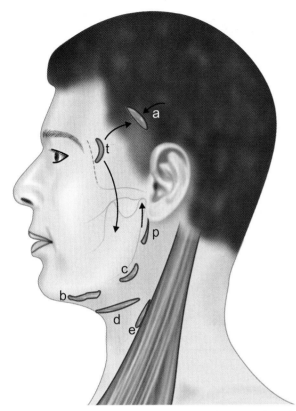

Fig. 40.32: Incisions for extraoral drainage of various deep fascial spaces infection: (a) Superficial or deep temporal, (b) Submental or submandibular, (c) Submandibular, submasseteric, or pterygoman-dibular, (d) Lateral pharyngeal and upper part of the retropharyngeal space, (e) Retropharyngeal space and carotid sheath, (t) Temporal space can be drained through this incision also, (p) Parotid abscess

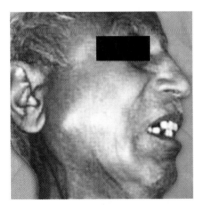

Fig. 40.33: Parotid space abscess

Clinical features:

i. Severe pain, which may be referred to the ear; and is accentuated by eating. Because of the pain associated with eating, these patients do not consume adequate

fluids, and hence, these patients may get severely dehydrated.

ii. Presence of swelling over the masseter muscle, extending from the level of zygomatic arch to lower border of mandible. Anteriorly, it ends at the anterior border of ramus of the mandible, and posteriorly, it extends into the retromandibular region. Ear lobe seems to be everted or lifted up.

iii. There is escape of pus from the Stenson's duct, when the gland is milked.

Incision and drainage: The drainage requires an external approach. A retromandibular incision is used, because the pus is usually not in a single pool, but is located in numerous loculations within glandular parenchyma and exploration of a wider area is often necessary to evaluate all the sites involved. An incision is placed in the skin behind the posterior border of mandible extending from the level of the inferior aspect of the lobule of the ear to just above the mandible. A sinus forceps is inserted, and with blunt dissection the parotid fascia is reached. The exploration of various parts of the gland is accomplished with the forceps. A rubber drain is inserted and secured to skin with a suture.

Spread: Communications between parotid space and submandibular space exist via anterior branches of posterior facial vein. Infection can spread to sub-masseteric, pterygomandibular and lateral pharyngeal spaces.

Masticatory Spaces (Figs 40.35 and 40.36)

Masticatory spaces comprise of the following spaces: (i) Pterygomandibular, (ii) Submasseteric, (iii) tempo-ral—superficial temporal, and (iv) deep temporal or subtemporal spaces. All these spaces are well differentiated, and communicate with other fascial spaces; such as buccal, submandibular, and para pharyngeal spaces. Infection from one compartment, may spread to any of the other compartments. Amongst the muscles of mastication, only the outer surface of masseter and inner surface of medial pterygoid muscles are covered by true fascia.

Masticatory spaces are divided into two by the ramus of mandible:

i. Lateral compartment
ii. Medial compartment.

Masticatory space is formed by splitting of investing fascia into superficial and deep layers; which define the lateral and medial extent of space.

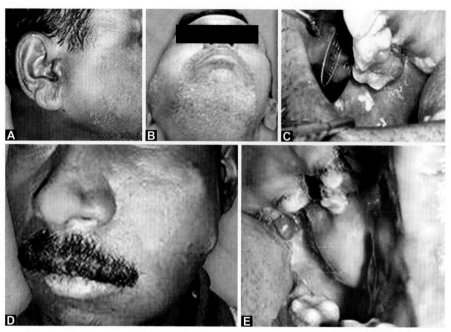

Figs 40.34A to E: Parotid space involvement: (A) Lateral view of the face, (B) Front view showing involvement of R parotid space, (C) Intraoral view showing R cheek swelling and pus discharge from parotid duct, (D and E) Extraoral and intraoral views of L parotid space involvement in another patient

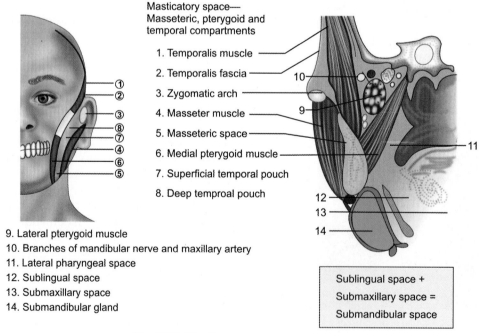

Masticatory space—
Masseteric, pterygoid and
temporal compartments

1. Temporalis muscle
2. Temporalis fascia
3. Zygomatic arch
4. Masseter muscle
5. Masseteric space
6. Medial pterygoid muscle
7. Superficial temporal pouch
8. Deep temproal pouch
9. Lateral pterygoid muscle
10. Branches of mandibular nerve and maxillary artery
11. Lateral pharyngeal space
12. Sublingual space
13. Submaxillary space
14. Submandibular gland

Sublingual space +
Submaxillary space =
Submandibular space

Fig. 40.35: Masticatory space surgical anatomy

The superficial layer lies along lateral surfaces of masseter and lower half of temporalis muscles. Superiorly, the superficial layer fuses with periosteum of zygoma and temporalis fascia. The deep layer passes along the medial surface of pterygoid muscles, before attaching to base of skull superiorly.

The masticatory space borders the number of other spaces, which include: the parotid space posteriorly,

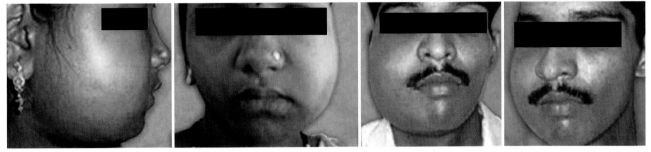

Fig. 40.36: Clinical extraoral picture of masticatory space odontogenic infection in two different patients

parapharyngeal space medially, and the submandibular and sublingual spaces inferiorly.

Submasseteric Space

Masseter consists of three layers, which are fused anteriorly, but can be easily separated posteriorly. There is potential space in the substance of the muscle between the middle and the deep heads, while the bony insertion is firm above and below, the intermediate fibers have only a loose attachment. It is possible for these fibers to be separated from bone relatively easily by the accumulation of pus at this site.

When the pus accumulates between the ramus of the mandible and the masseter muscle, it produces a submasseteric space abscess.

Involvement: Infection usually originates from the lower third molars; either resulting from (i) Pericoronitis related to vertical and distoangular third molars, or (ii) a periapical abscess spreads subperiosteally in a distal direction.

The presence of buccinator attachment probably discourages backward extension of pericoronal infection, where third molar crown is anterior to this muscle barrier.

The extension of abscess inferiorly is limited by the firm attachment of masseter to lower border of ramus of mandible. The forward spread beyond the anterior border of ramus is restricted by the anterior tail of the tendon of temporalis, which is inserted into the anterior border of the ramus.

Surgical anatomy—Boundaries:
- *Anterior:* Anterior border of masseter muscle and buccinator.
- *Posterior:* Parotid gland, and posterior part of masseter.

- *Inferior:* Attachment of the masseter to the lower border of mandible.
- *Medial:* Lateral surface of the ramus of mandible.
- *Lateral:* Medial surface of the masseter muscle.
- *Contents:* Masseteric nerve, superficial temporal artery, and transverse facial artery.

It contains muscles of mastication; masseter, lateral and medial pterygoids, and insertion of temporalis muscle. It also contains ramus and posterior part of mandible; and branches of mandibular division of trigeminal nerve. These branches include: buccal, lingual, and inferior alveolar nerves.

Clinical features: External facial swelling is moderate in size; and is confined to the outline of the masseter muscle, i.e. the swelling is seen extending from the lower border of the mandible to the zygomatic arch; and anteriorly to the anterior border of masseter; and posteriorly to the posterior border of the mandible.

There is tenderness over the angle of the mandible. There is almost complete limitation of mouth opening. Fluctuation may be absent; and if present, cannot be elicited, because the muscle lies between the pus and the surface. There is pyrexia and malaise.

The ramus of the mandible is more dependent upon blood supply from the overlying muscle than the body of the mandible, which is supplied by inferior alveolar artery. As a result, ischemic changes may take place in that part of bone denuded by periosteum by a submasseteric abscess so that a low-grade osteomyelitis of lateral cortical plate may occur with sequestrum formation. Often submasseteric infection leads to subperiosteal new bone deposition beneath the periosteum. Necrosis of the muscle can also occur.

Incision and drainage: There are two approaches:
1. *Intraoral approach:* An incision is made vertically over the lower part of anterior border of the ramus

of the mandible, deep to the bone. A sinus forceps are passed along the lateral surface of the ramus downwards and backwards and the pus is drained. The drain is inserted and secured with a suture. The abscess is usually situated below the level of incision, and not at a point of dependent drainage, and hence the drainage may be inefficient.

2. *Extraoral approach:* When the mouth cannot be opened, an incision is placed in the skin behind the angle of the mandible to open the abscess by Hilton's method. A rubber drain is inserted and secured in position with a suture. Dressing is applied.

Pterygomandibular Space (Table 40.4)

Involvement: (i) The situation most frequently responsible for involvement of this space, is the pericoronitis related to the mandibular third molar. (ii) Infection can also be produced by a contaminated needle used for an inferior alveolar nerve block. (iii) Infection, at times, can originate from a maxillary third molar, following a posterior superior alveolar nerve block injection.

Surgical anatomy (Fig. 40.37)—Boundaries:

- *Lateral:* Medial surface of ramus of mandible.
- *Medial:* Lateral surface of medial pterygoid muscle.
- *Posterior:* Parotid gland (deep portion).
- *Anterior:* Pterygomandibular raphae.
- *Superior:* Lateral pterygoid muscle forms roof to the pterygomandibular space. The space, just below the lateral pterygoid muscle communicates with the pharyngeal spaces.
- *Contents:* Lingual nerve, mandibular nerve, inferior alveolar or mandibular artery. Mylohyoid nerve and vessels. Loose areolar connective tissue.

Clinical features: Even the established cases of pterygomandibular space infections, do not cause much swelling of face over the submandibular region. However, there is severe degree of limitation of mouth opening. Tenderness can be elicited over the area of swollen soft tissues medial to anterior border of ramus of the mandible. Dysphagia is present. Medial displacement of the lateral wall of the pharynx, redness and edema of the area around the third molar. Midline of the palate is displaced to the unaffected side and the uvula is swollen. Difficulty in breathing.

Incision and drainage (Fig. 40.38): The abscess usually tends to point at the anterior border of the ramus of the mandible and drainage can be easily done by intraoral route.

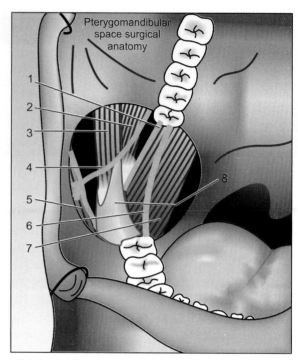

Fig. 40.37: (1) Inferior alveolar nerve, (2) Deep tendon temporalis, (3) Superficial tendon temporalis, (4) Buccal nerve, (5) Buccinator muscle (cut), (6) Lingual nerve, (7) Medial pterygoid muscle, (8) Ramus of the mandible

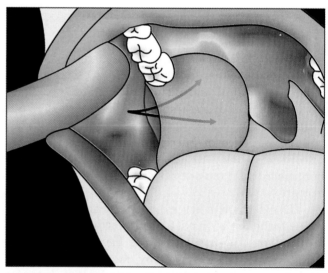

Fig. 40.38: Intraoral incision for draining the pterygomandibular or lateral pharyngeal space abscess. Dissection is done posteriorly for pterygomandibular space. For lateral pharyngeal space, dissection is done first medially and then posteriorly

a. *Intraoral:* A vertical incision, approximately 1.5 cm in length, is made on the anterior and medial aspect of the ramus of mandible. A sinus forceps in inserted in the abscess cavity, opened and closed and

Table 40.4: Main features of pterygomandibular, lateral pharyngeal and peritonsillar space			
	Pterygomandibular space	*Lateral pharyngeal space*	*Peritonsillar space*
Anatomy	Between mandible and medial pterygoid	Between medial pterygoid and superior constrictor	Between superior constrictor and mucous membrane
Limitation of opening	Extreme	Moderate	Some
External swelling	Little	None	None
Swelling in mouth and throat	Swelling over medial aspect of anterior border of ramus	Swelling over pillars of fauces, little swelling on superior constrictor	Swelling over pillars of fauces and most of superior constrictor

withdrawn. The pus is evacuated, a rubber drain is introduced and is secured in position with a suture.

b. *Extraoral:* An incision is taken in the skin below the angle of the mandible. A sinus forceps is inserted towards the medial side of the ramus in an upward and backward direction. Pus is evacuated and the drain is inserted from an intraoral approach and sutured in position.

Spread

i. Occasionally, infection may spread superiorly along the medial surface of ramus to involve the infratemporal fossa and beneath the temporal fascia.

ii. The infection can spread posteriorly to lateral pharyngeal space and then to retropharyngeal space.

iii. It can also spread around the front of the ramus of the mandible to involve the buccal space.

iv. It can also spread around the front of the ramus of the mandible extending anteroinferiorly below the lower border and under the superior constrictor to involve the submandibular space.

Parapharyngeal Spaces

They include lateral pharyngeal and retropharyngeal spaces. These are the major pathways for spread of head and neck infections.

These spaces form a "ring" around pharynx; and together form a pathway for spread of orofacial infections in neck and mediastinum. The parapharyngeal spaces communicate directly with both submandibular space, anteroinferiorly; and retromandibular space posteriorly.

Lateral Pharyngeal Space (Figs 40.39 and 40.40)

It is a potential cone shaped space or cleft with its base uppermost at the base of skull and its apex at the greater horn of the hyoid bone. The space is divided into two by the styloid process, as anterior and posterior compartments. Infection of this space is extremely serious owing to the intimate relationship with the carotid sheath.

Involvement

i. It is involved from an abscess extending backwards from mandibular third molar area

ii. By backward spread from sublingual, submandibular and pterygomandibular space infections.

iii. Lateral spread from tonsillar abscess.

iv. Surgical displacement of mandibular third molar distally under the lingual flap and backwards into the lateral pharyngeal space. Similarly, a third molar root may get dislodged into the space through a hole in the lingual plate.

The boundary walls of the space do not permit easy communication with the adjacent spaces. Infection passes most easily between lateral pharyngeal space and submandibular space by tracking along the styloglossus muscle.

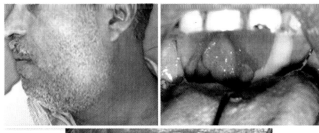
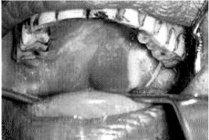

Fig. 40.39: Lateral pharyngeal space involvement along with peritonsillar abscess

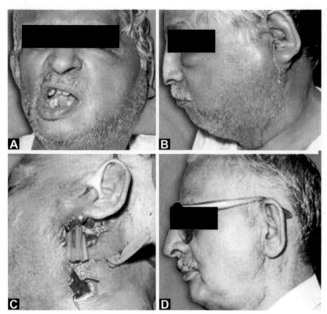

Figs 40.40A to D: (A and B) Clinical picture of a patient with lateral pharyngeal and pterygomandibular space infection (C) Extraoral drains are in place in the anterior and posterior compartments of lateral pharyngeal space, additional intraoral drain was put in the pterygomandibular space, (D) Patient after complete recovery

There is a weak zone in the posterior part of the fascia around the submandibular salivary gland, medial to stylomandibular ligament, and rupture of a submandibular abscess into the parapharyngeal space at this point may result in rapid onset of respiratory embarrassment.

Surgical anatomy:

a. *Boundaries:* Superiorly, base of the skull. Petrous portion of the temporal bone with foramen lacerum and jugular foramen.
    • Inferiorly, hyoid bone (submandibular gland and posterior belly of digastric).
    • Anteriorly, bounded by pterygomandibular raphe.
    • Laterally, bounded by the ascending ramus of mandible, insertion of medial pterygoid muscle, and medial surface of deep lobe of parotid gland along with their covering fascia.
    • Medially, bounded by pharyngeal wall, (palatal muscles at the level of nasopharynx; and pharyngeal constrictors (superior and middle) and stylopharyngeus; covered by buccopharyngeal fascia; at the level of oropharynx.

• Posteriorly, bounded by styloid muscle, and upper part of carotid sheath, prevertebral fascia, with foramen lacerum and jugular foramen.

These spaces separate the muscles of mastication from muscles of deglutition.

Some surgeons include a downward continuation of this compartment around carotid sheath; as far as the thoracic inlet. Thus, they include inferior constrictor and esophagus in the medial wall, the lateral lobe of thyroid gland as an anterior relation, and sternocleidomastoid and superior belly of omohyoid in the lateral wall.

b. *Contents:*
    i.   *Anterior compartment:* Lymph nodes, ascending pharyngeal, facial artery, loose areolar connective tissue.
    ii. *Posterior compartment:* Carotid sheath (internal jugular vein, internal carotid artery, and vagus nerve), glossopharyngeal nerve, spinal accessory nerve, hypoglossal nerve, and cervical sympathetic trunk.

Clinical features: Clinical picture is grave, because of generalized septicemia and respiratory embarrassment due to edema of the larynx.

General constitutional symptoms in the form of malaise and pyrexia are present.

a. *Anterior compartment:*
    i.   *Extraoral:* Brawny induration of the face, above the angle of the mandible. This induration may extend downward to the submandibular region, as well as, upwards to the parotid region on the ipsilateral side.
    ii. *Intraoral:* The anterior part of the lateral pharyngeal wall may be swollen; that pushes the soft palate and the palatine tonsil towards the midline. Marked trismus may be present. Severe pain arising from the collection of pus between the medial pterygoid and superior constrictor. Dysphagia is present.

b. *Posterior compartment:* The clinical picture is dominated by septicemia. Usually little or no trismus is present. Slight pain is present.

External swelling is less extensive. There is subtle swelling in lateral neck, just above the hyoid bone, between posterior belly of digastric and sternocleidomastoid muscle externally. This is the area where lateral pharyngeal space is closest to the skin.

Internal swelling involves the lateral wall of pharynx behind the palatopharyngeal arch.

Incision and drainage: Extraoral approach—An incision is made along the anterior border of sternocleidomastoid muscle, extending from below the angle of the mandible, to the middle third of submandibular gland. The fascia behind the gland is incised and a curved hemostat is inserted and carefully directed medially behind the mandible, as well as superiorly and slightly posteriorly until the abscess cavity is reached. A rubber drain is inserted and is secured to the skin with a suture.

A 3 to 5 cm incision is placed low over the submandibular space just superior and parallel to the hyoid bone. The posterior end should lie just over the anterior border of sternocleidomastoid muscle. The dissection is carried through skin, subcutaneous tissue, superficial fascia, and platysma muscle to expose the superficial or anterior layer of deep cervical fascia. The fascia is exposed sufficiently to identify submandibular gland and the posterior belly of digastric muscle. The surgeon will be able to identify by finger dissection and palpation, the angle of the mandible, hyoid bone, sternocleidomastoid muscle. The dissection is then carried further just posterior to the posterior belly of digastric muscle in a superior, medial, and posterior direction. The dissection of lateral pharyngeal space is completed when the surgeon is able to palpate the endotracheal tube medially, the ipsilateral transverse processes of the vertebrae posteromedially, and the carotid sheath posterolaterally. The surgeon should avoid rupturing the pharyngeal mucosa by using only gentle force during finger dissection, as the infected tissues are quite friable.

Intraoral approach. A vertical incision is placed over the pterygomandibular raphe. A sinus forceps or curved hemostat is passed through the pterygomandibular raphae along the medial surface of the mandible, medial to the medial pterygoid and just lateral to the superior constrictor is then divided posteriorly to the pus pocket.

Spread: Infection can spread in the following manner:
1. It can either spread upwards through various foramina such as, foramen ovale, foramen lacerum, and jugular foramen, present at the base of the skull, producing brain abscess, meningitis or sinus thrombosis.
2. It can also spread downwards into the carotid sheath towards the mediastinum; a pathway which Mosher called the "Lincoln's highway" of the neck.

Retropharyngeal Space: Prevertebral Space

It is a potential midline space between the pharyngo-basilar fascia, which attaches the pharyngeal constrictors to the base of skull, and prevertebral fascia.

Involvement: The space is involved by an extension of infection from the lateral pharyngeal space.

Surgical anatomy: Boundaries
- Laterally, carotid sheath.
- The retropharyngeal space is continuous with retro-esophageal space into the posterior mediastinum to the level of sixth thoracic vertebra.
- There are no midline attachments in the retropharyngeal space; thereby, permitting unimpeded inferior extension of inflammatory and neoplastic processes into mediastinum.

Clinical features: There is usually a preceding or concurrent acute infection of the throat. Patient will complain of painful deglutition, and if the swelling is marked or in the lower portion of the pharynx, obstructive symptoms such as snoring, choking or even dyspnea and stertorous breathing may occur. A unilateral cervical adenitis on the affected side is always seen. The voice is same as in quinsy.

Incision and drainage: The space can be safely divided into two for the convenience of description:
(a) Suprahyoid portion, and (b) Infrahyoid portion.
a. *Suprahyoid portion:* The suprahyoid portion of retropharyngeal space can be approached by using the same incision described for lateral pharyngeal space. The space is approached through the lateral pharyngeal space, hence the dissection is the same, until the lateral pharyngeal space is further explored by blunt finger dissection. The dissection is continued until the surgeon is able to palpate the contralateral transverse processes of the vertebrae, the endotracheal tube from its posterior aspect, and if necessary the opposite carotid artery.
b. *Infrahyoid portion:* If the space is involved below the hyoid bone, then the posterior end of the low submandibular incision described above is extended inferiorly along the anterior border of sternocleidomastoid muscle. As the dissection passes deep to anterior layer of deep cervical

fascia, the sternocleidomastoid muscle is retracted posterolaterally to expose the carotid sheath. The loose connective tissue lying between the carotid sheath and the esophagus is bluntly dissected medially and posteriorly to expose the visceral fascia, which surrounds the trachea, esophagus and thyroid gland. Blunt dissection with finger is used to follow the visceral fascia into the retropharyngeal space. Multiple soft drains are then placed in the superior and inferior portions of the retropharyngeal space as well as in the lateral pharyngeal space.

Peritonsillar Abscess (Quinsy) (see Fig. 40.39)

It is a localized infection in the connective tissue bed between the tonsil and the superior constrictor muscle, between the anterior and posterior pillars of fauces.

Involvement

i. Infection coming from the depth of the tonsillar crypt or supratonsillar fossa.
ii. As a complication of acute pericoronal abscess in which case the abscess points near the lower pole of the tonsil.

Clinical features:

i. Patient looks ill, anoxic and dehydrated.
ii. Pain on one side of the throat radiating to the ear.
iii. Dysphagia
iv. Limitation of mouth may not be pronounced.
v. Speech is difficult, especially, in bilateral cases and a peculiar muffled "hot potato in mouth" voice is characteristic.
vi. Drooling of saliva.
vii. When the abscess is fully developed; a large tense swelling of anterior pillar of fauces, and a bulge in the soft palate on the affected side, which in extreme cases reaches the midline; and pushes the uvula downwards and forwards, until it impinges against the opposite tonsil.
viii. Coated tongue with marked fetor oris.

Incision and drainage: It can be achieved by using a guarded knife and sinus forceps, which are inserted into the most prominent part of the soft palate, where the fluctuation is the maximal.

Spread: Edema may eventually affect the base of the tongue, epiglottis and aryepiglottic fold. In 3 to 5 days duration, the mass becomes fluctuant and ruptures by pointing usually through the anterior tonsillar pillar.

Pericoronitis/Pericoronal Abscess

The meaning of the word "peri" means, surrounding, "coronos" means pertaining to crown, and "itis" means inflammation. The meaning of the word would be inflammation of the surrounding tissues of the tooth.

Definition: The definition would be an inflammatory process involving the soft tissue covering of the crown of a partially erupted or unerupted teeth.

Etiology: It is usually seen in teeth, which are prevented from eruption for prolonged time, such as malpositioned or impacted teeth, mostly mandibular third molars.

Bilateral concurrent pericoronitis predisposes infectious mononucleosis, or Vincent's infection.

Trauma to the overlying gingivae from the cusps of an opposing tooth is the most common etiology associated with inflammation due to bacterial invasion.

It can be classified into following stages: (a) Acute, (b) Subacute, and (c) Chronic.

Many pericoronal infections are suppurative and some are ulcerative.

Classical ulcerative pericoronitis is due to Vincent's infection, acute herpetic gingivostomatitis may start around the lower 3rd molar and spread forward and backwards onto the fauces and soft palate.

Clinical features:

a. *Acute:* Well localized dull pain, swollen red tender gingival pad, pus discharge from underneath the gingival pad, fetor oris, indentations of cusps of upper teeth, slight discomfort on swallowing, restriction of oral opening, enlarged, tender submandibular lymph glands on the affected side.
   Facial swelling, limitation of oral opening, severe throbbing pain, interfering sleep, discomfort on swallowing.
   Constitutional symptoms: Pyrexia, malaise, and anorexia.
   Regional lymph nodes are palpable, enlarged and tender.
   If left untreated, most likely to spread to adjacent tissue spaces.
b. *Subacute—Clinical features:* Well localized dull pain, swollen, red, tender gum pad, pus discharge, fetor oris, indentations of cusps of upper teeth, slight discomfort on swallowing, difficulty in oral

opening, enlarged, tender submandibular lymph glands on the affected side.

c. *Chronic* recurrent episodes of infection. Clinical features: (i) Asymptomatic. (ii) Occasional mild discomfort/bad taste due to pus discharge, and (iii) Subacute or acute exacerbations.

Spread: The pericoronal infection, if left untreated can spread to the following regions:

i. It can extend submucosally and form a vestibular abscess against mandibular second or third molars; and may discharge as intraoral sinus.

ii. It can extend on the outer surface of buccinator causing buccal space abscess.

iii. It can extend into the submandibular, pterygomandibular and submasseteric spaces.

iv. Rarely, it can extend down to lower border of mandible behind the depressor anguli oris muscle; and burst through the skin (if not incised).

POSSIBLE UNTOWARD OR LIFE THREATENING COMPLICATIONS OF OROFACIAL INFECTION

Which may be classified as follows:

1. Those related to the lower jaw
   a. Ludwig's angina.
   b. Descending deep cellulitis of the neck, resulting in mediastinitis.
   c. Carotid sheath invasion.
2. Those related to the upper jaw
   a. Intracranial complications, with possibilities of cavernous sinus thrombosis, brain abscess, dural meningitis and osteomyelitis of the skull.
   b. Retrobulbar cellulitis with possibility of blindness.

Ludwig's Angina

Historical background and definition: It is the name given to a massive, firm, brawny cellulitis/induration, and acute, toxic stage, involving simultaneously, the submandibular, sublingual and submental spaces bilaterally. It was first described by Wilhelm Friedreich Von Ludwig (1836). As the definition suggests, only the bilateral involvement of above-mentioned spaces is considered to be classical, disease entity. All other types of presentations, though massive are not considered as Ludwig's angina.

The term 'Ludwig's angina' was coined by Camerer in 1837, who presented cases which included classic

description of the entity as done in the previous year by WF Ludwig. The word "angina" is derived from the Latin word "angere", meaning suffocation or choking sensation; and the word "Ludwig" comes from the person to whom the credit goes for its description. Interestingly, Ludwig died of throat inflammation in 1865.

Von Ludwig described the classical features of the disease and presented a case of Franklin N.N. whom he treated successfully.

The condition had established its unique identity in general medical personnel with three "F"s as: —it was to be feared, —it rarely becomes fluctuant, and —it was often fatal.

Many terminologies were used for this condition which include:

1. *Marbus strangulatorius:* It is so called, because of the choking effect, which the victim experiences
2. *Angina maligna*
3. *Garrotillo:* It is the Spanish version for Hangman's noose.

Etiology: The following causes can be attributed to Ludwig's angina:

1. *Odontogenic:* This is the cause in majority of cases (90% in some studies). It can cause infections in various other forms:
   - Acute dentoalveolar abscess
   - Acute periodontal abscess
   - Acute pericoronal abscess.
   - Acute dentoalveolar abscess: *The most common teeth involved are mandibular second and third molars.*
   - *Acute periodontal abscess:* Deep abscess may involve sublingual spaces.
   - *Pericoronal abscess:* in relation to erupting mandible third molars, which can extend to the following spaces:
     i. Submandibular space
     ii. Buccal space
     iii. Sublingual space
     iv. Pterygomandibular space.
   - Infected mandibular cyst also can spread to form Ludwig's angina.
2. *Iatrogenic:* Use of a contaminated needle for giving local anesthesia.
3. *Traumatic injuries to orofacial region:* These can be in the form of: (a) Mandibular fractures, the chances of developing Ludwig's angina are more, if the fracture is compounded and comminuted, (b) Deep

lacerations or penetrating injuries such as punctured wounds.

4. *Osteomyelitis* secondary to compound mandibular fractures; or acute exacerbation of chronic osteomyelitis of mandible may develop into Ludwig's angina.

5. *Submandibular and sublingual sialadenitis:* Acute or chronic infection from these glands.

6. *Secondary infections of oral malignancies:* The associated malignancies of the region may give rise to secondary infection, leading to the condition.

7. *Miscellaneous causes:* It includes rare causes such as:
   a. Infection in the tonsils or pharynx such as purulent tonsillitis, etc.
   b. Foreign bodies such as fish bone, etc.
   c. Oral soft tissue lacerations.

8. Cervical lymphoid tissues.

Pathology: The condition is a cellulitis—a diffuse inflammation of soft tissues which is not circumscribed or confined to one area, but in contrast to the abscess, tends to spread through tissue spaces and along fascial planes.

Such type of spreading infection occurs in the presence of organisms that produce significant amounts of hyaluronidase and fibrinolysins, which act to break down or dissolve, respectively hyaluronic acid and fibrin. Streptococci, being the potent producers of hyaluronidase are always associated with classical or true Ludwig's angina.

Microbiology: A plethora of micro-organisms has been implicated as the causative agents of this conditions. Previously, it was thought that, the streptococci and mixed oral flora, were the commonly reported micro-organisms. Contemporarily, the reports have demonstrated presence of staphylococci, streptococci, gram negative enteric micro-organisms, such as *E. coli* and Pseudomonas; and anaerobes including Bacteroides (*B. melaninogenicus, B. oralis,* and *B. corrodens*), anaerobic streptococci, Peptostreptococcus and fusospirochaetes.

The isolation of these organisms does not indicate that there is changing oral flora; but are due to employment of sophisticated and modern culture techniques.

In early stages, with almost no putrefaction, the disease shows mixed aerobic and anaerobic infection. In later stages, where frank putrefaction exists, when the infection gets localized, the infection becomes more anaerobic and the bacteria found are almost anaerobic.

Involvement: Most cases originate in association with mandibular second and third molars. A possible explanation to this can be given by evaluating the anatomical relationship of these teeth and the involved spaces.

The bone around these teeth is usually thicker on the buccal aspect than lingual side. The apices of these teeth are placed below the mylohyoid line of mylohyoid muscle, so that infection tends to spread primarily to submandibular space. Hence, the submandibular space plays a vital role in development and progress of the disease. The subsequent spread of the disease is determined by the muscles in the area.

The condition usually follows a submandibular space infection caused by a periapical infection, or pericoronitis around mandibular third molar. The infection then spreads to the sublingual space on the same side, around the deep part of the submandibular gland. The submental space is involved by lymphatic spread. The condition can also occur in converse manner, i.e. by spread from the sublingual spaces to the submandibular spaces (Fig. 40.41).

Clinical features: The following signs and symptoms are present with varying degree of severity (Fig. 40.42):
a. *General examination:* It includes: (i) General constitutional symptoms: Patient looks toxic, very ill and dehydrated. There is pyrexia, anorexia, chills, and malaise. (ii) Marked pyrexia (iii) Difficulty in swallowing (Dysphagia) (iv) Impaired speech, and hoarseness of voice.
b. *Regional examination:* Extraoral examination (Figs 40.43 and 40.44).
   i. Firm/Hard brawny (boardlike, woody hard) swelling in the bilateral submandibular and submental regions, which soon extends down the anterior part of the neck to the clavicles. Swelling is nonpitting, minimally or nonfluctuant associated with severe tenderness. Classically shows ill-defined borders with induration.
   ii. Severe muscle spasm may lead to trismus with restricted mouth opening and also jaw movements. Typically mouth remains open due to edema of sublingual tissues leading to raised tongue almost touching the palatal vault. In extreme circumstances, tongue may actually protrude from the mouth; the tongue movements are reduced.
   iii. Airway obstruction.

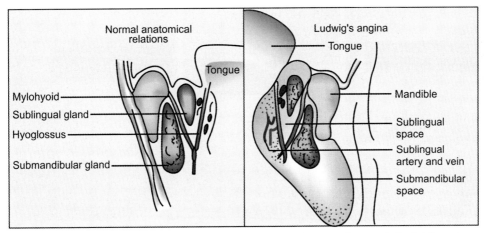

Fig. 40.41: Comparison of normal anatomical relations to involvement of spaces in Ludwig's angina

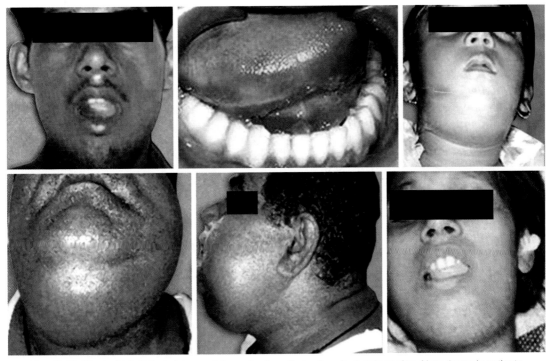

Fig. 40.42: The typical clinical pictures of the patients suffering from Ludwig's angina. Note the toxic patients, with firm, brawny induration with raised floor of the mouth, tongue protruding out and elevated

iv. Respiratory rate may be seen to be raised; breathing being shallow with accessory muscles of respiration being used.

v. There may be dilation of alae nasi, raising of thoracic inlet by the scalencs and sternocleidomastoid muscles and indrawing of the tissues above the clavicle. Respiratory rate may be seen to be raised; breathing being shallow with accessory muscles of respiration being used.

vi. Cyanosis may occur due the progressive hypoxia.

vii. Fatal death may occur in untreated case of Ludwig's angina within 10 to 24 hours due to asphyxia.

c. Intraorally, the swelling develops rapidly, which involves the sublingual tissues, and distends or

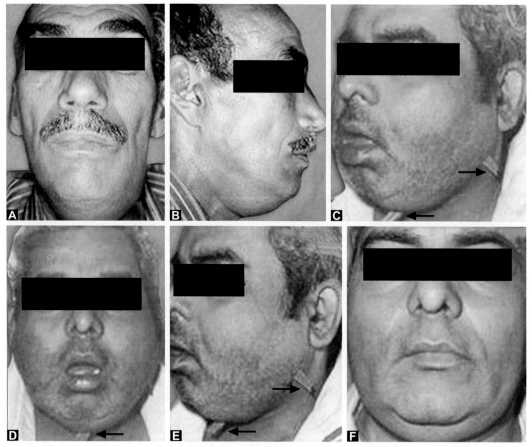

Figs 40.43A to F: (A and B) Clinical picture of Ludwig's angina (C to E) Drainage, decompression of Ludwig's angina patient with multiple corrugated rubber drains in place, (F) Patient after complete recovery

raises the floor of mouth, woody edema of the floor of the mouth and tongue (ii) Tongue may be raised against palate; (iii) Increased salivation, stiffness of tongue movements, difficulty in swallowing (iv) Backward spread of infection leads to edema of glottis, resulting in respiratory obstruction/embarrassment. Stridor being the alarming sign of this fatal extension needing emergency intervention to keep airway patent.

There is reduced control of muscles and jaw posture—salivation is excessive and saliva may be even seen drooling.

Part of the tongue may get pushed backward making swallowing even liquid very difficult or even impossible. Oral opening and jaw movements may be reduced.

Progressive dyspnea is caused by backward spread of infection, until in the untreated case, edema of the glottis causes a complete respiratory obstruction.

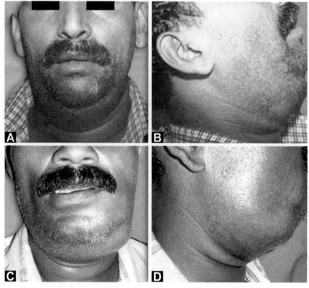

Figs 40.44A to D: Severe stage of Ludwig's angina

Spread

i. From the sublingual spaces, the infection may spread backwards in the substance of the tongue in the cleft between the hyoglossus and genioglossus muscles along the course of sublingual artery. By this route the infection reaches the region of epiglottis and produces swelling around the laryngeal inlet.

ii. Due to anatomical continuity of various spaces with submandibular space, the infection may track to submasseteric, and pterygomandibular spaces; and more posteriorly, parapharyngeal, paratonsillar spaces; and worsening airway compromise.

iii. Infection from the submandibular region, can spread downwards along and beneath the investing layer of deep cervical fascia, towards clavicle and subsequently to mediastinum (Fig. 40.45).

iv. Uncommonly, infection can spread below and reach close to carotid sheath, pterygopalatine fossa, leading to cavernous sinus thrombosis with subsequent meningitis.

Fate of Ludwig's angina: Ludwig's angina, if untreated, can be fatal within 12 to 24 hours; death arising from asphyxia. Established cases may become more complicated with involvement of other spaces. The other causes of death include: septicemia/septic shock, mediastinitis, and aspiration pneumonia, which are also caused by the complications of the disease.

With the introduction of newer antibiotics, the mortality rate has been significantly dropped, from almost 75 to 4 percent. However the possible fatal outcome of new cases cannot be ignored.

Principles of treatment: It should be taken as a life threatening emergency situation. It is best treated by aggressive intervention.

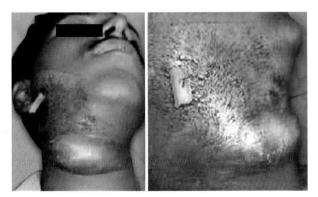

Fig. 40.45: Descending spread of infection in Ludwig's angina patient

The treatment is based on the combination of the following factors: (1) Early diagnosis, (2) Maintenance of patent airway, (3) Intense and prolonged antibiotic therapy, (4) Extraction of offending teeth, and (5) Surgical drainage or decompression of fascial spaces.

The general anesthesia should be given to such patients by a skilled and experienced anesthesiologist. The endotracheal tube should be passed with the help of fiberoptic laryngoscope, while the patient is conscious and wide awake.

With the use of IV anesthetic agents used for induction, the patient maintain airway by the vigorous use of voluntary muscles, together with the accessory muscles of respiration. When a general anesthetic is used, this voluntary control is lost. Further, when the patient becomes unconscious, there is a massive increase in the edema; the airway becomes occluded; and it becomes quite difficult to pass an endotracheal tube as the pharynx billows inwards.

A nasopharyngeal airway and a tracheostomy set should be kept ready by the side of the bed of the patient of Ludwig's angina. Evaluation of blood gases gives an indication of the degree of respiratory obstruction and may indicate the need for tracheostomy even if the patient is not in distress.

Airway maintenance: This condition is considered to be fatal. Death can occur from asphyxia rather than the infection itself, leading to septicemia and shock. Hence, it is advisable to observe the patient for respiratory obstruction and restlessness. In case of respiratory embarrassment the following points should be considered for using artificial airway.

1. It can cause trauma and resultant inflammation may worsen the edema and airway obstruction

2. Chances of inadvertently rupturing any pointing or superficial abscess in the pharyngeal wall are high as it is a blind procedure and may itself lead to aspiration of pus and instant death.

Intubation of the patient: Blind intubation should be avoided. Nasoendotracheal intubation is far more reliable and almost predictable and should be preferred.

Surgical airway: It may be required in case of severe upper respiratory obstruction.

Laryngotomy, cricothyroidotomy (tracheotomy) are always preferred over tracheostomy or rather emergency tracheostomy is avoided because of:

1. Identification of landmarks that may be required before it, is most of the time quite difficult due to associated massive edema and tissue distortion.

2. The surgery itself may lead to spread of infection to deeper tissues due to additional incision required.

3. There are high chances of getting pneumonia as a sequelae of tracheostomy which itself is a life threatening condition (Aird 1957).

4. Tracheal stenosis is observed in 25 to 50 percent of cases following tracheostomy.

Use of Cuffed Endotracheal Tube

• Avoid sedatives, narcotic agents that may deteriorate respiration.

• Degree of respiratory obstruction can be better evaluated using pulse oximeter and evaluating blood gases. It is better to rely on these parameters as clinical picture may vary from patient to patient and may even mask extreme airway obstruction.

• *Anesthesia:* As a general rule, it is always better to use local anesthesia for surgical intervention. Local infiltration with 2 percent lidocaine with adrenaline into skin and superficial tissues of neck is sufficient to fulfill the need for surgical intervention. In patients, who are already intubated, GA can be considered after evaluating its advantages over local anesthesia.

• Intravenous analgesics can be supplemented to relieve pain.

• **Surgical intervention:** It has two aims: (i) Remove the cause, (ii) Surgical decompression: Decompression of the spaces involved.

• *Removal of the cause:* Removing the offending tooth may facilitate evacuation of pus present in close vicinity of the tooth without any special surgical intervention.

• In most cases of Ludwig's angina, small amount of pus is always associated with the offending tooth close to its lingual cortex.

• The initial stage of Ludwig's angina or those cases which progress to Ludwig's angina are seen to be managed by simple extraction coupled with antibiotics.

Surgical Decompression

As Ludwig's angina is, in fact cellulitis, its treatment by aggressive surgical intervention is a debatable issue. The advantages of early surgical decompression include the following:

i. It reduces pressure of edematous tissues on the airway reducing respiratory embarrassment.

ii. It allows prompt drainage should suppuration develop.

iii. It allows obtaining specimen or samples for Gram staining, and culture and sensitivity, for identification of micro-organisms; and according adjustment of antibiotics later on.

iv. It allows placement of drains, which may be valuable to drain pus collection as time progresses, and irrigation of the tissues at regular intervals.

Bilateral submandibular incisions and if required a midline submental incision 1 cm below the inferior border of mandible are sufficient to drain the involved spaces.

Following aseptic technique and adequate local anesthesia, an incision is made, which divides skin, the superficial fascia, platysma, investing layer of deep fascia, geniohyoid and finally mylohyoid muscles.

To be effective, it is essential to divide deep fascia and the mylohyoid muscle, then only it will drain sublingual space. A through and through drain is placed to relieve the intense pressure of the edematous tissues on the airway. Sublingual space can be separately drained by intraoral approach if required and if oral opening permits it. Surgical drain should be secured by suturing to the margins of the incision.

In most of Ludwig's angina cases, little or no pus can be drained out by surgical intervention, as it is a cellulitis, but in later stages or during postsurgical period, profuse pus may be seen draining. Whatever may be the situation, bilateral and complete drainage or rather decompression is the key for success of surgical intervention.

Care: It should be taken to preserve or avoid trauma to: (i) Facial vessels near angle, (ii) lingual nerve, and (iii) Jugular vein, laterally below angle region.

Antibiotic Therapy

Antibiotics: Antibiotics play a vital role in managing Ludwig's angina. Usually, IV antibiotics with proper dosage and frequency are necessary.

Penicillin and its derivatives:

i. Penicillins are the first line of antibiotics in treating such infection as it covers the majority of aerobic gram positive microbial flora commonly associated with this infection. It is administered in the form of aqueous penicillin G, 2 to 4 million units, IV 4 to 6 hourly; or 500 mg six hourly orally.

ii. Semisynthetic derivatives of penicillin: Ampicillin/amoxycillin; 500 mg 6 and 8 hourly, IV and orally respectively.

iii. Cloxacillin; 500 mg orally, 8 hourly.

iv. In case of allergy to penicillin; Erythromycin 600 mg 6 to 8 hourly.

v. Gentamicin has activity against some resistant staphylococci and pseudomonas. 80 mg I.M, B.D.

vi. Clindamycin IV 300 to 600 mg 8 hourly, orally and intravenously. Its spectrum of activity includes gram positive cocci including penicillinase resistant staphylococci, and Bacteroides.

vii. Metronidazole: It is a useful antibiotic against anaerobic flora found in oral infections. It is administered in the form of 400 mg 8 hourly orally or intravenously.

viii. Cephalosporins: These are closely related to penicillin and have similar spectrum of their activity. These are usually reserved for resistant infections. Usually, a combination of antibiotic therapy is indicated for aggressive management of Ludwig's angina, a penicillin or it's derivative alongwith metronidazole or gentamicin.

Antibiotics should be changed subsequent to the result of bacterial culture and sensitivity testing. The therapy should also be changed, if favorable results are not observed after 48 to 72 hours of therapy.

Hydration: Most cases of Ludwig's angina are dehydrated, because of two reasons: (i) Diminished liquid intake due to pain, discomfort associated with swallowing (dysphagia). (ii) Due to the toxic nature of the condition, there is usually excessive urination and perspiration which further diminishes body fluids. For these reasons patients should be encouraged to have liquids frequently and if required intravenously, fluids can maintain hydration and even calories

Hydrotherapy: It is debatable issue till today. It was defined by Steward Mead (1939) and practiced routinely as an adjunct procedure. In contrast, cold application decreased inflammation, decreased exudates—edema formation and decreased swelling. It can be said that cold application in postsurgical cases of Ludwig's angina when given intermittently reduces edema, tissue tension and aids fast recovery. It is usually given by placing gauze pieces over the most indurated area and wetting them intermittently with cold water. Significant improvement from discomfort can be expected in initial 48 hours.

A Simple Prototype Protocol

A. *Preoperative:*

1. *Airway assessment:* Observe signs and symptoms of obstruction. Thorough examination including: mouth opening, tongue mobility or protrusion, uvula and faucial region. Evaluate need for endotracheal intubation; or surgical airway preferably using pulse oximeter monitoring. Lateral neck radiographs, CT scan, MRI (additional) for extensions beyond maxillofacial region.

2. *Etiological findings:* Further radiographs—OPG, and other radiographs.

3. *Risk factor consideration:* Diabetes, immunodeficiency status.

4. *Hydration:* Check with BP, pulse and urine output.

5. *Temperature:* Assess blood/urine cultures for septicemia. Apply cold packs. Use of antipyretics.

6. *Chest radiographs,* to rule out pneumonia.

7. *Evaluate laboratory data:* Blood count and proteins.

8. Consider emergency airway preparations.

B. *Perioperative:* (a) Intubation: Due care for surgical airway in emergency. (b) Removal of cause, and surgical drainage. (c) Antibiotics

C. *Postoperative:*

1. Extubate after confirming adequate airway.

2. Irrigation of drains periodically.

3. Culture reports: Adjust antibiotics accordingly.

4. Re-evaluate laboratory data: Blood count.

5. Monitoring course of infection: If necessary re-exploration or drainage.

6. Regular follow up.

Irrigation: Copious irrigation of the wound drains with an antibacterial solution. Typically, bacitracin in a mixture of H_2O_2 and normal saline is recommended. In an odontogenic infection, antibiotic regimen should be targeted to the micro-organism most likely to cause the infection, yet should cover a spectrum broad enough to sufficiently combat infrequent pathogens.

Complications: Ludwig's angina continues to be a cause of significant morbidity and mortality. The complications can be listed as follows: (1) Osteomyelitis (2) Maxillary sinusitis (3) Localized respiratory tract disturbances (4) Digestive tract disturbances.

More serious complications include: (1) Life-threatening airway obstruction (2) Septicemia (3) Distant metastatic foci, mediastinitis (4) Pericarditis (5) Internal jugular vein thrombosis (6) Neurological complications\ Intracranial involvement: includes, (a) Meningitis, (b) Epidural abscess/brain abscess (c) Cavernous sinus thrombosis (7) Involvement of carotid sheath: Carotid artery erosions, and (8) Death.

Signs and symptoms of these conditions should be looked for and recognized as early as possible, because some of the complications can be fatal.

Involvement of Carotid Sheath

Carotid sheath is a fascial condensation surrounding the internal jugular vein, the vagus nerve, the common and internal carotid arteries. It lies below the sterno-cleidomastoid muscle and the part most commonly affected lies above the posterior belly of the omohyoid muscle.

Involvement: Infection of the carotid sheath may be derived from the submaxillary space, the infratemporal space and the parapharyngeal space.

Clinical features: If lateral pharyngeal space is infected, the signs of involvement of carotid sheath should be looked for. Its involvement is frequently associated with thrombosis of the internal jugular vein, as the vessel may be adherent to the sheath. The patient usually takes a turn for the worse when this complication sets in. Chills, septicemia, fever is present. The swelling extends down the neck, with localized pain along the course of the vessels.

1. The most ominous of these signs is "herald bleeds", which are intermittent bleeding episodes from nose or pharynx that are caused by incipient erosions of carotid artery or internal jugular vein.
2. Other signs of involvement of carotid sheath include: palsies of cranial nerves IX, X, and XII, Horner's syndrome, and an enlarging hematoma in the neck.
3. Manifestations of septic shock.
4. History of persistent swelling after drainage of a peritonsillar abscess; and a protracted course.

Thrombophlebitis of internal jugular vein may occur as a complication; and if pus in the lateral pharyngeal space is undrained for any length of time, the common carotid artery, may become eroded with fatal consequence. Inequality of pupils due to involvement of cervical sympathetic can be a warning signal of such a disastrous sequel.

Management: If involvement of the carotid sheath is suspected, then vascular control of carotid artery should be established before the rest of the lateral pharyngeal space is dissected. Abscess of the carotid sheath is serious and early intervention is a must. The incision is made along the anterior border of the sternocleidomastoid muscle. Generally, the region above the omohyoid gives a satisfactory exposure, where the external jugular vein can be explored. If it is thrombosed, then it is ligated below the lowest level of its involvement to prevent further spread of infection.

Brain Abscess

Etiology: It can occur from bacteremia accompanying an odontogenic infection. The micro-organisms reaching the brain produce inflammation, localized edema and septic thrombosis. The abscess may be single or multiple.

Clinical features: The signs and symptoms vary depending upon the site of involvement. Headache is the most consistent symptom. Nausea and vomiting are common. Other signs and symptoms include: Hemiplegia, papilledema, aphasia, convulsions, hemisensory deficit, hemianopia and abducens palsy. Abscess of the frontal lobe may cause stupor, confusion and subtle changes in personality.

Treatment: (1) Drug therapy (antibiotics, steroids and mannitol to reduce edema). IV Chloramphenicol is an initial antibiotic of choice. The causative organism is identified and its antibiotic sensitivity is determined. Early diagnosis and treatment are important if the prognosis is to be favorable. (2) Surgery to provide drainage.

Meningitis

It is the most common neurological complication resulting for infection in orofacial region.

Clinical features: It is characterized by headache, fever, stiffness of the neck, and vomiting. Patient is often confused and eventually may become comatose. Convulsions may occur. Kernig's sign (strong passive resistance when an attempt is made to extend the knee from the flexed thigh position) and Brudzinski's sign (abrupt neck flexion in the supine resulting in involuntary flexion of the knees).

The diagnosis is based on the results of lumbar puncture and examination of increased pressure and is opalescent or cloudy. It contains numerous polymorphonuclear cells, the protein is generally high and glucose is almost always reduced. The treatment of meningitis is medical rather than surgical. A combination of chloramphenicol and penicillin G is the treatment of choice until the organism can be identified by culture and its antibiotic sensitivity determined. Antibiotics should be continued for at least a week after the fever subsides and CSF returns to normal. An addition to antibiotics a, attention should be given to maintain proper hydration and electrolyte balance, control of cerebral edema and avoidance of vascular collapse and shock.

Mediastinitis

Odontogenic infection spreading to the mediastinum is rare and is an ominous life threatening late complication and should be suspected in the patient who exhibits exacerbation of fever associated with substernal pain. Progressive septicemia, mediastinal abscesses, pleural effusion, empyema, compression of mediastinal veins with decreased venous return to the heart and pericarditis may occur, with death as the final step. A 40 percent mortality rate persists in the antibiotic era, often due to delayed diagnosis and inadequate surgical drainage (Fig. 40.46). *This is an infection involving the connective mediastinal tissue that fills the interpleural space and surrounds the median thoracic organs.* (The mediastinum is the central portion of the thorax. It is bounded bilaterally by the pleura, ventrally by the sternum, dorsally by the vertebrae and inferiorly by the diaphragm. Vital structures located within or coursing through the mediastinum include the heart, aortic arch, carotid and subclavian arteries, thoracic duct, vagus, phrenic and splanchnic nerves, superior and inferior vena cavae, trachea and esophagus).

This descending cervical cellulitis can arise from submandibular space infection, and parapharyngeal space which may get involved from pterygomandibular space or the zygomaticotemporal space or the buccal space. Respiratory dynamics also influence the spread of infection within the mediastinum. Fluctuations in the negative intrathoracic pressures tend to draw the contents of fascial spaces into the mediastinum. Further, oral contents (air, saliva, anaerobic oral organisms) are often forced into the mediastinum, which contribute to virulent necrotizing mediastinitis (Fig. 40.47). The fulminating infection can infiltrate diffusely across

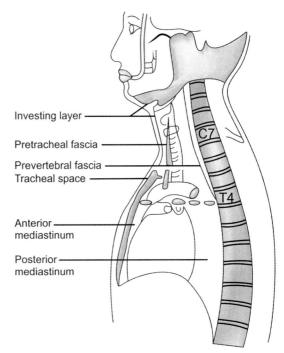

Fig. 40.46: Anterior mediastinum and posterior mediastinum

tissue barriers, taking the form of a descending necrotising mediastinitis (DNM). This most lethal form of descending infection spreads along fascial planes from an oropharyngeal source through the neck to gain access to the mediastinum, necrosis occurs because the infection is often polymicrobial and gas producing.

Clinical presentation (Fig. 40.48):

- *Age:* Most patients are in 3rd to 5th decade of life.
- *Sex:* Male to female predilection of 5:1.
- *Predisposing conditions:* Diabetes, alcoholism, obesity, malnutrition and immunosuppression.
- *Signs and symptoms:* Unremitting high fever, tachycardia, tachypnea and hypotension. Pleuritic chest pain, dyspnea and retrosternal discomfort may be also present. Brawny edema, induration of the neck and chest and crepitus may be palpable. An odontogenic, peritonsillar or retropharyngeal abscess may be visible, depending on the degree of trismus. A profound leukocytosis with a left shift is common.

Radiographic study: The chest X-ray will show typical widening of the mediastinum, pneumomediastinum, pleural effusion and obliteration of the retrosternal or retrocardiac clarity.

The lateral cervical film may demonstrate widening of the retropharyngeal space, loss of normal cervical lordosis and gas along the soft tissue planes of the neck (Fig. 40.49).

CT scan of the neck and chest will reveal the size and location of mediastinal fluid collection, with or without gas bubbles, pericardial effusion, empyema and airway patency (Fig. 40.50).

Microbiology: A mixed aerobic (alpha- and beta-hemolytic streptococcus, staphylococcus and gram negative bacilli) and anaerobic (Bacteroides, Peptostreptococcus

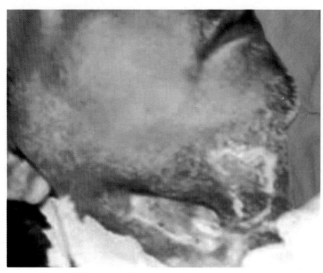

Fig. 40.47: Descending necrotizing mediastinitis (DNM)

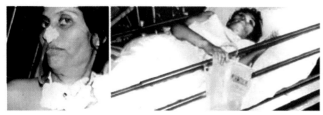

Fig. 40.48: Clinical presentation and management of a patient in intensive medical care unit, suffering from descending infection from lower right first molar, involving mediastinum and multiple organ failure

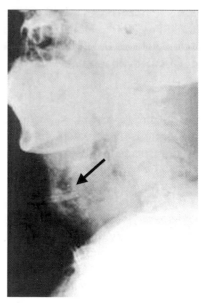

Fig. 40.49: Lateral cervical X-ray film showing widening of retropharyngeal space and gas formation along the soft tissue planes

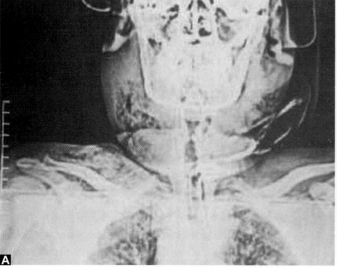

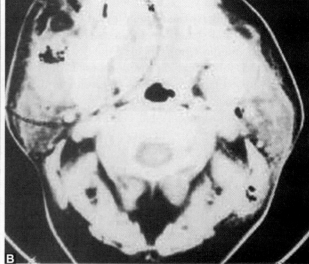

Figs 40.50A and B: (A) CT scan of chest and neck showing mediastinum fluid collection, pericardial effusion and massive involvement of the fascial spaces with gas formation, (B) Axial CT scan showing again extensive involvement with gas bubbles

and Fusobacterium) infection of polymicrobial nature has been implicated in the majority of cases.

Treatment: Early recognition, airway control, aggressive surgical intervention, appropriate antibiotic therapy, supportive systemic care and hyperbaric oxygen therapy, whenever indicated.

Cavernous Sinus Thrombophlebitis: Intracranial Complication (Figs 40.51A and B)

Involvement: It is a serious condition consisting of formation of thrombus in the cavernous sinus or its communicating branches. Infection of head, face and intraoral structures above the maxilla, particularly, lead to this disease. There are two routes by which infection may reach cavernous sinus. *External route-*Infection from the face and lip is carried by facial and angular veins and nasofrontal veins, (danger area of the face) to the superior ophthalmic vein, which enters the cavernous sinus through the superior orbital fissure, *while in internal system*, the dental infection is carried by the way of the pterygoid plexus from the posterior maxillary region, from here through the inferior orbital fissure into the terminal part of the inferior ophthalmic vein and then through the superior orbital fissure into cavernous sinus. The infection spreading by the facial or external route is very rapid with a short fulminating course because of the large, open system of the veins leading directly to cavernous sinus. In contrast infection spreading through the pterygoid or internal route reaches the cavernous sinus only through many small, twisting passages and has a much slower course. *The other pathway from the pterygoid plexus*, is an emissary vein, which connects the cavernous sinus with the pterygoid plexus of veins. It passes through an opening of the base of the greater sphenoid wing, the foramen of vesalius or through the fibrocartilage filling the foramen lacerum or foramen ovale.

Infection, usually involves one side initially, but can easily spread to the opposite side through the circular veins.

Rapid complications and occasionally death can result, from infections by virulent organisms from the upper part of the face, because:

i. The short distance from the facial regions to the sinuses of the brain through the superiorly draining venous system.

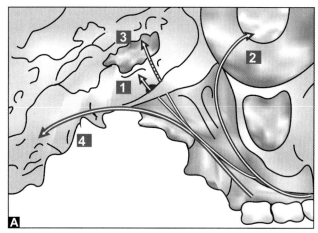

Venous tributaries of cavernous sinus

Figs 40.51A and B: Pathways of ascending infections from jaws to intracranial cavity. (A): (1) Foramen ovale, (2) Via orbital tissues, then via ophthalmic veins or superior orbital fissure, (3) Sphenoid sinus and overlying sella turcica, (4) Petrous portion of temporal bone. (B): (1) Superior ophthalmic vein, (2) Inferior ophthalmic vein, (3) Angular vein, (4) Superior labial vein, (5) Inferior labial vein, (6) Facial vein and common facial vein, (7) Carotid artery, (8) Cavernous sinus, (9) Pterygoid venous plexus

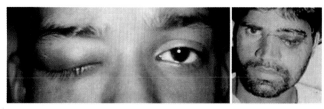

Fig. 40.52: Clinical presentation of cavernous sinus thrombophlebitis

ii. Frequent and complicated anastomoses of these veins leading to direct communications with the sinuses.

iii. The lack of protective valves that other venous system of the body possess and which factor is significantly absent in the facial vessels involved in this complication.

Microbiology: The various bacteria implicated are streptococci and staphylococci and some gram negative bacteria.

Clinical features (Fig. 40.52): Generalized constitutional symptoms; High fluctuating fever, chills, rapid pulse and sweating.

a. *Initial symptoms:* It presents with: (i) Swelling of the face, with edematous involvement of the eyelids. Pain in the eye and tenderness to pressure, (ii) Venous obstruction leading to marked edema and congestion of eyelids, (ii) Edema of conjunctiva due to impaired venous return, (iii) pulsating exophthalmos, where carotid pulse is transmitted through retrobulbar edema, (iv) Cranial nerve involvement: (oculomotor, trochlear, abducent, ophthalmic division of trigeminal nerve, and carotid sympathetic plexus. It results in ophthalmoplegia, paresis or paralysis of the abducent nerve is diagnosed by the weakness or paralysis of the lateral rectus muscle of the eye. The weakness of the other muscles of the eye, culminates in paralysis, diminished or absent corneal reflex, ptosis and dilation of pupil, exophthalmus, photophobia with profuse lacrimation and pain in the distribution of the ophthalmic division of the 5th nerve. (v) Papilledema with multiple retinal hemorrhages, (if retina can be visualized), and chemosis, epistaxis, due to increased intracranial pressure and decreased venous return.

b. *Late symptoms:* (vi) If left untreated, thrombophlebitis spreads to other side, and bilateral signs can be seen.

c. *Advanced stage:* There may be signs of advanced toxaemia and meningitis, producing stiffness of the neck, with positive Kernig's sign and Brudzinski's signs and Biot's respiration. Unless it is treated early, the prognosis is poor. Septicemia with leukocytosis and severe acidosis with a positive blood culture.

Treatment: (i) Antibiotic therapy: IV chloramphenicol 1 g six hourly. (ii) Heparinization, to prevent extension of thrombosis, Heparin 20,000 units in 1500 ml. Of 5 percent dextrose or Dicumarol 200 mg may be given orally, for the first day, and 100 mg daily, there after (iii) Neurosurgical consultation. (iv) Mannitol: It reduces edema, (v) Anticoagulants: It prevents venous thrombosis. (v) Surgical drainage.

41

Osteomyelitis and Osteoradionecrosis of the Jaw Bones

■ OSTEOMYELITIS OF THE JAW BONES

Definition

The words, "osseus" in Latin means bony, and "osteon" in Greek means ''bone'', and "myelos" means marrow; and "itis" in Greek means inflammation.

By meaning osteomyelitis **(OML) is an inflammation of medullary portion of bone or bone marrow or cancellous bone**. However, the process is rarely confined to medulla. It involves cortical bone and periosteum as well. Therefore, **OML may be defined as an inflammatory condition of bone, that begins as an infection of medullary cavity and haversian systems of the cortex and extends to involve the periosteum of the affected area**.

The inflammation may be *acute, subacute or chronic*. It may *be localized;* or may *involve a larger portion of bone*. It may be *suppurative or nonsuppurative*.

Osteomyelitis (OML) of the jaws was once a common and dreaded disease; because of its prolonged therapy and the resultant disfigurement and dysfunction, due to loss of major portion of the jaw bone.

In the contemporary world, the incidence of OML of the jaws has become less, because of the worldwide availability of newer antimicrobials, better awareness, and better dental health care. However, we do come across a few cases of OML; the causes can be attributed to the following: (i) development of certain strains of organisms, which are resistant to certain antibiotics, and (ii) presence of more cases of medically handicapped individuals in the present population. It is an opportunistic disease, as presented by the host to the pathogenic microbe.

Predisposing Factors (Table 41.1)

The factors that predispose to OML are: (1) Conditions affecting host resistance or defenses, (2) Compromised vascular integrity and perfusion in the host bone, at the local, regional or systemic level and (3) Virulence of microorganisms. These factors play an important role in the onset and severity of OML.

1. **Conditions that alter host defenses** would include chronic debilitating systemic diseases—such as diabetes mellitus, agranulocytosis, leukemia, severe anemia, malnutrition, drug abuse, chronic alcoholism, sickle cell disease, and febrile illnesses such as typhoid.

2. **Conditions that alter vascularity of bone**, include—therapeutic irradiation, osteoporosis, Paget's disease, fibrous dysplasia, bone malignancy, metallic bone

Table 41.1: Another group of risk factors predisposing to OML of jaws (Hudson-1993)
1. Noncompliant patients refractory to health care delivery
2. Systemic, metabolically compromised individuals who can be further categorized into the following subsets (a) Age of patients, (b) Malnutrition, (c) Immunosuppression, (d) Congenital or acquired pathophysiology disrupting microvascular perfusion of the calcified tissue structure and investing soft tissue envelope.
3. Inaccessibility to health care delivery.

necrosis (caused by mercury, bismuth, and arsenic). An intrinsic and extrinsic vascular component has a more profound influence, both in onset of occurrence as well as in resolution outcome.

3. **Virulence of organisms**: Certain organisms precipitate thrombi formation by virtue of their destructive lysosomal enzymes (Hudson 1993). Lysosomal and enzymatic degradation of host tissue, along with microvascular thrombosis brought about by pathogen-borne bioactive peptides and chemoattracted leukocytic purulence, forms a protective barrier for the infectious foci, allowing organisms to proliferate in an enriched host medium while protected from the host immunity.

Brodie's abscess of long bone osteomyelitis is the classic example of this isolational phenomenon, which can also occur in osteomyelitis of tooth bearing bone, but to a lesser extent.

The process of OML is initiated by invasion of bacteria into the cancellous bone, followed by acute inflammation hyperemia, increased capillary permeability; and infiltration of granulocytes. The failure of microcirculation in the cancellous bone is a critical factor in the establishment of the osteomyelitis. The infection spreads along the path of least resistance. Since the involved area becomes ischemic and bone becomes necrotic, bacteria can then proliferate, because normal bloodborne defenses do not reach the tissue and osteomyelitis spreads, until it is stopped by medical and surgical therapy.

Etiology

Osteomyelitis of the jaws is caused by:
1. *Odontogenic infections:* Primarily odontogenic infections originating from pulpal or periodontal tissues, pericoronitis, infected socket, infected cyst, tumor, etc.

2. *Trauma:* It is the second leading cause: (a) Especially, compound fracture, and (b) Surgery-iatrogenic
3. Infections of oro-facial regions derived from:
   a. Periostitis following gingival ulceration,
   b. Lymph nodes infected from furuncles, and
   c. Lacerations
   d. Peritonsillar abscess.
4. *Infections derived by hematogenous route:* Furuncle on face, wound on the skin, upper respiratory tract infection, middle ear infection, mastoiditis, systemic tuberculosis.

The infections from the last two groups account for a small percentage of cases.

Pathogenesis

Osteomyelitis is initiated from a contiguous focus of infection or by hematogenous spread.

Osteomyelitis is an infectious process of the medullary myeloid cavity of bone. In the craniofacial skeleton only the mandible and the calvarium have myeloid compartments.

The important factor in establishment of OML is the compromise in the blood supply. It is worth considering the blood supply and venous drainage of mandible (Figs 41.1 and 41.2).
1. (a) *Primary supply:* The mandible is supplied by inferior alveolar artery, except coronoid process, which is supplied by temporalis muscle vessels.
   (b) *Secondary supply:* It is the periosteal supply, which generally runs parallel to cortical surface of bone, giving off nutrient vessels those penetrate

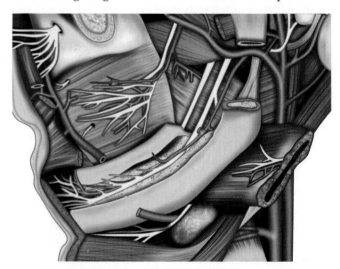

Fig. 41.1: Blood supply to mandible and its musculature

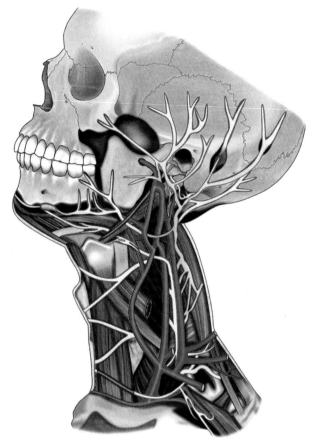

Fig. 41.2: Venous and lymphatic drainage of the head and neck region

cortical bone and anastomose with the branches of inferior alveolar artery.

2. *Venous drainage of mandible:* There are two routes: (i) Via inferior alveolar vein; it runs upwards, and joins pharyngeal plexus, and (ii) It runs downwards, and joins external jugular veins.

Waldron (1943), gave an exhaustive morphologic description of vascular morphology of mandible and associated structures to account for spread of OML. He described mandibular vascular support as being provided through multiple arterial loops from a single major vessel, which renders large portion of bone susceptible to necrosis with the occurrence of major vessel infectious thrombosis.

Waldervogel (1970), described, its relationship to vascular support of long bones of developing and adult human skeleton. He made several conclusions:

1. There tends to be segregation of vascular channels, which act like "end organs", due to lack of terminal collateral anastomosis, ultimately, leading to vascular plugging by bacteria, microthrombi or both.

2. When afferent vessels anastomose with medullary channels, there is a possibility of a decrease in venous flow with associated areas of greater turbulence.

3. There may be a reduction in host immune defense mechanism associated with these vascular channels in calcified tissue.

A true osteomyelitic infectious process does not occur in the maxilla despite the presence of tooth follicle or anatomic respiratory sinus cavities, including the nose.

Osteomyelitis in Maxilla

It is rare; due to: (i) Extensive blood supply and significant collateral blood flow in midface, (ii) Porous nature of membranous bone, (iii) Thin cortical plates, and (iv) Abundant medullary spaces. These preclude confinement of infections within bone; and permit dissipation of edema and pus into soft tissues and paranasal air sinuses.

The mechanism of formation and accumulation of pus is worth understanding.

The process leading to osteomyelitis is initiated by acute inflammation, hyperemia, increased capillary permeability and infiltration of granulocytes. Tissue necrosis occurs, as proteolytic enzymes are liberated and as destruction of bacteria and vascular thombosis continues, there is a pus formation. The pus is a combination of necrotic tissue and dead bacteria and WBC accumulate. When pus accumulates, the intramedullary pressure increases resulting in vascular collapse, venous stasis, and ischemia. Subsequently, pus travels through haversian and nutrient canals and accumulates beneath the periosteum, elevating it from the cortex; and thereby further reducing vascular supply. Compression of neurovascular bundle accelerates thrombosis, ischemia, and infarction, later resulting in paresthesia and sequestrum formation.

Extensive periosteal elevation is seen more frequently in children, since periosteum is presumed to be less firmly bound to bone. If pus continues to accumulate, the periosteum is penetrated; mucosal and cutaneous abscesses and fistulae develop. As natural host defenses and therapy begin to be effective, the process may become chronic, inflammation regresses, granulation tissue is formed; new blood vessels cause lysis of bone, thus separating fragments of necrotic bone (sequestrum) from viable bone.

Small sections of bone may be completely lyzed, whereas larger ones may be isolated by a bed of granulation tissue encased in a sheath of new bone (***Involucrum***). Sequestra, may be revascularized, remain quiescent, or continue to be chronically infected and require surgical removal. Occasionally, involucrum gets penetrated by channels, known as *cloacae*, through which pus escapes from sequestrum to an epithelial surface.

Radiographically, the bone surrounding sequestrum appears less densely mineralized than sequestrum itself, since vascularity of vital bone creates relative demineralization. Ischemia causes increase in CO_2 level, which attracts calcium due to change in pH. The calcium deposition leads to increase in mineralization of the sequestrum.

Microbiology

In the past, the etiology of OML was associated with skin surface bacteria; *S. aureus*; and to a lesser extent *S. epidermidis*, or hemolytic streptococci. However, the picture of *S. aureus* as primary offending pathogen does not hold true with regard to OML of tooth bearing bone. Sinus tract culture results, especially in the jaws, are often misleading, as they are usually contaminated with *Staphylococcus* organisms.

Most of the cases are caused by aerobic streptococci (α-hemolytic streptococci, *Streptococcus viridans*), anaerobic streptococci; and other anaerobes, such as Peptost-reptococci, Fusobacteria, and *Bacteroides* (Peterson 1999). Sometimes, anaerobic or microaerophilic cocci, Gram negative organisms such as *Klebsiella*, *Pseudomonas* and *Proteus* are also found. Other organisms such as *M. tuberculosis*, *T. pallidum*, and *Actinomyces* species produce their respective specific forms of OML. Hence, established acute OML is usually a polymicrobial disease and includes: Streptococci, *Bacteroides*, Peptostreptococci and Fusobacteria, as well as other opportunistic bacteria. Marx et al. (1992), identified Actinomycoses, *Eikenella* and *Arachnia* as pathogens in some of the more refractory forms of OML of jaws. Other unusual organisms such as *Coccidioides*, Tuberculous bacilli, *Treponema* and *Klebsiella* have also been implicated as causative agents. The change in bacterial pattern is not because of ecology. It is attributable to the employment of more sophisticated culture methods.

Classification and Staging

Due to the long standing existence of OML as a clinical entity, a variety of classifications of this disease process have evolved.

A variety of classifications of various forms of the disease are given, which are as follows:

1. *Historically accepted classification:* It is based on clinical course.

   (A) Acute, and (B) Chronic. The arbitrary time limit, to identify acute from chronic forms, is of one month. (Koorbusch et al; 1992, Marx; 1992, and Mercuri; 1992) (Table 41.2).

2. *Classification based on pathogenesis of altered vascular perfusion as a major contributing factor to the presence and persistence of OML as a clinical disease.* (Vibhagool et al. 1993): There are three types:
   - Hematogenous OML
   - OML secondary to a contiguous focus of infection
   - OML associated with or without peripheral vascular disease

3. *Classification based on presence or absence of suppuration (Table 41.3):*

4. Cierny et al. (1985) and Vibhagool (1993) developed a classification and staging system; based on
   i. Anatomic location of infectious process, and
   ii. Physiological status of the host (iii) Systemic or local factors affecting immune system, metabolism, and local vascularity (Table 41.4).

Table 41.2: Hudson's classification of OML of the jaws
A. **Acute forms of OML** (suppurative or nonsuppurative) include:
a. *Contiguous focus:* (i) Trauma, (ii) Surgery, and (iii) Odontogenic infections.
b. *Progressive:* (i) Burns, (ii) Sinusitis, and (iii) Vascular insufficiency.
c. *Hematogenous (metastatic):* Developing skeleton (children)
B. **Chronic forms of OML**
a. *Recurrent multifocal:* (i) Developing skeleton (children), (ii) Escalated osteogenic activity (< age 25 years)
b. Garre's: (i) Unique proliferative subperiosteal reaction, (ii) Developing skeleton (children to young adults)
c. *Suppurative or nonsuppurative:* (i) Inadequately treated forms, (ii) Systemically compromised forms, and (iii) Refractory forms (CROML: Chronic refractory OML).
d. *Diffuse sclerosing:* (i) Fastidious organisms, and (ii) Compromised host/ pathogen interface.

Table 41.3: Suppurative and nonsuppurative OML

Suppurative OML	Nonsuppurative OML
i. Acute suppurative (pyogenic) OML	i. Chronic sclerosing OML
ii. Chronic suppurative (pyogenic) OML	a. Focal sclerosing OML
a. Primary	b. Diffuse sclerosing OML
b. Secondary	ii. Garre's sclerosing OML
iii. Infantile OML	iii. Actinomycotic OML
	iv. Radiation OML (ORN)
	v. Specific infective OML
	a. Tuberculosis
	b. Syphilis

Table 41.4: Classification and staging system of OML developed by Cierny et al. and Vibhagool

I. Anatomic types:

Stage I	Medullary OML:	It involved medullary bone without cortical involvement; usually hematogenous.
Stage II	Superficial OML:	Less than 2 cm of bony defect without cancellous bone.
Stage III	Localized OML:	Less than 2 cm bony defect seen on radiograph, defect does not appear to involve both cortices.
Stage IV	Diffuse OML:	The defect is less than 2 cm, pathological fracture, infection, and nonunion.

II. Physiological types:

A Host:	Normal host
B Host:	Systemic compromise (Bs), local compromise (Bl)
C Host:	Treatment is worse than the disease.

III. Systemic or local factors that affect immune surveillance, metabolism, and local vascularity.

a. *Systemic (Bs):*	(i) Malnutrition, (ii) Renal or hepatic failure, (iii) Diabetes mellitus, (iv) Chronic hypoxia, (v) Immune deficiency or suppression, (vi) Malignancy, (vii) Extremes of age, (viii) Autoimmune disease, and (ix) Tobacco and Alcohol abuse
a. *Local (Bl):*	(i) Chronic lymphedema, (ii) Venous stasis, (iii) Major vessel disease, (iv) Arteritis, (v) Extensive scarring, (vi) Radiation fibrosis, (vii) Small vessel disease, and (viii) Loss of local sensation

Acute Pyogenic OML (Acute Suppurative OML)

It may have the appearance of a typical odontogenic infection.

It can be localized and widespread, with extensive sequestration and possible pathological fracture.

Microbiology

It is caused by pyogenic organisms. OML in the tooth bearing area is polymicrobial in nature. The most commonly found organisms in odontogenic OML is *Staphylococcus aureus*; and also *Streptococcus pyogenes*. Vincent's spirochetes may also be present. Gram negative bacilli may also be present (*E. coli*).

Etiology

(1) Odontogenic infections, (2) Local traumatic injuries, (3) Peritonsillar abscess, (4) Furunculosis, (5) Hematogenous infections, (6) Infected compounded odontoma (Romer, 1955), (7) Compound fractures of jaws are complicated by OML.

1. *Odontogenic infections (Figs 41.3A to F):* These are the common local cause of OML. These infections may result from
   i. Periapical disease secondary to pulp pathosis,
   ii. Periodontal disease, (Figs 41.4A to C)
   iii. Pericoronitis of long duration,
   iv. Infected odontogenic cyst, and
   v. Infection of an extraction wound or fracture site.
2. *Local traumatic injuries:* (a) Injuries of gingiva, are usually insignificant; however, may become serious in patients with low resistance (Ivy and Cook, 1942), and (b) Instruments used for extraction of teeth.
3. *Peritonsillar abscess:* It has been reported as a cause of OML of ascending ramus
4. *Furunculosis:* Of skin is a rare cause of OML. Hoenig et al. (1931) have reported such a case.
5. *Hematogenous infection:* It may cause multiple sites of OML. The organisms enter the blood stream through a minor wound in the skin, or infection of upper respiratory tract, or infection of middle ear. The predisposing factors include: (i) Undernourished children, (ii) Lowered general resistance of body, (iii) Generalized body diseases: such as; diabetes, leukemia, and agranulocytosis, and (iv) Acute illnesses, such as influenza, measles, scarlet fever, pertussis and pneumonia, etc. Blair et al. (1931), reported one case following tonsillitis, one following measles, and one following diphtheria. Galli, (1926) reported a case of OML of maxilla associated with renal complication. Recently, with the use of newer antibiotics and early institution of antibiotics hematogenous spread is not commonly seen.

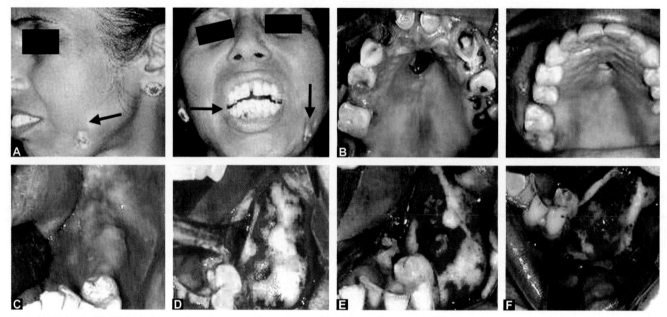

Figs 41.3A to F: (A) Clinical picture of acute suppurative osteomyelitis due to odontogenic infection. Note the decreased oral opening of the patient due to oral submucous fibrosis, (B) Intraoral palatal perforation and pus discharge in another patient chronic suppurative osteomyelitis due to odontogenic cause, (C) Intraoral picture showing swelling and pus discharge from lower left first, second and third molar region, (D) Surgical exposure showing presence of granulation tissue, (E) Curettage done, sequestras exposed, (F) Sequestrectomy and saucerization carried out

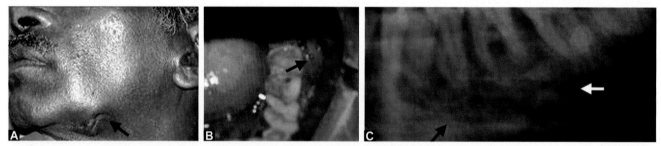

Figs 41.4A to C: Chronic osteomyelitis due to periodontal disease: (A) Extraoral sinus, (B) Chronic intraoral abscess in lower left first and second molar region, (C) OPG showing multiple sequestra

Clinical features: Occurrence: In adults, it is more common in mandible and involves alveolar process, angle of mandible, posterior part of ramus and coronoid process. OML of condyle is reportedly rare (Linsey, 1953).

A. *Early cases are characterized by:*
1. Generalized constitutional symptoms: High intermittent fever, malaise, nausea, vomiting, anorexia
2. Deep seated boring, continuous intense pain in the affected area
3. Intermittent paresthesia or anesthesia of the lower lip, which helps the clinician to differentiate this condition from alveolar abscess.

4. Facial cellulitis, or indurated swelling of moderate size, which is more confined to the periosteal envelop and its contents. (i) Thrombosis of inferior alveolar vasa nervorum, (ii) Rise in pressure from edema in inferior alveolar canal, (iii) Teeth are tender to percussion and loose, and
5. Trismus.

In children: (i) Fulminating. (ii) Severe and serious. (iii) Involvement of maxilla or mandible. (iv) Complicated by the presence of unerupted developing teeth buds, which become necrotic and act as foreign bodies and prolong the disease process. Long term involvement of TMJ can cause ankylosis of TMJ and subsequently affect the growth and development of facial structures.

Laboratory studies: Show mild leukocytosis (PMNL) and albuminuria.

B. *Established cases are characterized by:*
1. Deep pain, malaise, fever, dehydration, anorexia
2. Teeth in involved area begin to loosen and become sensitive to percussion.
3. Purulent discharge through sinuses: (a) Intraorally; (i) around gingival sulcus: or (ii) through buccal vestibule, and (b) Extraorally on the face, through cutaneous fistulae.
4. Fetid odor is often present.
5. Trismus may be present.
6. Dehydration, acidosis and toxemia.
7. Regional lymphadenopathy is usually pesent.

Laboratory studies show: (1) Moderate leukocytosis (PMNL), and (2) Slightly elevated ESR (3) Anemia, and (4) Albuminuria.

Blood cultures, wound culture and sensitivity, and complete blood count along with peaks and troughs on any antimicrobial prescribed should be assessed on a regular basis. Radiological changes are absent initially.

Chronic Osteomyelitis

It can be (a) *primary*: resulting from organisms which are less virulent, and (b) *secondary:* occurring after acute OML, when the treatment did not succeed in eliminating the infection.

The clinical features are usually limited to: (1) Pain and tenderness: the pain is minimal, (2) Non-healing bony and overlying soft tissue wounds with induration of soft tissues, (3) Intraoral or extraoral draining fistulae, (4) Thickened or "wooden" character of bone, (5) Enlargement of mandible, because of deposition of subperiosteal new bone. (6) Pathological fractures may occur, (Figs 41.5A to C) (7) Sterile abscess (Brodie's abscess), common to long bones is rare in jaws. (8)Teeth in the area tend to become loose and sensitive to palpation and percussion.

Radiographic findings: The radiological examination can be accomplished by the use of the following methods:
A. *Conventional radiography:* Radiographic changes occur only 3 weeks after initiation of OML process. It is generally accepted that 30 to 60 percent of mineralized portions of bone must be destroyed before significant radiographic changes are noted. This degree of bone alteration requires a minimum of 4 to 8 days after the onset of acute OML. Therefore, in early stages, history and clinical features constitute the sole data upon which diagnosis can be made.

In early stage, there is widening of marrow spaces, and enlargement of Volkmann's canals, which imparts a "mottled appearance".

The granulation tissue between living and dead bone produces irregular lines and zones of radiolucency. This results in characteristic "moth-eaten appearance" of established OML.

In later stages, the cortex gets involved and due to ischemia, an island of cortical bone becomes devitalized and becomes favorable for the precipitation of ionized calcium, mobilized by the surrounding osteolytic process. The gradual resorption around periphery of infarcted area of bone separates it off as a sequestrum. Such a devitalized piece of bone appears sclerosed and becomes a foreign body which is called as sequestrum. These segments appear highly calcified and therefore appear prominent. Large areas of bone destruction are seen as radiolucent areas.

Subperiosteal new bone, *the involucrum*, can be seen as a fine linear opacity, or as a series of laminated

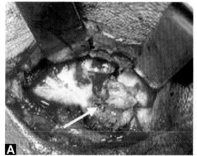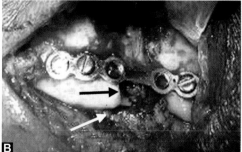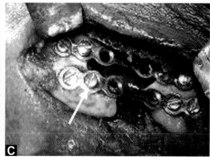

Figs 41.5A to C: Pathological fracture due to chronic osteomyelitis: (A) Pathological fracture exposed surgically, (B) Chronic unhealthy granulation tissue curettage done with freshening of bony margins, (C) Bony defect bridged and fragments stabilized using bone plate fixation

opacities, like an onion skin, parallel to surface of cortex. This is seen at the lower border; or may be best outlined on buccal cortex by an occlusal film. This adds to loss of radiological definition of original underlying bone structure. Where new bone is superimposed upon that of jaw, a delicate "fingerprint" or "orange-peel" appearance is seen.

The deposition of subperiosteal new bone-involucrum is particularly marked in children and adolescents, and absent in adults. Later, substantial fragments of dead bone, especially, thick cortical bone may be separated from adjacent bone by a well demarcated radiolucent zones and may even become displaced from their original position.

Sequestra often prevented from spontaneous discharge through sinus in overlying soft tissue by enveloping involucrum and come to lie in granulation tissue and pus filled cavities between involucrum and surviving mandibular bone. At this stage, there is a risk of pathological fracture.

Once OML is well established, radiographical changes usually demonstrate one of the following sets of characteristics, as suggested by Worth (1969) (Figs 41.6 to 41.9).

1. Scattered areas of bone destruction, separated by variable distances. The appearance is one of increased radiolucency, which may be uniform or patchy. There is a "moth-eaten" appearance, because of enlargement of medullary spaces and widening of Volkmann's canals.

2. Bone destruction of varied extent, in which there are "sequestra" with a trabecular pattern and marrow spaces. A sheath of new bone, "involucrum", is often found separated from sequestra by a zone of radiolucency. (There are areas of radiopacity within the radiolucency. The radiopaque areas represent islands of bone, that have not been resorbed-sequestrum).

3. Stippled or granular densifications of bone caused by subperiosteal depositions of new bone obscuring intrinsic bone structure or depositions of new bone on the surfaces of existing trabeculae, at the expense of marrow spaces (Fig. 41.10).

B. *Imaging:* Specialized radiographic techniques—the other radiographic techniques employed for diagnosis are: (1) Computerized tomography (CT), (2) Radio-isotope scanning, (3) Positron emission tomography (PET)

1. *Computerized tomography:* It gives a more definitive picture of calcified tissue involvement, especially with regard to disruptions of cortical plates.

2. *Radioisotope scanning:* Radioisotope Tc-99m methylene diphosphonate bone scanning can identify occult areas of involvement and has previously been used to identify margins or extent of calcified tissue involvement. However, due to poor resolutions, this has not been proved to be effective.

3. *Positron emission tomography (PET):* More recently, PET, using radioisotopes of physiologically active compounds such as glucose, ammonia, and fluoride has shown greater promise in mapping out varying margins of metabolic activity. Changes in the bone are seen as early as 3 days, after the onset of symptoms of osteomyelitis. (a) confirms the diagnosis of very early osteomyelitis. (b) early interceptive antibiotic and supportive therapy can be instituted. (c) establishment of the typical, fulminating disease

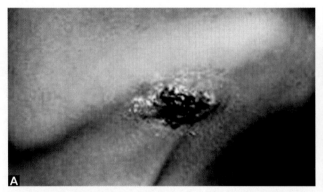
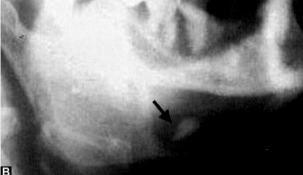

Figs 41.6A and B: (A) Extraoral draining sinus, (B) Lateral oblique view showing the radiopaque sequestrum

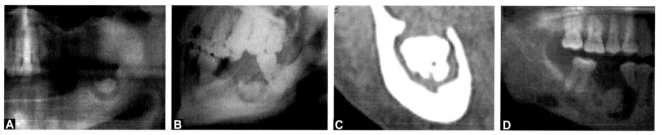

Figs 41.7A to D: OPG, lateral view X-ray and Dentascan image showing the sequestrum and involucrum

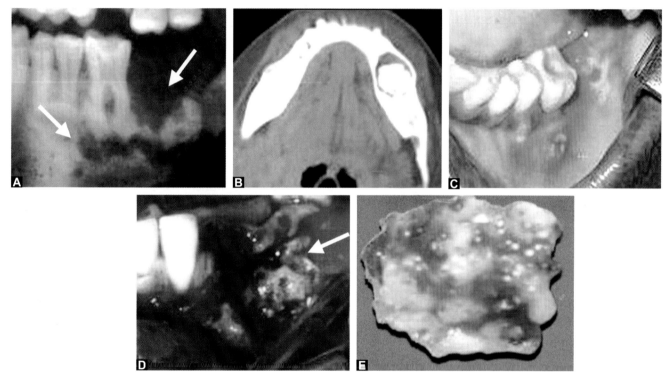

Figs 41.8A to E: (A) Lateral oblique view of L mandible showing chronic osteomyelitis due to odontogenic infection. Note that the extraction of (L) 2nd and 3rd lower molars has been done. 1st lower molar shows periapical pathology, (B) CT scan showing the presence of sequestrum, (C) Intraoral picture of the patient showing draining sinus and pus discharge, (D) Surgical exposure of sequestrum, (E) Big sequestrum removed

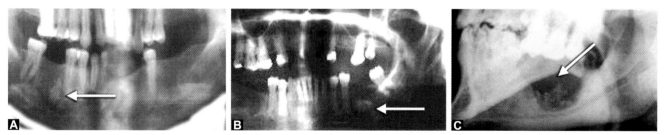

Figs 41.9A to C: Chronic osteomyelitis of the mandible due to odontogenic cause. Arrows on OPGs and lateral view is showing sequestrum formation with surrounding radiolucent zone

can be prevented. (d) useful in chronic osteomyelitis, when a decision is to be taken regarding the prolonged duration of antibiotic therapy. (A negative evidence indicates that bone activity has ceased and supports discontinuing therapy. (e) In those patients, who show early symptoms suggestive of relapse, a positive scan allows early diagnosis and immediate resumption of therapy, before symptoms worsen.

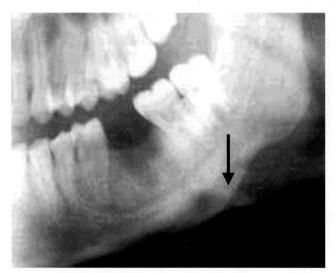

Fig. 41.10: Subperiosteal deposit of new bone

Table 41.5: The treatment guidelines for acute or chronic OML (Marx, 1992)
1.   Disrupt infectious foci
2.   Debride any foreign bodies, necrotic tissue, or sequestra
3.   Culture and identify specific pathogens for eventual definitive antibiotic treatment
4.   Drain and irrigate the region
5.   Begin empiric antibiotics based on Gram stain
6.   Stabilize calcified tissue regionally
7.   Consider adjunctive treatments to enhance microvascular reperfusion: (a) Trephination, and (b) Decortication. These may be accomplished during debridement, (c) Vascular flaps (muscle), and (d) Hyperbaric oxygen (HBO) therapy.
8.   *Reconstruction:* As necessary following resolution of infection.

Diagnosis: It is made on basis of: (i) Presence of sequestra, (ii) Areas of suppuration involving the tooth bearing area of jaw bone, not responding to debridement and conservative therapy, (iii) Regional or systemic compromise of immune response, microvascular decompensation or both.

Treatment: The treatment measures remain the same as for acute as well as for chronic OML.

In certain circumstances, after performing the necessary surgical procedures, where the soft tissues cannot be closed without leaving dead space, or because of rigid fibrosis; the wound may be packed with 2″ ribbon gauze soaked with Whiteheads varnish.

A differentiation has to be made between the types of bone encountered. The necrotic but unsequestrectomised bone, the cortex has dirty white color; while the living cortical bone has a yellowish hue. The viable cortex shows tiny red bleeding spots on cut surfaces.

Chronic external sinuses require irrigation.

Resection: It is rarely required. When full thickness of segment of jaw is involved and a conservative approach has failed to cure, resection of the involved part should be considered. However, the only soft tissue related to the necrotic bone should be elevated, to avoid devitalization of the adjoining cortex.

Secondary bone grafting: This should be considered when the wound has healed completely and is free of infection.

Management: The management includes: *(A) Conservative treatment, and (B) Surgical treatment*

The goal of the management is to: (i) Attenuate and eradicate proliferating pathological organisms, (ii) Promote healing, and (iii) Re-establish vascular permeability (Table 41.5).

Successful treatment is based on the following fundamental principles: (1) Early diagnosis, (2) Bacterial culture and sensitivity testing, (3) Adequate, appropriate, and prompt antibiotic therapy, (4) Adequate pain control, (5) Proper surgical intervention, (6) Reconstruction, where indicated.

A. *Conservative management:* It includes: (1) Complete bed rest, (2) Supportive therapy, (3) Dehydration, (4) Blood transfusion, (5) Control of pain, (6) IV antimicrobial agents, (7) Postoperative care, (8) Hyperbaric oxygen (HBO therapy), and (9) Special treatment for specific needs.

B. *Surgical management:* The various surgical treatment modalities reported in literature, are adjunct to medical treatment; and include: (1) Extraction of offending teeth, (2) Incision and drainage, (3) Continuous or intermittent indwelling closed catheter irrigation, (4) Sequestrectomy and saucerization, decortication. (5) Resection of jaw with or without immediate or delayed reconstruction with bone graft and (6) Postoperative care.

A. *Conservative management:*
1. Complete bed rest.
2. *Supportive therapy:* It includes, nutritional support, in the form of high protein and high caloric diet; and adequate multivitamins.
3. *Dehydration:* Hydration orally or through administration of IV fluids.
4. *Blood transfusion:* In case, RBCs and hemoglobin is low.

5. *Control of pain:* It is controlled with analgesics. Sedation may be employed for keeping patient comfortable and allow to sleep.

6. *IV antimicrobial agents:* Penicillin remains the time honoured empiric antibiotic of choice for OML of jaws (Vibhagool, 1993).

Since streptococci and penicillin sensitive anaerobes are organisms frequently involved. Antibiotics of value in treatment of OML include: penicillins, penicillinase-resistant penicillins, clindamycin, cephalosporins, and erythromycins. Some of the newer antibiotics which provide effective coverage include: metronidazole, clindamycin, ticarcillin, clavulanic acid, cephalosporins, vancomycin in combination with other antibiotics, and fluoroquinolones.

Another unique pharmacological measure that has been tried experimentally; is the use of prostaglandin-inhibiting salicylate therapy. This is in an attempt to diminish osteolytic destruction (Dekel and Francis, 1981).

Hudson (1993), in his 50 years perspective on OML of jaws, described various methods to augment systemic host immune response to reach the site of infection. (1) Intra-arterial antibiotic therapy, (2) Local implantation of antibiotic saturated beads [Nakajima et al. (1977), and Goodell et al. (1986)], and (3) HBO therapy.

Recommended Antibiotic Regimens for OML of jaws are as follows:

1. Regimen I (*1st choice*): As Empirical therapy, Penicillin (Penicillin V) is given.
   a. Aqueous Penicillin 2 million units IV every 4 hourly.
   b. Oxacillin–1 gm IV every 4 hourly.
      When the patient has been asymptomatic for 48 to 72 hours, then switch to—Penicillin V orally 500 mg. Every 4 hourly with Dicloxacilin 250 mg. Orally every 4 hourly for 2 to 4 weeks.

2. Regimen II is based on Culture and Sensitivity results. Penicillinase-resistant penicillins, such as oxacillin, cloxacillin, dicloxacillin, or flucloxacillin may be given.

In case of allergy to penicillin, the following antibiotics are prescribed, in order of preference: (i) Clindamycin 300 to 600 mg orally 6 hourly. (ii) Cephalosporin 250 to 500 mg orally every 6 hourly: (a) Cefazolin 500 mg 8 hourly, or (b) Cephalexin 500 mg 6 hourly. (iii) Erythromycin 2 g every 6 hourly IV, then 500 mg every 6 hourly orally.

2nd choice: Clindamycin: It is effective against penicillinase producing staphylococci, streptococci and anaerobic bacteria including *Bacteroides*. It is used because of its ability to diffuse widely in bone. It is not recommended as first choice; as it is bacteriostatic, and causes diarrhea due to pseudomembranous colitis.

3rd choice: Cefazolin or Cephalexin: It is effective against most cocci including penicillinase-producing staphylococci, Gram negative aerobic bacilli viz, *E. coli*, *Klebsiella*, and *Proteus*.

Cephalosporins are not recommended as first choice; because: (i) these are moderately effective against anaerobes, and (ii) because of broad spectrum coverage, which increases antibiotic complications (Bacterial resistance and superinfection).

4th choice: Erythromycin: These drugs cannot be used as first choice, as these are: (i) bacteriostatic, and (ii) rapidly develop resistant strains.

The dose and duration of antimicrobial therapy is dependent upon severity of infection and its response to treatment. Usually with the disruption of the organized foci and with potent, sustained, and penetrating bactericidal antimicrobial therapy, most cases of suppurative and nonsuppurative osteomyelitis will rapidly resolve.

7. Special treatment for specific needs: Anemia, diabetes mellitus, and malnutrition need specific treatment.

Specific infective forms of chronic OML include: tuberculosis, syphilis, and actinomycosis. Their management is the same, as in chronic OML; and in addition, their respective appropriate medications have to be instituted. Tuberculosis may require therapy for up to a year, while actinomycosis may require for 2 to 3 months.

Complications: Several sequalae/complications can occur as a result of OML of jaws.

1. *Neoplastic transformation:* With chronic OML, neoplastic conversion of inflammatory metaplasia to squamous cell carcinoma is noted. The incidence reported is 0.2 to 1.5 percent.

2. *Discontinuity defects:* The defects can be (a) spontaneous or (b) surgically induced; necessitating jaw reconstruction; once infection is resolved (Figs 41.11A to D).

3. *Progressive diffuse sclerosis:* It involves the medullary and cortical portions of maxillofacial skeleton; especially mandible, over a period of time.

A. Hyperbaric oxygen (HBO) in treatment of OML: (Fig. 41.12): Hyperbaric oxygen therapy involves the intermittent, usually daily, inhalation of 100 percent humidified oxygen under pressure, greater than one

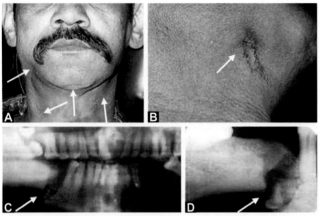

Figs 41.11A to D: (A) Front view of a patient with multiple facial scars due to trauma six months back, (B) Chronic draining extraoral sinus on the R side of the lower border of the mandible, (C) After multiple surgical exploration and prolonged antibiotic therapy also the chronic osteomyelitis with sequestrum formation is seen in OPG. The osteomyelitis is developed following compound fracture of R body mandible, (D) Intraoral periapical X-ray of the same area. Thorough curettage with extraction of lower R 1st premolar, excision of cutaneous tract and stabilization of fracture with reconstruction plate and stepping up of appropriate antibiotic cover resulted in good healing

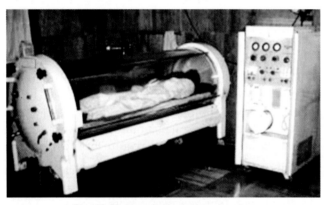

Fig. 41.12: Hyperbaric oxygen chamber

atmospheric absolute pressure (ATA). Patient is placed in a chamber; O_2 is given by mask or by hood. Each "dive" is 90 minutes in length. The treatment is given 5 days per week for 30, 60, or more dives in monoplace chamber at 2.4 ATA for 90 minutes while breathing 100 percent oxygen twice daily.

Over the last several decades, HBO therapy has emerged as (i) a potent alternative to surgical reperfusion; and (ii) as an adjunctive enhancement to host-immune response. Its use has increased in the treatment of OML and ORN (osteoradionecrosis).

HBO therapy increases a dose of oxygen dissolved in the plasma and delivered to the tissues. It reduces hypoxia within the affected tissues and stimulates angiogenesis in the hypovascular tissues. The mechanism of HBO on nonhealing wounds is complex. Regular, periodic elevation of the oxygen within hypoxic tissues has shown to enhance the phagocytic ability of leukocytes to stimulate fibroblast growth, increase collagen formation and promote growth of new capillaries.

Five aspects of the action of HBO are beneficial:

1. HBO therapy enhancement of lysosomal degradation potential of polymorphonuclear leukocytes and O_2 radicals; which are major components of catabolic enzymes of macrophage lysosome. Formation of these enzymes is decreased in hypoxic environment, as in OML.
2. Free radicals of O_2 are toxic to many pathogenic anaerobes (bactericidal).
3. Many exotoxins liberated by microorganisms are rendered inert by exposure to elevated partial pressure of O_2.
4. Tissue hypoxia is intermittently reversed by HBO therapy mimicking tissue level during wound healing.
5. Positive enhancement of neoangiogenesis, in the aerobic portion of proliferative phase of wound healing.

The beneficial effects presumably result from:

i. An increased vascular supply, and
ii. Increased O_2 perfusion to ischemic areas of infection,
iii. Bactericidal or bacteristatic action of increased O_2 levels [(Bornside, (1967); Gottlieb and Pakman (1968)].

Adequate tissue O_2 tension also facilitates fibroblast proliferation, new capillaries formation (Hunt et al. 1975), osteogenesis (Makley et al. 1967, Penttinen et al. 1971), and optimal polymorphonuclear leukocyte function (Mandell, 1974; McRiplet and Sbarra, 1967).

The therapeutic and detrimental effects result from features of this treatment: (i) The mechanical effects of increased pressure; and (ii) the physiological effects of hyperoxia (Grim et al. 1990). HBO therapy produces improved tissue oxygenation due to increased arterial oxygen tension and increased dissolved plasma oxygen content. The therapy also produces a vasoconstriction of arteries related to the degree of pressure (Ricci and Calogero 1988).

Clinical effects: It aids in healing of draining sinus, improves osteogenesis in lytic areas, reduces destruction of bone and soft tissues, sequestra undergo rapid dissolution without suppuration; and healing frequently eliminates the need for surgical intervention.

Clinical application: It has been described by Hart and Mainous, (1976) and Marx, (1983). The protocol they followed is as follows: the patients were treated with 2 ATA of O_2 for a total of 60 sessions (i.e. 120 hours), or until they are asymptomatic, and the defects are closed. Patients with ORN are subjected to second course of series of treatment six months later, consisting of twenty-two hours daily. Mansfield et al. (1981) have described a modified treatment regimen, with alternating 100 percent O_2 with intermittent O_2 followed by air. This is done to avoid possible O_2 toxicity (Hendricks et al, 1977).

The protocol of Marx (1983b) for ORN is divided into 3 stages. First stage comprises of 30 initial dives. If patient shows definite improvement clinically, then a full course of 60 dives is completed. Otherwise, sequestrectomy is done and then 30 additional dives are completed. If there is wound dehiscence, resection is done and 60 dives are completed. Then patient receives additional 20 dives, 10 weeks after resection, in preparation for reconstruction with bone graft. Patient with pathological fracture, oro-cutaneous fistula, and resorption of inferior border are given an initial 30 dives prior to undergoing resection.

Due to the effects of increased O_2 tension on cell mitosis and cell proliferation, patients with known as neoplastic disease should not be treated with HBO (Laskin, 1999).

Antioxidation supplementary therapy: Marx (1992) described cellular respiration in a discussion of superoxide dismutase scavenging ability of most aerobic organisms. There are periods of sustained ischemia and hypoxia, which are followed by reperfusion. This allows normal endogenous antioxidant capability resulting in tissue reperfusion injury to occur. The xanthine oxidase enzymatic pathways is responsible for liberation of superoxide radicals.

Control of this destructive activity is appreciated in soft tissue flap transfer, and organ transplantation, and is accomplished by using (i) allopurinol which blocks xanthine reduction, and (ii) tocopherol (vitamin E) antioxidant supplemental therapy.

Contraindications: The contraindications to HBO therapy; as considered by the HBO Committee of the Undersea Medical Society, Fisher et al. (1988), and Marx et al. (1985) are as follows: (i) Pneumothorax, (ii) Severe chronic obstructive pulmonary disease, (iii) Optic neuritis, (iv) Acute viral infection, (v) Congenital spherocytosis, (vi) Uncontrolled acute seizures disorders, (vii) Upper respiratory tract infection, (viii) Uncontrolled high fever, (ix) Pregnancy (questionable), (x) Psychiatric problems, (xi) History of prior thoracic or ear surgery. (xii) Malignant disease.

Potential complications: Some of the possible complications associated with HBO therapy are listed here. [Gabb and Robbin, (1987), Wirjosemito and Touhey (1988), and Giebfried et al. (1986)].

(i) Eustachian tube dysfunction, (ii) Tympanic membrane rupture, (iii) Oxygen toxicity, (iv) Ear, sinus or tooth pain, (v) Decompression sickness, (vi) Pneumothorax, (vii) Arterial gas embolism, (viii) Nitrogen emboli to CNS, lung or joints, (ix) Middle ear hemorrhage, (x) Deafness, (xi) Changes in vision, (xii) Certain hemolytic anemias, (xiii) Fire hazard, (xiv) Nausea, fatigue, claustrophobia, (xv) Equipment malfunction. These complications are rare. Toxic effects of oxygen in the central nervous system, eye, liver and tracheobronchial tree are reported.

B. Surgical management: The surgical treatment modalities include: (1) Incision and drainage (2) Extraction of loose or offending teeth (3) Debridement (4) Decortication (5) Continuous or Intermittent indwelling closed catheter irrigation (6) Sequestrectomy (7) Saucerization (8) Resection of jaw (Figs 41.13 and 41.14) (9) Trephination (10) Immediate or delayed reconstruction with bone graft.

Surgical intervention is done under antibiotic cover, started at least, 1 to 2 days prior to the procedure.

Immobilization of the part is advocated; generally, a bandage is sufficient. Hot moist compresses should be applied to promote localization of infection. Application of cold is contraindicated. The procedures are to be carried out with minimal trauma.

1. **Incision and drainage:** It should be done as soon as possible. It relieves the pressure and pain caused by the accumulation of pus. Incision of abscesses should be carried out intraorally or extraorally depending upon the location. Evacuation of pus, by drainage, lessens absorption of toxic products and prevents further spread of infection in the bone; thus helping in its localization. The consistency, color and odor of the pus may provide important clues to the diagnosis and initial treatment. Patients with compromised systemic conditions or toxemia, surgical interference may be postponed for 2 to 3 days.

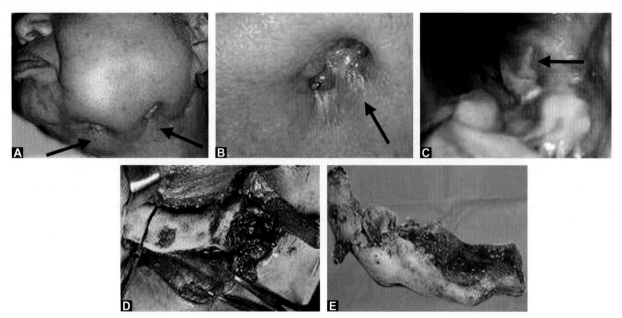

Figs 41.13A to E: (A) Extraoral clinical picture of a patient with uncontrolled diabetes mellitus. Multiple draining sinuses with pus discharge for 2 years, (B) Close-up view of one of the draining sinuses, (C) Intraoral picture showing the exposed sequestrum in the oral cavity, (D) After controlling the diabetes, surgical resection (Hemimandibulectomy) was planned. Extraoral surgical picture of resection of hemimandible being carried out, (E) Resected specimen

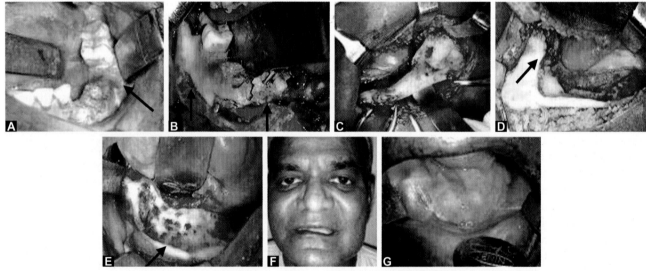

Figs 41.14A to G: Unusual case of osteonecrosis: (A) A 60-year-old patient came with C/O foul smell and chronic pus discharge intraorally and dull pain in left mandibular region. Intraoral examination revealed the presence of dead, necrosed bone from midline to left angle mandible. Patient gave H/O stroke on the left side one year back, for which he received treatment and recovered. No other systemic cause could be attributed to avascular necrosis of left hemimandible, (B) Surgical resection of the necrosed bone was planned, using both extraoral and intraoral incisions. Intraorally, clear demarcation between the necrosed and normal bone was seen, (C) Extraorally, the necrosed bone was separated from normal bone, (D) and (E) Peripheral osteotomy and saucerization was carried out (F) and (G) Extraoral and intraoral clinical picture of the patient postoperatively

The various methods employed for causing drainage from the bone include: (i) Opening up the pulp chamber, (ii) By making fenestration through cortical plate over the apical area with a drill, (iii) In an edentulous area, especially, posterior maxilla or maxillary tuberosity region, by making an incision over the alveolar crest, and by making a window, pus is evacuated, and (iv) OML at the angle of mandible, or ascending ramus, drainage can be achieved by a small incision made over the point of greatest tenderness, or just below the mandible.

2. **Extraction of loose or offending teeth:** Sometimes, drainage is achieved by extraction of offending teeth.

3. **Debridement:** Followed by I/D, through debridement of affected area should be carried out. The area may be irrigated with hydrogen peroxide and saline. Any foreign body, necrotic tissue or small sequestrum should be removed.

4. **Decortication:** Removal of chronically infected lateral and inferior cortical plates of bone 1 to 2 cm beyond the area of involvement. Thus an access is provided to medullary cavity. Obwegeser, (1960) advocated this procedure, as it shortens healing time.

   Decortication and mobilization of muscle flaps to achieve or improve regional and systemic vascular supply to the involved area have been used to bring the overlying vascular soft tissue envelope to a closer proximity to infected spongiosa.

   Decortication should be performed in subacute or chronic stage. It is based on the principle, that the involved cortical bone is avascular and harbors microorganisms, while an abscess exists within the medullary cavity, where antibiotics cannot penetrate. This procedure should be performed, where initial conservative regimes have failed. The steps in decortication are:

   i. Creation of buccal flap by crestal incision extending along the necks of the teeth.
   ii. Reflection of mucoperiosteal flap to the inferior border.
   iii. Removal of teeth in the involved area.
   iv. Removal of cortical plates-lateral and inferior border, with chisel in one piece. Bone must be cut back to uninvolved areas.
   v. Bony bed should be thoroughly debrided and flap should be closed primarily and dead space is eliminated by applying pressure bandage placed to keep vascularized soft tissue in contact with bony bed.
   vi. Irrigation tubes should be placed through separate stab incision and closed suction should be employed.

5. **Continuous or intermittent indwelling closed catheter irrigation:** After intraoral sequestrectomy and saucerization or decortication, 2 small pediatric nasogastric feeding tubes, catheters or polythelene drain tubes, 3 to 4 mm in diameter and 6 to 10 inches long in length are placed against the bony bed through separate skin incisions at some distance and secured with sutures. One tube is connected to the low pressure suction to allow drainage of pus and serum and another is kept patent to provide a route through which locally antibiotics may be instilled in very high concentrations. Daily, first saline irrigation followed by antibiotic instillation should be repeated, until negative cultures are obtained. Systemic antibiotics are also continued for atleast 2 to 3 months following cessation of clinical evidence of disease.

6. **Sequestrectomy:** An integral part of definitive therapy. It helps in establishment of local microvascular proliferation. It should be undertaken through an intraoral incision; or extraoral (submandibular) approach, depending upon the site of sequestrum.

   Sequestra, are (i) usually cortical; and may be (ii) cancellous, or (iii) corticocancellous. Usually, are not seen until 2 weeks after onset of infection. These are avascular and therefore, poorly penetrated by antibiotics (Khosla, 1970). Small sequestra may undergo resorption or may get expelled spontaneously from the mucosal or skin surface. Resorption occurs by lytic activity of osteoclasts contained within the granulation tissue, which can ingrow sequestra. Sequestra are avascular, therefore are not penetrated by antibiotics. Pathological fractures can occur in the region of the sequestrum due to bone loss or because of diminution in bone strength.

   In chronic form, the involucrum is perforated by tracts (cloacae), through which pus escapes to epithelial surfaces. Rarely, sterile abscesses (Brodie's abscesses) common to long bones occur in jaws. Once the sequestrum is formed, it should be removed with minimum amount of surgical trauma.

   Prior to sequestrectomy; an assessment should be done for the need to splint and immobilize the mandible to support it, so as to avoid a surgical fracture; or to avoid displacement of fragments if pathological fracture is already present. The form of fixation is decided on the basis of dentition and site of fracture. Feeding the patient with a nasogastric tube, should be considered; if jaw movements are restricted.

   The preoperative radiograph showing the location of sequestrum is an important guide for deciding the site of incision, which may be intraoral or extraoral. The sequestrum can be clssified as— (a) small and accessible—intraoral approach, (b) large and inaccessible—extraoral approach.

Involved teeth should be removed at the same time. Intraoral wounds should be packed with iodoform gauze soaked in betadine to permit observation, as the defect fills up with granulation tissue and to allow the removal of small sequestrum, if it forms again. Extraoral submandibular incision is needed to expose the inferior border and posterior parts of the mandibular ramus. Condyle, if involved can be reached via preauricular incision. Generally, the sequestrum lies on the surface of the bone and can be removed with little effort after the periosteum has been incised and retracted. If the sequestrum is encased by the involucrum, a window must be made to allow it to be taken out. The window is cut with a sharp curette, chisel or drill may be used to outline the natural perforation created by the disease process. The cavity that is exposed almost always contains granulation tissue in which the sequestrum lies. The contents are carefully curetted out until the healthy bone is exposed to the view. If the suppuration is present, then the wound is partly closed with sutures and a rubber drain is inserted through the skin. Otherwise the wound is completely closed and antibiotic therapy is continued fo atleast 2 weeks.

7. **Saucerization:** Excision of margins of necrotic bone overlying a focus of osteomyelitis. It is useful in chronic form, since it permits removal of formed and forming sequestra with better visualization. It is performed when removal of sequestrum leaves a large cavity; and to eliminate the dead space to avoid reinfection of extensive clot. It is performed with a large round bur, so that when wound is closed, the soft tissues eliminate a dead space. The buccal cortex is reduced to the level of unattached mucosa, producing a saucer like defect.

Sequestrectomy and saucerization are to be carried out after the acute phase has subsided; and the defense mechanism of host and antimicrobial therapy have overcome the virulence of organisms.

8. **Trephination** or fenestration is the creation of bony holes or windows in the overlying cortical bone adjacent to the infectious process for tissue ammoniation and decompression of the medullary compartment. Drilling of holes into cortex and reaching medulla provide multiple surgical transcortical ports, that allow vascular communication between the periosteum and the medullary cavity.

Table 41.6: Hudson, 2000: Osteomyelitis treatment plan	
Acute osteomyelitis healthy host	***Acute osteomyelitis compromised host***
1. Conservative decompression and debridement of infection with extractions	1. Stabilize condition of host especially nutrition status
2. Drainage and irrigation, if pus present	2. Aggressive debridement and decompression with disruption of the involved periosteal rind
3. Culture and sensitivity of infected foci	3. Culture and sensitivity of infected foci
4. Antibiotic treatment for 3–4 weeks, duration based on Gram's stain, culture and sensitivity, blood culture, and ESR	4. Sustained antibiotic treatment 6–12 weeks, duration based on Gram's stain, culture and sensitivity, blood culture findings
5. Regional bony stabilization, if necessary	5. Regional bony stabilization, if necessary.

Chronic Osteomyelitis

Chronic infection present more than 1 month.

1. Host almost always compromised, if only by infectious process.
2. CT, nuclear medicine scan, perfusion studies.
3. Stabilize condition of host, especially nutrition status.
4. Wide bony sequestrectomy and decortication to normal bleeding bone and disruption of the involved periosteal rind, core out sinus tracts with extended culture and sensitivity of sequestrum specimen.
5. If purulent, consider drainage and irrigation.
6. Sustained antibiotic therapy 3–6 months, possibly longer, via central line as necessary. Duration based on Gram's stain, culture and sensitivity findings.
7. Consider nonsteroidals versus steroids.
8. Regional bony stabilization.
9. Perioperative hyperbaric oxygen therapy 20–40 dives b. i. d. on 100% O_2 for 90 @2.5 ATA.
10. Reconstruction as necessary.

9. **Resection:** When extensive portion of the bone is involved in the disease process, then resection of the jaw bone is advocated. Following resection, reconstruction is advocated: (a) to maintain the continuity of the fragments, (b) to prevent pathological fracture. (c) to prevent facial deformity and (d) to provide attachment of the soft tissues.

10. **Immediate and/or delayed reconstruction:** It is controversial. It has been used successfully in cases of (i) pathological fracture, (ii) persistence of infection after decortication, and (iii) when both cortical plates are markedly diseased. Iliac crest is a desirable graft. A block of corticocancellous iliac crest can be used or cancellous marrow is used. Stabilization may be achieved with vitallium or titanium mesh that also serves as a tray to contain the graft. Immediate reconstruction offers the obvious advantage of shortening the period of illness and speeding recovery and rehabilitation. In cases, where immediate bone grafting is contraindicated, a reconstruction plate is fixed as a spacer.

11. **Postoperative care:** It includes the following: (i) Continued use of antibiotics, analgesics, and hot saline mouth rinses, (ii) Adequate hydration, complete rest, removal of sequestrae, in case they are in the alveolar part of bone. The wound is closed preferably primarily, with a drain.

Prognosis: If proper aggressive and comprehensive therapy is instituted on time, then the recovery of acute and chronic osteomyelitis is always good. But, in cases of chronic refractory or diffuse sclerosing osteomyelitis, associated with regional or systemic disease, such as microvascular or immunosuppressive disorders, the treatment may be worse than the disease itself. In these cases attempt should be done to provide long term conservative therapy than major surgical debridement. Long term use of salicylates, nonsteroidals or steroids with laboratory monitoring is advised in some of these cases.

The treatment regime will have to be modified depending on the status of general health of the patient (Figs 41.15 to 41.21) and (Table 41.6).

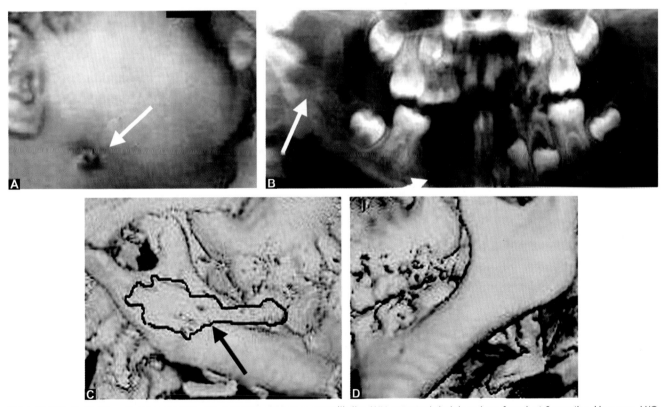

Figs 41.15A to D: Chronic osteomyelitis. (A) A 6-year-old boy came with the C/O extraoral draining sinus from last 3 months. He gave H/O high fever following swelling of R body mandibular region. He also gave H/O extraction of right side lower teeth with surgical curettage. He had pathologic fracture in R body mandible, which was treated conservatively, six months back, (B) Present OPG showed healed pathological fracture and multiple radiolucent areas in the ascending ramus right side, (C) 3D CT scan of R mandible showing the sequestrum at the ascending ramus and external oblique ridge, (D) L side 3D CT scan picture of healthy ascending ramus for comparison

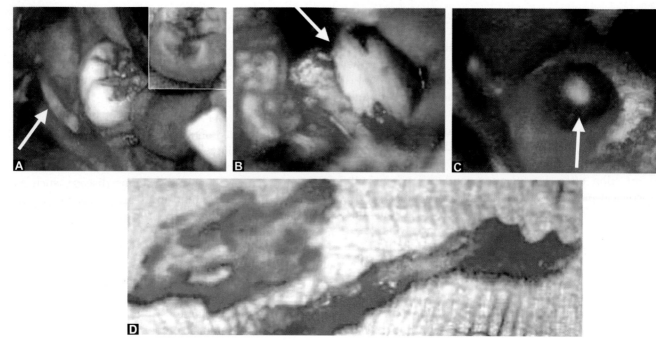

Figs 41.16A to D: Chronic osteomyelitis due to systemic high fever. Surgical sequestrectomy procedure for the boy seen in Figure 41.15: (A) Intraoral exposure of the sequestrum, (B) Extraoral postramal incision to expose the sequestrum involving the external cortex of the ascending ramus (white in color), (C) Developing tooth bud of right 2nd molar was removed (inset in 1) as it was leading to cutaneous tract and was enveloped in granulation tissue, (D) Large pieces of sequestrum were removed

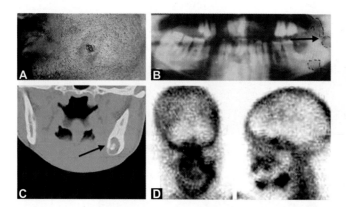

Figs 41.17A to D: Chronic osteomyelitis of odontogenic origin: (A) 50-years-old male patient C/O draining persistent cutaneous sinus and on and off swelling L mandible. H/O persistent sinus since last 8 months, following extraction of L lower third molar. Earlier multiple times extraoral curettage was done by private practitioner, (B) OPG showing multiple radiolucent areas in the ascending ramus and at the angle of L mandible. Poor periodontal status of the teeth, (C) CT scan showing the involvement at the angle region with sequestrum formation, (D) Bone scan is showing increased uptake at the left side of the mandible, suggestive of increased vascularity, inflammatory, infective pathology. Extraoral submandibular approach for sequestrectomy and saucerization was taken. Excision of the extraoral sinus tract with curettage was done

■ TYPES OF OSTEOMYELITIS

Infantile OML (OML Maxillaries Neonatorum, Maxillitis of Infancy)

It is a rare type of osteomyelitis seen in infants involving maxilla.

Wilensky, (1932) described OML in infants in a comprehensive manner. Subsequently, cases have been reported by Hitchin and Naylor, (1957), Cavanagh, (1960) and Norgaard and Pindborg (1959). It deserves special mention because of its seriousness and potential for facial deformities resulting from delayed or inappropriate treatment.

Etiology: (1) Trauma: The access may be through a break in the mucosa. Perinatal trauma caused to oral mucosa during delivery. When obstetrician's finger is inserted into child's mouth, or injury to the mucosa caused by mucous suction bulb, used to clear airway soon after birth. (2) Infection of maxillary sinus. (3) Contaminated human or artificial nipples. (4) Paunz, (1926) and Ramon et al. (1977) believe that the disease is caused by

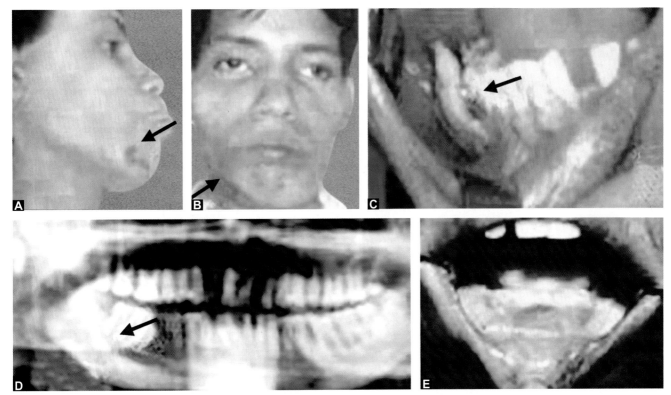

Figs 41.18A to E: Osteomyelitis secondary to sickle cell thalassemia minor. In this disorder the sickle red cell become adherent to vascular endothelium and erythrostasis is seen, which increases blood viscosity and decreases the blood flow. This brings about hypoxia to the affected region: (A and B) Extraoral draining sinus in a male patient aged 21 years, (C) Exposed large sequestrum on the right side body of the mandible. Poor oral hygiene, (D) OPG showing radiopaque sequestrum involving right ascending ramus and body, (E) Total mandibular extractions with sequestrectomy resulted in good healing

infections from the nose. (5) Hematogenous invasion by streptococci and pneumococci is also reported.

Clinical features: Almost seen a few weeks after birth. The disease shows considerable variation in severity. There is sudden onset and acute course. The disease may also have slow onset and a chronic course. In acute stage, severe pain and high fever; and with chronic course there is moderate pain and slight fever.

a. *General constitutional manifestations:* Pyrexia, anorexia, dehydration, convulsions, or vomiting may occur.

b. *Extraoral examination:* Facial cellulitis seen centered around orbit. Inner canthal swelling, palpebral edema, closure of eye, conjunctivitis, and proptosis may result.

c. *Intraoral examination would reveal:* (i) Maxilla usually affected; especially molar region, (ii) Subperiosteal abscesses in alveolar region. These are seen as buccal or palatal swellings. (iii) Fluctuation is often present, (iv) Fistulae or pus draining tracts may exist in alveolar mucosa.

d. *Laboratory findings:* Leukocytosis is generally present.

e. *Microbiology:* Organisms implicated are *S. aureus* and also streptococci.

f. *Radiological findings:* In early stage, the radiographs are of a little value, as there is minimal bone involvement. In late stages, intraoral films help to locate sequestra and necrotic tooth germs.

g. *Risks:* Prior to pre antibiotic era, mortality and morbidity was very high. With the advent of the antibiotics, it is considerably reduced. Death usually occurs due to spread of infection to brain (Cavernous sinus thrombophlebitis).

The risks involved are: (i) Permanent optic damage, (ii) Neurological complications, (iii) Loss of tooth buds and bone. Instances of extension into dural sinuses has been reported.

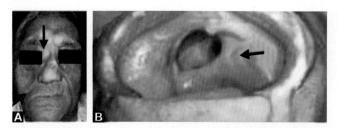

Figs 41.19A and B: Extensive bone loss due to osteomyelitis following aspergillosis infection of the right upper jaw: (A) An 80 years old male gave H/O on and off swelling on the right upper jaw and purulent discharge from right nostril, fever and general debility. Intraoral draining sinuses were present through which small sequestras used to come out. For six months patient was treated by various doctors. At our center, patient was diagnosed having aspergillosis infection. Extraoral Weber Fergusson incision was taken. Large pieces of sequestrae were removed. Postoperative photo showing the extensive bone loss in right maxilla and nasal bones, (B) Intraoral healing showing the defect following sequestrectomy

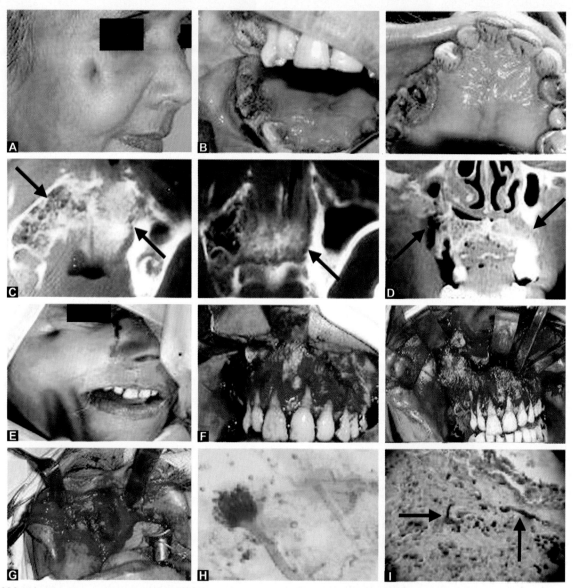

Figs 41.20A to I: (A) A 65-year-old lady came with C/O draining extraoral sinus in the R cheek area and pus discharge from R tuberosity region, (B) Intraoral picture shows the extensive sequestrum exposed in the oral cavity in R maxillary region from R tuberosity to R canine region, (C) CT scan-occlusal view shows much more extensive destruction of maxillary bone from R tuberosity till L premolar area involving complete palatal vault, (D) Coronal view CT scan shows pathological fracture of R infraorbital rim, involvement of R maxillary sinus and separation of sequestrum from the nasal floor, (E) Extraoral Weber Fergusson incision was planned, (F) Complete maxilla along with the teeth showed necrotic bone and its separation from the normal bone. Downfracturing of maxillary sequestrum carried out, (G) Surgical defect after sequestrectomy, (H) Tissue was sent for fungal culture-report was aspergillus fumigatus infection. Fungal hyphae were seen, (I) Fungal hyphae seen in GMS (Gomori's methenamine silver) stained slide

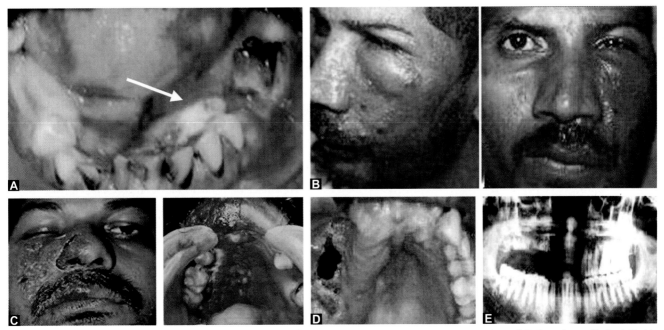

Figs 41.21A to E: Osteomyelitis following herpes zoster infection of face: (A) Intraoral picture showing the exfoliation of mandibular left side teeth and sequestrum in the body, (B) Extraoral picture of the patient, (C) Another patient with herpes zoster infection of the face, (D) Intraoral exfoliation of right maxillary teeth with sequestration of bone, (E) OPG showing the bone and teeth loss on right side maxilla

Differential diagnosis: (1) Dacrocystitis neonatorum, (2) Orbital cellulitis, (3) Ophthalmia neonatorum, and (4) Infantile cortical hyperostosis. The oral manifestations help to distinguish the early condition from these conditions.

Treatment: The treatment should be prompt and aggressive.

1. Antibiotics, be preferably given by IV route. Penicillins or penicillinase-resistant penicillins like flucloxacillin, or broad spectrum antibiotics may be given for 2 to 4 weeks.
2. *Culture and sensitivity testing:* Culture is taken from the discharge from sinus tracts; and sensitivity testing should be done. The antibiotic regimen is to be modified accordingly. Many cases of acute OML, are cured by antibiotics only. Schenk (1948) was the first to report five cases treated with penicillin. All his patients were cured without loss of tooth germs.
3. *Incision and drainage of fluctuant areas:* It is indicated in the presence of periosteal or palatal abscesses.
4. *Irrigations:* In case of sinus tracts, irrigations are done frequently.
5. *Supportive therapy:* (i) Analgesics and antipyretics, (ii) Fluids, (iii) Proper diet. Proteins and multivitamins should be supplied abundantly.

6. *Sequestrectomy or removal of necrotic tooth germs:* Removal of sequestra is undertaken when they are completely separated, and on the basis of clinical and radiological findings. Surgical interference should be conservative; as loss of bone and teeth leads to severe deformities later in life.
7. Children who have undergone sequestrectomies, should be followed up by an orthodontist to aid in the development of the arch and maintenance of occlusion.

The development of adult dentition gets disturbed. Teeth may show hypoplasia, similar to those in Turner's syndrome. Some degree of decreased development of affected maxilla is expected.

Garre's Sclerosing Osteomyelitis

Also known as chronic nonsuppurative sclerosing OML, chronic OML with proliferative periostitis, and periostitis ossificans.

It was first described by Carl Garre (1893), as irritation induced focal thickening of periosteum and cortical bone of tibia. It is a nonsuppurative inflammatory process; where there is peripheral subperiosteal bone deposition caused by mild irritation and infection.

Pathogenesis: The etiological agents can be a carious tooth, or the overlying soft tissue infection (Ellis et al. 1977). The infectious process localizes in periosteum or beneath the periosteal covering of cortex and spreads slightly into the interior of bone.

In case of persistence of the causative agent, it causes bony thickening, visible on radiograph (Smith and Farmann, 1977).

Pell et al. (1955) reported the first case in jaws. It generally involves mandible (Lichty et al, 1980). The disease primarily occurs in children and young adults; and occasionally in older individuals.

Clinical features: It is characterized by: (i) localized hard, nontender bony swelling of lateral and inferior aspects of mandible, (ii) lymphadenopathy, hyperpyrexia and leukocytosis usually not found.

Radiography: A focal area of well calcified bone proliferation may be seen that is smooth and that often has a laminated or "onion skin" appearance.

The radiographic appearance is typical. There is condensation of cortical bone, and overgrowth of bony tissue beneath the periosteum. The increase in mass of bone is due to several factors: (i) Mild toxic stimulation of fibroblasts by attenuated infection, (ii) Compensatory thickening of bone as a mechanical adaptation to reinforce the area weakened through disease; and (iii) An exuberant attempt at repair.

When no dental disease exists; or when lesion persists after treatment of dental pathology, biopsy should be considered to establish diagnosis.

Differential diagnosis: It should be differentiated from infantile cortical hyperostosis, or Caffey's disease. It occurs in young infants and involves a number of bones. The clavicles and ulnae are usually, and mandible invariably involved. Caffey, (1950) believed that the disease was of infectious origin because of high fever and increased ESR.

No bacteria could be cultured from the tissues. The condition is uninfluenced with antibiotics. The disease usually is self-limiting and eventually regresses.

Treatment: It is directed towards removing sources of inflammation: (a) Removal of infected tooth and curettage of socket, (b) Surgical recontouring: This is done to recontour the cortical expansion of the jaw. This is attempted only if there is obvious expansion, (c) Endodontic therapy, (d) Antibiotics: if signs of infection are present, and (e) Follow up.

Chronic Sclerosing OML (Focal and Diffuse)

The various other names are sclerosing osteitis, ossifying OML, sclerosing cementoma, gigantiform cementoma, and sclerotic cemental masses.

Radiographically: There are two forms: (i) Focal (condensing osteitis), (ii) Diffuse (multiple condensing osteitis). Nonexpansile radiopaque lesion.

1. *Focal form:* (i) Below the age of twenty, (ii) More common in mandible, (iii) Associated with infected pulp of lower molars/premolars, (iv) Appears as circumscribed radiopaque mass of sclerotic bone associated with tooth roots. (v) Margins may be distinct or may blend into surrounding bone.

   It is thought that sclerotic /condensed bone is the body's response to irritation.

   Histopathologically: There is dense mass of bone trabeculae with little interstitial marrow and few lymphocytes.

   Treatment: (i) Endodontic therapy, and/or (ii) Extraction

2. *Multilple form:* These occur in both maxilla and mandible (resembles chronic suppurative OML). Pain is a prominent feature. Suppuration is usually absent.

   Radiographically: It shows dense radiopaque masses.

   Treatment: Much depends upon presentation: debridement, antibiotic therapy, alveolectomy, and HBO_2, etc.

Actinomycotic OML of Jaws

Definition: It is a chronic infection manifesting both granulomatous and suppurative features; and usually involves soft tissues and occasionally bone.

Types: There are three types: (1) Cervicofacial, (2) Thoracic, and (3) Abdominal.

Cervicofacial: About 2/3rd of cases are cervicofacial. It involves mandible, overlying soft tissues, parotid gland, tongue and maxillary sinuses. Secondary spread to other areas of head may occur.

Historical background: J Israel in 1877, isolated an organism belonging to genus *Actinomyces.* Historically, such organisms were considered to be fungi and are associated with a disease in humans analogous to lumpy jaw disease of cattle.

At least three types of *Actinomyces* have been related to the disease. (i) *A. israelii:* It is responsible for disease in humans. (ii) *A. bovis:* It is responsible for disease in cattle, but rarely in humans. (iii) *A. baudetti:* It is responsible for diseases in cats and dogs.

Several species of Actinomyces are found as normal saprophytes in human oral cavity; including: *A. israelii, A. naeslundii, A. propionicus,* and *A. eriksonii.* Except for *A. Israelii,* the role of these organisms in the disease is not established.

These are endogenous in origin, and are found in (i) Tonsillar crypts, (ii) Salivary and dental calculus, and (iii) Mucosa of oropharyngeal and gastrointestinal regions.

Pathogenecity is attributed to changes in local or general environment.

Characteristic features: It is now recognized that *Actinomyces* are not fungi; but are Gram positive, microaerophilic, nonsporeforming, and non-acid-fast bacteria.

Like *Nocardia* and Mycobacteria, Actinomycetes, share characteristics of both bacteria and fungi. However, they are not sensitive to antifungal drugs; and unlike fungi, are sensitive to antibiotics.

Cell-wall: Electron microscopy and other studies confirm their bacterial nature.

Pathogenesis: Organisms gain entry into soft tissues directly or by extension from bone through (i) Periapical, or (ii) Periodontal lesions, and (iii) Fractures, or (iv) Extraction sites.

When established, infection spreads without regard to fascial planes and typically appears on cutaneous rather than mucosal surfaces.

Clinical features: Patients present with the following:
  i. Soft or firm tissue masses on the skin; which have purplish, dark red, oily areas with occasional small zones of fluctuation.
 ii. Spontaneous drainage of serous fluid containing granular material. These granules are yellowish substances called sulfur granules, and represent colonies of bacteria.
iii. Regional lymph nodes are occasionally enlarged.
 iv. Trismus: Not common; unless secondary infection.
  v. Pyrexia: Usually the patient is not febrile; and does not feel ill.
     Microscopically, it shows closely packed branching filaments 1 μ in diameter.

Radiography: The common findings are (i) radiolucent areas of varying sizes, and (ii) delay in healing of extraction sites.

Periostitis: Diffuse mandibular radiolucencies and marked bone sclerosis.

Sequestra formation is occasionally present.

Laboratory studies: ESR and WBCC may be slightly elevated.

Whenever, a firm mass/infections, which does not respond to conventional antibiotic therapy, then actinomycosis, mycosis, mycobacterial infection, and neoplasms should be considered in diagnosis.

Differential diagnosis of actinomycosis: The following conditions should be considered: Parotitis, parotid tumors, cervical tuberculosis, and pyogenic OML.

Diagnosis is based on (1) Culture and sensitivity testing, and (2) Biopsy.
1. Culture: Aerobic and anaerobic organisms, and (2) Direct fluorescent antibody test. It is shown to be specific for *A. israelii.*
2. Biopsy of the wall of abscess or fistula is useful when material is not available for smear and culture, or laboratory data.

Management: In the past, many therapeutic agents and techniques were used including: (i) Iodides, (ii) Radiation, (iii) Incision and drainage, and (iv) Excision of soft tissues and bone. Currently, iodides and radiotherapy are considered to be ineffective.

Incision and drainage: All abscesses, regardless of how small they are, should be surgically disrupted with a hemostat and all loculations penetrated.

Hospitalization is required; because, antibiotics are administered parenterally: (i) in high doses, (ii) for protracted periods of time, and (iii) shows temporary resolution and recurrence.

Penicillin is the antibiotic of choice. The dose depends on severity of the disease. 10 to 20 million units daily for 3 to 4 months; 3 million units IV every 4 hourly for 2 weeks or longer.

Subsequently; 0. 5 gm probenecid orally four times daily. This daily 2 gm probenecid will increase blood concentration of penicillin 2 to 3 folds by inhibiting its renal excretion.

In patients allergic to penicillin:
 a. Tetracycline (especially Minocycline 250 mg 4 times daily for 8 to 16 weeks, may be prescribed (Martin, 1985).
 b. Erythromycin 500 mg 4 times daily for 6 months. The dosages and durations for therapy used are effective for most infections; and result in temporary resolution, only to be

followed by recurrence. Therefore, high doses for extended periods are recommended.

c. Sequestrectomy and saucerization may be necessary.

Follow-up: Radiographs are taken periodically to monitor changes in bone.

TUBERCULOUS OSTEOMYELITIS OF THE JAW BONES

Tuberculosis, or the king of diseases, as it was known, was rampant in the Third World Countries way back in the early 1900's. A chronic infectious disease caused by *Mycobacterium tuberculosis*, it was considered to be the single most common cause for death in those days.

Advances in chemotherapy, inoculation with BCG vaccines and improvement in public health and nutritional status led to a drop in the incidence of the disease in the 1980s. But again there has been a resurgence of the disease in the 1990s.

According to the World Health Organization's Survey in 1998, one-third of the world's population is suffering from tuberculosis. Every year 10 to 12 million new cases are developing worldwide, with approximately 2 to 2.5 million cases in India alone.

The disease once considered to be nonexistent in developed countries is now being diagnosed more commonly in those countries also. Surprisingly, now it is the musculoskeletal system that is more commonly affected as compared to the respiratory system (Lachenauer CS, Constentinos, 1991). This resurgence of tuberculosis has been attributed to:

1. Population explosion in the world leading to poor sanitation and hygiene.
2. Failure of patients to complete the long term Antikoch's therapy, thereby acting as carriers of the disease.
3. Complacency of the pharmaceutical companies to develop a new drug in the past two decades leading to the development of drug resistant strains of *Mycobacterium tuberculosis*.
4. Increase in the number of AIDS patients.

Tuberculous osteomyelitis of the maxilla and mandible was earlier considered as a rare disease. But, of late, the incidence is on the rise with isolated presentation in the jaws. The supposed rarity of the disease in the jaws seldom arouses clinical suspicion, especially, when a positive history of systemic infection is absent. The diagnosis is established only after a careful biopsy and microbiological study.

Etiopathogenesis

The tuberculous microorganism belongs to the *Mycobacterium* genus. This genus includes a group of aerobic, nonsporulating, nonmotile bacilli with a high cell wall lipid content and a slow growth rate. *M. tuberculosis* is classified as an acid fast *Bacillus*, because it retains the carbol fuchsin red dye after washing with acid, alcohol or both. It is transmitted from person to person by inhalation of infective droplets that result from aerosolization of respiratory secretions.

In tuberculous osteomyelitis of the maxilla and the mandible, there are three possible methods of inoculation of the bacteria into the bone.

1. Direct inoculation of the bacilli into the oral mucosa through an ulcer or break in the continuity of the mucosa.
2. Spread to the bone via an extraction socket or an infected fracture line.
3. Hematogenous or lymphatic spread from a primary focus elsewhere in the body.

The disease progresses slowly, with the formation of a tubercle in the bone marrow. There is an increased vascularity of the periosteum with initial subperiosteal resorption of bone, followed by laying down of a new layer of reactive bone. As the disease progresses, there is caseation in the central portion of the bone. Ultimately, the pus extends peripherally and a subperiosteal abscess is formed. If the disease progresses, the periosteum gives way and the tuberculous debris are expelled into the soft tissues, from where they follow the path of least resistance. The infection tracks along the fascial planes to the surface of the skin. The abscess reddens, but is not warm and is therefore called a "cold abscess". The skin becomes progressively thinner and ultimately yields in such a way that a tuberculous sinus is formed.

Clinical Presentation of Tuberculous Osteomyelitis of the Jaw Bones

The sites most commonly involved are the ramus and body of the mandible. The age group is around 15 to 40 years. The patient may show clinical features similar to a subperiosteal abscess, which may have initially be drained resulting in a non healing sinus tract formation. There may be two types of presentation of tuberculous osteomyelitis of the jaw bones.

Closed Lesions (Lumpy Jaw) (Fig. 41.22)

The lesion is located centrally in the bone. The patient will present only with a swelling and no draining sinuses. There is usually an absence of any oral septic focus. This lesion is usually seen in the ramus of the mandible. When the lesion is in the ramus, it may mimic a parotid swelling or submasseteric abscess.

Open Lesions (Fig. 41.23)

There is a presence of multiple extraoral and intraoral sinuses with mucopurulent discharge. Oral septic focus may or may not be present.

Diagnosis and Treatment

10-point Protocol Formulated for the Management of Tuberculous Osteomyelitis of the Jaw Bones (Figs 41.24 and 41.25)

1. *Aspiration for smear and culture studies:* In cases of closed lesions in the jaws, in the absence of an oral septic focus, aspiration is a must to identify and differentiate between a cystic lesion, neoplasm, odontogenic infection, and cold abscess. Aspiration is done using a 5 cc syringe and a disposable 18G needle. Using aseptic precautions, the skin is pierced to enter the abscess cavity. The aspirate is then collected in a sterile test tube and sent to the microbiology laboratory for smear and culture studies. The smear is tested for acid fast bacilli. Culture is done on Lowenstein Jensen medium. The time taken for the colonies to develop varies from 48 hours to 8 weeks.

2. *Radiographs:* The commonly used views to visualize the mandible and the maxilla are:
   - Orthopantomogram
   - PA Mandible
   - PA Waters
   - Lateral Oblique view of the mandible closed lesions of the jaws are usually seen as a small well defined radiolucency, usually in the ascending ramus with destruction of the buccal or medial cortical plate.

   Chest radiographs are a must to rule out pulmonary involvement. Both PA and lateral views are indicated. Full body radiographs are taken, only when a scintigram shows a 'hotspot' in any other area of the body apart from the affected site.

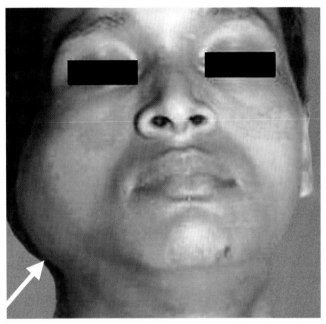

Fig. 41.22: Tuberculous osteomyelitis—closed lesion or lumpy jaw

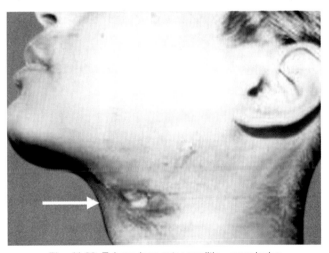

Fig. 41.23: Tuberculous osteomyelitis—open lesion

3. *Scintigraphy:* It is indicative of the metabolic changes within the bone. These metabolic changes preceed the changes seen on the radiograph. Scintigraphy though not specific, is a sensitive indicator of bone disease with a range of 89 to 100 percent sensitivity. A full body scan with technetium-99m diphosphonate dye is done to rule out systemic involvement.
   Areas of increased activity are seen as 'Hot spots' on the scan.

4. *Computed tomography:* This is a very useful and accurate imaging system, which shows not only

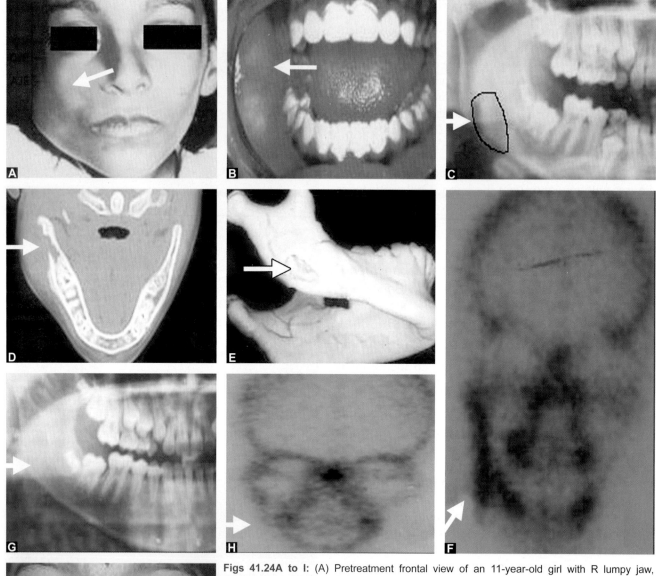

Figs 41.24A to I: (A) Pretreatment frontal view of an 11-year-old girl with R lumpy jaw, (B) Pretreatment intraoral view. Note the swelling on the right side and fair oral hygiene, (C) Pre-OPG showing unicystic radiolucency at R angle and ramus mandible, (D) Pre-axial CT scan—destruction of the buccal cortex of ascending ramus, (E) Pre-3D reconstruction CT scan perforation of buccal cortex, (F) Pretreatment bone scan. Increased uptake in right ramus mandible, (G) Post-AKT regime-16 months later. Regeneration of bone seen in OPG, (H) Post-AKT regime-16 months later. Decreased uptake in R ramus mandible, (I) Post-AKT front view after 16 months

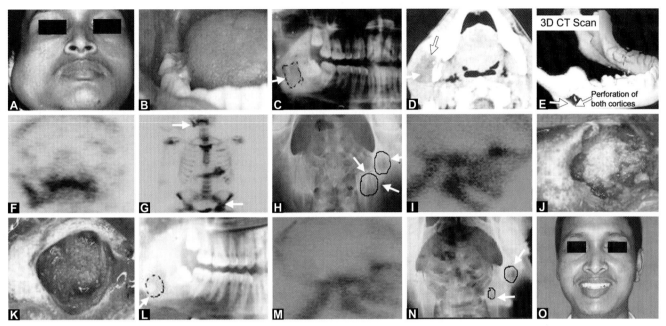

Figs 41.25A to O: (A) Preoperative front view showing right ramus swelling: Lumpy jaw, (B) Preoperative intraoral view showing fair oral hygiene, (C) Preoperative OPG—unicystic radiolucent lesion in R ramus, (D) Preoperative axial CT scan: Note the abscess in masseter muscle and destruction of buccal and lingual cortices, (E) 3D CT scan showing perforation of both cortices, (F) Preoperative bone scan: Hot spot in R ramus, (G) Preoperative whole body bone scan: Hot spot in R ramus and L pelvic region, (H) Preoperative X-ray pelvis—radiolucencies in L pelvic region, (I) Preoperative bone scan mandible, (J) Intraoperative caseated necrotic tissue, perforation of buccal and lingual cortex, (K) Intraoperative picture after complete curettage. Medial pterygoid muscle is seen through the perforation, (L) Postoperative OPG-after 6 months of AKT following surgery. Note the decrease in size of the lesion, (M) Postoperative and post-AKT bone scan after 6 months, (N) Post-AKT (after 6 months) X-ray of pelvis showing regression of the radiolucencies, (O) Postoperative post-AKT (after 6 months) front view of the face

bony, but also soft tissue changes. The advantages over routine radiographs are:

- The extent of the disease can be accurately determined.
- Medullary involvement can be identified.
- A medial rotation of the mandible can be done to visualize the medial cortex (which is very often the site for involvement for closed lesions.)
- Diagnosis of subperiosteal abscess, muscle involvement and lymph node involvement is facilitated.

5. *Mantoux testing:* An intradermal injection of 5 tuberculin units (5TU) in a 0.1 ml solution of purified protein derivative is given using a 27 G needle.

   A positive reaction may be seen clinically after 48 hours as erythema and induration measuring > 5 to 10 mm.

   A negative mantoux test does not exclude tuberculosis. Similarly a positive mantoux is not confirmatory for tuberculosis.

6. *Sputum for AFB:* Early morning sputum samples are collected on three consecutive days and sent to the laboratory for smear and culture. A positive report may indicate involvement of the lungs or the nasopharynx. A nasopharyngeal swab and scraping may be required to rule out involvement of the latter. Detection of sputum AFB under fluorescent microscopy is a more sensitive test.

7. *Biopsy:* An incisional biopsy is done only for open cases. Aspiration is done for closed cases.

   Tissue curetted from the sinus tract and deeper tissues is sent immediately in normal saline for smear and culture. Tissue is also sent in 5 percent formalin for histopathological evaluation to identify tuberculoma, early caeseation, Langhans giant cells, and lymphoid activity. These features are pathognomonic of tuberculosis. A positive biopsy is confirmatory for tuberculous infection.

8. *Surgical treatment*
   a. *Closed lesions:* Usually no oral septic focus is present.

i. *Aspirate positive for AFB:* In these cases, the patient is started on a suitable antikoch's regimen. After 6 to 8 weeks the lesion is reviewed both clinically and radiographically to evaluate the need for surgical debridement.

ii. *Aspirate negative for AFB:* If the aspirate is negative for AFB, no incisional biopsy is indicated. A complete excisional biopsy and debridement of the tissues is done. The tissue is sent for histopathological studies. If positive for tuberculosis, the patient is started on Antikoch's therapy.

b. *Open lesions:* For open lesions, a biopsy of the tissue from the sinus tract and the deeper tissues is sent for histopathological studies. If the tissue is positive for tuberculosis, a suitable Antikoch's regimen is started, and no surgery is performed immediately. This to prevent dissemination of the disease, that is, milliary spread of tuberculosis by the hematogenous route.

After 6 to 8 weeks of Antikoch's treatment, the patient is reassessed clinically as well as radiographically to decide upon the need for surgery.

9. *Antikoch's treatment:* Depending on the severity of the disease, and the patient's body weight, the physician starts on a suitable Antikoch's therapy. Usually a six months regimen with four drugs is advised.

Intensive treatment: In the first four months, all four drugs, that is, isoniazide, rifampicin, ethambutol, and pyrizinamide are given.

Continuation phase: Isoniazide and rifampicin are given for the next four months.

In addition, ciprofloxacin may be added to the regimen as it is known to be extremely effective in bone tuberculosis.

During the therapy, the patient is advised to have high protein and carbohydrate diet. As these drugs are hepatotoxic, the patient is monitored for signs of hepatotoxicity. Liver function tests are done every six weeks.

10. *Long term follow up:* It is advised to ensure patient compliance in taking the drugs. A periodic monitoring of the patient clinically and radiographically to assess the course of the disease is a must. Adjustments in the AKT regimen must be done accordingly. The patients must be followed up for reccurence.

OSTEORADIONECROSIS OF THE FACIAL BONES

Osteoradionecrosis (ORN) is also known as radiation OML. It is known as the most serious, late complication of therapeutic radiotherapy (RT) for head and neck (H and N) cancer, as it produces considerable morbidity.

The cancers of oral and maxillofacial region are treated by (i) Radiation therapy, and (ii) Surgery, or (iii) Both. This complication of ORN is seen to be dependent on the technique of the RT used, in particular— the radiation dose to the bone. A total dosage of approximately 6500 to 7000 uGy or greater, particularly to the floor of the mouth and mandible significantly show elevated incidence of ORN of the mandible. Dose rates in excess of 0. 55 uGy/hour have also been seen to elevate the risk of ORN. Increased dosages and dose rates are usually given in the treatment of T2, T3 and T4 neoplastic lesions. Radioactive implants given within a tissue tumor also shows a higher incidence of ORN.

Ionizing radiation destroys malignant neoplasms by damaging the chromosomes; so that, the cell division is impaired. Irradiation induces inflammatory response in soft tissue with erythema, desquamation and pigmentation of overlying skin. Radiation injuries include hard and soft tissues, because of the damage to tissue cells and the vascular system. These changes are progressive and may result in gradual devitalization of bone tissue, which may lead to bone and/or soft tissue necrosis in a small percent of patients.

Major salivary glands—which are within the field of irradiation show changes in the salivary function. Fractionated irradiation impairs the flow of saliva by slowly destroying salivary gland tissue. Salivation is suppressed; the saliva is scanty and sticky. Xerostomia is the principal long term symptom of impairment of salivary flow in irradiated tissue. Decreases of 83 percent or more of mean whole salivary flow rates have been recorded. Possible sequelae to xerostomia include an alteration of the chemical composition of saliva and increased potential for traumatic injury due to dry oral mucosa.

Periodontal disease: It is exacerbated; some degree of atrophy of periodontal membrane, gingival recession occurs without pocketing, exposing the necks of teeth.

Widespread radiation caries: Affecting smooth surfaces of the crowns of teeth. The most damaging effect of xerostomia, is the rapid shift of the oral microflora to highly cariogenic bacteria. This is because of decreased salivary flow, which compromises the body's defenses against increased growth rates of cariogenic microorganisms. Many of the patients develop a highly destructive type of dental caries and saliva recalcification of early (white spot) enamel lesions cannot occur.

Definition

Osteoradionecrosis (ORN) is an exposure of nonviable, non-healing, nonseptic lesion in the irradiated bone, which fails to heal without intervention. It is a sequelae of irradiation induced tissue injury, in which hypocellularity, hypovascularity and hypoxia are the underlying causes.

Clinically, ORN may appear as a sequestrum or dead bone, osteopenic and fibrotic in nature. Although ORN lesions may be infected, this is usually a secondary event to the true pathophysiologic process of radiation necrosis, which provides a host medium opportunity for the infecting bacteria. Role of microorganisms is that of, not the causative factor, but they complicate the process and the extent of the treatment.

Exposed bone, however, is not necessarily radiation compromised or dead. It may be due to the soft tissue envelope insult and if conservatively supported, may heal without bone debridement. This is generally seen in cases, in which the total radiation dosage is below 500 uGy. Glabrous skin is a reliable sign of atleast radiation induced soft tissue injury and should promote suspicion of underlying bony sequestrum.

Incidence

The reported incidence of ORN of the facial bones varies widely. Incidence of involvement of the mandible ranges from 2 to 3 percent. A key factor in ORN, particularly of the mandible refers to trauma, especially tooth extraction. Extraction has been reported as the trigger for ORN in 60 to 89 percent of cases. Osteoradionecrosis of the maxilla is extremely rare. The second most common facial bone involved with ORN is the temporal bone, in which it usually develops spontaneously with a long latency period.

The time period between the RT and the development of ORN has been reported as a mean of 7. 5 years and up to 20 years.

Etiopathology (Pathological Changes)

1. Marx, (1983) described its causes, as the 'Three H' principle of irradiated tissue. (i) Hypocellularity, (ii) Hypovascularity of the irradiated tissues and (iii) Hypoxia. This comprises of all the elements of bone; including marrow and periosteum, as well as the investing soft tissues. 2. Failure of osteoclastic activity. The hypoxic tissue, when damaged, is unable to respond metabolically to the injury. Due to hypoxia, the injured tissue macrophages are unable to phagocytose bacteria or dead tissue in wounds, fibroblasts fail to lay down new collagen and a chronic non healing wound develops. (Wound, whose oxygen and metabolic requirements for healing exceed the available supply).

Mechanism

Therapeutic doses of irradiation cause endothelial death, thrombosis and hyalinization of blood vessels. It is described as progressive obliterative endarteritis, periarteritis, hyalinization; and fibrosis, and thrombosis of vessels that leads to a decreased microcirculation (ischemia and reduction in viable osteocyte population). Periosteum undergoes fibrosis, osteoblasts and osteocytes are destroyed and marrow spaces in bone become filled with fibrous tissue. There is a decrease of cellularity of all tissues and vascularity is markedly decreased. These changes lead to a measurable hypoxia in irradiated tissues compared with normal.

Pathological Changes

Effects of radiation on soft and hard tissue: (i) Mucositis, (ii) Atrophic mucosa, (iii) Xerostomia, and (iv) Radiation caries. Bone absorbs more energy than soft tissues, because of it's mineral composition; and is more susceptible to secondary radiation.

Effects of radiation on bone depend upon: (i) Quality and quantity of radiation, (ii) Size of portals used, (iii) Location and extent of lesion, and (iv) Condition of teeth and periosteum.

The irradiated bone may become necrotic (aseptic necrosis), and the regenerative capacity of bone forming tissues is destroyed. The effects are: (i) Direct effects on the osteoblasts and osteoclasts, (ii) Occlusion of blood vessels by thrombosis or by fibrosis of surrounding structures.

The mandible is more commonly subjected to thrombosis, because inferior alveolar artery is the main arterial supply. Maxilla has multiple blood supply, hence it develops aseptic necrosis less frequently. The presence of aseptic necrosis predisposes to ORN; which can be initiated by trauma, infection or both. The trauma is usually the result of extraction of teeth after irradiation; or the result of ulceration from a denture.

The preradiation extraction of teeth in a neglected mouth in the affected segment is strongly recommended.

It is advisable to delay irradiation for 7 to 10 days to allow healing of extraction sockets. If necessary, the patient may be hospitalized and the teeth should be removed in one session preferably under antibiotic cover.

Alveoloplasty, at this stage is also recommended to allow proper wound closure. All prominent interdental septa are ground off and sharp bony margins are removed or filed off.

Factors Involved in Reduction of ORN

Problems caused by irradiation of tumors

1. In children, it can cause: (i) Interference with normal growth and development of jaws, (ii) Irregularities in the formation and eruption of teeth (Pietrokovski and Menczel; 1966).
2. *In adults, it causes:* (i) Demineralization of teeth; known as "irradiation caries". It usually affects the cervical margins of teeth. del Regato et al. (1985) and Meyer, (1958 and 1970) have discussed the effects of irradiation caries.
3. Decreased salivary flow and reduced salivary pH have been implicated and contributes to irradiation caries.
4. *Mucositis:* (i) This leads to poor oral hygiene, and predisposes to infection of periodontal structures. (ii) The integrity and resistance of oral mucosa to injury is impaired, especially gingivae. (iii) Bone-forming and protective function of periosteum is lost if it has been destroyed. (v) Pressure from a denture may cause ulceration. This may destroy the continuity of gingivae of alveolar process. The failure to heal, the exposed bone is subject to infection and may lead to sequestration.
5. Secondary candidiasis.
6. *Skin:* It becomes inflamed, resulting in dermatitis; which is extremely painful. When recovery occurs, there is destruction of hair follicles resulting in partial baldness of the face. The subcutaneous tissues along with the skin; also undergo breakdown similar to mucosa; this may complicate the situation, if infection develops, and if surgical procedures are undertaken.

With the modern methods of therapeutic irradiation, ORN is less frequent now. (i) Recently, megavoltage has replaced orthovoltage. The megavol-tage is thought to be bone-sparing. Other factors are effective in reduction of its occurrence. (ii) Dose fractionation, (iii) Meticulous collimation, (iv) Shielding normal tissues, and (v) Maintaining pre and post-irradiation dental health.

Clinical Features

Osteoradionecrosis (ORN) has a varied clinical and radiographic presentation and there is no single diagnostic sign or test. ORN is painful, debilitating and frequently refractory to treatment: (1) Severe, deep, boring pain which may continue for weeks or months. (2) Swelling of face when infection develops, (3) Soft tissue abscesses and persistently draining sinuses, (4) Exposed bone; in association with intraoral or extraoral fistulae (Figs 41.26 to 41.30), (5) Trismus, (6) Fetid odor, (7) Pyrexia, (8) Pathological fracture may be present.

The signs and symptoms would vary depending upon the cause: (i) If extraction of tooth is the cause, an area of denuded bone may be seen on alveolar process, which may be viable. The mucosa may show sloughing, and the area of exposed bone shows tendency to become larger.

There is slow sequestration; because not only the osteoblastic, but also osteoclastic activity is destroyed. When sequestration occurs, generally, a large piece of bone is separated from unaffected vital part of mandible.

Involvement of fascial spaces of face and neck leading to deep cellulitis. There may be sloughing of adjoining skin and mucosa. Pathological fracture may also occur.

Radiological Features

In the early stage, there is little change. It may appear as radiolucent, modeling with indefinite nonsclerotic borders and occasional areas of radiopacity associated with bony sequestrum. Sequestra and involucra occur late or not at all; because of severely compromised blood supply. Initial blood flow assays with nuclear isotope technetium-99 methylene diphosphate scanning can be of some benefit in assessing regional perfusion of the afflicted areas.

Treatment

There is no universally accepted treatment for ORN of the jaws. The management of ORN remains controversial, both radical and conservative treatments have been reported. *Conservative treatment*—systemic antibiotics, selective rinsing with topical antiseptics, selective removal of small sequestra, curetting and

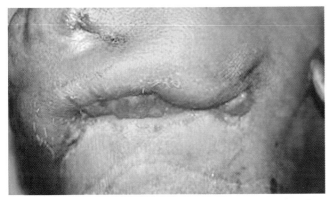

Fig. 41.26: Clinical picture of chronic osteoradionecrosis. Note the multiple draining sinuses with exposure of bone

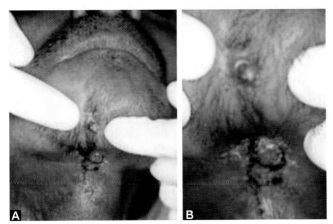

Figs 41.27A and B: Chronic osteoradionecrosis following radiation which was given following surgery for malignancy of lower jaw

local debridement and/or burring it out until normal bleeding bone appears.

Radical treatment is indicated, where acute and progressive ORN is refractory to conservative treatment.

Recent treatment is directed to supporting and salvaging viable but compromised tissue and not attempting to resurrect dead tissue and is aimed at reversing the hypoxia and increasing the vascularity and cellularity of the tissues. It is focused on revascularization of irradiated bone by certain techniques, such as HBO and microvascular free flaps. However, the choice depends on the general condition of the host, severity and location of the disease and availability of the techniques (Tables 41.7 and 41.8).

In general, the treatment comprises of:

1. Debridement.
2. *Control of infection:* Antibiotics are administered to control acute infection, if present. However, since there is no circulation in the necrotic bone, antibiotics do not penetrate it.
3. Hospitalization.
4. *Other supportive treatment:* (i) Hydration: fluid therapy, (ii) High protein and vitamin diet.
5. Analgesics: Narcotic and non-narcotic analgesics. Bupivacaine (Marcaine), alcohol nerve blocks, nerve avulsion, rhizotomy.
6. *Good oral hygiene:* Oral rinses, such as 1 percent sodium fluoride gel, 1 percent chlorhexidine gluconate and plain water help to prevent radiation induced caries from the xerostomia and mucositis by providing some local augmentation of the host immune antimicrobial activity.
7. Frequent irrigations of wounds.
8. Exposed dead bone: (i) Small pieces of bone may become loose and can be removed easily.

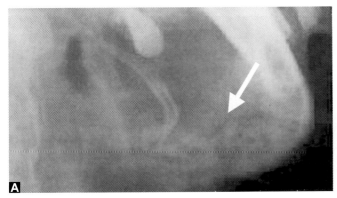

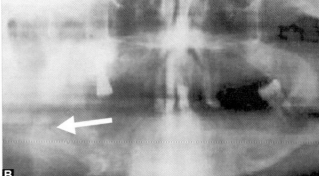

Figs 41.28A and B: Osteoradionecrosis, X-ray picture of the patient seen in Figure 41.27: (A) Lateral oblique view mandible showing moth-eaten appearance of the bone all over, (B) OPG showing pathological fracture

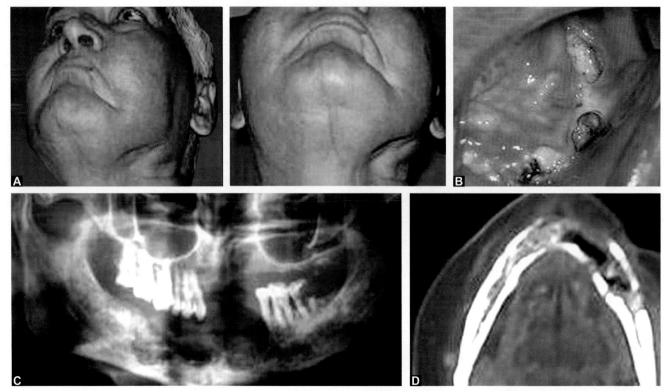

Figs 41.29A to D: (A) Clinical extraoral pictures of 60-year-old patient, who underwent neck dissection and surgery for tongue lesion, followed by radiation 3 years back, (B) He C/O multiple draining sinuses and dull pain in the left side of the jaw, (C) OPG showing moth-eaten destruction of body mandible, (D) CT scan picture also showing extensive osteoradionecrosis changes in the body mandible

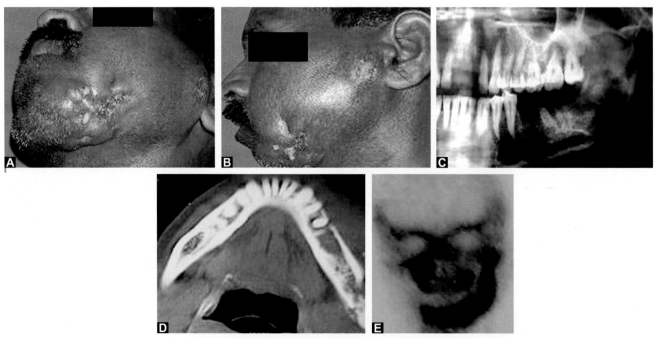

Figs 41.30A to E: Typical presentation of osteoradionecrosis: (A and B) Extraoral nonhealing, chronic multiple draining sinuses, nonresponsive to medication, (C) OPG showing complete involvement of left body and ramus of the mandible, (D) CT scan confirms the destruction, involvement of left hemimandibular bone, (E) Bone scan shows the "Hot spot" involving the hemimandible

Table 41.7: Recent development in treatment plan of ORN

1973	Greenwood and Gilchrist—1st reported the benefits of HBO in postirradiated patients.
1975	Mainous and Hart—14 cases of refractory ORN of mandible treated with HBO and hemimandibulectomy.
1981	Mansfield—reported complete healing with HBO in 12 patients.
1993	Mckenzie— reported resolution of ORN following HBO in 69% of patients.

Table 41.8: Hudson, 2000: Treatment of radionecrotic wounds

1. Rule out recurrence of neoplastic disease.
2. Stabilize patient condition metabolically, especially nutritional status.
3. Administer preoperative hyperbaric oxygen treatment.
4. Debride soft and bony radionecrotic tissues as necessary.
5. Provide postoperative hyperbaric oxygen treatment.
6. Consider soft tissue vascular flap support.
7. Perform bony reconstruction as warranted.

9. Treatment of small areas by drilling multiple holes into vital bone is recommended by Hahn and Corgill, (1967) as a means to encourage sequestration.
10. Sequestrectomy, is preferrably performed intra-orally, because of skin and vascular damage resulting from irradiation.
11. Pathological fractures are not so common. These may occur from minor injuries. The fractures do not heal readily. The best form of treatment is excision of necrotic ends of both fragments and replacement with a large graft. Reconstruction of bone defects usually warrants major soft tissue flap revascularization support.
12. Bone resection is performed, if there is persistent pain, infection or pathological fracture. It is preferrably done intraorally, to avoid possibility of orocutaneous fistula in radiation-compromised skin.
13. HBO therapy is a useful adjunct. It may not be sufficient alone, in its neovascularization influence to recruit the vascular support, necessary for sustaining bone graft healing, but may be useful in supporting soft tissue graft healing while minimizing compartmentalization.

Rationale for the use of HBO in association with surgery in irradiated tissues is to increase blood to tissue oxygen tension, which enhances the diffusion of oxygen into the tissues. This revascularizes the irradiated tissue and improves the fibroblastic cellular density, thus limiting the amount of nonviable tissue to be surgically removed.

Staging and Treatment Algorithm

This is a dynamic process with staging and treatment decisions being made on clinical response grounds. The number of HBO treatments is recommended minimum and more are given if the response is slow. (Royal Adelaide Hospital, Australia, modification of the MARX protocol (Flow chart 41.1).

S Vudiniabola, AN Goss et al. modified MARX protocol for the treatment of ORN and proposed staging of ORN depending on its clinical presentation and progression or on a clinical presentation plus response to treatment with hyperbaric oxygen (HBO) with or without surgery. They advocated clinical response based treatment.

Stage I: Exposed bone with non healing wound-30 HBO treatment and review. Those patients, who have responded well—further 10 HBO.

Stage I: Nonrespondent—considered as Stage II ORN.

Stage II: Local debridement to induce fresh bleeding, followed by 10 HBO.

Stage III: Nonrespondent stage II ORN or those patients with cutaneous fistula, pathologic fracture or inferior border resorption. Total 30 HBO treatment followed by surgical resection with stabilization of the remaining jaw by external fixation or IMF.

Stage III R: If reconstruction is required, then they enter Stage III R. —further 10 HBO.

Reconstruction with a free bone graft followed by 10 HBO.

They have recommended to rely on clinical observation to ensure optimum treatment, rather than strictly follow a fixed number of protocol treatment.

Daland, (1949) advised: (i) Electrocoagulation of exposed bone to expedite sequestration, (ii) Drainage of subcutaneous abscesses, to prevent sloughing of skin. These should possibly be drained intraorally, (iii) Control of pain by judicious use of analgesics. Alcohol block to nerve; in case of severe pain.

OML (i) may follow months or years after radiotherapy, but 30 percent of cases develop within six months, (ii) OML heralded by pain and swelling, (iii) Area of bone involved is often small (less than 2 cms in diameter), (iv) With antibiotics, the signs and symptoms of inflammation may subside within a few weeks, and (v) Complete resolution: It takes 2 or more years in spite of intensive treatment with antimicrobials.

Prevention of ORN

Pre-irradiation Dental Care

1. *Extraction of teeth:* The teeth in direct beam of radiation should be extracted; which include: (i) nonrestorable teeth, (ii) teeth with considerable periodontal disease, (iii) patients with poor oral health and motivation. The radiation therapy is delayed by 10 to 14 days to allow for initial healing.
2. The prominent interdental septa, sharp socket margins should be trimmed as remodeling

resorption of alveolar process will not occur after irradiation.

3. Unerupted and deeply buried teeth are best left *in situ.*
4. *Restoration of teeth:* The remaining teeth should be restored and periodontal therapy should be completed in this two week period. Oral hygiene instructions are given. The application of topical fluoride is carried out 0.4% stannous fluoride gel, or 1% acidulated fluorophosphates gel is applied for 15 minutes twice a day for two weeks, followed by once daily thereafter.
5. *During therapy:* (i) Mouthwash: 0.2 percent aqueous chlorhexidine decreases secondary infection of any ulcerated mucosa, reduces plaque accumulation and caries. (ii) Supervised cleaning of all the teeth by an hygienist on regular basis. (iii) Oral hygiene instructions: with fluoride toothpaste is essential,

Flow chart 41.1: Staging and treatment algorithm

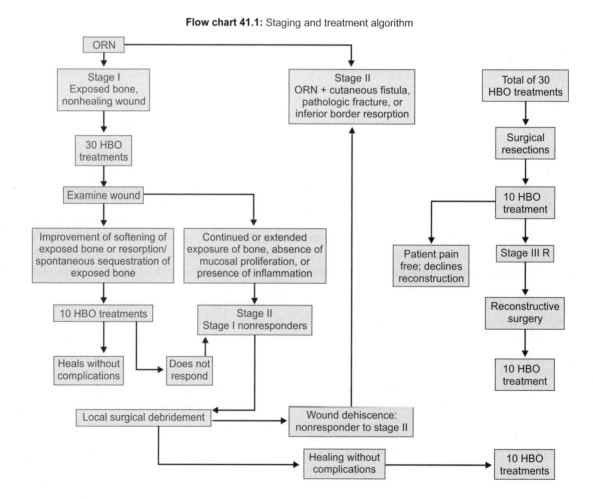

and use of daily fluoride mouthwash is important. (iv) Dietary advice: reduce the intake of characteristic in food and drinks (v) Improve general health of the patient.

Post-irradiation Dental Care

1. Avoidance of dentures: The dentures should not be worn in the irradiated jaw for one year after therapy.
2. Maintenance of oral hygiene.
3. Application of topical fluoride as for pre-irradiation care.
4. Saliva substitutes. They perform the following functions: (i) Lubricate mucosa to replace diminished flow from irradiated mucous and salivary glands, (ii) Facilitate rehardening of tooth surfaces, (iii) Minimize xerostomia-induced soft tissue disorders (Shannon, 1977).
5. Restoration of teeth with post-irradiation pulpitis. Patients requiring endodontic treatment for post-irradiation pulpitis, caution should be exercised not to introduce organisms beyond the apex by instrumentation. It is advisable to carry out such treatment under antibiotic prophylaxis.
6. Extraction as a last resort: The number of necessary extraction should be limited to a minimum of one or two per appointment. Teeth should be removed atraumatically. Sharp bony margins should be trimmed off, without raising extensive flaps. Extractions to be done under antibiotic prophylaxis.

Beumer et al. reported that the most common factors associated with ORN were postradiation extractions (26.5%), spontaneous bone exposure associated directly with the dentition secondary to dental disease (22.8%). Marx et al. proposed prophylaxis with hyperbaric oxygen HBO before postradiation dental extractions. But, some clinicians believe that the high cost and limited availability of HBO precludes recommending its universal application for ORN prophylaxis. The risk of ORN though highest during first 4 to 12 months after RT, has been found to persist for the remainder of the patient's life. Therefore, atraumatic extractions are advocated.

S E C T I O N

Facial Neuropathology

12

42 The Trigeminal Nerve (V)

FUNCTIONS

The trigeminal nerve supplies sensation to meninges, skin of anterior part of the head, nasal and oral cavities and the teeth. It provides motor innervation to the muscles of mastication, which are derived from the first branchial arch.

ATTACHMENT

Trigeminal nerve is attached to the lateral aspect of pons, near middle cerebellar peduncle (Fig. 42.1).

COURSE

Trigeminal nerve passes below tentorium cerebelli over the apex of petrous temporal bone, into middle cranial fossa (MCF). The trigeminal (sensory) ganglion is in a small depression on the temporal bone (Meckel's cave).

DIVISIONS

Trigeminal nerve divides into three branches:
1. Ophthalmic (V_1)
2. Maxillary (V_2)
3. Mandibular (V_3)

Type of Fibers

The sensory fibers are present in all three divisions of trigeminal nerve; only the mandibular division (V_3) contains motor fibers.

TRIGEMINAL GANGLION

Trigeminal ganglion contains the cell bodies of all primary sensory neurons in all three divisions of trigeminal nerve, except those neurons carrying proprioceptive impulses. It is partially surrounded by cerebrospinal fluid, in an extensions of subarachnoid space below superior petrosal sinus; the trigeminal cave (or Meckel's cave).

Trigeminal nerve is the largest cranial nerve composed of the following:
1. Small motor root
2. Large sensory root.

Motor root supplies muscles of mastication and other muscles in the region.

Sensory root has three branches and supplies:
1. Skin of entire face
2. Mucous membrane of cranial viscera, and
3. Oral cavity (except of pharynx and base of tongue).

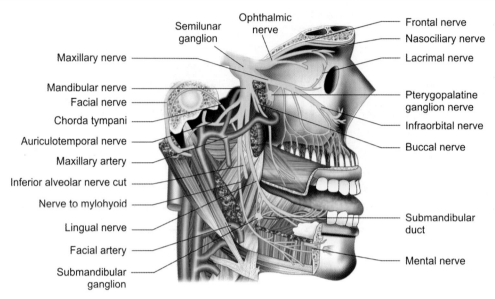

Maxillary nerve

Mandibular nerve

Facial nerve

Chorda tympani

Auriculotemporal nerve

Maxillary artery

Inferior alveolar nerve cut

Nerve to mylohyoid

Lingual nerve

Facial artery

Submandibular ganglion

Semilunar ganglion

Ophthalmic nerve

Frontal nerve

Nasociliary nerve

Lacrimal nerve

Pterygopalatine ganglion nerve

Infraorbital nerve

Buccal nerve

Submandibular duct

Mental nerve

Fig. 42.1: Course of the trigeminal nerve and its branches

Motor Root

Motor root arises separately from sensory root, originating in main nucleus with pons and medulla oblongata.

Its fibers (as a small nerve root), travel anteriorly along with, but separately, the sensory root to the region of semilunar ganglion/gasserian ganglion.

1. At the sensory ganglion, the motor root passes in a lateral and inferior direction under the ganglion towards foramen ovale, through which it leaves middle cranial fossa, along with the sensory root of the mandibular nerve.

2. Just after leaving the skull, the motor root unites with sensory root of mandibular division to form a single trunk.

3. Motor fibers of trigeminal nerve supply the following muscles:
   i. Masticatory muscles—temporalis, masseter, medial pterygoid and lateral pterygoid.
   ii. Mylohyoid.
   iii. Anterior belly of digastric.
   iv. Tensor tympani.
   v. Tensor veli palatini.

Sensory Root

- Sensory root fibers of trigeminal nerve comprises of the central processes of ganglion cells located in trigeminal ganglion (or semilunar/gasserian ganglion)

- There are two ganglia; one innervating each side of face

- They are located in Meckel's cave, on anterior surface of petrous temporal area

- Ganglia are flat and crescent shaped, their convexities facing anteriorly and downwards; they measure 1.0 x 2.0 cm

- Sensory root fibers enter the concave portion of each crescent and the three sensory divisions of trigeminal nerve exit from the convexity.
   i. *Ophthalmic nerve (V_1):* It travels anteriorly in lateral wall of cavernous sinus to medial part of superior orbital fissure, through which it exists the skull into the orbit.
   ii. *Maxillary division (V_2):* It travels anteriorly and downwards to exit cranium, through foramen rotundum into upper portion of pterygopalatine fossa.
   iii. *Mandibular division (V_3):* It travels almost directly downwards to exit the skull, along with the motor root, through foramen ovale. These two roots then intermingle, forming one nerve trunk, then enter infratemporal fossa.

Ophthalmic Nerve (V_1)

Functions

The ophthalmic nerve transmits sensory innervation from eyeballs, skin of upper face and anterior scalp, the lining of upper part of nasal cavity and air cells and the meninges of anterior cranial fossa.

Its branches also convey parasympathetic fibers to the ciliary and iris muscles for accommodation and pupillary constriction and to the lacrimal gland.

Origin, Course and Branches

It originates from trigeminal ganglion in middle cranial fossa. It passes anteriorly through lateral wall of cavernous sinus. It divides into three branches:
1. Frontal
2. Nasociliary
3. Lacrimal.

All these branches pass through superior orbital fissure into the orbit.

Frontal branch: It is the largest branch; supplies frontal sinus and skin of forehead and scalp. It passes through superior orbital fissure outside common tendinous ring. It passes forwards above levator palpebrae superioris just below frontal bone. It divides into two branches:
1. *Supraorbital:* It is the larger and lateral branch.
2. *Supratrochlear:* It is the smaller and medial branch.

Supraorbital nerve: It crosses supraorbital margin in the notch or foramen (with supraorbital branch of ophthalmic artery), turns upwards to supply skin of forehead and scalp as far posterior as the vertex.
NB: The nerves and vessels in scalp lie superficial to fronto-occipital aponeurosis.

Nasociliary branch: It supplies meninges, eyeball, upper part of nasal cavity and ethmoidal air cells and anterior nasal skin. It passes the superior orbital fissure, medially within the common tendinous ring.
It divides into the following:
a. Short ciliary nerve.
b. Long ciliary nerve.
These nerves pass to eyeball to innervate ocular structures including cornea:
a. Short ciliary nerve contains preganglionic parasympathetic fibers from Edinger-Westphal nucleus and oculomotor nerve passing to ciliary ganglion (synapse).
b. Long and short ciliary nerves also contain sympathetic fibers.

Anterior ethmoid nerve. It gives sensory fibers to the meninges of anterior cranial fossa; and enters nasal cavity.

It supplies along with posterior ethmoidal, upper part of nasal cavity and sphenoid and ethmoid cells. It

turns towards bridge of nose and becomes superficial at the junction of nasal bone and cartilage of nasal bridge.

Now called as external nasal nerve, supplies cutaneous sensation to anterior aspect and tip of nose.

Lacrimal nerve: It supplies lacrimal gland and a small area of adjacent skin and conjunctiva. It passes through superior orbital fissure lateral to and outside common tendinous ring. It receives postganglionic parasympathetic fibers from pterygopalatine ganglion which enters orbit with zygomatic nerve for distribution to lacrimal gland.

Nerve fibers: Central connections
a. *Somatic sensory fibers* sensory nuclei of trigeminal nerve are present in all branches of ophthalmic nerve. The axons pass centrally to trigeminal ganglion where cell bodies are situated. The central axonal processes pass to pons and trigeminal sensory nuclei.
b. *Parasympathetic fibers*
   i. Edinger-Westphal nucleus to muscles of ciliary body and iris
   ii. Superior salivatory nucleus to lacrimal gland.

Maxillary Nerve (V₂)

It is the nerve of maxillary process, that differentiates from first pharyngeal arch. It is purely sensory; and is intermediate in size between ophthalmic and mandibular nerve.

Functions

The maxillary nerve transmits sensory fibers from the skin of face between the lower eyelid and the mouth from the nasal cavity and sinuses, from the maxillary teeth.

At its origin from the pons, it contains only sensory fibers some of its branches receive postganglionic parasympathetic fibers from pterygopalatine ganglion which pass to the lacrimal, nasal and palatine glands, and others convey taste (visceral sensory) fibers from the palate to the nucleus of the solitary tract.

Origin, Course and Branches

It originates from the middle part of trigeminal ganglion in middle cranial fossa. It gives off meningeal branch in middle cranial fossa which is sensory. The nerve runs forwards through lower part of lateral wall of cavernous sinus (below the ophthalmic division). The lateral wall here fuses with endosteal layer of dura mater at lateral margin of foramen rotundum; so maxillary division is directed through the foramen rotundum into the uppermost part of pterygopalatine fossa between pterygoid plates of sphenoid bone and the palatine bone. It has a short course below the root of pterygopalatine fossa to inferior orbital fissure. As it crosses pterygopalatine fossa, it gives off its main branches to pterygopalatine ganglion, posterior superior alveolar nerve and zygomatic branches. It then angles laterally in a groove on posterior surface of maxilla, entering the orbit through inferior orbital fissure. Within the orbit it occupies the infraorbital groove and becomes infraorbital nerve which courses anteriorly into the infraorbital canal. The maxillary nerve emerges on anterior surface of face through infraorbital foramen where it divides into its terminal branches, supplying skin of middle portion of face, nose, lower eyelid and upper lip.

Maxillary nerve innervates:
1. Skin of:
   i. Middle portion of face
   ii. Lower eyelid
   iii. Side of nose
   iv. Upper lip.
2. Mucous membrane of:
   i. Nasopharynx
   ii. Maxillary sinus
   iii. Soft palate
   iv. Tonsil
   v. Hard palate.
3. Maxillary teeth and periodontal tissues.

Branches

Maxillary nerve gives off branches in four regions:
1. Within the cranium
2. In the pterygopalatine ganglion
3. In the infraorbital canal
4. On the face.

Branches Within the Cranium: Middle Meningeal Nerve

Immediately after separating from trigeminal ganglion, the maxillary nerve gives off a small branch, middle meningeal nerve. It travels with middle meningeal artery. It provides sensory innervation to the dura mater of anterior half of middle cranial fossa.

Branches in the Pterygopalatine Fossa

i. Pterygopalatine nerves
ii. Zygomatic nerves
iii. Posterosuperior alveolar nerves.

Pterygopalatine nerves: Two short nerves, that suspend the pterygopalatine ganglion. They pass through the ganglion into its branches. They also serve as a communication between pterygopalatine ganglion and maxillary nerve.

These branches mingle with postganglionic secretomotor fibers of greater petrosal nerve and sympathetic fibers of deep petrosal nerve.

By way of ganglion, the maxillary nerve has the following branches: All of which carry sensory, secretomotor and sympathetic fibers. The branches of pterygopalatine nerve include those that supply four areas: orbit, nose, palate and pharynx.

1. *Orbital branches:* Supply periosteum of orbit.
2. *Nasal branches:* Supply mucous membranes superior and middle conchae, the lining of posterior ethmoidal sinus and posterior portion of nasal septum.

These convey postganglionic parasympathetic fibers from pterygopalatine ganglion to nasal glands.

   a. Nasopalatine nerve (long sphenopalatine nerve)—a significant branch. It enters sphenopalatine foramen, crosses the roof of nasal cavity and slopes downwards and forwards where it lies between mucous membrane and periosteum of nasal septum (passes over the roof of nasal cavity to reach septum). Here, it supplies its posteroinferior half. The nasopalatine nerve continues downwards reaching the floor of nasal cavity and giving off its branches to anterior part of nasal septum and the floor of nose. It enters incisive canal through which it passes into the oral cavity via the incisive foramen located in the midline of hard palate, about one centimeter posterior to maxillary central incisors. The right and left nasopalatine nerves emerge together through this foramen and provide sensory innervation to palatal mucosa in the region of premaxilla (central and lateral incisors and canines).

   b. Posterior superior lateral nasal nerves (short sphenopalatine nerves)—enter the sphenopalatine foramen and supply the posterosuperior quadrant of lateral wall of nose.

3. *Palatine branches*:
   a. Greater palatine nerves (or anterior palatine nerves)
   b. Lesser palatine nerves (or middle and posterior palatine nerves).

   These branches provide sensory innervation to hard and soft palate. These branches also convey postganglionic parasympathetic fibers from pterygopalatine ganglion to palatal glands.
   a. *Greater palatine nerve:* It is necessary for hard palate. It descends down through pterygopalatine canal (greater palatine canal) of maxilla. It emerges on hard palate through greater palatine foramen, which is usually located about one centimeter towards the palatal midline, just distal to second molar. Multiple branches supply the posteroinferior quadrant of lateral wall of nose and adjacent floor of nose, others supply maxillary sinus nearby.

      The nerve courses anteriorly, after emerging from greater palatine foramen between mucoperiosteum and osseous hard palate supplying sensory innervation to palatal soft tissues and bone anterior to first premolar, where it communicates with terminal fibers of nasopalatine nerve. It also provides sensory innervation to some parts of soft palate. It supplies all the hard palate except incisor gingiva.
   b. *Lesser palatine nerve:* These are sensory to soft palate. They descend through lesser palatine foramina in palatine bone and pass backwards to supply mucous membrane on both surfaces of soft palate.
4. *Pharyngeal branch*: It provides sensory innervation to nasopharynx. It is a small nerve, leaving posterior part of pterygopalatine ganglion, passes backward, through the pharyngeal canal and supplies mucous membrane of nasopharynx, posterior to auditory (Eustachian) tube; down to the level of Passavant's muscle.

Zygomatic nerves: It provides sensory innervation to skin over zygomatic region. These nerves also convey postganglionic parasympathetic fibers from pterygopalatine ganglion to lacrimal nerve and glands. It is a terminal branch. It carries out of pterygopalatine fossa and travels anteriorly entering the orbit through inferior orbital fissure and runs along the lower part of lateral wall of orbit.

The zygomatic nerve enters zygomatic bone and divides into two branches (some authors mention that in inferior orbital fissure, it divides into two branches).
1. *Zygomaticotemporal nerve:* It perforates temporal surface of zygomatic bone, pierces temporalis fascia and supplies skin above zygomatic arch (skin of side of forehead or the "hairless" skin of temple).
2. *Zygomaticofacial nerve:* It perforates the facial surface of zygomatic bone and supplies skin over the bone (skin over the prominence of cheek.) Just before leaving orbit, zygomatic nerve sends a branch which communicates with lacrimal nerve of ophthalmic nerve. It carries secretomotor fibers from pterygopalatine ganglion for lacrimal gland. These leave zygomatic nerve and go up the lateral wall of orbit to join lacrimal nerve.

Posterosuperior alveolar nerves: These nerves are two to three in number, descend from the main trunk of the maxillary nerve in the pterygopalatine fossa just before the mandibular division enter inferior alveolar canal. They emerge through the pterygomaxillary fissure. They pass downwards through the pterygopalatine fossa and reach the posterior surface of maxilla (or infratemporal surface of maxilla). When more than two; one branch remains external to bone, continuing downward on posterior surface of maxilla, to provide sensory innervation to buccal gingiva in maxillary molar region; and adjacent facial mucosal surfaces. Other branch enters maxilla (along with a branch of internal maxillary artery) through the posterior or posterolateral wall of maxillary sinus, and provides sensory innervation to mucous membrane of sinus. Continuing downward, this second branch provides sensory innervation to alveoli, periodontal ligaments and pulpal tissues of maxillary molars, with the exception of (25%) patients of mesiobuccal root of first molar.

Branches in the Infraorbital Canal

In the infraorbital canal, the maxillary division gives two branches of significance to dentistry.
1. Middle superior alveolar nerve.
2. Anterior superior alveolar nerve.

   While in infraorbital groove and canal the maxillary division is known as infraorbital nerve.

The nerve passes forwards along the floor of orbit, sinks into a groove then enters a canal and emerges on the face through infraorbital foramen.

It supplies multiple small branches through orbital plate of maxilla to roof of maxillary sinus. In the infraorbital groove it gives off middle superior alveolar nerve and in the infraorbital canal it gives off the anterior superior alveolar nerve.

Middle superior alveolar nerve: Site of origin: anywhere in the infraorbital canal, from posterior part in the canal to anterior portion. The nerve runs down, supplying adjacent mucosa of maxillary sinus; two premolars and mesiobuccal root of first molar, periodontal tissues, buccal soft tissue and bone in premolar region.

Anterior superior alveolar nerve: Relatively large branch, is given off the infraorbital nerve approximately 6 to 10 mm before the latter's exit from the infraorbital foramen. It descends first lateral and then inferior to infraorbital canal. Within the anterior wall of maxillary sinus, provides innervation to central and lateral incisors and the canines as well as sensory innervation to periodontal tissues, buccal bone and buccal gingiva of these teeth.

It reaches anteroinferior quadrant of lateral wall of nose (including nasolacrimal duct) and adjacent floor of nose. It ends on nasal septum.

In patients where middle superior alveolar nerve is absent, the anterior superior alveolar nerve provides sensory innervation to premolars and occasionally the mesiobuccal root of first molar.

The innervation of roots of all teeth, bone and periodontal structures are derived from terminal branches of larger nerves. These nerves make network; termed as dental plexus.

The superior dental plexus: These plexuses are composed of small nerve fibers from the three superior alveolar nerves anterior, middle and posterior superior alveolar nerves.

Three types of nerves emerge from these plexuses are as follows:
1. Dental nerves
2. Interdental branches and
3. Inter radicular branches.

And each accompanied along its pathway by corresponding artery.

 i. *Dental nerves*—enter a tooth through apical foramen dividing into many branches within the pulp.

 ii. *Interdental nerves*—also known as perforating branches travel through the entire height of inter-radicular septum providing sensory innervation to periodontal ligaments of adjacent teeth through alveolar bone. They emerge at the height of the crest of interalveolar septum and enter the gingiva to innervate the interdental papilla and buccal gingiva.

 iii. *Inter radicular branches*—traverse the entire height of inter radicular or interalveolar septum, providing sensory innervation to periodontal ligaments of adjacent roots. They terminate in the periodontal ligament at root furcations.

Branches on the Face

Infraorbital nerve emerges on the face through infraorbital foramen, lies between levator labii superioris and levator anguli oris, divides into its terminal branches.

 i. Inferior palpebral supply skin of lower eyelid with sensory innervation to both surfaces of conjunctiva.
 ii. External nasal/lateral nasal provides sensory innervation to skin on lateral aspect of nose.
 iii. Superior labial provides sensory innervation to skin and mucous membrane of whole of upper lip (and sometimes also the adjacent gingiva from midline to second premolar teeth).

Infraorbital nerve has many communications with local branches of 7th cranial nerve, i.e. facial nerve, these are for proprioceptive supply of nearby facial muscles.

Mandibular Nerve (V₃)

Mandibular nerve is the nerve of first (mandibular) branchial arch. The first arch gives rise to the following:
• Precursor of mandible (Meckel's cartilage)
• Spine of sphenoid
• Sphenomandibular ligament
• Muscles of mastication.

It is the largest branch of trigeminal nerve.

It transmits sensory fibers from the skin over the mandible, side of the cheek and temple, the oral cavity and its contents, external ear, tympanic membrane and temporomandibular joint. It also supplies the meninges of cranial vault.

It is motor supply to the muscles derived from first branchial arch:
• Temporalis and masseter
• Medial and lateral pterygoid

- Mylohyoid and anterior belly of digastric
- Tensor tympani and tensor palati.

Note the four groups of two—two tensors, two pterygoids, two big chewing muscles and two in floor of mouth.

Some of its distal branches also convey parasympathic secretomotor fibers to salivary glands and taste fibers from anterior portion of tongue.

Origin, Course and Branches

Sensory root of the mandibular division—It originates at the inferior part of trigeminal ganglion in the middle cranial fossa; whereas motor root arises in motor cells located in pons and medulla oblongata.

The two roots emerge from the cranium, separately through the foramen ovale, the small motor root lying medial to sensory root. They unite just outside or at the foramen ovale, and form the main trunk of mandibular nerve.

The main trunk remains undivided only for a short distance of 2 to 4 mm and then it divides into a "cat of nine tails." The branches are:
  i. Small anterior trunk—all motor except one
  ii. Large posterior trunk—all sensory except one.

The mixed nerve, emerging from foramen ovale, into infratemporal fossa between upper head of lateral pterygoid muscle and tensor palati (which lies on the side wall of nasopharynx).

Branches

In infratemporal fossa, it gives branches in three areas:
1. From undivided nerve
2. From anterior trunk
3. From posterior trunk.

Branches from Undivided Nerve

These are two branches: (1) meningeal branch; (2) nerve to medial pterygoid.

Meningeal branch (nervus spinosus): It is the nerve of first pharyngeal arch. It passes upwards and re-enters the cranium through foramen ovale (sometimes through foramen spinosum along with middle meningeal artery). Here it supplies:
  i. Cartilaginous part of eustachian tube
  ii. Middle cranial fossa; it supplies dura mater in the posterior half, then passes between squamous and

petrous parts of temporal bone to supply mastoid air cells/antrum that extend from it.

Nerve to medial pterygoid: It sinks into the deep surface of muscle. It has a branch that passes close to otic ganglion and supplies the two tensor muscles, tensor velli palati and tensor tympani.

Branches from Anterior Trunk

Branches from anterior trunk significantly smaller than the posterior trunk. The branches provide:
  i. Motor innervations to the muscles of mastication
  ii. Sensory innervations to mucous membrane of cheek and buccal gingiva of mandibular molars.

The trunk runs forwards under lateral pterygoid muscle for a short distance and then reaches the external surface of that muscle by either passing between its two heads or less frequently, winding over its upper border. From this point it is known as long buccal nerve.

While under the lateral pterygoid muscle, the nerve gives off several branches providing motor innervation to respective muscles.
a. Deep temporal nerves—pass above the upper head of lateral pterygoid turn above. Infratemporal crest and sink into deep surface of temporalis.
b. Nerve to masseter—likewise passes above the upper head of lateral pterygoid, proceeds laterally behind temporalis and through mandibular notch to sink into masseter. It gives off branch to temporomandibular joint.
c. Nerves to lateral pterygoid—one to each head.

Buccal nerve (also long buccal nerve/buccinator nerve)

- The only sensory branch of anterior trunk
- The only nerve to pass between two heads of lateral pterygoid
- It passes down, deep to temporalis, on lower head of lateral pterygoid
- Emerges under the anterior border of masseter muscle, continuing in anterolateral direction
- At the level of occlusal plane of mandibular third or second molar, it crosses in front of anterior border of ramus and enters cheek through buccinator muscle
- It gives off a cutaneous branch, a sensory branch to the thumb print area of skin over the soft cheek immediately between zygomatic bone
- After piercing the buccinator, it supplies the mucous membrane adherent to deep surface of

muscle, passes into retromolar triangle and ends by supplying sensory innervation to buccal gingiva of mandibular molars and adjoining mucobuccal fold

- It carries secretomotor fibers from otic ganglion for molars and buccal glands.

NB: (i) Buccal nerve does not innervate buccinator, which is supplied by the seventh, i.e. facial nerve, (ii) Anesthesia of buccal nerve is important for dental procedures, requiring soft tissue manipulation on buccal surface of mandibular molars.

Branches of Posterior Trunk

- Primarily sensory, with a small motor component.
- It descends for a short distance downwards and medially to lateral pterygoid muscle, at which point its branches into the following:
  - i. Auriculotemporal
  - ii. Lingual
  - iii. Inferior alveolar nerve.

Auriculotemporal nerve: It supplies temporomandibular joint, parotid fascia, skin of temple, most of the skin of external auditory meatus and tympanic membrane. For a short distance between foramen ovale and parotid gland, it carries parasympathetic fibers originating in inferior solitary nucleus to otic ganglion and parotid gland. It arises immediately beneath foramen ovale by two roots that pass back around middle meningeal artery. It transverses upper part of parotid gland, between the temporomandibular joint and external auditory meatus, crosses posterior part of zygomatic arch and ascends close to superficial temporal artery.

It gives off a number of branches, all of which are sensory. These include the following:

- i. A communication with facial nerve, providing sensory fibers to the skin over the areas of innervation of the following motor branches of facial nerve, the zygomatic, the buccal and mandibular.
- ii. Curving around the neck of mandible a communication with otic ganglion, providing sensory, secretory and vasomotor fibers to parotid gland.
- iii. The anterior auricular branches supplying skin over the helix and tragus of ear.
- iv. Branches to external auditory meatus and tympanic membrane.
- v. Articular branches to posterior portion of temporomandibular joint and it passes back deep to neck of mandible.

- vi. The superficial temporal branches, supplying hairy skin over temporal region or scalp (the hair that first turn gray). It runs upwards over the root of zygomatic process of temporal bone behind superficial temporal vessels.

Lingual nerve: Second branch of posterior trunk of mandibular division. It passes downward medial to lateral pterygoid muscle and as it descends, it lies between the ramus and the medial pterygoid muscle in the pterygomandibular space. It runs anterior and medial to inferior alveolar nerve, whose path it parallels. It then continues downwards and forwards, deep to pterygomandibular raphe and below the attachment of superior constrictor of pharynx, to reach the side of the base of tongue, slightly below and behind and medial to mandibular third molar. Here it lies just below the mucous membrane in the lateral lingual sulcus. It then proceeds anteriorly in the floor of the mouth winding around the submandibular (Wharton's) duct, passing lateral, than beneath, then medial to the duct, across the muscles of tongue to the deep surface of sublingual gland, where it breaks up into its terminal branches.

It is sensory to anterior two-third of the tongue, for both general sensation and gustation (taste) for this region.

It is joined by chorda tympani, a branch of facial nerve about 2 cm below base of skull deep to lower border of lateral pterygoid muscle. It carries visceral sensory and parasympathetic fibers. The parasympathetic fibers originate in superior solitary nucleus and visceral sensory fibers pass to the facial nerve. It also provides sensory innervation to mucous membrane of floor of mouth and gingiva on lingual side of mandible.

Inferior alveolar nerve: Largest branch of mandibular division, it descends medial or deep to the lower part of lateral pterygoid muscle and lateroposterior to lingual nerve to the region between sphenomandibular ligament and medial surface of ramus of mandible, where it enters mandibular canal at the level of mandibular foramen. Throughout its path, it is accompanied by inferior alveolar artery (a branch of internal maxillary artery) and inferior alveolar vein. The artery lies just anterior to the nerve. The nerve, artery and vein travel anteriorly in mandibular canal as forwards as mental foramen, where the nerve divides into terminal branches:

i. Incisive nerve, and

ii. Mental nerve.

Rarely, (i) sensory innervation to b uccal periodontal tissues of same teeth.

i. Incisive nerve—remains within the mandibular canal.

ii. Mental nerve—emerges the canal through the mental foramen and divides into three branches that innervate:

1. Skin of chin
2. Skin
3. Mucous membrane of lower lip.

Mylohyoid Nerve

Branches from inferior alveolar nerve prior to its entry into the mandibular canal. It runs downwards and forwards in mylohyoid groove on medial surface of ramus and along the body of mandible to reach the mylohyoid muscle. It is a mixed nerve being motor to mylohyoid muscle and anterior belly of digastric. It is thought to contain sensory fibers for the skin on inferior and anterior surfaces of mental protruberance.

Rarely, sensory innervation to mandibular incisors and molars (usually mesial root of mandibular first molar).

43 Orofacial Region Pain

When the word *pain* is uttered, it brings to the mind a picture of agony and suffering. Pain is an unpleasant sensation as perceived by the patient and in simple terms described by the patient, as that sensation which hurts. Pain, truly, is a very personal experience. The original English meaning of *pain* signified punishment, whilst bodily suffering was described by the Latin word *dolor*. The word pain implies for both these meanings. Pain can be measured only in terms of the patient's verbalization of the problem. Pain can be modified by psychological, emotional, biological, ethnic, social and environmental factors. One of the major concerns of any branch of health sciences is pain control. Lot of controversies and confusion exist while diagnosing and treating pain, as it is personal and always subjective and is because of the neuroanatomical complexity and the absence of the standard objective method of measuring pain.

Pain in the orofacial region has special significance. Face and oral cavity serve key functions of eating and communicating, therefore orofacial pain disorders have a major impact on the quality and functioning of life.

INCIDENCE

Incidence is estimated that head and facial pain accounts for up to 35 percent of all pain disorders.

DEFINITION

1. *Subjective definition:* International Association for study of pain: Pain is an unpleasant sensory and emotional experience associated with actual or potential tissue damage or described in terms of such a damage.
2. *Objective definition:* Pain is an unpleasant emotional experience, usually initiated by a noxious stimulus (that injure or threaten to destroy the tissue) and transmitted over a specialized neural network to the central nervous system, where it is interpreted as pain.
3. *Shetrington definition:* A psychical adjunct of an imperative protective reflex, i.e. pain causes withdrawal response and at the same time, pain unlike the other sensations, has a large emotional component.

4. *International Association for study of pain, 1994*: Pain is defined as 'the subject's conscious perception of modulated nociceptive impulses that generate an unpleasant sensory and emotional experience associated with actual tissue damage or described in terms of such damage.

BASIC CLASSIFICATION OF PAIN

1. *Acute pain:* It is of short duration from noxious disease or recent injury. The severity of acute pain will differ. It may be of mild, severe, dull type. It will have an obvious definite treatable etiology associated with pain.

2. *Chronic pain:* When the pain persists for longer duration, i.e. 3 to 6 months or more, then it is labelled as chronic type. Unlike acute pain, chronic pain occurs spontaneously, without evidence of any organic cause on many occasions and is often associated with feelings of suffering and depression. Therefore, it may be associated with neurophysiologic and behavioral changes.

   Chronic pain in the suffering patients is associated with: (i) Lowered pain thresholds, (ii) Spontaneous and elicited (triggered) pain activity, (iii) Central behavioral changes, (iv) Refractoriness to therapies.

3. *Nociceptive type pain:* Final conduit of pain is an activation of a specific class of neural receptors, known as nociceptors, irrespective of the site and the cause of the initiating noxious stimulus.

   Pain of non neural origin, in which normal peripheral nerve endings are activated by inflammation or trauma that is affecting the tissues like skin, teeth, muscles, glands, blood vessels. A transition from acute to chronic pain may occur, if underlying causes of non neural pain or trauma are not controlled.

4. *Neuropathic pain:* It is a chronic state, in which the central nervous system has been sensitized by repetitive direct or indirect injury or uncontrolled nociceptive disease. This is seen due to a series of changes in the nervous system, thereby nociceptive pain induces neuropathic pain through a process known as 'sensitization."

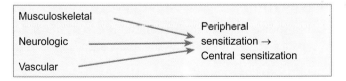

On the basis of differential diagnosis, the orofacial pain has been classified into five broad categories.

1. *Typical orofacial pain of extracranial origin*
   a. Dental cause—pulpitis, dentin hypersensitivity, periapical lesion.
   b. Periodontal—primary herpetic gingivostomatitis, acute necrotising ulcerative gingivitis, desquamative gingivitis.
   c. Mucosal—ulceration—aphthous or traumatic, herpetic, etc.
   d. Salivary gland—bacterial sialadenitis.
   e. Temporomandibular joint—dysfunction and others.
   f. Paranasal sinuses—sinusitis, malignancy.

2. *Primary neuralgias*
   a. Trigeminal neuralgia and variants.
   b. Glossopharyngeal neuralgia.
   c. Ramsay Hunt syndrome.
   d. Postherpetic neuralgia.

3. *Vascular origin:*
   a. Migraine and variants.
   b. Cluster headache, chronic paroxysmal hemicranial headaches and others.
   c. Giant cell arteritis and variants.

4. *Referred pain*
   a. Ocular pain
   b. Anginal pain
   c. ENT pain
   d. Myofacial pain dysfunction syndrome.

5. *Psychogenic origin*
   a. Atypical facial pain
   b. Burning mouth syndrome and variants.

NEUROPHYSIOLOGY OF PAIN

A knowledge of the neuroanatomical pathways and chemical mediators that either enhance or diminish the perception of pain is essential for successful management of pain.

There are two aspects of pain:
1. Pain perception, 2. Pain reaction.

Pain Perception

Pain perception is the physioanatomical process by which pain is received and transmitted by neural structures from the end organs or pain receptors, through the conductive and perceptive mechanism. The continuing ability to perceive pain depends on the neural mechanisms involved remaining intact. Pain perception is localized with the cortex and the brain, but to a certain degree, it is also dependent on other anatomical structures such as free nerve endings or pain receptors and afferent sensory fibers for conducting the impulses from the site of the original stimulus.

Pain Reaction

Pain reaction is a psychophysiological phenomenon. It represents the individual's manifestation of unpleasant reaction and involves complex neuroanatomical and psychological factors. The pain reaction, therefore, varies from person to person, depending on individual pain threshold.

The structural unit of the nervous system is the neuron, which consists of a nerve cell body and protoplasmic processes—axons and dendrites. Axon forms the essential conducting part of a nerve fiber. Nociception is the mechanism that provides for reception and conversion of noxious or potentially noxious stimuli into neural impulses and transmission into CNS. Nociceptors are receptors sensitive to noxious stimuli. These are the free nerve endings mostly of myelinated fibers. They may be in the form of delicate loops or a long naked hair like network. These nociceptors are found in orofacial skin, oral mucosa, TMJ, periodontium, tooth pulp, periosteum and muscles, etc.

These nociceptors are attached to first order neurons of afferents. The two major classes of afferent nerves that provide input to brain are:

1. *A delta fibers*—large, myelinated, 3 to 20 m in diameter. Mechanothermal, nociceptive afferent. They respond to intense thermal, mechanical stimuli. Conduct pain fast or first which is sharp and localized at a rate of upto 100 m/s.
2. *C fibers*—small, polymodal, unmyelinated nociceptive afferents. 0.5 to 1 m in diameter. They get excited by strong mechanical, thermal, chemical stimuli. They conduct slow/second pain at a rate of 0.5 to 2 m/s, carry touch sensation.

Noxious Stimuli Causing Pain

In order to cause pain, there must be an environmental change in excitable tissue. This change is called stimulus. It may be electrical, thermal, chemical or mechanical in nature of sufficient intensity (threshold stimulus) to excite the free nerve endings.

> Once the nerve endings are excited
> ↓
> Creation of an impulse
> ↓
> Self-propagating wave of excitation (impulse)
> along the nerve fibers

1. Pain detection and transmission is done in the orofacial region chiefly by fibers of trigeminal nerve.
   i. The ophthalmic division supplies skin of parietal, frontal region, eyes, nose, orbit and upper part of the nasal cavity.
   ii. The maxillary division supplies anterior portion of temple, malar and maxillary and nasal cavity, palate, maxillary sinus and maxillary teeth and gums.
   iii. The mandibular division supplies posterior temple, tragus, preauricular area, masseter area and mandibular region. It also supplies sensory innervation to anterior two-thirds of tongue, mandibular teeth and gums as well as masticatory muscles, tensor muscles of soft palate and tympanic membrane.
2. Upper second and third cervical nerves innervate superficial structures of head and neck posterior to trigeminal area and below the lower border of mandible and provide deep sensibility in cervical areas.
3. Facial nerve provides deep sensibility of facial skin in mastoid region and external auditory meatus.
4. Glossopharyngeal nerve provides for sensory function to back of tongue, tonsillar region, tympanic cavity and antrum.

■ TRANSMISSION OF IMPULSES IN THE CNS

Nerves supplying facial and oral tissues carry information of pain predominantly through gasserian ganglion, where primary afferent cell bodies are located. They, then enter brainstem and ascend or descend in the trigeminospinal tract before entering the trigeminal sensory nuclear complex. By the process of synaptic transmission, neurons in the complex are excited by the incoming afferent information.

Pain Pathways

Once impulse reaches the thalamus, it is sent not only to sensory cortex, but simultaneously, signals are sent to limbic structure and hypothalamus. The sensory cortex then recognizes impulse as pain. At this point, cortex reaches back into memory for evaluation of this experience and accordingly, meaning (such as suffering) is given to pain.

The limbic system centers (associated with behavior) influence affective nature of sensory sensation. The hypothalamus also influences other responses of pain. As a result, the subject is driven to a behavior that eliminates pain. The limbic system affects the subject's response to pain.

Certain neurochemicals and neuropeptides play a role in nociception. Damage to tissues results in release of potassium, histamine, bradykinin, which sensitize the nerve endings. Also, prostaglandins, a metabolic product of arachidonic acid is released and sensitizes nociceptive nerve endings.

In chronic pain—sensitization appears to occur at both the peripheral and central nervous system levels. In *the peripheral sensitization* of trigeminal nerves, small A-delta-fibers and C fibers nociceptors become chronically hyperactive to all stimuli, because of at least three interacting processes.

1. The first mechanism of peripheral sensitization is the sustained release of inflammatory chemical mediators such as 5-hydroxytryptamine (5-HT), bradykinin and prostaglandins at the nociceptor surface receptor. Because of this nociceptor threshold decreases and even stimuli such as touch or pressure, which are not painful, are transmitted to CNS through the sensitized nociceptors and perceived as pain.

2. The second mechanism of peripheral sensitization appears to be the induction of pathologic ectopic electrophysiologic activity at specific sites, on injured nerve trunks (neuromas) or at the trigeminal ganglion itself.

3. The third mechanism of nerve sensitization has been linked to pathologic changes in autonomic nerves, which become neurochemically linked to injured peripheral somatosensory nerves through up regulation of autonomic receptors. A final basis for chronic central sensitization appears to be a failure in the normal pain inhibition systems that originate in forebrain-hypothalamic centers and descend to spinal cord—brainstem levels to modulate pain through neurochemical mediators such as 5-HT and norepinephrine and GABAergic and encephalonergic interneurons.

The sensitization which results in lowering of threshold can occur centrally also. When nociceptive input is continuous, i.e. when second order neurons constantly receive nociceptive input, specific receptors that increase sensitization of that neurons are activated. This sensitization can result in normal impulses being misinterpreted as noxious. This is called neuroplasticity, which explains for chronic neuropathic pains.

Thus pain modulation can occur anywhere in trigeminospinal tract, nucleus, reticular formation by endorphine, as well as by psychologic factors.

44 Trigeminal Neuralgia and its Management

It is a truly agonizing condition, in which patient may clutch the hand over the face and experience severe, lancinating pain associated with spasmodic contractions of the facial muscles during attacks—a feature that led to the use of the term (its archaic name) 'Tic Douloureux' (painful jerking) (Figs 44.1A and B).

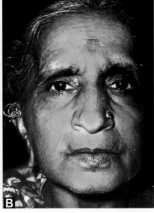

Figs 44.1A and B: (A) Patient's photograph during the attack of trigeminal neuralgic pain, (B) Patient's photograph after diagnostic injection with local anesthetic agent

DEFINITION

Trigeminal neuralgia (TN) is defined as sudden, usually unilateral, severe, brief, stabbing, lancinating, paroxysmal, recurring pain in the distribution of one or more branches of 5th cranial nerve.

- John Locke in 1677, gave the first full description with its treatment.
- Nicholaus Andre in 1756, coined the term 'Tic Douloureux.'
- John Fothergill in 1773, published detailed description of TN, since then, it has been referred to as 'Fothergill's disease'.

In spite of the condition being known since centuries, it still continues to baffle the clinician and its pathogenesis remains as enigma to the medical profession. Multiple views have been hypothecated regarding its etiology generating nothing, but confusion, and simultaneously opting for many different therapies in an effort to treat this ongoing condition.

ETIOLOGY AND PATHOGENESIS

The cause of this disease process is unknown. It is usually idiopathic. However, the fact that benign tumors and vascular anomalies that compress the trigeminal nerve root can produce symptoms clinically indistinguishable from classic TN stongly implies that injury to the nerve root is an important initiating factor in the disease.

Vascular factors such as transient ischemia and autoimmune hypersensitivity responses have been proposed as causes of the demyelination of the nerve.

Mechanical factors have also been postulated, such as the pressure of aneurysms of the intrapetrous portion of the internal carotid artery that may erode through the floor of the intracranial fossa to exert a pulsatile irritation on the ventral side of the trigeminal ganglion.

Anomaly of the superior cerebellar artery has been more recently blamed for causing TN. The artery lies in contact with the sensory root of the trigeminal nerve and its anomaly has been implicated as a cause of demyelination. Surgical elevation of the artery or decompression of the sensory root has been highly successful in relieving paroxysmal pain in cases of idiopathic TN.

The probable etiologic factors are listed below:

i. *Dental etiology:* According to Westrum and Black (1976), differentiation from loss of teeth and degeneration of nerve is not restricted to peripheral parts of the ganglia, but proceeds proximally to involve areas of spinal nucleus. This can partly explain the affliction in the maxillary and mandibular divisions of 5th cranial nerve.

ii. *Infections:* Various granulomatous and non-granulomatous infections involving the 5th cranial nerve can bring about neuralgic pain.

iii. *Ratner's jaw bone cavities (1979):* Cavities found in the alveolar and jaw bones are the causative factor. Patients with neuralgia inducing cavitational osteonecrosis also can be candidates.

iv. *Multiple sclerosis:* Olfson (1966), suggested the presence of sclerotic plaque located at the root entry zone of the trigeminal nerve. Usually patients will have an established diagnosis of multiple sclerosis with demyelinating disease.

v. *Petrous ridge (basilar) compression:* Lee (1937), suggested that trigeminal neuralgia may be caused by compression of the nerve at the dural foramen or over the petrous tip and advocated decompression by performing removal of the bony rim of petrous bone.

vi. *Post traumatic neuralgia:* The most common types of traumatic neuromas involving the trigeminal branch, are those following trauma and those resulting from some dental procedures. These may lead towards neuralgic pain.

Based on the morphologic and physiologic changes following partial nerve injury, Devor et al proposed an 'ignition hypothesis' to explain the main signs and symptoms of TN. In this model, a trigeminal injury induces physiologic changes that result in a population of hyper excitable and functionally linked primary sensory neurons. The discharge of any individual neuron in this group can quickly spread to activate the entire population. Such a sudden synchronous discharge could underlie the sudden jolt of pain characteristic of a TN pain attack.

vii. *Intracranial tumors:* Many lesions such as epidermoid tumors, meningiomas of cerebellopontine angle and Meckel's cave, arteriovenous malformations, aneurysms and vascular compression have been suggested as the causes. Trigeminal neuromas in the middle cranial or the posterior fossa may be also the causative factor. These intracranial tumors or vascular malformations may impinge on the nerve.

viii. *Intracranial vascular abnormalities:* Compression – Jannetta et al showed that vascular compression is a common finding in patients with TN and that surgical decompression of the nerve root often effectively alleviates TN symptoms.

Distortion of the root entry zone of the trigeminal nerve at the pons by an arterial loop, usually of the superior cerebellar artery, or by venous compression by arteriovenous malformations, etc. Compression of the intracranial retrogasserian portion of the 5th cranial nerve by a displaced vein or artery may be also a cause. Aneurysm of the internal carotid artery may cause TN

ix. *Viral etiology:* Postherpetic neuralgia is seen in elderly patients. History of a previous episode of infection by varicella zoster virus may be present in these patients. Viral lesions of the ganglion can be the etiological factor.

GENERAL CHARACTERISTICS

- *Incidence:* It is a rare affliction, seen in about 4 in 100,000 persons.
- *Age of occurrence:* Late middle age or later in life (5th or 6th decade)
- *Sex predilection:* With female predisposition (58%).

- *Affliction for sides:* Predilection for the right side is noted (60%).
- *Division of trigeminal nerve involvement:* V_3 is more commonly involved than V_2 division. Very rarely V_1 ophthalmic division is involved in about 5 percent of cases (Only sensory division is affected).

CLINICAL CHARACTERISTICS

Trigeminal neuralgic pain typically arises in the persons, who have no abnormal neurologic deficit such as loss of corneal reflexes, anesthesia, paresthesia, muscular atrophy or weakness, etc.

- TN typically manifests as a sudden, unilateral, intermittent paroxysmal, sharp, shooting, lancinating, shock like pain, elicited by slight touching superficial 'trigger points' which radiates from that point, across the distribution of one or more branches of the trigeminal nerve
- Pain is usually confined to one part of one division of trigeminal nerve—mandibular or maxillary, but may occasionally spread to an adjacent division or rarely involve all three divisions
- *Pain rarely crosses the midline:* The pain is of short duration and lasts for a few seconds, but may recur with variable frequency. Even though there is a refractory period (complete lack of pain) between the attacks, some patients report a dull ache in between the attacks
- During an attack, the patient grimaces with pain, clutches his hands over the affected side of the face, stopping all the activities and holds or rubs his face, which may redden or the eyes water until the attack subsides. Male patients avoid shaving. The oral hygiene is poor, as patient avoids brushing of teeth
- The paroxysms occur in cycles, each cycle lasting for weeks or months and with time, the cycle appears closer and closer. With each attack, the pain seems to become more intense and unbearable.
- In extreme cases, the patient will have a motionless face—the 'frozen or mask like face'
- Presence of an intraoral or extraoral trigger points provocable by obvious stimuli is seen in TN. Trigger zone is an area of facial skin or oral mucosa,where low intensity mechanical stimulation such as light touch, an air puff, or even touching face at a particular site or by chewing or even by speaking or smiling, brushing, shaving or even washing the face, etc. can elicit a typical pain attack.

- The location of the trigger points depends on which division of trigeminal nerve is involved.
    i. In V_2—points are located on the skin of the upper lip, ala nasi or cheek or on the upper gums.
    ii. In V_3—this is the most frequently involved branch. Trigger points are seen over the lower lip, teeth or gums of the lower jaw. Tongue is rarely involved.
    iii. In V_1—the trigger zone usually lies over the supraorbital ridge of the affected side.
- It is characteristic of the disorder, that attacks do not occur during sleep.
- Many patients will lead a very poor quality of life, because of excruciating pain.
- It is very common for these patients to undergo indiscriminate dental extractions on the affected side without any relief from pain, because the pain of the trigger zone and pain fiber distributions often mimic pain of odontogenic origin.
- More than 50 percent of patients experience early remissions of greater than 6 months before return of active pain.

DIAGNOSIS

The diagnosis of TN rests on the clinician's ability in recognizing a distinctive series of signs and symptoms that define this disorder. Although the hallmark findings of TN were known for centuries, White and Sweet made a significant contribution by articulating precise diagnostic criteria for TN. These "Sweet Criteria" are used worldwide (Table 44.1).

The White and Sweet criteria were incorporated into the official research by the International Association for the Study of Pain-IASP and the International Headache Society-IHS. The current IHS recommended classification for TN is listed in "International Classification of Headache Disorders II-ICHD-II". It subdivides TN into "Classic idiopathic TN" and "Symptomatic TN". (Tables 44.2 and 44.3).

Diagnosis is made from a well taken history. The classic clinical pattern will lead towards the diagnosis. Sometimes, if symptoms may be less classic and may

Table 44.1: Sweet diagnostic 5 major criteria for TN
1. The pain is paroxysmal
2. The pain may be provoked by light touch to the face (trigger zones)
3. The pain is confined to trigeminal distribution
4. The pain is unilateral
5. The clinical sensory examination is normal

Table 44.2: International classification of headache disorders ICHD criteria for classical TN

A. Paroxysmal attacks of pain,lasting from a fraction of a second to two minutes, affecting
   One or more divisions of the trigeminal nerve and fulfilling criteria B and C.
B. Pain has at least one of the following characteristics:
   1. Intense, sharp, superficial or stabbing
   2. Precipitated from trigger areas or by trigger factors
C. Attacks are stereotyped in the individual patient
D. There is no clinically evident neurological deficit
E. Not attributed to another disorder.

Table 44.3: ICHD criteria for symptomatic TN

A. Paroxysmal attacks of pain lasting from a fraction of a second to two minutes, with or without persistence of aching between paroxysms, affecting one or more divisions of the trigeminal nerve and fulfilling criteria B and C
B. Pain has at least one of the following characteristics:
   1. Intense, sharp, superficial or stabbing
   2. Precipitated from trigger areas or by trigger factors
C. Attacks are stereotyped in the individual patient
D. A causative lesion, other than vascular compression, has been demonstrated by special investigations and/or posterior fossa exploration

mimic toothache, sinusitis, stomatitis or other inflammatory conditions. Proper clinical examination along with history is mandatory. The neuralgic symptoms in younger group of patients (< 35 years of age) should alert the clinician to a possible intracranial space occupying lesion or intracranial arteriovenous anomalies. Other differential diagnosis should include acaustic neurilemoma, multiple sclerosis, postherpetic neuroma or post traumatic neuralgias. All patients should ideally have MRI scanning or at least a CT scan. Preoperative localization of compressive vessels at the root entry zone is done by MRI scanning.

Response to treatment with tablet carbamazepine is universal in trigeminal neuralgia, as in other types of facial pain it is not useful. Many clinicians use this response as a step in definitive diagnosis of the condition. Failure to obtain any improvement with this treatment should bring the diagnosis into question.

Diagnostic injections of a local anesthetic agent into the patient's trigger zone should temporarily eliminate all pain. Mathews and Scrivani have proposed a simple algorithm for the differential diagnosis and management of TN (Flow chart 44.1).

Flow chart 44.1: Diagnostic algorithm for TN by Scrivani, Mathews

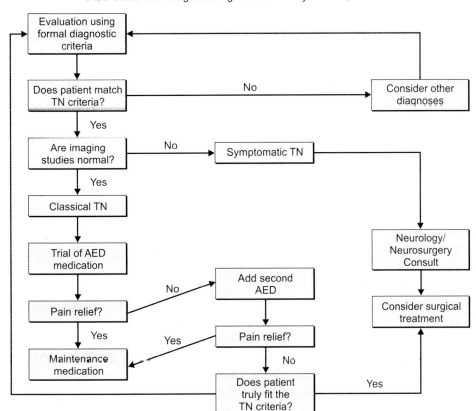

Protocol for Diagnostic Local Anesthetic Peripheral Nerve Blocks

Majority of TN patients have an extremely sensitive trigger zone in the perioral region. A standard local block that anesthetizes the facial region containing the trigger often results in an immediate reduction in TN attacks. This allows the patient to talk and provides a practical way for the clinician to get a full history before making decisions regarding definitive treatment. Local anesthetic blocks have also been reported to eliminate the bouts of pain for prolonged time, outlasting the duration of the particular anesthetic agent utilized.

Material Required

- 3–1 cc syringes
- 3–25 gauge needles
- Sterile normal saline
- Two percent lignocaine without adrenaline.
- Several alcohol wipes

Procedure

- Always begin injections at surface site of pain and then move proximally. For example, if the pain is perceived in the lower lip, then inject lower lip, then mental nerve and then inferior alveolar nerve.
- Inject 0.5 cc of normal saline at test site. Wait for 5 minutes. If pain is relieved, then psychogenic pain is likely.
- If the pain persists, then inject 0.5 ml of 2 percent lignocaine without adrenaline at surface site and wait for 5 minutes. If pain is relieved, then direct therapy at small nociceptor fibers.
- If the pain persists–inject little deeper and wait for 5 minutes. If pain is relieved, then consider musculoskeletal origin of pain.
- If pain is not relieved, inject at more proximal portion of nerve—If pain is relieved, direct therapy at site, when relief occurred.
- Thus, selective inferior alveolar, lingual, buccal, infraorbital, posterior superior alveolar blocks can be given to know the involvement of the branch of the trigeminal nerve.

▌ TREATMENT

Once the diagnosis of trigeminal neuralgia is established, then the treatment regime is started. First medicinal management is advocated. If the patient does not respond to it, then only surgical management is opted (Flow chart 44.2).

Medicinal Management

Medicinal Line of Treatment (Modification of the Paroxysmal Pain at Cortical Level)

This is the first line approach for most of the patients. TN does not respond to analgesics including opiates.

The attacks of pain in TN are probably caused by a group of pathologically "hyper excitable" sensory trigeminal neurons that discharge spontaneously, exhibit abnormal after discharges, and demonstrate abnormal spread of excitation to adjacent primary afferents. Similar mechanisms occur in epilepsy, therefore, many antiepileptic drugs-AEDs are used to suppress pain attacks in TN.

Bourguignon (1942), used anticonvulsant phenytoin to effectively control attacks of pain in TN.

Blom (1962), showed a response to anticonvulsants (Table 44.4).

Carbamazepine is highly specific in only relieving pain of TN and not any other type of facial pain. It has, therefore, suggested that its response can be used as a diagnostic indicator.

In TN, most clinitians usually initiate AED therapy with a low dose of a single AED. This dose is gradually escalated over subsequent days until the patient achieves satisfactory pain relief or until significant drug-related side effects emerge.

- Carbamazepine (Tegretol) and phenytoin (Dilantin) are the traditional anticonvulsants used primarily, as soon as the diagnosis is done. This therapy consists of titration and maintenance with anticonvulsant drugs.
- Carbamazepine 100 mg three times a day is introduced and titrated over 1 to 5 weeks period until either remission is achieved or side effects or toxicity are unacceptable. (Commercially, tegretol 100 mg, 200 mg or 400 mg tabs are available. Controlled or slow release tablets are available.)

The dosage of the drug used initially should be kept small to minimum especially in elderly patients to avoid nausea, vomiting and gastric irritation. More of daily drug dosage should be taken at night, so that adequate serum concentration can be present in early morning, when pain most occurs. Complete blood count with platelet count, liver function screening should be done prior to treatment, a month after treatment and at 3 to 4 months intervals, particularly, if patient continues to receive a high dose (1000 to 1500 mg/day).

Flow chart 44.2: Various treatment modalities implicated for the treatment of trigeminal neuralgia

Table 44.4: Drug Therapy for TN

Drug	Initial Dose	Maintenance Dose
Gabapentin	300 mg TID	1800 mg
Baclofen	5 mg BID-TID	80 mg maximum dose
Clonazepam	0.5 mg TID	4 mg, maximum 20 mg
Lamotrigine	50 mg QD	300-500 mg
Oxcarbazepine	300 mg BID	1200 mg BID
Toprimate	50 mg QD	200 mg BID
Carbamazepine	100 mg BID	1200-2400 mg

Side effects: Visual blurring, dizziness, somnolence, skin rashes and ataxia and in rare cases hepatic dysfunction, leukopenia, thrombocytopenia—aplastic anemia (It is known to suppress the bone marrow. Patients should be monitored to avoid agranulocytosis). Whenever the side effects appear, a reduction of 200 mg of drug will often eliminate them. Once the pain remission has been achieved, the drug dose should be kept at maintenance level or withdrawn and restarted if symptoms appear.

If carbamazepine does not control symptoms adequately, then another anticonvulsant like sodium valproate 600 mg/day can be added or amitriptyline can be added. Co-administration of phenytoin or baclofen is also advocated.

When carbamazepine is contraindicated, clonazepam 1.5 mg/day can be used.

Clonazepam side effects: Drowsiness, fatigue, lethargy.
- Tab. Phenytoin: Dose—100 mg three times a day.
  Side effects: Slurred speech, abnormal movements, swelling of lymph glands, gingival hypertrophy, hirsutism, folate deficiency.
- Tab. Oxcarbazepine—1200 mg/day.
  Side effects: Hyponatremia, double vision.
- Valproic acid—600 mg/day.
  Side effects: irritability, tremors, confusion, hepatoxicity, weight gain.
- Mephenesin Carbamate (Tolceram)—5 to 15 ml/ 5 times a day to every 3 hours.

- Other less toxic agents:
  - Baclofen (Lioresal)—10 mg tds
    Side effects: fatigue, vomiting
  - Gabapentin (Neurontin) recently introduced drug.
  - Lamotrigine
  - Felbamate
  - Topiramate
  - Vigabatrin
  - Clonazepam
  - Levetiracetam
  - Zonisamide

Multiple Drug Therapy

- When a patient only partially responds to single drug therapy at dosages that evoke side effects, adding a second AED may enhance the therapeutic response. Because AEDs have differing mechanisms of action as well as differing side effect patterns, combining

agents is a good approach. However, when patient do not satisfactorily responds to 2 AEDs, there is little chance of success for additional third drug.

- A better strategy entails a careful reappraisal of the case, including a critical reevaluation of the TN diagnosis.If the diagnosis of TN is confirmed, such patients should be considered for surgical interventions.

Surgical Treatments (Fig. 44.2)
(Peripheral Nerve Surgical Treatments)

Peripheral Nerve Injections

For several years, it has been known that injections of destructive substances into peripheral branches of trigeminal nerve, produce anesthesia in the trigger zones or in areas of distribution of spontaneous pain, and this procedure can be effective in relieving this syndrome, usually as long as the anesthesia persists. Care should

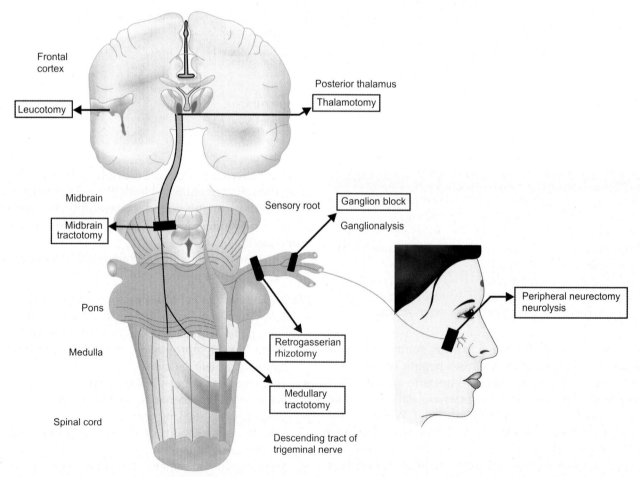

Fig. 44.2: Various sites of surgical control for maxillofacial pain

be taken to ensure that IV injections are avoided. This method is successful, when there is well localized trigger area.

a. *Long acting anesthetic agents* without adrenaline such as bupivacaine with or without corticosteroids may be injected at the most proximal possible nerve site. The selective nerve blocks can be given as an emergency measure, where the patient is suffering quite a lot, but the pain free period will be very short lived. The injection can be repeated, when the pain recurs.

b. *Alcohol injections*—peripheral branches of trigeminal nerve can be blocked by the intraoral injection of 95 percent absolute alcohol in small quantities (0.5 to 2 ml). This produces anesthesia of the region, supplied by the branch. Repeated alcohol injections should be avoided, as it causes local tissue toxicity, inflammation and fibrosis. It can also cause a complication of burning alcohol neuritis. The results are variable. Sometimes it provides relief for a period of 6 to 12 months or sometimes patient comes back with pain immediately within short time span. Extraoral injections into maxillary and mandibular division of the trigeminal nerve at the level of the base of the skull also can be given. Peripheral injections—infraorbital, mental, inferior alveolar nerve blocks can be given depending on the involvement.

Peripheral Neurectomy (Nerve Avulsion)

- Oldest and most effective peripheral nerve destructive technique
- Simple procedure can be repeated and relatively reliable technique
- It acts by interrupting the flow of a significant number of afferent impulses to central trigeminal apparatus
- Indicated in patients, in whom craniotomy, a more extensive procedure is contraindicated, because of age, debility or significant systemic diseases, limited life expectancy
- Performed most commonly on infraorbital, inferior alveolar mental and rarely lingual nerves
- It has a disadvantage of producing full anesthesia or deep hypoesthesia related dysfunction
- There is also the expected eventual return of pain with proliferation of amputed nerve stump neuromas
- To achieve better results, the peripheral nerve is always avulsed both from the bone as well as from the soft tissues

- The duration of pain remission after neurectomy may be lengthened, if the cut nerve end is cauterized or redirected and sutured into viable muscle, periosteum or bone tissue to prevent active neuroma formation
- The bony foramen may be plugged with nonabsorbable material or by the bone piece itself
- The procedure is carried out under general anesthesia to ensure successful avulsion.

Infraorbital neurectomy: It can be performed through (i) conventional intraoral approach or (ii) through Braun's transantral approach.

i. *Intraoral conventional approach* (Figs 44.3 and 44.4)—a U-shaped Caldwell-Luc incision is made in the upper buccal vestibule in the canine fossa region. Mucoperiosteal flap is reflected superiorly to locate the infraorbital foramen. Once the nerve is exposed, all the peripheral branches are held with the hemostat and avulsed from the skin surface intraorally. Then, the entire trunk is separated from the skin surface, is held with the hemostat at the exit point from the foramen and is removed by winding it around a hemostat and pulling it out from the foramen. The infraorbital foramen may be plugged with polyethylene plug and wound is closed with interrupted sutures.

ii. *Braun's transantral approach (1977)*—It has got the potential to have sound treatment for intractable V_2 neuralgia, because of the direct access and visualization it provides. The key to this approach is a thorough knowledge of anatomy. With sectioning of the maxillary nerve, anesthesia is created over its entire distribution.

An intraoral incision is made from the maxillary tuberosity to the midline in the maxillary vestibule. The mucoperiosteal flap is reflected to expose the anterior and lateral maxillary antral wall, the zygoma and the infraorbital nerve. A 3 cm window is made in the anterolateral wall of the maxillary sinus (Fig. 44.5). The operating microscope is usually required for the remainder of the procedure. The lining in the posterosuperior portion of the antrum is carefully excised and bone is removed to create a posterior window. Careful dissection is now performed to expose the descending palatine branches of V_2, which are then traced superiorly to the sphenopalatine ganglion (Fig. 44.6). In order to provide anatomical verification, the infraorbital nerve is identified in the roof of the maxillary sinus and is carefully followed posteriorly to the trunk of V_2 near the sphenopalatine ganglion. Dissection is then completed by

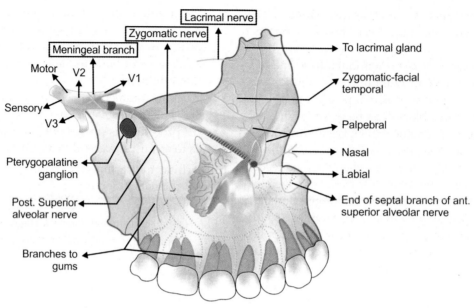

Fig. 44.3: Course of maxillary nerve

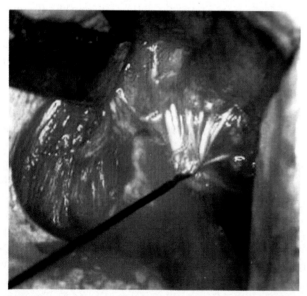

Fig. 44.4: Intraoral conventional neurectomy procedure for infraorbital nerve: exposure of infraorbital nerve at the infraorbital foramen

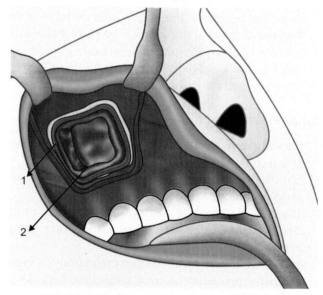

Fig. 44.5: Surgical approach to pterygomaxillary fossa (1) Anterior antral wall, (2) Posterior antral wall

isolating and identifying the trunk of V_2 superiorly and posteriorly to the sphenopalatine ganglion. The trunk of the maxillary nerve (V_2) is then sectioned posterior to the sphenopalatine ganglion near the foramen rotundum and close to the inferior orbital fissure (Figs 44.7A and B). The antral mucoperiosteal flap in the vestibule is repositioned and sutured back.

Complications (i) inadvertent section of the vessels in the pterygopalatine fossa (ii) inadvertent sectioning of the branches of the sphenopalatine ganglion or the vidian nerve, entering the posterior aspect of the ganglion.

Inferior alveolar neurectomy: It can be performed via intraoral or extraoral approach. The intraoral approach is preferred, as it is simple and more cosmetic.

1. *The extraoral approach*—is through Risdon's incision, where after reflection of masseter, a bony window is drilled in outer cortex and nerve is lifted with nerve hook and avulsed from its superior attachment and mental nerve is avulsed anteriorly through the same approach.

2. *Intraoral approach* –**Via Dr Ginwalla's incision** (Figs 44.8A to D)—it is mainly used in dentulous cases.

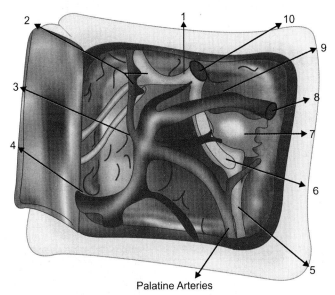

Palatine Arteries

Fig. 44.6: View of the contents of pterygomaxillary fossa (1) Maxillary nerve, (2) Infraorbital nerve and artery, (3) Maxillary artery, (4) Posterior superior alveolar artery, (5) Palatine nerves, (6) Vidian nerve, (7) Sphenopalatine ganglion, (8) Sphenopalatine foramen, (9) Sphenopalatine artery, (10) Foramen rotundum

Incision is made along the anterior border of ascending ramus, extending lingually and buccally and ending in a fork like an inverted Y (Dr Ginwalla's incision). Such incision provides better exposure of the field. The incision is then deepened on the medial aspect of the ascending ramus by means of blunt and sharp dissection. The temporalis and medial pterygoid muscles are split, rather than divided at their insertion and the inferior alveolar nerve is located. Two heavy black linen threads are then looped around the nerve using nerve hook and then divided between the 2 threads. This is done as high as possible and the upper end is cauterized, while dividing and lower end is held with the hemostat. Another linear incision is made in the buccal vestibule overlying the mental foramen. A mucoperiosteal flap is reflected to expose the mental nerve. It is then tied with heavy black linen just little away from the foramen. The nerve is then caught with the hemostat distal to the knot and is divided between the two. The distal part held between the hemostat and is wound around it and the peripheral branches entering the mucosa are avulsed out. There is puckering of the skin surface seen during this procedure.

Now after the mental nerve is freed, then at the mandibular foramen, the distal part of the nerve which is held with the hemostat is pulled until the entire nerve length of the canal is avulsed out. If any obstruction is encountered, a window may be made in the buccal cortex posterior to the mental foramen, along the level of the inferior alveolar canal and the nerve is lifted out

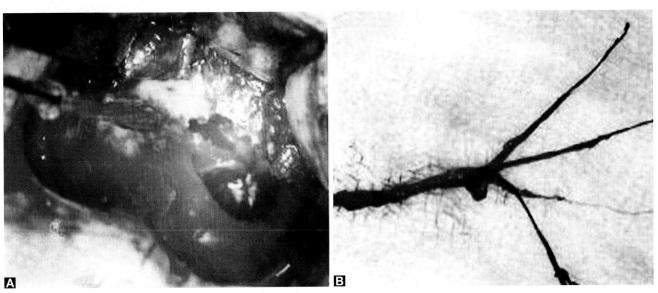

Figs 44.7A and B: (A) Surgical exposure of infraorbital nerve via transantral approach, (B) Avulsed nerve

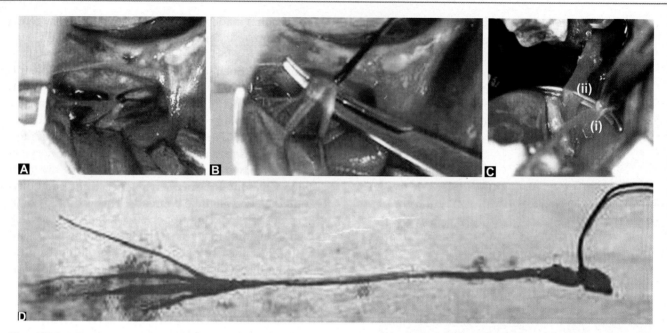

Figs 44.8A to D: Inferior alveolar neurectomy. Dr Ginwalla's procedure—(A) Exposure of mental nerve, (B) Peripheral branches of mental nerve ready for avulsion, (C) Exposure of (i) inferior alveolar nerve and (ii) Lingual nerve, via Dr. Ginwalla's intraoral incision, (D) Inferior alveolar nerve avulsed

of the canal through the window. The wound is closed with interrupted sutures.

Lingual neurectomy (Fig. 44.9): A vertical incision is made at the inner border of the ascending ramus, extending from the coronoid process down the level of the floor of the mouth. Keeping the two sides of the incision retracted, the dissection is continued downwards until the lingual nerve comes into view at the border of the medial pterygoid muscle. In the region of the floor of the mouth, the nerve lies even more superficially and it can be easily found between the anterior pillar of the fauces at the root of the tongue. After dissection, the nerve is grasped with a hemostat and is then either avulsed or cauterized and cut. The wound is closed with interrupted sutures.

Cryotherapy or Cryoneurolysis for Peripheral Nerves

Direct applications of cryotherapy probe at temperatures colder than –60°C are known to produce Wallerian degeneration without destroying the nerve sheath itself. For this procedure the nerve is exposed as described in peripheral neurectomy procedure and is frozen with

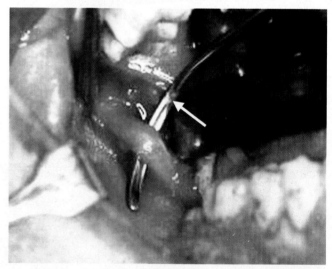

Fig. 44.9: Exposure of the lingual nerve. Arrow—nerve hook

a cryoprobe (Nitrous oxide probe) for a period of 1 to 2 minutes followed by 3 minutes thaw, to be repeated three times. The pain remission follows the procedure. But regeneration of axons is expected. No large series are available for comparison with peripheral cryotherapy techniques. But the procedure is relatively simple.

Peripheral Radiofrequency Neurolysis (Thermocoagulation)

Gregg and Small in 1986, reported surgical management of trigeminal pain with radiofrequency lesions of the peripheral nerves. A radiofrequency electrode that has the capacity to definitely destroy the pain fibers is used in this procedure. The use of radiofrequency (RF) lesioning of trigeminal nerve has been used sparingly, but with success. RF neurolysis has been shown to induce pain remission in 80 percent of cases with a 20 percent/year recurrence rate.

Procedure: Topical anesthesia with mild sedation is used. The patient is grounded in an electronic circuit and the 22 gauge lesion probe is positioned adjacent to nerve to be lesioned. Paresthesias are elicited to ensure proximity to the nerve and tissue temperature is measured with the probe tip through the probe thermocouple. Lesioning is then carried out at 65 to 75°C for 1 to 2 minutes. Repositioning may be required to ensure adequate RF wave effect on the nerve fibers.

Advantages: Low morbidity in high risk/elderly patients.

Disadvantages: Needs specific electronic armamentarium and reasonable patient cooperation. In case of inaccessibility of some pain triggering nerve trunks, the technique will fail to achieve pain relief.

Gasserian Ganglion Procedures

Around 1900—first open surgeries were performed on the gasserian ganglion for TN. These were recorded as hazardous procedures

- 1910—Harris, Tapatas and Hartel separately introduced percutaneous approaches to the ganglion via the foramen ovale. Absolute alcohol or phenol-glycerol mixture was used as the neurolytic agent.
- 1931—Kirschner introduced percutaneous electrocoagulation of the gasserian ganglion.
- Since then, three main percutaneous gasserian ganglion procedures are being used with variable success rate: (i) glycerol injection, (ii) thermocoagulation, (iii) balloon compression.

The technique of needle placement is common to all of these. Initial pioneering procedures were performed free hand, but now hard copy X-ray or image intensification on monitors is used first for visualization of position of the foramen ovale and then for confirmation of the depth of penetration of the needle and the position of any contrast medium used.

Technique for Percutaneous Approach to the Gasserian Ganglion: Anesthesia Protocol

Patient is admitted on the day of surgery and kept nil by mouth for at least 4 hours prior to surgery. Injection atropine (0.6 mg IM) is given one hour prior to surgery to reduce oral secretions and to prevent intraoperative bradycardia.

Injection methahexitone: Ultrashort acting barbiturate (Brevital) is administered intravenously in dose of 1.5 to 2 mg/kg body weight in increments, so as to maintain an adequate level of unconsciousness during lesion production and during painful part of the procedure, like when needle/electrode comes in contact with the base of the skull, when it penetrates foramen ovale. Pulse oximeter, oxygen saturation, vital signs including systolic and diastolic blood pressure, respiratory rate, pulse rates as well as ECGs are monitored throughout the procedure. The duration of procedure is usually of one hour. Patient should be given intranasal oxygen and intravenous fluids.

Procedure: The patient is made to lie on a table with neck well extended. The foramen ovale is best visualized with the X-ray tube placed for a submentovertex position. Infiltration of the skin and cheek is done with local anesthetic agent on the affected side. Three points of Hartel are marked on the side of the face using marking ink (Fig. 44.10).

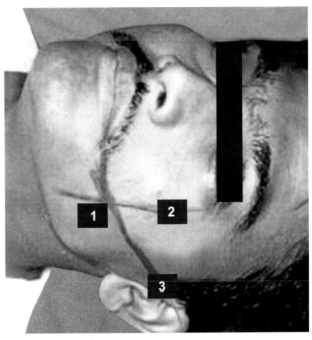

Fig. 44.10: Hartel's 3 point markings

First point is marked at lateral orbital rim and a perpendicular line is drawn till the inferior border of the mandible.

Second point is marked at about 15 mm (3 inches) lateral to the angle of the mouth on the perpendicular first line. This is a point of penetration of needle/electrode.

Third point is marked at the level of TMJ. 2.5 cm from the center of external auditory meatus. This point is joined with the 2nd point of Hartel. This line will form a plane, which is the plane of elevation. When the patient is positioned in supine position with head extended, the plane of elevation is perpendicular to the floor (a flat pillow is kept under the shoulder). The needle/electrode is passed through the cheek from the point of penetration (2nd point). The finger of gloved hand is placed inside the oral cavity to prevent inadvertent penetration of needle/electrode in the oral cavity (Fig. 44.11).

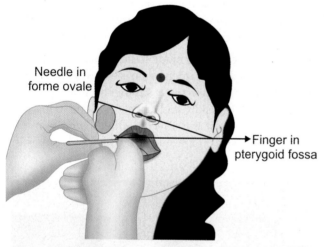

Needle in forme ovale

Finger in pterygoid fossa

Fig. 44.11: Prevention of inadevertent penetration of needle in the oral cavity, while injecting into the gasserian ganglion

Pass the needle/electrode along the plane of elevation till it reaches the anterior border of ramus of mandible, then turn the needle medial to ramus, pass it upwards to the base of the skull in pupillary plane.

During this phase, the needle/electrode lies below the orbit, medial to ramus of the mandible and lateral to maxilla. Engagement of the needle/electrode in the foramen ovale is best confirmed by biplanar radiology or image intensifier (Figs 44.12A and B).

The final position of the needle/electrode is then pushed for another half a centimeter.

Glycerol injection: Glycerol or absolute alcohol can be used for percutaneous ganglion neurolysis. The agent is injected into Meckel's cave or in the ganglion (Fig. 44.13). The agent then diffuses throughout the ventral ganglion, producing low grade damage to nerve cells, presumably through dehydration. This technique induces pain relief in around 80 percent of cases, it can be repeated if required and it prevents gross facial sensation with lower levels of anesthesia. It also spares the important ophthalmic division and the motor root.

For this injection, a 16 gauge spinal needle is used and inserted through the foramen ovale into the ganglion till CSF is obtained on withdrawal of the stylet (Fig. 44.14). Contrast medium is injected to check the position of the needle. The contrast is evacuated and replaced by 0.5 to 0.75 ml of pure glycerol or 0.5 ml of absolute alcohol. The patient is sent to ward and kept there with head extended for 2 hours. The relief obtained varies from six months to two years. In this procedure patient cooperation is needed, if it is done under local anesthesia.

Controlled radiofrequency thermocoagulation (Fig. 44.15): A radiofrequency electrode that has the capacity to definitely destroy pain fibers is now used.

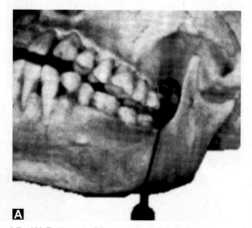

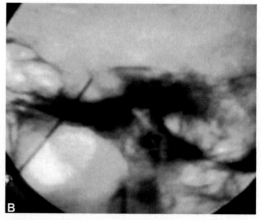

Figs 44.12A and B: (A) Pathway of the needle towards foramen ovale, (B) Needle/Electrode point at the clivus seen on image intensifier screen

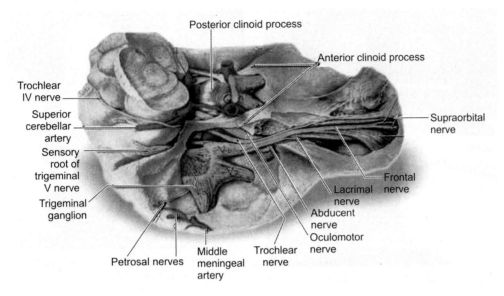

Fig. 44.13: Gasserian ganglion and its relations

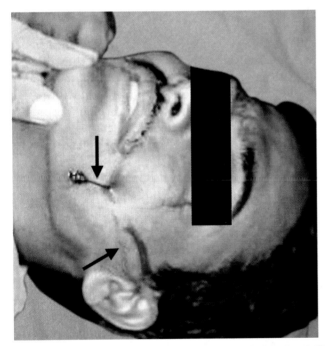

Fig. 44.14: Gasserian ganglion injection technique preparation. A 16 gauge spinal needle is inserted through the foramen ovale into the ganglion. Arrow—CSF flow

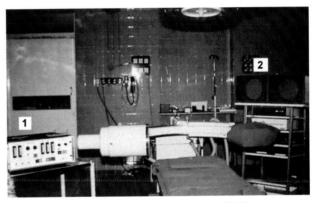

Fig. 44.15: (1) Owl's radiofrequency system, (2) C-arm image intensifier screen

Advantages

1. Avoidance of denervation of cornea.
2. Comparative lower rate of recurrence.
3. Procedure can be repeated in case of recurrence.
4. Zero mortality.
5. Well tolerated by elderly and medically compromised patient.
6. Patient will prefer thermocoagulation rather than opting for neurectomy, which leads to facial numbness.
7. Where facilities permit, it can be performed on outpatient basis.

Electrocoagulation of gasserian ganglion was introduced first by Kirschner (1931) and later modified by Sweet (1970).

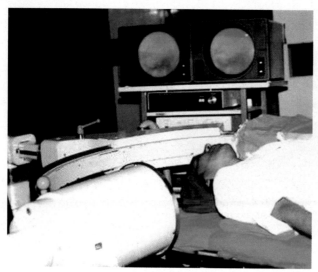

Fig. 44.16: Patient in position for radiofrequency thermocoagulation procedure

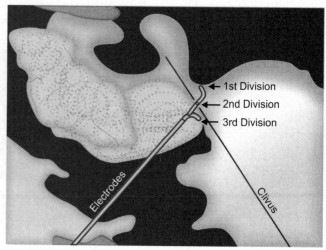

Fig. 44.17: Position of the electrode is adjusted as per the division of the trigeminal nerve involved on clival plane

8. Thermocoagulation preserves the motor function of trigeminal nerve.
9. Simple, accurate procedure, less time consuming and less expensive, and comfortable for the patient.

Indications

- Toxicity of drugs
- Failure of response to other modalities
- Dependence on drug for lifetime
- Elderly patients
- Medically compromised patients
- Recurrence cases—previously treated by intracranial surgery, neurectomies, etc.

Procedure

The trigeminal ganglion may be approached through the foramen ovale by percutaneously placing a 22 gauge probe under fluoroscopic guidance. The image intensifier is used and middle cranial fossa is focussed in the center of screen, the contrast is adjusted to sharpen the bony landmarks (Fig. 44.16). Clear visualization of foramen ovale is obtained by adjusting the position. The probe used should have an insulated shaft and a bore sufficient for the passage of a radiofrequency electrode (Fig. 44.17). When the probe is placed correctly in the foramen ovale and advanced into the trigeminal ganglion, CSF should emerge on removal of the stylet as the ganglion contains CSF (in patients who have undergone previous surgeries or chemical injections you will not get CSF flow). The electrode is inserted then just beyond the tip of the probe and a low amplitude current is applied using a lesion generator (Figs 44.18A and B).

Patient at this stage should be awake and cooperative, is asked whether on the face the stimulation is felt (electric like impulse). The position of the probe is adjusted until stimulation is experienced by the patient in the area where trigeminal neuralgia pain was present. Stimulation is initiated utilizing square wave pulses at 50 cycles per second slowly raising the voltage until full areas of pain covered.

Lesion production: Patient at this stage should be given neurolept anesthesia. Thermal lesions of 30 to 90 second duration are then made at 65 to 75°C using RF generator of microwave energies.

Power 25 watts, voltage 40 to 45 volts. Current 120 to 140 mA. With these parameters a temperature range of 65 to 75°C is achieved. A 5 mm bare tip electrode with 2 mm diameter will produce a lesion of 10 x 6 mm within the trigeminal root at 75°C.

A radiofrequency current when an alternating current of high frequency is passed through the electrode, it produces ionization in biological tissues. Heat results from *ionic friction,* which leads to coagulation of tissues. Great care is exercised to avoid over shooting to preserve the sense of touch. After partial result is produced, it is mostly possible to complete the lesion without additional short acting anesthetic agent. A facial blush usually appears at this point and helps to localize the region of nerve root undergoing thermal destruction.

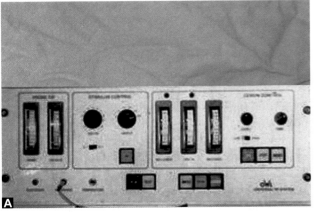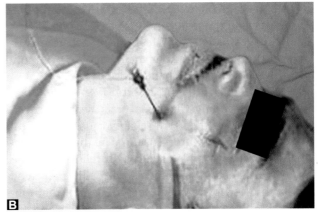

Figs 44.18A and B: (A) Owl's radiofrequency system, (B) Electrode with generator cable attached

This is due to the vasodilator system emerging from the brainstem and passing to the facial vasculature with trigeminal nerve.

At the end of the procedure, patient is asked to perform those manoeuvers that characteristically trigger the TN. Once the patient and operator satisfied with the desired RF lesion production, the electrode is removed and patient is sent to recovery room.

Balloon compression: It is done under general anesthesia. It is a mechanical technique to destroy root fibers partially by advancing 4FG Fogarty catheter 1 to 2 cm within Meckel's cave and inflating the balloon at the ventral aspect of the ganglion root.

A 12 gauge spinal needle is passed first to the foramen ovale and the balloon catheter is passed through it. Once it is in position the balloon is inflated with X-ray contrast medium upto 0.75 ml. When inflated, the balloon should take up the pear shape of Meckel's cave and it should remain inflated for 1 minute.

Open Procedures (Intracranial Procedures)

Microvascular decompression of the sensory root (Posterior Fossa Decompression-PFD)
- Procedure popularized in 1967-1976 by Jannetta
- Most commonly performed intracranial open procedure
- Open craniotomy approach is used to gain access to the trigeminal root entry zone and adjacent brain stem
- The root is examined under the microscope. A compressing branch of the superior cerebellar artery

will be seen medial to the nerve at the root entry zone
- The artery is carefully separated from the nerve and interpositioned by using sponge or Teflon wool
- Patient usually retains good facial sensation without anesthetic dysfunction.
- 75 to 80 percent of patients are pain free for at least 5 years
- Overall mortality rate is 2 percent. It can be associated with infrequent hearing loss, vertigo, cranial nerve VII weakness
- Contraindicated in elderly patients and medically compromised patients.

Trigeminal Root Section

a. *Extradural sensory root section: Frazier's approach (1901)*
   The subtemporal extradural route retrogasserian rhizotomy (root sectioning).

   Here sensory root is divided, sparing the motor root, as close to the brainstem as possible.

   This procedure is rarely used now and it is of historical value, because of the profound sensory loss and high incidence of anesthesia dolorosa. Sensory loss involving ophthalmic division leads to keratitis.

b. *Intradural root section* Described by Wilkins (1966), is superior to extradural approach, as it has less chances of damage to superior petrosal nerve and facial nerve, less chance of bleeding.

   In 1932, Dandy recommended posterior fossa surgery, but technique is more difficult than Frazier's approach and it can damage 5th, 7th or 8th cranial nerves, because of excessive retraction or manipulation, vascular damage, etc.

Advantages of posterior fossa approach is unsuspected tumors or vascular malformation are more readily delineated and handled.

c. *Trigeminal tractotomy (Medullary Tractotomy)* Incision of descending trigeminal tract near the cervicomedullary junction will reliably cause the loss of pain and temperature sensation in the ipsilateral face and pharynx and usually will relieve the pain of TN. It is helpful in patients with pain perceived in both glossopharyngeal and trigeminal distribution. It can be also used for intractable facial pain and should not be routinely used.

Update

Three surgical approaches are commonly used at present to treat TN. All of these techniques produce relief of TN symptoms in large majority of patients—80 to 90 percent. The incidence of complications is low.

1. Percutaneous stereotactic radiofrequency thermal lesioning of the trigeminal ganglion and/or root (RFL).

    This technique produce mild injury to the sensory fibers in the trigeminal root. It is minimally invasive and successfully controls pain in over 85 percent of TN cases and can be performed as day care procedure. Specific side effect is sensory loss and occasional dysesthesia in the distribution of the damaged trigeminal fibers.

    Recommended for patients, who are elderly and medically frail.

2. Posterior fossa exploration and microvascular decompression MVD of the trigeminal root.

    It is a more complex and invasive therapy. But, this directly treats a hypothetical cause of the disorder (nerve compression) while minimizing any trigeminal sensory damage.

    Recommended for young patients, who can tolerate longer, invasive surgical procedure.

3. Gamma knife radiation to the trigeminal root entry zone-GKR

    Relatively recent procedure, that employs computerized stereotactic methods to concentrate gamma radiation on the trigeminal root entry zone. It has gained wide acceptance, however long term results of GKR in TN remain to be established. Advocated in old, frail patients.

▮ BIBLIOGRAPHY

1. Adams CB. Trigeminal neuralgia:pathogenesis and treatment. Br J Neurosurg. 1997;11;493-5.
2. Bayer DB, Stenger TG. Trigeminal neuralgia:an overview. Oral Surg Oral Med Oral Patho Oral Radiol Endod. 1979; 48;393-9.
3. Scrivani SJ, Mathews ES, Maciewicz RJ. Trigeminal neuralgia. Oral Surg Oral Med Oral Pathol Oral Radiol Endod 2005;100;527-38.
4. Smyth P, Greenough G, Stommel E. Familial trigeminal neuralgia: case reports and review of the literature. Headache 2003;43;910-5.

Sensory Disturbances of Face and Jaws

Injuries to peripheral branches of the fifth (trigeminal) nerve is ever present risk during surgical procedures performed in the oral cavity and associated maxillofacial region. Sensory disturbances of the face due to trigeminal nerve branches injury, usually undergo spontaneous regeneration and sensory recovery, but some will result in incomplete regeneration with *paresthesia* or will result in a painful neuropathy—*dysesthesia*. The resulting loss of sensory function can be distressing to those patients in whom spontaneous return of nerve function does not occur. As per older belief, nerve injuries do not always heal spontaneously. Advances in microsurgical techniques and better understanding of neuroanatomy have made possible, the surgical repair of selected maxillofacial peripheral nerve injuries, when carried out timely by a skilled surgeon (Fig. 45.1).

IMPAIRED SENSATION

Sometimes, one or more or all forms of sensation may be impaired. In some cases, the sense of pain is only disturbed, in others the tactile or temperature sense is also affected.

The various terminologies, which are used for expressing the neurological disturbances are listed below:

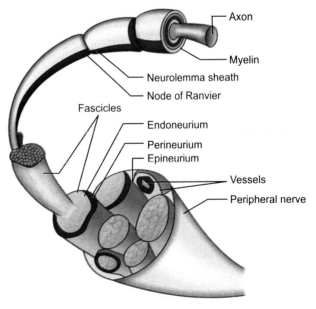

Fig. 45.1: Structure of a myelinated peripheral nerve

i. *Allodynia*: Pain due to a stimulus that does not normally provoke pain.
ii. *Analgesia*: Absence of pain in response to stimulation, that would normally be painful.

iii. *Anesthesia*: Total loss of all types of sensation in response to the stimulation, that would normally be painful or nonpainful. (Total numbness in the distribution of the injured nerve).

iv. *Paresthesia*: An altered sensation, which is not pleasant, like tingling, crawling, burning, pricking, itching, etc. The area supplied by the nerve is numb. This is due to injury or severance of a nerve. The abnormal sensations are produced by an irritation of the nerve at the site of injury or because of the neuroma formation at the severed end.

v. *Dysesthesia*: An unpleasant painful abnormal sensation, either spontaneous or evoked. Patient complains of numbness associated with burning, stabbing or burrowing type or a phantom pain.

vi. *Hyperesthesia*: An increased sensitivity to stimulus.

vii. *Hypoesthesia*: Decreased sensitivity to stimulation.

viii. *Hypo and hypergesia*: Decreased or increased response to a stimulus that is normally painful.

ix. *Ageusia*: Loss of taste.

x. *Neuritis*: Designates an inflammation of a nerve.

xi. *Neuralgia*: Transmission of a pain impulse passed along the course of the nerve.

ETIOLOGY

Due to the injury to the sensory nerve branches, there can be *temporary deficit* or *permanent deficit*.

Maxillofacial surgical procedures that run the risk of injury to one of the peripheral branches of the trigeminal nerve:

A. *Inferior alveolar nerve*: Mandibular impacted third molar or any impacted mandibular tooth removal, mandibular molar endodontics, endosteal implant placement, visor osteotomies, alveolectomy, man-dibular body/ramus/subapical osteotomies, mandibular cyst or tumor removal, mandibular resection, fractures of mandibular body and angle region, preprosthetic surgery, genioplasty, gun shot wounds, osteomyelitis can lead towards anesthesia.

B. *Lingual nerve*: Mandibular third molar removal, excision of the sublingual or submandibular gland, iatrogenic instrumentation of floor of the mouth, sulcoplasties of lingual vestibule, mandibular tumor removal, mandibular ramus osteotomies.

C. *Infraorbital nerve*: LeFort II, III level osteotomies, Caldwell Luc procedure, orbital osteotomies, fractures of the midface and orbits.

INCIDENCE

American Association of Oral and Maxillofacial Surgeons in 1993, reported the removal of impacted third molars is associated with inferior alveolar nerve injury in 1.0 to 7.1 percent of patients, whereas the incidence of injury to the lingual nerve is estimated at 0.02 to 0.06 percent.

CLASSIFICATION OF MECHANICAL NERVE INJURIES

Classification of nerve injuries helps the clinician in making a diagnosis, developing a rational plan of management, determining the need for and timing of surgical intervention and estimating the prognosis of an injury (Figs 45.2A to E).

Seddon (1943) and *Sunderland* (1978), have proposed nerve injury classifications, which are most commonly used. *It is applied to both motor as well as sensory nerves.*

Seddon's Classification (Table 45.1)

1. *Neuropraxia*: Mild, temporary injury caused by compression or retraction of the nerve. There is no axonal degeneration distal to the area of injury.

Table 45.1: Seddon's classification of nerve injuries			
	Neuropraxia	Axonotmesis	Neurotmesis
1. Sunderland classification	1°	2°, 3°, 4°	5°
2. Nerve sheath	Intact	Intact	Interrupted
3. Axons	Intact	Interrupted	Interrupted
4. Wallerian degeneration	None	Yes, partial	Yes, complete
5. Conduction failure	Transitory	Prolonged	Permanent
6. Spontaneous recovery	Complete	Partial	Poor to none
7. Time of recovery	Within 4 weeks	Months	Begins by 3 months, if any

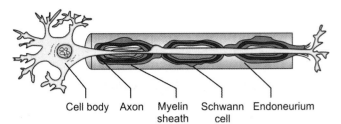

Fig. 45.2A: Stages of peripheral nerve healing. Normal nerve cell and axon

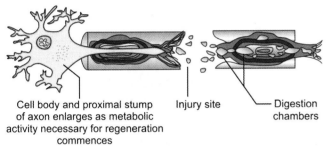

Cell body and proximal stump of axon enlarges as metabolic activity necessary for regeneration commences   Injury site   Digestion chambers

Fig. 45.2B: Early Wallerian degeneration

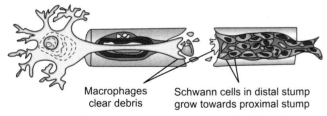

Macrophages clear debris   Schwann cells in distal stump grow towards proximal stump

Fig. 45.2C: Phagocytosis and Schwann cell proliferation

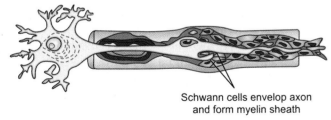

Schwann cells envelop axon and form myelin sheath

Fig. 45.2D: Growth

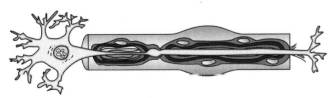

Fig. 45.2E: Repaired nerve fibre

There is a temporary conduction block—sensory loss. Spontaneous recovery usually occurs within 4 weeks or less time. No surgical intervention is required.

2. *Axonotmesis—more significant injury*: There is disruption or loss of continuity of some axons, which undergo Wallerian degeneration distal to the site of injury. The general structure of the nerve remains intact. There is prolonged conduction failure. Initial signs of recovery of nerve function do not appear for 1 to 3 months after injury. Eventual recovery is often less than normal (paresis, hypoesthesia). Sensory nerve injuries may develop persistent painful sensation (dysesthesias).

3. *Neurotmesis*: It is complete severance or internal physiologic disruption of all layers of the nerve. Wallerian degeneration of all axons occurs distal to the injury. There is a total permanent conduction block of all impulses (paralysis, anesthesia). The discontinuity gap between proximal and distal nerve stumps becomes filled up with scar tissue and proximal axonal sprouts are prevented from recannulating distal endoneurial tubules. No recovery is expected without surgical intervention.

Tinel's Sign

It was used earlier as an indication of the start of nerve regeneration. It is elicited by percussion over the divided nerve, which results in a tingling sensation in the part supplied by the peripheral section.

Now *electroneurography diagnostic studies* are carried out serially for evidence of reinnervation.

Sunderland's classification is based on detailed description of pathophysiology and anatomy of the injured nerve. It also incorporates the features of Seddon's scheme that includes the amount of nerve tissue damaged and tissue still intact.

1. *A neuropraxia (Seddon)/First degree lesion (Sunderland) (Fig. 45.3A)*: It is characterized by a conduction block, the rapid and virtually complete return of sensation or function and no degeneration of axon. There are three types of first degree nerve injuries based on the proposed mechanism of conduction block.

   a. *$1°$ type I injury*: It may be the result of nerve trunk manipulation, mild traction or mild compression, such as during sagittal split ramus osteotomy, inferior alveolar nerve repositioning or lingual nerve manipulation during excision of

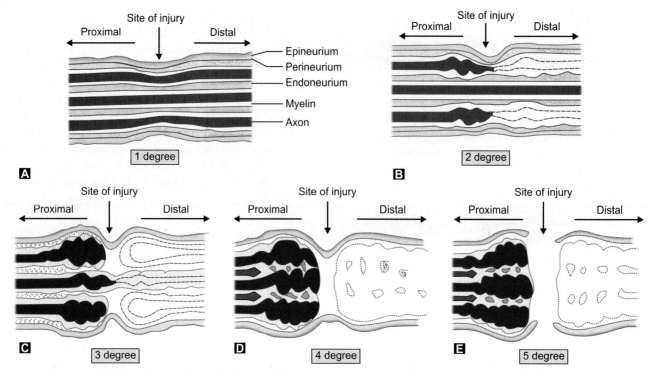

Figs 45.3A to E: (A) Neuropraxia—first degree lesion, (B) Axonotmesis—second degree lesion,
(C) Axonotmesis—third degree lesion, (D) Axonotmesis—fourth degree lesion, (E) Neurotmesis—fifth degree lesion

sublingual or submandibular salivary gland. The mechanism of conduction block is presumed to be anoxia from interruption of the segmental or epineurial blood vessels, but there is no axonal degeneration or demyelination. There is a rapid return of normal sensation and function within 24 hours following the restoration of circulation.

b. *1° type II injury*: It may be caused by moderate manipulation, traction or compression of a nerve. Trauma of sufficient magnitude to injure the endoneurial capillaries cause intrafasicular edema and results in a conduction block. Normal sensation or function returns within 1 to 2 days following the resolution of intrafasicular edema, generally 1 week following nerve injury.

c. *1° type III injury*: It results from severe nerve manipulation, traction or compression pressure on the nerve, which may result in segmental demyelination or mechanical disruption of the myelin sheath. Sensory and functional recovery are complete within 1 to 2 months, far earlier than can be explained by axonal regeneration. The psychophysical response to this type of injury is paresthesia. Surgery is not indicated for first degree nerve injuries.

2. a. *Axonotmesis (Seddon)/2° Sunderland nerve injury*: It is characterized by axonal injury with subsequent degeneration and regeneration. Traction, compression are the usual mechanism of this type of nerve injury and may cause severe ischemia, intrafascicular edema or demyelination. Even though the axons are damaged, there is no disruption of the endoneurial sheath, perineurium or epineurium. Within 2 to 4 months following injury, there are signs of sensation or function, which continue to improve over the next 8 to 10 months. The psychophysical response to an axonotmesis or 2° injury is an initial anesthesia and Tinel's sign followed by a paresthesia as recovery begins. Complete recovery may take as long as 12 months. Unless there is an extraneurial irritant inhibiting complete recovery, microreconstructive surgery is not indicated for 2° nerve injuries (Fig. 45.3B).

b. *Axonotmesis (Seddon)/3° Sunderland nerve injury*: The etiology of a 3° nerve injury is typically traction or compression. Not only is the axon damaged, but the endoneurial sheath is breached resulting in intrafascicular disorganization, while the perineurium and epineurium remain intact. The first signs of sensation or function are evident within 2 to 5 months and may take another 10 months or so (Fig. 45.3C).

Recovery is never complete. There is cross shunting of axons as they enter the distal endoneurial tubes and there is inaccurate localization of cutaneous stimuli. Endoneurial fibrosis may prevent the regeneration of axons to their original targets resulting in an intrafascicular neuroma.

c. *Axonotmesis (Seddon)/4°Sunderland nerve injury*: The etiology of a 4° nerve injury may include traction, compression, injection injury and chemical injury. The injection of chemical agents into the nerve trunk may cause irreversible damage to the axons and connective tissue components of the nerve trunk. 4° nerve injuries are characterized by disruption of the axon, endoneurium and perineurium with preservation of the continuity of the epineurium, resulting in severe fascicular disorganization. There is poor prognosis for recovery and a high probability of development of a central neuroma incontinuity (Fig. 45.3D).

3. *Neurotmesis (Seddon) or 5° Sunderland nerve injury*: It is characterized by severe disruption of connective tissue components of the nerve trunks with compromised sensory and functional recovery. There is considerable amount of tissue loss also. The mechanisms of this injury include laceration, avulsion and chemical injury. There is damage to all components of the nerve trunk: axon, endoneurium, perineurium and epineurium (Fig. 45.3E).

Useful sensory or functional recovery is unlikely and the development of extensive fibrosis and amputation (stump) neuroma is highly likely. The psychophysical response to this group of nerve injuries is an immediate anesthesia. This may be followed by a Tinel's sign and paresthesia or possibly neuropathic responses like allodynia, hyperesthesia, hyperalgesia or sympathetic mediated pain, which may develop into a chronic pain state (Figs 45.4A to E).

The indications for microreconstructive surgery are strongest for neurotmesis or 5° nerve injuries, since the prognosis for useful recovery is poor and the probability of getting symptomatic neuromas are high.

Not all nerve fibers have the same susceptibility to compression injuries and ischemia. Nerve fi-

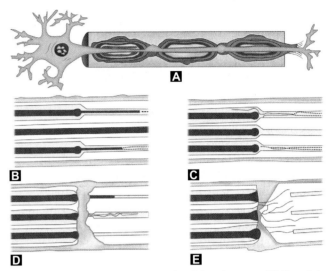

Figs 45.4A to E: Recovery group of peripheral nerves: (A) Complete recovery, (B) Satisfactory recovery, (C) Incomplete recovery, (D) Weak recovery, (E) No recovery

bers responsible for mechanoception (touch) are more susceptible to compression and ischemia than the A-δ and C fibers. Following a mild to moderate compression injury, it is quite possible to have a deficit in mechanoception (light touch and moving touch), but intact nociception (pin prick) and thermal discrimination.

Neuritis

Neuritis designates an inflammation, a disease of a nerve due to variety of conditions like traumatic neuritis, if the nerve is torn, pinched or lacerated and especially if the injury is associated with infection. Inflammation of the nerve also can be caused due to an infectious process-osteomyelitis, etc. Neuritis also occurs in herpes zoster. Toxic neuritis may be seen in arsenic, lead, mercury and alcohol poisoning and in vitamin deficiencies.

Clinical symptoms: There is deep seated pain, diffuse in character and relatively continuous, varying in intensity and functional loss is seen, if a motor nerve is involved. The area supplied by sensory nerves becomes hyperesthetic, unless the affected branch passes through a bony canal causing compression of the nerve due to edema, when hypoesthesia or anesthesia results. The pain or dysfunction may last for several weeks and is treated symptomatically by means of analgesics, narcotics, physiotherapy and vitamin B_1, B_6, B_{12} therapy. Hot, moist towels, heated sand bags and more modern electric pads can be used. Infrared lamp also can be used.

Neuropathic events following nerve injury: There are four basic neuropathic events that can occur:
1. Collateral macrosprouting.
2. Peripheral neuroma.
3. Cervical sympathetic pathosis.
4. Central pathosis.

These neuropathic events may be manifested clinically as anesthesia dolorosa, causalgia or sympathetic mediated pain, allodynia and hyperpathia.

Collateral macrosprouting from the injured or more commonly from adjacent uninjured nerves will produce a dysesthetic patterns due to neuroma like collaterals involving the injured zone.

Neuromas

Neuromas are characterized by disorganized microsprouting and formation of a disorganized mass of collagen and randomly oriented small neural fascicles. Peripheral neuromas may be classified as amputation/stump, central, eccentric:
a. *Amputation/stump neuromas:* It is a knobby, disorganized mass of axons and collagen associated with the proximal nerve stump and completely separated from the distal nerve stump. It is the result of 5° injury.
b. *The central neuroma:* It is a neuroma in continuity. It is a result of 4° injury or 5° injury, in which the continuity between the proximal and distal stump is established and there is no breach of the epineurium. It is a fusiform expansion or fibrotic narrowing of the nerve with varying degrees of fascicular disruption and disorganization.
c. *Eccentric neuromas:* Two types of neuromas of inferior alveolar nerves are seen.
  i. *Lateral exophytic:* Outgrowth of axons and collagen forming a terminal knoblike structure on an intact nerve. Only a few superficial fascicles are disrupted owing to incomplete transection of the nerve or form a poor coaptation of distal and proximal nerve stumps. There is a recognizable breach of epineurium at the site of lateral exophytic neuroma.
  ii. *Stellate neuroma:* It has two or more branches at the site of injury ending in adjacent soft tissue or mucosa. The epineurium is intact. Eighty percent of painful neuromas are refractory to any treatment.

▌ EVALUATION

1. First step is to ascertain the patient's main complaint—regarding loss of sensation, pain, abnormal sensation or functional impairment.
2. Patient's history:
   a. Trauma or surgical procedure associated with injury.
   b. The date of the incident.
   c. The progress of symptoms or functional complaints.
   d. Progress of recovery—return of sensation within the first 4 weeks—excellent prognosis and indicates neuropraxia. Later onset of sensation (1 to 3 months) is usually associated with axanotmesis. Total lack of recovery for 12 weeks or longer indicates neurotmesis and a poor prognosis for significant spontaneous recovery.
3. Clinical neurosensory examination of the trigeminal nerve consists of four tests (Figs 45.5 and 45.6)
   a. Static light touch
   b. Brush directional discrimination
   c. Two point discrimination
   d. Pin pressure nociceptive discrimination.

The first step is to map the area of sensory disturbance (Fig. 45.5). This is done by brushing the skin with a camel hair brush from an unaffected region of the face toward the affected area. The patient is instructed to raise his or her hand, when the brush can no longer be detected or the sensation of the brush changes significantly. The area of transition is marked on the skin using an eyebrow pencil and divided into grids to allow topographic recording of the test results. Next, a dot is marked in the center of each grid to aid in the assessment of localization of stimuli.
a. *Static light touch detection:* The test is performed using the Semmes-Weinstein filaments, which are nylon filaments of identical lengths, but variable diameter mounted in plastic handles.

The stiffness of each filament is calculated and calibrated by the manufacturer, so a known force can be applied to the skin.

The patient is instructed to close the eyes and to say 'touch', whenever a light touch on the face is felt and asked to point the exact spot where the touch was felt. The filament is vertically oriented and placed on the skin and in 1 to 1.5 seconds continue the descent until the filament is bowed but the side is not in contact with the skin. Continue pressure without movement for 1 second and in 1 to 1.5 seconds slowly raise the filament. The patient should be questioned as to perception of the stimulus relative to the unaffected side.

b. *Brush directional discrimination:* With the patients eyes closed, a (00) camel hair brush is gently stroked over a 1 cm. area of skin at a constant rate. The patient is asked if any sensation is detected and which direction the brush moved. The correct number of responses for total number of trends is recorded.

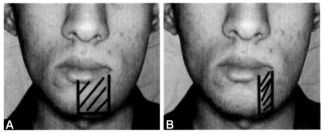

Figs 45.5A and B: Mapping of the areas of sensory disturbance: (A) Area of total anesthesia in a patient one week after bilateral sagittal split ramus osteotomy, (B) Same patient after 8 weeks. Note the decrease in the area of altered sensation

c. *Two point discrimination:* It is measured with any instrument which allows the distance between the points to be altered. Two point anesthesiometer is used. A sharp and blunt point is used.

d. *Pin pressure nociception:* A pressure algesimeter is used, made from a number 4 tailor's needle and an orthodontic strain gauge (15-150 g). The force is gradually increased on the affected area, until the sharpness of pain is identical to that of unaffected area is tested. If there is no response at 100 g of pin pressure, then the area is considered as anesthesia.

Thermal discrimination is assessed with a cotton swab saturated with ethyl chloride spray and immediately applied to the skin.

Photographs or diagrams of the affected area while testing are helpful in documentation and for comparison with results of subsequent testing. Local anesthetic nerve blocks are indicated in evaluating painful nerve injuries. Failure to relieve pain in the presence of effective nerve block suggests a central sympathetic or psychological rather than peripheral cause of dysesthesia.

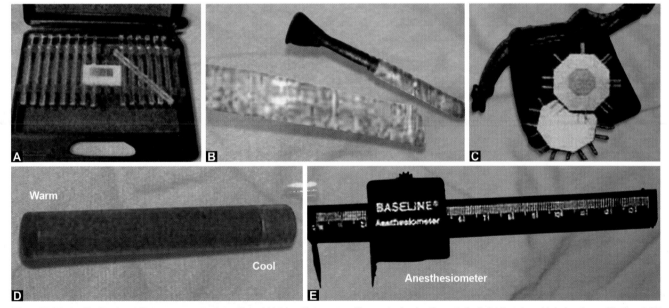

Figs 45.6A to E: Devices for neurosensory testing: (A) Von Frey monofilaments for testing static light touch, which begins with the 1.65 monofilament (B) Ultra soft brush for light touch testing brush directional stroke (C) Two points discriminator—The instrument is the two point anesthesiometer. It is capable of applying a standardized amount of pressure at bending of approximately 3.6 gm. This device consists of two parallel von Frey monofilaments attached to an acrylic bar at specific millimeter distances from each other 8 mm, 10 mm, 12 mm anesthesiometer can be selected, which is applied perpendicular to the skin surface, with both the filaments touching simultaneously until they bend. A normal response is considered 2 of 3 correct responses of feeling two points. (D) Thermal discrimination—the device selected is a cotton tipped applicator saturated with ethyl chloride. The applicator applied rapidly, lightly to each facial zone. This is randomly repeated 3 times using ethyl chloride or placebo. A normal response is considered 2 of the 3 correct answers of a cool/normal/or not cold feeling, (E) Anesthesiometer

■ MANAGEMENT

Nerve regeneration in bony canals frequently occurs without surgical aid because the canal acts as a guide to growth and union.

But, if the bony canal is obstructed by displaced bone or a fragment of a tooth or soft tissue/muscle interposition, then the nerve regeneration is not possible without surgical intervention.

   i. Neurorrhaphy should not be performed until infection has subsided.

  ii. All pathologic conditions of the nerve ends must be resected (neuromas)

 iii. The nerve must be properly coapted.

Indications for microneurosurgery:
1. Observed nerve severance.
2. Total anesthesia beyond 3 months.
3. Dysesthesia beyond 4 months.
4. Severe hypoesthesia without improvement beyond 4 months.

Contraindications for microneurosurgery:
1. Central neuropathic pain.
2. Dysesthesia not abolished by LA nerve block.
3. Improving sensation.
4. Sensory deficit acceptable to the patient.
5. Metabolic neuropathy.
6. Medially compromised patient.
7. Excessive delay after injury.

Principles of repair of injuries of the peripheral branches of the trigeminal nerve (microneurosurgery):

    i. Controlled general anesthesia.

   ii. Visualization.

  iii. Magnification of the surgical field.

  iv. Good hemostasis.

   v. Removal of pathologic tissue or foreign material.

  vi. Proper alignment.

 vii. Coaptation of proximal and distal nerve stumps.

viii. Suturing without tension.

Surgical Approach

- The inferior alveolar nerve is exposed by either a transoral or a submandibular approach depending on the location and circumstances (intentional or unintentional) of the injury and the preference of the surgeon.

- The mental nerve is approached by a buccal sulcus incision

- The lingual nerve is operated through an incision around the lingual aspects of the premolar and molars that extends posteriorly along the superior border of the ascending mandibular ramus.

- The infraorbital nerve is visualized through intraoral maxillary labiobuccal vestibular approach or extraoral subciliary, transconjunctival incisions.

- Magnification of the nerve is provided by surgical loops and operating microscope.

- The nerve is exposed, impinging scar tissue, bone or foreign material is removed, (external decompression)

- The epineurium may be opened and inter fascicular scarring relieved (Internal neurolysis)

- Internal inspection of the nerve is also necessary to detect neuromas or discontinuity of individual fascicles (Fig. 45.7)

- When neuromas are excised, the existing pathology or its removal may create a discontinuity defect.

- The proximal and distal nerve ends are assessed and serial 1 mm sections are removed if indicated until viable fascicles are visualized or identified on frozen sections.

- The nerve stumps are then fully mobilized and advanced to close the gap (Pre existing gaps of

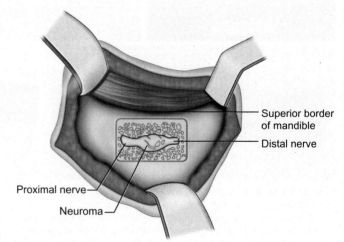

Fig. 45.7: Extraoral Risdon's incision to expose the inferior alveolar nerve. Window is created by removing the buccal cortical bony plate. Inspection of the nerve to detect neuroma is done

1 to 1.5 cm can be closed in the lingual nerve, but not possible in the infraorbital, mental or inferior alveolar nerves) (Fig. 45.8)

- The coapted nerve ends are secured with tension free sutures (neurorraphy) of fine 10-0 nonreactive material.
- The sutures are generally placed through the epineurium only. In pure sensory nerves polyfascicular, perineural suturing provides no special advantage.
- In case of wider gap, an autogenous nerve graft is interposed between the nerve stumps to eliminate tension and facilitate healing potential and regeneration equal to that of a tension free neurorrhaphy (Fig. 45.9)

- The great auricular (neck) and sural (lower extremity) nerves are common donors. The medial antebrachial cutaneous nerve (forearm) is also advocated.

Planned repositioning of the inferior alveolar or mental nerves is helpful in preventing injury, when surgeries like dental implant placement, screw fixation, alloplastic augmentations are to be carried out.

Short span (1 to 3 cm) nerve gaps may be repaired without autogenous nerve grafting by the technique called 'guided nerve regene-ration'. Axonal growth is directed across the discontinuity by a tube made of alloplastic materials (Polytetrafluoroethylene, polyglycolic acid, collagen with laminin gel) or autogenous tissue like vein graft which prevents in growth of the scar tissue (Figs 45.10 and 45.11).

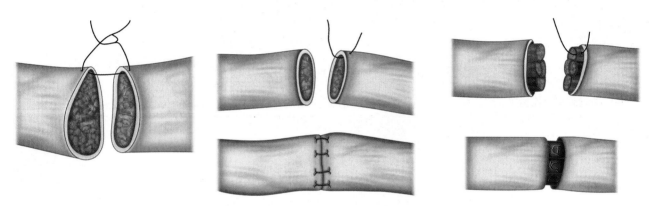

Fig. 45.8: Approximation of the nerve stumps and suturing

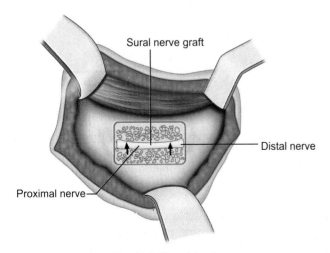

Fig. 45.9: Neurorrhaphy

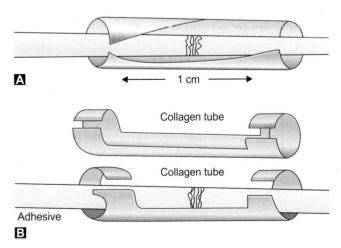

Figs 45.10A and B: (A) Silastic sleeve wrapped around the severed nerve for guided nerve regeneration, (B) Collagen tube or sheath is used along with collagen adhesive for guided nerve regeneration

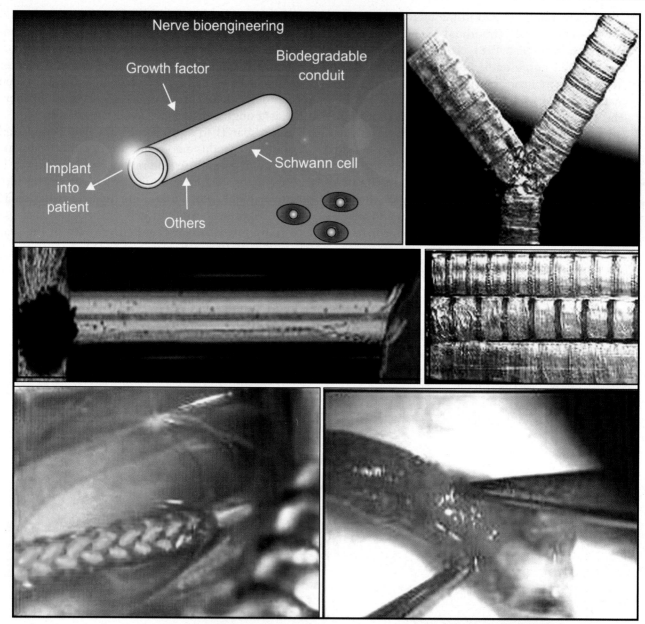

Fig. 45.11: Nerve guidance conduits (NGC) with jetted reinforcing rings

Nerve Regeneration: New Concept (Fig. 45.12)

If a traumatic injury takes place causing a loss of nerve tissue, the clinician has the option of taking nerve from another portion of the patient's body to replace the "more important" nerve deficit. While up to 80 percent successful, autologous nerve grafts create further trauma to the patient. Tissue engineers have recognized the need for an artificial means to facilitate nerve regeneration and have pursued bioabsorbable nerve guidance conduits as a solution. "Bioabsorbable nerve conduits" are designed to facilitate nerve regeneration by optimizing growth conditions at the wound site in a number of ways. When a peripheral nerve guidance conduit is surgically implanted, the proximal and distal nerve stumps are sutured into the conduit. This creates a physical guiding pathway for nerve growth, as well as a reservoir that sequesters important growth factors

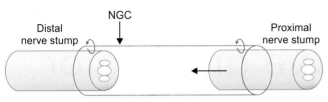

Fig. 45.12: Nerve regeneration—new concept

that further guide the sprouting daughter axons in the proximal nerve stump. Finally, by building the conduit with development of a tissue engineered device to aid nerve tissue regeneration involves synthesis of novel biodegradable polymers, controlled release of pharmaceutical agents from biodegradable polymers, and micropatterning polymer surfaces with extra-cellular matrix proteins or peptides, hence defining cell adhesion, spreading and axonal outgrowth.

Postoperative Management

The patient must be mentally prepared for anesthesia in the nerve distribution to be operated on:

- Standard protocols are followed regarding antibiotics, analgesics, fluids and discharge.
- The neck sutures are removed at 5 to 7 days post-surgery. Leg sutures are removed at 10 days post surgery.

Long Term Prognosis

Best prognosis for an anesthetic nerve operated on within 3 months. 75 to 80 percent of patients show significant subjective and objective return by 4 months and about 10 percent more by 6 months. The usual waiting period is of 6 months. Return of sensation in large defects may take 1 year.

46

Facial Nerve and Motor Disturbances of Face and Jaws

■ FACIAL NERVE

- It is the 7th cranial nerve
- It is the nerve of second branchial arch
- Facial nerve possesses a motor and a sensory root
- The sensory root is called the nerves intermedius
- It supplies the motor innervation to muscles of facial expressions and also for elevation of the hyoid bone (special visceral [branchial] efferent).
- The motor root supplies to the muscles of the face, scalp, and auricle, the buccinator, platysma, stapedius, stylohyoid and posterior belly of diagastric muscle.
- General visceral efferent (parasympathetic) fibers: It is believed to transmit the preganglionic parasympathetic (secretomotor) fibers to the submandibular and sublingual salivary glands, the lacrimal gland and glands of the nose, the palate and the pharynx.
- The sensory root conveys from the chorda tympani nerve, the fibers of taste for the anterior two-third of the tongue and from the palatine and greater petrosal nerves, the fibers of taste from the soft palate (Fig. 46.1).

Anatomical Course and Relationship (Fig. 46.2)

- The two roots of the facial nerve, i.e. a motor and a sensory root, both appear at the lateral part of the lower border of the pons, just medial to the 8th cranial (auditory) nerve. The motor part lies more medial and sensory root laterally, just adjacent to auditory nerve. From their attachment to the brain, the two roots of the facial nerve pass laterally and forward with the 8th cranial nerve to the opening of the internal auditory meatus.

- In the internal auditory meatus, the motor root lies in a groove on the upper and anterior surface of the auditory nerve, the sensory root being placed between them (there 7th and 8th nerves are accompanied by the labyrinthine vessels).

- At the bottom of the meatus, the two roots (sensory and motor) fuse to form a single trunk, which lies in the petrous temporal bone—the facial nerve enters the facial canal.

- Within the canal, the course of the nerve is divided into 3 parts by two bends (Fig. 46.3):
  a. The first part is directed laterally above the vestibule.
  b. The second part runs backwards in relation to the medial wall of the middle ear, just above the promontory. The first bend is sharp at the junction of the first and second part and is called the genu. It presents a reddish gangliform swelling—named *the ganglion of the facial nerve or geniculate ganglion.*
  c. The third part is directed vertically downwards behind the promontory. This second bend is gradual and lies between the promontory and the aditus to the mastoid antrum.

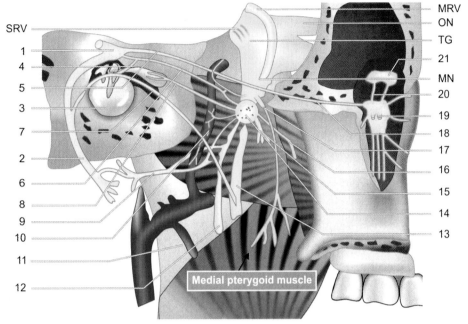

Fig. 46.1: (1) Geniculate ganglion of facial nerve, (2) Facial nerve, (3) Tympanic membrane, (4) Tympanic branch of IX, (5) Greater (major) petrosal nerve, (6) Lesser (minor) petrosal nerve, (7) Chorda tympani, (8) N of tensor tympani, (9) Auriculotemporal nerve, (10) Sympathetic plexus, (11) Inferior alveolar artery, (12) Inferior alveolar nerve, (13) Lingual nerve, (14) Otic ganglion, (15) Anterior division of mandibular nerve, (16) Nerve to tensor veli palatini, (17) Nerve to medial pterygoid muscle, (18) Nerve of pterygoid canal, (19) Pterygopalatine ganglion, (20) Ganglionic branches, (21) Maxillary nerve SRV—Sensory root of V nerve, MRV—Motor root of V nerve, TG—Trigeminal ganglion, ON—Ophthalmic nerve, MN—Mandibular nerve

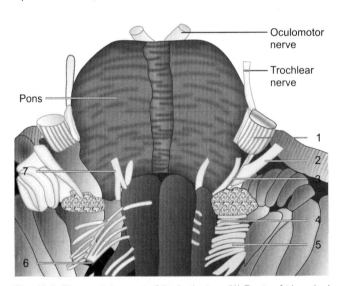

Fig. 46.2: The ventral aspect of the brainstem: (1) Roots of trigeminal nerve, (2) Auditory nerve, (3) Roots of facial nerve, (4) Glosso-pharyngeal nerve, (5) Rootlets of vagus nerve, (6) Hypoglossal nerve roots, (7) Abducent nerve

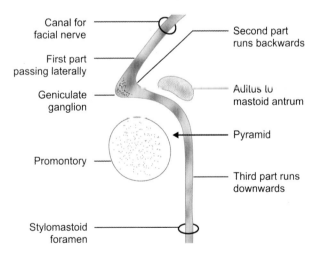

Fig. 46.3: Diagram to show intrapetrous part of the facial nerve

- The facial nerve leaves the skull by passing through the stylomastoid foramen
- As it emerges from the stylomastoid foramen, the facial nerve lies about 2 cm deep to the middle of the anterior border of the mastoid process

- *The extracranial course of the facial nerve.* It crosses the lateral side of the base of the styloid process. It enters the posteromedial surface of the parotid gland, runs forward through the gland crossing the retromandibular vein and the external carotid artery. Behind the neck of the mandible, it divides into its five terminal branches, which emerge along the anterior border of the parotid gland (Fig. 46.4).

Branches of Distribution of the Facial Nerve

A. Within the facial canal :
1. Greater petrosal nerve
2. The nerves to the stapedius
3. The chorda tympani

B. As it exits from the stylomastoid foramen :
1. Posterior auricular
2. Digastric, posterior belly
3. Stylohyoid

C. Terminal branches within the parotid gland- on the face (Fig. 46.5) :
1. Temporal
2. Zygomatic
3. Buccal
4. Mandibular
5. Cervical

D. Communicating branches with the adjacent cranial and spinal nerves—the motor nerves of first, second and third branchial arches communicate with each other. The facial nerve also communicates with the sensory nerves distributed over its motor territory.

Ganglia

There are three ganglia associated with the facial nerve:
1. *The geniculate ganglion:* It is a sensory ganglion and is located on the first bend of the facial nerve, in relation to the medial wall of the middle ear. The taste fibers present in the nerve are peripheral processes of pseudounipolar neurons present in the geniculate ganglion.

2. *Submandibular ganglion* (Fig. 46.6): It is a parasympathetic peripheral ganglion. It relays secretomotor fibers to the submandibular and sublingual glands. Functionally, it is connected to the facial nerve (chorda tympani), but topographically, it is related to the lingual nerve. The fusiform ganglion lies on the hyoglossus muscle just above the deep part of the submandibular salivary gland, suspended from the lingual nerve by two roots.

3. *The pterygopalatine ganglion (sphenopalatine ganglion):* It is the largest parasympathetic peripheral ganglion. It serves as a relay station for secretomotor fibers to the lacrimal gland and to the mucous glands of the nose, the paranasal sinuses, the palate and the pharynx. Topographically it is related to the

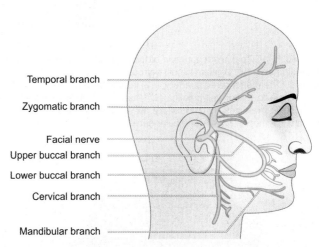

Fig. 46.5: Terminal branches of facial nerve within the parotid gland (on the face)

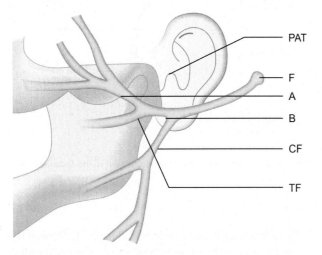

Fig. 46.4: Extracranial course of facial nerve. TF—Temporofacial division; CF—Cervicofacial division; PAT—Post aspect of tragus of the ear; A to PAT = 22.5 mm; B to PAT = 23 mm

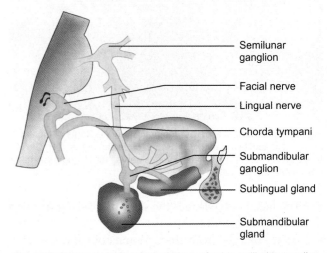

Fig. 46.6: Diagram: Anatomical relations of submandibular ganglion

maxillary nerve, but functionally it is connected to the facial nerve through its greater petrosal branch.

The flattened ganglion lies just below the maxillary nerve, in the pterygopalatine fossa, close to the spheno-palatine foramen and in front of the pterygoid canal. The branches which appear to arise from the sphenopalatine ganglion include:

1. Orbital branches.
2. The palatine branches: The greater palatine and lesser palatine nerves.
3. Nasal branches—long and short sphenopalatine nerves.
4. Pharyngeal branches.

Applied Anatomy

Facial palsy is commonly unilateral. It may be either:

1. Peripheral—from lesion of the facial nerve.
2. Nuclear—from destruction of the facial nucleus.
3. Central or cerebral or supranuclear—from injury to the brain to the fibers passing from the cortex through the internal capsule to the facial nucleus or from the injury to the face area of the motor cortex itself.

Motor Control

The motor centers controlling the muscles of the face are situated in the lowest portion of the motor area, whereas centers affecting the foot muscles are situated high on the brain. The control of skeletal muscles of the maxillofacial region originates in cerebral cortex. These nerve tracts controlling the extraocular, masticatory, lingual, palatal, pharyngeal and facial group of muscles are labelled as upper motor neurons. From the cerebral cortex, these neurons travel both in crossed and uncrossed tracts to terminate at various levels of the brainstem. From there the lower motor neurons send cranial nerves to the skeletal muscles. It is because of these tracts and their crossed and uncrossed courses the various types of palsies are seen.

It is important to know that the lower motor neurons of all cranial nerves except trochlear nerve do not cross the midline. Therefore, the lesions of the facial nerve lower motor neurons cause paralysis of all facial muscles on the same side, whereas the lesions of the upper motor neurons of the facial nerve cause palsy of the lower facial muscles only.

Supranuclear Facial Paralysis

Supranuclear facial paralysis which is usually a part of hemiplegia—is the lower part of the face that is chiefly affected, while the upper part remains unaffected, i.e. the frontalis and orbicularis oculi muscles escape.

Nuclear Paralysis

Nuclear lesions may vary in extent. Several types may be distinguished according to the point in its course at which the facial nerve is injured.

1. A lesion in the pons may involve the motor nucleus of the facial nerve along with the abducent nerve, as the fibers of the facial nerve loop around its nucleus in the pons.
2. When the nerve is paralyzed in the petrous temporal in addition to the paralysis of the motor nucleus, there is loss of taste in the anterior part of the tongue. The sense of hearing is affected from paralysis of the stapedius.
3. When the cause of the paralysis is fracture of the base of the skull, the auditory and petrosal nerves are usually involved.
4. The most common cause of facial palsy is injury at or after facial nerves exit from the stylomastoid foramen (Bell's palsy).

   In these cases:
   - The face looks asymmetrical even at rest and more so in the old patient than in the young.
   - The affected side of the face and the forehead remains motionless, when voluntary or emotional movement is attempted (Fig. 46.7).
   - The creases of the forehead are smoothened out
   - The eyes can be shut only by hand. Efforts to close the eye merely cause the eyeball to roll upwards until the cornea lies under the upper lid (Figs 46.8 and 46.9).
   - The tip of the nose is drawn over towards the unaffected side.
   - The nasolabial fold is partially obliterated on the affected side.
   - The ala nasi does not move properly on respiration.
   - The lips remain in contact on the paralyzed side, but cannot be pursed for whistling (Fig. 46.10).
   - When a smile is attempted, the angle of the mouth is drawn up on the unaffected side, but on the affected side the lips remain nearly closed and

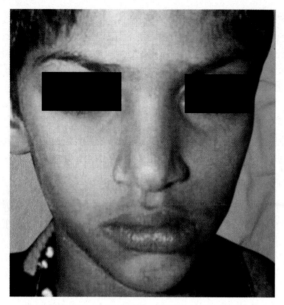

Fig. 46.7: Note the left side of the face is motionless

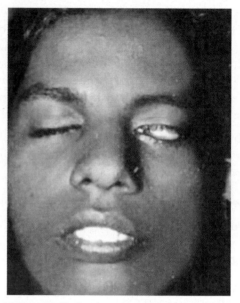

Fig. 46.8: Bell's palsy. Patient is making efforts to close the eyes. Note that on the left side, the eyeball is rolled up and there is inability to close the left eye

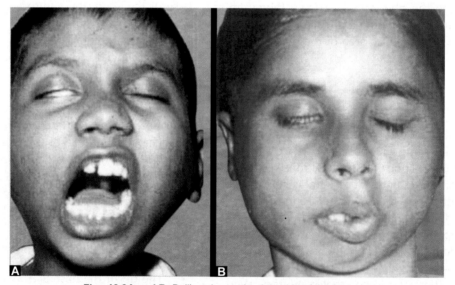

Figs 46.9A and B: Bell's palsy on the right side of the face

the mouth assumes a characteristic triangular form (Fig. 46.11).

- During mastication food accumulates in the cheek, from paralysis of the buccinator, and dribbles or is pushed out from in between the paralyzed lips.
- On protrusion, the tongue is thrust over towards the paralyzed side.

In *histrionic spasm* because of the dysfunction of the facial nerve, there is almost constant and uncontrollable twitching of some or all of the muscles of the face. This twitching is sometimes so severe as to cause great discomfort and annoyance and embarrassment to the patient and it may also interfere with sleep. Many a times a tonic contractions of orbicularis oculi muscles only will be seen and there will be constant blinking of the eye.

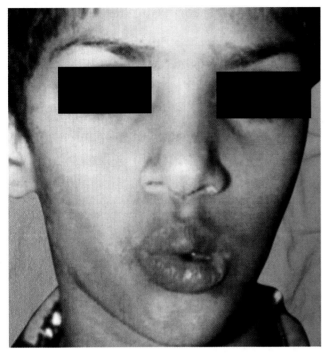

Fig. 46.10: Bell's palsy. Lips cannot be pursed to whistle

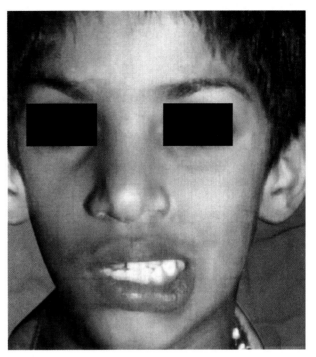

Fig. 46.11: Bell's palsy. Patient is attempting to smile. Note the drooping of the L side of lower lip

Melkersson-Rosenthal Syndrome (Orofacial Granulomatosis)

In this syndrome, there is a presence of nontender persistent swelling, which may involve one or both lips. Sometimes amber vesicles resembling lymphangiomas are found. In addition, to this there is facial paralysis and presence of fissured tongue.

Crocodile Tear Syndrome

Due to the injury to the facial nerve proximal to the geniculate ganglion, there may be a misdirection of the nerve fibers to the lacrimal gland instead of going to submandibular gland, through the greater petrosal nerve. As a result the patient lacrimates while eating. This paroxysmal lacrimation is termed as 'crocodile tear syndrome' and can be treated by dividing the greater petrosal nerve.

▌MOTOR DISTURBANCES OF FACE AND JAWS

Weakness of facial muscles to perform motor functions is called *paresis* (partial dysfunction).

Total flaccidity of facial muscles to perform motor functions is called *facial paralysis*.

- Paresis or paralysis of the facial muscles is a dreaded functional and esthetic complication
- Altered motor function of the lips, cheeks, forehead and eyelids produces significant problems in the affected individual.
  a. Loss of motor control of the lips and cheeks makes the drinking of fluids and mastication of food difficult or clumsy.
  b. There can be drooling of saliva outside the mouth.
  c. Loss of protection for cornea of the eye can lead to pain, infection and reduced visual acuity (corneal ulceration).
  d. Facial expression becomes asymmetric and is socially embarrassing—serious disturbance in social life.

Etiology Classification

The various etiological factors for facial paralysis may be broadly classified into three major groups:

1. *Intracranial (central cause)*
   i. Vascular abnormalities
   ii. CNS degenerative diseases
   iii. Tumors of the intracranial cavity
   iv. Trauma to the brain
   v. Congenital abnormalities and agenesis.

2. *Intratemporal*
    i.   Bacterial and viral infection
    ii. Cholesteatoma
    iii. Trauma
         a. Blunt temporal bone trauma
         b. Longitudinal and horizontal fractures of the temporal bone
         c. Gunshot wounds
    iv. Tumors invading the middle ear, mastoid and facial nerve
    v.   Iatrogenic causes.
3. *Extracranial*
    i.   Malignant tumors of the parotid gland
    ii. Trauma—lacerations, gunshot wounds
    iii. Iatrogenic causes
    iv. Primary tumors of the facial nerve
    v.   Malignant tumors of the ascending ramus of the mandible, pterygoid region and skin.

Extracranial iatrogenic causes, in which facial nerve is at risk in oral and maxillofacial surgical procedures:
    i.   Facial trauma—lacerations, fractures
    ii. Orthognathic surgery
    iii. TMJ arthrotomy, arthroscopy
    iv. Parotid gland surgery
    v.   Facial esthetic surgery.

Such injuries report range from 1 to 55 percent in TMJ surgeries. Most of the injuries, however, produce only temporary motor dysfunction that resolves within 6 months. The overall risk of permanent motor deficit from facial nerve injuries during surgical procedures is much less than 1 percent excluding those in which the nerve must be intentionally sacrificed as in malignancies.

The facial paralysis following injection of local anesthetic agent is occasionally seen after pterygomandibular block technique. If the needle is inserted too far backwards, causing deposition of local anesthetic solution in the parotid gland, disturbs the function of the peripheral branches of the facial nerve. In other instance, it is the result of a vascular reflex caused by the vasoconstrictor, which produces an ischemic paralysis in the region of the stylomastoid foramen. In the first instance the duration of the paralysis equals to that of the duration of the anesthesia, whereas in the latter, it may be much longer, depending on the degree of damage to the nerve.

Management

i.   Reassure the patient—explain that it resolves without residual effect.
ii. Eye patch to prevent corneal ulceration—topical ointment and eye closure with the cotton pad is used.

iii. Instruct to avoid wearing of contact lenses till the effect is worn off.
iv. Record the incidence on the patient's chart.
v.   Further care in future.

Rainer Schmelzeisen et al. reported following causes of facial nerve palsy in 1999:
1. *Congenital:*
    i.   Rare—due to congenital nuclear aplasia-Moebius' syndrome
    ii. Myotonic dystrophy
    iii. Melkersson-Rosenthal syndrome + lingua plicata
    iv. Congenital cholesteatoma/congenital facial nerve palsy.
2. *Neurologic:*
    i.   Myasthenia gravis
    ii. Multiple sclerosis
    iii. Guillain-Barré syndrome.
3. *Neoplastic:*
    i.   Facial nerve tumors—Schwannoma, neurofibroma, neurogenic sarcoma
    ii. Glomus tumors
    iii. Meningiomas, acaustic neuroma
    iv. Parotid tumors
    v.   Temporal bone/external auditory canal tumors (carcinomas).
4. *Infectious:*
    i.   Otitis media, mastoiditis
    ii. Bacterial causes (diphtheria, tuberculosis)
    iii. Viral causes (herpes zoster oticus, lyme disease, cat scratch disease, mumps, infectious mononucleosis).
5. *Other causes:*
    i.   Toxic
    ii. Metabolic
    iii. Idiopathic—Bell's palsy brainstem infarction.
6. *Iatrogenic:*
    i.   Parotidectomy
    ii. Rhytidectomy
    iii. Lateral skull base surgery
7. *Traumatic:*
    i.   Temporal bone fractures
    ii. Penetrating trauma (gunshot)
    iii. Facial lacerations
    iv. High altitude palsy.

Goals in the Treatment

1. To achieve normal appearance at rest.
2. Symmetry with voluntary motion.
3. Control of the ocular, oral and nasal sphincters.
4. Symmetry with involuntary emotion and controlled balance when expressing emotion.

5. No significant functional deficit secondary to the reconstructive surgery.

The fact remains that the totally paralyzed face can never be made normal, as some of the treatment methods for facial paralysis are controversial and still under evolution. The facial rehabilitation requires expertise of many disciplines—neurosurgeon, neurologist, ophthalmologist, otolaryngologist, plastic surgeon, oral and maxillofacial surgeon, physiotherapist, etc.

Evaluation of Facial Nerve Functions

The patient who exhibits facial nerve dysfunction requires prompt evaluation.

1. A careful history for the onset characteristics is important and duration of the condition and the degree of recovery.

    An acute onset on awakening in the morning is typical of Bell's palsy. Sudden onset may be also of infectious or inflammatory etiology (herpes zoster oticus, multiple sclerosis). Patients with neoplasm usually demonstrate progressive paresis over long period with initial mild symptoms. In trauma, there is definite history given by the patient. Delayed onset of facial palsy has better prognosis. Temporal bone neoplasms may show involvement of other cranial nerves—9th, 10th, 11th nerve, etc.

    A history of trauma, surgery or infection or rashes should be investigated and a full otologic history is obtained.

2. Examination of face at rest and in motion, noting muscular tone and symmetry and analyzing the various mimetic muscles. It is important to differentiate weakness (paresis) from total flaccidity (paralysis).
    i. The symmetry of the forehead wrinkling—patient is asked to raise the brows.
    ii. A functioning orbicularis oculi muscle allows for a complete closure of the eyelid and absence of visible upward rotation and exposure of sclera.
    iii. A forced smile allows the detection of asymmetries of the perioral muscles depending on the buccal and marginal mandibular branches. Patient is also asked to blow.
    iv. The side comparisons of the depth of the nasolabial fold and the symmetric contraction of the platysma muscle are important.
    v. Pure taste sensation is carried out using samples of sweat, bitter, acid and salty substances on the anterior tongue.
    vi. CT scan for skull base fracture, if history is obtained.
    vii. MRI to detect intracranial lesions, if suspected.
    viii. Electromyography (EMG), evoked electromyography as well as electroneurography are employed.
    ix. In case of acute injury—nerve excitability tests are used (NET)
    x. Magnetic transcranial and electrical stylomastoidal stimulation allows the differentiation of lesions and enables distinction to be made between central and peripheral facial nerve palsy.

Prognosis

Facial nerve injuries are also classified according to Seddon or Sunderland. *Neuropraxia* resolves promptly with return of facial mobility within few weeks. *Axonotmesis* exhibits prolonged weakness with gradual return of function after several months. Total and prolonged paralysis of affected facial musculature with little or no return of function is the usual fate of untreated *neurotmesis*.

House-Brackmann (1985) Classification

The House-Brackmann (1985) classification is used for the classification of facial palsy:

Grade I : Normal function without weakness.
Grade II : Mild dysfunction with slight facial asymmetry with a minor degree of synkinesis.
Grade III : Moderate dysfunctions—obvious, but not disfiguring, asymmetry with contracture and/or hemifacial spasm, but residual forehead movement.
Grade IV : Moderately severe dysfunction–obvious, disfiguring asymmetry with lack of forehead motion and incomplete eye closure.
Grade V : Severe dysfunction—asymmetry at rest and only slight facial movement.
Grade VI : Total paralysis—complete absence of tone or motion.

Prognosis is dependent on grade of severity.

Treatment

Open injuries of the facial nerve should be repaired surgically as soon as possible. Immediate primary repair at the time of intentional or unintentional transection (neurotmesis) gives the best result.

Delayed primary repair or early secondary repair is acceptable, when delay is necessary for certain reasons like contaminated wound, compromised medical status, extensive tissue destruction, etc.

Because of progressive distal nerve degeneration and muscle atrophy, 12 months is often considered as the limit for successful facial nerve repair.

Neurorrhaphy Procedures

i. Surgical repair of the transected facial nerve is done with direct end to end approximation and suturing (lacerations, iatrogenic injuries, benign conditions) (Figs 46.12A and B).
ii. If there is a gap between the proximal and distal part of the nerve with some part of the nerve loss—then autogenous nerve grafting is done (Figs 46.13A and B).
   a. The hypoglossal nerve has been a very effective autogenous graft for facial nerve reconstruction.
   b. The sural nerve is an alternative donor (Fig. 46.14).
   c. Branches from the cervical plexus, from the ipsilateral or contralateral side are also most frequently used for facial nerve autografting (Fig. 46.15).
   d. A great auricular nerve can be used.

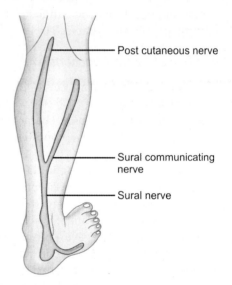

Fig. 46.14: For cross face nerve grafting a sural nerve graft of 30–40 cm length can be obtained

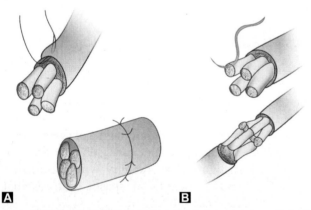

Figs 46.12A and B: Neurorrhaphy: (A) Epineural suture. Only the outer connective tissue sheath, the epineurium is sutured together with interrupted sutures, (B) Perineurium is sutured individually

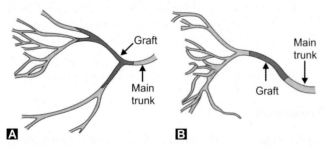

Figs 46.13A and B: Variations in nerve grafting: (A) Main trunk and three peripheral branches, (B) Single graft is interposed between the main trunk and the dominant peripheral division

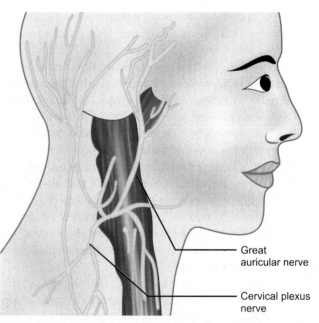

Fig. 46.15: A cervical plexus nerve graft from the ipsilateral side of the face can be obtained. Usually a 9–12 cm graft with a main trunk and 4–5 branches can be obtained with good physical match

Factors Influencing the Results of Extracranial Facial Nerve Repair

a. Level of the injury.
b. The prevailing biologic condition of the wound
c. The technique of repair.
d. The amount of tissue damage or loss, scar formation, vascular supply in the area of repair, patient's age and general health also have direct effect on the healing.
   • The graft must lie in a healthy, well vascularized area, free of scar tissue.
   • There should be no tension on the neuror-rhaphies.
   • Because of slight shrinkage of a graft, about 20 percent longer nerve than the actual defect is used.
   • When treating long standing facial paralysis, it is important to resect fibrotic tissue in addition to any neuroma of the proximal stump.
   • Placement of a minimum number of small diameter sutures are critical.

Technique of Nerve Grafting

Microsurgical techniques:

1. In primary or early secondary nerve reconstruction following injury, direct identification and preparation of the nerve stump is possible.
2. In secondary microsurgical nerve repair, exploration of the site of the lesion and the stumps of the facial nerve is done. The identification of the nerve at the stylomastoid foramen is the best choice.

At least 2 mm thick facial nerve stump is identified with the help of a nerve stimulator.

The main facial nerve and small distal branches are repaired by epineural sutures, which are technically easier and provide less surgical trauma to the inner nerve structures. Depending on the nerve diameter, two, four or six 10.0 nylon sutures are given.

End-to-end anastomosis can be only performed immediately following sharp injury of the facial nerve.

Reanimation technique: Using hypoglossal and/or contralateral facial nerve anastomosis or surgical redirection of the accessory nerve into the degenerate 7th nerve tissues has been effective in restoring some facial muscle function (Fig. 46.16).

Masking procedures (Repair of facial drooping due to facial paralysis): In long standing facial nerve palsy, the results of micronerve reconstruction are unfavorable due to the atrophy of the facial muscles.

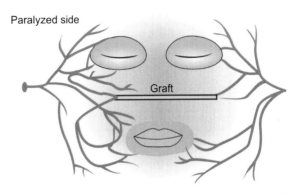

Paralyzed side

Fig. 46.16: Reanimation or cross face nerve grafting technique—Fisch technique—On the nonparalyzed side intact buccal branch can be connected to the paralyzed stem of the facial nerve with a sural nerve graft. The graft is passed over the upper lip

In these patients, regional muscle transpositions with temporal, masseter or platysma muscles may be considered (Figs 46.17 and 46.18).

These muscles are transposed and passed through the incisions in the lip/cheek groove and then sutured to the dermis. Alternately, the strips of fascia lata may be looped through the cheek and anchored to the temporal and parotid fascia at one end and to the angle of the mouth and lips at the other end.

Blair's 4 strips of fascia lata procedure—one strip to engage the upper lip, another the lower, a third is attached just external to the angle of the mouth and a fourth grips the tissue in the region of the nasolabial fold.

Surgical correction of the eyelids (Figs 46.19A to D): Medical treatment for protection of the cornea (ointment, taping) often fails and surgical procedures such as tarsorrhaphy, magnetic implants and springs may be associated with infections. Insertion of gold weight implants has been also tried.

Use of prosthesis to give support to the buccal sulcus is also tried. The rim of the prosthesis distends the lateral part of vestibule of mouth, chiefly in front of the zygomatic process. This bulk is attached to a denture. Such buccal support does a great deal to improve the appearance of the patient.

Postoperative care: Prevention of disturbance of the nerve repair area during recovery from anesthesia and in the first few postoperative days is important for successful nerve regeneration.

Avoidance of talking and intake of solid food in the first 48 hours followed by minimal facial movement for the next 5 days is emphasized.

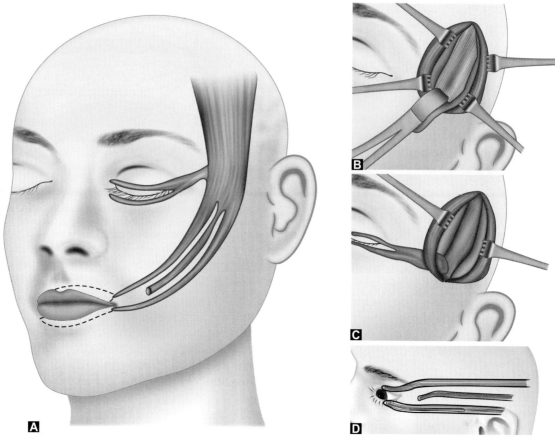

Figs 46.17A to D: Temporalis transposition—muscle slings are transposed to the upper and lower eyelids, upper and lower lips, nasolabial fold and commissure. Undermined tunneling is done to transfer the slings to the desired destination. The ends of the slings are then sutured

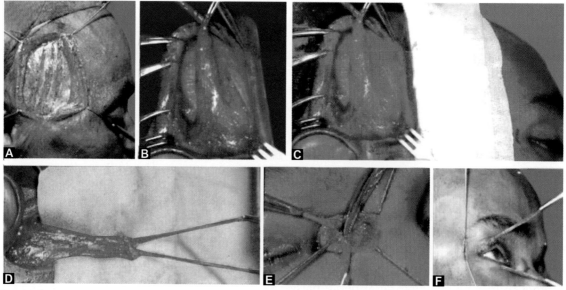

Figs 46.18A to F: Temporalis muscle transposition—intraoperative photographs: (A) Exposure of temporalis muscle through extended preauricular incision, (B and C) Elevation of temporalis muscle slings, (D) Temporalis muscle slings brought forwards through the tunnel to the commissure, (E) Tunneling near the outer canthus of the eye, (F) The slings are transposed to the upper and lower eyelids

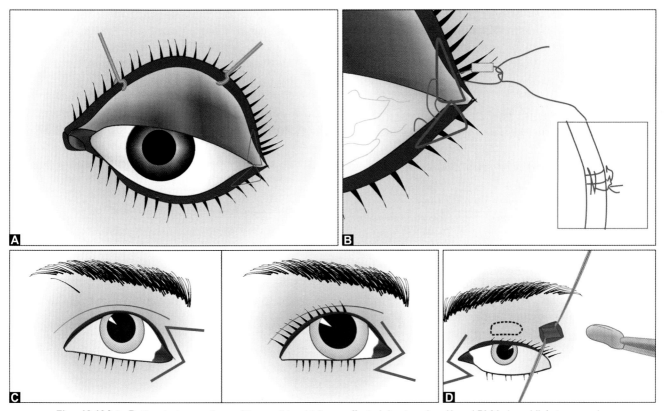

Figs 46.19A to D: Surgical corrections of the eyelids which are affected due to palsy: (A and B) Mc Laughlin's tarsorraphy (C) Other tarsorraphy incisions, (D) Insertion of gold weight implant in the upper eyelid

Supportive care: A tarsorrhaphy or eye patch and methylcellulose drops are provided, when eyelid closure is inadequate to protect the cornea from injury. Application of heat to the face, massage to facial muscles and attempted facial exercises are helpful to maintain the muscle tone and to prevent muscle atrophy.

Electrodiagnostic studies are carried out serially, until there is evidence of reinnervation. Once this has occurred, then intensive physical therapy is begun to stimulate and facilitate coordinated movements of the facial muscles. Patient should be followed up for minimum 3 years.

Bell's Palsy

Definition is defined as an idiopathic paresis or paralysis of the facial nerve of sudden onset (Unilateral lower motor neuron paralysis of sudden onset, not related to any other disease elsewhere in the body). The name was ascribed to Sir Charles Bell, who in 1821, demonstrated the separation of the motor and sensory innervation of the face.

Incidence—15 to 40 cases per 1 lac cases.

Sex predilection: Women are more affected than men. The disease is 3.3 times more common in pregnant women and is especially prevalent in the third trimester or within the first week of postpartum.

Age: It can occur at any age. But more seen in the middle-aged people. Thirty-one percent of patients with recurrent Bell's palsy are diabetics.

Side involvement: It can be equally seen involving the right or left nerves. It is unilateral but in 1 percent of cases bilateral involvement can be seen. Positive family history is reported in about 8 percent of patients.

Etiology: Although Bell's palsy by definition is idiopathic condition, there are abundant etiological theories put forward from abnormal immune response to reactivated herpes simplex virus in the geniculate ganglion.

Five hypotheses have been proposed regarding etiology, but many times a combination of factors may be in the play.

1. *Rheumatic hypothesis:* Berard (1936), proposed that rheumatic swelling may press the nerve against the walls of the fallopian canal (Obsolete theory).
2. *Cold hypothesis:* Proposed by Charles Bell. Exposure to extreme cold or cold draught can bring about the disorder.
3. *Ischemic hypothesis:* The ischemia from disturbed circulation in the vasoneurosum causes facial paralysis.

   Factors producing vasospasm: (i) cold, (ii) anoxia, (iii) CO_2 excess (iv) vasomotor instability (v) injury, (vi) toxic, allergic, hormonal influence.
4. *Immunological hypothesis:* This theory has gained acceptance in recent years. There is similarily between Bell's palsy and Guillian-Barre' syndrome, which is more widespread, but also a neurological condition. It is postulated that *in vivo* sensitization of lymphocytes to peripheral nerve myelin gives rise to a cell mediated autoimmune response in both conditions.
5. *Viral hypothesis:* The proponents believe that Bell's palsy is caused by subclinical herpes zoster or herpes simplex infection. Herpes simplex virus hypothesis has gained much attention, because of the high frequency of elevated viral antibody titers, as well as elevated levels of interferon in these patients. The combination of facial paralysis and herpes is known as the *Ramsay-Hunt syndrome*. Herpetic eruptions may occur on the skin, ear, tympanic membrane, palate, fauces, soft palate and tongue. The eighth nerve involvement will have vertigo, deafness, vomiting and tinnitus (Figs 46.20A and B).

Histologically patients with Bell's palsy have a thickened, edematous perineurium and associated normal blood vessels. There is a diffuse infiltrate of small round inflammatory cells between nerve bundles. Myelin sheaths undergo degeneration. These changes are seen throughout the bony course of the facial nerve.

Clinical Features

- There is sudden onset, usually patient gives history of occurrence after awakening early in the morning
- Unilateral involvement of the entire side of the face is seen
- Abrupt loss of muscular control on one side of the face
- Inability to smile, close the eye or wink or raise the eyebrow on the affected side
- Whistling is impossible
- The corner of the mouth droops, causing drooling of saliva
- In an attempt to close the eyelid, the eyeball rolls upward, so that the pupil is covered and only the white sclera is visible (*Bell's sign*).

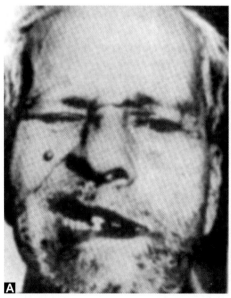 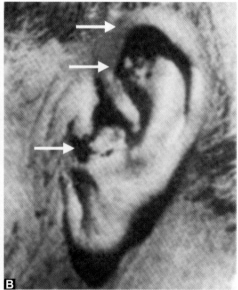

Figs 46.20A and B: Ramsay-Hunt syndrome: Ramsay-Hunt in 1907 described a clinical syndrome comprising of herpes zoster oticus, lower motor facial nerve paralysis with or without deafness, tinnitus and vertigo due to geniculate ganglionitis: (A) Patient with lower motor neuron facial palsy, (B) Vesicular eruptions over concha and external auditory meatus

- Inability to wrinkle the forehead or elevate the upper or lower lip
- The eye waters due to inability to close
- There is widening of the palpebral fissure, loss of blinking reflex
- There is obliteration of the nasolabial fold
- The face appears distorted and mask like appearance to the facial features
- Speech becomes slurred
- Occasionally there is loss or alteration of taste.

Prognosis: Initially unilateral facial weakness affecting all parts of the facial musculature is noticed. This gradually worsens over 2 to 3 days, reaching a maximum in about 2 weeks. Remission begins within three weeks of onset in 85 percent of cases with remainder taking as long as six months. Spontaneous recovery is known to occur in Bell's palsy.

Differential diagnosis should be made in the facial paralysis due to other etiological factors and idiopathic Bell's palsy.

Management: Physiotherapy—the effect of facial paralysis or Bell's palsy is wasting or muscle atrophy. Physiotherapy is therefore indicated to maintain the muscle tone and should be instituted as early as possible. It consists of electrical stimuli by galvanism, gentle massage and facial exercises.

Medication: If the patient is seen within 2 to 3 weeks of onset of symptoms—tab prednisolone in doses of 1 mg/kg/d for 10 to 14 days has been recommended with a gradual tapering.

Example: Dosage for a 60 kg person—prednisolone 10 mg tablets—3 tablets twice daily for 4 days, then 2 tablets twice daily for 4 days, then 1 tab twice daily for 4 days, then 1 tablet daily for 4 days and stop.

Vitamins B_1, B_6, B_{12} may be administered.

If the patient is seen after 3 to 4 weeks, then steroid therapy is of no use.

An audiogram should be performed, a CT or MRI and an EMG should be considered.

If incomplete eye closure is present, artificial lubrication, taping the eye or perhaps the placement of a spring, gold weight or tarsorrhaphy might prevent visual loss from exposure keratitis.

A baseline ophthalmologic examination is often helpful to determine further therapy.

Chronic sequelae—may be in the form of hyperkinesias or hypokinesia.

In hyperkinesias—offending muscle groups are denervated or botulinum toxin can be used.

Clostridium botulinum toxin (Botax) is a neurotoxin, that temporarily interferes with acetylcholine release from motor nerve end-plates, causing skeletal muscle paralysis. The effect lasts 4 to 6 months. Botulium toxin has been useful in the treatment of facial paralysis by weakening the contralateral side to allow centering of the mouth, more symmetry on smiling and treatment of hypertrophic platysmal bands.

Hypokinesia may require nerve transfers, muscle transfer or static slings.

If electroneurography reveals a greater than 90 percent loss of compound action potential within first 2 weeks following onset of paralysis, facial nerve decompression is recommended. After this period, surgery is not beneficial.

- *Nerve decompression*—can be carried out internally or externally.
- *Internal decompression*—the nerve is exposed in the fallopian canal and pressure in the canal is relieved by exposing the nerve and the epineural sheath is opened to visualize the nerve fibers and release adhesions or re-establish continuity.
- *External decompression*—is done by releasing of epineural sheath from surrounding scar tissue, bone or a foreign body.
- *Nerve anastomosis—reanimation*—anastomosis of the central end of hypoglossal or spinal accessory nerve with the distal end of the facial nerve is done.
- *Nerve grafting*—whenever there is evidence of neuroma or loss of portion of a nerve, nerve grafting can be considered.

Oral Malignancies

47

Oral Cancer

The oral cavity is the most predominant location in the head and neck region for primary malignant tumors. The oral cancers are the leading cause of morbidity and mortality amongst all cancers in India. The higher rates in India are attributed to the differences in lifestyle, habits, poverty, lack of education and less access to medical care. The malignant tumors of the oral cavity can arise from either mesenchymal or epithelial tissues.

Squamous cell carcinoma can arise from oral epithelium itself and from the terminal portions of the ducts of the salivary glands, minor and major. Salivary tumors arise from the minor salivary glands. Malignant melanoma arises from the melanocytes distributed in the basal layer of the oral epithelium. Sarcoma can arise from cartilage, bone, muscle, fibrous tissue and fat (osteosarcoma, chondroma, chondrosarcoma). Lymphoma also occurs in and around the mouth.

The term "Oral Cancer" is nearly synonymous with squamous cell carcinoma, because of its predominance seen in the oral cavity. In all primary oral malignant tumors, 92 percent are the squamous cell carcinomas.

INCIDENCE

Cancer of the oral cavity is a major public health problem with approximately 300,000 new cases reported annually worldwide. Two-thirds of these occur in developing countries, the majority within the Indian subcontinent, where these account for up to 20 percent of all cancers. The majority present with locally advanced disease (stage III and IV) with dismal 5-year survival rates of 20 to 50 percent. There are 145,000 deaths worldwide and 45,000 deaths in India per year. The oral cavity includes various subsites namely, the lip, buccal mucosa, alveolar bone (including upper and lower gums), hard palate, retromolar trigone, anterior two-thirds of the tongue and floor of the mouth. The involvement of each of these cancers has a different and distinct global incidence, patterns of spread and prognosis. However, they are broadly clubbed into two groups- tongue and floor of the mouth cancers and buccal mucosa, alveolus cancers. In the west, due to the high consumption of smoked tobacco and alcohol, tongue and floor of the mouth are the predominant oral cancers. In contrast, buccal mucosa, lower alveolus and retromolar trigone are the predominant sites in India, owing to the high consumption of chewed tobacco and areca nut chewing habit. (In South Asia, tobacco and areca nut chewing habit results in chronic lesions and the majority of the oral cancers arise from such lesions). These cancers are together called 'Gingivo-Buccal cancers' and have aptly been defined as the 'Indian oral cancer'. Discussion of the details of each individual oral cavity subsite is beyond the scope of this chapter. However, the broad principles governing the diagnosis and management of these patients are discussed below.

ANATOMICAL SUBSITES OF CANCER IN THE ORAL CAVITY

The oral cavity consists of the following subsites (Fig. 47.1):
- Lip mucosa
- Buccal mucosa
- Lower alveolar ridge
- Upper alveolar ridge
- Retromolar gingiva (trigone)
- Floor of the mouth
- Hard palate
- Anterior two-thirds of the tongue (oral tongue)

Lip Mucosa

It begins at the vermilion border of the lip and includes only that surface which comes in contact with the opposing lip.

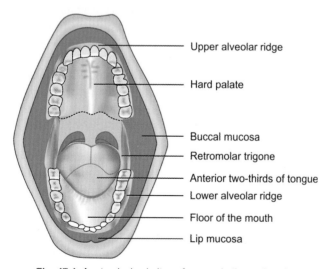

Fig. 47.1: Anatomical subsites of cancer in the oral cavity

Buccal Mucosa

This includes all the lining of the inner surface of the cheeks and the lips from the line of contact of the opposing lip to the line of attachment of the mucosa of the alveolar ridge (upper and lower) and pterygo-mandibular raphe.

Lower Alveolar Ridge

This refers to the mucosa overlying the alveolar process of the mandible, which extends from the line of attachment of the mucosa in the buccal gutter to the line of free mucosa of the floor of the mouth. Posteriorly, it extends to the ascending ramus of the mandible.

Upper Alveolar Ridge

This refers to the mucosa overlying the alveolar process of the maxilla, which extends from the line of attachment of the mucosa in the upper gingival gutter to the junction of the hard palate.

Retromolar Gingiva (Retromolar Trigone)

This is the attached mucosa overlying the ascending ramus of the mandible from the level of the posterior surface of the last molar tooth to the apex superiorly, adjacent to the tuberosity of the maxilla.

Floor of the Mouth

This is a semilunar space over the mylohyoid and hyoglossus muscles, extending from the inner surface of the lower alveolar ridge to the undersurface of the tongue. Its posterior boundary is the base of the anterior pillar of the tonsil.

Hard Palate

This is the semilunar area between the upper alveolar ridge and the mucous membrane covering the palatine process of the maxillary palatine bones.

Anterior Two-thirds of the Tongue

This is the freely mobile portion of the tongue that extends anteriorly from the line of the circumvallate papillae to the undersurface of the tongue at the junction with the floor of the mouth.

ETIOLOGY

Various etiological factors have been implicated in the causation of oral cancer. Case control and cohort studies have revealed that the *consumption of tobacco* and *alcohol* are the two most important of these risk factors.

Tobacco

Nitrosamines derived from nicotine are the main carcinogens implicated. It has been shown that those smoking 40 or more cigarettes/day are 5 to 7 times more at risk of developing cancer than nonsmokers.

The type of tobacco, curing methods (e.g. bidi) and method of smoking (e.g. reverse smoking) may influence risk of oral cancer. Paan chewing (betel quid) is an important factor in our nation. It consists of betel nut and lime wrapped in a betel leaf, tobacco, catechu and spices. This induces leukoplakia, which can undergo malignant transformation. Use of areca nut has been implicated in the causation of oral submucous fibrosis of the oral cavity.

Alcohol

This possibly acts as irritant or solvent which facilitates penetration of mucosa by other carcinogens. It may also suppress efficiency of DNA repair after exposure to nitrosamines.

Tobacco and Alcohol Synergism

The harmful effects of the two etiological agents are enhanced when they are used in combination.

Viruses

Oral human papilloma virus (HPV) infection has now been recognized to play a role in the pathogenesis of head and neck squamous cell carcinomas. The high risk prototypes HPV-16 and HPV-18 are found to be capable of transforming epithelial cells into cancer in the upper respiratory tract. Although HPV infection is a predominant factor in causation of cancers of the oropharynx, it has also been implicated as a cause of cancer in the oral cavity.

Poor Dental Hygiene, Constant Chronic Trauma to Mucosa Due to Dental Cause

Poor oral and dental hygiene, sharp teeth, ill fitting dentures, sharp crown and bridges, etc. are factors which may contribute to oral cancer.

The above mentioned factors probably result in cancer due to altered cell growth control processes, together with changes in interaction between the cell and it is surrounding, which give rise to invasion and metastasis. A well-described tumor progression cycle has been described for oral cancers implicating various genetic changes. However, in brief, the genes involved in carcinogenic process are oncogenes, tumor suppressor genes, DNA repair genes and those controlling apoptosis (programmed cell death). Imbalance in the interaction between these, can cause increased cell proliferation or reduced apoptosis. If DNA repair does not occur, cells accumulate abnormalities and cancer develops.

SPREAD OF SQUAMOUS CELL CARCINOMAS OF THE ORAL CAVITY

The major mechanisms of squamous cell carcinoma spread are by
A. Local infiltration.
  1. Invasion of local soft tissues.
  2. Invasion of perineural spaces.
  3. Invasion of vessels–(The internal jugular vein is often involved by direct spread from adjacent nodal metastasis).
  4. Invasion of bone.
B. Lymphatic spread—metastasis in regional lymph nodes (Fig. 47.2)

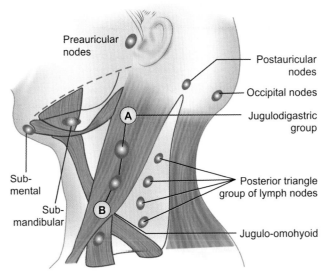

Fig. 47.2: Cervical lymphatic system. A to B level deep to sternocleidomastoid—deep jugular chain of nodes

Lindberg in 1972, described spread of tumor in lymphatics by tumor emboli from primary passing into deep lymphatics and then to regional nodes.

C. Blood borne metastasis. (Distant spread)

1. Cancers of the tongue, floor of the mouth and alveolar ridges metastasize primarily to the ipsilateral submandibular, jugulodigastric and middle deep cervical groups-the 'submaxillary', 'subdigastric and midjugular' groups of Lindberg.
2. Retromolar trigone lesions metastasize into submandibular, jugulodigastric and upper and middle deep cervical nodes.
3. Lip and tongue lesions metastasize to submental and submandibular nodes.
4. Lesions of tongue, lip, floor of the mouth, close to the midline metastasize to nodes bilaterally.
5. Once in deep jugular chain, tumor spreads from node to node in downward direction towards mediastinal nodes.

ORAL PRECANCER

There are well defined oral premalignant lesions/conditions that often precede oral cancer. These potentially malignant lesions and conditions are associated with mucosal atrophy and altered mucosal homeostasis. It is important to identify these lesions/conditions as the carcinogenesis process can be reversed at this stage, thus avoiding the morbidity and mortality associated with oral cancers.

Definitions (WHO, 1972)

Premalignant Lesion

A morphologically altered tissue, in which a cancer is more likely to occur than in its apparently normal counterpart, e.g. leukoplakia, erythroplakia, erythroleukoplakia, erosive lichen planus.

Precancerous Condition

A generalized state associated with a significantly increased risk of cancer, e.g. oral submucous fibrosis, sideropenic dysphagia, (mucosal atrophy associated with chronic iron deficiency anemia).

RISK OF MALIGNANT TRANSFORMATION OF ORAL PREMALIGNANT LESIONS

The overall incidence of progression of premalignant lesions of the oral cavity, to invasive squamous cell carcinoma has been quoted in the range of 2.7 to 17.5 percent.

Erythroplakia are more ominous than leukoplakia and have a higher risk of malignant transformation which may be as high as 50 percent. Also important is the site of involvement within the oral cavity. High-risk sites for change into dysplasia and Ca *in situ* as identified by Waldron and colleagues, are floor of mouth, tongue and lip leukoplakia.

Leukoplakia: A predominantly white lesion of the oral mucosa, which cannot be rubbed or dislodged or scraped off easily, and that cannot be characterized (clinically or histopathologically) as any other definable lesion (Fig. 47.3).

Erythroplakia: Red patches or plaques that cannot be characterized clinically or pathologically as any other definable lesion.

Erythroleukoplakia: A clinically mixed lesion which is a combination of the above two types of lesions (Figs 47.4A to C).

Classification of Leukoplakia

There are the number of classifications for oral leukoplakia, but the two most widely used are (Figs 47.5A to C):

1. ***Sugar and Banoczy***

   Leukoplakia simplex: White homogeneous keratinized lesion, slightly elevated.

   Leukoplakia verrucosa: White verrucous lesion with wrinkled surface.

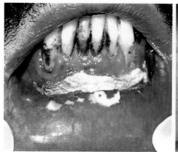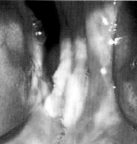

Fig. 47.3: Leukoplakia of the gingivobuccal sulcus

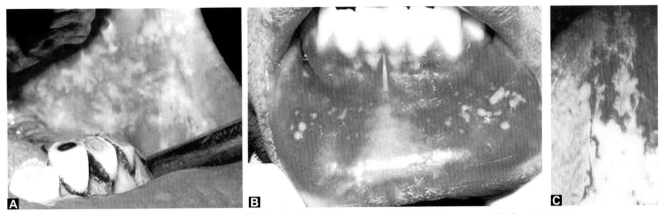

Figs 47.4A to C: Erythroleukoplakia: (A) On the cheek mucosa, (B) On the lip mucosa, (C) On the tongue

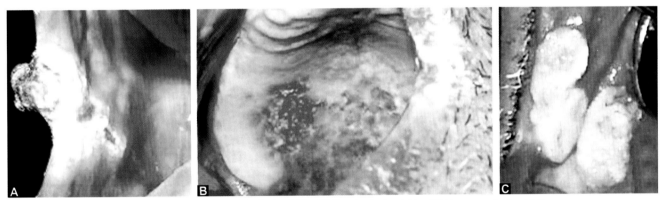

Figs 47.5A to C: (A) Nodular leukoplakia, (B) Erosive leukoplakia, (C) Verrucous leukoplakia

Leukoplakia erosive: White lesion with erythematous erosions, fissures.

? *Pindborg and associates*

Homogeneous: White patch with a variable appearance, smooth or wrinkled; smooth areas may have small cracks or fissures.

Speckled or nodular: Erythematous base with white patches or nodular excrescences.

Treatment of Leukoplakia

The treatment for oral leukoplakia is dictated by its risk to progress to malignancy.

Homogeneous leukoplakia, at sites other than the high risk sites, may be conservatively managed by close observation. Heterogeneous leukoplakia and leukoplakia at high risk sites and erythroleukoplakia needs to be treated. The general principles of management of leukoplakia are:

1. Removal of offending agent
   - Stop use of tobacco, alcohol, etc.
   - Attention to sharp teeth and ill fitting dentures
2. Chemoprevention.

3. Surgical management—heterogeneous leukoplakia, erythroplakia and lesions at high risk sites are usually excised surgically in view of their high propensity for malignant change. This can be accomplished either with conventional surgical methods (knife, electrocautery) or with the use of a carbon dioxide laser. If the laser is used, every effort should be made to excise rather than fulgurate the lesion as this provides tissue for histopathological examination, which may occasionally reveal foci of invasive squamous cancer.

Oral Submucous Fibrosis

Oral submucous fibrosis (OSMF), first described in the early 1950s, is a potentially malignant disease predominantly seen in people of Asian descent. It is a chronic progressive disorder and its clinical presentation depends on the stage of the disease at detection. The pathogenesis has been attributed primarily to the use of areca nut, the risk increasing with the duration and amount of its use. The majority of patients present with an intolerance to spicy food, rigidity of lip, tongue and

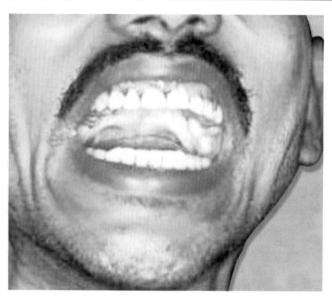

Fig. 47.6: Oral submucous fibrosis

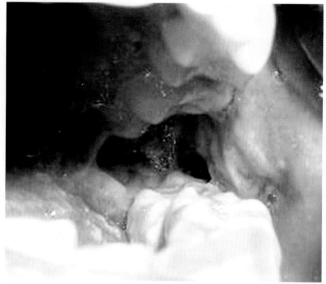

Fig. 47.7: Malignant lesion in retromolar region in OSMF patient

palate leading to varying degrees of limitation of mouth opening (trismus) (Fig. 47.6).

Trismus can Present in One of the Following Four Groups

Group I refers to the earliest stage with no limitation in mouth opening and interincisal distance greater than 35 mm.

Group II refers to patients with interincisal distances of 26 to 35 mm.

Group III patients are moderately advanced cases with interincisal distances of 15 to 25 mm.

For group IVA patients, trismus is more severe with interincisal distance of less than 15 mm. There is extensive fibrosis of all oral mucosa.

Group IVB is even more advanced with premalignant or malignant changes.

The hallmark of the disease is oral submucosal fibrosis that affects most parts of the oral cavity, pharynx and upper third of the esophagus.

Recent epidemiological data indicates that the number of cases of OSMF have risen rapidly in India. The reasons for the rapid increase in the incidence of this disease are, an upsurge in the popularity of commercially prepared areca nut preparations (pan masala) in India and an increased uptake of this habit by young people.

Malignant Transformation Rate of OSMF (Fig. 47.7)

This was found to be in the range of 7 to 13 percent. According to a long term follow up study, the transformation rate of 7.6 percent over a period of 17 years was reported. (OSMF is caused by areca nut chewing in genetically predisposed individuals. Malignant transformation is enhanced by traditional risk factors for oral cancer, but can occur in their absence).

Management of OSMF

Nonsurgical measures like local steroids, hyaluronidase injections, vitamin supplements have poor results. In the trismus group (groups III, IVA), surgical release of fibrous bands in the oral mucosa and temporalis muscle myotomy may be performed. However, surgical procedures only partially relieve the trismus and do not have an effect on the underlying pathology. Therefore, as in the management of leukoplakia, aggressive counseling needs to be done with regards the cessation of areca nut consumption.

Chemoprevention for Oral Premalignant Lesions (Table 47.1)

Chemoprevention has been defined as the administration of agents, either biologic or synthetic, to reverse or suppress premalignant changes.

Table 47.1: Limitations of chemoprevention
• Costly
• Side effects-dry skin, cheilitis (with retinoid use)
• Not available commercially (retinoids)
• Lesions recur on stoppage
• Exact combination, agent and duration of use not known

The most widely studied agents are retinoids, carotenoids, vitamin C, E, natural agents (green tea) and nonsteroidal anti-inflammatory agents. The retinoids are a group of naturally occurring synthetic vitamin A like compounds, which promote the resolution of cellular dysplasia and oncogenesis. Retinoids are used in the cis retinoic form. Beta-carotene is a provitamin A that is converted into the active form in the body and overcomes the limitations of retinoid use. In controlled clinical trials in patients with premalignant lesions, both beta-carotene and 13-cis-retinoic acid have shown regression of leukoplakia. However, upon cessation of therapy, lesions generally recur. Hence, long term preventive therapy is needed. This long term preventive therapy is not without drawbacks, due to the toxicity associated with retinoid administration and the high costs of such therapy.

Therefore, the routine use of chemopreventive agents is not advocated today in the treatment of premalignant lesions/condition. A large number of studies are now focusing on naturally occurring agents such as curcumin (turmeric/haldi), which overcome the limitations of retinoids and have shown great promise in laboratory and early human trials.

DIAGNOSIS AND STAGING OF ORAL CAVITY CANCER

Clinical Features (Fig. 47.8)

Cancer of the oral cavity can present in a variety of ways depending on the subsite involved. Classically they present either as a non healing ulcer, with varying degrees of pain and occasional episodes of bleeding from the lesion or an exophytic growth of duration may be several weeks to a few months before patient seeks treatment. Ulcerative lesions usually have an irregular edge and induration of the underlying soft tissues. Exophytic growth may present as a cauliflower like irregular growth or may be flat. Occasionally they may also present as a submucosal growth with surrounding induration. More advanced lesions can present with pain, bleeding or fixity to surrounding structures. Buccal mucosa cancers that involve the infratemporal fossa present with recent onset of trismus. This must be distinguished from long standing trismus, which is a sign of oral submucous fibrosis. Advanced tongue cancers present with hypoglossal palsy and restriction of mobility of tongue, progressive difficulty in mastication and speech, pooling of saliva, friability and surface bleeding. Lesions can also present with metastatic disease to the regional draining cervical nodes. It is important to remember that occasionally lesions of the alveolus in and around the non healing tooth extraction sockets can manifest with unexplained loosening of the involved teeth

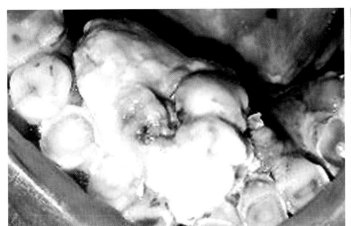 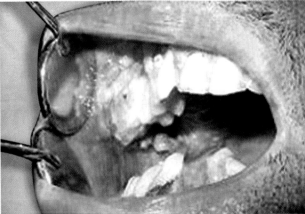

Fig. 47.8: Clinical intraoral pictures of oral cancer

The cancer may affect the nutritional status by preventing the alimentation. Functional impairment may be caused by the obstruction from a large mass or from other associated condition like trismus. Malnutrition results in impaired wound healing, reduced immunocompetence and decreased tolerance to chemotherapy, radiotherapy and surgery.

Biopsy

A biopsy is the minimum investigation required for diagnosis. Biopsy of the lesion should be in the form of a punch biopsy or an incisional biopsy, if the lesion is largely submucosal. The biopsy should not be taken from the edge of the lesion as this may be very painful. Avoid taking biopsy from obviously necrotic areas in the lesion. There is no role for scrape cytology in the diagnosis of squamous cell cancer of the oral cavity.

Imaging for Oral Cavity Cancers

Clinical examination is fairly accurate for evaluation of early oral cancers. However, with larger tumors, clinical examination alone is inadequate. Accurate assessment of the extent of these cancers requires proper imaging studies. Important treatment decisions are based upon the exact extent of spread of disease to areas such as the mandible, the floor of mouth, the infratemporal region, base of tongue, soft tissue, etc. When choosing the ideal imaging modality, our decision is guided by the clinical findings.

Imaging for Assessing Mandibular Involvement (Table 47.2)

The orthopantomogram can be used to identify gross involvement of bone; however it has its limitations. It cannot identify subtle erosions of mandible and is not reliable for midline lesions of the oral cavity. A comparison of the sensitivity and specificity of all other investigations, for imaging of the mandible, is outlined in the Table 47.3.

Table 47.2: Guidelines for the selection of imaging modality

a. Imaging to assess mandibular involvement—orthopanto-mogram or CT scan
b. Imaging to assess extent of soft tissue spread and recurrent tumors—MRI scan
c. Imaging for involvement of infratemporal fossa—CT scan
d. Imaging for tongue lesions—MRI scan

Table 47.3: Summary and comparison of the imaging techniques and clinical examination

Imaging technique	Number of reports	Specificity (mean)	Sensitivity (mean)
1. Clinical examination	9	61	82
2. Plain radiography	18	81	76
3. Bone scintigraphy	15	74	93
4. SPECT*	3	76	97
5. Computerized tomography	7	86	75
6. Dentascan	3	–	–
7. Magnetic resonance imaging	4	72	85

* Single photon emission computed tomography

As can be seen SPECT has the highest sensitivity in identifying bone involvement. However, this is an expensive investigation and is not readily available. A contrast enhanced CT scan using the puffed cheek technique, is the recommended investigation for identifying early mandibular invasion and involvement of bones of the paranasal sinuses.

Imaging to Assess the Extent of Soft Tissue Spread

A CT scan is the imaging modality of choice. Involvement of the infratemporal fossa must be closely evaluated, particularly, if the patient gives a history of recent onset of trismus. Involvement of the infratemporal fossa is a sign of relative inoperability as lesion clearance in this area is difficult (Fig. 47.9).

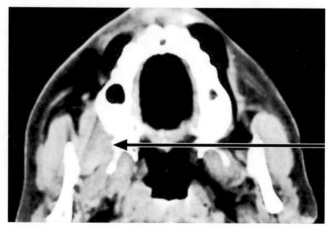

Fig. 47.9: CT scan showing involvement of the infratemporal fossa

FNAC of Neck Nodes

Fine needle aspiration cytology (FNAC) can be used to diagnose metastatic neck nodes to help in treatment planning. Open biopsies should never be performed as it violates the field and can cause seeding of cancer.

TNM Staging (Table 47.4)

T staging

Tx   Primary lesion cannot be assessed
T0   No evidence of primary lesion
Tis Carcinoma *in situ*
T1   Lesion 2 cm or less in the greatest diameter
T2   Lesion >2 cm but <4 cm in the greatest diameter
T3   Lesion >4 cm in the greatest diameter
T4   T4 lesions have been divided into

 T4 A—Lesion invades through cortical bone, into deep/extrinsic muscles of the tongue (genioglossus, hypoglossus, palatoglossus and styloglossus), maxillary sinus or skin of face
 T4 B—Lesion invades masticatory space, pterygoid plates, or skull base and/or encases internal carotid artery.

N Staging

Nx   Regional LN cannot be assessed
N0   No regional LN metastasis
N1   Metastasis to a single ipsilateral lymph node <3 cm in greatest dimension
N2 A Metastasis to a single ipsilateral node, >3 cm but not more than 6 cm in greatest dimension
N2 B Metastasis in multiple ipsilateral nodes none more than 6 cm in greatest dimension
N2 C Metastasis in bilateral or contralateral nodes, none more than 6 cm in greatest dimension
N3   Metastasis in a lymph node more than 6 cm in greatest dimension.

M stage

Mx   distant metastasis cannot be assessed
M0   no distant metastasis
M1   distant metastasis present.

■ MANAGEMENT

Management of oral cavity cancers presents unique problems to clinicians as treatment has a bearing on esthetics as well as it affects critical functions like mastication, swallowing and speech. Treatment of oral cancer requires a multimodal approach with a team comprising of oncosurgeons, radiotherapists, and medical oncologists. In addition to these, supportive specialities such as radiology, pathology, speech therapy, dental and physiotherapy play an equally important and critical role.

Treatment of oral cancer depends upon the stage of cancer at diagnosis. The broad guidelines are as follows:

Early stage oral cancer (Stage I and II) can be treated with single modality treatment. **Locally advanced and operable cancers** (Stage III and IVA) need to be treated with combined modality treatment.

Locally advanced, inoperable cancers or metastatic cancers (Stage IVB and IVC) are treated with palliative intent (Radiotherapy-RT or Chemotherapy-CT) or only symptomatic treatment if the patient's performance status is low.

Principles of Management of Early Stage Cancer

Oral cancer and its treatment often expose the patient to considerable physiologic and psychologic strain.

Early oral cavity cancer can be treated with surgery or radiotherapy or a combination of both. There is no difference in survival with either modality of treatment. However, even within early oral cancers, both modalities have their specific indications.

Advantages of Surgery

- Simple
- Fast

Table 47.4: Staging of oral cavity cancer

	N₀	N₁	N₂	N₃	
T₅	Stage 0				
T₁	Stage I				
T₂	Stage II	Stage III			
T₃			Stage IVA		MO
T₄				Stage IVB	
T₄					

Stage IVC   Any T any N N1

Stage IV has been divided into

Stage IVA operable cancer
Stage IVB inoperable cancer
Stage IVC metastatic cancer

- No significant cosmetic and functional defects
- Repeated procedures possible
- Cost effective.

Disadvantages of Radiotherapy

- Prolonged treatment
- Significant side effects like xerostomia, dental caries, osteoradionecrosis
- Can usually be given only once
- Not suitable for treatment, if lesion involves or is close to the bone

Keeping the above in mind, for early oral cavity lesions, surgery is the treatment of choice. Radiotherapy is reserved for patients who are not willing for surgery or when surgery will cause significant cosmetic or functional defects or if patients are unfit for anesthesia.

Radiotherapy in Early Oral Cavity Cancer

Radiotherapy can be given either as brachytherapy (see below) or as external beam radiotherapy. External beam radiotherapy is given with radiation sources external to the patient. Telecobalt machines emitting gamma rays or linear accelerators producing photons are commonly used.

Brachytherapy

In this form of radiotherapy, radiation is administered interstitially through catheters surgically placed across the lesion. Brachytherapy spares normal tissues such as bone, salivary glands and spinal cord. Lymph nodes are under dosed with brachytherapy alone and hence external beam radiotherapy is also used in addition in such cases. The ideal lesions suitable for brachytherapy should be less than 3 cm, superficially invasive and not close to the bone.

For interstitial implants alone or as a part of treatment, median local control rates for T1, T2 lesions of 86 and 80 percent, respectively, have been reported. These control rates are comparable to surgery for early oral cavity cancers.

Postoperative Radiation Therapy to the Neck is Indicated

1. Multiple positive lymph nodes in the neck.
2. Extracapsular extension by metastatic disease.
3. Perivascular or perineural invasion.
4. Gross residual disease following surgery.
5. Cranial nerve involvement or extension to the base of skull, tumor emboli in lymphatics, etc.

Surgical Technique for Resection of Early Oral Cancers

1. *Margins:* All lesions should be excised with a margin of at least one cm in all dimensions (mucosa and soft tissue) when feasible. Any margin less than 0.5 cm is a compromised margin.
2. *Modality used:* Excisions can be done using the cautery, laser (CO_2) or knife. The results are the same with any of the modality as far as cancer control is concerned. There have been some reports of better healing using lasers, but this has not been very well documented (Figs 47.10A and B).

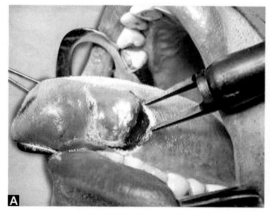 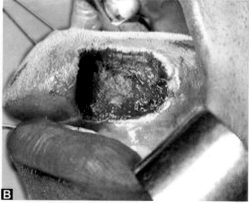

Figs 47.10A and B: (A) Lesion suited for laser excision, (B) Post laser excision minimal charring

Approaches to Oral Cavity

1. Peroral—restricted to small anteriorly placed lesions.
2. Lip split—to raise a cheek flap for posteriorly based gingivobuccal complex lesions and for performing marginal mandibulectomy.
3. Pull through approach—this approach is used for tongue and floor mouth lesions particularly when the posterior margin is an issue with peroral excision (Fig. 47.11).

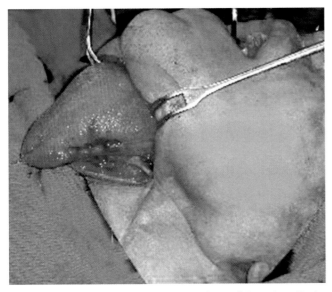

Fig. 47.11: Approach for tongue cancer via a pull through method

4. Mandibulotomy (median or paramedian)—for tongue and floor of mouth lesions close to the mandible to help achieve a lateral margin of clearance (Figs 47.12A and B).

Marginal Mandibulectomy

Marginal mandibulectomy involves the removal of the rim of the mandible and is done for lesions reaching close to the mandible, but not grossly involving it. It can be done for lesions superficially eroding the bone, but this should be done judiciously and in selected cases only. A margin of 0.5 to 1 cm should be achieved on the bone and a minimum of 1 cm of the mandible should be preserved to prevent postoperative fractures.

Types and Indications for Marginal Mandibulectomy

1. *Horizontal mandibulectomy/alveolectomy:* Patients with gingivobuccal cancer reaching close to the mandible, but not grossly involving the mandible.
2. *Lingual plate excision:* For lesions of the floor of mouth or tongue.
3. *Buccal plate excision:* For lesions of the gingivobuccal complex with minimal paramandibular spread.

Table 47.5: Contraindications for marginal mandibulectomy
• Edentulous mandible (as the height of an edentulous mandible is reduced)
• Post radiotherapy setting
• Gross paramandibular spread

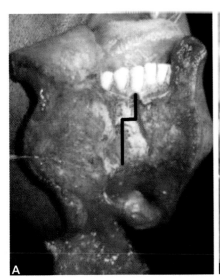
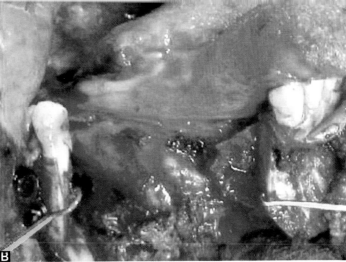

Figs 47.12A and B: (A) Paramedian mandibulotomy osteotomy cuts, (B) Apporoach via paramedian mandibulotomy demonstrating exposure

Principles of Management of Locally Advanced Oral Cavity Cancers

Locally advanced cancers (Stage III and Stage IV) require multimodality treatment. A flow chart showing the principles of management of these cancers is given in Flow chart 47.1 and Table 47.6.

Surgery for Locally Advanced Cancer

Composite resections are the surgical procedures performed for most patients with locally advanced oral cavity cancers. As in early oral cancers, all lesions should be excised with a margin of at least 1 cm in all dimensions. Adequate margin should be achieved on mucosa, soft tissue and bone. Any margin less than 0.5 cm is a compromised margin (Fig. 47.13).

Composite resections involve removal of,
- The entire lesion with involved areas like the mucosa, skin, and mandible.
- Removal of neck nodes
  These are usually done in continuity.

Types of Segmental Resections of the Mandible

- Hemimandibulectomy
- Segmental mandibulectomy
  – Posterior segmental mandibulectomy
  – Middle-third mandibulectomy

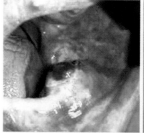
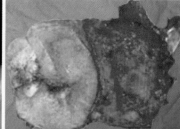
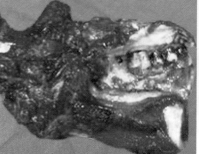
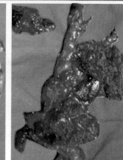

Fig. 47.13: Composite resection for oral cancer

Principles of Reconstruction (Table 47.7)

An attempt should be made to reconstruct all excised tissues with similar tissues. Mucosa, skin, soft tissue and bone should be reconstructed in all patients after composite resections. This will help to restore good function and cosmesis of the patient.

Mucosal Defects can be Delt with Following Modalities

- Leave raw areas, allow it to granulate on its own.
- Primary closure.
- Cover with split thickness skin graft (STSG).
- Microvascular reconstruction (Figs 47.14A to C).

Reconstruction of Mandibular Defects

Mandibular defects can be reconstructed using external material (plates, silastic implants, etc.), allografts (cadaveric bone) or autografts. Of these, the autografts

Flow chart 47.1: Principles of management of locally advanced oral cancer

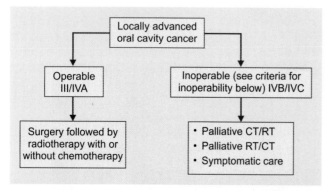

Table 47.6: Criteria suggesting inoperability

- Fixed neck nodal adenopathy
- Recent onset of trismus (gross infratemporal fossa invasion)
- Base skull involvement
- Extensive soft tissue involvement
- Distant metastasis

Table 47.7: Reconstruction after surgery for oral cavity cancers

Objectives
- Achieve primary healing
- Maintain oral competence
- Facilitate swallowing
- Prevent aspiration
- Preserve speech

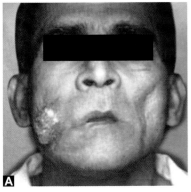 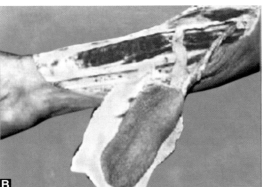 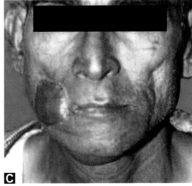

Figs 47.14A to C: Reconstruction of mucosa and skin after excision of a buccal mucosa cancer

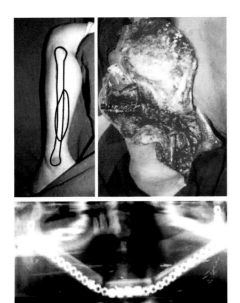

Fig. 47.15: Reconstruction using a free fibular osteocutaneous flap

are the preferred form of reconstruction using the microvascular free tissue transfer method.

Anterior mandibular defects should be reconstructed by free osteocutaneous flaps using microvascular anastomosis. The bone can be harvested from any one of the following areas of the body:

1. Fibular osteocutaneous flap (preferred, because of long bone length, easy contouring and dual blood supply), (Fig. 47.15)
2. Radial osteocutaneous flap
3. Scapular osteocutaneous flap
4. Iliac osteocutaneous flap

Of these flaps, the fibular osteocutaneous flap is the workhorse and the most preferred flap (>90% cases).

This is because it has the advantages of being reliable, gives a long bone length (up to 25 cm), has minimal or no donor site morbidity and provides for easy contouring due to its segmental blood supply.

Lateral mandibular defects usually do not require bone replacement and may be adequately reconstructed with soft tissue replacement using myocutaneous flaps. e.g. pectoralis major myocutaneous flap. This should be complemented by proper use of guide bite prosthesis and appropriate postoperative isometric exercises.

MANAGEMENT OF THE NECK LYMPH NODES

Clinical Examination of Neck Lymph Nodes

In a comprehensive examination, the patient should be seated with the head and shoulders in the position of anatomical rest. This gives a relaxed and balanced posture for the patient. Palpation of the neck is best conducted from the rear of the patient. The palpation should begin at the base of the posterior cervical triangles and then moves upwards within the anatomical confines of this triangle to the apex at the superior nuchal line. Anterior triangles are next palpated, with their apex below the sternoclavicular joint and suprasternal notch up to the base located at the inferior border of mandible.

Then, the simultaneous bilateral manual palpation is interrupted to displace the sternocleidomastoid muscle posteriorly and laterally. This displacement is done by having the nonexploring hand flex and laterally rotate the cervical spine, so that the palpating hand can feel the area under sternocleidomastoid muscle. The accessory group of lymph nodes is deep to the middle third of this muscle. Order of palpating the lymph nodes should be supraclavicular group, posterior triangle group, jugulo-omohyoid group, jugulodigastric group, submandibular, submental, preauricular, postauricular and occipital group of nodes.

The location, size, consistency and number of palpable lymph nodes should be noted.

Clinical Signs of Extracapsular Spread

- Invasion of the overlying skin.
- Fixation to deeper soft tissues.
- Paralysis of cranial nerves.

Assessment of the Extend of Involvement of Clinically Negative Lymph Nodes

- USG guided fine needle aspiration biopsy for histological diagnosis of metastasis.
- CT scan with intravenous contrast.
- MRI with gadolinium contrast.

▮ LYMPH NODE LEVELS (FIGS 47.16A AND B)

As per American Joint Committee Staging Manual, 1998.

Level I A—nodes in submental triangle (Submental group).

Level I B—nodes in submandibular triangle (Submandibular group).

Level II—upper deep jugular nodes (skull base to carotid bifurcation).

These are subdivided by spinal accessory nerve into IIA lying posterosuperior and IIB, lying anteroinferior to the nerve.

Level III—mid jugular group of nodes (carotid bifurcation to omohyoid)

Level IV—lower jugular group of nodes (omohyoid to clavicle)

Level V—nodes in posterior triangle

Level VI—nodes in anterior triangle (Central compartment group)

Level VII—upper mediastinal group of nodes.

For primary lesions in the oral cavity, the regional lymph nodes at highest risk of early dissemination by metastatic cancer are limited to levels I, II and III. Therefore, if the neck is clinically negative, levels IV and V lymph nodes are generally not considered for micrometastasis from primary oral cancers.

Nodal Metastasis

Involvement of regional lymph nodes by oral cancer is dependent on following factors:

1. Site and location of primary lesion, 2. Size, 3. T stage, 4. Histomorphologic feature.

Tongue and floor of the mouth lesions show more increased risk of nodal metastasis than hard palate lesion. Increasing T stage will increase the risk of nodal metastasis, irrespective to site. Endophytic lesions are more prone than exophytic lesions, similarly

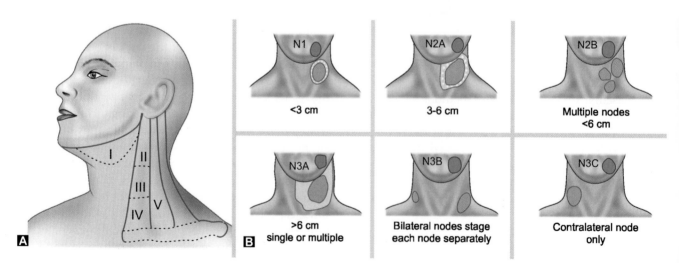

Figs 47.16A and B: (A) Lymph node levels, (B) Lymph nodes-N staging

poorly differentiated carcinoma have increased risk of metastasis than well differentiated carcinoma.

The management of neck nodes depends upon
- Staging of the neck
- T size of the oral cancer
- Type of treatment for the primary (surgery, radiotherapy).

Minimal gross metastasis or micrometastasis may be controlled by radiotherapy alone.

Surgical treatment: Comprehensive surgical clearance of all grossly enlarged lymph nodes offers accurate histological information for micrometastasis in the clinically negative neck. Whenever a significant risk of micrometastasis to regional lymph node is anticipated, based on the features of the primary lesion of the oral cancer, an elective dissection of regional lymph nodes is undertaken.

The principles for management of the neck are shown in Flow chart 47.2 and 47.3.

CLASSIFICATION OF NECK DISSECTION (FIGS 47.17A TO C)

The current classification of neck dissections is as follows:

Flow chart 47.2: Principles for management of the neck

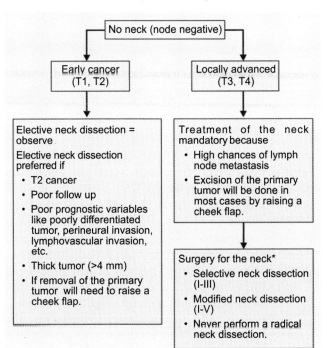

Radical Neck Dissection (RND)

Removal of all cervical lymphatics and lymph nodes from level I-V, with sacrifice of the spinal accessory nerve, the sternocleidomastoid muscle and the internal jugular vein.

Modified Radical Neck Dissection (MRND)

Involves the removal of cervical lymphatics and lymph nodes from levels I-V along with one or more of the non lymphatic structures mentioned below:
- The spinal accessory nerve (SAN)
- The internal jugular vein (IJV)
- The sternocleidomastoid muscle (SCM)

Nomenclature of MRNDs: The structures preserved should be specifically named along with the MRND, e.g. when the internal jugular vein and the spinal accessory nerve are preserved the denotation will be *"MRND (preserving the IJV and the SAN)"*.

The earlier nomenclature of MND Type I, II III is no longer to be used.

Selective Neck Dissection (SND)

This refers to a cervical lymphadenectomy in which there is preservation of one or more lymph node groups that are routinely removed in a MRND along with preservation of the SAN, IJV and the SCM. The lymph node groups removed depend upon the patterns of metastasis relative to the primary site of the tumor. This procedure is generally performed for staging of the neck and is rarely used as a therapeutic procedure.

Nomenclature of SNDs: Each variation of SND is denoted by "SND (denote levels and sublevels), e.g.

Flow chart 47.3: Principles for management of neck

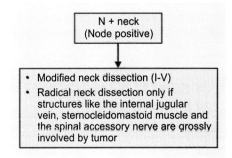

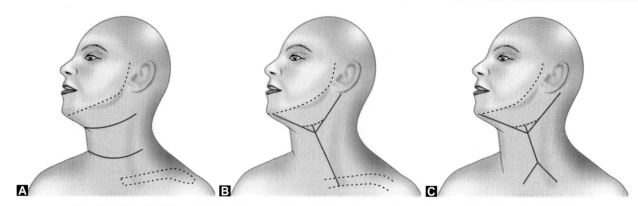

Figs 47.17A to C: Different skin incisions used in neck dissection, carried out in association with the surgery for the management of oral cancer: (A) MacFee's incision, (B) Triradiate incision, (C) Hayes Martin's incision

for oral cavity cancers, lymph node levels I-III are at highest risk for metastasis, therefore *"SND (I-III)"* will be performed as a staging procedure.

Extended Neck Dissection

When lymph node groups or non lymphatic structures other than the ones removed in a RND need to be removed, e.g. external carotid artery, level VI lymph nodes, etc. it is called an extended neck dissection.

Adjuvant Treatment

As outlined above, patients with Stage III and Stage IV cancers need adjuvant treatment with radiotherapy. Current standards of care dictate, that patients with high risk tumors (see below) within stage III and IV need to be treated with radiotherapy and chemotherapy (Flow chart 47.4).

Flow chart 47.4: Adjuvant therapies for stage III and stage IV oral cancer

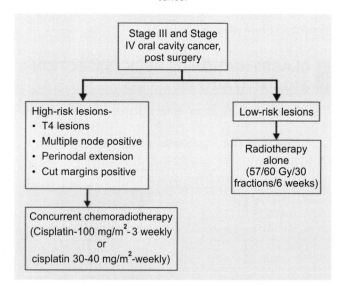

SURVIVAL AND PROGNOSIS

The stage of disease at presentation is the most important factor. Stage I and II disease has better prognosis (5 years survival 31–100%) whereas advanced stages III, IV have poor prognosis (5 years survival 7–41%) depending upon site.

ROLE OF DENTAL PRACTITIONER IN ORAL CANCER MANAGEMENT

This traditionally neglected area is assuming an increasing importance with the modern multidisciplinary management concept. Dental oncology is the discipline within dentistry that combines general dentistry, oral and maxillofacial surgery, maxillofacial prosthetics, oral medicine and oral pathology.

1. Prevention and early detection—dentists are often likely to be consulted for premalignant or early malignant lesions. Here they can encourage patients to quit tobacco and refer suspicious lesions to specialist. It is important for practicing dentists to examine the entire oral cavity when performing routine dental care to pick up suspicious lesions.

2. Dental care prior to commencing radiation—this is very important and involves oral prophylaxis, fluoride application, extract hopeless teeth and restore carious teeth.

3. Patient education post radiotherapy to maintain good oral health.
4. Maxillofacial prosthesis fabrication—both intra and extra-oral prosthesis can be fabricated to replace teeth, nose, ear and eye, etc. This has become possible due to the advent of osseointegrated implants.

Preoperative Dental Work-up

- Many patients with primary cancer of oral cavity have extremely poor oral hygiene.
- Optimum status of oral hygiene should be achieved prior to surgery.
- All grossly septic teeth should be extracted except teeth involved within the lesion or its near vicinity.
- Oral prophylaxis should be carried out.
- All dental restoration work can be postponed until adequate surgical treatment.
- Planning dental impression taking for the fabrication of mandibular splint or obturator should be done prior to surgery.

Implantology in Oral and Maxillofacial Surgery

48 Dental Implants

Implants for rehabilitation and retention of dental and facial prostheses have graduated from a phase of wishful thinking to one of the most gratifying experiences for patients and treating fraternity alike.

This magnificent journey began about 3000 years ago, when a copper stud was nailed into an Egyptian's mouth. This was documented by Dr and Mrs Popenoe, after their excavations in 1931, in Honduras. They found a mandible of Mayan skull with tooth shaped pieces of shells in the sockets of missing teeth. In the recent history, Magiolo (1809), Edmunds (1886) and Harns (1887), attempted similar things using a variety of metals in different shapes after a certain period of post-extraction healing.

Dahl (1940), proposed intramucosal implants or button implants. The subperiosteal implants were suggested in 1941.

There was a period of lull in the implant activity all over the world till 1952, when Bränemark demonstrated that under controlled conditions, titanium could be structurally integrated into living bone with a high degree of predictability of success.

Thereafter, the expedition moved to Linkow's blade vent implants (1967), followed by Robert and Roberts, ramus frame implants (1970). The first screw shaped implant, however, was placed in a patient in 1965.

Bränemark coined the term **"Osseointegration"** which has, probably been, derived from Latin 'Os' (meaning 'bone') and integration (meaning 'being contained').

Osseointegration as defined by Bränemark and co-workers (1989) is "total integration of an implant in bone" specially after the bone is healing after trauma of implant placement in bone.

Osseointegration logically, should be better known as **Osteointegration**. This phenomenon has also been called as "ankylotic bond".

IMPLANT MATERIALS

Many metals and nonmetals have been used as implants materials. These could broadly be classified as:

A. *Metal and alloys:*

a.	Titanium (Pure)	100% pure (cpTi)
b.	Titanium alloy	Titanium 90%
		Chromium 2%
		Molybdenum 7%

c. Chromium cobalt   Cobalt 66%
    alloy   Chromium 37%
    Molybdenum 7%
d. Stainless steel   Iron 70%
    Chromium 18%
    Nickel 12%
e. Tantalum   100% Pure
f. Zirconium   100% Pure
g. Gold   100% Pure
h. Platinum   100% Pure

B. *Inert ceramics*
    a. Aluminium oxide Al_2O_3
       i. Polycrystalline
       ii. Single crystal
    b. Zirconium oxide ZrO_2
       Zircona
    c. Titanium oxide TiO_2

C. *Calcium phosphate* $CaPO_4$
    ceramics

D. *Bioactive and biodegradable ceramics:*
    a. Hydroxyapatite $Ca_{10}(PO_4)_6(OH)_2$
    b. Tricalcium phosphate $Ca_3(PO_4)_2$
    c. Bioglass $CaPO_4$
    d. Calcium aluminates
    e. Carbon
    f. Carbon silicone
    g. Polycrystalline glassy carbon

E. *Polymers:*
    a. Polymethyl methacrylate
    b. Polytetra fluoroethylene
    c. Polyethylene
    d. Polyethylene terephthalate
    e. Polypropylene
    f. Silicon rubber
    g. Polysulfone

Out of the above, pure titanium is highly reactive, but when it comes in contact with air or body fluids, becomes 'titanium oxide', which is probably the most bioinert. Pure titanium, when exposed to environment quickly undergoes oxidation and forms a thin layer (5 to 20 μm thick) of titanium oxide, this titanium oxide is almost totally inert. Even this metal is considered to release some amount of titanium in the patient's body. This titanium 'load' is considerably less (about 10,000 times as per rough estimates) than the total ingestion of titanium via various foods. Therefore, it will be seen that this 'release' appears to be non significant. Furthermore, the biologic half-life of titanium is 320 days, far too short to accumulate in human body to any levels of clinical importance.

Titanium, in its implanted form offers considerable strength (both crushing and shearing) to withstand the occlusal or functional load that would be put on the final prosthesis ultimately. This coupled with Osteointegration makes it, so far, the closest to ideal implants materials.

■ TITANIUM IMPLANTS

These are either 'plasma coated' or are surface 'etched' (by sand blasting or LASER) to further help in Osteointegration, but the rough surface of the implant, so prepared is unsuitable for soft tissue (gingival cuff) and leads to inflammation in the gingiva, much in the same way as the plaque and calculus on the natural teeth.

To overcome this difficulty, the neck of the implant, (the portion which is above the alveolar crest of bone but is encompassed by the gingiva) is highly polished which obviates gingival irritation and ensures a healthy interface between implants and the gingiva.

■ CLASSIFICATIONS OF DENTAL IMPLANTS (FIG. 48.2A)

Based on Shape and Form

Post or root form implants

    i. Solid tapering types
    ii. Solid cylinder type
    iii. Pin types
    iv. Screw shaped implant type
    v. Basket design
    vi. Hollow cylinder design

Blade implants

    i. Conventional blade design
    ii. Vented blade design

Based on Surface Characteristics

a. Titanium plasma—Sprayed coating
b. Sand blasting—Surface etching
c. Laser induced surface roughening
d. Hydroxyapatite coating

Based on Implant Tissue Interface

a. Osseointegration
b. Fibrointegration

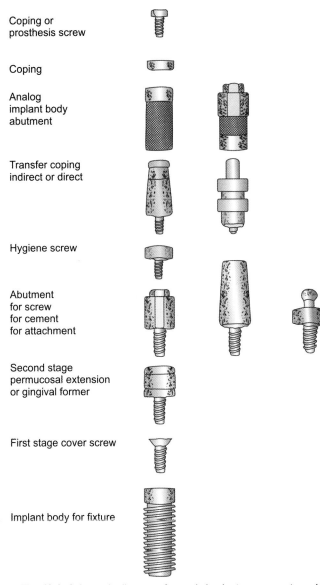

Coping or prosthesis screw

Coping

Analog implant body abutment

Transfer coping indirect or direct

Hygiene screw

Abutment
for screw
for cement
for attachment

Second stage permucosal extension or gingival former

First stage cover screw

Implant body for fixture

Fig. 48.1: Schematic diagram of generic implant components and terminology developed by C.E. Misch and C.M. Misch

Based on Foundation

a. Implant supported
b. Implant assisted

Based on Mode of Retention of Prosthesis

a. Removable
b. Fixed
  i. Screw retained
  ii. Cement retained

Based on Various Systems

a. Branemark implant system (Nobel Biocare System)
b. International Team for oral Implant (ITI) System
c. Implant Innovations system
d. Astra Dental Implant System
e. IMZ implant system (Interpore IMZ)
f. Corevent system
g. Sterri-Oss System
h. Endosteal Hollow Basket System

Immediate Implants

Immediate implants are those which are inserted into the freshly extracted teeth sockets.

Transient Implants for Immediate Loading

As the name suggests, these are temporary and are suitable to carry prostheses during the period of Osteointegration of regular Implants.

Parts of Implant

A generic language for endosteal implants has been developed by Misch and Misch. It is presented in an order following the chronology of insertion and restoration. In formulating the terminology, five commonly used systems were referenced.

The endosteal implants have segmented portions placed in different phases. At the time of insertion of the implant body or first stage surgery, a cover is placed into the top of implant to prevent bone, soft tissue, or debris from invading the abutment connection area during healing. If the first stage, cover is screwed into place, the term *cover screw* is used (Fig. 48.1).

After a prescribed healing period sufficient to allow a supporting interface to develop, a second stage procedure may be performed to expose the implants and/or attach a transepithelial portion. This transepithelial portion is termed as *permucosal extension* or *gingival former*, because it extends the implant above the soft tissue and results in the development of a permucosal seal around the implant. This implant component is also called a healing cap. Another name given to this implant component is healing abutment, because in stage II to uncover implant, often this device is used for initial soft tissue healing.

The *abutment* is the portion of the implant that supports and/or retains prosthesis or implant superstructure. *A superstructure* is defined as a metal framework that fits the implant abutment(s) and provides retention for a fixed prosthesis. Three main categories of implant abutment are described, according to the method by which the prosthesis or superstructure is retained to the abutment.

1. An abutment for screw retention uses a screw to retain the prosthesis or superstructure.
2. An abutment for cement retention uses dental cement to retain the prosthesis or superstructure.
3. An abutment for attachment uses an attachment device to retain a removable prosthesis.

The prosthesis may be classified as fixed, whenever cement retains the prostheses, fixed/removable when screws retain a fixed prosthesis and removable when the prosthesis is removed by the patient.

Each of the three abutment types may be further classified as straight or angled abutments, describing the axial relationship between the implant body and the abutment (Figs 48.2A and B). An abutment for screw retention uses a hygiene cover screw placed over the abutment to prevent debris and calculus from invading the internally threaded portion of the abutment during prosthesis fabrication.

An impression is necessary to transfer the position and design of the implant or abutment to a master cast for prosthesis fabrication. A *transfer coping* is used in traditional prosthesis to position a *die* in air impression. Most implant manufactures use the terms transfer and/ or coping to describe the component used for the final impression. Therefore, a transfer coping is used to position an analog in an impression and is defined by the portion of the implant it transfers to the master cast, either the implant body transfer coping or the abutment transfer coping.

Two basic implant restorative techniques are used to make a master impression and each uses a different design transfer coping, based on the transfer technique performed. An indirect transfer coping uses the impression material requiring elastic properties. The indirect transfer coping is screwed into the abutment or implant body and remains in place when the set impression is removed from the mouth. The indirect transfer coping is parallel sided or slightly tapered to allow ease in removal of the impression and often has flat sides or smooth undercuts to facilitate reorientation in the impression after it is removed.

A direct transfer coping usually consists of a hollow transfer component, often square, and a long central screw to secure it to the abutment of implant body.

After the impression material is set, the direct transfer coping screw is unthreaded to allow removal of the impression from the mouth. Direct transfer coping takes advantage of impression materials having rigid properties and eliminates the error of permanent deformation, because it remains within the impression until the master model is poured and separated. An analog is something that is analogous or similar to something else. An implant analog is used in the fabrication of the master cast to replicate the retentive portion of the implant body or abutment (implant body analog, implant abutment analog). After the master cast obtained, the corresponding analog (e.g. implant body, abutment for screw) is attached to the transfer coping and the assembly is poured in stone to fabricate the master cast.

A prosthetic coping is a thin covering, usually design to fit the implant abutment for screw retention and serve as the connection between the abutment and the prosthesis as superstructure.

A prefabricated coping is a metal component machined precisely to fit the abutment.

■ BIOLOGIC PARAMETERS FOR IMPLANTS ACCEPTANCE

The parameters that are considered for evaluation of implant viz a viz its success:

Material Biocompatibility

The implant material should be biocompatible (as discussed earlier) and in this category titanium screws score over all other materials for making an implant.

Implant Design

Various designs have been employed with varying degrees of success. We already know that at present the most suitable design is that of a cylinder. This has further been improved to make it a screw and then on to tapering screw implant. But then there is yet another cylindrical implant which has small spheroids attached to the surface, which not only facilitates Osteointegration by making it rough but also increases the surface area of bone to implant contact. This is classically seen in 'endopore' implants. These implants are screwed into the drill hole in the bone but have to tapped into it for tight fit.

Of the screw type cylindrical implants the bone has to be either 'tapped' prior to implant insertion or

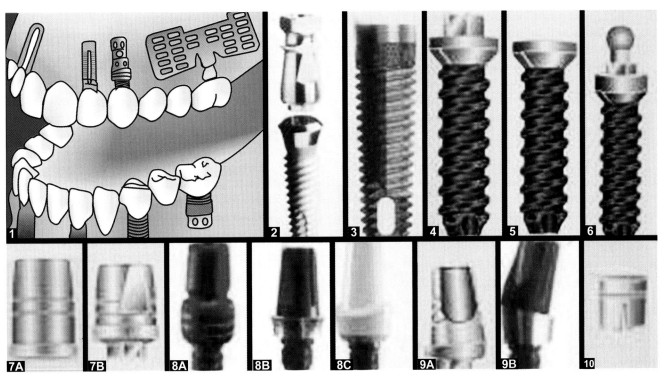

Fig. 48.2A: (1) Different forms and shapes of implant, (2) One stage implant, (3) Two stage implant, (4) External Hex implant, (5) Internal Hex implant, (6) Ball and socket implant, (7A and B) External straight Hex abutment, (8A to C) Internal straight Hex abutment, (9A and B) Internal angulated Hex abutment, (10) Abutment for ball and socket implant

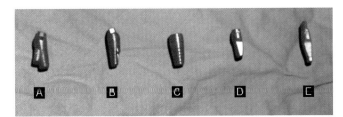

Fig. 48.2B: Different forms of abutments: (A and B) Screw abutment, (C) External hexagon abutment, (D and E) Angulated abutment

the other variety are self-tapping types, which cut the thread in the bone as it is inserted into the bone.

Implant Surface

The surface (that part which is in the bone) has to be made 'rough' by either plasma spraying or surface etching also spheroids can be attached on to the surface as mentioned above.

That part of implant which is above the bone level but within the soft tissue is also known as neck of the implant and therefore has to be highly polished to prevent soft tissue inflammation, so as to promote water tight gingival cuff.

Host Site

The host site plays an important role in the ultimate success of implant as quality of bone is of paramount importance for Osteointegration, e.g. if the bone is dense, then primary stability of implant would be achieved but long term stability (achieved by Osteo-integration) may not be forthcoming easily and may take longer time.

■ INDICATIONS AND CONTRAINDICATIONS

The implants have a very wide range of indications to their use. They may be employed to provide and retain single tooth replacements to a few teeth as implant supported bridges as also for providing complete denture prostheses in either or both the jaws.

Apart from this, the titanium implants have also been used for other applications like craniofacial implants (for retaining maxillofacial prosthesis) and in orthodontic treatment for skeletal anchorage (micro or mini implants).

As regarding contraindications, it can be safely said that there are no specific absolute contraindications.

The implants may be inserted in any jaw except the patient who is still in growing stages (i.e. prepuberty) but then it is a relative contraindication.

It would be prudent, in debilitating systemic disease, to control the condition and maintain the patient in as optimal health as is possible, a good example would be diabetes mellitus.

However, the radiated bone for cancer treatment would not be a good site for implant success.

The shape and type of jaw bones, their relationship with inferior alveolar nerve as in severely atrophied, alveolar ridges, where the inferior dental canal becomes very close to the alveolar crest; similarly in maxillary arch, the proximity of maxillary sinus and also in some cases, the relative height of alveolus in relation to pyriform fossa should be kept in mind. In all such cases appropriate implant sizes (length) should be used.

Sometimes, in these cases procedures like 'sinus lift for maxilla; or alveolar bone graft for the mandible may be undertaken.

Lately bone alternatives like hydroxyapatite and lyophilized bone may be considered but autogenous bone graft still remains the choice of graft material.

When selecting a small length of implant, it is advisable to select an implant of the widest circumference that the recipient bone would accept. Thereby increasing the so important surface area contact of bone to implant. The *rule of thumb* is to select the largest implant size that would be suitable for the particular region in that patient.

PRESURGICAL INVESTIGATIONS

a. To assess the general health of the patient, routine blood tests and tests for HbsAg and HIV may be asked for to rule out hepatitis B and HIV-AIDS (even though they are no contraindications)
b. Study dental casts
c. Imaging:
   1. Intraoral periapical X-rays of the concerned region to assess the bone quality viz a viz density, quantity and also ruling out of any residual pathology.
   2. *Orthopantomogram (OPG):* It gives a general view of both jaws and bone condition, therein as also the jaw relationship, the location of inferior dental canal, mental foramen, maxillary sinus and nasal floor. It is helpful in establishing the length of implant that can be used. However, this does not give information regarding the width of the bone.
   3. *Computerized tomogram (CT)/dentascan:* This imaging enables differentiation and quantification of both soft and hard tissues in all three dimensions.

      Dentascan visualizes true cross-section of mandible and maxilla thereby allowing visualization of body structures preoperatively and is therefore a tremendous help in deciding location, size and angulation if any of implants.
   4. 3D reconstruction and StereoLithoGraphic Models, is newer facility to locate anatomical structures but needs SIMPLANT software, for optimal utilization, therefore is expensive.

ANESTHESIA

Most implants can be very conveniently placed under local analgesia suitable for the region. Regional nerve blocks are often frowned upon as they take away the initial information of pain when drilling in close vicinity of the nerve and moreover the local infiltration provides enough analgesia for implant placements. In some cases on surgeon's or patient's choice, general anesthesia may be employed.

INSERTION OF IMPLANT

The patient should be so prepared and draped, that it would facilitate aseptic technique with complete sterility of equipment.

The implant is provided by the manufacturers in a double sealed sterile container and is sterile. Each manufacturer provides its own surgical kit containing drills, ratchets, depth gauge, etc. (Figs 48.3 to 48.5).

Surgical Steps

The surgical site is thoroughly cleansed and painted with 1 percent povidone iodine solution to bring down the bacterial colony count in the mouth.

It is worth while to note that mouth or oral cavity cannot be made sterile.

Incision

Standard trapezoidal incision—or any other suitable incision as in case of Brānemark system buccal incision is made midway between the crest and depth of the vestibule and then flap is reflected lingually so that the implant, after insertion, is completely covered by mucoperiosteum to prevent leakage of oral fluid on to the implant site (Fig. 48.6).

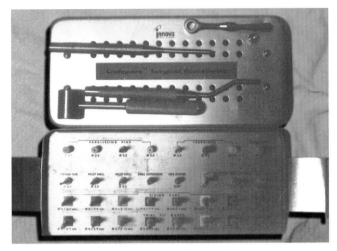

Fig. 48.3: 'Innova' implant kit

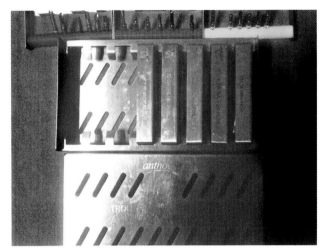

Fig. 48.5: Anthrogyr implant kit

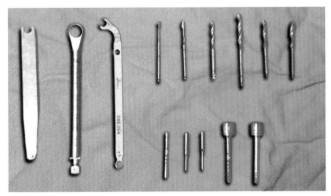

Fig. 48.4: ITI implant kit by Straumann

Drilling into Bone

The manufacturer gives a guide to the sequence of drills (sizes) to be used in order to make proper sized drill hole for a particular implant (Figs 48.7 and 48.8).

Drilling

The first drill invariably is the round one, to perforate the cortex at crest thereafter the drills are used in ascending order of thickness (diameter).

Drilling Speed

Bone must be drilled at a low speed. Generally, a speed less than 800 rpm is recommended. The slower the better, as higher speed tends to raise the local temperature in bone and may be detrimental for the bone to remain viable and creep into the implant surface (roughened by plasma spraying or etching) to ultimately bring about osteointegration.

The drills are marked for depth (Figs 48.7 and 48.8A) to guide the surgeon as to how deep is the hole. Finally, when the required depth is reached it is checked by the provided depth gauge. A little (1 mm or so) over drilling is better than under, as it prevents crushing of bone 'apical' to implant.

If the implant is not self tapping, the required bone tap is used to cut 'thread' in bone and then the implant is screwed in.

Insertion

Implants are provided in sterile pre-packed container with an implant carrier, which is gently taken to the drilled site and hand twisted to engage a few threads and then a special ratchet is used to screw the implant up to its required depth. The implant carrier is removed at this stage and the 'healing cap' or 'cover screw is screwed on to the visible implant top.

Irrigation

It is one of the most important steps during the entire drilling process to keep the local bone temperature at normal body temperature and also to flush out the bone debris from the drill hole.

Normal saline at room temperature is ideal for this purpose. 'Very cold' saline should be avoided as this might cause 'Thermal shock' in the local area in a restricted sense and it may be injurious to bone.

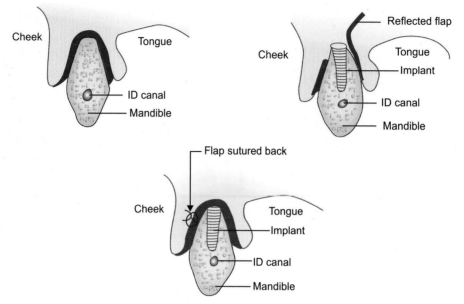

Fig. 48.6: Diagrammatic representation of flap reflection for Bränemark implants

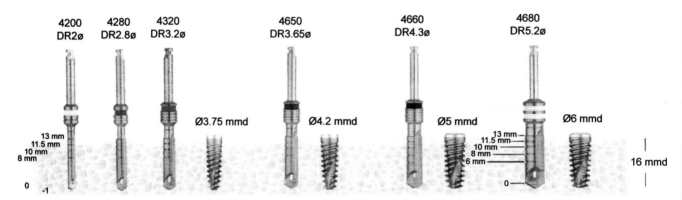

Fig. 48.7: Schematic representation of sequence in implant placement

Various types of 'Physiodispensers' are available commercially', generally the manufacturer either provides one of their own or recommends a particular model (Figs 48.8B and C).

Closing the Wound

3'0 black silk is the preferred suture material with atraumatic curved needle. Interrupted sutures are placed and are removed 5 to 7 days postoperatively.

Suitable antibiotics and nonsteroidal analgesics are prescribed for 3 to 7 postoperative days.

Chlorhexidine 0.2 percent w/v mouth wash is added to the prescription at least 3 to 6 times daily for 7 to 20 days or even longer. This may be alternated with warm saline mouth rinses.

■ COMPLICATIONS

Intraoperative

    i. Tear of flap
   ii. Lack of irrigation or insufficient irrigation
  iii. Perforation of buccal or lingual cortex
  iv. Implant/drill impinges on the inferior dental nerve
   v. Implant/drill impinges on the neighbouring tooth root

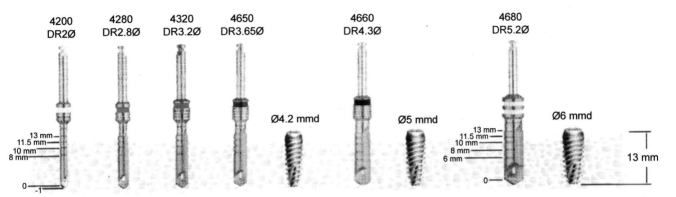

Fig. 48.8A: Schematic representation of sequence in implant placement

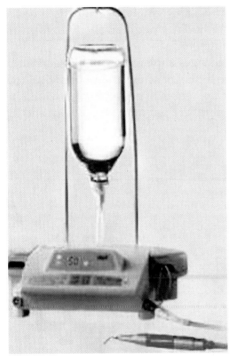

Fig. 48.8B: Piezo ultrasonic physiodispenser unit

vi. Perforation of maxillary sinus
vii. Perforation of pyriform fossa base
viii. Lack of primary stability of implants
ix. Rarely fracture of implant.

Immediate postoperative

i. Pain (Unusual)
ii. Hemorrhage (rarely)
iii. Swelling
iv. Nerve injuries.

Delayed

i. Infection
ii. Secondary hemorrhage
iii. Nerve injury
iv. Loosening of implant
v. Loss of implant.

AILING V/S FAILING IMPLANT

Ailing implant is where there a radiolucent line like the periodontal ligament shadow in normal tooth

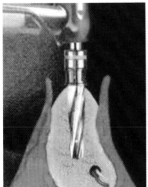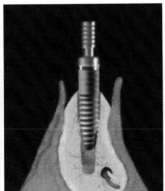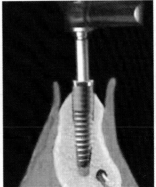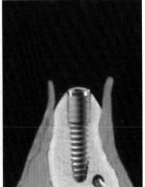

Fig. 48.8C: Diagrammatic representation of sequence in implant placement

(radiologically, best seen in intraoral periapical X-rays), this implant is likely to fail but has a chance to survive if remedial measures are undertaken in time like local curettage to remove soft tissue from in between the implant and host bone (Fig. 48.9).

A failing implant is one with the above alongwith 1° or 2° mobility. The chances of salvaging such an implant are bleak (Fig. 48.9).

Healing Period

A period of 12 to 16 weeks is allowed of Osteointegration to take place. Only after this period has lapsed and the implant does not show any sign of ailing/failing should the loading be undertaken.

Impressions for Loading

In single stage implant (where no second surgery is required to remove the healing caps), the healing cap is unscrewed and gingival former is screwed in and left for 7 to 17 days for gingival cuff to form around the future abutment.

In two stages implants, second surgery is undertaken to remove the cover screw and put gingival former.

After the requisite period, the provided impression posts (coping) are put onto the implant and impression is taken.

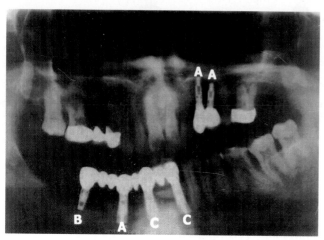

Fig. 48.9: (A) Ailing implant, (B) Failing implant, (C) Healthy (osteointegrated) implant

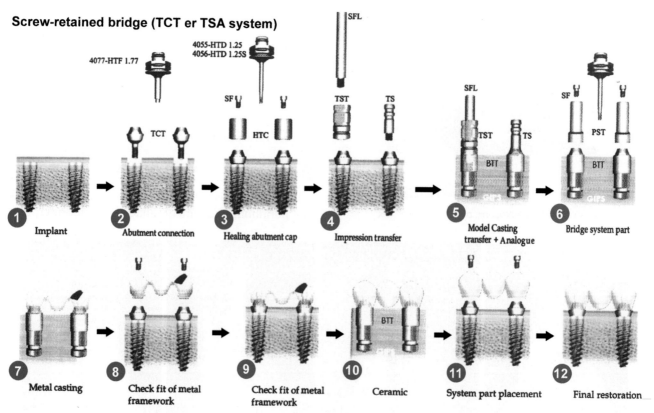

Fig. 48.10: Schematic representation of stages of screw retained prosthesis

Cemented restoration

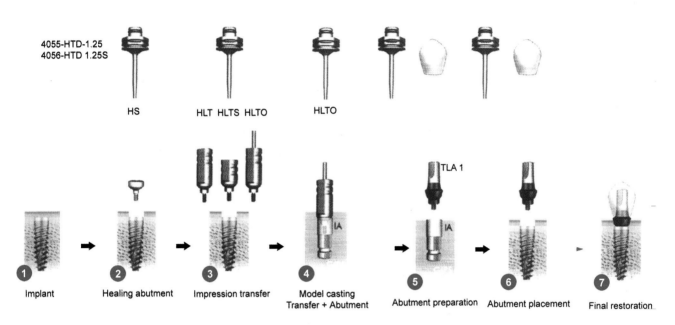

Fig. 48.11: Schematic representation of stages of cemented restorations

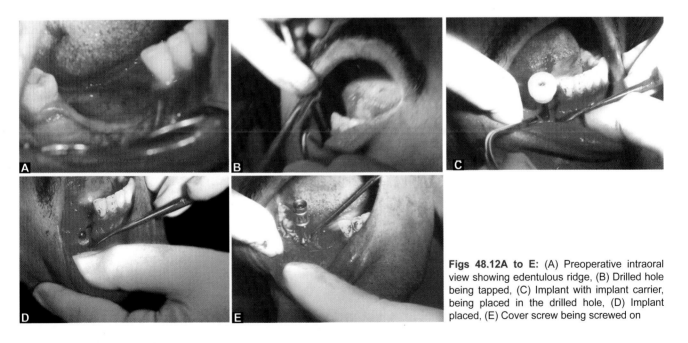

Figs 48.12A to E: (A) Preoperative intraoral view showing edentulous ridge, (B) Drilled hole being tapped, (C) Implant with implant carrier, being placed in the drilled hole, (D) Implant placed, (E) Cover screw being screwed on

Then implant analog is fixed on to the impression posts (coping) and the impression is poured in die stone.

Once the plaster is set, the post is removed and abutments are placed.

The cast can then be sent to the laboratory for fabrication of prosthesis (crown).

The abutment is taken off the cast leaving the implant analogue in the cast. This abutment can now be

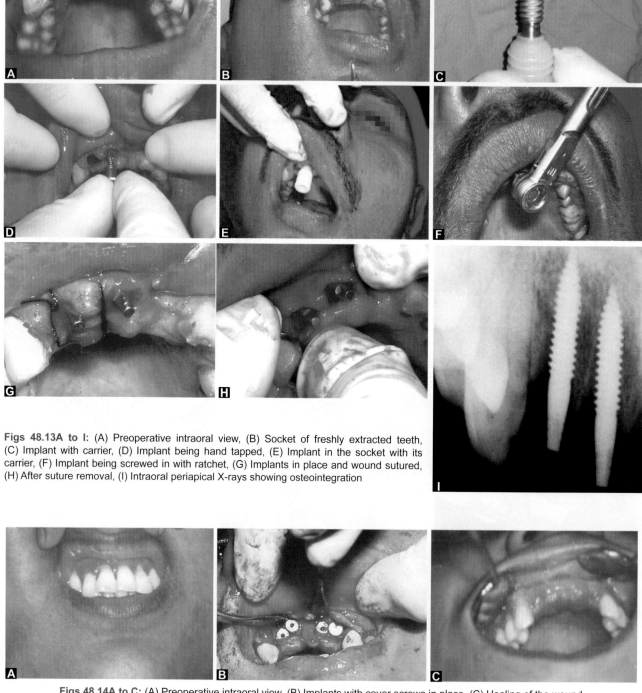

Figs 48.13A to I: (A) Preoperative intraoral view, (B) Socket of freshly extracted teeth, (C) Implant with carrier, (D) Implant being hand tapped, (E) Implant in the socket with its carrier, (F) Implant being screwed in with ratchet, (G) Implants in place and wound sutured, (H) After suture removal, (I) Intraoral periapical X-rays showing osteointegration

Figs 48.14A to C: (A) Preoperative intraoral view, (B) Implants with cover screws in place, (C) Healing of the wound

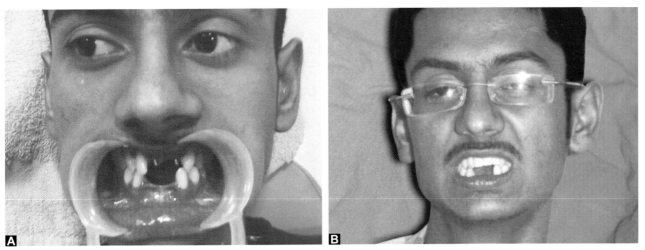

Figs 48.15A and B: (A) Implants in place, (B) Post prosthesis

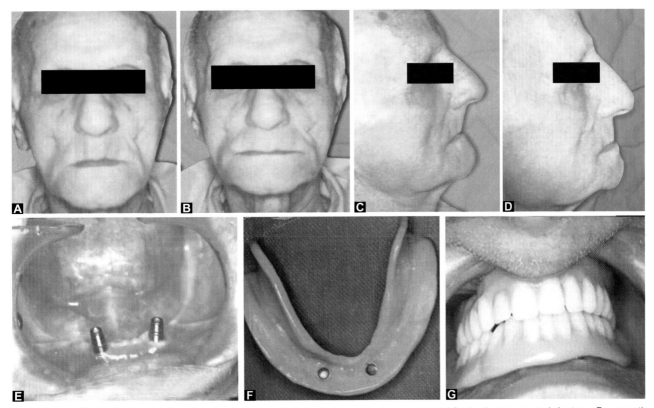

Figs 48.16A to G: (A) A 72-year-old male patient could not retain his lower denture, requested for implant supported denture. Preoperative frontal view, (B) Frontal view of the same patient, after the delivery of upper normal full denture and lower implant supported denture, (C) Predenture delivery profile, (D) Postdenture delivery profile, (E) Two implants seen in mandibular canine region bilaterally, (F) Lower denture inner aspect—implant sockets in position, (G) Full denture *in situ*

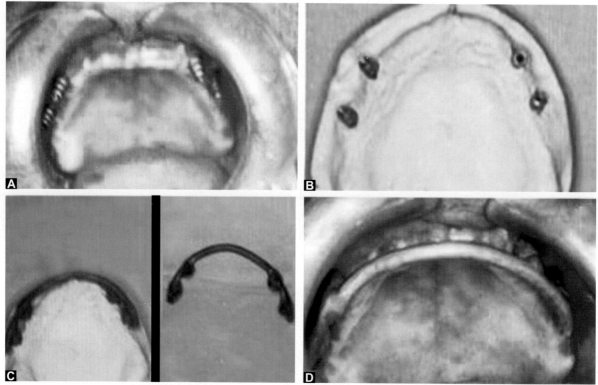

Figs 48.17A to D: (A) Four implants in place in maxillary edentulous ridge, (B) Plaster model with implant analogs, (C) Castable dolder bar pattern prepared on the model, (D) Checking for the fit of the dolder bar in the mouth, before final finish

transferred and screwed onto the implant and prosthesis affixed to it (either cemented or screwed to the abutment).

Occlusal adjustment is undertaken if required, (Figs 48.10 and 48.11).

■ CLINICAL PHOTOGRAPHS

Figures 48.12 to 48.17.

■ BIBLIOGRAPHY

1. Babbush, Charles A. Dental Implants the Art and Science, WB Saunders, Co. 2001.
2. Bränemark PI, Adell R, Albrektsson T, et al. An experimental and clinical study of osseointegrated implants penetrating the nasal cavity and maxillary sinus. J Oral Maxillofacial Surgery 1984; 42:497-505.
3. Bränemark PI, Tolman DE. Osseointegration in craniofacial reconstruction. Quintessence publishing Co. Inc. 1998.
4. Linkow LI, Donath K. Retrieval analysis of blade implant after 231 months of clinical function. Implant Dent 1992;1:37.
5. Misch Carl E. Contemporary implant dentistry 2 edn, Mosby 1999.
6. Misch CE. Bone density its effects on surgery healing and progressive bone loading. Int J Oral and Maxillofacial Implant 1990;6:23-31.
7. Schroeder A, Sutter F, Buser D, Krekeler G. Oral Implantology Basics, ITI Hollow Cylinder System, George Thieme Verlag Stuttgart, New York, 1996.

49 Implants—An Overview

IMPLANTATION

It is defined as insertion of any object or material, which is alloplastic in nature, either partially or completely into the body for therapeutic, experimental, diagnostic or prosthetic purpose.

Dental Implant (According to Glossary of Prosthodontic Terms, 8th Edition)

It is a prosthetic device of alloplastic material(s) implanted into oral tissues beneath the mucosal and/or periosteal layer, and a substance that is placed into and/or upon the jaw bone to provide retention and support for a fixed or removable prosthesis. Dental implants may be classified by their silhouette or geometrical form (fin, screw, cylinder, blade, basket, root form, etc.) Generally, dental implants are classified based on their anchorage

component (the dental implant body), as it relates to the bone that provides support and stability. Thus, there are three types of basic dental implants: epiosteal, endosteal and transosteal dental implants. Some dental implants possess both epiosteal and endosteal components (by design or subsequent anchorage change); the decision as to what anchorage system provides the most support at initial placement, determines which category is used to best describe the dental implant.

OSSEOINTEGRATION OR OSSEOUS INTEGRATION (1993) GLOSSARY OF PROSTHODONTIC TERMS-8 (FIGS 49.1A AND B)

1. It is the apparent direct attachment or connection of osseous tissue to an inert, alloplastic material without intervening connective tissue.

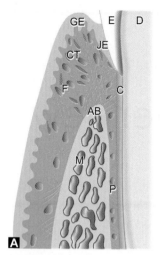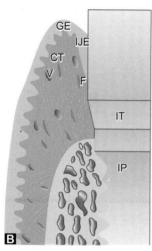

Figs 49.1A and B: In the normal periodontium at (A) Collegen fibers are highlighted extending from the gingival alveolar bone (AB) crest to the cementum (C) gingiva and periodontal ligament (P) to form a cross-hatch pattern at the connective attachment. The rich blood supply (V) and fibroblastic (F) components can be seen to a lesser extent in the cervical peri-implant connective tissue (CT), (B) Bundles of collagen fibers in the peri-implant cervical connective attachment to run parallel to the surface of the intermediate prosthesis (IT). GE—gingival epithelium; JE—junctional epithelium, IJE—implant junctional epithelium, D—dentin; M—marrow space, IP—implant

2. The process and resultant direct connection of an exogenous material's surface and the host's bone tissue without intervening fibrous connective tissue present.
3. The interface between alloplastic material and bone. *Osseointegration is also defined as: "the formation of a direct interface between an implant and bone, without intervening soft tissue".*
   A. Osseointegrated implant is a type of implant defined as "an endosteal implant containing pores into which osteoblasts and supporting connective tissue can migrate".
   B. Applied to oral implantology, this refers to bone grown right up to the implant surface without interposed soft tissue layer. No scar tissues, cartilages or ligament fibers are present between the bone and implant surface. The direct contact of bone and implant surface can be verified microscopically.

Two theories regarding the chemical mechanism by which endosteal implants integrate with bone have been proposed. That type of integration contrasts with fibrosseous integration, in which soft tissues such as fibers and/or cells are interposed between the two surfaces.

1. Brånemark's Theory of Osseointegration

Brånemark proposed that implants integrate such that the bone is laid very close to the implant without any intervening connective tissue. The titanium oxide permanently fuses with the bone, as Brånemark showed in 1950s.

2. Weiss' Theory of Fibro-osseous Integration

Weiss' theory states that there is a fibro-osseous ligament formed between the implant and the bone and this ligament can be considered as equivalent of the periodontal ligament found in the gomphosis. He defends the presence of collagen fibers at the bone-implant interface. He interpreted it as the peri-implantal ligament with an osteogenic effect. He advocates the early loading of an implant.

Osseointegration Process

For osseointegrated dental implants, metallic, ceramic, and polymeric materials have been used, in particular, *titanium*. To be termed osseointegration, the connection between the bone and the implant needs not be 100% and the essence of osseointegration derives more from the stability of the fixation than the degree of contact in histologic terms. In short, it represents a process, whereby, clinically asymptomatic rigid fixation of alloplastic material is achieved, and maintained in bone during functional loading. When osseointegration occurs, the implant is tightly held in place by the bone. The process typically takes several weeks or months to occur, which is well enough for the implant dentist to complete the restorations. The fact is that the degree of Osseointegration of implants is a matter of time. First evidence of integration occurs after a few weeks, while more robust connection is progressively effected over the next months or years. Though the osseointegrated interface becomes resistant to external shocks over the time, it may be damaged by prolonged adverse stimuli and overload, which may result in implant failure. In studies performed on dental implants, it was noted that the absence of micromotion at the bone-implant interface was necessary to enable proper osseointegration. Further, it was noted that there is a critical threshold of micromotion, above which a fibrous encapsulation process occurs, rather than osseointegration. Already Brånemark stated that the implant should not be loaded and left out of function during the healing period for osseous integration to occur (Figs 49.2 and 49.3).

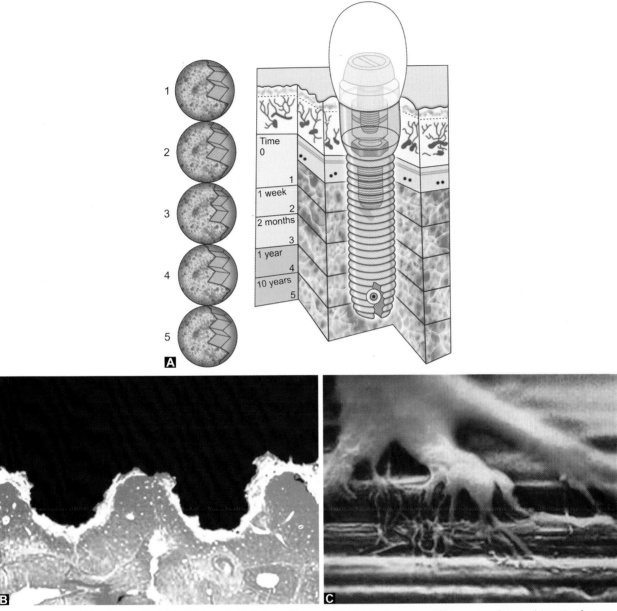

Figs 49.2A to C: (A) Titanium implant (Blue) integrated into bone (Brown), (B) Histologic section, (C) Its comparison to the roots of a tree

RATIONALE FOR IMPLANT TREATMENT

There is an increased need for implant supported prosthesis due to the following factors:
1. An aging population; longer life span.
2. Age related tooth loss.
3. As a consequence of failure of fixed prosthesis.
4. Unacceptability or poor performance of removable prosthesis.
5. Psychological aspects of tooth loss.
6. Anatomical consequences of edentulism.
7. Advantages of implant prosthesis such as conservation of adjacent tooth structure and bone loss.
8. Predictable long term results.

CLASSIFICATIONS FOR IMPLANT TREATMENT

1. **Based on placement within the tissues:**
   A. *Epiosteal:* When the dental implant receives its primary support by resting on the bone, e.g. subperiosteal implants.

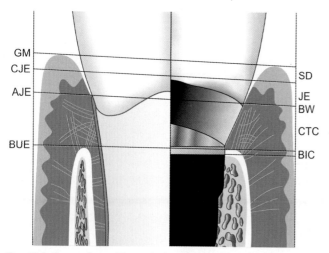
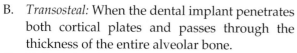

Fig. 49.3: Comparison of the periodontal structures in the natural tooth and in the implant. GM—gingival margin, CJE—coronal junctional epithelium, AJE—apical junctional epithelium, BUE—bone upper edge, BIC—bone implant contact, SD—sulcus depth between GM and CJE, JE—junctional epithelium between CJE and AJE, CTC—connective tissue contact between AJE and BIC, BW—biological width between GM and BIC

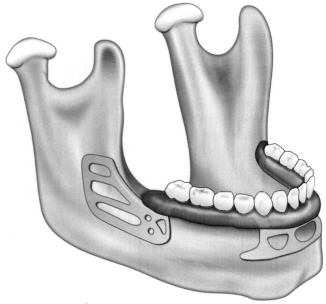

Fig. 49.4: Blade implants

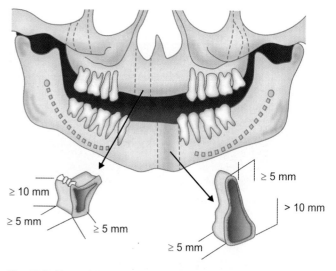

Fig. 49.5: Kennedy's class I division A bone. > 10 mm bone height. 7 mm bone length. Crown implant ratio < 1

B. *Transosteal:* When the dental implant penetrates both cortical plates and passes through the thickness of the entire alveolar bone.
C. *Endosteal:* When the dental implant extends into the basal bone for support. It transects only one cortical plate and is further classified into:
    i. *Root form:* Used over a vertical collar of bone. Available forms: cylindrical/press fit, screw root form, combination
    ii. *Plate/blade form (Fig. 49.4):* Used for a horizontal column of bone, which is flat and narrow in the faciolingual direction

2. **Based on classification of edentulous spaces:**
    Misch and Judy classified implant bone volume based on Kennedy-Applegate's classification of partially edentulous spaces. Accordingly, each of Kennedy's classification is divided into four divisions of varying bone volume:
    i. *Kennedy's class I div A bone (Fig. 49.5):* Greater than 10 mm bone height, greater than 5 to 7 mm bone length, crown to implant ratio of less than 1. Rootform implants and independent prosthesis is indicated
    ii. *Kennedy's class I div B bone (Fig. 49.6):* Moderate bone width (2.5-5 mm), adequate bone height >10 mm, adequate bone length >15 mm, crown to implant ratio <1. Direction of load is within 20 degrees of implant body axis. Surgical options include osteoplasty, small diameter implants, and augmentation.
    iii. *Kennedy's class I div C bone (Fig. 49.7):* Inadequate bone height and width for endosteal implant placement, too little bone width (c-w), length, height (c-h), or angulation of load (c-a), crown height is >15 mm. Crown implant ratio is > 1, Surgical options for c-w include osteoplasty and augmentation: for c-h, subperiosteal implants

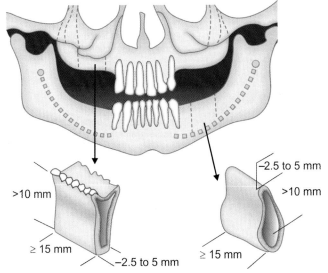

Fig. 49.6: Kennedy's class I division B bone: Moderate bone width (2.5 to 5 mm). Adequate bone height (>10 mm). Adequate bone length (>15mm). Crown implant ratio is <1

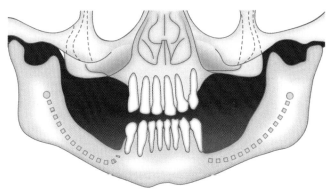

Fig. 49.7: Kennedy's class I division C bone: Inadequate bone width, height and thickness not sufficient for endosteal implant placement, crown implant ratio is >1

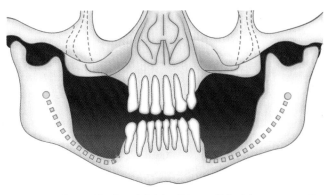

Fig. 49.8: Kennedy's class I division D bone: Edentulous areas with severely resorbed ridges. Crown implant ratio is >5

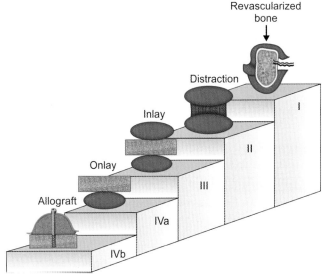

Fig. 49.9: Classification of absolute alveolar ridge augmentation. The assessment is based on vascularization and hence the ability to form new bone or resorb and remodel foreign material

and augmentation. Rootform implants may be considered after augmentation and/or nerve repositioning.

iv. *Kennedy's class I div D bone (Fig. 49.8):* Edentulous areas with severely resorbed ridges, involving a portion of basal or cortical supporting bone. Crown to implant ratio >5. Surgical options usually require augmentation before implants can be inserted (Fig. 49.9).

v. Kennedys class II div A bone in upper arch and div B in lower arch.

vi. Kennedy's class II with div C bone in upper arch and div D in lower arch.

vii. Kennedy's class III with div A bone in upper arch and div B bone in lower arch.

viii. Kennedy's class III with div C in upper arch and div D in the lower arch.

ix. Kennedy's class IV with div A in upper arch and B in lower arch.

x. Kennedy's class IV with div C in upper arch and D in lower arch.

3. **In case of completely edentulous ridges:** Misch divided each arch into 3 segments (Fig. 49.10):

(A) Anterior

(B) Right posterior

(C) Left posterior

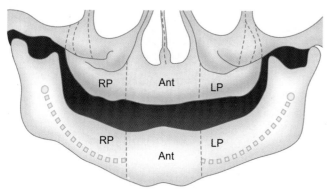

Fig. 49.10: Completely edentulous jaw is divided into three segments for convenience. Anterior component (Ant) is between the mental foramen. Right posterior (RP) and left posterior (LP) segments correspond to patient's righy and left sides

The clinical conditions are divided according to bone density present in different locations in each segments (Table 49.1, Figs 49.11 and 49.12)

The clinical conditions are grouped as:

Type 1/D1: Dense compact bone—offers excellent stability to implant.

Type 2/D2: Dense to porous compact bone—coarse trabecular bone inside, dense bone outside. Threaded or cylinder implants are indicated.

Type 3/D3: Porous compact, coarse trabecular bone-implants coated with hydroxyapatite are indicated with gradual loading.

Type4/D4: Fine trabecular bone—very less density and no cortical crestal bone. Larger implant should be used with bone graft.

4. **Based on mode of retention of prosthesis:**
   i. Removable prosthesis
   ii. Fixed prosthesis
      – Screw retained
      – Cement retained
   iii. Hybrid prosthesis

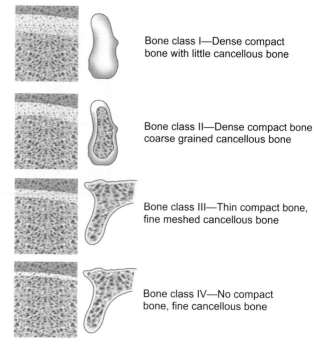

Fig. 49.11: Macroscopic description of the four densities

Bone class I—Dense compact bone with little cancellous bone

Bone class II—Dense compact bone coarse grained cancellous bone

Bone class III—Thin compact bone, fine meshed cancellous bone

Bone class IV—No compact bone, fine cancellous bone

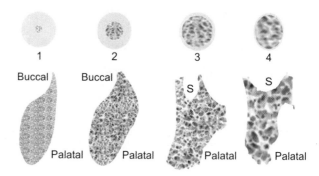

Fig. 49.12: Qualitative bone supply based on the Lekholm and Zarb, (1985) classification

Table 49.1: Misch bone density classification			
Bone density	Description	Tactile analog	Typical anatomical location
D1	Dense cortical	Oak or maple wood	Anterior mandible
D2	Porous cortical and coarse trabecular	White pine or spruce wood	Anterior mandible
			Posterior mandible
			Anterior maxilla
D3	Porous cortical (thin) and fine trabecular	Balsa wood	Anterior maxilla
			Posterior maxilla
			Posterior mandible
D4	Fine trabeculur	Styrofoam	Posterior maxilla

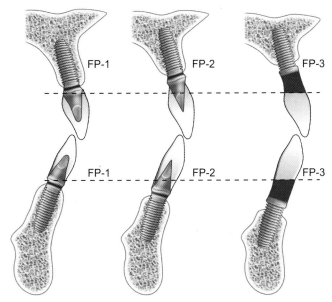

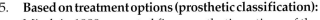

Fig. 49.13: Misch prosthetic options

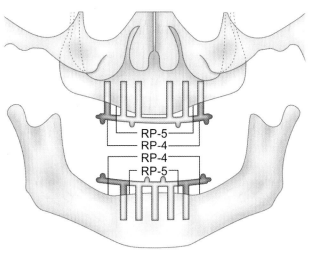

Fig. 49.14: Options for implant supported removable prosthesis

5. **Based on treatment options (prosthetic classification):**
Misch in 1989, reported five prosthetic options of the implants. The fixed prosthesis are classified based on the amount of hard and soft tissue structures to be replaced. Removable prosthesis are derived based on the support derived (Fig. 49.13).

FP1: Fixed prosthesis replaces only the crown and looks like a natural tooth

FP2: Fixed prosthesis replaces the crown and a portion of the root

FP3: Fixed prosthesis replaces missing crown and gingiva, prosthesis most often uses denture teeth with acrylic gingiva, but may also be made of metal or porcelain.

Removable restorations have two categories based on implant support (Fig. 49.14).

RP4: Implant supported over denture removable prosthesis. Complete support, anterior and posterior is on implants. In mandible, the superstructure bar is often cantilevered from implants positioned between the mental foramen. The maxillary prosthesis usually has more implants and little or no cantilever.

RP5: This type of restoration has primarily anterior implant support and posterior soft tissue support in the maxilla or mandible. Often fewer implants are required and bone grafting is less indicated.

6. **Based on loading protocols:**
i. *Conventional loading/delayed loading or two-stage protocol:* Where in first stage, implants are surgically placed and the patient is made to wait for 6 months for osseointegration; 2nd stage surgery is then performed, where the healing cap is placed and after a week of satisfactory formation of a gingival collar for emergence profile is achieved, impressions are made for implant prosthesis, which may be cement or screw retained.
ii. *One stage protocol*—further divided into *immediate loading* and early loading:
   A. *Immediate loading:* is when a provisional prosthesis is placed during the same session as the surgery.
   Immediate loading is further divided based on the biomechanical definition:
   • Immediate loading with provisional Prosthesis out of or shy of occlusion.
   • Immediate loading with provisional prosthesis in occlusion.
   B. *Early loading:* When the implant prosthesis is placed after a delay of 48 to 72 hours.

ADVANTAGES OF DENTAL IMPLANTS

1. Aids in bone maintenance—prevents the progress of residual ridge resorption.
2. Restoration and maintenance of occlusal vertical dimension.

3. Maintenance of facial esthetics (muscle tone) Implants also provide a natural emergence profile.
4. Improved phonetics
5. Improved occlusion
6. Improved occlusal awareness
7. Improved masticatory performance, maintenance of masticatory muscles and muscles of facial expression
8. Reduced size of prosthesis (elimination of palate or flanges)
9. Provision for fixed or removable prosthesis
10. Improved stability and retention of fixed prosthesis-implants provide stable retention due to osseointegration
11. Eliminates need to alter adjacent teeth
12. More permanent replacement
13. Improved psychological health
14. Improved comfort level.

ANATOMY OR PARTS OF AN IMPLANT (FIG. 49.15)

1. *Implant body/fixture screw:* Portion of the implant system placed within the bone.
2. *Cover screw/sealing screw/healing screw/1st stage cover screw:* Seals the occlusal surface of the implant during osseointegration. Prevents the overgrowth of the tissues over and in the implant.

3. *Healing abutment/temporary gingival cuff/healing collar/ healing cap:* A dome-shaped screw that is attached to the implant in the second stage, to maintain the opening through the tissue until the restoration is completed. Length varies from 2 to 10 mm (Fig. 49.16).
4. *Healing cap/comfort cap/temporary screw/abutment healing cap (Fig. 49.17):* A cover that is attached to the top of a transmucosal abutment protecting the internal threads and interface surfaces of the abutment.
5. *Standard abutment/tissue extension/per mucosal extension/transmucosal extension (Fig. 49.18):* An intermediate component placed between the implant and metal framework/restoration providing support and retention for a fixed removable restoration.
6. *Tapered abutment/conical abutment/trans or per mucosal abutment:* An intermediate component placed between the implant and restoration, providing support and restoration for a fixed removable restoration.
7. *Hex driver/hex tool/screw driver (Fig. 49.19):* Used for placing and removing all hex screws (abutment fastening screws, impression post and healing abutments).
   Available in two lengths short for posterior and long for anterior.
8. *Abutment driver/seating tool:* Used to seat abutments directly into implants.

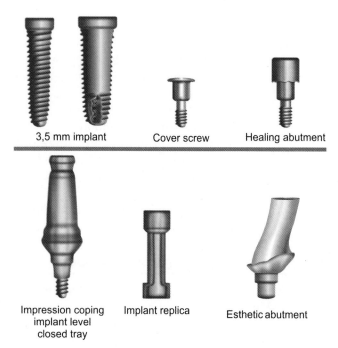

3,5 mm implant   Cover screw   Healing abutment

Impression coping implant level closed tray   Implant replica   Esthetic abutment

Fig. 49.15: Various parts for implant fixture

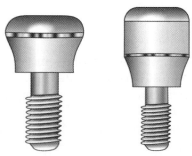

Fig. 49.16: Healing cap

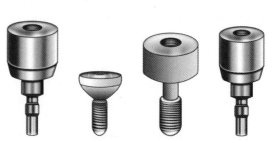

Fig. 49.17: Abutment healing cap

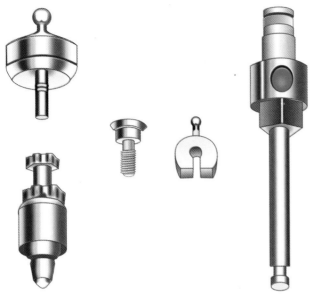

Fig. 49.18: Transmucosal extension

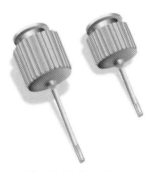

Fig. 49.19: Hex driver

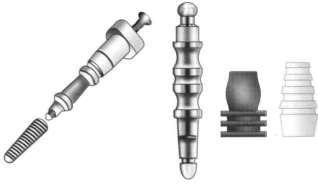

Fig. 49.20: Post and lab analog

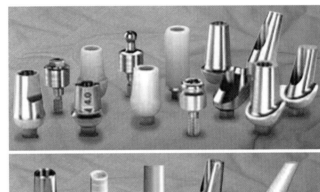

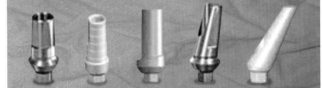

Fig. 49.21: Prosthetic abutments

9. *Impression post/impression pin/transfer pin/post/impression coping:* Component used during the impression procedure to transfer the intraoral position of the implant to the same position on the cast.

10. *Laboratory analogue/implant/abutment analogue/fixture replica/implant body analogue (Fig. 49.20):* Replicates the implant for use in the laboratory cast in order to fabricate an implant supported prosthesis.

11. *Temporary coping/cylinder or provisional abutment:* Provides support and retention for acrylic temporary and provisional restorations.

12. *Fixed abutment/straight abutment/coping abutment/ abutment post (Fig. 49.21):* An abutment used for cement retained restorations available in 15 and 25 degrees.

13. *Plastic sleeve/waxing sleeve/castable/plastic coping (Fig. 49.22):* A castable wax pattern used to form an abutment during the laboratory waxing procedure.

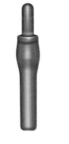

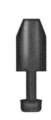

2.0 mm impression post titanium

2.0 mm impression sleeve plastic

2.0 mm implant analog titanium

Fig. 49.22: Plastic coping

14. *Gold cylinder/gold sleeve/gold coping:* Premachined abutment that is waxed and cast to its interfaces directly on to the transmucosal abutment.

15. *Prothesis retaining screw/coping screw:* Screw used to secure a screw retained metal bar framework or restoration onto transmucosal abutments (conical or standard).

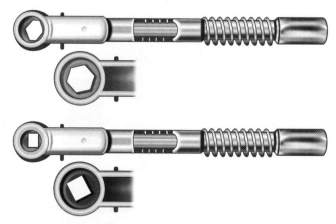

Fig. 49.23: Universal ratchet or torque wrench 10-45 Ncm

16. *Universal ratchet or torque wrench:* Used for torquing the implant and abutment (Fig. 49.23).

■ PATIENT SELECTION CRITERIA

It includes an extensive medical and dental examination, as to whether the patient is an ideal candidate for implant therapy.

Indications (Adell, Zarb and Lindquist)

1. Patients who do not accept removable prosthesis
2. Patients who lack neuromuscular control
3. Single tooth replacements
4. Where complete denture has deleterious effect on tissues
5. High gag reflex
6. Long edentulous span
7. Low tissue tolerance
8. Unfavorable number and location of abutments
9. Unrealistic expectations from complete dentures
10. When it offers to solve psychological problems associated with edentulism
11. In situations, where it can achieve superior results in terms of function and esthetics.

Absolute Contraindications/Medical/Systemic Factors

1. Boxers and wrestlers
2. Cerebral palsy patients
3. Irradiated tissues
4. Psychogenic disorders
5. Drug or alcohol dependence
6. Immunocompromised patients
7. Patients on bisphosphonate therapy
8. Uncontrolled diabetes mellitus
9. Blood dyscrasias
10. Patients who lack manual dexterity
11. Ischemic heart disease
12. Musculoskeletal disorders
13. Limited mouth opening as a sequel to oral submucous fibrosis.

Relative Contraindications

1. Smokers (smoking cessation protocol to be followed prior and after surgery)
2. Well controlled diabetes
3. Cardiac patients with stable condition
4. Patients on antidepressants or anticoagulants
5. Bruxism and tongue thrust (night guards and habit breaking appliance prior to implant therapy)
6. Trismus
7. Endocrine disorders
8. Chronic sinusitis (for implant therapy in the maxilla which may require sinus lift procedures—direct or indirect).

Intraoral Examination of a Partially Edentulous Patient

1. Length of the edentulous span.
2. Periodontal health.
3. Adequate access to edentulous areas (fixture mount connector + hand piece = 4 cm).
4. Adequate distance between adjacent teeth 2 mm on either side of the implant and sufficient bone volume.
5. Palpation and inspection of ridge crest, buccal or lingual fossa may be concave, narrow crest may require augmentation/bone splitting, knife edge or uneven crest may require mild alveoloplasty.
6. Inspection of covering mucosa whether it is normal, atrophic, thick, dense or loose crestal mucosa.
7. Bone mapping or bone sounding
8. Comparison of position of adjacent natural tooth crown to determine likely position of artificial tooth crown by a wax up (prosthetically driven implant placement).
9. Interocclusal clearance
10. Parafunctional habits (wear facets on natural teeth).

Evaluation of Occlusion

1. Freeway space path of mandibular closure
2. Absence of tooth wear facets

3. Areas of natural tooth contact to determine occlusal stability
4. Occlusal derangements or discrepancies
5. Occlusal plane/supraeruption of teeth
6. Sufficient space for abutment and prosthesis.

Intraoral Examination for Completely Edentulous Patients

1. Inspection of ridges and volume of bone
2. Palpation of ridges for sharp crest or remnants of teeth
3. Palpation for fibrous or flabby ridges and buccal and lingual concavities
4. Ridge relationship
5. Interocclusal space
6. Examination of previous dentures for short comings.

Radiographic Assessment

1. It is complementary to clinical examination
2. Provides a comprehensive analysis of the edentulous space, dentition and supporting structures
3. Reveals pathological conditions of the dentoalveolar region
4. Reveals pathological conditions of the basal bone, maxillary sinus and TMJ
5. Enables assessment of the available bone volume in three dimensions
6. Enables assessment of bone quality to some extent
7. Precisely, locates anatomical structures and boundaries such as inferior alveolar nerve, incisive canal, nasal cavity, maxillary sinus
8. Enables measurement of limiting bone height and width
9. Enables selection of optimal site and angulation for implant placement
10. Enables selection of implant system, length and width of the implant
11. Minimizes risk during surgery.

Periapical Radiographs Aids in Assessing

1. Interradicular space
2. Infection in adjacent teeth or bone
3. Identifying critical structures
4. Limited value in determining quantity of bone and bone density
5. Used primarily for single tooth implant therapy in regions of abundant bone height and width.

Cephalometric Radiograph

1. Demonstrates the geometry of the alveolus in the anterior region and the relationship of the lingual plate to the patients skeletal anatomy.
2. Loss of vertical dimension, skeletal interarch relation and crown to implant ratio may be ascertained.

Panoramic Radiographs

1. Opposing landmarks can be identified
2. Vertical height of bone can be assessed
3. Gross anatomy of the jaws and related pathological findings
4. General dental status
5. Can be used to identify implant location
6. Monitor prosthetic outcome.

◼ COMPUTED TOMOGRAPHY

It provides imaging analysis of the proposed surgery by enabling the exact evaluation of the proposed implant site in relation to height, width, bone density, distance from vital structures, position and orientation of implants. As implant surgery must be prosthetically driven, a diagnostic template may be used during imaging—these diagnostic templates may be an acrylic reproduction of a diagnostic wax up using radiopaque denture teeth or coated with a thin film of barium sulfate or by filling a hole drilled with gutta percha through the occlusal surface of denture teeth, thus rendering them radiopaque. This procedure results in a natural tooth like appearance to the proposed restoration in the CT scan, which helps to precisely identify the position and orientation of the proposed implant. This diagnostic template may latter be modified into a surgical template.

Cone Beam Computer Tomography

Cone beam computer tomography (CBCT) is a medical imaging technique, that has become increasingly important in treatment planning and diagnosis in implant dentistry. The advantage over the regular CT scan is that the patient is in a seated position and sectional areas may be scanned, thus reducing radiation exposure to the patients. During CBCT, the scanner rotates around the patients head obtaining up to 600 distinct images. The scanning software collects the data and reconstructs it composed of three dimensional voxels of anatomic data that can then be manipulated and visualized using specialized software.

Interactive Computer Tomography

It is a technique, which enables the practitioner to view and interact with the images received either from CT or CBCT scans. There are specialized softwares, which can convert the dentascan images, so that the dentist can perform electronic surgery by selecting and placing arbitrary size cylinders that simulate root form implants, enables determination of bone quality, quantity, critical structures, prospective occlusion and esthetics, implant position and orientation. The number and size of implants can be accurately determined using the interactive software. A three dimensional computer generated surgical template may be constructed from a steriolithographic model based on this digital data (Figs 49.24A and B).

Basic Treatment Order

Decision regarding the treatment order may vary, based on the degree of difficulty. But, for cases involving a traditional plan, the following may be used.

1. Examination—clinical and radiographic/medical history/pathological test, etc.
2. Diagnostic set up, provisional restoration and specialized radiographs (CBCT), if required
3. Discussion of treatment options with the patient and mutual consent on final restoration
4. Completion of any adjunctive necessary treatment such as extraction of hopeless teeth, periodontal treatment, restorative or endodontic treatment
5. Fabrication of provisional or transitional restorations
6. Fabrication of surgical guide or stent
7. Surgical placement of implants
8. Allow adequate time for osseointegration based on bone quality and loading protocol
9. Prosthodontics phase
10. Maintenance phase

■ ARMAMENTARIUM FOR IMPLANT SURGERY (FIG. 49.25)

- Operator gowns/patient gowns/head cap/masks/sterile gloves
- Suction apparatus
- Blood pressure apparatus and pulse oximeter
- Disposable needles and syringes.
- Autoclaved implant surgical kit
- LA cartridges, needles
- Mouth retractors
- Mosquito forceps
- Periodontal probe
- mouth mirror, explorer
- Periosteal elevator
- scissor
- Tissue holding forceps
- Curettes
- Suction tips
- Needle holder
- BP blade handle and blades no 11, 15
- Bone gauge

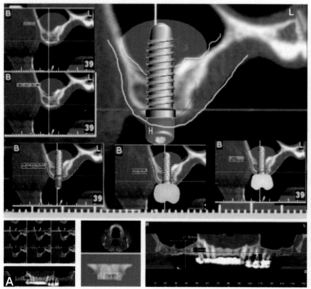
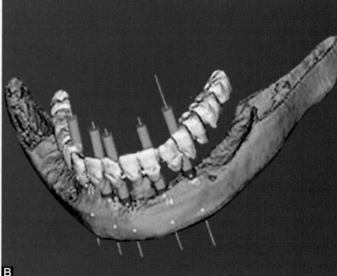

Figs 49.24A and B: Clinical use of interactive computer tomography

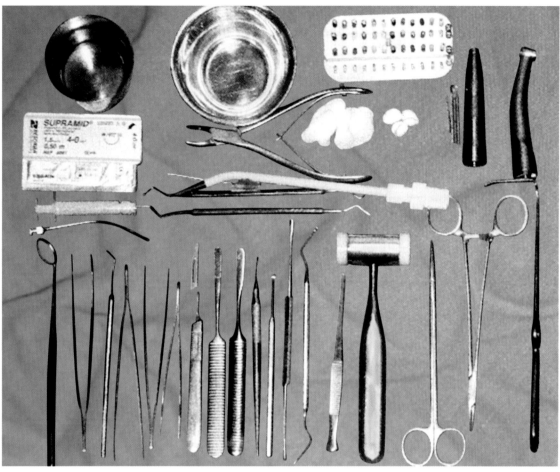

Fig. 49.25: Instruments/armamentarium for implants surgery

- Osteotomes
- Suture material (vicryl/polypropylene)
- Physiodispensor and reduction handpiece (20:1)—a physiodispensor is a must. The basic requirements are minimum torque of 70 Ncm to 1500 rpm speed, reduction gear of 16:1, integrated pulsating pump for sterile solution, stand for saline solution bottle.

BASIC FACTORS IN IMPLANT SURGERY

1. A sterile technique, avoiding any contamination of the implant surface.
2. Avoid damage to the bone by thermal injury during the drilling process.
3. Careful preparation of the osteotomy, so that the implant is stable on placement.
4. Placement of the implant in an esthetic and prosthetically driven position.
5. Avoidance of excessive loading during the healing period depending on the type of implant used and the loading protocol followed.

Avoidance of Thermal Injury to the Bone

Bone cells are irreversibly damaged if the temperature of the bone is raised above 47 degrees for more than 1 minute, resulting in bone necrosis, extensive resorption and failure of osseointegration.

This may be avoided by:
1. Careful cooling of bone and drills with copious sterile saline solution using internal or external irrigation through a physiodispenser.
2. Use of sharp drills
3. Control of cutting speeds (1500-2000 rpm)
4. In all implant systems, the implant site is first prepared using a pilot drill to mark the position

of the implant and then the site is gradually made larger with increasing diameter drills of the ascertained length. In addition to minimizing heat production, the initial use of small diameter drills allows for small changes in implant position and modification of angle if required.

Ensuring good initial or primary stability is one of the main aims of surgical preparation. This can be judged by:

1. Clinical examination
2. Minimum torque insertion of 45 N-cm
3. Perio test where the mobility is measured using an electronic device
4. Resonance frequency analysis—is one of the latest devices that measures the stability of the implant within the bone through vibration and recording.

An implant which is loose in the prepared site will never osseointegrate. In the initial healing phase the implant must not be subjected to movement, micromovement of 100 micron meter may lead to osseointegration, but beyond that there will be fibrous encapsulation and implant failure.

Initial primary stability of an implant depends on the:

1. Length of the implant
2. Diameter of the implant
3. Design of the implant
4. Surface characteristics of the implant
5. Thickness of the bone cortex and how many cortices the implant engages
6. Density of the medullary bone trabeculation
7. Dimension of the preparation site compared to the implant size.

PLACEMENT OF THE IMPLANT IN AN ACCEPTABLE POSITION

1. Careful treatment planning/case selection
2. Use of surgical stents
3. Reviewing each stage of the preparation process
4. Surgical templates/stents (Figs 49.26A to D) should be constructed using diagnostic set ups or provisional prosthesis. They should be rigid and stable. The stent helps the surgeon to ascertain the mesio-distal, buccolingual position and angulation. When replacing anterior teeth, it is important to profile the buccal aspect of the prosthesis, to plan emergence profile and optimize esthetics.

The surgical stents may be bone supported, teeth supported, tissue supported.

5. The stages of implant placement can be reviewed using indicator posts in the prepared sites for determination of the length of the osteotomy.
6. Paralleling pins may also be used to review parallism of multiple implants prior to the final osteotomy drill. Failure to do so may result in surprising errors.
7. The indicator post should also be reviewed in relation to opposing dentition, e.g. in patients with normal buccopalatal relation. The maxillary indicator should be directed towards the buccal cusp of the lower teeth and mandibular indicators towards the palatal cusp of maxillary teeth. This ensures that the implant is placed in the central fossa of the opposing tooth and forces are directed along the long axis of the implant.

PREOPERATIVE CARE

1. Oral prophylaxis and antiseptic rinsing of the oral cavity with the solution such as chlorhexidine gluconate 1.2/2 percent for 1 minute and perioral skin preparation with betadine scrub.
2. Administration of antibiotics standard protocol of 3 g of amoxicillin preoperatively followed by a 5 days course
3. Oral analgesics (200-400 mg) of Ibuprofen or comparable alternatives.

ANESTHESIA

Local anesthesia is generally sufficient, depending on the skill of the clinician and attitude of the patient.

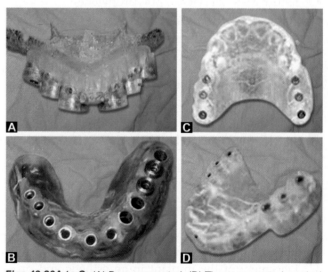

Figs 49.26A to C: (A) Bone supported, (B) Tissue supported surgical stents (C and D) Teeth supported

Sedation techniques may also be considered. The advantage of local anesthesia, is that the conscious patient is able to co-operate by performing normal jaw movements in centric and lateral excursions to verify appropriate implant positioning. The vasoconstrictor in local anesthesia provides local hemostasis. Full mouth rehabilitation or extensive grafting procedures may warrant the use of general anesthesia.

INCISIONS

1. A midcrestal incision is employed in most cases. The incision can be extended within the gingival crevices of adjacent teeth and mucoperiosteum elevated in an apical direction to allow adequate visualization of the bone contour.
2. Relieving incisions may aid flap reflection, they must be kept vertical and parallel to the overlying sound bone, so that on closure, blood supply is not compromised.
3. Obliquely inclined relieving incisions should be avoided over prominent root surfaces as it could lead to wound dehiscence and gingival recession.
4. Relieving incisions must also be done carefully over anatomical structures as injury to vital nerves could result in bleeding or paresthesia.
5. The crestal incision may be located palatally in the maxillary arch, where there is more keratinized tissue and also in cases, where bone augmentation and graft material or membranes have to be placed on the labial aspect.
6. In single tooth implants, it is prudent to preserve the papilla for the sake of esthetics, but if the mesiodistal space is narrow, then elevation of the papilla becomes unavoidable hence the following is recommended.
   i. In sites less than or equal to 7 mm mesiodistally, reflect the papilla
   ii. In sites 8 mm or greater, a mesiodistal crestal incision of 5 to 6 mm, will allow nonreflection of an adequate width of papillary tissue
   iii. If anatomical structures are present, such as incisive nerve or augmentation techniques are indicated then a wider flap design involving the papilla is indicated.
7. In edentulous maxilla or mandible, a midline labial relieving incision extending into the sulcus enables the surgeon to elevate under the periosteum more easily, especially when the crest of the ridge is knife edged or uneven. The relieving incision also reduces tension on the buccal flap and makes retraction easier.

BASIC FLAP DESIGN AND SOFT TISSUE HANDLING

Some operators recommend implant placement without flap elevation, but this can readily lead to lateral perforation of the bone in inexperienced hands. Flapless procedure is more suited to single implants in extraction sockets or when using tissue supported surgical templates which have been derived accurately via CAD/CAM from steriolithographic models.

i. Flap design and elevation should achieve complete exposure of the edentulous ridge including bone concavities and identification of anatomic structures.
ii. Elevation of flaps is best accomplished using periosteal elevator with a flat sharp edge. Fibrous and muscle attachments that tether the flap margins, may need to be relieved by sharp dissection.
iii. Good flap reflection on the lingual side of the lower premolars is advised, as implant preparation may perforate the lingual plate in a natural concavity and damage a branch of the sublingual artery.
iv. Before closure of the flap, it is important to check that there is no residual bone debris, by careful irrigation with sterile saline and inspection with suction.
v. Flap should be closed with minimum tension with resorbable or nonresorbable sutures. 4-0 vicryl sutures may be used. Vertical mattress sutures over grafted sites for a more secure seal, can be used. Gortex, poly propylene 5-0 or 6-0, 7-0 sutures are also recommended, but require special micro-surgical instruments and use of dental loops by the operator.

POSTOPERATIVE INSTRUCTIONS

1. No spitting or gargling, drinking with a straw (in case of maxillary sinus lift procedures)
2. No smoking or alcohol consumption
3. Fingers and tongue should be kept away from the surgical area
4. Follow the antibiotic and anti-inflammatory regimen
5. Ice pack application extraorally
6. Sleep with the head slightly elevated to reduce swelling
7. Avoid brushing in the surgical area
8. A fairly soft diet must be maintained, avoid hard and crusty food

9. Addition of multivitamin supplements and 500 mg of vitamin C
10. Rinsing with chlorhexidine or saline after meals from the 2nd postoperative day
11. In case of maxillary posterior implants, avoid swimming and blowing through the nose
12. Temporary prosthesis may require periodic adjust. ments; old dentures may be worn after adequate soft lining procedures.

ABUTMENT CONNECTION

The abutment connection surgery in a two stage protocol it is carried out after three months in the mandible and 6 months in the maxilla (Brånemark):

The fixture may be exposed by
- Scalpel technique
- Tissue punch technique
- Laser technique

A long incision along the crest, exposing all fixtures in case of multiple implants or a smaller individual incision over each fixture, where there is ample keratinized tissue. On exposure, the cover screw is removed and healing caps are placed for one week or until there is a good formation of gingival cuff for good emergence profile of the prosthesis. This is then followed by the prosthetic phase, wherein the healing cap is removed and impression post is placed during the impression procedures either by the open or closed tray technique.

SURGICAL COMPLICATIONS OF IMPLANT THERAPY

I. **Preoperative conditions that may lead to complications:**
   - Inadequate vertical and horizontal restorative space
   - Limited jaw opening and interarch distance
   - Inadequate alveolar width for optimal buccolingual position.

II. **Intraoperative complications in implant placement**
   - Incorrect angulations (buccolingual and mesiodistal)
   - Malalignment
   - Nerve injury
   - Irregular sharp or too narrow crestal ridge
   - Extensive resorption of mandibular alveolar bone, curved extraction socket
   - Acute or chronic infection at insertion site
   - Overheating the bone at the time of implant preparation
   - Sinus and nasal floor perforation
   - Accidental, partial or complete displacement of dental implants in the maxillary sinus, maxillary incisive canal.
   - Deep or shallow implant placement.

   Complications in flapless implant placement
   - Implant fracture
   - Excessive torque during insertion/compression leading to necrosis
   - Inadequate primary stability or loose implant.

III. **Postoperative complications**
   - Postoperative pain and its management
   - Incision line opening. (improper suture technique)
   - Cover screw exposure during healing period
   - Bone loss during healing period/thread exposure
   - Implant mobility during second stage surgery
   - Implant periapical lesion and retrograde periimplantitis, radiotherapy and dental implants/osteoradionecrosis
   - Shallow vestibule secondary to ridge augmentation.

Diagnosis and Management of Complications

Wound Dehiscense

If the cover screw is exposed or a portion of the implant head, the area must be kept clean with 0.2-0.12 percent chlorhexidine rinse to prevent inflammation and marginal bone loss. The situation may be improved by changing the cover screw to a healing abutment.

Early Implant Failure

Most surgical failures of osseointegration are due to poor surgical technique or placement of implants into bone of poor density or lack of bone volume.

Damage to bone, resulting in necrosis, pain and subsequent infection is more likely, where dense bone has been prepared with inadequate cooling and blunt drills. It is more likely in preparations deeper than 13 mm. The resultant pain can be severe and can lead to a deep seated track through soft tissues.

Damage to Neurovascular Structures

Loss of sensation to the lower lip caused by trauma to the inferior dental or mental nerve (Fig. 49.27).

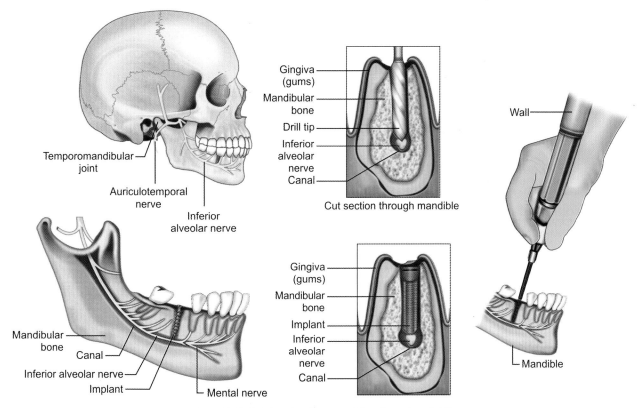

Fig. 49.27: Inferior alveolar nerve injury from dental drill

To avoid this complication:
- Infiltration rather than block anesthesia
- Avoid relieving incisions in the region of the mental nerve
- No crestal incisions over superficially located mental foramen in severely resorbed mandible
- Adequately expose, identify and protect the nerve when operating close to it
- Check for anterior loops of the nerve, by radiography
- Careful planning through CT scan
- Careful measurement of height and width of bone above the canal
- Avoid thermal damage to the bone left between the implant tip and nerve canal.

Fractures

Severely resorbed mandible may be compromised by implant placement, such that a fracture occurs at the time of surgery or a short time thereafter. CT scans must be used to assess severity of the resorbed mandible to avoid placement of too many implants within the zones of low bone volume (e.g. mandibular 1st premolar region)

Soft Tissue Complications

The mucosa around the abutments should be free from inflammation and bleeding or exudate, probing depth must be evaluated at regular intervals with clinical examination along with radiographic evaluation (Figs 49.28 and 49.29).

Surgical correction of soft tissue problems may be required in case of:
- Soft tissue overgrowth
- Soft tissue deficiency
- Persistent inflammation/infection
- Continuing bone loss

In case of soft tissue hyperplasia: Simple excision may be required to thin out the excess tissue, but preserve the keratinized tissue to produce a zone of attached mucosa around the abutments. This may occur around poorly designed embrasures or bar attachments in over dentures.

Soft tissue deficiency: In cases of severe bone loss, non-keratinized mucosa appears redder and delicate and may lack attachment to underlying bone. Persistent soreness and inflammation can be overcome by grafting

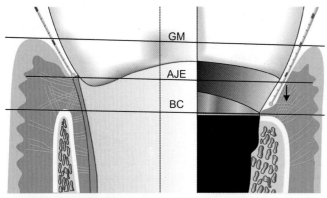

Fig. 49.28: Different probe depths in the natural tooth and in the implant, caused by the absence of direct fiber insertion into the titanium. GM—gingival margin, AJE—apical junctional epithelium, BC—bone crest

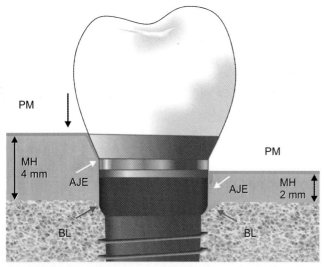

Fig. 49.29: Comparison of the normal peri-implant gingival condition with a peri-implant mucosa that is too thin, resulting in peri-implant bone resorption. PM—marginal portion of the peri-implant mucosa, MH—mucosal height in mm. AJE—apical junctional epithelium, BL—degree of wedge shaped peri-implant bone loss

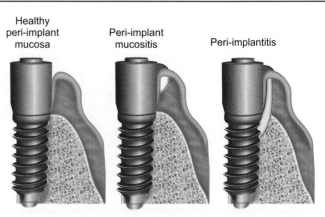

Fig. 49.30: Soft tissue problems following implant surgery

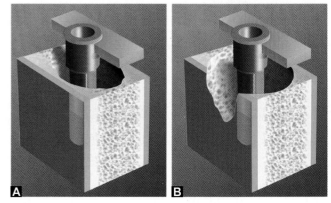

Figs 49.31A and B: (A) Bowl shaped defect, (B) Funnel-shaped defect

keratinized mucosa such as a free gingival graft from the palate.

Persistant inflammation: May arise due to poor implant positioning. This may require soft tissue recontouring to allow patient hygiene and soft tissue esthetics.

Peri-implantitis (Fig. 49.30): It is an inflammatory lesion which has caused obvious bone loss, the marginal soft tissue will appear inflamed. Bacterial colonization is one of the prime factors which may be induced due to:
- Poor oral hygiene
- Cement retained in the subgingival area
- Microscopic gaps between implant components
- Inflammation, exudation and soft tissue proliferation
- Wide saucerization areas of bone loss on the radiograph.

Spiekermann's Classification of Defects Following Periimplantitis (Figs 49.31A and B)

Class I—Horizontal defect
Class II—Bowl shaped defect
Class III—Funnel shaped defect

NONSURGICAL MANAGEMENT OF PERIMPLANTITIS

- Mechanical cleaning of implant surface—with curettes of titanium or steel or prophy jets.
  Local medicaments:
  - Chlorhexidine chips (perio chips)

– Chlorhexidine lavage/citric acid or powder jet devices
– Local doxycycline or metronidazole gel application
– Ligosan—260 mg slow release ligosan or 12 days direct delivery
- *Laser decontamination*—with either CO_2 or erbium – Yag laser of 1.5 w frequency.
- *Photodynamic therapy*—Photochemical decontamination of peri-implant tissues and implant surface with a photosensitizer dye in combination with laser light.
- Ozone therapy
- *Systemic antibiotics:* Metronidazole 400 mg TDS + Amoxicillin 500 mg TDS for 7 days or clindamycin 300/600 mg 4 times a day for 7 days.

SURGICAL MANAGEMENT OF PERIMPLANTITIS

- Resective therapy—Clean the exposed implant surface with the above mentioned chemical agents. Polish the implant surface with Arkansas stone. Resection of periimplant soft tissue and readapt the mucosal flap with connective tissue attachment.
- Regenerative therapy (as yet only experimental)— Guided bone regeneration, autologous bone, bone substitute and membrane.

ABSOLUTE INDICATION FOR EXPLANTATION (TABLE 49.2)

- Mobility of implant with advanced bone depletion
- Therapy resistant peri-implantitis

Prosthetic Complications

Screw loosening, fixture fracture, abutment loosening may be a sign of implant overload due to:
- Poorly fitting prosthesis
- Poorly designed cantilevers
- Poor implant to crown ratio
- Inadequate occlusal adjustments
- Too few number of implants to establish adequate occlusal table
- Uncontrolled parafunctional activity.

Table 49.2: Statistical review of implant failure causes

Reason for implant failure	
Periimplantitis	75%
Insufficient maintenance by patient	58%
Insufficient maxillary bone	44%
Prosthetic difficulties [other than premature loading]	33%
Premature loading	29%
Illness/systemic disease	29%
Insufficient maintenance by doctor	28%
Insufficient mandibular bone	19%
Increased periodontal involvement throughout mouth	16%
Bone augmentation needed but not initially provided	15%

LONG TERM MAINTENANCE PROTOCOL FOR IMPLANTS

Patient's Role

- Maintain plaque control
- Use interdental brush, waterpik, etc.
- Dip brush in 0.12 percent solution of chlorhexidine
- Use floss/yarn/tapes dipped in chlorhexidine at night
- Use cotton swab dipped in chlorhexidine for implants with tooth color materials or composites.

Dental Hygienist's Role

- Check for effectiveness of plaque control
- Check for inflammatory changes
- If pathological conditions are present, probe gently with plastic probe (sensor)
- Scale supragingivally or slightly subgingivally with impla care, implant prophy
- Check for loose suprastructure, broken screw or sore spots.

Dentist's Role

- Check patient every 4 months
- Check for 85 percent plaque control effectiveness
- Radiographs every 12 to 18 months, if no pathological condition is present or as required, if pathology is present

- If implant needs repair, degranulate, detoxify and graft with guided bone regeneration if required. Wait for 10 to 12 weeks before loading implant into function
- Document all data.

▋ BIBLIOGRAPHY

1. Branemark PI, Zarb GA, Albrektsson T. Osseointegration in clinical dentistry. Chicago: Quintessence Publishing.
2. Carl E Misch. Dental implant prosthetics.
3. Grondhal K, Lekholm U. Predictive value of radiographic diagnosis of implant stability. Int J Oral Maxillofacial implants 1997;12:59-64.
4. Implant in clinical dentistry-Martin Dunitz.
5. Mombelli A, Lang NP. Diagnosis and treatment of peri-implantitis, periodontal 2000;17:63-76.
6. Shillingburg HT, Hobo S, Whitsett LD. Fundamentals of fixed prosthodontics. Chicago: Quintessence Publishing.
7. Smith RA, Berger Dodson TB (1992). Risk factors associated with dental implants in healthy and medically compromised patients. Int J Oral Maxillofacial implants 1992;7:367-72.

Hemorrhage and Shock

50

Hemorrhage and Shock: Its Management in Oral Surgery

HEMORRHAGE

Hemorrhage (Hemo + rrhage) denotes the escape of blood from a blood vessel. The word hemorrhage is synonymous with bleeding. Any damage to the vasculature leads to outflow of blood. Blood carries oxygen and nutrients to the tissues and is vital for body functions. Loss of blood due to any reason beyond a certain point is potentially life threatening and may lead to exsanguination.

This chapter provides an overview of the coagulation system, with emphasis on control of bleeding in oral surgery patients, who are otherwise normal or are having acquired or hereditary bleeding disorders. In this section, shock occurring as a result of blood loss and its management is also described.

Types of Hemorrhage

Depending on the Type of Blood Vessel Involved

Depending on the type of blood vessel involved, hemorrhage can be arterial, venous or capillary.
1. *In arterial hemorrhage*, there is bleeding from a ruptured artery. Arterial bleeding is pulsatile, brisk and bright red in color.
2. Loss of blood from a vein is known as *venous hemorrhage*. Bleeding from veins is dark in color and blood flows in a even stream. Due to lack of valves in veins of the facial region and extensive communication, there is relatively more flow from these veins as compared to other parts of body.
3. Oozing from the capillaries is known as *capillary hemorrhage*. In capillary hemorrhage, blood oozes from the area and no bleeding point can be made out. The blood is bluish bright red in color as compared to arterial and venous blood. Bleeding is not severe and is easily controlled by simple pressure with gauze pads. In coagulation disorders, there can be extensive blood loss from capillaries.

Primary, Reactionary, Intermediate Bleeding and Secondary Bleeding

1. *Primary bleeding* occurs at the time of injury. Hemostatic mechanisms in the body attempt to stop the bleeding by formation of a clot.
2. If the primary bleeding has stopped once, and wound starts to bleed again after 24 hours to several days, it is known as *secondary bleeding*. It may be due to: (a) dislodgement of clot or (b) secondary trauma to the wound, (c) infection is also the most common reason for secondary bleeding. Infection causes softening of the blood clot or even erosion of the vessel wall. Attempt to control bleeding by

ligating the bleeding vessel may fail as the ligature may easily cut through softened infected tissues, (d) elevation of patient's blood pressure enough to overcome pressure external to blood vessel is another common reason for secondary bleeding.

3. According to some authors bleeding occurring within eight hours after stoppage of primary bleeding is labeled as *intermediate bleeding*. Loose foreign body in the wound like calculus, broken bone piece, and pre-existing extensive granulation tissues in the extraction socket are the most common causes for the intermediate bleeding.

Internal or External Bleeding

Bleeding that is confined within the body cavity and is not apparent on the surface is known as (i) *internal or concealed bleeding*. Whereas, blood escaping through a wound in the skin is known as (ii) *external bleeding*.

Spontaneous Bleeding

Sometimes bleeding can occur without any provocation, e.g. in acquired (patients on oral hypoglycemic agents—decreased platelets count) and hereditary coagulopathies, such type of bleeding is labeled as *spontaneous bleeding*.

Hemostasis

It is important to understand the mechanism of stoppage of bleeding. There are four important steps in hemostasis:

1. First of all, the injured blood vessel, in an attempt to reduce blood flow undergoes constriction due to spasm in the vessel wall.
2. In the second step, there is activation of platelets and formation of platelet plug. This leads to primary hemostasis.
3. In the third step, there is activation of clotting mechanism and formation of clot leading to completion of secondary hemostasis.
4. In the final step, there is fibrous organization of the clot or retraction of clot.

Primary Hemostasis

Primary hemostasis is the process of platelet plug formation at the site of injury. It occurs within seconds of injury and is important in stoppage of blood from small arterioles, venules and capillaries. There is platelet adhesion, release of granules and platelet aggregation resulting in formation of a primary hemostatic plug.

Secondary Hemostasis

Secondary hemostasis is the activation of clotting process in plasma, that ultimately results in the formation of fibrin, which strengthens the primary hemostatic plug. It is completed in several minutes and is important in bleeding from larger vessels. Coagulation mechanism is a continuous process and there are approximately 40 substances, which affect clotting, some promote clotting called procoagulants and others prevent clotting called anticoagulants. Normally, there is fine balance between these factors and blood usually does not coagulate inside the body. Whenever there is an injury to the vessels these procoagulant factors are activated and balance tilts in favor of coagulation and there is formation of a clot. There is a complex interaction of various factors of coagulation in the formation of a clot (Table 50.1) (Flow chart 50.1).

For the purpose of simplicity and understanding, coagulation mechanism can be broken into a series of 4 reactions:

Reaction 1: This is intrinsic or contact phase of coagulation. In this phase, mainly factors VIII, IX, XI, XII along with calcium and plasma proteins take part. Partial thromboplastin time (PTT) screens this intrinsic limb of the coagulation.

Reaction 2: This is extrinsic pathway for initiation of coagulation. In this phase, there is release of tissue thromboplastin from injured tissues. A protease complex is formed between factor VII, calcium and tissue thromboplastin, which activates factor X and takes part in reaction III—the common pathway. Prothrombin time (PT) {laboratory test} screens the extrinsic limb of coagulation.

Reaction 3: In this phase, factor X is activated by proteases generated in previous two reactions.

Reaction 4: In this phase, prothrombin is converted into thrombin in the presence of factor V, calcium and phospholipids. Thrombin has got multiple functions in hemostasis. Its main role is conversion of fibrinogen into fibrin, but it also further activates factor V, VIII and XIII and helps in platelet aggregation and secretion. Flow chart 50.1 summarizes all these reactions of coagulation cascade.

	Table 50.1: List of coagulation factors and their important features			
	Factors name	*Half-life*	*Biosynthesis*	*Vitamin K dependency*
I	Fibrinogen	1.5–6.3 days	Liver	No
II	Prothrombin	2–4 days	Liver, brain	Yes
III	Tissue factor	Unknown	—	No
IV	Calcium	—	—	No
V	Proaccelerin, labile	12–24 hours	Liver, megakaryocytes	No
VII	Proconvertin	1–5 hours	Liver	Yes
VIII	Antihemophilic factor	8–12 hours	Liver, spleen, endothelium, reticuloendothelial cells	No
IX	Christmas factor	15–24 hours	Liver	Yes
X	Stuart-Prower factor	2–9 hours	Liver	Yes
XI	Plasma thromboplastin antecedent	40–84 hours	Liver	No
XII	Hageman factor	48–52 hours	Liver	No
XIII	Fibrin-stabilizing factor	4.5–12 days	Liver, megakaryocytes	No

Flow chart 50.1: Coagulation cascade

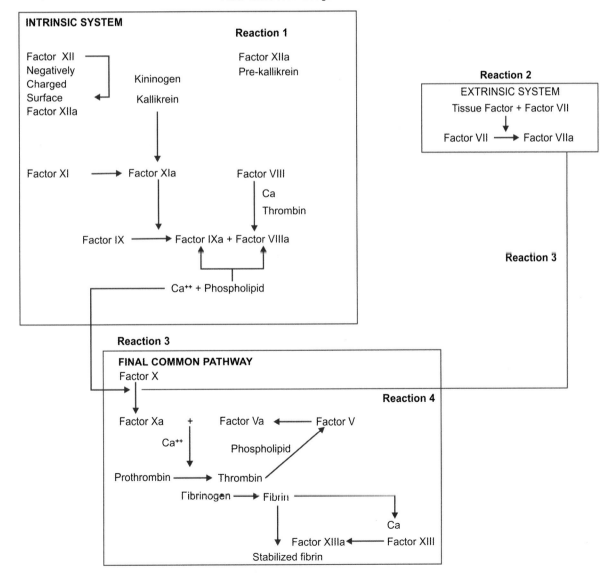

Clinical Evaluation of the Bleeding Patient

Careful evaluation of the patient with co-ordinated history and physical examination provides valuable clues as to whether the bleeding abnormality resides in: (a) the vessels walls, (b) platelets or (c) in the process of coagulation. Laboratory tests should supplement and not supersede a careful review of history and physical examination. The history should include the following questions:

1. Is there any personal or family history of a bleeding tendency?
2. Has the patient undergone surgery or dental extractions previously?
3. Is there any history of hematuria, gastrointestinal hemorrhage, easy bruising, hemarthrosis, menorrhagia, or epistaxis?
4. Is there any history of cancer or collagen vascular disease?
5. What medications is the patient taking or has taken recently?
6. Is the patient on any special diet?

A careful physical examination should note any adenopathy, splenomegaly, or hepatomegaly. Hepatic insufficiency should be assessed by seeking signs of jaundice, telangiectasias, gynecomastia, testicular atrophy, or any other stigma of liver disease. Assessment of the skin and mucosal surface is mandatory.

Bleeding into superficial skin and soft tissues usually seen as small capillary hemorrhages ranging from size of pinhead (petechia) to large areas of ecchymoses is usually characteristic of abnormalities of the vessels or the platelets. Hemorrhage into synovial joints is virtually diagnostic of a severe hereditary coagulation disorder.

Laboratory Tests for Screening

Majority of defects of hemostasis can be screened by four basic tests.

Bleeding Time

Bleeding time (BT) is a sensitive measure of platelet function. Usually there is a linear relationship between platelet count and bleeding time. Patients with bleeding time more than 10 minutes have increased risk of bleeding. There are various methods of measuring bleeding time, e.g. Ivy, Duke and template. It should be performed by expert technicians and small differences in technique have, a big effect on outcome. BT is prolonged in thrombocytopenia, Von Willebrand's disease and platelet dysfunction.

Platelet Count

Normal platelet count is 1,50,000 to 4,50,000 per cumm of the blood. When count becomes 50,000 to 1,00,000 per cumm, there is mild prolongation of bleeding time, so that bleeding occurs after severe trauma, or surgery. Patients with count less than 50,000 per cumm have easy bruising manifested as petechia and ecchymoses during trauma or surgery. Patients with platelet count below 20,000 per cumm have an appreciable incidence of spontaneous bleeding, which may be intracranial or any other internal bleeding.

Minor oral surgical procedure can be safely done, if platelet count is above 80,000 to 1,00,000 per cumm, otherwise patient needs transfusion of platelet rich plasma.

Prothrombin Time

Prothrombin time (PT) screens the extrinsic limb of coagulation pathway (Factors V, VII and X) and factors I, II and V of the common pathway. It is prolonged in patients, who are on warfarin anticoagulant therapy, vitamin K deficiency or deficiency of factor V, VII, X, prothrombin or fibrinogen. The results obtained from prothrombin time must be related to control value. Normal PT is usually 12 to 14 seconds. As a general guideline for dental procedures, the PT should be less than 1½ of the control value.

Partial Thromboplastin Time

Partial thromboplastin time (PTT) screens the intrinsic limb of coagulation pathway and tests for the adequacy of factors VIII, IX, X, XI, XII of intrinsic system and factors I, II, V of the common pathway. It is prolonged in hemophiliacs.

Both the tests PT and PTT together also screen the common coagulation pathway involving all the reactions, that occur after activation of factor X. If both the tests are prolonged, then factor II, V, X or vitamin K deficiency and liver disease are suspected. Normal PTT is less than 45 seconds. It is important to note that PTT is relatively insensitive to changes in the intrinsic coagulation system. A 70 percent decrease in factor levels may still provide normal results; small changes in PTT therefore, may be of great significance.

When abnormalities are noted in any of the screening tests, further specific tests (like bioassays of coagulation factors) are carried out in consultation with the hematologist to get the exact diagnosis.

Hemostatic agents can be (i) local and (ii) systemic.

Local Hemostatic Measures

In a patient with normal coagulation mechanism, the control of hemorrhage is dependent on vessel contraction, retraction, and clot formation. During any surgical procedure, complete hemostasis must be achieved before closure of the wound. Direct control of bleeding at the site of injury is the best method to achieve hemostasis. Surgical bleeding most of the times is caused by ineffective local hemostasis. The techniques for local hemostasis may be classified as (i) mechanical, (ii) thermal or (iii) chemical.

Mechanical Methods

Pressure: Application of pressure basically counteracts the hydrostatic pressure within the bleeding vessel until such time, that a clot can form and occlude the bleeding orifice. Pressure is usually able to control most of the hemorrhages. Pressure should be applied directly over the bleeding site firmly over a gauze pack for at least five minutes. One should not be in a hurry and should not lift pack every minute to see whether bleeding has stopped or not. Post-traumatic nasopharyngeal bleeding or pharyngeal bleeding due to maxillofacial trauma can be controlled by nasal packing. Sometimes posterior nasopharyngeal pack is required. This can be easily achieved with the use of a no. 20 Foley's catheter. The catheter is inserted through one nostril into the nasopharynx and balloon is inflated with approximately 30 ml of saline. When traction is applied, the balloon will lodge in the nasopharynx and tamponade the bleeding. Along with this, anterior nasal packing can be done, if bleeding point is located anterior to the pressure area. In fractures of mandible, bleeding from inferior dental artery usually stops spontaneously or with the help of pressure packs. Severe maxillofacial bleeding due to facial fractures, may be tamponaded with temporary or definitive reduction and fixation of the fractures.

Use of hemostats: Hemostat (Mosquito, artery) forceps are specially designed to catch bleeding points in the surgical area. These can be straight or curved. Curved hemostats are used more frequently, because of their versatility and ease in tying the ligature around the tip of forceps. Usually electrosurgical thermocoagulation is done after catching the bleeding point with artery forceps, if the vessel is small. The large vessels are ligated with suture.

Sutures and ligation: Transected blood vessel may need to be tied with the help of ligature. When large pulsatile artery needs to be tied, nonabsorbable material like 3-0 black silk is preferred. Smaller vessels can be ligated with 3-0 catgut, or polygalactin. The presence of nonabsorbable material in an infected wound can lead to extrusion or sinus tract formation. Large arteries with pulsation, such as external carotid artery, should have double transfixion suture passed through the wall of vessel to prevent chances of slipping of ligature. Ligation of major vessels in maxillofacial region is further described in detail in the subsequent text.

Embolization of the vessels: With the help of angiography, the exact bleeding point can be localized. Agents which can be used for embolization include steel coils, polyvinyl alcohol foam, gel foam, silicon spheres and methyl methacrylate. These particles are placed via a catheter superselectively into the bleeding vessel usually via femoral artery. The femoral artery is percutaneously punctured. A guidewire is then inserted into the vessel followed by a 100 cm long catheter. This catheter can be maneuvered into various branches of the external carotid artery under constant fluoroscopic control. Vessels that are usually investigated and catheterized for treatment of oral and perioral lesions include the facial, lingual, transverse facial and internal maxillary arteries. After the individual vessels are identified, contrast media is injected via the catheter and films are obtained. After the lesions are completely mapped angiographically, the angiograms are studied and embolization of the bleeding vessel can be carried out by various agents. The major risk is deposition of stray particles into normal territories via transcranial collaterals including internal carotid system and vertebral arteries. Careful mapping of the involved vessels and superselective technique reduces the risk of misplaced embolic material significantly.

Thermal Agents

Cautery: Heat achieves hemostasis by denaturation of proteins which results in coagulation of large areas of tissue. In cauterization, heat is transmitted from the instrument by conduction directly to the tissues. Electrocautery has replaced direct heat application. When an electrosurgery unit is not available, dental burnisher like instrument can be directly heated over a flame and applied directly to the bleeding point in the oral cavity.

Electrosurgery: In electrocautery, heating occurs by induction from an alternating current source. It is an effective and convenient way of controlling hemorrhage. Electrocautery can be applied directly to bleeding point or after catching the bleeding point with hemostat. Then cautery point is touched to the hemostat, causing sealing of the vessel through the action of heat. It causes tissue destruction producing a burning smell and smoke during application. This cannot control hemorrhage from large vessels, which need to be ligated.

Cryosurgery: Extreme cooling has been used for hemostasis. Temperature ranging from –20°C to –180°C are used. At these temperatures, the tissues, capillaries, small arterioles, and venules undergo cryogenic necrosis. This is caused by dehydration and denaturation of lipid molecules. Cryosurgery is specially used to treat superficial hemangiomas.

Argon-beam coagulator: It represents a new form of electrocautery, shown to be more effective than standard electrocautery. In this, coagulator, monopolar current is transmitted to tissues through the flow of argon gas. This allows bleeding from vessels that are smaller than 3 mm in diameter to be controlled without the use of hemostats or ligatures. The tip of the coagulator is held approximately 1 cm from the tissue. A flow of argon gas clears the surgical site of fluids to allow current to be focused directly on tissue, with reduced carbonization. There is formation of 1 to 2 mm of Escher, that covers the bleeding surface and remains attached to the tissues with less tendency to rebleed. There is possibility of gas embolism, as there is stream of gas in direct contact with tissues. This risk can be eliminated by not placing handpiece tip in direct contact with tissues.

Lasers: Lasers usually result in bloodless surgery, as these effectively coagulate the small blood vessels during cutting of tissues.

Chemical Methods

Local agents

a. *Astringent agents and styptics:* Chemical agents vary in their hemostatic action. Monsel's solution contains ferric subsulfate and it acts by precipitating proteins. It is quite effective in arresting the capillary bleeding and post extraction bleeding in medullary bone.

Tannic acid also helps in precipitating proteins and causes clot formation. This is more helpful as a home remedy or prescription over phone until patient reaches the clinician. Patient can be asked to bite over a folded tea bag in case of post extraction bleeding. Mann hemostatic is a mixture of tannic acid, alum and chlorobutamol.

Silver nitrate and ferric chloride are other agents, which can be used in case of minimal capillary bleeding.

b. *Bone wax:* When bleeding is occurring from a bony canal, it can be troublesome, because of inability to occlude the vessel that is confined within bony canal In such a case, small quantity of bone wax can be applied to the bleeding bone. It acts by mechanical occlusion of the bony canal. Large quantity of bone wax can lead to foreign body granuloma and infection. Therefore, it should be used judiciously.

c. *Thrombin:* Topical use of thrombin acts by converting fibrinogen into fibrin clot. It is very kind to tissues and quite effective. It is applied to the bleeding surface via a pack, gelatin sponge or surgicel.

d. *Gelfoam:* It is made from gelatin and is sponge like. Gelfoam has no intrinsic hemostatic action. Its main hemostatic activity is related to large surface area, which comes in contact with blood and further swells on absorbing blood. It exerts pressure along with acting as scaffold for fibrin network. It is absorbed by phagocytosis. Gelfoam should be moistened in saline or thrombin solution prior to application and all the air should be removed from interstices.

e. *Oxycel:* It is oxidized cellulose and on application releases cellulosic acid, which has marked affinity for hemoglobin, leading to formation of artificial clot. It should be applied dry, because acid formed during wetting process inactivates the thrombin or other hemostatic agent. Acid produced also inhibit epithelialization, therefore, it is not recommended for use over epithelial surfaces.

f. *Surgicel:* It is glucose polymer based sterile knitted fabric prepared by the controlled oxidation of regenerated cellulose. Its local hemostatic mechanism depends on binding of hemoglobin to oxycellulose, allowing the dressing to expand into a gelatinous mass, which in turn acts as scaffold for clot formation and clot stabilization. Surgicel can be applied dry or it can be soaked in thrombin solution.

It is removed by liquefaction and phagocytosis over a period of one week to one month. This product does not inhibit epithelialization and can be used over epithelial surfaces.

g. *Fibrin glue*: It is a biological adhesive containing thrombin, fibrinogen, factor XIII and aprotinin. Thrombin converts fibrinogen to unstable fibrin clot, factor XIII stabilizes the clot and aprotinin prevents its degradation. During wound healing, fibroblasts move through the fibrin meshwork forming more permanent framework composed of collagen fibers. The product poses virtually no risk of transmission of viral infections because of pasteurization of the plasma components and has little or no antigenic potential. This product has been recently allowed for clinical use in UK and USA.

h. *Adrenaline*: Adrenaline or epinephrine, applied topically induces vasoconstriction and thus helps in achieving hemostasis. Extensive application or undiluted preparation can cause systemic effects, therefore, one should be careful while using adrenaline. The drug is applied with the help of gauze pack in a concentration 1:1000 over oozing sites. It can also be injected along with local anesthetic in concentration of 1:80,000 to 1:2,00,000. This drug should not be used in patients who have hypertension or previously existing cardiac disease. The vasoconstrictor effect is reversible and one should be careful to watch for recurrence of bleeding when its effect wears off.

Systemic agents

a. *Whole blood*: When there is excessive blood loss due to hemorrhage, and there are symptoms of hypovolemic shock, whole blood transfusion may be indicated. Fresh whole blood contains all the factors for coagulation. When specific blood components are not available to treat the patient's hemostatic defect, whole blood may be used. It is necessary to type and cross-match the blood before transfusion. Blood must be checked for hepatitis B, C and HIV viruses before transfusion. Banked blood is a poor source of platelets. Factors II, VII, IX and XI are stable in banked blood. Fresh whole blood refers to blood that is administered within 24 hours of its donation. Fresh whole blood is rarely indicated because of specific component therapy available these days. One unit of platelet concentrates has

more viable platelets than one unit of fresh whole blood, but it is an inadequate source of factor VIII.

b. *Platelet rich plasma*: It is advisable to elevate the platelet levels to the range of 50,000 to 1,00,000 cells per cu mm to provide continued protection. Platelets can be collected from donated whole blood or directly from the patient via plasmapheresis. Platelet concentrates are viable for three days when stored at room temperature. If they are refrigerated viability decreases. They must be infused quickly via a short IV transfusion set with no filter. One unit of platelet rich plasma raises the platelet count approximately by 7,000 to 10,000 cells per cu mm.

c. *Fresh frozen plasma*: A unit (150 ml) of fresh frozen plasma is usually collected from one donor and contains all coagulation factors including 200 u factor VIII, 200 u factor IX and 400 mg fibrinogen. Fresh frozen plasma is stored at –30°C and should be infused within two hours once defrosted.

d. *Cryoprecipitate*: A 15 ml vial of cryoprecipitate contains approximately 100 u factor VIII, 250 mg fibrinogen, factor XIII and von Willebrand factor and is stored at –30°C. Each bag of cryoprecipitate is derived from a single donor and is not treated to inactivate viruses. Therefore, the use of cryoprecipitate is associated with a substantial risk of viral transmission.

e. *Adrenochrome monosemicarbazon and ethamsylate*: These systemic chemical agents are of doubtful efficacy. Adrenochrome monosemicarbazon (1 mg/ml injection) is given 2 ml/6 hourly before the surgical procedure. Ethamsylate reduces capillary bleeding in the presence of normal number of platelets. It probably acts by correcting abnormal platelet adhesion.

Control of Hemorrhage from Major Arteries

The best control of hemorrhage is directly at injured site and in majority of cases local measures can adequately control hemorrhage. One must always be prepared to tie off a major vessel, if bleeding cannot be controlled locally. Major vessels should be ligated in a planned surgical manner. If one is dealing with a vascular tumor, hemangioma or arteriovenous malformation, major vessels should be exposed and ligature passed around the concerned vessels before proceeding for the surgery of the tumor, so that in case of inadvertent bleeding major vessel can be tied without any delay.

In order to control bleeding, the clinician must be able to visualize clearly the exact point of bleeding. This can be achieved with the help of good light source, adequate suction, adequate anesthesia and sound workable knowledge of the anatomy of the area concerned. One should approach bleeding problem with utmost confidence. Majority of times, the problem arises from inadequate preparation on the part of clinician before surgery, poor visibility in the operative field, poor co-operation from the patient, and incomplete armamentarium to implement the procedure.

Greater Palatine Artery

Greater palatine artery runs anteriorly from the greater palatine foramen in the submucosa of the hard palate in a groove between the horizontal palatine process of the maxilla and the inner plate of the alveolar process. The incisions over the palate should be made parallel, rather than perpendicular to this vessel. If accidental injury occurs, bleeding is copious and application of clamp is difficult. Most of the times, the hemorrhage can be controlled by a pressure pack. A round bolus of gauze is made of adequate size, so that it does not cause gagging. It is kept in place by tie over sutures for 24 to 48 hours. Pressure pack can be safely removed after 48 hours.

Sublingual Artery

Injury to sublingual artery can occur accidentally by rotating disks or slipping of sharp instrument, while working on mandibular teeth. Injury to this artery during mandibular implant placement has been reported and it may lead to large sublingual hematoma which, if not controlled, can compromise airway and may be life-threatening.

It is a small artery and local clamping of the artery and application of electrocautery usually controls the bleeding. There is anatomic variation in the origin of this artery. In most of the cases it is a branch of lingual artery, but in significant number of cases it is a branch of submental artery, which is a further branch of facial artery. So, sometimes ligation of lingual artery may not stop bleeding from sublingual artery. In that case facial artery needs to be ligated.

Ligation of Lingual Artery

Lingual artery is second anterior branch of external carotid artery. It arises just below the facial artery or it can arise as a common linguofacial trunk, from the external carotid artery. Its exposure is done in submandibular triangle. Submandibular curvilinear incision is taken from the gonial angle to mental region, extending inferolaterally overlying hyoid bone. The skin, platysma and deep fascia are incised and lower pole of the submandibular gland is exposed. The gland is lifted upwards and tendon of digastric muscle is exposed. Mylohyoid and hyoglossus muscles are identified forming floor of digastric triangle.

Hypoglossal nerve is identified at the posterior border of mylohyoid muscle. Lingual triangle or Lesser's triangle is formed by digastric tendon, posterior mylohyoid border and the hypoglossal nerve. Within the triangle, vertical fibers of hyoglossus muscle are separated bluntly and in the gap between these fibers, lingual artery is identified and ligated.

Control of bleeding can also be achieved by ligating lingual artery at its origin from external carotid artery. Even by ligating external carotid artery bleeding can still continue because of rich venous supply and anastomosing arteries from opposite side. Expanding hematoma from lingual artery can compromise airway and sometimes tracheostomy is required.

Ligation of Facial Artery

Facial artery is third anterior branch of external carotid artery. It can be easily ligated at the point where it crosses lower border of mandible just anterior to masseter muscle. If patient is asked to clench the teeth, the pulsations of facial artery can be easily felt externally.

Facial vein accompanies the facial artery and lies posterior to it in majority of cases. Marginal mandibular branch of facial nerve crosses superficially over facial artery and vein. To prevent damage to this nerve submandibular incision is given one to two cm below the lower border of mandible. The skin, subcutaneous tissue, platysma and deep fascia are cut. These tissues are retracted upwards and here artery lies just anterior to masseter muscle. It is isolated, tied and cut.

Ligation of Maxillary Artery

The maxillary artery is terminal branch of external carotid artery. It is situated deep and direct ligation is difficult. Transantral approach for ligation of maxillary artery has been described. This artery is at risk during surgery of temporomandibular joint, as it lies medial to condylar neck. Ligation is difficult due to limited access. Direct pressure with packing can control the bleeding in majority of cases. If direct packing cannot achieve hemorrhage control, the ligation of external carotid artery becomes necessary.

Superficial Temporal Artery

It is also one of the terminal branches of the external carotid artery. Bleeding from temporal region (scalp) can be best managed by direct identification of the bleeding point and electrocoagulation. The pulsations of superficial temporal artery can be felt just anterior to preauricular region. This artery is usually encountered during surgery of the temporomandibular joint through the preauricular incision. The artery can be exposed through same incision as used for exposure of temporomandibular joint.

External Carotid Artery

The common carotid artery divides into internal and external carotid artery at the level of superior border of the thyroid cartilage. However, sometimes this division can take place at the level of hyoid bone or slightly superior. The internal carotid artery is branchless in its vertical course in the carotid triangle. This point helps in differentiating of external carotid artery from the internal one.

The external carotid artery gives rise to three anterior branches, two posterior branches, one medial branch and two terminal branches. Superior thyroid artery, lingual artery and facial artery are anterior branches. Occipital artery and posterior auricular artery are posterior branches. Ascending pharyngeal artery is the medial branch. Maxillary artery and superficial temporal artery are the terminal branches. There is extensive anastomosis of all the branches of external carotid artery and the anastomoses of right and left arteries, across the midline. This means that unilateral ligation of these vessels will not stop the hemorrhage completely or will not allow dry bloodless surgery.

The external carotid artery can be ligated at two places depending on the site of bleeding. Firstly, external carotid artery can be ligated just above the origin of superior thyroid artery in carotid triangle. This will eliminate bleeding from all the branches of external carotid artery except the superior thyroid artery. Secondly, external carotid artery can be ligated

higher up in retromandibular fossa, when bleeding is exclusively from the maxillary artery or its branches.

Ligation of External Carotid Artery in Carotid Triangle

The patient is placed supine and neck is extended and rotated towards contralateral side by placing a pillow below the shoulders. An incision is placed through skin and superficial fascia at the level of the hyoid bone. Next the platysma muscle and superficial layer of deep investing fascia is cut gaining an entry into the carotid triangle. Sternocleidomastoid muscle is retracted back and blunt dissection is done to expose the contents of carotid sheath. Pulsations of carotid artery can be felt and help in direction of dissection. Blue internal jugular vein covers the common carotid artery superficially. Lying between the two vessels and deep to them, there is yellow vagus nerve. External carotid artery is identified by its branching. Umbilical tape is passed and fixed superior to superior thyroid artery and its effect seen by occluding the artery. If need be, ligatures and transfixion sutures are passed.

Ligation of External Carotid Artery in Retromandibular Fossa

Retromandibular incision is planned. Skin is incised behind the ramus and angle of mandible starting at tip of mastoid process continued till just below the mandibular angle. Skin and platysma muscle are incised. Retromandibular vein, external jugular vein and branches of great auricular nerve are encountered and these are sectioned. Parotid gland is separated from anterior border of sternocleidomastoid muscle by sharp dissection and retracted. Posterior belly of digastric and above it stylohyoid muscle becomes visible. The mandible is pulled forward to widen the retromandibular fossa. Here pulsations of external carotid artery can be felt. Blunt dissection is done to expose the external carotid artery. Here it can be ligated.

Hereditary Coagulopathies

Ninety percent of inherited hemostatic disorders consist of hemophilia A, B and von Willebrand's disease. Hemophilias are inherited disorders caused by a decreased activity or absence of coagulation factor VIII or IX. Hemophilia A is factor VIII deficiency and is most common. It occurs in 70 to 80 percent of the affected persons with hereditary coagulopathies, whereas, hemophilia B (Christmas disease, or factor IX deficiency) accounts for 6 percent.

Hemophilia A

The severity of the disease is dependent on the amount of factor present in the blood stream. Normal plasma contains 1.0 unit of a factor per milliliter or level that is defined as 100 percent. Deficiency of a factor is expressed as percentage (0.25 unit/ml = 25%). There is a close correlation between plasma factor VIII levels and severity of disease. Patients with less than 1 percent factor VIII activity have severe disease. They bleed frequently into soft tissues, muscles and weight-bearing joints even without discernible trauma. Patients with levels between 1 and 5 percent have moderate disease with less severe bleeding episodes. Those with levels above 5 percent have mild disease with infrequent bleeding usually secondary to trauma or surgery. Majority of patients of hemophilia A have levels of factor VIII below 5 percent.

The recommended level of replacement therapy of factor VIII varies from 30 to 75 percent. For extensive surgical procedure, the levels of factor should be raised to 50 to 75 percent. Factor VIII has half-life of 8 to 12 hours, uncomplicated procedure may not require further replacement therapy. Each unit of factor VIII transfused is estimated to raise factor VIII levels 2 percent per kilogram of body weight. The following formula can be used to calculate the dose of Factor VIII needed to achieve desired plasma concentration:

Dose of factor VIII in units =
$$(\text{desired \% activity} - \text{initial \% activity}) \times \frac{\text{weight in kg}}{2}$$

The more extensive procedures like surgical extraction or major oral surgery may require further infusion at 12 to 24 hours intervals and adequate levels of factor VIII may have to be maintained until healing is complete. Table 50.2 summarizes the sources of factor VIII. Local hemostatic measures such as application of topical thrombin, surgicel or gelfoam is indicated. Stabilization of clot with antifibrinolytic drugs such as epsilon-aminocaproic acid (EACA) and tranexamic acid (5%) mouthwash 4 to 6 times daily is indicated. Analgesics such as aspirin and NSAIDs are contraindicated as they alter platelet function. Routine comprehensive dental care can be provided to the patients with

Table 50.2: Sources of factor VIII

Sources	Concentration of factor VIII
Fresh frozen plasma (Blood bank)	1 unit/ml
Cryoprecipitate (Blood bank)	5 to 10 units/ml or 80 to 100 units/bag of 10 to 15 ml
Plasma derived lyophilized factor VIII concentrate (Commercially available)	250 to 500 units/vial
Genetically engineered factor VIII (Commercially available)	250 to 500 units/vial

hemophilia on an outpatient basis, if the practitioner is familiar with the type and severity of factor deficiency and plans accordingly. Surgical procedures should be done after admitting the patient and a minimum of 50 percent of normal levels should be maintained by daily monitoring of the patient. Supragingival scaling can be managed by a single infusion of cryoprecipitate or factor VIII concentrate coupled with administration of 4 to 6 gm of EACA four to six times daily for 72 to 96 hours after the dental procedure. Inferior alveolar nerve block and posterior superior alveolar nerve block injections should be administered only after replacement therapy of factor VIII, because of possibility of a dissecting hematoma. EACA is a potent antifibrinolytic agent that inhibits plasminogen activators present in oral secretions and stabilizes clot formation in the oral tissues.

Tranexamic acid is a more potent and longer acting antifibrinolytic drug. It is available as both oral and parenteral forms. Intravenous dose is 10 mg/kg body weight, the dose being repeated 4 to 6 hourly. It can be used as 5 percent mouthwash (500 mg tablet dissolved in 10 ml of water) and this solution can be swallowed.

Development of antibodies to factor VIII occurs in 5 to 20 percent of the patients with deficiency of factor VIII and presents a major problem in treatment. These antibodies are generally IgG antibodies and act as inhibitors, because these rapidly neutralize factor VIII activity. Control of bleeding in patients with inhibitors may require either infusion of porcine factor VIII, which may not cross react with inhibitors, or prothrombin complex concentrates, which contains trace quantities of activated factors and can bypass the inhibitor. This prothrombin complex is administered over a 30 to 60 minutes period and exhibits short duration of action. Local hemostatic measures are indicated; however, systemic EACA or tranexamic acid is contraindicated. Other methods of treating patients with inhibitors include plasmapheresis, which has been advocated in patients to reduce antibody titer, and a synthetic vasopressin analog desmopressin, which has been shown to produce increase in vWF and factor VIII activity. Conventionally, it is given in a dose of 0.3 microgram/kg in 100 ml normal saline by intravenous infusion over 30 minutes.

Hemophilia B

Factor IX deficiency is clinically indistinguishable from factor VIII deficiency, therefore, accurate laboratory diagnosis is critical. It requires therapy with fresh frozen plasma or factor IX concentrates. Unlike factor VIII, which is maintained within the circulatory system, factor IX enters the extravascular space, from where it is released slowly. Therefore, there is more biologic half-life (32 hours) as compared to factor VIII. Replacement therapy consists of raising the plasma level factor IX to 30 to 50 percent of normal by using fresh frozen plasma (FFP) or prothrombin complex concentrates. Plasma infusion can begin 24 to 36 hours before the scheduled procedure due to long half-life of factor IX. This allows multiple units of plasma transfusion to be given without overloading the circulating system. Use of cryoprecipitate offers no advantage over plasma since it is not concentrated in plasma. The lyophilized factor IX concentrates have significant quantities of factors II and X and variable amount of factor VII, and have the potential for inappropriate thrombosis as well as risk of transmitting hepatitis. Local hemostatic measures are indicated. Systemic use of EACA or tranexamic acid can be done with plasma replacement therapy, but it is contraindicated with prothrombin complex concentrates.

Management of Patients with Von Willebrand's Disease

Von Willebrand's disease (VWD) is an autosomal dominant inherited disorder of coagulation, that results from a quantitative or qualitative abnormality of the plasma protein, i.e. Von Willebrand's factor (VWF). It is a glycosylated protein which is synthesized in endothelial cells of blood vessel and megakaryocytes.

Three Main Roles of VWF in Hemostasis

1. It enables the binding of platelets to the subendothelial collagen matrix at the sites of vascular injury.
2. It mediates subsequent platelet aggregation allowing the formation of platelet plug.
3. It acts as carrier protein for factor VIII protecting it from proteolytic degradation.

The most common bleeding manifestations are easy bruising, epistaxis, gingival bleeding, menorrhagia and excessive bleeding postoperatively or after dental extractions. Patients with severe Von Willebrand's disease may have hemophilic bleeding pattern with spontaneous bleed into joints and muscles. VWF activity can be measured by specific enzyme-linked immunosorbent assay.

There are three different types of VWD, which have been described depending upon quantitative, qualitative or complete deficiency of VWF.

Type I—which accounts for approximately 70 percent of VWD, typically mild decrease in quantity of VWF.

Type II—VWD results from qualitative abnormalities in the VWF. It has got four subtypes depending on defect in VWF protein. These subtypes are type IIA, type II B, type II M, and type II N.

Type III VWD—in this type patients have severe quantitative deficiency of VWF.

Patient with mild VWD respond favorably to desmopressin in a dose of 0.3 microgram/kg in 100 ml; normal saline infused over 30 minutes. The response is rapid with maximum concentration reaching within one hour of administration. It results in 2 to 10 fold rise in plasma concentration of VWF and F VIII with a mean rise of three fold. People with baseline concentration greater than 10 iu/dl should respond favorably to desmopressin. Concentration usually fall to baseline within 12 to 24 hours. Further, daily dose of desmopressin can be given, if necessary. Patients undergoing minor surgery and dental extraction should be adequately covered with single infusion of desmopressin. To cover major soft tissue and hard tissue surgery, VWF and factor VIII concentration should be checked after infusion of desmopressin prior to surgery to ensure adequate response. It should be given postoperatively daily for at least 5 days and VWF activity and F VIII concentrations monitored daily after surgical procedure.

Type II B and type III of VWD do not respond to desmopressin and these patients can be managed by blood product replacement therapy. Fractionated virally inactivated factor VIII concentrates have good concentration of VWF and provide adequate hemostasis. When these products are not available fresh frozen plasma and cryoprecipitate can be used.

Local hemostatic measures and use of antifibrinolytic agents such as tranexamic acid can be used. An appropriate antibiotic should also be given to minimize risk of infection that may cause secondary hemorrhage. Aspirin and other NSAIDs should not be prescribed for pain relief because they exacerbate hemorrhage by disturbing platelet function.

Acquired Coagulation Factor Disorders

Vitamin K Deficiency

Vitamin K is a necessary cofactor for carboxylation of factors II, VII, IX, X. Vitamin K deficiency results in abnormal blood coagulation and bleeding. Vitamin K deficiency can occur in biliary obstruction, malabsorption syndrome, prolonged antibiotic therapy, nutritional deficiency and warfarin ingestion. Hospitalized patients who are unable to eat and are receiving antibiotics that suppress intestinal flora may become vitamin K deficient in 1 to 2 weeks. Prothrombin time (PT) is usually prolonged.

Deficiency can be usually corrected by administration of vitamin K injection 10 mg for 1 to 3 days. Intravenous administration of vitamin K has been associated with anaphylaxis in rare patients; therefore, it should be given in a closely monitored setting. Patients with severe hemorrhage due to vitamin K deficiency can be managed by transfusing fresh frozen plasma.

Coagulopathy Associated with Liver Diseases

Severe liver disease causes decreased synthesis of fibrinogen, prothrombin and factors V, VII, IX, X and XI. Thrombocytopenia due to accompanying hypersplenism may complicate the hemostatic defect. Bleeding in a patient with liver disease presents a difficult therapeutic problem. Empirical therapy with vitamin K injection may be tried, although majority of patients will not respond. Replacement therapy with fresh frozen plasma is indicated in such a patient, and platelet transfusion may be considered if thrombocytopenia is present.

Concept of International Normalized Ratio and Management of a Patient on Oral Anticoagulants

Many patients seeking dental treatment are on oral anticoagulant therapy. Most common indications for anticoagulant therapy are prevention of thromboembolism from prosthetic heart valves and arrhythmias, prevention of stroke, and prevention of deep venous thrombosis. The prothrombin time (PT) has been the conventional means used to monitor the degree of anticoagulation. Prothrombin ratio (PTR) is the ratio of patient's PT divided by control PT from the laboratory. A PTR of 2 to 2.5 is considered to be the therapeutic range. World Health Organization (WHO) has recently recommended monitoring of these patients with international normalized ratio (INR), because PT has been shown to be imprecise and variable. There is little comparability of PT values taken in different laboratories. These differences are primarily due to the thromboplastin used in performing the test as thromboplastin can be obtained from different sources and the type of instrumentation used in performing the test.

In an effort to standardize the results of the PT, World Health Organization introduced the concept of INR. INR is the PTR that would have been obtained if a standard thromboplastins reagent had been used. The INR relates all thromboplastins to the standard of human brain thromboplastin with the use of internal sensitivity index (ISI). The ISI established the reference standard of 1.0 to human brain derived thromboplastin.

$$INR = (patient's\ PT/control\ PT)^{ISI}$$

With the use of INR variations due to differences in nature of source and potency of thromboplastin has been standardized. INR for a normal healthy adult is 1.0. Recommended intensity of INR for patients on oral anticoagulants varies form 2.0 to 4.5 depending on indication for use. For example recommended INR for deep vein thrombosis, valvular heart disease, pulmonary embolism, myocardial infarction is 2.0 to 3.0 and in case of artificial mechanical heart value is 3.0 to 4.5.

Extraction of teeth is generally considered a good test of the efficacy of the hemostatic mechanism, as both hard and soft tissues are torn during the process, and usually there is no primary closure of soft tissues. The clinician who is faced with warfarinized patients requiring extraction has to balance the risk of reducing or stopping the anticoagulant therapy with that of excessive bleeding from the extraction sockets. Bleeding can be troublesome and excessive bleeding into the soft tissues particularly sublingual, retropharyngeal areas can compromise the upper airway. On the other hand stoppage of anticoagulation therapy puts the patients on greater risk of thromboembolism, which is potentially life threatening.

There is no current consensus on how to manage these patients. Each patient has to be individually assessed and risks and benefits of stoppage of therapy or altering the therapy are assessed in consultation with the treating cardiologist or physician.

In patients, where stoppage of anticoagulant therapy can lead to significant risk of thromboembolism, they are shifted to heparin therapy after stoppage of the oral anticoagulant and then surgical procedures are carried out. Current literature suggests that, if international normalized ratio (INR) of prothrombin is below 3.5 then simple extractions can be done safely without altering the oral anticoagulant therapy. Hemostasis can be achieved with the use of local hemostatic measures and use of topical antifibrinolytic agent such as 5 percent tranexamic acid mouthwash.

SHOCK

Shock is a pathophysiologic condition, clinically recognized as a state of inadequate perfusion. Due to inadequate blood flow, there is inadequate delivery of nutrients to the tissues and inadequate removal of cellular waste products from the tissue cells, which results in disruption of vital organ functions. In late stage, even the cardiovascular system itself begins to deteriorate, so that the shock becomes progressively worse. Early identification and elimination of the underlying cause of shock usually reverses the chain of events resulting from cellular dysfunction. Delay in treatment may result in permanent cellular and organ damage leading to irreversible shock and ultimately death. Shock can be classified mainly into four types based on pathophysiology and hemodynamic changes.

Classification

- Hypovolemic shock
- Cardiogenic shock
- Septic shock
- Neurogenic shock.

Hypovolemic Shock

Hypovolemic shock results from a decrease in the circulating or effective intravascular volume. It is the most common type of shock in the victim of maxillofacial trauma. Hypovolemic shock can be further classified into hemorrhagic and nonhemorrhagic.

1. Hemorrhagic shock is due to loss of blood from the body as a result of injury. Hemorrhage decreases the mean systemic filling pressure and a resultant decrease of venous return and there is fall of cardiac output. Approximately 10 to 15 percent of the total blood volume loss will have no significant effect on arterial pressure or cardiac output. 15 to 25 percent loss of blood volume may not cause hemodynamic change, if the blood loss is not rapid, but the metabolic changes associated with shock may be initiated. Rapid loss of 30 to 40 percent of the blood volume causes shock and if not treated becomes progressive and may lead to death.

2. In nonhemorrhagic shock, there is massive fluid shift from intravascular compartment to extravascular compartment. This can result from burns, crush injuries, pancreatitis, peritonitis, pleural effusion and ascites. Water loss due to severe diarrhea, vomiting, diabetes insipidus, hyperglycemia, nephritis and excessive diuretic use can also lead to nonhemorrhagic hypovolemic shock.

Decrease in arterial pressure caused by blood loss, stimulates powerful sympathetic reflexes, that result in constriction of arterioles, veins and venous reservoirs and there is increase in heart activity. The body tries to maintain cardiac output and arterial pressure to normal levels. There is formation of angiotensin and vasopressin, which constricts the peripheral arteries and cause increased conservation of water and salt by the kidneys. If body reflex mechanisms are not able to raise the arterial pressure sufficiently and no urgent intervention is done by replacement of fluids, there is depression of myocardium and vasomotor center. Blood flow through the tissues becomes sluggish, there is accumulation of acids due to continued tissue metabolism. These acids and other deterioration products from the ischemic tissues, cause blood agglutination in the capillaries. Due to prolonged hypoxia, the permeability of capillaries gradually increases and large quantities of fluid transudes into the tissues. This further decreases blood volume and there is generalized cellular deterioration, generalized and local tissue acidosis and tissue necrosis in vital organs. This leads to a vicious cycle, i.e. each increase in degree of shock causes a further increase in the shock. After the shock has progressed to a certain stage, transfusion or any other therapy becomes incapable of saving the life of the person. Therefore, the person is said to be in irreversible stage of shock.

Therefore, it is prudent that the oral surgeon *should be able to recognize early features of shock*. Physiologic response to hemorrhage range from tachycardia, poor capillary perfusion, and a decrease in pulse pressure to hypotension, tachypnea, and delirium. Serum hematocrit and

Table 50.3: Clinical manifestations of shock	
Blood loss	Clinical manifestations
Mild < 20 percent	Postural hypotension; patient feeling cold; tachycardia; cool, pale, moist skin; collapsed neck veins; concentrated urine
Moderate > 20-40 percent	Thirst; supine hypotension and tachycardia; oliguria or anuria
Severe > 40 percent	Agitation, confusion; supine hypotension and tachycardia are invariably present; rapid deep respiration

hemoglobin concentrations are not accurate indicators of acute blood loss. *The degree of hypotension* on presentation to emergency room and operating room *correlates strongly with mortality rate.*

Table 50.3 gives clinical manifestation of shock depending on loss of blood volume.

Monitoring

Whenever possible, patient should be treated in intensive care unit. Vital signs should be monitored periodically. Continuous electrocardiography, pulse oxymetry should be performed. Blood pressure and heart rate should remain stable. Tachypnea, worsening of hypotension and tachycardia indicate inadequately treated shock.

Urine output should be measured and it should be greater than 40 ml/hour. Arterial blood gases, pH and electrolyte levels are monitored.

Central venous pressure should be monitored. In patients with moderate and severe shock, fluid therapy is monitored by right heart catheterization with a balloon tipped, flow directed (Swan-Ganz) catheter. This not only provides diagnostic hemodynamic assessment of pulmonary capillary wedge pressure and cardiac output, but also helps in monitoring the response to therapy.

Treatment

Replacement of fluids and tissue perfusion are the mainstay of the treatment of shock. Volume resuscitation must be undertaken promptly. The legs raised and body supine is the preferred posture, as this increases venous return and cardiac index. In addition to this the patient should be kept warm.

Fluid replacement: When hemorrhage is massive, type specified matched transfused blood is the preferred method to correct hypovolemia. Typing and cross-matching of blood takes time sometimes. Uncrossed type O –ve blood should be reserved for life threatening blood loss that cannot be adequately replaced by other fluids. Initial resuscitation is done with crystalloids, such as normal saline or Ringer lactate. It requires up to several liters of fluids, but replacement of interstitial fluid with crystalloids is preferred. After initial resuscitation, colloids such as albumin or starch solution can be used, as these restore intravascular volume more effectively. All these fluids should be warmed before transfusion, because hypothermia worsens acid-base disorders, and myocardial function. The amount of fluid administration is based upon improvement of clinical signs, particularly blood pressure, pulse pressure and heart rate. Central venous pressure and urinary output also provide indication of restoration of vital organ perfusion. Hypotension in patients with hypovolemic shock should be aggressively treated with intravenous fluids and not vasopressors. Exception to this dictum include cardiogenic shock, severe hypotension unresponsive to fluid replacement and cardiac arrest. The role of vasopressors is further discussed in septic shock.

Cardiogenic Shock

Cardiogenic shock occurs as a result of inadequate cardiac output, impaired oxygen delivery, and reduced tissue perfusion, caused by loss of effective contractile function of myocardium (acute myocardial infarction, hemodynamically significant brady or tachyarrhythmias, cardiomyopathy) or from mechanical processes, reducing adequate forward output (acute valvular regurgitation, acute ventricular septal defect, critical aortic stenosis). Pulmonary artery wedge pressure is elevated (> 18 mm Hg), cardiac output is decreased (cardiac index < 2.0 l/min/m^2), peripheral vascular resistance is increased, and mean arterial pressure is less (< 60 mm Hg). Initial treatment is directed towards identifying the cause, maintaining adequate systemic blood pressure, cardiac output and tissue perfusion with volume expansion and inotropic drugs. Dopamine is the vasopressor of first choice. It is diluted in normal saline or 5 percent dextrose drip and given at 5 to 10 microgram/kg/min. Other drugs like norepinephrine and dobutamine can be used.

Septic Shock

Septic shock describes the clinical syndrome corresponding to acute circulatory failure resulting from serious infection. Mostly, it is provoked by gram-negative bacteria, but fungi, viruses and parasites can also lead to septic shock. This presents as arterial hypotension (systolic blood pressure below 90 mm Hg or mean arterial pressure below 60 mm Hg) associated with altered mental status, changes in organ perfusion and signs of organ failure, such as reduction in urine output, increased blood lactate levels (>2 mEq/l) reflect alteration in cellular metabolism. Septic shock is extremely important to the clinician, because it is this type of shock, which has higher mortality in the hospital.

Development of sepsis is related to complex interplay between endotoxins, release of pro- and anti-inflammatory mediators, like tumor necrosis factor-alpha, interleukins and prostaglandins. The pathophysiology of septic shock involves an extremely complex interplay between tissue hypoxia and the host's immune response. Most frequent cause of death, is sepsis induced multiorgan failure, e.g. acute respiratory distress syndrome, renal failure, and disseminated intravascular coagulopathy. Due to severe sepsis, there is increased oxygen demand, because of direct cellular activation, hormonal stress response and hyperthermia. There is altered oxygen extraction and oxygen transport.

Management of septic shock should be based on: (i) early and effective volume replacement; (ii) restoration of tissue perfusion; (iii) adequate oxygen supply to cells and; (iv) control of infection with antibiotic therapy and control of source of infection.

In most patients, systolic blood pressure of 90 to 100 mm Hg or a mean arterial pressure of 70 to 75 mm Hg is acceptable. In minor cases, fluid administration alone can be sufficient to restore hemodynamic stability. In majority of cases, administration of a vasopressor is required to increase arterial pressure. Dopamine or noradrenaline should be selected for this purpose. Dopamine is usually the first choice, because it can better maintain organ blood flow, preserving renal and mesenteric circulation. If hypotension still persists, despite dopamine administration at doses of 20 to 25 microgram/kg/min, noradrenaline should be added to regimen. Once minimal tissue prefusion pressure has been restored, attention should focus on the restoration of a sufficient oxygen delivery to the tissues. The maintenance of a hemoglobin saturation in the arterial blood (SaO_2) above 95 percent is a fundamental goal in any type of acute circulatory failure. This implies that arterial oxygen tension (PaO_2) should be above 60 mm Hg. Hematocrit should be maintained above 30 percent. Myocardial depression can limit oxygen supply to tissues, even when cardiac output is normal or elevated. The addition of dobutamine, in this condition has been shown to be effective. Use of dobutamine should result in increase in cardiac output, but no change in arterial pressure, so that systemic vascular resistance will decline resulting in restoration of oxygen delivery to tissues.

Neurogenic Shock

Occasionally shock results without any loss of blood volume what so ever. Instead, the vascular capacity increases so much that even the normal amount of blood becomes incapable of adequately filling the circulatory system. One of the major cause of this, is loss of vasomotor tone throughout the body, causing massive dilatation of veins, and the resulting condition is known as neurogenic shock. *Vasovagal syncope* or emotional fainting most commonly seen in dental clinics, is caused by excitation of the parasympathetic nerves to the heart and vasodilator nerves to the skeletal muscle, thereby slowing the heart and reducing the arterial pressure. There is a decrease in cerebral blood flow below a critical level and the patient usually falls down. Consciousness returns almost immediately, and within a short period of time, the victim appears to be completely recovered. The early signs and symptoms include pale or ashen gray skin, heavy perspiration, nausea, tachycardia, feeling of warmth in neck or face. The late symptoms show coldness in hands and feet, hypotension, bradycardia, dizziness, visual disturbance, pupillary dilation, hyperpnea and loss of consciousness. Duration of the syncope is extremely brief, once the patient is placed in supine position. Placing the patient in supine position is the most important and first step in the management. This increases the blood flow from the periphery to the cerebral tissues thus aiding in recovery.

Miscellaneous

HIV Disease—
An Overview

In India, the current dramatic spread of blood-borne infections from HIV/AIDS and hepatitis C is increasing the morbidity and mortality and hence aggravating the suffering of the community.

Therefore, concerted efforts are required to reach people and practitioners before they join the ranks of the HIV positive. This is where we can make a significant difference. As it is easier to attack a problem before it spins out of control, initiatives and resources need to be channelized appropriately.

However, two important aspects are identified to be taken care of. Firstly, all necessary measures should be taken during management to prevent further transmission of HIV in the community.

An equally important aspect is to protect health care providers from affliction of HIV. In this context, dental professionals merit separate and specific contemplation as they stand at risk while performing dental procedures.

Pathogenesis and natural history of the disease:

Acquired immunodeficiency syndrome (AIDS) is caused by the human immunodeficiency virus (HIV). It is a serious disorder of the immune system in which the body's normal defenses against infection breakdown, leaving it vulnerable to a host of life threatening infections/conditions including unusual malignancies.

HISTORY AND ORIGIN

AIDS was officially recognized for the first time in June, 1981, at the Centres for Disease Control, USA, in previously healthy homosexual men dying with *Pneumocystis carinii* pneumonia and candidiasis. Since then, AIDS has been reported from all the continents. The virus causing AIDS was independently identified by a team of French Scientists led by Dr Lue Montagnier of Pasteur Institute and American Scientists led by Dr Robert C Gallo of National Cancer Institute in 1983. The virus has been called by different names LAV, i.e. lymphadenopathy associated virus by the French and HLTV–III, i.e. Human T-lymphocytotropic virus type III by the Americans.

The international committee on nomenclature of viruses named it the human immunodeficiency virus (HIV) and two types, HIV-1 and HIV-2 are identified.

Structure

HIV is a 120 mm icosahedral, enveloped, RNA virus. HIV comprises of an outer envelope consisting of a lipid bilayer with uniformly arranged 72 spikes of knobs of gp 120 and gp 41.

Glycoprotein (gp) 120 protrudes out of the surface of the virus and gp 41 is embedded in the lipid matrix. Inside is the protein cell surrounding 2 copies of RNA.

Cell also contains various enzymes like reverse transcriptase, integrase and protease, all essential for viral replication and maturation. Proteins p7 and p9 are bound to the RNA and are believed to be involved in regulation of gene expression.

Human Cells/Cell Lines and Tissue Susceptibility to HIV

HIV practically multiplies in all cells, but the extent of replication varies in different cells.

- *Hematopoietic system*: Lymphocytes, B lymphocytes, macrophage, natural killer cells, megakaryocytes, dendritic cells, promyelocytes, stem cells. Thymic epithelium, follicular dendritic cells.
- *Brain*: Capillary endothelial cell, astrocytes, macrophages (microglia), oligodendrocytes, choroid plexus ganglia, neuroblastoma cells, glioma cell lines and neurons.
- *Bowel*: Columnar and goblet cells enterochromaffin cells and colonic carcinoma cells.
- *Others*: Myocardium, renal tubular cells, synovial membrane, hepatic sinusoid epithelium, hepatic carcinoma cell, kupffer cell, fetal adrenal cell, retina, prostate cells and placental trophoblast cells.

Susceptibility

Fortunately, HIV is a very fragile virus. It is susceptible to heat, a temperature of 56°C for 30 minutes or boiling for a few seconds kills the virus. Most of the chemical germicides used in hospitals/casualties and health care settings kill HIV at much lower concentrations. Thus, 0.5 percent to 1 percent sodium hypochlorite, 70 percent ethanol, 2 percent glutaraldehyde, acetone, ether, beta propiolactone (1:400 dilutions) and sodium hydroxide (40 mmol/liter) inactivate the virus.

Global Scenario

The HIV/AIDS epidemic continues to grow world wide. In the year 2005, about 40.3 million people are estimated to be living with HIV/AIDS, including 2.3 million children. Eight million of these are young people in the age group of 15 to 24 years. The highest burden of HIV/AIDS is in Sub-Saharan Africa, followed by South East Asia (6.7 million). India, Thailand, Myanamar and Indonesia account for the majority of the estimated HIV burden.

Indian Scenario

India has the second largest population of HIV infected individuals, at an estimated 5.1 million. Since the first case of HIV was detected in Chennai in 1986, cases of HIV infection have been detected in all states across the country.

In most of the infectious diseases, the immune system is capable of mounting resistance in the human body, which brings about the complete destruction of the invading pathogen. The invading pathogen is not only eliminated from the body, but the immune system retains the memory of the pathogen, which can be tackled more efficiently when encountered in future.

HIV infects CD_4 helper lymphocytes in the immune apparatus. The HIV envelope glycoproteins (gp 120), bind the CD_4 molecules on the surface of the CD_4 lymphocytes and gains entry into the cell. Inside the cell, the virus uses the cellular machinery of the host to produce innumerable new virions and this ultimately leads to the death of the cell.

Inspite of this attack on the key cell of the immune system, the body is capable of mounting an immune response to HIV. However, the immune response is not capable of eliminating the virus from the body.

HIV is also capable of reproducing in very large quantities, at times larger than the immune system seems prepared to handle. Over many years, as the immune system gradually loses its own cells faster than it can replace them, and as more of the body's organs and systems are disrupted by HIV, overall health begins to decline.

As HIV gains a strong hold in the body, CD_4 cells, the primary target of HIV, begin to decline. When the

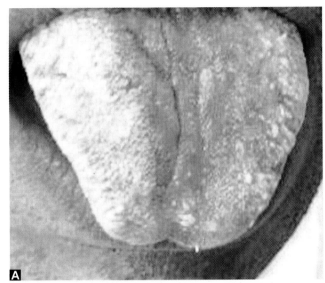

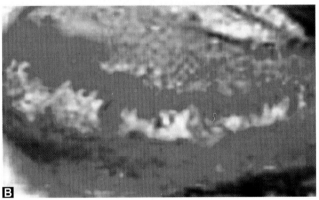

Figs 51.4A and B: Hairy leukoplakia on the lateral border of the tongue

Treatment

Hairy leukoplakia is asymptomatic and does not require treatment. HL is almost always a manifestation of HIV infection and clinicians should arrange evaluation of HIV disease and appropriate treatment for patients with HL. HL has disappeared in patients receiving high dose of acyclovir for herpes zoster because of the anti-EBV activity of acyclovir. Doses of acyclovir (2.5 to 3 mg per kg body weight) usually eliminate HL, but the lesion usually recurs with cessation of treatment.

Elimination or almost complete clinical resolution of the lesion has occurred in patients treated with agents such as desciclovir, an analog of acyclovir, phosphonoformate, Retin A and podophyllin resin, although lesions tend to recur within few months. Case reports describe HL disappearing during treatment with ganciclovir and aerosolized pentamidine.

Occasionally, *Candida albicans* may be found in HL lesions. Treatment consists of antifungal medications.

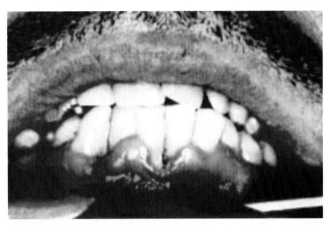

Fig. 51.5: Necrotizing ulcerative periodontitis in lower anterior teeth region

■ BACTERIAL LESIONS

Periodontal Disease

Periodontal disease is a fairly common problem in both symptomatic and asymptomatic HIV infected patients. It can take two forms: The rapid and severe condition called *necrotizing ulcerative periodontitis* (NUP) (Fig. 51.5) and its associated and possibly precursor condition called *linear gingival erythema* (LGE) (Fig. 51.6). The presenting clinical features of this disease often differ from those in non-HIV infected persons.

Clinical Features

Linear gingival erythema (LGE) and NUP often occur in a clean mouth, where there is very little plaque or calculus to account for the gingivitis. The onset is often sudden, with rapid loss of bone and soft tissue. In LGE, the gingiva may be reddened and edematous. Patients sometimes complains of spontaneous bleeding. In acute onset, ulcerative gingivitis ulcers occur at the tips of the inter dental papilla and along the gingival margins and often elicit complaints of severe pain. The ulcers heal, leaving the gingival papillae with a characteristic cratered appearance.

Necrotizing ulcerative periodontitis (NUP) may present as rapid loss of supporting bone and soft tissue. Typically, these losses occur simultaneously with no formation of gingival pockets. Sometimes involving only isolated areas of the mouth. Teeth may loosen and eventually fall out, but uninvolved sites can appear healthy. Necrotizing stomatitis may develop and areas of necrotic bone may appear along with the gingival margin. The bone may eventually sequestrate.

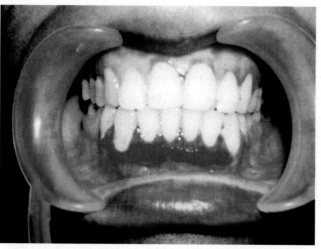

Fig. 51.6: Linear gingival erythema associated with HIV disease

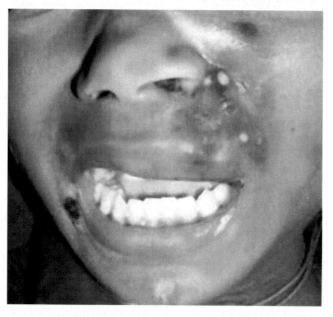

Fig. 51.7: Cancrum oris in HIV patient

Patients with NUP and necrotizing stomatitis frequently complain of extreme pain and spontaneous bleeding.

Cancrum oris or noma is a gangrenous affection of the mouth; especially attacking children, in whom the constitution is altered by bad hygiene and serious illness, especially from the eruptive fevers, beginning as an ulcer of the mucous membrane with edema of the face, destroying the soft tissues and the bone and it can be almost fatal (Fig. 51.7).

Differential Diagnosis

The patient's history and clinical appearance lead to the diagnosis. It is sometimes difficult to distinguish this type of periodontal disease from non-HIV related periodontal disease. However, the complaints of severe pain, rapid onset and rapid destruction in an often extremely clean mouth are unusual for non-HIV related periodontal disease.

Treatment

Clinicians should refer patients to a periodontist or dentist for management. The following protocol has achieved reasonable success—plaque removal, local debridement, irrigation with povidone-iodine, scaling and maintenance. Chlorhexidine mouthrinse once or twice daily are recommended. Studies show that the addition of chlorhexidine for this regimen produce significant improvement in periodontal condition. In case of NUP, metronidazole (one 250 mg tablet four times daily), Amoxicillin/clavulanate (one 625 mg tablet TDS) or clindamycin (one 300 mg tablets TDS) should be added to treatment regimen.

Different Course in HIV Infection

The microbiology of periodontal disease in HIV infected patients has not been fully described. Oral flora associated with LGE and NUP appear to be similar to those associated with periodontal disease seen in non-HIV infected persons. Recurrences of acute episodes are common and response to conventional treatment may be poor. However, therapeutic strategies and frequent recall appointments can produce effective local treatment of LGE and NUP. There is as yet no known relationship between these conditions and the progression of HIV disease.

MYCOBACTERIUM AVIUM-INTRACELLULARE

Mycobacterium avium-intracellulare is common etiological agent for palatal and gingival granulomatous masses in the oral cavity of HIV infected patient. A diagnosis of acid-fast bacilli (AFB) can be made from specially stained (acid-fast) biopsy specimen.

■ NEOPLASTIC LESIONS

Kaposi's Sarcoma

Kaposi's sarcoma (KS) may occur intraorally either alone or in association with skin and disseminated lesions. Intraoral lesions have been reported at other sites and may be the 1st manifestation of late stage HIV disease (AIDS).

Kaposi's sarcoma (KS) occurs most commonly in men, but also has been observed in women.

Clinical Features

Kaposi's sarcoma (KS) can appear as a red, blue or purplish lesion. It may be flat or raised and solitary or multiple. The most common oral site is the hard palate, but lesion may occur on any part of the oral mucosa including the gingiva, soft palate and buccal mucosa and in the oropharynx occasionally yellowish mucosa surrounds the KS lesion (Fig. 51.8). Oral KS lesions may enlarge, ulcerate and become infected. Good oral hygiene is essential to minimize these complications.

Differential Diagnosis

Kaposi's sarcoma (KS) must be distinguished from vascular lesions such as hematomas, hemangiomas, other vascular tumors, pyogenic granulomas, bacillary angiomatosis and pigmented lesions such as oral melanotic macules. Diagnosis is made from histological examination. These are usually no bleeding problems associated with a biopsy of oral KS. However, aspiration of a lesion prior to biopsy may be useful to rule out a hemangioma, small, flat lesions are probably in early stages and the histologic appearance is different from

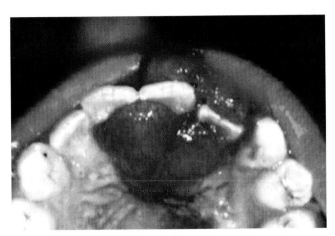

Fig. 51.8: Kaposi's sarcoma in maxillary anterior region

the larger, nodular lesions that are probably more advanced. Early lesions may be difficult to diagnose histologically, because they resemble endothelial proliferation. KS may appear suddenly within days of a normal oral examination in previously uninvolved areas of the mouth.

Providers should ensure that a patient with KS receives evaluation and follow up care for the underlying HIV disease.

Treatment

Treatment is determined on the basis of the number, size and location of the oral KS lesions. The choice of therapy depends on the effect of treatment on adjacent mucosa, pain associated with treatment, interference with eating and speaking and the patients preference. It is important to perform thorough dental prophylaxis before initiating therapy for KS lesions involving the gingiva. Response to therapy is improved if all local plaque and calculus are removed. Local application of sclerosing agents may reduce the size of oral lesions.

Local treatment is appropriate for longer oral KS lesions that interfere with eating and talking. Oral KS can be treated surgically or with localized intralesional chemotherapy, surgical removal is suitable for small, well circumscribed lesions such as gingival or tongue lesions. Surgical removal can be performed under local anesthesia with a blade or with the carbon dioxide laser. Intralesional vinblastine is useful for breaking small lesions, particularly on the palate or gingiva. Several studies have documented the effectiveness of one or two injections of 0.1 to 0.2 mg per ml 33 percent of vinblastine. Post treatment pain is fairly common, but systemic effects are rare. The pain usually disappears several days after therapy.

Radiation therapy may be indicated for large, multiple lesions. A single dose of 800 cGy or an equivalent fractionation is frequently used and produces a good response. Side effects include xerostomia and mucositis, although both conditions usually improve with cessation of radiation therapy.

■ LYMPHOMA

Clinical Features

Diffuse, undifferentiated non-Hodgkin's lymphoma (NHL) is a frequent HIV associated malignancy. Most are of β cell origin and Ebstein-Barr virus occurs in cells from several cases. Lymphoma can occur anywhere in the oral cavity and there may be soft tissue involvement with or without involvement of underlying bone. The lesion may present as a firm, painless swelling that may be ulcerated. Some oral lesions may appear as shallow ulcerations. Oral NHL may appear as solitary lesions with no evidence of disseminated disease.

Differential Diagnosis

Oral NHL may be confused with major apthous ulcers and rarely as a pericoronitis associated with an erupting third molar. Diagnosis of NHL must be made by histologic examination of biopsy specimens.

Treatment

After diagnosis of the oral lesions, the patient must be referred for further evaluation for disseminated disease and its subsequent treatment.

OTHER LESIONS ASSOCIATED WITH HIV DISEASE

Oral Ulceration

Oral ulcers resembling recurrent apthous ulcers (RAU) in HIV infected persons are reported with increasing frequency. The cause of these ulcers is unknown. Proposed causes include stress and unidentified infectious agents. The ulcers of the minor RAU type may appear as solitary lesions of about 0.5 to 1.0 cm. The herpetiform type appears as clusters of small ulcers (1 to 2 mm), usually on the soft palate and oropharynx. The major RAU type appears as extremely large (2 to 4 cm) necrotic ulcers. The major RAUs are very painful and may persist for several weeks.

Diagnosis

The ulcers may become a diagnostic dilemma. Herpetic form RAUs may resemble the lesions of coxsackie virus infection and major RAUs may require biopsy to exclude malignancy, such as lymphoma or opportunistic infection such as histoplasmosis. The ulcers usually occur on nonkeratinized mucosa; this characteristic differentiates them from those caused by herpes simplex.

Treatment

The RAU type ulcers usually respond well to topical steroids such as fluocinolone (0.05%) ointment mixed

with equal parts orabase applied six times daily or clobetasol (0.05%) ointment mixed with equal parts or a base applies three times per day. Dexamethasone elixir (0.5 mg/5 ml) used as a mouthrinse and then expectorated two to three times daily is helpful in multiple ulcers and for those where topical ointments are hard to apply for HIV infected persons with oral and gastrointestinal apthous like ulcers, systemic steroid therapy (predinisolone 40 to 60 mg/day for 7 to 10 days) has been reported as helpful. The risks of steroid therapy, however, must be considered before administration to individuals in this population. Thalidomide (50 to 200 mg) has been used in Europe and is the subject of many clinical trials.

Idiopathic Thrombocytopenic Purpura

Idiopathic thrombocytopenic purpura (ITP) can be seen in HIV infected patients. Oral lesions may be the first manifestation of this condition.

Clinical Features

Petechiae, ecchymoses and hematoma can occur anywhere on the oral mucosa, spontaneous bleeding from the gingiva can occur and patient may report finding blood in their mouths on waking.

Differential Diagnosis

The clinician must distinguish ITP from other vascular lesions and KS. Because of potential bleeding risk, no clinician should obtain blood and platelet counts before performing other diagnostic procedures.

SALIVARY GLAND DISEASE AND XEROSTOMIA

Salivary gland disease-associated with HIV infection (HIV-SGD) can present as xerostomia with or without salivary gland enlargement. Reports describe salivary gland enlargement in children and adults with HIV infection usually involving the parotid gland. The enlarged salivary glands are soft, but not fluctuant. In some cases, enlarged salivary glands may be due to lymphoepithelial cysts. Schiodt et al found that 9 of 12 patients (11 adults and 1 child) with HIV-SGD had salivary gland enlargement and three had xerostomia. Labial salivary gland biopsy revealed histologic features similar to those in Sjögren's syndrome. In HIV-SGD, however, the lymphocytic infiltrate is predominantly CD cells, unlike that in Sjögren's syndrome, which are predominantly CD_4 cells.

No evidence of Epstein-Barr virus or cytomegalovirus has been found in biopsies of salivary glands. One report describes an association between HIV-SGD and HLA-DR5 and HLA-B35 cell surface antigen.

The etiology of HIV-SGD patients are yet unknown but the enlarged parotid glands can be a source of annoyance and discomfort.

Xerostomia: It is sometimes seen in individuals with HIV-SGD. HIV infected patients may also experience dry mouth in association with taking certain medications that can hinder salivary secretion, such as anti-depressants, antihistamines and antianxiety drugs.

Management

Removal of the enlarged parotid glands is rarely recommended for individuals with xerostomia, the use of salivary stimulants such as sugarless gum or sugarless candies may provide relief. Candies that are acidic should be avoided as frequent use may lead to loss of tooth enamel. The use of salivary substitutes may also be helpful. An increase in caries can occur, so fluoride rinses should be used daily and visits to dentists should be scheduled 2 to 3 times per year.

■ MANAGEMENT OF OCCUPATIONAL EXPOSURE AND POST EXPOSURE PROPHYLAXIS

In anticipation of accidental exposure of health care workers (HCW) its necessary to have a comprehensive program in place, for postexposure prophylaxis (PEP). The risk of infection varies with types of exposure and other factors such as:
- The amount of blood involved in the exposure
- The amount of virus in the patient's blood at the time of exposure
- Whether postexposure prophylaxis was taken within the recommended time

Steps to be taken on exposure to HIV infected blood/body fluids and contaminated sharps, etc. immediately following exposure:
- Needle stick injuries and cuts should be washed with soap and water
- Splashes to the noses, mouth or skin should be flushed with water

- Eyes should be irrigated with clean water, saline or sterile irrigants
- Pricked finger should not be put into the mouth by reflex.

Reporting of the Exposure

Report the exposure to the appropriate authority and treat as an emergency. PEP should be started within 2 hours. Initiating treatment after 72 hours of exposure is not recommended.

Determination of HIV Status Code

The main purpose of determining HIV status code (HIV SC) is to know the HIV status of source of exposure.

No PEP is required in case, the source was HIV negative.

If the source was HIV positive, but it was a low titer exposure, the status is HIV SC_1. If it was a high titer exposure then status is HIV SC_2.

If the status of the source is unknown or if the source is unknown, then the status is HIV SC unknown.

Basic Regimen

Zidovudine (AZT)—600 mg in divided doses. (300 mg/twice a day or 200 mg/thrice a day for 4 weeks + lamivudine (3TC)—150 mg twice a day for 4 weeks).

Four weeks of drug therapy is usually sufficient to provide protection against HIV.

Expanded Regimen

Basic regimen + Indinavir—500 mg/thrice a day or any other protease inhibitor.

Testing and Counseling

Testing should be done at time of exposure, at six weeks following exposure and at twelve weeks following exposure.

Pregnancy and PEP

Antiretroviral therapy taken during 2nd and 3rd trimester usually does not cause serious side effects.

Side Effects of these Drugs

Most drugs are well tolerated except for nausea, vomiting, tiredness or headache.

■ HIV TESTING AND COUNSELING

Early diagnosis of HIV infection is critical to control the spread of the virus. Persons infected with HIV are more likely to adopt behavioral changes to reduce transmission of virus. Diagnosis is also the first step into medical care for HIV infected patients.

Different HIV Antibody Assays

ELISA: HIV antibodies in the test serum are detected using an antibody sandwich capture technique. Essentially, HIV antibodies, if present, in the test serum are 'sandwiched' between HIV antigen, which is fixed to the test well and to 'enzymes' that are added to the test well following addition of the test serum. The test well is washed thoroughly to remove any unbound enzyme. A color reagent is then added to the well following addition of the test serum. Any bound enzyme will catalyze a change in color which is read colorimetrically.

Rapid Tests

Varieties of rapid tests are available including particle agglutination, lateral flow membrane, through flow membrane and comb or dipstick—basal assay systems. Rapid tests are most appropriate for the smaller health institutions, where only a few samples are processed each day. Rapid tests are quicker and do not require specialized equipment. Most are dot-blot immunoassays or agglutination assays requiring no instrumentation or specialized training and take 10 to 20 minutes to perform. Most rapid test have sensitivities and specificities equal to ELISA test, which has sensitivity equal to almost 100 percent and specificity to 99 percent or more respectively.

Western Blot

HIV antibodies in the test serum are detected by reacting to a variety of viral proteins. Viral proteins are initially separated into bands according to their molecular weight on an electrophoresis gel. These proteins are then transferred or "blotted" to nitrocellulose paper. The paper is then incubated with the patient's serum. HIV antibodies to specific HIV proteins bind to the nitrocellulose paper at precisely the point to which the target protein migrated. Bound antibodies are detected by colorimetric techniques.

The major advantage of the rapid HIV test is that it allows results to be given on the same day, thus reducing the number of visits made by clients. There is also an increased likelihood of clients receiving test results on the same day.

Transfusion Safety

A single ERS (ELISA Rapid Simple) test is sufficient to ensure transfusion safely with the provision of simple test in places without electricity. The objective of the transfusion safety does not require identification of donor of the infected unit of blood and in low prevalence settings of HIV, single ERS would detect at least 56 percent samples falsely positive. However the same test gives more than 99.9 percent surity that blood found negative is actually free of infection. Therefore, while we can label blood as safe, it is risky to label any donor HIV positive on such test result.

Diagnosis of HIV in the Newborn

HIV antibody assays cannot be used to diagnose HIV infection in the neonate, due to secondary transmission of maternal antibodies via the placenta or breast milk. Maternal antibodies may be present in the neonate for up to 18 months. Neonates will test HIV antibody positive, whether they have HIV infection or not during this period. Antenatal diagnosis is confirmed at 18 months of age by a persistently positive HIV antibody test. HIV can be diagnosed in the newborn before this point of time by using a variety of non-antibody based assays. These assays include HIV p24 antigen, viral culture or HIV PCR tests which may be quantitative, or qualitative. The sensitivities of these assays ranges from 8 to 32 percent, from 95 to 100 percent and to > 99 percent respectively.

Goals of HIV Pretest Counseling

1. To help the patient make an informed choice
2. To explore the patient's knowledge on HIV/AIDS and provide correct information
3. To assess the patient's potential exposure to HIV
4. To explain the process of testing
5. To help patients prepare themselves for the test result and the issues that may arise after learning their HIV status
6. To bring about behavior change in order to prevent further transmission
7. To refer patients for medical and nonmedical care and support, if necessary.

Aims of Post test Counseling

1. To help patient understand and cope with the HIV test results
2. To provide the patient with any further information required
3. To help the patient make immediate and short term and long term future plans to improve the quality of life
4. To help the patient decide what to do about disclosing their test result to partners and others.

Reproductive Health Services

Female patients who are pregnant or of child bearing age should receive or be referred to reproductive health services. HIV infected pregnant women should be referred to PPTCT (Prevention of parent to child transmission of HIV) program.

Transmission of HIV from parent to child can occur during pregnancy, at the time of delivery or through breastfeeding. There is a 25 to 30 percent chance that the child of an HIV positive mother will also be infected with HIV in India. Parent-to-child transmission of HIV (perinatal transmission) accounts for more than 2 percent of the country's HIV/AIDS cases. HIV transmission from parent-to-child can be prevented with a combination of low cost, short term preventive drug treatment, safe delivery practices, counseling and support and safe infant feeding methods.

■ PROTOCOL FOR TREATING HIV POSITIVE PATIENTS

Theatre

1. The posting of the patient should be at the end of the operating list and to allow ample time for the theatre and scrub room to clean after surgery. The patient should be induced in the theatre and should recover fully in the theatre, so that contamination is contained within that theatre room.
2. All nonessential items should be removed from the theatre, but leave enough on trolley.
3. The operating table should be covered with waterproof sheet.
4. All equipment needed for observing precautions should be available within the theatre before the case is started. This include:
   a. Adequate quantities of a suitable disinfectant, e.g. freshly prepared 2 percent gluteraldehyde or 1 percent spdoi, hypochlorite solution.
   b. Plastic apron to be worn under the gowns by all personnel.
   c. Eye protective should be worn.
   d. Specimen bottles to be labeled with "Biohazard" and outer plastic bag for safe transport of specimen.
   e. Linen and plastic bags for transporting linen and instruments.
5. After surgery, the operating room and all equipment must be throughly cleaned with hot soapy water and sodium hypochlorite.
   (N.B. sodium hypochlorite must not be used on stainless steel).

Personnel

Nonessential personnel should not be admitted into the operating room during surgery and those inside should be kept to a minimum. This means that an extra nurse and technician will be required to be stationed outside the operating room door to fetch any equipment or drugs needed for the scrub nurse, surgeon or anesthetist during surgery. This is to prevent infection spreading to the rest of the theatre block.

Spillage

Should there be spillage of body fluids or blood, this should be dealt with as follows:
a. The area should be covered with sodium hypochlorite 1 percent and left for 30 minutes.
b. It should be mopped up by a knowledgeable person using gloves and old linen paper towels (newspaper) and sent for incineration (In plastic bag).

Instruments

Procedure for autoclavable instruments:
a. These should be autoclaved before washing
b. Allow to cool
c. Wash in soapy water
d. Rinse
e. Reautoclave
f. Brushes used for washing instruments.

Procedure for nonautoclavable instruments:
a. Immerse in gluteraldehyde 2 percent for one hour
b. Discard this solution
c. Instruments should be physically cleaned in warm water and detergent
d. Rinse in gluteraldehyde 2 percent and leave to soak for 3 hours.

Procedure for suction bottles:

These should contain 30 ml of gluteraldehyde 2 percent or 60 ml of hypochlorite 2 percent.

After surgery they should be carefully emptied, rinsed and autoclaved.

Procedure for anesthetic equipment:

Ventilator tubes should be rinsed with running tap water for 5 minutes and subsequently immersed in gluteraldehyde 2 percent solution for 6 hours.

Sharps

Special care required when dealing with needles and sharps. Needles should be decontaminated before disposal.

Laboratory Specimens

These should be clearly labeled and double bagged in plastic bags for transportation.

■ DISINFECTANTS

a.	Fresh sodium hypochlorite	1% 30 min
b.	Gluteraldehyde	2% 60 min
c.	Formaldehyde	5% min 60 min
d.	Ethyl alcohol	70% 60 min
e.	Isopropyl alcohol	50% 60 min
f.	Lysol	1% 60 min
g.	Fresh hydrogen peroxide	3% 60 min

Recent Advances in Oral
and Maxillofacial Surgery

52 Recent Advances in Oral and Maxillofacial Surgery

Innovations and discoveries in the field of science are happening rapidly. The emerging technologies are rapidly changing the nature of dental, medical, and surgical practice. As clinicians involved in direct patient care, it is our fundamental duty to keep abreast with latest advances in the field of medical sciences and use these technologies judiciously for the benefit of the patients. On the other hand, clinician must be prudent enough to adopt the new technology, and should not put the patients to increased risk, in the name of advanced technology. This chapter will cover the latest trends and changes in the field of oral and maxillofacial surgery under the following heads.

—Advances in the field of radiology and imaging

Positron emission tomography scan and its application in Head and neck region.

- Stereophotogrammetry and laser surface scanning
- Intraoperative navigation and robotic surgery
- Rapid prototyping and stereolithography
- Surgical guides and custom made implants
- Tissue engineering and stem cell research as applicable to oral and maxillofacial surgery
- Minimal invasive surgery and role of endoscopes in oral and maxillofacial region
- Advances in local anesthesia and general anesthesia

- Advances in TMJ surgery
- Advances in maxillofacial trauma management
- Advances in topical hemostatic agents

Advances in the Field of Radiology and Imaging

Over the last two decades, there have been tremendous improvements in the field radiology and imaging. There are faster and powerful computed tomography (CT) and magnetic resonance imaging (MRI) machines backed by advanced softwares and graphics, which have given the capability to capture images of any part of the body in great detail. With the use of digital radiography it is possible to see images instantaneously with decreased dose of ionizing radiation. The images can be stored, manipulated, and retrieved easily.

CT scan has become an invaluable tool in assessment of craniofacial morphology. It gives better details of bone as compared to the soft tissues. With advanced multi slice scanners it is possible to capture images in great detail in all the three planes in a few seconds. CT angiograms give accurate pictures of vascular anatomy in vascular lesions. Further, data generated by CT in the form of 'Digital imaging and communication in medicine' (DICOM) files can be used to construct actual 3 dimensional (3D) models.

Advances in the field of MRI technology have produced faster machines with no need to lie in closed chambers for long time. MRI is an important tool in the diagnosis of head and neck pathologies. Major advantage is that it does not use ionizing radiations and gives excellent soft tissue details. It is useful in evaluation of head and neck malignancies, temporomandibular joint (TMJ) pathologies and vascular lesions. MRI angiograms are helpful in differentiation between high flow and low flow vascular malformation. DICOM data generated from MRI can also be used for production of stereolithographic models.

Positron Emission Tomography (PET) and PET/CT

Advent of PET and combined PET/CT is a promising development. These modalities have the potential to help in staging, identifying responses to nonsurgical therapy and allowing early detection of recurrence of patients with head and neck cancer. The positron emission tomography is used to study *in vivo* metabolic processes by using physiologically active compounds labelled with short acting positron emitting isotopes. Positron emitting tracers, e.g. oxygen-15, nitrogen-13, and fluorine-18 can bound to a variety of molecules, which are used in the human metabolic pathways. Fluorodeoxyglucose (FDG) is the most widely used tracer with PET imaging. When administered intravenously, FDG is trapped as 2-deoxyglucose-6-phosphate within cells. The unstable photon rich fluoro nucleus rids itself of excessive charge with emission of a positively charged electron, becoming a more stable nucleus. These positrons travel a millimetre or less in the tissues before interacting with electron resulting in an annihilation reaction, which results in release of two photons at approximately 180 degrees to one another (gamma photons). Detection of these photons by detectors is used to build-up three dimensional representations of these events. The data are displayed in a manner similar to conventional sectional imaging. These images produced reflect glucose uptake within various tissues.

The application of PET-FDG in detection of malignancy arises because of the hallmark of the malignant cells, which is increased glucose metabolism. One of the disadvantages of PET is that the areas of abnormality on PET imaging cannot be perfectly correlated with the anatomy. To overcome this problem PET scans are increasingly read alongside CT or MRI scans, the combination giving both anatomic and metabolic information. The fusion of PET and CT technology (PET/CT) taken on a single device offers excellent localization and improved detection of head and neck pathologies.

One of the main advantages of PET/CT is that, it can pick-up the lesions in early stage before these are morphological evident, which leads to earlier diagnosis of tumors. It is helpful in head and neck malignancy to detect metastatic or recurrent disease and occult primary unknown cancer. In addition, it can demarcate tumor margins at sites, where it is difficult to evaluate the tumor clinically. It is particularly helpful in areas, where it is difficult to separate recurrence from changes resulting from previous treatment, such as surgery and radiotherapy. It can establish whether enlarged lymph nodes contain tumor or are reactive and it can detect small foci of disease (Fig. 52. 1) and assess the whole body in one step with a much lower dose of radiation than whole body CT. Other use of PET/CT is in evaluating growth abnormalities of the temporomandibular joint such as condylar hyperplasia (Fig. 52. 2).

Many benign causes and several artefacts can simulate physiologic or pathologic FDG uptake in the head and neck, e.g. tuberculous cervical lymph nodes may mimic malignancy on PET. Therefore, interpreting

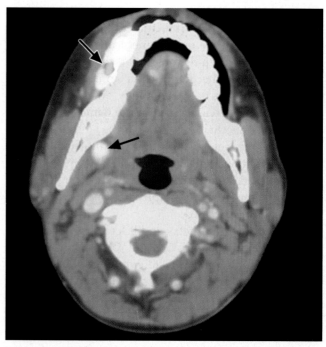

Fig. 52.1: PET/CT fusion image in a patient with oral squamous cell carcinoma of buccal mucosa, showing metastasis to ipsilateral submandibular lymph nodes

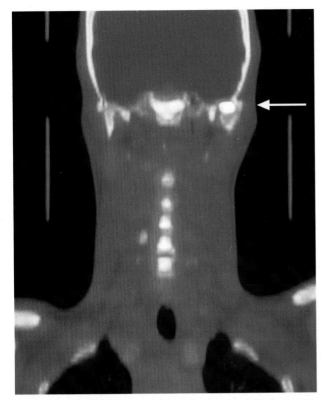

Fig. 52.2: PET/CT fusion image showing hyperactivity (hot spot) in left TMJ in a case of condylar hyperplasia

radiologists and nuclear medicine physicians must be familiar with the patterns of FDG uptake in the head and neck to avoid misinterpretation or misdiagnosis.

Stereophotogrammetry and Laser Surface Scanning

These are the two most commonly used techniques to capture the three dimensional surface images of face. Stereophotogrammetry uses two or three cameras configured to a computer to capture a stereo image of face by means of triangulation. In laser surface scanning the light and camera technology is used to capture the image exact position of surface point on the object. Then computer software is used to synchronize the data and generate a 3D image. These images can be used for diagnosis, treatment planning and comparison of surgical outcome, as these images are highly accurate (up to 0.5 mm accuracy). The maxillofacial applications of these 3D cameras are growing, especially in orthognathic surgery, orthodontics and evaluation of craniofacial deformities. It is possible to superimpose photographic soft tissue data over the bony data set obtained from CT or CBCT. This fusion of hard tissue images and surface images of face provides opportunities for diagnosis and planning corrective surgeries and postoperative comparisons. 3D cephalometric measurements can be done on these images.

Rapid Prototyping and Stereolithography

Rapid prototyping is the process of creation of physical models from medical scan data. The physical model is built in a layered manner and it reproduces internal and external anatomy accurately. Medical scan data can be obtained from CT, CBCT or MRI. There are many technologies for manufacturing of medical models. All of these technologies were basically developed for industrial purposes and later on adopted for production of medical models. These include stereolithography, selective laser sintering, 3D printing, fused deposition modelling, digital light processing and polyjet modelling. Stereolithography is the most commonly used technology and involves selectively solidifying an ultra-violet sensitive liquid medical resin using laser beam. Stereolithographic models (Figs 52.3A to D) can be used for diagnosis, surgical planning, teaching, custom made implants and prosthetic devices. The models allow for wax replacement of avulsed structures or generation of mirror-image structures, prebending of osteosynthesis bone plates, fabrication of templates, choosing of stock alloplasts. These technologies are also used for making surgical guides (Fig. 52.4), and scaffolds for tissue engineering.

Surgical Guides and Custom made Implants

Special interactive computer softwares are available for maxillofacial surgery and oral implant planning (Figs 52.5A to C) and (Fig. 52.6).

Scanned data from CT or CBCT is converted into virtual 3D models. These virtual models can be used for surgical planning in cases of orthognathic surgery, distraction osteogenesis and dental implant placement. This virtual planning can be used for production of surgical guides, stents or customised implants. With the help of surgical guides, operation can be performed exactly according to the plan with reduced operating time.. Surgical guides are quite popular for dental implant placement (Fig. 52.4). In implantology, surgery is no longer restricted to the imagination of operator, but can be visualized in 3D. Template systems designed to

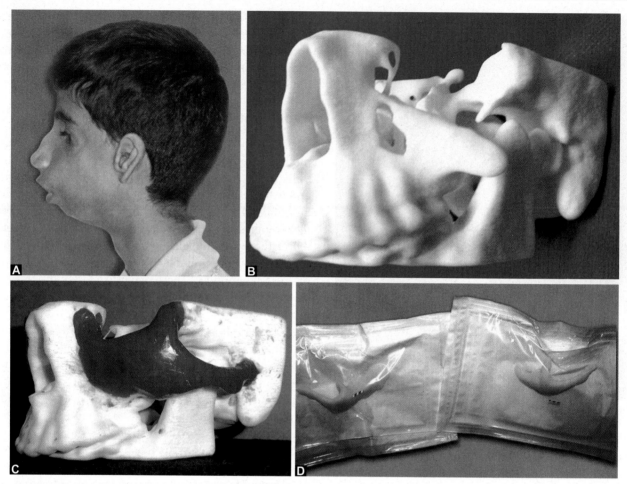

Figs 52.3A to D: (A) Profile of a patient suffering from Treacher collin syndrome, (B) Stereolithographic model of the patient suffering from Treacher Collin Syndrome. Model was generated from scanned CT data, (C) Wax-up was done on this model for planned malar reconstruction with customised porous polyethylene implant, (D) Customised implant for correction of missing malar prominence was manufactured by the company biopore. (Nobel guide implant planning software was used. Virtual 3D model generated from scanned CT data is being used for placement of zygoma implants. surgery was done as per the planning.)

transfer a preoperative desired implant position on to the surgical site are reported to produce accuracy, eliminate errors in manual insertion and complications like damage to inferior alveolar nerve canal can be avoided.

Its applications for osteotomy guide, distractor placement guide and occlusal wafer guide for orthognathic surgery are increasing. Surgical guides have been shown to provide an accurate reliable physical alternative to computer guided navigation.

Softwares can also be used to capture the anatomy of normal side and produce mirror image to be used as guide for reconstruction on the abnormal side. Rapid prototyping techniques can be used to construct customized implants. These customized implants reproduce the exact details as needed by the patient (Fig. 52.3).

INTRAOPERATIVE NAVIGATION AND ROBOTIC SURGERY

Surgery in the cranial area includes complex anatomic situations with high risk vital structures and high demands for functional and esthetic results. Conventional surgery requires that the surgeon transfers complex anatomic and surgical planning information, using spatial sense and experience. The surgical procedure depends entirely on the manual skills of the operator. The development of image-guided surgery provides new revolutionary opportunities by integrating presurgical 3D imaging and intraoperative manipulation.

Integration of imaging with surgical field allows visualization of different types of images and simultaneously shows structures that are normally visible intraoperatively and permit navigation in areas of anatomical sensitivity. This enables preoperative surgical planning to be incorporated directly into the procedure. Clinical benefits of image guided surgery include use of smaller incisions, direct access to targeted areas and consequently less invasive procedures.

Computer aided surgery systems are commonly used in neurosurgery, endoscopic sinus surgery, and some orthopedic procedures. Because of the complex nature of maxillofacial reconstruction procedures, these systems are now being used for maxillofacial surgery. Intra-operative navigation gives the surgeon control in difficult access areas and complex procedures, thus reducing the chances of human error.

In computer aided surgical systems a virtual patient is generated from the preoperative scans. Certain stable landmarks are identified on both the virtual patient and actual patient. In technical language, these markers are known as 'Fiducial markers'. These markers serve as a guide for tracking of the patient and surgical instrument in space. Tracking is mainly done with the help of transmitters, which uses an optical source or electromagnetic source. There are two transmitters, one to be placed on the patient and other to be placed on surgical instrument. Computer with the help of fiducial markers integrates the information from the actual

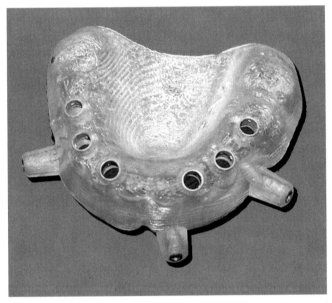

Fig. 52.4: Custom made surgical guide for dental implant placement manufactured through rapid prototyping. Planning was done on Interactive Implant planning software (Nobel biocare)

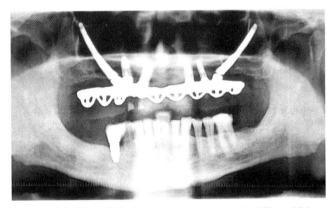

Fig. 52.6: Final OPG of zygomatic bone supported (R) and (I) implants

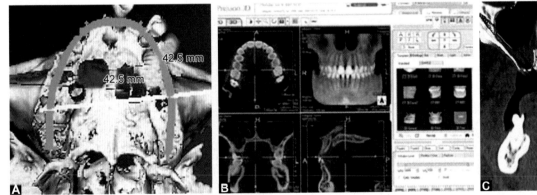
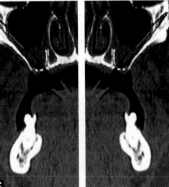

Figs 52.5A to C: (A) Nobel guide implant planning software. Virtual 3D model generated from scanned CT data is being used for placement of zygoma Implants. Surgery was done as per the planning; (B) Different softwares for construction of 3D models; (C) Zygomatic bone supported (R) and (L) implants placement planning

patient with the virtual patient to precisely locate the patient and surgical instrument in space.

Further step in the advancement with fusion of these technologies is robotic surgery. In robotic surgery, a robotic arm controlled by the surgeon, sitting far away from the operation table, actually performs the procedure. Surgery with great precision in difficult areas through minimal access is possible with the help of robotic arm. Many advanced hospitals in the world have robotic surgery suites to perform difficult surgeries in head and neck with the help of robotic arm (Trans-oral robotic system—TORS based on Da Vinci robotic arm) (Figs 52.7A and B). TORS has the benefits of being less invasive, with fewer complications and shorter hospital stays. There is less blood loss, little scarring, and fewer temporary and permanent side effects, such as loss of speech or swallowing ability. Surgeons operate with greater precision and control using the TORS approach, minimizing the pain, and reducing the risk of possible nerve and tissue damage linked to large incisions.

Minimal Invasive Surgery and Role of Endoscopes in Oral and Maxillofacial Region

Minimally invasive surgery, with the use of the endoscope has improved in recent years, because of technological advancements in optics and associated instrumentation. Flexible endoscopes have revolutionized many fields of surgery including maxillofacial surgery. First application of endoscopic surgery was in sinus surgery and functional endoscopic sinus surgery has become a standard of care. Endoscopic surgery has been applied to many areas of craniomaxillofacial surgery, which includes

correction of cranial synostosis, esthetic procedures like brow lift, forehead contoring, frontal sinus fracture repair, orbital decompression, various osteotomies and fracture repair including mandibular condyle fractures. Trauma, orthognathic, sialoendoscopy, and TMJ surgery are commonly performed with the assistance of the endoscope. From an educational standpoint, surgical anatomy and various other principles can easily be taught to trainees with the assistance of the endoscope. The operating surgeon can visualize an area via the endoscope, and instruct regarding the surgical maneuvres on the monitor, without obstructions to view. This technique also allows others in and out of the room to view the image. Endoscopically assisted surgery is gaining popularity and is becoming a tool frequently used by surgeons to assist in and simplify some of the more difficult techniques that often require more extensive surgical exposure for visualization. In this way, difficult deeply located areas can be accessed easily through small incisions ,thus reducing morbidity and hospital stay. Flexible endoscope is especially available for TMJ arthroscopy, and salivary gland endoscopy. Endoscopically assisted approaches have been advocated for open reduction and internal fixation of condylar fractures (Fig. 52.8). This approach allows fracture treatment with limited transoral incision. In conjunction with transoral approach, scars are invisible and risk of facial nerve damage is minimal.

With the advent of sialoendoscope (Figs 52.9A toC) nonsurgical removal of stones has become possible. Sialoendoscopy has been used for obstructive sialadenitis. Its use is recommended in all cases where stone has not been visualised radiologically. It is also useful

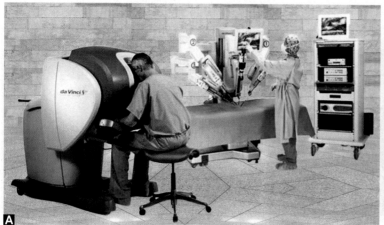
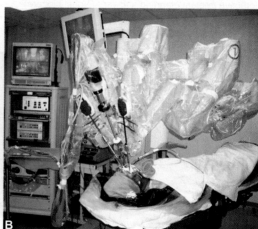

Figs 52. 7A and B: (A) Robotic surgery—da Vinci operation suite for performing robotic surgery; (B) Transoral robotic surgery with the help of robotic arm in a head and neck cancer patient

for balloon dilation of ductal strictures, basket retrieval of stones and washing of mucosal plugs.

Fiberoptic assisted intubation for general anesthesia also has made the job of anesthetist easy in difficult airway cases.

Tissue Regeneration/Engineering in Oral and Maxilla-Facial Surgery

An oral and maxillofacial surgeon is constantly facing the difficult task of reconstruction of missing tissues as a result of ablative surgery, post traumatic or congenital defects. Each different anatomic area offers a different challenge in terms of specific need for bone reconstruction in terms of esthetics, form and function.

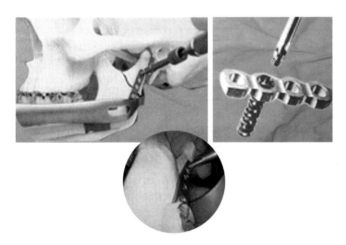

Fig. 52.8: Instrumentation and technique for endoscopic assisted reduction and fixation of condylar fracture

Autogenous bone grafting, regional or free microvascular flaps have been the main stay for reconstruction, but this causes possible donor and recipient site morbidity. The development of effective reconstructive procedures using tissue engineering techniques without the need for conventional tissue transplantation procedures can have a tremendous impact on surgery of head and neck area.

Tissue engineering is an interdisciplinary field comprising of cell biologists, bio-chemists, material scientists, engineers, and clinicians, and an understanding of the complex role of the various components with the aim to create limitless and readily available supply of off- the- shelf tissue regenerates. Tissue engineering involves the vital collaboration between the three key components, stem cells, resorbable scaffolds and bioactive molecules such as growth factors. The combination of scaffolds and cells is often referred to as a construct. Constructs may be fashioned ex *vivo*, and then implanted into an individual.

Approaches to Tissue Engineering

(a) Growth factors/Bone Morphogenic Proteins: BMPs are a group of osteoinductive sequentially arranged amino acids and polypeptides that are capable of stimulating adult mesenchymal cells to become osteoblasts and form bone. Adult mesenchymal cells are supplied by periosteum and paraperiosteal connective tissue. Recombinant human BMP-2 (rh-BMP-2) (Infuse, medi-tronics) was approved as an alternative to autogenous bone graft for sinus augmentations and for localized

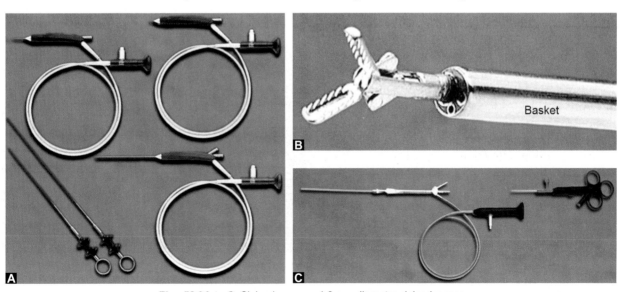

Figs 52.9A to C: Sialendoscope—1.3 mm diameter sialendoscope

alveolar ridge defects associated with extraction sockets. It has been used for reconstruction of mandibular continuity defects as well. Tissue engineered osteo-inductive grafts may someday eliminate the need for harvesting cortico-cancellous grafts. At present rh-BMP-2 is very costly. However, there is no need to harvest autologous bone graft, the cost of surgery and duration of hospital stay is less, thereby reducing the cost difference with non BMP cases.

(b) Stem Cells: Stem cells can dedifferentiate in the correct setting into simple, unspecified forms. They, then have the ability to form new structures based on the stimulus and chemical factors that are present in the matrix. There are two types of stem cells – adult stem cells and embryonic stem cells. Human embryonic stem cells are pluripotent stem cells isolated from the inner mass of human blastocysts. At this time, embryonic stem cells are not usually used in the clinical setting and are used for only research purpose in some countries. Embryonic stem cells have great potential because of their capacity for differentiation. However, before human embryonic stem cells can be used clinically for tissue engineering, problems, such as culturing them without exposure to animal proteins as well as avoiding teratoma formation and immune rejection by the recipient's host, must be solved.

The source of cells for tissue engineering depends on the structure to be replaced. Currently, adult stem cells used in clinical setting are autologous cells. For the tissue engineering of bone, cells from the bone marrow and adipose tissue have been used as autologous cells, These have the ability to dedifferentiate from mesenchymal cells to osteoblasts and then to osteocytes, which have the ability to lay bone in a laminated form. Harvesting adipose tissue or bone marrow is not morbid. These cells are then used to seed a resorbable scaffold made with CAD/CAM technology to the precise dimensions of a missing segment of bone. The seeded cells can be stimulated physically with magnetic or galvanic stimulation, ultrasound, hypoxic or hyperoxic gradients, growth factors such as transforming growth factor beta-1 (TGFB-1), bone morphogenetic proteins (BMPs) or vascular endothelial growth factor (VEGF), to guide the differentiation and growth of the cells.

Despite some success in areas of bone tissue engineering, limitation of these techniques, methods and strategies are evident in the clinical arena. The central issue is how to generate a blood supply within any bone construct such that new bone functions as normal bone. Blood supply allows bone to fight infection and to receive nutrition that aid in its incorporation and remodeling at the site of implantation. Without a method of generating an adequate blood supply, bone regeneration cannot become the method of choice. Although use of tissue engineering for reconstruction of mandible has been reported at present, the technology is very expensive and at experimental stage.

Stem cells from dental pulp from developing teeth, shed deciduous teeth and dental follicle provide other source of adult epithelial and mesenchymal stem cells (Fig. 52.10).

Third molar removal also presents some opportunity for harvesting follicular cells, cementoblast-like cells and dental pulp stem cells, which have been cultured and studied. The receptors of these cells can be characterized, an important first step in understanding these cells and their potential future use.

There is a hope to create synthetic form of bone, skin, cartilage and muscle that can function as well as normal tissues depends on ability to effectively integrate multiple technologies and components that are capable of meeting the complex demands of reconstruction in head and neck area. No single scientific field can generate the ideal method of engineering tissues. However, through collaboration and expansion of progression in tissue engineering the right combination of materials, cells and growth factors may be found, so as to make taking tissues from other sites of body a thing of past.

Fig. 52.10: Stem cell cultured from dental pulp at Department of Regenerative Medicine, Postgraduate Institute of Medical Education and Research, Chandigarh

Advances in Local Anesthetics

In oral surgery, local pain management is the most critical aspect of patient care. Improvement in local anesthetic agents and their delivery system are the most significant advances that have occurred in last decade. Today's anesthetics are safe, effective and can be reversed and are associated with minimal risk of allergic reactions.

Articaine

It is a new aminoamide class of local anesthetic, approved by FDA in 2000 for clinical use. It is available in 4% strength with 1: 100,000 o 1: 200,000 epinephrine. It has thiopentone ring instead of benzene ring, which makes it more lipid soluble. Therefore, it has got better tissue penetration and diffusion than the lidocaine. Because of better bone penetration and diffusion it can anesthetise palatal side and anterior lingual sides with buccal infiltration only. Because of the presence of additional ester group it can undergo biotransformation in plasma as well as in liver. Its lower systemic toxicity and wide therapeutic range allows its use for in higher concentration than other amide type local anesthetic. The maximum dose of 4% articaine should not exceed 7 mg/kg body weight. 4% articaine is as efficient as 2% lidocaine in achieving anesthesia for various dental and oral surgical procedures.

Reversing Effects of Local Anesthesia

Soft tissue anesthesia after local anaesthetic infiltration or block may linger on for several hours. This may not be desirable in certain case especially in children. In 2009, FDA approved phentolamine mesylate (Oraverse, Novalar Pharmaceuticals Inc. USA) for the reversal of the local anesthetic. This can be used both in adults and children, but not recommended below six years of age or weight <15 kg. Phentolamine is an α adrenergic agonist, it acts by providing vasodilatation, thus allowing the faster diffusion of local anesthetic into vascular system. It is injected in same volume as the local anesthetic and it accelerates the reversal of soft tissue anesthesia.

Local Anesthesia Delivery Devices

Fear of needle prick and pain during injection of local anesthetic are the main problems of local anesthesia delivery. Newer local anesthetic delivery devices not only provide reduction in pain on injection and failure rates, but also produce more precise anesthetised area.

Vibrotactile, Vibraject, dental vibe, accupal, compudent are the few local anesthetic delivery devices which uses vibration technology to decrease the pain on injection.

Advances in General Anesthesia Technique

Submental Intubation in Maxillofacial Trauma Patients

Airway management during surgery in patients with complex craniomaxillofacial trauma has always been a challenge for anesthesiologists, as the surgeon and the anesthesiologist share the same limited space. Intraoperative assessment of occlusion and maxillomandibular fixation is often required for exact reduction of facial fractures. Conventional oral tracheal intubation does not allow intraoperative assessment of the occlusion and maxillomandibular wiring. Most oral surgical procedures are undertaken with the nasotracheal tube in place. In certain circumstances where access to both the nose and oral cavity is required, the endotracheal tube has to be shifted intraoperatively from the nose to the oral cavity or vice versa.

Submental intubation is a procedure in which endotracheal tube is passed through a surgically created opening in submental region (Fig. 52.11).

It allows free intraoperative access to the dental occlusion and the nasal pyramid. Therefore, simultaneous treatment of all the facial fractures, without interference of the tube or the need of switching tube from nasal to oral or vice versa during surgery. Usually there are no additional problems in passing the tube through the floor of the mouth. Complications of submental intubation

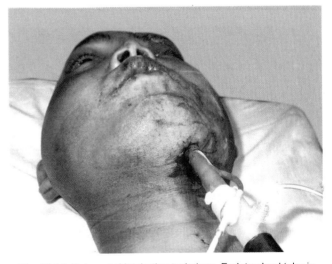

Fig. 52.11: Submental intubation technique. Endotracheal tube is brought out through a surgically created opening in submental region

could include damage to the cuff balloon, infection of submental wound, abscess formation in the floor of the mouth, salivary fistula, development of mucocele, and hypertrophic scarring. All these complications are relatively rare and avoidable with meticulous technique.

Retromolar Intubation Technique

To avoid invasive nature and complications associated with submental intubation the technique of retromolar intubation can be used in selected cases. In this technique, the endotracheal tube is placed in the retromolar space behind the last erupted teeth (Fig. 52.12). Arora and Rattan, for the first time demonstrated that there is sufficient space in retromolar region for successful placement of the endotracheal tube in children and certain adults. In some adults this space can be created by extracting nonfunctional third molars. Intermaxillary fixation of teeth is possible with endotracheal tube exiting through retromolar space. This technique has the potential of replacing more invasive techniques such as tracheostomy and submental intubation in some cases..

Advances in TMJ Surgery

Advances in TMJ Arthroscopy and One Point Arthroscopy

The improvements in optics and lens technology have advanced the ability to diagnose and treat various pathologic conditions of TMJ through arthroscopy. The TMJ arthroscope is a small, tube like camera that projects the image of the joint onto a monitor, allowing the surgeon to view the inside the joint without making any

large incisions. Over the last decade TMJ arthroscopy and arthrocentesis have gained popularity because of its minimal invasive nature and low complication rates. Now it is possible to use lasers instead of conventional cutting instruments through the arthroscope. This allows the surgeon to cut and ablate tissues without causing iatrogenic tissue damage.

Standard TMJ arthroscopy involves two arthroscopy portal punctures over the TMJ. One is for the arthroscope and other for the blunt probe, which is used for lysis and lavage. Recently one puncture arthroscope has been introduced for visualisation of TMJ. The OnPoint™ 1.2 mm Scope System (Biomet Microfixation, USA) is an innovative breakthrough that provides minimally invasive visualization of the TMJ in the comfort and convenience of an office based setting. It uses disposable 1.2 mm fiberoptic scope (Fig. 52.13). With a scope diameter no larger than an 18 gauge needle, this state-of-the-art imaging system allows for an accurate and less invasive procedure.

BUCCAL PAD OF FAT IN TMJ RECONSTRUCTION

This technique has been invented by Rattan V, in year 2004. In this technique dead space created after gap

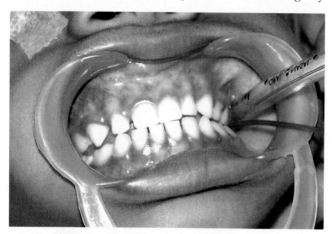

Fig. 52.12: Retromolar intubation technique. Endotracheal tube is brought out through the retromolar space. Occlusion can be achieved without any hindrance

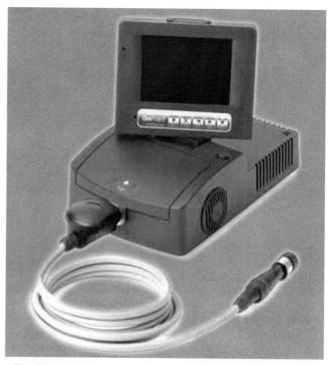

Fig. 52.13: Single port 1.2 mm flexible TMJ arthroscope (Onpoint)

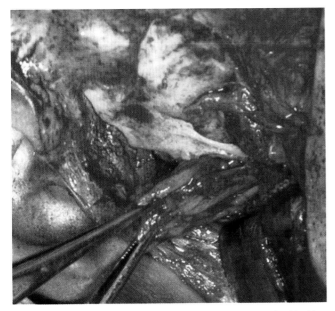

Fig. 52.14: Buccal pad of fat flap can easily reach TMJ for blocking the dead space and prevents heterotopic bone formation. Technique developed by Dr Vidya Rattan

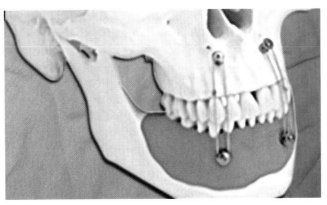

Fig. 52.15: Intermaxillary fixation with the help of screws (Synthes)

arthroplasty is blocked with the help of buccal pad of fat. Buccal pad of fat is harvested through the same preauricular approach as used for TMJ surgery. Blunt dissection is done anteromedial to the coronoid process, where buccal pad of fat is located and it is transposed to TMJ area (Fig. 52.14). This fat can completely block the dead space as compared to any other tissue, because of its fluidity. This prevents formation of blood clot, which is primary factor for heterotopic bone formation and reankylosis of TMJ. Long term viability of this flap has been established by the author in a MRI study. This technique has totally eliminated chances of reankylosis of TMJ. In a follow up of 60 cases, ranging from 1 to 7 years, treated by this technique, none of the patients had reankylosis.

Recent Advances in Maxillofacial Trauma Management

High velocity trauma leads to badly comminuted and displaced fractures. To manage these complex fractures, there have been improvements in techniques of fracture fixation and reduction. Other advances in the field of surgery are also applicable to trauma management. This include improved diagnostic imaging, minimal access surgery and endoscopic surgery, biomaterial advances, intra-operative imaging, rapid prototyping techniques, computer assisted surgery, and customised implants.

Intermaxillary Fixation Screws

Special screws for intermaxillary fixation are available, which have a hole for passage of wire below the screw head. The screws are inserted above the root apices in maxilla and mandible, and wire is passed through the holes to close the mouth in occlusion (Fig. 52.15). These are temporary fixation devices and once the fractures are fixed screws can be removed intraoperatively or a later date under local anesthesia. Screws are quick to place, maintain better oral hygiene, and there is no risk of prick injury, as compared to fixation with arch bars and wires. There is risk of injury to tooth roots so these should be placed away from roots of teeth.

Rapid IMF

Rapid IMF (Synthes, Switzerland) is an adjustable flexible plastic band that wraps around the tooth to create an anchorage point for temporary maxillomandibular fixation and immobilization. These have been developed to reduce the risk of needle-stick injury. Intermaxillary fixation is done with the help of elastic chain (Fig. 52.16). These anchorage points can retain intermaxillary fixation up to three weeks.

A recent and significant advancement has been the development of resorbable implants. Drawbacks of currently used titanium implants may include soft tissue irritation and cold intolerance, creation of distortion artefact on computed tomography and magnetic resonance imaging, weakening of bone from excessively rigid fixation, "stress shielding" possible interference with facial growth, implant migration over time, and the possible need for subsequent implant removal. Resorbable plates provide initial osseous fixation strength for direct bone healing and then they disappear over a period of time leaving behind no foreign body.

Resorbable plates and screws typically feature one or a combination of the esters of polylactic acid (PLA) or polyglycolic acid (PGA). PLA occurs in the stereoisomer polylevolactic acid (PLLA) and the stereocopolymer polydextrolactic acid (PLDA). The strength of plates depends on the biomechanical properties of polymer used. PLLA is the strongest with least tissue reaction and bulk, although not as resorbable. PLLA plates have 50% yield strength required to break a titanium miniplate—champy type. PLDA is the weaker polymer that degrades rapidly. The alloy of PLLA and PLDA can achieve a balance between strength, lack of bulkiness, crystallinity and optimal resorption rate. The manufacturing process technique is also important for optimization of biomechanical properties of the plates.

PLA and PGA are degraded by hydrolytic destruction of the polymer via citric acid cycle in the liver followed by metabolism of single lactic or glycolic acid molecules through corresponding biochemical pathways and elimination primarily through respiration. The rate of degradation depends upon blended composition of the PLA and PGA components. Complete resorption may take 12—24 months depending on the composition.

Potential problems of biodegradable plating systems include decreased strength; screws require tapping, water bath for heating to aid adaptation, and increased bulk as compared to titanium. These plates are costly than titanium plates. These materials have been successfully used for fixation of fractured and osteotomised segments in craniomaxillofacial region.

The strength of these plates has been improved by self reinforcing technique in which polymeric fibers of same material are added to the binding matrix of the plates and screws. These (BioSorb FXs, Conmed Linvatec, Finland) plates can be bent at room temperature and do not require heat to become malleable (Fig. 52.17).

SonicWeld Treatment

The SonicWeld Rx (KLS Martin, USA) system is a further improvement to overcome the limitations of resorbable screw. The SonicWeld Rx process takes advantage of polymer characteristics instead of adapting titanium screw designs. A completely resorbable SonicPin Rx is inserted into a predrilled hole. The user activates the SonicWelder, creating ultrasound vibration while driving the pin into the pilot hole (Fig. 52.18). The SonicPin penetrates into all bone cavities and welds to

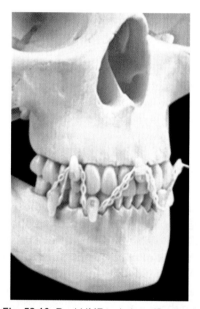

Fig. 52.16: Rapid IMF technique (Synthes)

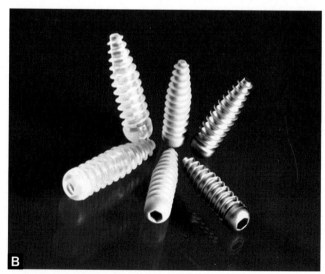

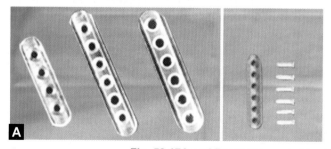

Fig. 52.17A and B: (A) Bioresorbable plates and screws, (B) Bioresorbable screws

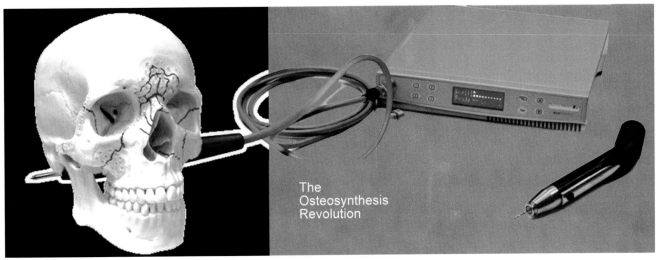

Fig. 52.18: SonicWeld treatment concept (KLS Martin)

the resorbable plate. The SonicPin is allowed to return to a solid, and then the process is complete. The result is a three dimensionally stable construct. Implant insertion takes only a few seconds and there is minimal possibility of stripping in the hone or shearing of the pin as with screw fixation. SonicPin is comprised of the same material as PDLLA implants (Resorb-X). Resorb-X implants are a homogenous blend of D and L isomers of poly lactic acid and are an inherently amorphous, totally non crystalline polymer.

Biological, mechanical and histological testing and clinical validation have proven the biocompatibility of SonicWeld Rx implants. It maintains its strength for approximately 10 weeks, and safely degrades through hydrolysis and the metabolic process. SonicWeld Rx is not indicated for fully load bearing situations or for patients with conditions including blood supply limitations, insufficient quantity or quality of bone, or latent infections.

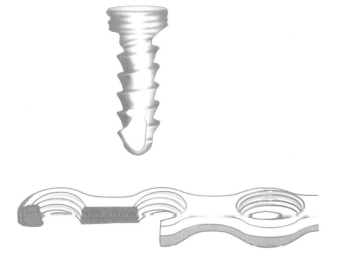

Fig. 52.19: Locking plate and screw concept (AO).

Self-Drilling, Self-Tapping Screws

The self-drilling principle has the advantage of avoiding the necessity to drill a hole, thus shortening the process of osteosynthesis and requiring less instrumentation. Preclinical investigations at the AO center utilizing cadaver cortical bone in 1 to 3 mm thickness as well as cancellous bone block have demonstrated that in thin bone, (1 to 3 mm thickness), pull out strength of the self-drilling, self-tapping screws was similar to conventional self-tapping screws. With cancellous bone blocks, the self-drilling screws had a three fold increase in retentiveness, when compared to the self-tapping variety. Thus the self-drilling, self-tapping screws were essentially equal to the retentiveness of self-tapping screws in thin bone, but were much superior in cancellous bone. This is presumably due to self-drilling screws compressing rather than cutting the cancellous bone around the threads of the screws. The clinical implication is that self-drilling, self-tapping screws are much superior when fixing screws into a cancellous bone graft. It should be noted that self-drilling screws may be difficult to apply in extremely dense bone such as the mandible.

◼ LOCKING PLATES AND SCREWS SYSTEM

In locking plates, the screw locks not only to the bone, but to the bone plate as well. This is accomplished by having a screw with a double thread. One thread will engage the bone; another will engage a threaded area of the bone plate (Fig. 52.19). The result is a locking plate system, which in effect provides a mini internal fixator. This avoids problem of loosening of one or more screws during the convalescent period following miniplate osteosynthesis.

Since the plate locks to the screw rather than gaining its rigidity by being compressed against the bone, it also avoids the cortical necrosis, which is sometimes seen under a plate ,which is compressed against the bone.

Locking plate and screw systems have several advantages over the conventional screw systems. It becomes unnecessary for the plate to intimately contact the underlying bone in all areas. Conventional plate/screw systems require precise adaptation of the plate to the underlying bone. Without this intimate contact, tightening of the screws will draw the bone segments toward the plate, resulting in alterations in the position of the osseous segments and the occlusal relationship. As the screws are tightened, they "lock" to the plate, thus stabilizing the segments without the need to compress the bone to the plate. This makes it impossible for the screw insertion to alter the reduction. Another possible advantage to this property of a locking plate/screw system is a decreased incidence of inflammatory complications from loosening of the hardware. It is known that loose hardware propagates an inflammatory response and promotes infection. Locking plate/screw systems have been shown to provide more stable fixation than conventional nonlocking plate/screw systems. The locking screws need to be in alignment to the threads on plate meaning that axis of insertion need to be guided with the help of a guiding sleeve.

Another advancement in locking technology is multidirectional fixation. TriLock technology (Medartis, Basel, Switzerland) represents a significant step forward in multidirectional and angular stable fixation. The spherical three-point wedge-locking creates a connection between the head of the screw and the plate hole which is stable in angle and axial plane (Fig. 52.20). The locking can be adjusted up to three times within ± 15° without loss of stability.

However, locking plates are not without problems. The locking plates can fatigue or fail in long unsupported

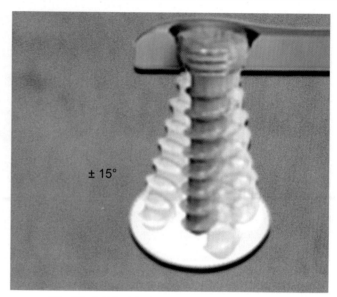

± 15°

Fig. 52.20: Trilock locking screw concept (Medartis)

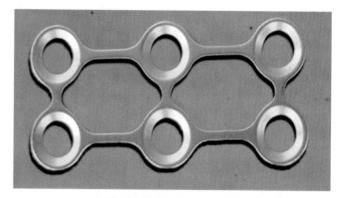

Fig. 52.21: 3D plate concept

sections or if it is stressed too much at one level. Locking plate failures can be mechanical—bending stresses on the plate, the screw-to-plate junction or biological—the screw-to-bone interface, bone quality.

3D plates

In 1992, Farmand developed 3D plate with quadrangular design formed by joining two miniplates with interconnecting crossbars. In 3-dimensional plates, whose stability, unlike traditional plates, do not depend on the thickness of the plate, but depends on its format. The stabilization of plates with monocortical screws forms a cuboid that gives to the system tridimensional stability (Fig. 52.21). This stability is shown in biomechanical studies. These plates can be inserted through intraoral techniques and have shown low complication rates. Because of smaller size, these are easy to handle and adjust. To overcome the disadvantages of loosening of hardware and need of perfect adaptation of miniplates, a new internal mini-locking- 3D system was developed in collaboration with the AO/ASIF-Institute.

Trapezoidal Condylar Plates

These plates are specially designed on the concepts of Christopher Meyer and colleagues from France, who did experimental studies on photoelastic analysis of bone deformation in the region of the mandibular condyle during mastication. They consistently found compressive stress patterns along the posterior border of the ramus and tensile stress patterns along the anterior border of the ramus and in the zone situated below the siqmoid notch. Therefore, there is need of osteosynthesis plates in the condylar region, close to the tensile strain lines, as has been recommended also for other parts of the mandible when applying semi-rigid internal fixation. Trapezoidal condylar plates (TCPs) fulfil these biomechanically required principles of functionally stable osteosynthesis (Figs 52.22A and B). The primary stability achieved by TCPs is superior to that obtained by single plating techniques, by axial lag-screw osteosynthesis, and by rectangular plates in the sagittal plane. This is due both to the 3D concept and to the trapezoidal shape itself.

Delta Plate Fixation for Condylar Fractures

The design of the new delta-shaped miniplate (Modus Trauma 2.0 Condylus Fragment Plate; Medartis, Basel, Switzerland) takes into account previous in vitro analysis on load, strain, and bone deformation at the condylar neck region, as well as finite-element analysis. Tensile strains occur mainly at the anterior and lateral borders of the condyle; compressive strains, at the posterior and medial borders. The plate is 1 mm thick, 20 mm long and 5 mm wide at the top and 12 mm wide at the base. Each side of the plate has a cross-section of 1×2.5 mm, considerably greater than that of an adaptation miniplate. The plate has the base oriented toward the angle of the mandible; thus, the lines of tensile and compressive stress distribution run parallel to both sides of the plate. At the top of the plate is an arm with 2 longitudinally arranged holes, the lower of which has a gliding design. Two more gliding holes form the 2 corners of the base of the plate. The design of the plate allows for treatment of even high condylar neck fractures (Fig. 52.23). The plate's delta shape can handle changing loads, with the highest tensile strain occurring at the anterior and lateral surfaces and the highest compressive strains on the posterior surface. The plate can be easily placed in the confined space at the condylar neck. In cases, when it is desired to avoid

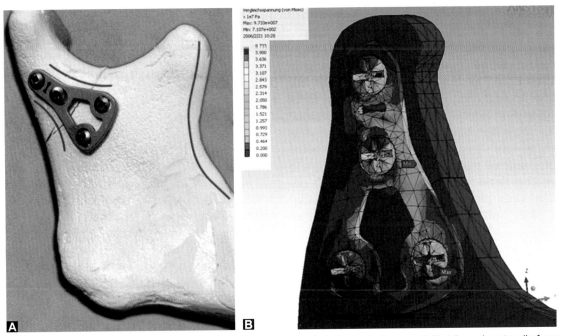

Figs 52.22A and B: Trapezoidal plate for fixation of condylar fracture, based on the Meyer's concept. Red lines show tensile forces during chewing. Osteosynthesis plates should be placed on these lines to counteract functional forces

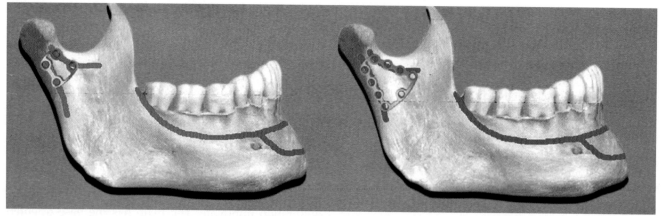

Fig. 52.23: Delta plate for fixation of condylar fracture (Medartis)

visible scars on the face and neck, endoscopic-assisted transoral fracture reduction and stabilization using the delta-shaped miniplate can be done. Taking into account the advantages in biomechanics and handling of the locking miniplate system and the advantages of the delta plate for fixation of condylar neck and subcondylar fractures, a locking delta-plate has been developed, i.e. the TriLock delta condyle trauma plate (Medartis, Switzerland). These plates are made of pure 1.3-mm-thick titanium and are fixed with 2.0-mm TriLock titanium monocortical screws.

Porous Polyethylene Implants (Figs 52.24A to D)

This carbon base polymer is a linear high density polyethylene sintered synthetic alloplastic implant. It has become one of the most popular alloplastic material (Medpore, Porex, Biopore, Synpore) for facial augmentation, for correcting contor deformities, orbital floor repair and enophthalmos correction. The implants are manufactured from an inert, nonabsorbable polymer, formulated to contain a network of open and interconnecting pores approximately 100 to 250 μm in size. The large pore size allows for fibrovascular ingrowth, thus substantially decreasing chances of extrusion and rejection.

Various preformed implants of various standard shapes and sizes are readily available. Orbital floor implants are available with channel for miniplate or titanium orbital mesh aiding in fixation and stability (Fig. 52.25). One side of the implant facing orbital floor can be made smooth to decrease the risk of orbital soft tissue adhesion. In complex deformities customised

implants can be made to order by utilising rapid prototyping techniques.

Advances in Topical Hemostatic Agents

Hemostatic agents provide control of bleeding by enhancing or accelerating the natural clotting process. Although pressure, ligation of vessels and use of electrocautery are the main techniques to control bleeding, the role of hemostatic agents may be secondary, but of great importance in certain cases. Hemostatic agents can facilitate clot formation through enzymatic reactions with host factors, mechanical compression, or a combination of the two. Tissue sealants and bioadhesives act through polymerization between themselves and adjacent tissues. Many new products have been introduced as hemostatic agents. These will be discussed in this section.

Ostene

Ostene (Baxter, USA) is a Wax-like and malleable sterile mixture of water-soluble alkylene oxide copolymers developed as an affordable, easy-to-handle synthetic bone hemostasis material, that reduces the overall risk of post surgical infections. It is a replacement for bone wax which remains indefinitely at the site of application, inhibits bone healing and increases inflammation and infection. In contrast, ostene is water soluble, gets dissolved within 48 hours, and reduces bacterial adhesion. The material is used in cardiac, orthopedic, oral and maxillofacial, and neurosurgery. Other applications under development include the use of Ostene as a safe, soluble delivery vehicle for a variety

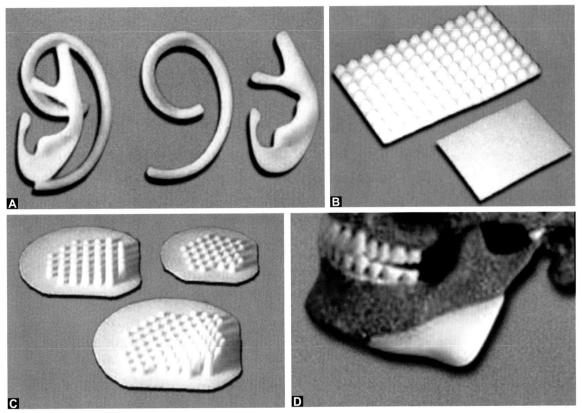

Figs 52.24A to D: (A) Medpore Prefabricated Implant for ear reconstruction; (B and C) Medpore sheets and blocks; (D) Medpore for angle reconstuction

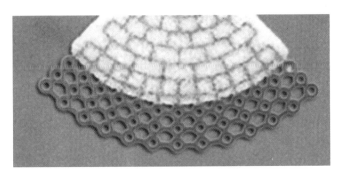

Fig. 52.25: Porous polypropylene with titanium mesh for orbital floor repair (Synpore, Synthes)

of therapeutic agents, from antibiotics to bone growth factors.

ActCel

ActCel hemostatic gauze (Coreva health sciences, USA) is a collagen-like natural substance, created from chemically treated cellulose. ActCel hemostatic gauze is hypoallergenic and contains no chemical additives, thrombin or collagen. When hemostatic gauze contacts blood and other body fluids, it expands three to four times, the original size. ActCel gauze will convert to a gel that self dissolves into glucose and saline over a one to two week period, if not removed. ActCel effectively reduces clotting time by accelerating the formation of fibrin cross-linkages, while increasing blood viscosity. This biological reaction promotes the aggregation of red blood cells acting as a clotting agent. ActCel hemostatic gauze may be easily removed from a wound, if necessary, by simply applying water to the gauze; the dressing will dissolve immediately.

Gelitacel

Gelitacel (Gelita Medical, Netherlands) is a fast working oxidized resorbable cellulose hemostatic gauze of natural origin made from highest alpha grade selected cotton. Gelitacel is absorbed in 96 hours, thus reducing risk of encapsulation. It is approved for dental use in Europe. It can be cut to the desired size and adapts easily to anatomical structures. Specifically when soaked with blood, gelitacel is easy to use. It can be sutured to ensure position. It does not stick to the instruments or to the surgical gloves. It can be removed easily to check the bleeding, without falling apart. Gelitacel maintains its original consistency as gauze and does not immediately change into an amorphous mass during the surgical procedure. Extensive tests on gelitacel have proven that the gauze has outstanding strength in longitudinal direction, under both dry as well under fluid/blood saturated conditions.

Chitosan Products

Chitosan is a naturally occurring positively charged polysaccharide derivative of deacetylated chitin. Chitin can be obtained from a variety of sources including the exoskeletal structure of crustaceans (crabs, shrimps, diatoms, etc.). Chitosan is derived from chitin, using various processes of sodium hydroxide washing to obtain the desired degree of deacetylation and molecular weight. The positive charge attracts the negatively charged red blood cells forming a coagulum that seals the bleeding vessel. It is able to act as a hemostatic independent of coagulation factors. It does not have toxicity and side effects to the human body except for very low risk of allergic reaction. The biological functions of chitosan are antibiosis and bacteriostasis, hemostasis, and promoting wound healing. It is available in sponge, bandages (e.g. Hemcon), and granular form for use on external wounds, nasal packing and dental use.

HemoStase

HemoStase (Cryolife, USA) is a natural hemostatic product used for the control of surgical bleeding. It is a plant based powder that rapidly dehydrates blood and promotes clotting on contact by controlling the clotting factors. The HemoStase got FDA premarket approval in 2006. It is available in a convenient ready-to-use applicator. HemoStase rapidly absorbs fluids from the blood and accelerates the natural, physiologic clotting process for both diffuse and profuse bleeding, and in the presence of anticoagulants. HemoStase, unlike many hemostatic agents, does not require additional operating room preparation or special storage conditions. In addition, preclinical studies have shown that HemoStase does not promote infection and absorbs within 24 to 48 hours of application at the wound site, compared to other surgical hemostats which can take three to eight weeks or more to fully break down.

Quikclot

QuikClot (Z-medica, USA) is a granular hemostatic agent, that saves lives by rapidly stopping severe bleeding. It is being promoted as prehospital hemostatic agent. It is composed of an inert mineral derivative of volcanic rock with active substance Koline. It meets a variety of medical needs and application is nonallergenic. It is applied on the wound and then pressure dressing is given to achieve hemostasis. It acts by activating the intrinsic pathway of coagulation by way of activating factor XI and XII.

Floseal

Floseal basically consists of bovine thrombin plus cross-linked gelatin granules mixed together. The bovine thrombin directly activates fibrinogen and converts it into fibrin monomers. It works on the common pathway bypassing all of the other necessary clotting factors. Only requirement is to have functional fibrinogen in order for it to work. The product floseal itself is a little bit different from just using topical thrombin plus Gelfoam, because the gelatin granules are cross linked in such a way, that they do not swell to nearly the same extent. It is absorbed in approximately 6 to 8 weeks. Because it is Gelfoam beads it can cause arterial embolization, if it is used near a larger vessel. It contains bovine antigens; therefore, it can lead to antibody formation.

Fibrin Sealants

Fibrin sealant [Tisseal (Baxter) and hemaseel (Angiotech Inc. Canada), crosseal (Omrix Biopharmaceuticals)] is a natural or synthetic combination of hemostatic and tissue adhesive. It is available in two separate tubes/vials and these need to be mixed before application. The basic idea is that pure human fibrinogen is combined with bovine thrombin and aprotonin. The bovine thrombin converts exogenous human fibrinogen to fibrin monomers. The patient's own factor XIII and calcium, then converts it into fibrin polymer. There are two vials and these need to be prepared by mixing, just before application. Fibrin sealants are absorbed within 10 to 14 days and need a relatively dry field in order to work. Some of the fibrin sealants use pooled human fibrinogen, in which there is always the potential for transmission of infectious agents. There is, risks of arterial embolization and antibody formation, when used near large torn vessels. The fibrin sealants are expensive and most efficacious, of all the topical hemostatics.

Artiss

Artiss (Baxter) is a human fibrin sealant, which is used to cause blood clotting during surgery or due to trauma when natural blood clotting processes are deficient. Artiss is the only premixed, ready-to-use fibrin sealant specifically indicated for tissue adherence in face-lift and burn surgeries. It was first approved by the FDA in 2008, to adhere autologous skin grafts to surgically prepared wound beds resulting from burns in adult and pediatric populations of one year of age or older.

Feracrylum

Feracrylum (e.g. Sepagard, Themis Medicare, India) is a biocompatible, biodegradable water-soluble polymer of polyacrylic acid. This polymer is hygroscopic in nature, soluble in water, nonabsorbable in the system. Its mode of action is via activation of thrombin, which subsequently causes conversion of fibrinogen to fibrin and thus clots formation. Feracrylum has a high molecular weight of 5,00,000 to 8,00,000 Daltons, thus has no adverse systemic effects. On coming in contact with serum proteins, it forms a thin film, thus acting as a mechanical barrier preventing exogenous contamination. The unique inherent antimicrobial property of these synthetic polyacrylates simultaneously prevents bacterial growth on and near the wound site. It is available in gel form and 1 percent solution. Solution can be irrigated or sprayed onto tissues or applied soaked in a gauze over the wound.

53 Cone Beam Computed Tomography

Also known as CBVS—Cone Beam Volumetric Scanning OR Volumetric CT/Volumetric Computed Tomography OR Dental 3D CT OR CBVI—Cone Beam Volumetric Imaging, CBVT—Cone Beam Volumetric Tomography.

A relatively new diagnostic imaging modality, which promises to revolutionize the practice of oral and maxillofacial radiology. It is used as a dedicated 3D imaging tool in dentistry, which has improved the maxillofacial surgeon's access to advanced imaging. The advent of CBCT as a contemporary diagnostic aid, in craniofacial imaging has brought in a paradigm shift in the diagnosis and management in the field of oral and maxillofacial surgery.

HISTORY

Medical CT was available since early 1970s, but it was only in late 1980s its use in Dentistry came into practice.

Original cone beam algorithm was developed by Feldkamp L.A., Davis L.C., and Kress J.W. in 1984. (Feldkamp et al).

This technique was used in different industries and biomedical applications such as micro CT. Among the first original clinical application of CBCT was in 1982, at the Mayo clinic Biodynamics Research Laboratory, primarily for angiography. In 1992, it was used for image – guided radiation therapy and later for Single Photon Emission Computerized Tomography (SPECT), etc.

Dedicated CBCT scanners for oral and maxillofacial region were pioneered in 1998, by Mozzo P, Procacci E, Tacconi A, Martini P.T., Andreis I.A. in Italy and in 1999, independently by Arai Y, Tammisalo E, Iwai K, Hashimoto K and Shimoda K in Japan. CBCT was originally devised as a cost-effective, giving better image quality with much lower radiation dose device and efficient method for obtaining cross-sectional 3-dimensional images.

It arrived in North America in 2001 and its use in maxillofacial imaging was approved by U.S. FDA, since then it has been rapidly embraced by the dental profession. Increasing number of dental hospitals and clinics are adding CBCT machines or replacing orthopantomograph machines with CBCT.

Cone beam computed tomography (CBCT) is a medical image acquisition technique based on a cone-shaped X-ray beam centered on a two dimensional (2D) detector. [**This modality uses a cone beam instead of a fan-shaped beam, as used in computed tomography—medical CT**] (Fig. 53.1).

Craniofacial CBCTs were designed to counter some of the limitations of the conventional CT scanning devices. The object to be evaluated is captured as the radiation source falls onto a two-dimensional detector. This allows a single radiation source, to capture an entire region of interest, as compared to conventional CT devices, where multiple slices (axial slices) are captured by multiple exposures around an object to reveal the internal architecture of the object (Figs 53.2A and B).

Thus, in CBCT, the area to be imaged can be covered in single 360 degrees rotation of the machine around the patient to acquire images of entire volume with significant reduction of radiation dose in comparison to medical CT scan.

It produces a series of 2D images, which can be reconstructed in a three-dimensional (3D) data.

In comparison to conventional plane radiography, the potential for obtaining substantial additional information from a CBCT volume is tremendous. The clinician is freed from the constraints of cephalometry orientation, the problems of geometric distortion and many of the challenges separating cephalometric landmarks from structure noise. In addition, new ways of observing data (maximum intensity projection multiplanar reconstructions, rotation in 3D) may provide diagnostic insights that were not possible. (it overcomes the limitations of routine radiography, like 2D projections, magnifications, distortion, superimpositions and misrepresentation of structures).

It acquires data, which can be reformatted to show sequential slices through the oral and maxillofacial complex, in the axial, coronal and sagittal planes (Fig. 53.3).

This data, with the help of software, can be further be manipulated to produce precise 3D reconstruction of the area of interest, giving a clear images of highly contrasted structures, such as bone and its relation to the adjacent anatomic structures,and can be viewed on a computer workstation. It offers high resolution, isotropic images for effective evaluation and allows us to accurately plan the treatment strategy, as the visualization to the proximity of vital structures is very clear (Fig. 53.4).

In addition, panoramic reconstruction of data from CBCT, can be performed at various slice thicknesses, giving a familiar radiographic environment to evaluate, without distortion, magnification or superimposition, which is usually seen in 2D panoramic images (Figs 53.5A to E).

TECHNICAL BASIS OF CBCT

The two principle differences that distinguish CBCT from traditional CT, are the type of imaging source detector complex and the method of data acquisition.

Figures 53.2A and B illustrate the basic difference between these two technologies. The X-ray source for CT is a high output rotating anode generator, while that

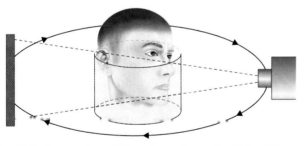

Fig. 53.1: A cone-shaped X-ray beam is used, which orbits once around the patient gaining information in a cylindrical volume.This is the basic concept of CBCT

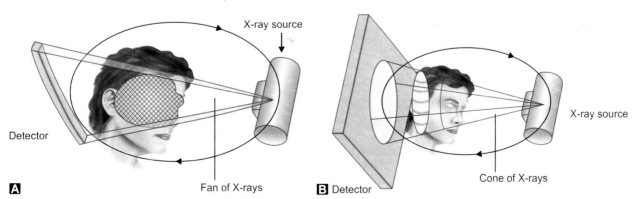

Figs 53.2A and B: X-ray beam projection scheme comparing a single detector array fan-beam CT: (A) and cone-beam CT, (B) geometry

for CBCT can be a low energy fixed anode tube. The X-ray energy of CBCT is similar to that of panoramic radiography with a typical operating range of 1 to 15 mA at 90 to 120 kVp, while that of medical CT is significantly higher at 120 to 150 mA, at 220 kVp. Medical CT employs a fan shaped X-ray beam, in a helical progression, from

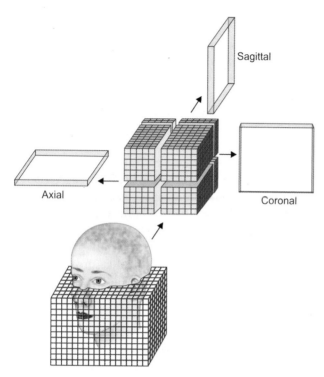

Fig. 53.3: The patient's maxillofacial skeleton is positioned within the cylinder and is divided up into tiny cubes or voxels. Computer manipulation (multiplanar reconstruction) of the data obtained, allows separate images in the sagittal, coronal and axial planes to be created

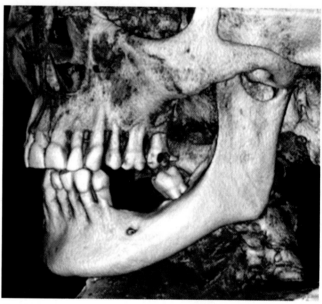

Fig 53.4: A 3D color reconstruction of the patient rotated to show left mandible. Note the detail of the bony anatomy

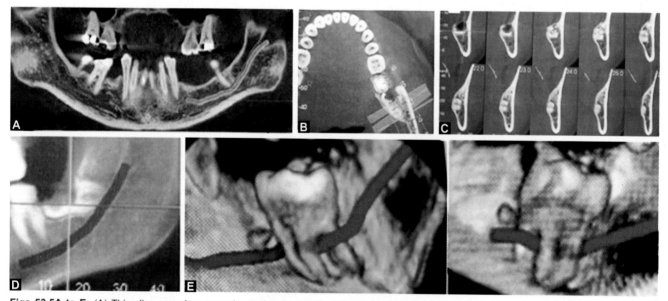

Figs 53.5A to E: (A) This slice pseudopanoramic used to "paint" the inferior alveolar nerve canal, allows reconstruction of the implant site showing the canal painted in yellow exiting the mental foramen, (B) Selection of a region for CBCT, (C) Cross sectional images showing the position of the nerve (red dot), (D) Cropped panoramic reconstruction for the position of nerve in relation to impacted left lower third molar, (E) 3D reconstruction indicating the inferior alveolar nerve position in relation to mandibular impacted third molar. (Nerve is passing between the roots.)

its source for imaging and records the data, on a solid state image detectors arranged in a 360 degree array around the patient. (Each slice requires a separate scan and separate image reconstuction) CBCT technology uses a cone-shaped X-ray beam with a special image intensifier and a solid state sensor or an amorphous silicon plate for capturing the image.

Depending on the device, the patient is in the sitting, standing or supine position during CBCT scanning. During imaging, the X-ray source and the detector move around the patient's head, which is stabilized with a head holder (Fig 53.6A to F).

During rotation, multiple from 150 to more than 600–sequential planar projection images/Frames of the entire field of view-FOV are acquired. This series of basis projection images is referred to as projection data. The height and diameter of the beam's cylindrical FOV can vary from small fields for dental imaging to large fields for other facial examinations. Some machines allow the FOV to be selected to suit the particular examination.

FOV mode options may include facial, panoramic, implant and dental, etc.

In CBCT machine, there is a rotating gantry to which an X-ray source and 2D detector are fixed. CBCT scanners use a tightly collimated narrow cone-shaped X-ray beam, resulting in a scan range with a more restricted FOV in the axial dimension than in medical CT [image data can be collected for either a complete dental/maxillofacial volume or limited regional area of interest]. Image data is collected/recorded in single one rotation sweep of the patient, similar to that of panoramic radiography [180–360 degrees gantry rotation by a 2D detector] (Figs 53.7A and B).

Multiplanar Reformation

Due to its isotropic nature of the volumetric data sets, CBCT units can reconstruct oblique, curved or cross-sectional reconstructions from it, known as Multiplanar Reconstruction-MPR.

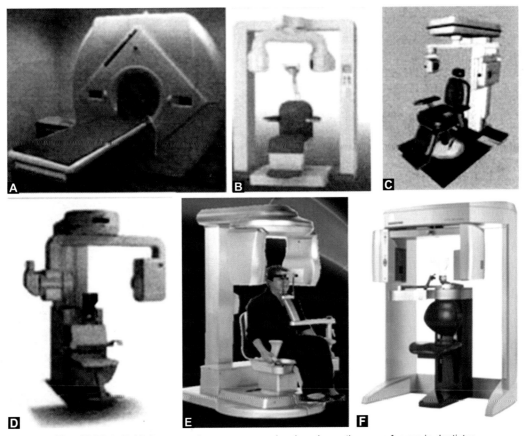

Figs 53.6A to F: Various cone beam scanners developed over the years for use in dentistry

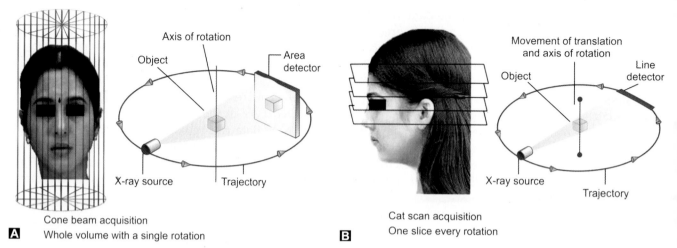

Figs 53.7A and B: Differences in image acquisition between cone beam volume tomography (A) and traditional computed tomography-CT (B)

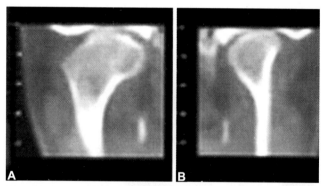

Figs 53.8A and B: Oblique planar reformation image through lateral and medical poles of mandibular condyle demonstrating right condylar hyperplasia

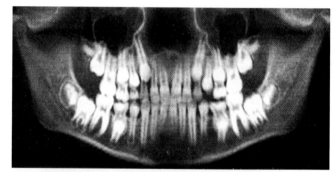

Fig. 53.9: Curved planar reformatted panoramic image

1. **Oblique planar reformation (Figs 53.8A and B):** This creates nonaxial 2D images by transecting a set or stack of axial images. This mode is useful for evaluating specific structures e.g. TMJ, impacted third molars, as certain features may not be readily apparent on perpendicular MPR images.

2. **Curved planar reformation (Fig. 53.9):** This is the type of MPR, obtained by aligning the long axis of the imaging plane with a specific anatomic structure. It is useful in displaying the dental arch, providing familiar panoramic like thin slice images.

3. **Serial transplanar reformation (Fig. 53.10):** A series of stacked sequential cross-sectional images orthogonal to the oblique or curved planar reformation is produced. Images are usually thin slices- 1 mm thick and 1 mm apart. They are useful in the assessment of specific morphologic features, such

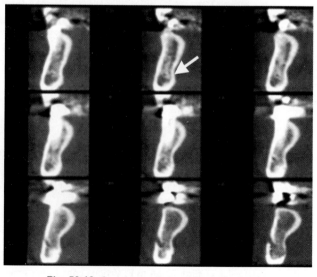

Fig. 53.10: Serial transplanar reformation image

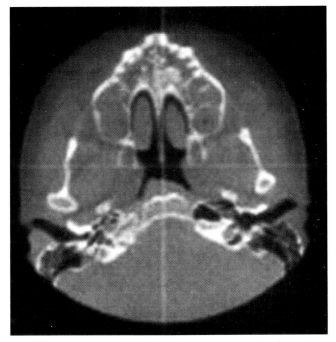

Fig. 53.11: Multiplanar volume reformation image, showing axial section slice

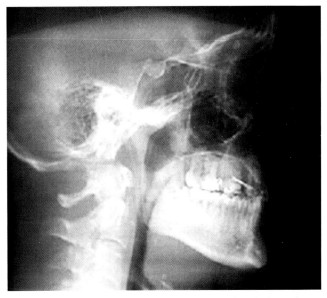

Fig. 53.12: "Ray sum" image simulated lateral cephalometric projection

as alveolar bone height and width for implant site assessment, the inferior alveolar canal in relation to impacted mandibular molars, TMJ evaluation, as well as evaluation of pathological conditions affecting the jaw bones.

4. **Multiplanar volume reformation (Fig. 53.11):** Multiplanar image can be obtained by increasing the number of adjacent voxels included in the slice. This gives us an image that represents a specific volume of the patient. The technique, by adding the absorption values of adjacent voxels, produces a 'ray sum' image (Fig. 53.12).

Radiation doses for CBCT

Studies indicate that the effective dose of radiation (average range 36.9–50.3 μSv) is significantly reduced up to 98 percent compared to medical CT.

CBCT technology allows scan time to vary, typically from 5 to 40/70 seconds, with an exposure dose in the range of 40 to 135 μSv, a fraction of the radiation dose of an equivalent CT scan (Approx. 15 times less than medical CT).

Currently, patient exposure effective absorbed radiation dose has been determined only for the Newton 9000 complete volume system. This can be as low as 50 μSv or in a similar range to that for a periapical

Table 53.1: Effective absorbed radiation doses from dental imaging	
Panoramic film	3-11 μSv
Lateral cephalograph	5-7 μSv
PA cephalograph	5-7 μSv
Occlusal film	5 μSv
Full mouth series	30-80 μSv
TMJ series	20-30 μSv
CBCT	18-135 μSv

full mouth series. For the purpose of comparison, the effective absorbed radiation doses for dental images are listed in Table 53.1

3D image construction in CBCT

1st Step—Thresholding Step

Here, a Hounsfield range (HU) of the desired anatomy is specified, e.g mandibular segment, threshold between 300 HU and 1800 HU is selected. This specific thresholding excludes soft tissue and air from the images. CBCT allows collimation of X–ray beam, *only to the area of interest, i.e. field of view–FOV,* which further enhances benefit of reduced radiation exposure to the patient [collimation device helps us to expose only the area to be imaged as it restricts the size and shape of X-ray beam and protects the adjacent structures against radiation exposure and damage].

During the active capture phase, in which the X-ray generator rotates or moves around the patient's head in approximately 10, 20 or 40 seconds, the device is capturing hundreds of raw X-ray images (from 150 to more than 600 sequential planar projection images of the FOV, e.g. the Hitachi Mercu Ray captures raw images in a 9.8 seconds and the Suni captures 280 raw images in 8.3 seconds). Scan times vary from 75 to 40 seconds for the complete volume to 17 seconds for the regional. A full volume scan encompasses the entire volume of anatomy from approximately the lower orbital rim to just below the inferior border of the mandible, while the regional is confined to a portion of one dental quadrant or regional area of interest. Some machines are restricted to either one of the methods, while others offer full or regional options.

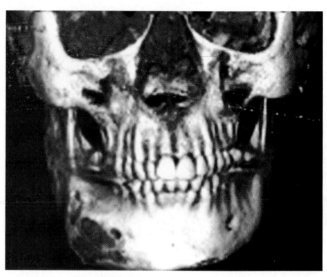

Fig. 53.13: 3D reconstruction in CBCT

2nd Step

From the first step, resulting segmentation will contain some artefact due to scatter from metal objects and fillings, etc. The operator goes through the images and cleans up the artefacts and extraneous objects from the images in this step.

3rd Step—Acquisition Stage—Image Collection

It's called 'Region Growing'. In this step the operator selects a 'seed point' within the structure of interest that has been already segmented in the first 2 steps. This will give the complete region of interest–ROI.

4th Step

Basic projection frames data processed to create the volumetric data set. Use of CBCT technology provides unique and valuable information that is unobtainable in any other format. This information can benefit practitioners in all aspects of dental treatment. Using computer mathematical algorithms, these images are pieced together and reconstructed into 3D volume.

Image Formatting/reporting

Most clinically useful aspect of CBCT imaging is the highly sophisticated software, that allows the huge volume of the data collected to be broken down and processed or reconstructed into a format, that closely resembles that produced by medical CT scan. This process of reconstruction into 3D volume can take anywhere from 5 to 6 minutes to 30 minutes, depending

on the device and amount of image data generated during the scan (Fig. 53.13).

After the secondary reconstruction, in which the 3D volume is exported as a series of small Digital Imaging and Communications in Medicine (DICOM) files,and the 3D volume is available for analysis. All CBCT devices come with imaging software for capturing and analyzing the information. Measuring the distances, angles and object segmentation is also possible. With the introduction of large (12″) imaging fields, there has been a surge of interest in the use of CBCT, as a substitute for conventional panoramic and cephalometric images.

Rapid prototyping models can also be generated using CBCT data. CBCT has excellent high contrast resolution as a result of the small size and geometry of its isotropic voxels. Poor soft tissue contrast of CBCT imaging is not usually a problem in dental and maxillofacial imaging, because the main subjects of interest are generally mineralized tissues, i.e. teeth and bones.

CBCT Indications (Table 53.5)

Cone beam computed tomography is an accurate and useful tool for many clinical oral-maxillofacial indications,including the identification of anatomical structures and locations prior to implant placement, and other oral surgical procedures, prior to and during endodontic procedures and when planning orthodontic treatment. CBCT also plays a role in the identification, diagnosis, and determination of the severity of diseases.

APPLICATION OF CBCT IMAGING TO CLINICAL DENTAL PRACTICE (TABLE 53.2)

Unlike conventional CT scanners, which are large and expensive to purchase and maintain, CBCT is suited for use in clinical dental practice, where cost and dose considerations are important, space is often at a premium and scanning requirements are limited to the head region.

All CBCT units initially provide correlated axial, coronal and sagittal perpendicular MPR images (Fig. 53.3).

Table 53.2: Clinical application of CBCT in Denstistry	
Clinician	*Clinical Application For CBCT*
General Dentist	Implant site assessment
	TMJ evaluation
	Paranasal sinus evaluation
	Airway analysis (sleep disorders)
Endodontist	Root form/morphology, pulp/root canal assessment (number, etc.)
	Periapical lesion assessment
	Quality of root canal fillings
	"Retreatment"
Orthodontist	Space analysis,cephalometry
	Impactions/Supernumerary tooth assessment
	Treatment "records"
	Craniofacial anomaly assessment
	Bone volume determination
	Root resorption/periodontal bone support
	Planning of orthodontic anchorage, implants, pins, mini screws
	TMJ evaluation
	Cleft patients
Oral And	Third molar assessment–Impacted Teeth/ supernumerary teeth/neurovascular proximity
Maxillofacial	Orthognathic surgery-planning, obtaining 3D data of craniofacial skeleton
Surgeon	Presurgical planning for lesions/pathologies
	Paranasal sinus evaluation
	TMJ evaluation-Visualization
	Surgical extraction planning
	Foreign body location
	Obstructive sleep apnea study
	Facial trauma evaluation
	Graft recipient and donar site status
	Intraoperative navigation and imaging
Pediatric dentist	Tooth development
	Supernumerary teeth assessment
Periodontist	Bone grafting
	Implant site assessment
Prosthodontist	Impalnt site assessment

Basic enhancements include zoom or magnification and visual adjustments to narrow the range of displayed grey-scales (window) and contrast level within this window, the capability to add annotation and cursor-driven measurement.

The value of CBCT imaging in implant planning, surgical assessment of pathology, TMJ assessment and pre and postoperative assessment of craniofacial fractures has been reported. In orthodontics, CBCT imaging is useful in the assessment of growth and development, and such imaging is becoming common place.

Perhaps the greatest practical advantage of CBCT in maxillofacial imaging is the ability it provides to interact with the data and generate images replicating those commonly used in clinical practice. All proprietary software is capable of various real-time advanced image display techniques, easily derived from the volumetric data set.

ROLE OF CBCT IN DENTAL IMPLANTLOGY (FIGS 53.14 TO 53.17)

CBCT allows to visualize cross sectional, axial, pan-oramic scans views for more precise planning of implant therapy.

Information about bone height,regional width,bone ridge thickness/concavities, and morphology, (bone quality) and inferior alveolar nerve canal location is essential for selection of the correct implant location,

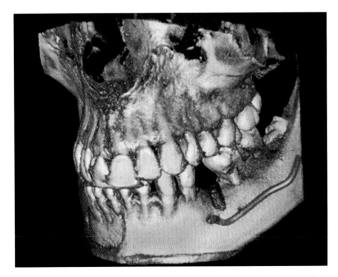

Fig. 53.14: Virtual implant planning

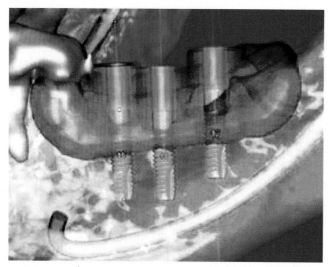

Fig. 53.15: The design of the CBCT generated surgical template

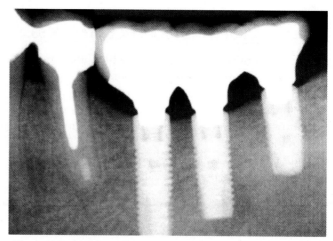

Fig. 53.17: Periapical radiograph of the implants one year after the implant placement

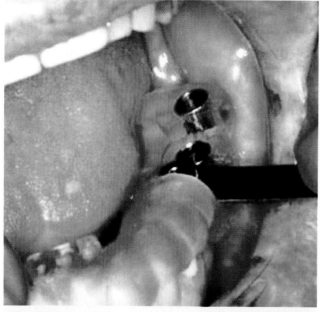

Fig. 53.16: Placement of tooth-supported CBCT generated surgical template to guide the drilling procedure

size and length. CBCT provides the clinician with more precise and accurate imaging, providing better preoperative information and thereby helping to avoid problems associated with any surgical sites, close to vital structures or where compromising factors are present. CBCT accurately detects differences in the loop length and diameter of mandibular canals in the interforamental region, and large variations in these structures, which occur in different individuals. Bone quality assessment also can be done accurately, which is the most important factor for primary implant stability.

The presurgical CBCT scan is used for implant selection and precise implant positioning. Virtual placement of dental implants in optimum positions and final treatment plan regarding exact implant size, depth and angulation.

Currently, a small number of implant planning software systems utilize CBCT scans to facilitate the creation of surgical drilling templates. These CBCT generated surgical templates are manufactured in such a way, that they match the location, trajectory and depth of the planned implant with a high degree of precision thus, allowing transfer of planning information to implant placement.

As the clinician places the implants, the guides stabilize drilling by restricting degrees of freedom for drill trajectory and depth. Studies have shown that utilization of 3D implant planning software resulted in implant positioning with improved biomechanics and esthetics.

Use of CBCT scans, implant planning software, and CBCT generated surgical templates usually avoid complications such as mandibular nerve damage, sinus perforation, fenestrations, or dehiscences and other iatrogenic sequelae of placement of dental implant (Table 53.3).

Table 53.3: Implant planning and anatomical considerations

Planning of exact implant position
Sinus lift planning
Intra-alveolar distraction osteogenesis
Reduced vertical bone height
Reduced horizontal bone width
Anatomical variations of the nerve
Preparation of templates

Table 53.4: Major benefits and limitations of CBCT imaging in the OMF region

Benefits

- 3D dataset
- Real-size data
- Potential for generating all 2D images (e.g. orthopantomogram, lateral cephalogram, TMJ)
- Potential for vertical scanning in a natural seated position
- isotropic voxel size
- High resolution (e. g. bone trabeculae, Periodontal ligament (PDL), root formation)
- Lower radiation dose than MSCT
- Less disturbance from metal artefacts
- Lower costs compared with MSCT
- Easy accessibility
- In-office imaging
- Easy handling
- Small footprint
- Digital Imaging and Communications in Medicine (DICOM) compatible
- User-friendly post-processing and viewing software
- Energy saving compared with MSCT

Limitations

- Low contrast range (dependent on the type of X-ray detector)
- Limited, small detector size causes limited field of view and limited scanned volume
- Limited inner soft tissue information
- Increased noise from scatter radiation and concomitant loss of contrast resolution
- Movement artefacts affecting the whole data set
- Cannot be used for estimation of Hounsfield units (HU)
- Truncation artefacts, caused by the fact that projections acquired with region of interest selection do not contain the entire object.

ADVANTAGES OF CBCT (TABLE 53.4)

Alternative to conventional medical CT, with easy accessibility in dental clinics. Costs less than medical scanning machine-(one-third to one-fourth). Less space requirement.

1. **Rapid, quick scanning time**, less than 4.8 to 30 seconds (less time for image acquisition) for producing high volume images.
2. **Radiation dose reduction** in comparison to medical CT scan, due to reduction in the number of rotation of X-ray beam. A radiation dose of one-sixth that of traditional spiral CT. Patient radiation can be further reduced using collimator, which allows the clinicians to limit the size of the image to the area of interest. This dose-controlling adaptable feature fully restricts radiation at the X-ray source to scan only the preselected areas of interest thereby eliminating exposure to the anatomy outside the field of view.
   CBCT 52- 1025 µSv, CT 1400- 2100 µSv. (microsievert)
3. **Reduction in the number of radiographic images.**
4. **Image accuracy:** The images are rendered in a precise 1:1 ratio in reconstruction. It provides submillimeter pixel resolution, ranging from 0.4 mm to as low as 0.125 mm, which is required for maxillofacial imaging.
5. **Reduced image artifacts:** Elimination of artifacts as blurring and overlapping of the adjacent teeth is possible, with manufacturer's artifact suppression algorithms.
6. **Unlimited number of views**: Chair side image display and real time analysis.
7. **Imaging can be obtained at any angle**, thus offering maximum viewing and eliminating superimpositions.
8. **Superior representation of bony structures** in comparison to conventional X-ray tomography.
9. **Ease of use/handling**
10. **Quick availability.**
11. Interactive display modes available in CBCT, by using its special software allows its multifield use in dentistry. Multiplanar reformation.
12. The use of orthogonal beam projection and computer reconstruction yields a volume that has no magnification error and provides true linear and angular measurements. (Distortion free 3D data, no magnification-inherent in traditional radiograph).
13. **Powerful diagnostic 3D planning tools**. The technology offers 3-dimensional visualization and more accurate imaging compared to analog and digital radiographs.
14. 3D determination of the patient's jaw anatomy and fabrication of both anatomical models and surgical template.

15. CAD/CAM software allows the transfer of planning information to implant placement.
16. Rapid prototyping using stereolithographic modeling-Dicom Data Format.
17. Visual treatment objectives VTO to digital casts to 3D cephalometric analysis.

Drawbacks

Drawbacks are mainly due to cone-shaped geometry of beam, flat panel detector and contrast resolution. CBCT exposes the patients to considerably more [about 4 to 5 times] dosage than a regular 2D radiographs, be it a panoramic, lateral or posteroanterior view. It has low contrast resolution and limited capability of visualizing the internal soft tissues. It cannot be used as a single imaging modality in polytrauma patients, because intra cerebral pathology could be easily missed.

1. Grainy image
2. **Cone beam effect:** Areas which are present in central position of beam are better recorded than the areas in peripheral portion of the beam as in this portion of X-ray beam is less attenuated.
3. **Cone beam streak artifacts:** Radiation is sometimes attenuated, when passing through dense metallic objects and does not reach the receptor. When this radiation-less information is reconstructed, streak artifacts in images are formed, that can obstruct the surrounding anatomy. Because CBCT beam has a range of wavelengths and low KVP, this artifact is more pronounced than medical CT.
4. **Image noise:** Because radiation from the source is transmitted through tissues in the body, the receptor receives nonuniform information from radiation scattered in many directions-which is termed as noise. This noise is 0.05 to 0.15 with conventional CT and can be as large as 0.4 to 2 in CBCT.
5. Poor soft tissue contrast. Only useful for hard tissue imaging.
6. Contrast enhancement facility is not available with present CBCT to detect soft tissue details (limited representation of soft tissues due to the lower radiation dose). Cannot be used for soft tissue pathologies and pathologies of mixed tissues.
7. Spatial resolution of subtle structures that is slightly inferior to that of spiral CT.

▮ WORD OF CAUTION! (TABLE 53.5)

Cone beam computed tomography (CBCT), which provides a lower dose, lower cost alternative to conventional CT is being used with increasing frequency in the practice of oral and maxillofacial radiology. Adapting to ALARA (As Low As Reasonably Achievable) principle, the radiation dosage from CBCT has been reduced through the process of collimation, and reduction in scan time. Radiation dose for a facial scan is similar to that of 10 dental radiographs. The dose of radiation can be further reduced by adjusting beam collimation to the field of view of interest.

With the introduction of large (12") imaging fields, there has been surge of interest in the use of CBCT, as a substitute for conventional panoramic and cephalometric images by various disciplines of endodontics, oral

Table 53.5: Special indications for cross-sectional imaging		
Maxilla	Single Tooth	a. Incisive canal
		b. Descent of maxillary sinus
		c. Clinical doubt about shape of alveolar ridge
		d. Descent of maxillary sinus
		e. Clinical doubt about shape of alveolar ridge
	Partially Dentate	a. Descent of maxillary sinus
		b. Clinical doubt about shape of alveolar ridge
	Edentulous	a. Descent of maxillary sinus
		b. Clinical doubt about shape of alveolar ridge
Mandible	Single tooth	a. Clinical doubt about position of mandibular canal
		b. clinical doubt about shape of alveolar ridge
	Partially Dentate	a. Clinical doubt about position of mandibular canal or mental foramen
		c. Clinical doubt about shape of alveolar ridge
	Edentulous	a. Severe resporation
		b. clinical doubt about shape of alveolar ridge
		c. Clinical doubt about position of mandibular canal if posterior implants are to be placed

and maxillofacial surgery, oral medicine, periodontology, restorative dentistry and orthodontics.

If CBCT is used as a substitute for medical CT, patients will benefit from dose reduction. However, in the case, where CBCT is substituted for lower dose conventional imaging alternatives, an increase in dose detriment, is imparted to the patient. **This is of particular concern in cases of children, because they carry any radiation burden for a longer period of time than adults and because developing organs are more sensitive to radiation effects.**

It is critical for health care providers, to weigh the potential benefit of diagnostic information against expense and risk of the imaging procedure. Radiation from the dental CBCT units, which is reported in the literature, is 2 to 23 percent of dose of comparable conventional CT examination. *But, it is several to hundreds of times greater than single panoramic image exposure.*

Requisite for Clinicians

Sufficient anatomical knowledge and experience to interpret the scanned data. CBCT will improve more patient care, but users have to be aware of their responsibility to interpret the data properly.

3D C arm

Based on CBCT technology 3D C arm has been developed for intraoperative imaging in operation theater. This C arm provides the surgeon control over bone fragments reduction, implant positioning, and bone grafting in complex craniofacial procedures, where visual judgement alone may not be sufficient.

BASIC PRINCIPLES FOR USE OF DENTAL CONE BEAM CT

EUROPEAN ACADEMY DENTOMAXILLOFACIAL RADIOLOGY (EADMFR)

Consensus Guidelines of the European Academy of Dental and Maxillofacial Radiology, January 2009

1.	CBCT examinations must not be carried out unless a history and clinical examination have been performed
2.	CBCT examinations must be justified for each patient to demonstrate that the benefits outweigh the risks
3.	CBCT examinations should potentially add new information to aid the patient's management
4.	CBCT should not be repeated 'routinely' on a patient without a new risk/benefit assessment having been performed
5.	When accepting referrals from other dentists for CBCT examinations, the referring dentist must supply sufficient clinical information (results of a history and examination) to allow the CBCT person to perform the justification process.
6.	CBCT should only be used when the question for which imaging is required cannot be answered adequately by lower dose conventional (traditional) radiography
7.	CBCT images must undergo a thorough clinical evaluation ('radiological report') of the entire image dataset
8.	Where it is likely that evaluation of soft tissues will be required as part of the patient's radiological assessment, the appropriate imaging should be conventional medical CT or MR, rather than CBCT.
9.	CBCT equipment should offer a choice of volume sizes and examinations must use the smallest that is compatible with the clinical situation if this provides less radiation dose to the patient
10.	Where CBCT equipment offers a choice of resolution, the resolution compatible with adequate diagnosis and the lowest achievable dose should be used
11.	A quality assurance program must be established and implemented for each CBCT facility, including equipment, techniques and quality control procedures.
12.	Aids to accurate positioning (light beam markers) must always be used
13.	All new installations of CBCT equipment should undergo a critical examination and detailed acceptance tests before use to ensure that radiation protection for staff, members of the public and patient are optimal.
14.	CBCT equipment should undergo regular routine tests to ensure that radiation protection, for both practice/facility users and patients, has not significantly deteriorated
15.	For staff protection from CBCT equipment, the guidelines detailed in Section 6 of the European Commission document 'Radiation Protection 136. European Guidelines on Radiation Protection in Dental Radiology' should be followed

16.	All those involved with CBCT must have received adequate theoretical and practical training for the purpose of radiological practices and relevant competence in radiation protection
17.	Continuing education and training after qualification are required, particularly when new CBCT equipment or techniques are adopted
18.	Dentists responsible for CBCT facilities who have not previously received 'adequate theoretical and practical training' should undergo a period of additional theoretical and practical training that has been validated by an academic institution (University or equivalent). Where national specialist qualifications in DMFR exist, the design and delivery of CBCT training programmes should involve a DMF Radiologist
19.	For dentoalveolar CBCT images of the teeth, their supporting structures, the mandible and the maxilla up to the floor of the nose (e.g. 8 cm x 8 cm or smaller fields of view), clinical evaluation ('radiological report') should be made by a specially trained DMF Radiologist or, where this is impracticable, an adequately trained general dental practitioner
20.	For nondentoalveolar small fields of view (e.g. temporal bone) and all craniofacial CBCT images (fields of view extending beyond the teeth, their supporting structures, the mandible, including the TMJ, and the maxilla up to the floor of the nose), clinical evaluation ('radiological report') should be made by a specially trained DMF Radiologist or by a Clinical Radiologist (Medical Radiologist)

Lasers in Oral and Maxillofacial Surgery

INTRODUCTION

The term "laser" is an acronym for *Light Amplification by Stimulated Emission of Radiation*. Laser energy released is based on the concept of Albert Einstein's (1917) quantum theory of radiation hypothesis, in which activated electrons of an atom, when return to a lower state, release electromagnetic energy, in the form of photons or light. The first working laser used on extracted tooth was developed by Maiman in 1960, by exciting a ruby rod with intense pulses of light from a flash lamp (Table 54.1).

Since then, its medical and photobiological applications have been expanding. Over the past two decades lasers are being used as a niche tool as a direct replacement for electrosurgery and other conventional approaches, e.g. scalpel blades, etc. and is beginning to replace the dental handpiece. Lasers of various types offer major advantages over scalpel and electrosurgery are in terms of increased precision, invasiveness of the procedure and patient postoperative experience (Tables 54.2 and 54.3).

Table 54.1: Time table reflecting the development of laser technology		
Year	*Contributor*	*Development*
1913	Bhor	Quantum theory
1917	Einstein	Theory of stimulated emission
1955	Townes	Maser production
1958	Townes and Schawlow	Laser principles
1960	Maiman	Developed the ruby laser
1961	Javan et al	Mixture of helium and neon (He-Ne) laser
1961	Johnson and Nassau laser	First solid state neodymium laser—neodymium ion in calcium tungstate ($CaWO_4$)
1961	Johnson	Neodymium ion-doped yttrium-aluminum-garnet (Nd:YAG) rod
1964	Patel	Developed carbon dioxide (molecular) gas laser. 1st most practical laser in oral and maxillofacial surgery
1964	Bridges	Argon laser (gas)—for angiodysplasias
1970	Polanyl	Clinically applied the carbon dioxide laser
1977	Shafir	First documented case in the oral and maxillofacial surgical literature
1989	Terr Myers	First dental laser—Nd:YAG was developed

Table 54.2: Comparisons of three common modalities used for surgery			
	Laser	Scalpel	Electrosurgery
Incision into tissue	Yes—focused	Yes	Yes
Recontouring	Yes—defocused	Yes	Yes (Loop)
Need for LA	No—erbium No—comfort pulse Yes—other lasers	Yes	Yes
Control of hemostasis	Yes	No	Yes (mode)
Control of coagulation	Yes	No	Yes (mode)
Collateral injury to bone	No	No	Yes
Sterilizing action	Yes	No	Yes
Low bacteremia	Yes	No	Yes
Safe near implants	Yes	Yes	No
Safe near other metals	Yes	Yes	No
Stimulates oral muscles	No	No	Yes
Low postoperative pain	Yes	No	No
Fast healing of incisions	Yes	Yes	No
Fast healing of excisions	Yes	No	No

Table 54.3: Treatment options		
Procedure	Conventional	Lasers
	Scalpel	Diode lasers
Soft tissue surgery	Ceramic burs	KTP and CO_2 lasers
	Electrosurgery	Erbium (Er) lasers
	Trichloroacetic acid	Diode lasers
Bone resection	Bone chisels	Erbium lasers
	Bone burs	
	Piezosurgery	

Early applications of lasers in oral and maxillofacial surgery began to appear in the mid to late 1970s. Laser device in dentistry is a unique, nonionizing form of electromagnetic radiation, that can be employed as a controlled source of tissue stimulation, cutting or ablation, depending on specific parameters of wavelength, power and target tissue.

Fundamentals of Laser Operation

Laser Physics

Lasers consist of a small number of basic components as shown in Figures 54.1A and B.

An *active lasing medium*, which can be a solid, liquid, or gas, is enclosed within a laser cavity bounded by two perfectly parallel reflectors (mirrors). High energy radiation is pumped into the active medium by means of a *pump source*. The pump source is energy generally provided by an intense optical or electrical discharge (It can be internal or external energy source).

The energy from the pump source, is absorbed by the active medium until the majority of atoms, ions, or molecules are raised to their upper energy state and it produces an excited population of atoms, molecules and rare gas (Photon). This is a condition known as a *population inversion* and is a necessary condition to generate laser light. The two parallel reflectors are situated at the ends of the laser cavity and act to constrain the light along and within the axis of the cavity. Thus, the light is repeatedly bounced between the reflectors. This will stimulate the emission of even more photons (**amplification**) in that axial direction. Light traveling in other directions escapes the cavity and is lost as heat. One of the mirrors is only partially reflective, enabling some of the light to escape the cavity as a beam of laser light (Figs 54.2 and 54.3).

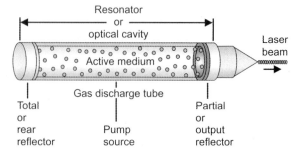

Fig. 54.1A: The basic components of a laser. The lasant is composed of a laser medium consisting of ions, atoms or molecules

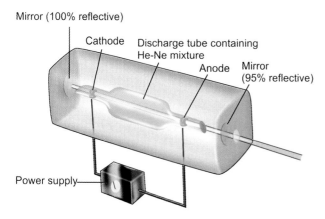

Fig. 54.1B: The basic components of a He-Ne (Helium/Neon) laser

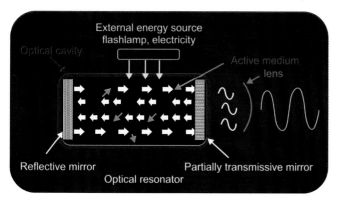

Fig. 54.2: Population inversion

Components of Laser System (Figs 54.1 A and B)

In order to understand the generation of laser radiation, it is essential to consider the fundamental design of the laser system.

1. *Active medium:* Every laser device has a laser medium. A material or laser medium, either naturally occurring or man made that when stimulated, emits laser light. This material may be a solid, liquid or gas. The active medium is positioned within the laser cavity, an internally-polished tube, with mirrors coaxially positioned at each end and surrounded by the external energizing input, or pumping mechanism. The 'active medium', may be solid crystals such as ruby or neodymium ion-doped yttrium-aluminium garnet (Nd:YAG) rod, holmium (HO:YAG) or liquid dyes, Erbium(Er). Diode-solid state semiconductor uses a combination of gallium, aluminum and arsenide. CO_2 or (He-Ne)Helium/Neon, Argon are the gases used as active medium. The active medium defines the type of laser and the emission wavelength of the laser (10,600 nm and 1,064 nm respectively) (Table 54.4). Atoms of the active medium are absorbed by the process of light emission.

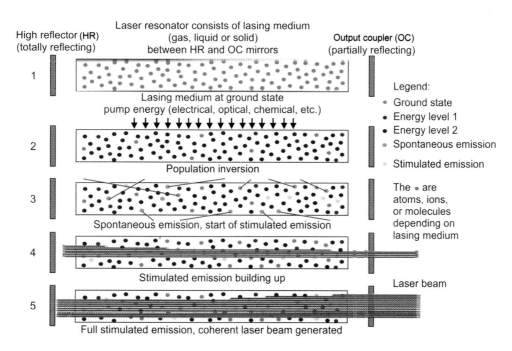

Fig. 54.3: Basic laser operation: Generation of laser energy

Table 54.4: Wavelengths of most common lasers			
Argon fluoride (Excimer-UV)	0.193	Ruby (CrAlO₃) (red)	0.694
Krypton chloride (Excimer-UV)	0.222	Gallium arsenide (diode-NIR)	0.840
Krypton fluoride (Excimer-UV)	0.248	Nd:YAG (NIR)	1.064
Xenon chloride (Excimer-UV)	0.308	Helium neon (NIR)	1.15
Xenon fluoride (Excimer-UV)	0.351	Erbium (NIR)	1.504
Helium cadmium (UV)	0.325	Helium neon (NIR)	3.39
Nitrogen (UV)	0.337	Hydrogen fluoride (NIR)	2.70
Helium cadmium (violet)	0.441	Carbon dioxide (FIR)	9.6
Krypton (blue)	0.476	Carbon dioxide (FIR)	10.6
Argon (blue)	0.488		
Copper vapor (green)	0.510		
Argon (green)	0.514		
Krypton (green)	0.528		
Frequency doubled Nd:YAG (green)	0.532		
Helium neon (green)	0.543		
Krypton (yellow)	0.568		
Copper vapor (yellow)	0.570		
Helium neon (yellow)	0.594		
Helium neon (orange)	0.610		
Gold vapor (red)	0.627		
Helium neon (red)	0.633		
Krypton (red)	0.647		
Rhodamine 6G dye (tunable)	0.570-0.650		

Key: UV = Ultraviolet (0.200–0.400 μm)
VIS = Visible (0.400–0.700 μm)
NIR = Near infrared (0.700–1.400 μm)

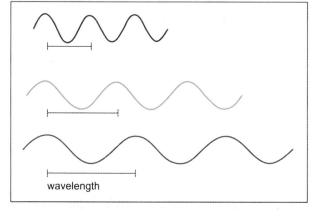

Wavelengths of most common lasers

2. *Pumping/Excitation mechanism:* This represents a man made source of primary energy that excites the active medium. This is usually a light source, either a flash light or arc light, but can be a diode laser unit or an electromagnetic coil. Energy from this primary source is absorbed by the active medium; resulting in the production of laser light. The dynamics of incident energy with time has a fundamental bearing on the emission mode characteristics of a given laser. A continuous feed electrical discharge will result in a similar continuous feed of laser light emission.

3. *Optical resonator:* (A) High reflectance mirror reflects essentially 100 percent of the laser light. (B) Partially transmissive mirror reflects less than 100 percent of the laser light and transmits the remainder.

   These mirrors are designed to reflect photons completely on one end.

   Laser light produced by the stimulated active medium is bounced back and forth through the axis of the laser cavity, using two mirrors placed at either end, thus amplifying the power. The distal mirror is partly transmissive, so that at a given energy density, laser light will escape to be transmitted to the target tissue.

4. *Laser delivery systems:* Early attempts to produce delivery systems relied upon the use of fixed mirror and/or lens apparatus. It was soon apparent that the use of a fine silica quartz fiberoptic cable maximized the feasibility for medical and dental lasers to reach their target site. However, the suitability of this delivery system is conditional upon the emission wavelength being poorly absorbed by water (hydroxyl groups), present in the quartz fiber. Therefore, shorter wavelengths (Er, Cr:YSGG, Er:YAG and carbon dioxide) give rise to severe power losses through quartz fiber and hence require alternative delivery systems. Examples of such alternatives are articulated arms incorporating internal mirrors and prisms, and hollow waveguides, where the light is reflected along internally polished tubes. Newer, water free fiber compounds, e.g. zirconium fluoride, are being developed to overcome this problem.

5. *Cooling system:* Heat production is a by product of laser light propagation. It increases with the power output of the laser, hence, with heavy duty tissue cutting lasers, the cooling system represents the bulkiest component. Coaxial coolant systems may be air or water assisted.

6. *Control panel:* This allows variation in power output with time, above that defined by the pumping mechanism frequency. Other facilities may allow wavelength change (multilaser) instruments and print out of delivered laser energy during clinical use.

PHYSICAL PROPERTIES OF LASER

There are several important properties of laser light, which distinguish it from white light.

These properties make it useful for surgery (Fig. 54.4). These are as follows:
1. Monochromaticity
2. Unidirectionality
3. Coherence
4. Brightness.

Monochromaticity

Lasers emit light that is monochromatic, that it is of a single color or wavelength.

In contrast, ordinary white light is a combination of many colors of light or wavelengths. Monochromaticty, is the property of a laser device to selectively destroy tumor cells that absorb a particular dye such as hematoporphyrin derivative (HPD), while not injuring the adjoining or overlying tissue cells. Lasers of varying types emit an individual wavelength or specified wavelengths, each type of target tissue absorbs a given wavelength far better than others.

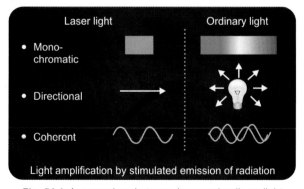

Fig. 54.4: A comparison between laser and ordinary light

Directionality

Laser light is emitted as a relatively narrow beam in a specific direction. Ordinary light (light bulb) is emitted in many directions away from the source. There is little diversion of the laser as it exits the laser device, and the beam can travel a considerable distance with very little movement away from parallelism. Lasers used clinically are unidirectional.

Coherence

The ability to direct the monochromatic, collimated photons is called coherence. This allows the laser to be focused to a precise point via the delivery system.

Laser light which is produced is coherent. It means that its wavelengths are in phase in space and time. Ordinary light can be a mixture of many wavelengths. It is the property of laser light that occurs when there is some fixed phase relationship between two waves of laser light. There are two types of coherence of laser light, longitudinal and transverse. The longitudinal coherence represents a time or temporal coherence along the longitudinal beam axis, where a transverse or spatial coherence refers to coherence across the beam. Laser light can deposit a lot of energy within a small area.

Brightness

This property arises from the parallelism or collimation of the laser light, as it moves through space, maintaining the concentration and the characteristic brightness.

CHARACTERISTICS OF LASER

Lasers are also characterized by the duration of laser emission—continuous wave or pulsed laser. A Q-switched laser is a pulsed laser, which contains a shutter like device that does not allow emission of laser light until opened. Energy is built up in a Q-switched laser and released by opening the device to produce a single, intense laser pulse (Fig. 54.5).

Continuous wave (CW): Lasers operate with a stable average beam power. In higher power systems, one is able to adjust the power. In low power gas lasers, such as He-Ne, the power level is fixed by the design, and performance usually degrades with long term use.

Single pulsed: (Normal mode) Lasers generally have pulse durations of a few hundred microseconds to a

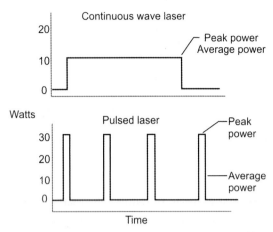

Fig. 54.5: Laser emission—continuous wave or pulsed laser

few milliseconds. This mode of operation is sometimes referred to as long pulse or normal mode.

Single pulsed Q-switched: Lasers are the result of an intracavity delay (Q-switch cell) which allows the laser media to store a maximum of potential energy. Under optimum gain conditions, emission occurs in single pulses; typically of 10(-8) second time domain. These pulses will have high peak powers often in the range from 10(6) to 10(9) Watts peak.

Repetitively pulsed: Scanning lasers generally involve the operation of pulsed laser performance operating at a fixed (or variable) pulse rates which may range from a few pulses per second to as high as 20,000 pulses per second. The direction of a CW laser can be scanned rapidly using optical scanning systems to produce the equivalent of a repetitively pulsed output at a given location.

Mode locked: Lasers operate as a result of the resonant modes of an optical cavity which can affect the characteristics of the output beam. When the phases of different frequency modes are synchronized, i.e. "locked together", the different modes will interfere with one another to generate a beat effect. The result is a laser output which is observed as regularly spaced pulsations. Lasers operating in this mode locked fashion, usually produce a train of regularly spaced pulses, each having a duration of 10(-15) (femto) to 10(-12) (pico) sec. A mode locked laser can deliver extremely high peak powers than the same laser operating in the Q-switched mode. These pulses will have enormous peak powers often in the range from 10(12) Watts.

Electromagnetic Spectrum

The laser functions within an optical spectrum, which is the portion of electromagnetic (EM) spectrum. Laser radiation is an intense beam of light, that generates energy in the wavelengths, that range from the near ultraviolet to the near infrared frequencies. The energy, thus generated by a laser beam and its position within the EM spectrum are determined by the wavelength and frequency of the light waves (Fig. 54.6).

Longer wavelength in the EM spectrum, such as infrared, produce lower energy, and they include not only infrared but microwaves, TV waves and radio waves. Shorter wavelengths have higher energy and include UV, X-ray, and gamma radiation.

The wavelength of photon, depends upon the active medium used and state of electron's energy, when the photon is released. Therefore, different types of lasers are wavelength specific. The wavelength of the laser determines the depth of tissue penetration, amount of scatter, and amount of energy absorbed. Different active mediums are used to produce required wavelength as per the need of procedure. Most commonly used mediums are Nd:YAG, Erbium:YAG, CO_2, Er, CR:YSGG (Waterlase MD, Biolase Technology Inc.) and argon ion. Recently, diode lasers have become popular because of compact nature and low cost, since the penetration of these diodes is between 2 and 4 mm, it could be hazardous to underlying bone or root cementum. The diode lasers are best used as a low level laser therapy (LLLT) in a non-cutting mode and out of contact for bacterial debridement after flap debridement, endodontic disinfection after manual biomechanical debridement, socket disinfection after extraction, and aphthous ulcer dissimulation.

Photobiology of Lasers

The interactions of nonionizing EM radiations with biomolecules and the resulting biologic reactions, is known as photobiology. All photobiologic effects are both wavelength and dose dependent (Fig. 54.7).

The consequences of the incident laser radiant energy on biological tissues, including skin, mucosa, odontogenic structures, and bone, is as a result of a photobiologic tissue reaction and a photophysical reaction. The outcome of the photophysical event can be apparent in a microsecond; however, the final long term reaction of laser radiated tissue may be apparent

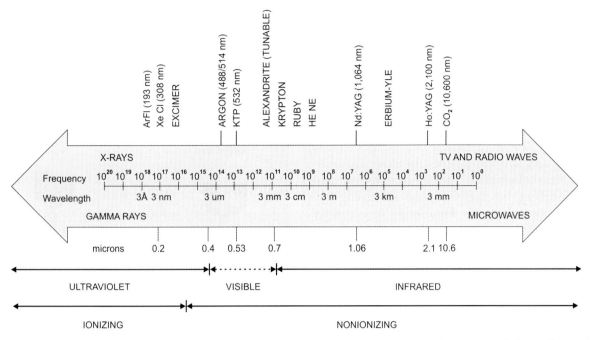

Fig. 54.6: The accepted electromagnetic (EM) spectrum. All lasers are represented on EM spectrum, depending on their specific wavelengths

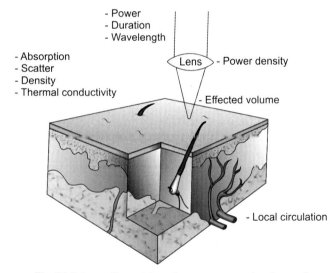

Fig. 54.7: Laser-tissue interactions are power, duration and wavelength dependent

only after some months. Tissue reactions to laser radiation can be considered to be thermal or non-thermal processes. Thermal laser effects are known as photocoagulation and photovaporization. Nonthermal laser effects are related to a photomechanical response or to a photochemical phenomenon.

Thus, the major reactions of laser radiant energy with target living tissues involve: (1) Photochemical, (2) photothermal, (3) photomechanical and (4) photo-electrical interaction.

1. *Photo chemical* interaction include
   a. *Biostimulation*-stimulatory effects of laser on biochemical and molecular processes, that normally occur in tissues, such as healing and repair.
   b. *Photodynamic therapy*, which is the therapeutic use of lasers to induce reactions in tissues for the treatment of pathologic conditions.
   c. *Photorescent re-emission or tissue fluorescence*, which may be used as a diagnostic method to detect light reactive substances in tissues.

2. *Photo thermal interactions* manifest clinically as
   a. *Photo ablation*, or removal of tissue by vaporization (Photovaporization) and super heating of tissue fluids, coagulation and hemostasis.
   b. Photopyrolysis or burning away of tissues.

3. *Photomechanical* interaction include
   a. *Photodisruption or photodisasociation*, which is breaking apart of structures by laser light, and
   b. *Photoacoustic interactions*, which involve the removal of tissue with shock wave generation.

4. *Photoelectrical interactions* include photoplasmolysis, which describes how tissue is removed through the formation of electrically charged ions and particles that exist in a semi gaseous, high energy state.

LASER INTERACTION WITH ORAL BIOLOGIC TISSUES

The oral cavity is a unique and complex environment, where hard and soft tissues exist in close proximity, within bacteria laden saliva. All oral tissues are receptive to laser treatment, but the biophysics governing laser tissue interaction demands knowledge of all factors involved in delivery of this modality. Through this knowledge, appropriate treatment can be delivered in a predictable manner. The biologic factors that influence laser-tissue interactions are more extensive. Included among these are the optical properties of various tissue elements that govern how specific molecular and chemical components in tissue react with light energy. The optical properties of tissue elements determine the nature and extent of the tissue response through the processes of *absorption, transmission, reflection, and scattering of the laser beam* (Dederich, 1991) (Figs 54.8A and B).

Other factors involve the various types of physiologic and mechanical processes that occur as a result of energy transformations within tissue mass, the inflammatory response of tissues to noxious stimuli, tissue vascularity, and repair mechanisms. The incident light energy interacts with a medium (e.g. oral tissue) that is denser than air, in one of the four ways as listed below.

Absorption

It is obvious that to exert laser energy effect upon a given tissue, it must first be absorbed. The amount of energy absorbed by a tissue depends on its characteristics, such as pigmentation and water content, laser wavelength and emission mode. The incident energy of the beam is attenuated by the medium and transferred into another form. Precise removal of specific kinds of tissue is based on tissue's inherent absorption of particular wavelengths. Chromophores are the compounds within the tissues, which absorb the wavelength of light. The absorption is dependent on the amount of chromophores within the tissue (Figs 54.9 and 54.10).

Hemoglobin reflects red wavelengths, imparting color to the arterial blood. It is therefore strongly

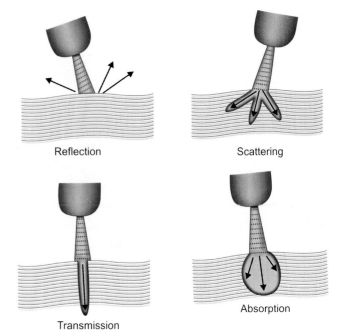

Fig. 54.8A: Various laser-tissue interactions

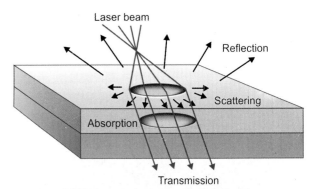

Fig. 54.8B: Laser interaction with biological tissues

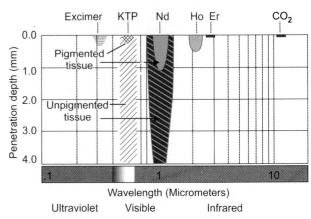

Fig. 54.9: A comparison of the carbon dioxide laser with other popular surgical lasers. Laser penetration in pigmented and unpigmented tissue

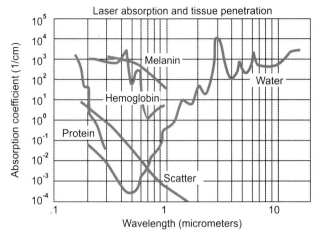

Fig. 54.10: Laser penetration is related to the presence of tissue chromophores. The absorption coefficient is plotted against the wavelength in micrometers (courtesy of coherent laser, Palo Alto, California)

absorbed by blue and green wavelengths. Venous blood, containing less oxygen, absorbs more red lights and appears darker. The pigment melanin, which imparts color to the skin, is strongly absorbed by short wavelengths, and water, the universally present molecule, has varying degrees of absorption by different wavelengths. Dental tissues have different amounts of water content by weight. A ranking from lowest to highest would show enamel (with 2% to 3%), dentin, bone, calculus, caries, and soft tissue (about 70%). In general, the shorter wavelengths (from about 500–1000 nm) are readily absorbed in pigmented tissue and blood elements.

Transmission

Transmission through the tissues results in no observable laser-tissue reaction.

The inverse of absorption, wherein laser energy passes directly through the tissue with no interaction between the incident beam and the medium. The beam will emerge distally, unchanged or partially refracted. This effect is highly dependent on the wavelength of laser light.

Reflection

The beam redirects itself off the surface, producing no effect on the target tissue. The density of the medium, or angle of incidence being less than the refractive angle, results in a total reflection of the beam. In true reflection,

the incident and emergence angles will be the same or, if the medium interface is rough or non homogenous, some scatter may occur, as seen in caries detection, which uses reflected light to measure the degree of sound tooth structure.

Scatter

Scattered laser energy is absorbed over a broader area or volume of tissue, thus diffusing the effects of the energy. There is some interaction, but this is insufficient to cause complete attenuation of the beam. Scatter will cause some diminution of light energy with distance, together with a distortion in the beam, whereby rays proceed in an uncontrolled direction through the medium. Back scatter of the laser beam can occur as it hits the tissue; this is seen most in short wavelengths, e.g. Diode, Nd: YAG (> 50 % back scatter).

Photocoagulation

If a laser incident to tissues with a normal body temperature of 37°C heats the tissues to 60°C, for a limited time, there is no alteration in the appearance of the tissue structure. However, biological tissues heated to temperatures over 60°C undergo coagulation. This coagulation phenomenon is the basis of most of the surgical application of lasers. As a result of photocoagulation, proteins, enzymes, cytokines, and other bioactive molecules are heated to temperatures over 60°C, the result being instant denaturation. The phenomenon of photocoagulation is dependent on the rate of energy transfer and is termed a thermo-chemical rate process. If radiant energy is delivered at a high intensity per unit of time (high irradiance), the result is high temperature. Higher irradiances produce a more rapid increase in temperature and faster tissue coagulation, exceeding 100°C. When this temperature is exceeded, the phenomenon of photovaporization is observed (Figs 54.11A and B and Tables 54.5 and 54.6).

Photocoagulation by inspection, appears as a whitening of the tissue surface. This surface change is the result of an alteration in the molecular structure of the tissue constituents, mainly collagen. Collagen has long been known to be a trihelical structure made up of long polypeptide protein chain linked in groups. When temperatures greater than 60°C are reached, the helical polymer is disrupted and the coils become randomized. The result is that the collagen fibers undergo significant shrinkage following photocoagulation. This physical

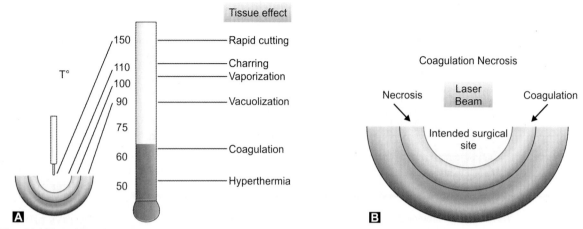

Figs 54.11A and B: (A) As the laser strikes the target, series of concentric circles form within the tissue, as the heat dissipates laterally, (B) The zone of coagulation necrosis surrounding the surgical site

Table 54.5: Laser energy temperature and its effects on biological tissues	
Tissue temperature	*Observed effects*
< 60°	Hyperthermia
60-70°	Coagulation
70-80°	Tissue welding
> 100°	Tissue ablation
> 200°	Carbonization

Fig. 54.12: Different tissue effects seen in laser incision technique. Different zones created are—vaporization, ablation as well as zone of coagulation. Tissue necrosis can be seen adjacent to the ablated zone

Table 54.6: The visual and biological effects on tissues as a function of temperature change		
Temperature	*Visual change*	*Biological change*
42.5 °C	None	Malignant cells are functionally damaged and die
44 °C	None	Normal cells are functionally damaged and die
60° C	Blanching	Warming, welding
65 °C	Hemostasis	Coagulation
65-90 °C	Tissue coloration to white or gray	Protein denaturization
90-100 °C	Topographic shrinkage	Desiccation of tissue
100 °C	Water vaporization, smoke plume	Vaporization of tissue, ablation
300 °C	Char formation	Burning tissue
700 °C	Iridescence	
3652 °C	Smoke plume	Carbon sublimation

event affecting collagen has a practical value during laser surgery: the lased tissues constrict against the proximal vasculature and the vessels shrink as a result of the collagen configuration of their walls, which results in the enhanced hemostasis associated with the use of the laser. Laser damage to erythrocytes attracts a population of platelets, which encourage intraluminal thrombosis, further decreasing blood loss. *This latter mechanism which appears to be the primary hemostatic phenomenon; while thrombosis is a secondary effect.* Photocoagulation is said to be ideal after the radiant energy generates temperatures within the range of 50° to 100°C. At temperatures of 45° to 50°C, actual photocoagulation is seen after several seconds; in contrast, at temperatures near or greater than 100°C, the phenomenon of photocoagulation occurs within fractions of a second (Figs 54.12 and 54.13).

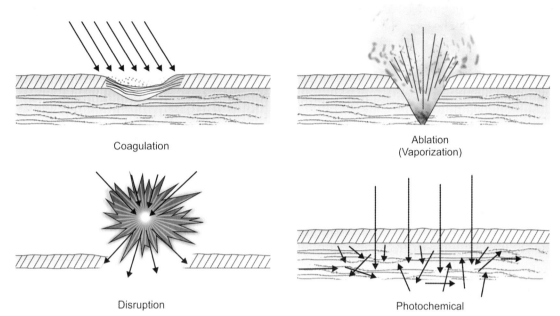

Coagulation

Ablation
(Vaporization)

Disruption

Photochemical

Fig. 54.13: Photothermal and photochemical interaction of laser on target tissue

The carbon dioxide laser is very useful in oral and maxillofacial surgery, and through its photobiologic effects on tissues, it can be used effectively in laser facial resurfacing. This is because the carbon dioxide laser provides photocoagulation in deeper tissues through heat conduction, because the absorption coefficient of its 10.6 micron wavelength is very high and it is, therefore, absorbed in the first 20 microns of tissues. Its energy is 90 percent absorbed within a depth of 100 microns, which is equivalent to a few cell diameters. The lateral necrosis of tissue observed with this laser is 41 to 85 microns.

It has been demonstrated in mammalian tissues that the peak temperature achieved by the carbon dioxide laser is 145°C, the heat of which is mostly lost in cell vaporization. There was an observed decrease in temperature to 45°C at 0.5 mm lateral to the laser beam, which may account for the comparative lack of extensive lateral thermal trauma.

Photodynamic Therapy (PDT) with Lasers

Photodynamic Theory (PDT) involves the activation of a normally inert substance by means of light energy, converting it into an active substance. It involves IV injection of a chemosensitizing agent, which is preferentially absorbed by malignant tissue or reticuloendothelial tissue. When these tissues are exposed to light energy, a photochemical reaction is catalyzed, releasing the toxic agents responsible for cellular death and tumor necrosis. The most commonly used chemosensitizing agents are *porphyrins* and more specifically, *hematoporphyrin derivatives (HPD)*.

HPD, in addition to localizing in malignant noeplasms, it also concentrates in inflamed tissues. PDT can be delivered to any neoplasm that is accessible by endoscopes, intravenous catheters, or hypodermic needles.

PDT, requires adequate tissue levels of photosensitiser, O_2, and laser energy. Photofrin II is administered in doses of 1.5–2.5 mg/kg, 48 to 72 hours before lasing a specific lesion. Following the loading dose of dihematoporphyrin ethers or esters-DHE, laser energy within the red spectrum (wavelength 630 nm) is applied for 5 to 15 minutes to a total dose of 25 to 250 joules/sq cm in the malignant disease. The range of DHE doses for treatment of head and neck malignancies has been about 3 to 5 mg/kg BW.

The laser light is delivered from the laser chamber to the tissues in various ways:

i. Through quartz fiberoptic cable
ii. Through an articulated arm system, consisting of a series of tubes, containing partially reflective mirrors to direct the beam

iii. A hollow flexible wave guide, which utilizes a hollow tube with inner reflective surface. Wave guide system is more cheaper. But its kinking or bending should be avoided as laser light can escape from the damaged area and become a hazard

iv. A handpiece containing laser unit—at present only for low powered lasers.

Final Laser Delivery Mechanisms to the Tissues (Figs 54.14 to 54.16)

Noncontact Laser System (Free Beam Lasers)

Free beam (sometimes referred to as noncontact) lasers are devices that permit laser energy alone (without influence by the delivery device) to interact with tissue, causing the final clinical result. The interactions between laser light and tissue described here are specific for free-beam lasers. They result from interactions between the native laser wavelength and tissue alone. Characteristic of these devices is that the effect on tissue is principally that of the laser emission alone. This is typically what occurs when there is no contact between the fiber optic end of the delivery device and the target tissue. Consider the laser beam exiting a laser delivery system used in a free beam mode. The beam will converge (or diverge) as it exits the focusing lens and some portion of the energy will be reflected from the tissue on impact. Should the distance from the fiber to the tissue be altered, the power density at the tissue will change, changing the clinical effect. Substantial energy is reflected or lost as heat and in smoke. The free beam method of delivery provides certain advantages over conventional surgery by providing a method for "nontouch" surgery, but suffers from the loss of tactile feedback. The techniques for learning and using the free beam laser are substantially different from those of conventional instruments. Perhaps the most limiting feature of the free beam laser is that different laser sources are required for different surgical maneuvers, e.g. Nd:YAG for coagulation and hemostasis and CO_2 for incision and excision.

Typical free beam delivery systems include articulating arm delivery systems, micromanipulators used in conjunction with surgical microscopes, and conventional fiber optics (i.e. the handpiece or its attachments do not come into contact with the target tissue).

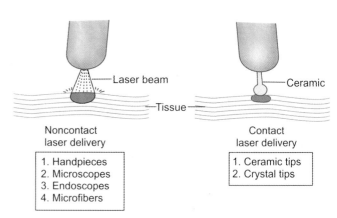

Fig. 54.15: Different types of laser delivery systems, which can be used in oral and maxillofacial surgeries

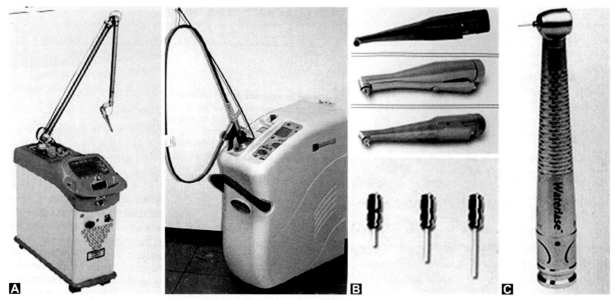

Figs 54.14A to C: (A) Er:YAG laser units, (B) Handpieces with tips, (C) Different fiber tips

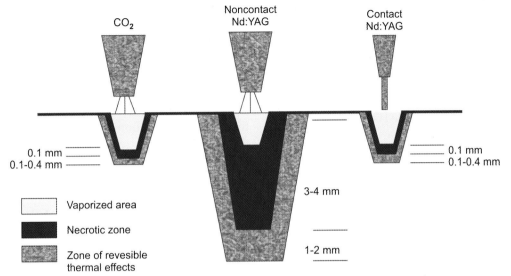

Fig. 54.16: Diagrammatic representation of free beam and contact laser tissue reaction

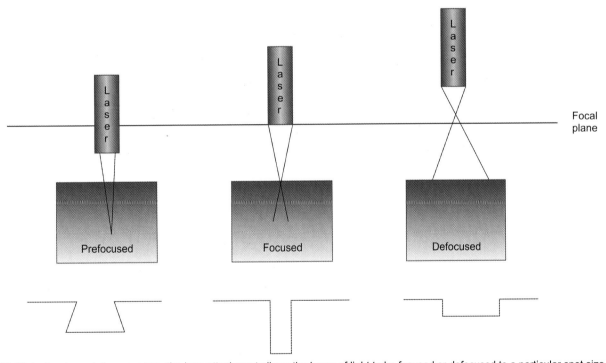

Fig. 54.17: In free laser delivery system, the lens attachment allows the beam of light to be focused or defocused to a particular spot size. The spot size of the beam varies on the distance that the operator holds it from the target tissue. On some systems, a pointing blade or guide pin is provided at the end of the handpiece to guide the operator. If the beam is focused to a smaller spot size, the power density is increased

(a) Handpiece, (b) Microscope-free beam lasers for surgical microscopes for dissection and anastomosis, (c) Endoscope and (d) Microfibers (Figs 54.14 to 54.16). Some noncontact or free beam laser systems have angled mirrors to direct the beam either at 90° or 120°. Safety checks should be carried out while using these type of lasers.

Carbon dioxide lasers work primarily in a noncontact mode. They can also be used either in a focused or defocused mode (Fig. 54.17).

Focused mode: It is when the laser beam hits the tissue at its focal point or the smallest diameter. This diameter is dependent on the size of the lens used. Most CO_2 laser systems today have a lens that can focus the beam down to spot sizes ranging from 0.1 to 0.35 mm or larger. This focused mode can also be referred to as a cut mode. For example, the cut mode is used when performing biopsies.

Defocused mode: By defocusing the laser beam or moving the focal spot away from the tissue plane, the beam size that hits the tissue has a greater diameter, thus causing a wider area of tissue to be vaporized. By defocusing the beam, however, laser intensity or power density is reduced. A defocused beam, for example, is used when performing frenectomies, or for the removal of inflammatory papillary hyperplasia.

Because all optical fibers have a high absorptive index for CO_2 laser light, true fiberoptic delivery cannot be used. Instead, some CO_2 lasers use articulating arms with properly aligned mirrors at knuckle joints and then a handpiece with a specific lens is used to create the desired spot size in the focused mode. Because of their sometimes cumbersome nature, CO_2 laser systems that use articulated arms are often difficult to use within the oral cavity. With articulated arm systems and those that use hand held technology, the focal distance to tissue can vary from 1 to 3 cm.

Modification of Free Beam Laser Surgery

Contact Laser System

Despite the benefits of free beam laser surgery, certain limitations and drawbacks exist. Perhaps the most significant is that to substantially change the tissue's temperature gradient (Clinical effect), one must choose different laser sources, an expensive and intraoperatively difficult task. Contact laser surgery has been developed to augment and overcome this and other fundamental deficiencies in free beam surgery. Contact laser surgery works by altering the tissue temperature gradient through changes in the laser delivery system, rather than by alteration in wavelength. A decade ago researchers developed a delivery system in which, an optical device is placed in direct contact with the tissue during laser surgery to increase the delivered power density and reduce changes in power density due to changes in distance to the tissue. This is accomplished by use of interchangeable contact laser probes and scalpels (tips) made from synthetic sapphire or fused silica. It uses tactile sensation during use. (Some Nd:YAG lasers have

a handpiece with specially designed interchangeable sapphire crystal tips or ceramic tips).

The tips have several different sizes and shapes and can be easily affixed to the end of fiber optics. The tip is heated when the laser is activated, enabling tissues to be cut and coagulated simultaneously with a precision. Several benefits result from the use of these tips. In addition to providing the surgeon with tactile feedback, a sense lost in free beam surgery, and controlling power density, the reflection of light from the tissue is significantly reduced. The improved efficiency in coupling of light into the tissue results in the requirement of less power, in most cases a reduction of 40 to 50 percent. Altering the tip configuration of a probe and scalpel makes it possible to change not only the spot size (and thus power density), but the angle of divergence of the beam. A frustroconical tip, for example, concentrates the laser light on a small, precisely defined distal area from which light plays out at a wide angle, creating a region of high power density that drops rapidly with distance. Alterations in the tip's shape can result in a low divergence angle. In addition to placing tips onto the ends of fiber optics, the ends of fiberoptics themselves can also be shaped, although they lack the mechanical strength and thermal resistance required for extended and precision use.

The contact laser attributes thus far described, still result in a tissue effect that is solely dependent on the absorption of the laser emission by the tissue to generate the temperature gradient. It is a major attribute of contact laser surgery to have the temperature gradient altered by the contact laser tip. By placing a small amount of light absorbing material integrally between the contact tip and the tissue, a portion of the energy will be absorbed by that material. The energy absorbed will be converted to heat and will result in a very high temperature. Since the absorbing material is in contact with the probe and the tissue, it will elevate the temperature of the tissue by thermal combustion in addition to the radiation heating, caused by the native wavelength. Thus, by use of this absorbing material, the tissue temperature gradient induced by the laser emission has been altered. Depending upon the quantity and distribution of the absorbing material, the contact tip can mimic the effect of other laser wavelengths. This event is referred to **as the wavelength conversion effect. The wavelength conversion effect does not result in changing the wavelength of the laser; rather, it changes the effect, the wavelength has in the surgical situation.** By adjusting the wavelength conversion effect material on the probe tip, one can titrate the amount of laser light exiting the tip in comparison to the amount of heat generated by absorption at the tip. This means, in essence, that a single laser in combination with different interchangeable tips can mimic the tissue temperature profile and effect of various lasers.

The American dental laser dLase Nd:YAG system was the first such instrument to use a fiberoptic delivery system. This fiberoptic technology allows for contact with the target tissue. The fiberoptic cables are attached to a small handpiece similar in size to a dental turbine and are available in sizes ranging from 200 to 1000 μm in diameter. They also are relatively flexible which allows easy transmission of the laser energy throughout the oral cavity, including periodontal pockets. Fiberoptic delivery and articulated arm systems are not the only two delivery systems currently in the market. One manufacturer has developed a hollow waveguide delivery system. In contrast to an articulated arm system, this waveguide is a single long, semiflexible tube, without knuckles or mirrors. The laser energy is transmitted along the reflective inner lumen of this tube and exits through a hand piece at the end of the tube. This hand piece comes with various attachments that the dentist may select, depending on the procedure to be performed, and may be used either in contact or out of contact with the target tissue. The final delivery system is the air cooled fiberoptic delivery system. This type of delivery system is unique to the erbium family of lasers. A conventional fiberoptic delivery system cannot transmit the wavelength of the erbium family of lasers, owing to the specific characteristics of the erbium wavelength. These special air cooled fibers terminate in a hand piece with quartz or sapphire tips. These tips are used slightly (1–2 mm) out of contact with the target tissue. Since the introduction of the dLase 300, general practitioners have seen the number of wavelengths and manufacturers available to them increased by leaps and bounds. It has increased from one manufacturer of one wavelength to eight different manufacturers offering six different wavelengths.

CLASSIFICATION OF LASERS

Lasers are divided into a number of classes depending upon the power or energy of the beam and the wavelength of the emitted radiation. *Laser classification is based on the laser's potential for causing immediate injury to the eye or skin and/or potential for causing fires from direct exposure to the beam or from reflections from diffuse reflective surfaces.* Since August 1, 1976, commercially produced lasers have been classified and identified by labels affixed to the laser. *Lasers are classified using physical parameters of the laser, power, wavelength, and exposure duration.* Currently, there are two classification systems available—the 'old system' used before 2002, and the 'revised system' being phased in since 2002. The classification of a laser is based on the concept of 'accessible emission limits' AEL that are defined for each laser class. This is usually a maximum power (in W) or energy (in J) that can be emitted in a specified wavelength range and exposure time that passes through a specified aperture stop at a specified distance.

It is the duty of the manufacturer of the laser to classify the product and consequently to place warning labels on the product and to realise safety features as prescribed by the regulations. Safety measures used with more powerful lasers include key controlled operations, warning lights to indicate laser light emission, a beam stop or attenuator, and an electrical contact that the user can connect to an emergency stop or interlock. However, if the user manipulates the laser product, so that the class is changed, the user becomes responsible for a reclassification.

1. General Classification of Lasers

Class 1 Laser

It is considered safe based upon current medical knowledge. Under normal operating conditions, Class 1 lasers cannot produce a hazard and no safety measures are required. A Class 1 laser could also be a higher-class laser that is completely enclosed to prevent personnel exposure to the laser beam.

Example: Laser telescope or microscope.

Class 1 M Laser

It is safe for all conditions of use, except when passed through magnifying optics such as microscopes and telescopes. Class 1M lasers produce large diameter beams or beams that are divergent. In this, the power that can pass through the pupil of the naked eye is less than AEL for Class 1 but the power that can be collected into the eye by typical magnifying optics is higher than the AEL for Class 1 and lower than the AEL for Class 3B. *Class 2 Laser.* It is defined as operating in the visible region (400–700 nm). These lasers are not inherently safe, but protection against eye damage will normally be afforded by aversion responses including the blink reflex. It is safe, because the blink reflex will limit the exposure to no more than 0.25 seconds, intentional extended viewing, however, is considered hazardous.

Example: Laser pointers, surveying lasers.

Class 2 M Laser

It is safe, because of the blink reflex, if not viewed through optical instruments. As with Class 1 M, this applies to laser beams with a large diameter or large divergence, for which the amount of light passing through the pupil cannot exceed the limits for Class 2.

Class 3 R Laser: It is considered safe, if handled carefully, with restricted beam viewing. With a Class 3 R laser, the MPE (maximum permissible exposure) can be exceeded but with a low risk of injury. Visible continuous lasers in Class 3 R are limited to 5 mW.

Class 3B

Class 3B lasers can emit either invisible or visible radiation and direct viewing is hazardous to the eye. Class 3B lasers are capable of causing eye injury either because their output is invisible and therefore aversion responses are not activated, or because the beam power is such that damage is done in a time shorter than the blink reflex (0.25s). Higher power lasers in this class may also cause skin burns. However, with laser wavelengths other than those in the ultraviolet region, the pain produced by rapid heating of the skin will usually evoke an aversion response sufficient to avoid such burns. Class 3B represents maximal power output of 0.5 W. Examples include soft medical lasers (LLLT), laser light show equipment and laser measuring devices. Protective eyewear is required, where direct viewing of Class 3 B laser is used. These also must be equipped with a key switch and a safety interlock.

Class 4 Lasers

Class 4 lasers are high power lasers with power levels greater than 500 mW radiant power, that pose a serious potential for injury of the eye and skin and require that users follow specific safety precautions and wear laser protective eyewear. They may operate in any part of the spectrum, as with the 3B. Class 4 laser systems can produce a hazard not only from direct or specular reflections, but also from a diffuse reflection. A fire risk may also be associated with the use of such high powered systems and their use requires extreme caution.

Example: Most Nd:YAG lasers of these classifications, only Class 4 lasers are incorporated into systems used for material processing such as cutting, heat treatment, surfacing and welding. A Class 4 laser may be part of a system designed in such a manner as to be considered a Class 1 laser system. Such a system cannot under normal operating conditions, produce a hazard. This can be achieved using engineering controls such as enclosures, interlocks, and other mechanisms.

2. Laser Classification as per the Medium Used

There are many types of lasers available for research, medical, industrial, and commercial uses. Lasers are often described by the kind of lasing medium they use—*solid state, gas, excimer, dye, or semiconductor.*

Solid state lasers: Have lasing material distributed in a solid matrix, e.g. the ruby or neodymium-YAG (yttrium aluminium garnet) lasers. The neodymium-YAG laser emits infrared light at 1.064 micrometers (1,064 nanometers(nm).

Gas lasers: Helium and Helium-Neon (He-Ne) are the most common gas lasers, which have a primary output of a visible red light. CO_2 lasers emit energy in the far-infrared, 10.6 micrometres, used for cutting hard materials.

Excimer lasers: (Derived from the terms excited and dimers) Use reactive gases such as chlorine and fluorine, mixed with inert gases such as argon, krypton, or xenon. When electrically stimulated, a pseudomolecule or dimer is produced and when lased, produces light in the ultraviolet range.

Dye lasers: Use complex organic dyes like Rhodamine 6G in liquid solutions or a suspension as lasing media. They are tunable over a broad range of wavelengths.

3. Semiconductor Lasers

Sometimes called diode lasers, are not solid-state lasers. These electronic devices are generally very small and use low power. They may be built into larger arrays, e.g. the writing source in some laser printers or CD players.

Diode lasers (Fig. 54.18): The diode laser was developed in 1960, and now represent 99 percent of all the lasers sold.

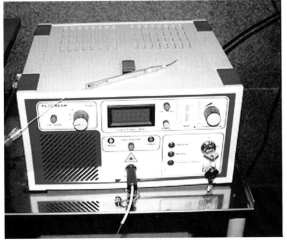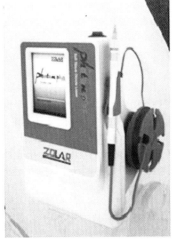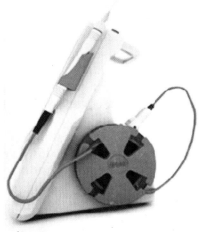

Fig. 54.18: Soft tissue diode laser unit machines

The medical use of diode laser was suggested in 1984 and first applied in 1987. The diode laser is a solid state semiconductor laser, that typically uses a combination of Gallium (Ga), Arsenide (As), and other elements such as Aluminum (Al) and Indium (In) to change electrical energy into light energy. The wavelength range is about 800 to 980 nm. The laser is emitted in continuous-wave and gated-pulsed modes, and is usually operated in a contact method using a flexible fiber optic delivery system. Laser light at 800 to 980 nm is poorly absorbed in water, but highly absorbed in hemoglobin and other pigments.

Since the diode basically does not interact with dental hard tissues, the laser is an excellent soft tissue surgical laser, indicated for cutting and coagulating gingiva and oral mucosa, for soft tissue curettage or sulcular debridement. The Food and Drug Administration (FDA) approved oral soft tissue surgery in 1995 and sulcular debridement in 1998 by means of a diode laser (GaAlAs 810 nm).

The diode laser exhibits thermal effects using the 'hot-tip' effect caused by heat accumulation at the end of the fiber, and produces a relatively thick coagulation layer on the treated surface. The usage is quite similar to electro cauterization.

Tissue penetration of a diode laser is less than that of the Nd:YAG laser, while the rate of heat generation is higher, resulting in deeper coagulation and more charring on the surface compared to the Nd:YAG laser. The width of the coagulation layer was reported to be in excess of 1.0 mm in an incision of bovine oral soft tissue *in vitro*. The advantages of diode lasers are the smaller size of the units, as well as the lower financial costs.

Surgery is usually performed in continuous mode, but the recently produced super pulsed diode laser allows the surgeon to perform interventions with very high energy levels up to 20,000 Hz. With a pulse duration in millisecond range. In this way, the thermal damage to the tissues does not progress deeper than 50 micron meters and carbonization is reduced to a minimum. The super pulsed 809 nm gaAlAs laser allows the excision of oral lesions of various consistency.

4. Classification Based on Applications

- Soft tissue laser, e.g. Argon, CO_2, Diode, Nd:YAG
- Hard tissue laser, e.g. Er:YAG
- Resin curing laser, e.g. Argon

5. Classification Based on Mode of Action

- Contact mode—focused or defocused, e.g. Ho:YAG; Nd:YAG
- Noncontact mode—focused or defocused, e.g. CO_2

6. Classification Based on Radiant Energy Generation

- Continuous wave or continuous form (CW)
- Discreet or single pulses
- Multiple timed pulses (Pulse modes)

7. Classification Based on Wavelength and Medium (Table 54.7)

Dental laser wavelengths are for diodes 830 to 1064 nm, Nd:YAG 1064 nm, Erbium 2790 to 2940 nm and CO_2 9.3 to 10.6 nm. Every wavelength has a specific thermal output and specific tissue interaction that is always predictable. The different wavelengths for dental lasers perform different procedures. Nd:YAG, diode lasers and CO_2 are used for soft tissues. These lasers give good coagulation. The laser energy of the diode and Nd:YAG lasers can penetrate a few millimeters into the tissue. A CO_2 laser can penetrate less than a millimeter and produce excellent coagulation and a very precise cut. Erbium wavelength can cut tooth, bone and soft tissue. They have affinity for water. They are not good for hemostasis, but are kind to tissues, as they only penetrate microns into the tissues.

8. Medical Laser Classification Based on Level of Energy Emission

Medical lasers can be divided into two main types: *the high-power (hard) lasers used for surgical purposes, and the low-power (soft) lasers used mainly to promote tissue regeneration.*

Soft tissue laser surgery is differentiated from hard tissue laser surgery (bone and teeth) by the type of laser used. A laser beam has a natural sterilization effect—it evaporates bacteria, viruses and fungi, which leads to a decrease in local infections. Probably most important,

the laser decreases postoperative pain by sealing nerve endings. Surgical laser systems are differentiated not only by the wavelength, but also by the light delivery system: flexible fiber or articulated arm, as well as by other factors. Different wavelengths react with tissues in different ways. The laser light from diode laser (980 nm, 810 nm wavelength) is most efficiently absorbed in pigmented tissues and melanin, which makes it effective for cutting soft tissues. The YSGG laser (2780 nm) is absorbed in water and hydroxyapatite, which makes it excellent tool for cutting enamel, dentin, bone and soft tissue.

High-energy lasers have a detrimental effect on tissues. The conversion of the absorbed energy into heat in the irradiated tissue is the reason for this destruction. Free-radical formation, pressure and shock-wave phenomenon, and electromagnetic and photochemical changes are the other aspects of high-energy lasers. High-energy lasers are useful in cutting biologic materials and in producing coagulation necrosis in target tissues with a subsequent reaction in the surrounding tissues. *Hard tissue surgical lasers are dominated by Er:YAG lasers* operating at the wavelengths around 3,000 nm. Er, Cr:YSGG laser can be used for both hard tissue as well as soft tissue surgery. It has got wavelength of 2780 nm.

Table 54.7: Classification based on wavelength and medium			
Laser type	*Medium*	*Wavelength*	*Color*
Excimer lasers	Argon fluoride (ArF)	193 nm	Ultraviolet
	Xenon chloride (XeCl)	308 nm	Ultraviolet
Gas lasers	Argon	488 nm	Blue
		514 nm	Blue-green
	Helium neon (He-Ne)	637 nm	Red
	Carbon dioxide (CO_2)	10,600 nm	Infrared
Diode lasers	In GaAsP	655 nm	Red
	GaAlAs	670–830 nm	Red-infrared
	GaAs	840 nm	Infrared
	In GaAs	980 nm	Infrared
Solid state lasers	Frequency-doubled Alexandrite	337 nm	Ultraviolet
	Potassium Titanyl Phosphate (KTP)	532 nm	Green
	Neodymium:YAG	1,064 nm	Infrared
	Holmium:YAG	2,100 nm	Infrared
	Erbium, chromium:YSGG	2,780 nm	Infrared
	Erbium:YSGG	2,790 nm	Infrared
	Erbium:YAG	2,940 nm	Infrared

In GaAsP—Indium gallium arsenide phosphorus, GaAlAs—Gallium aluminum Arsenide, GaAs—Gallium arsenide, In GaAs—Indium gallium arsenide

Low-energy lasers therapeutic success of low energy lasers in the treatment of wounds was first reported by Mester. CO_2 lasers remain the dominant soft tissue surgical lasers. Low energy lasers stimulate tissues, but have no thermal effect in contrast to high energy lasers that vaporizes tissues. It emits a visible light at 630 to 640 nm that easily passes through the dermal layers and is used to relieve pain, reduce inflammation and edema, and accelerate healing. Low energy laser therapy stimulates cell activation processes that intensify physiologic activity at the cellular level. It is thought that laser energy facilitates reactions between the cell membrane through the cytoplasm to the cell nucleus in a process called *cellular amplification*. It has been revealed in several studies, that low energy laser possesses the ability to stimulate the respiratory chain located in the mitochondrion; specifically, it is believed that nearinfrared light stimulation targets cytochrome c oxidase, a terminal enzyme, whose role is to transfer electrons between complex III and IV within the respiratory chain. It is believed that cytochrome c oxidase stimulation accelerates the transfer of electrons and promotes an up-regulation of oxidative phosphorylation, producing more adenosine triphosphate (ATP) molecules. This stimulation promotes intracellular signaling as well as extracellular signaling, which it is believed to reduce edema and pain. Low-intensity laser irradiation has been shown to increase the amount of growth factors, which in turn cause an increase in cellular matrix production, angiogenesis, and cytokine release. Numerous related studies showed fibroblasts and keratinocytes activation, which is critical to wound healing with low-level laser irradiation. Cell processes such as DNA replication, proliferation of cell lines, and promotion of microcirculation occur between 630 to 640 nm. Lyosomal stimulation can start at 670 nm, so band width is to be tightly controlled, e.g. He-Neon, Ga-Arsenide.

The principle of using low level laser therapy (LLLT) is to supply direct biosimulative light energy to the body's cells. Cellular photoreceptors (e.g. cytochromophores and antenna pigments) can absorb low level laser light and pass it on to mitochondria, which promptly produce the cells' fuel, ATP.

The most popularly described treatment benefit of LLLT is wound healing. Electron microscope examination showed evidence of accumulated collagen fibrils and electron dense vesicles intracytoplasmatically within the laser stimulated fibroblasts as compared with untreated areas. The mechanisms of action underlying the analgesic effects remain unclear, despite the implicit treatment benefits. There is evidence suggesting that LLLT may have significant neuropharmacology effects on the synthesis, release, and metabolism of a range of neurochemicals, including serotonin and acetylcholine at the central level and histamine and prostaglandin at the peripheral level. Enhanced synthesis of endorphin, decreased c-fiber activity, bradykinin, and altered pain threshold. By understanding the basic cellular effects of the lasers and the intended treatment goal of reducing inflammation, accelerating the healing process, and providing pain relief, the general principles of application for various clinical, conditions become clear.

ADVANTAGES OF LASER

Lasers transmit energy to the cells causing warming, welding, coagulation, protein denaturization, drying, vaporization and carbonization.

1. Laser unit is compact, portable surgical unit with efficient and reliable benefits like easy and safe to handle.
2. Improved surgical versatility over other conventional methods. Ability to coagulate, vaporize, or incise tissue.
3. Laser reduce or eliminate bleeding intraoperatively. It also seals the blood vessels (Instant coagulation).
   a. Spot coagulation and vaporization—excellent hemostasis.
   b. Improve visibility—precise and accurate surgery.
   c. Reduce operating time.
4. No need for using local anesthesia for minor surgical procedures. Anesthesia free hard and soft tissue cutting.
5. No need for antibiotic, analgesics, anti-inflammatory medication. Unique analgesic effect is created by the laser pulses and the conduction of these effects through both hard and soft tissues (a function of neuron sealing and decreased pain mediator release).
6. No need for suturing.
7. Instant sterilization of surgical site–production of a sterile surgical field, bactericidal, and viricidal.

   It also prevents bacterial infection of the wound and laser treated wounds give reduced bacteremia. Noncontact lasers can give zero bacteremia. (offer special bactericidal effect).
8. Economic because of above four.

9. Lasers can be used to create open wounds, which rapidly undergo secondary intention healing. No postoperative bleeding, or pain or discomfort as laser seals the nerve endings. Laser produces reduced mechanical trauma. No/less/minimum postoperative pain/discomfort/swelling. Reduce inflammation. Decreased swelling allows for increased safety, when performing surgery within the airway and increases the range of surgery, that oral and maxillofacial surgeons can perform safely without fear of airway compromise. This effect allows the surgeon to perform many procedures in an office or outpatient facility that previously would have required hospitalization for airway observation, postoperative nursing care, and parenteral pain management.

10. Decreased lateral tissue damage, less traumatic surgery, more precise control of depth of tissue damage and fewer myofibroblasts in laser wound, brings about excellent tissue healing compared to scalpel.

11. The surface layer created by lasing, serves as a scaffold for healing and as a wound dressing and offers excellent healing due to its biostimulating. Minimal cicatrix (scar) formation/wound contraction (decreased wound contraction-less scarring is due to reduction in stimulation of tissue myoepithelial and fibroblastic cellular elements).

12. No sensory disturbance.

13. No functional and/or mobility disorder post operatively.

14. More rapid repair and stronger healed tissue structure.

15. Lasers do not pose a risk of thermal injury to soft tissues and to teeth with metallic restorations or to the bone adjacent to implants. (no bone necrosis). Minimum collateral tissue damage. (no conduction of current in oral fluids, metallic dental materials and metal instruments).

16. Lasers do not rely on the flow of electrical current and thus do not pose a risk to patients with unshielded pacemakers, nor do they cause neuromuscular stimulation.

17. Access to difficult to reach anatomic sites by reflection or through waveguides.

18. Minimized tumor cell dispersion by lymphatic sealing.

19. Precise delivery of energy to diseased tissue via microscopes for reduced damage to surrounding structure.

20. Electrosurgery requires high powers (upwards of 350 watts), but laser can achieve tissue incision at 100 times lower average power.

21. High degree of patient comfort and acceptability. Operator comfort due to high degree of precision (reduced surgical stress for both the patient and the operator).

Disadvantages: Although oral and maxillofacial surgeons would be delighted at using lasers for osseous surgery (e.g. extraction of impacted teeth and osteotomies).

- The speed of the Er:YAG for osseous tissue removal does not yet compare favorably with conventional techniques.
- The speed of healing usually is prolonged compared with other types of wounds. This delay in healing undoubtedly is due to the sealing of blood vessels and lymphatic's and the subsequent need for neovascularization for healing. Typical intraoral healing takes 2 to 3 weeks for wounds that normally would take 7 to 10 days, and this must be taken into account, when considering suture removal (assuming that sutures have been placed) and obtaining patient consent.

    i. Specialized didactic and clinically oriented instructions required for laser use by the surgeon and assistants
    ii. Hazards to patient, operating and assisting team, and anesthesia personnel from misdirected and inadvertent laser radiation
    iii. Expense of laser equipment
    iv. Specialized wiring and plumbing connection
    v. Maintenance requirements
    vi. Fire hazard as related to anesthesia risk
    vii. Electrical hazards of laser equipment.

APPLICATIONS OF LASER IN ORAL AND MAXILLOFACIAL SURGERY AND DENTISTRY (TABLE 54.8)

Currently, most applications of lasers in Oral and Maxillofacial Surgery (OMS) are restricted to soft tissues of the face and oral cavity. The most commonly used lasers are the CO_2 and Er:YAG, both of which are absorbed primarily by water. Absorption into the target tissue results in four effects: *photoacoustic, photochemical, photoablation, and photothermal.* The photothermal effect, or the generation of heat, plays the most significant role.

Control of lateral thermal damage is paramount to the use of lasers in OMS. This is the area, surrounding

Table 54.8: Current and potential applications of lasers in dentistry	
Laser type	*Current/potential dental application*
Excimer lasers	
Argon fluoride (ArF) Xenon chloride (XeCl)	Hard tissue ablation, dental calculus removal
Gas lasers	
Argon (Ar)	Curing of composite materials, tooth whitening, intraoral soft tissue surgery, sulcular debridement (subgingivally), curettage in periodontitis and peri-implantitis
Helium Neon (He-Ne)	Analgesia, treatment of dentin hypersensitivity, aphthous ulcer treatment
Carbon dioxide (CO_2)	Intraoral and implant soft tissue surgery, aphthous ulcer, melanin pigmentation
Diode lasers Indium Gallium Arsenide Phosphorus (InGaAsP)	Caries and calculus detection
Gallium Aluminum	Intraoral general and implant soft tissue surgery, sulcular debridement
Arsenide (GaAlAs) and	Gallium Arsenide (GaAs) (subgingival curettage in periodontitis and peri-implantitis), analgesia, treatment of dentin hypersensitivity, pulpotomy, root canal disinfection, aphthous ulcer treatment, removal of gingival melanin pigmentation
Solid state lasers	
Frequency-doubled	Selective ablation of dental plaque and calculus
Alexandrite	
Neodymium:YAG (Nd:YAG)	Intraoral soft tissue surgery, sulcular debridement (subgingival curettage in periodontitis), analgesia, treatment of dentin hypersensitivity, pulpotomy, root canal disinfection, removal of enamel caries, aphthous ulcer treatment, removal of gingival melanin pigmentation
Erbium group	Caries removal and cavity preparation,
Erbium:YAG (Er:YAG),	modification of enamel and dentin surfaces, intraoral general and implant soft tissue surgery, sulcular debridement (subgingival curettage in periodontitis and peri-implantitis), scaling of root surfaces, osseous surgery, treatment of dentin hypersensitivity, analgesia, pulpotomy, root canal treatment and disinfection, aphthous ulcer treatment, removal of gingival melanin/metal/tattoo pigmentation
Erbium:YSGG (Er:YSGG), Erbium, chromium:YSGG (Er,Cr:YSGG)	

the incision site, damaged by lateral heat conduction into the tissues.

Factors Affecting the Lateral Zone of Necrosis Include

1. *The wavelength of the laser.*
2. *The target tissue:* The zone of thermal necrosis depends on the varying ability of different tissues to absorb and transmit the thermal effect.
3. *The energy density applied:* The longer the laser is applied, the greater the total energy density and, hence, the extent of lateral damage.
4. *The spot size:* Obviously, to have the least total width of thermal effect on the surface, one should minimize the initial spot size. This is accomplished by using the smallest spot size possible when making incisions.

5. *The speed of the laser application:* the faster the pulse, the less time available for conduction into adjacent tissues.

Three parameters controllable by the surgeon, function to control the laser's effect on tissues: *power, time on target, and effective spot size of the beam.* It is generally ideal to keep the spot size to whatever is the smallest practical spot size possible with the particular laser (usually 0.1–0.5 mm), because this will result in the thinnest cut, closely replicating the cut made with a standard scalpel blade. This approach is called focused mode because the smallest possible spot size occurs at the focal length of any particular laser, which varies from 1 mm to about 1 cm from the end of the hand piece. By adjusting these parameters, one can create a deep thin cut into tissue for incision or excision or a wide superficial surface vaporization for tissue ablation.

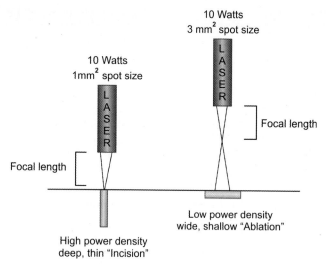

Fig. 54.19: Power density. When the same power is applied to a smaller spot size, the resultant increase in power density causes a deeper but thinner cut tissue, when compared with a larger spot size

Manipulation of these parameters becomes important when performing procedures, in which minimizing lateral damage is crucial to prevent scarring (e.g. skin resurfacing) (Fig. 54.19).

Therapeutic lasers are classified as class III medical devices, and surgical lasers are classified as class IV. Some phrases and phenomena describing the biologic effects of the therapeutic lasers are:

- Laser photobiostimulation
- Bioinhibition, which can increase and decrease the physiologic functions to reach normalization
- Laser photobiomodulation
- Laser bioactivation.

TECHNIQUES FOR USE OF LASERS IN ORAL AND MAXILLOFACIAL SURGERY

There are basically three photothermal techniques for laser use on soft tissues within the oral cavity. A common use of lasers in OMS is to use the device essentially as a light scalpel, using the laser to make relatively deep, thin cuts much as one would do with a scalpel blade. This technique allows the surgeon to perform almost any intraoral procedure that normally would be done with a scalpel.

- Incisional/excisional procedures
- Vaporization procedures–biopsy, lesion removal
- *Hemostasis:* This is specially important when performing incision/excision biopsy on lesions with high vascularity or lesions with blood loss potential, such as pyogenic granuloma, Kaposi's sarcoma, or hemangioma. (Figs 54.20A and B).

Technique for Incisional Biopsy (Figs 54.21A to C)

1. *Provide local or general anesthesia as indicated:* Nerve block or deep infiltration: If injected superficially into the tissues, the water content in the tissues caused by the anesthetic solution may, in some cases, lead to inconsistent tissue cutting.

2. *Outline the intended superficial incision line, without deep penetration:* It is a good practice to outline the biopsy area, in a slow, controlled fashion. It is advisable to include an additional 0.3 to 0.5 mm around the intended biopsy site to compensate for the zone of

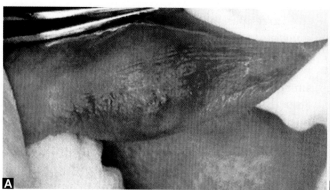
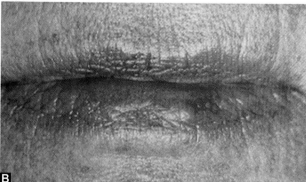

Figs 54.20A and B: (A) Hemangioma of the lip, (B) Laser treatment and postoperative result

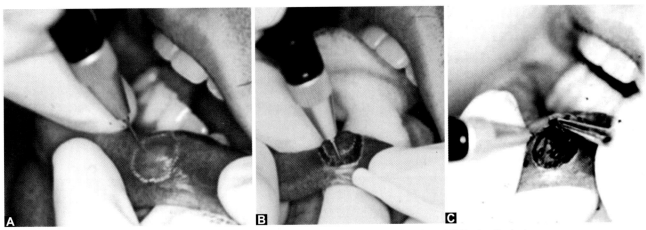

Figs 54.21A to C: (A) Outline the incision, (B) Connect the outline dots, (C) Excise the lesion

adjacent thermal coagulation (intermittent, pulsed or gated mode with rate of 10–20 pulses/second).

3. *Connect the outline marks:* Connect the outline marks made previously. This incision is carried into the tissues to the desired depth of the biopsy (on continuous mode, single depth cut).

4. *Excise the specimen:* Grasp the biopsy specimen with a forceps and using the laser in focused mode, undermine the specimen along its entire length by directing the laser into the margin at an angle parallel to the base of the lesion. Care is taken while the specimen is being removed to protect the surrounding tissue from inadvertently aimed laser beams. This is accomplished by always aiming the beam towards the center of the lesion.

5. *Obtain hemostasis, if necessary:* Sometimes bleeding may occur during the procedure, despite the intrinsic hemostatic effect of the laser. This is more likely with the CO_2 laser than with the Nd:YAG or argon laser. It is usually related to vessels greater than 0.5 mm or too rapid movement of the laser handpiece, not allowing sufficient time for the lateral thermal diffusion and coagulation.

6. *Consider the need for suturing:* In rare cases, in which suturing is desired, appropriate undermining, which can be done by laser, and suturing in layers may be performed in the usual manner. Sutures are absolutely required only for cosmesis, when leaving the wound to granulate slowly would present an unacceptable cosmetic situation.

7. If desired, leave a light char layer.

8. *Consider tagging the biopsy margins:* The margins of the pathological specimens, may be tagged for orientation by the pathologist.

Any soft tissue lesion that requires excision for histologic examination is best treated using this technique. Typical lesions treated by excision and incision include the following:

- Fibroma
- Mucocele
- Papilloma
- Gingival lesions
- Benign salivary gland lesions
- Salivary stones
- Malignancy removal
- Incisional biopsy
- Excisional biopsy
- Vestibuloplasty
- Epulis fissurata (Fig. 54.22)
- Hyperplastic tissue excision/Frenectomy (Fig. 54.23)
- Implant uncovering
- Peri-implantitis treatment
- Laser-assisted uvulopalatoplasty (LAUP)
- Tongue lesions treatment.

Ablation and Vaporization Procedures (Figs 54.24A to D)

Intraoral surface lesions: The laser excels in performing vaporization procedures. Tissue ablation (also called vaporization) is used when the surgeon wishes to remove only the surface of the target or to perform a superficial removal of tissue. In these situations, the lesion usually is confined to the epithelium.

Laser vaporization is an effective, nonmorbid, inexpensive, quick, and relatively painless method of managing premalignant lesions. Many clinicians believe

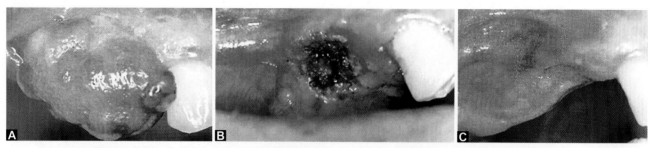

Figs 54.22A to C: (A) Epulis in the upper edentulous jaw, (B) Laser excision, (C) Postoperative result

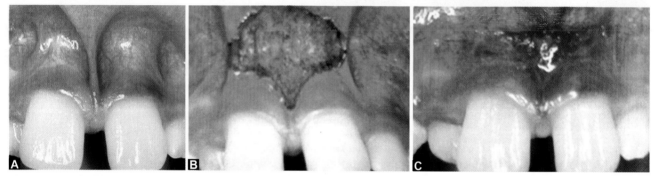

Figs 54.23A to C: (A) High frenum attachment, (B) Frenectomy with laser, (C) Immediate postoperative result

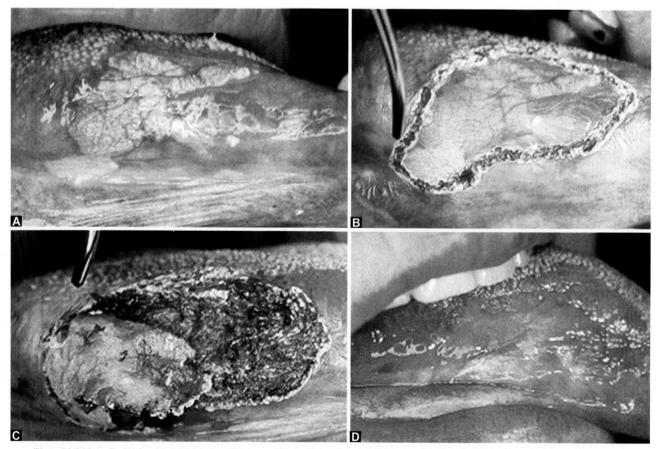

Figs 54.24A to D: (A) Leukoplakial lesion of tongue, (B) Outlining the excision area, (C) Excision with CO_2 laser in focused mode, (D) No recurrence one year postoperatively

that the hemostatic effect of the laser results in decreased tendency for hematogenous or lymphatic seeding of the malignant cells.

- A spot size of 1.5 to 3 mm is typical for most intraoral vaporization procedures and provides a reasonable area of coverage. The defocused beam is traversed along the lesion in a series of vertical strokes, represented as side-by-side "U's"
- A constant speed must be maintained to create uniform depth. 4 to 10 W with a spot size of 1.5 to 3 mm usually provides an acceptable starting point for most tissues. Increasing depth can be accomplished by increasing power or decreasing spot size.
- This technique allows for removal of a surface lesion in layers of a few hundred microns to 1 to 2 mm at a time.

Laser ablation technology is used for treating following:
- Solar chelitis
- Leukoplakias/Erythroplakia—precancerous mucosal lesions
- Dysplasia
- Lichen planus
- Papillary hyperplasia
- Focal hyperkeratosis (Frictional hyperkeratosis)
- Oral melanosis
- Nicotine stomatitis, smokeless tobacco-induced mucosal white lesions
- Oral papillomatosis
- Tissue hyperplasia
- Actinic cheilitis.

Use of the Holmium Laser in Temporomandibular Joint Surgery

The holmium:yttrium-aluminium-garnet (Ho:YAG) lasers are among the recently developed rare earth solid state lasers. These are pulsed, mid-infrared wavelength lasers and transmitted fiberoptically in a fluid environment, which makes it appropriate for use in arthroscopic joint surgery. Fanton and Dillingham (1986), clinically developed the holmium laser for use in orthopedic arthroscopic surgery. Koslin (1990) was the first to use holmium laser in the human temporo-mandibular (TM) Joint.

Lasers have several advantages for arthroscopic surgery of TM Joint:

- Diseased tissues can be removed without mechanical contact.

- Significantly decreasing trauma to the articular cartilage and synovial surfaces.
- Lasers also provide hemostasis within the joint without causing thermal damage.
- The technical precision of laser surgery is far superior and eliminates the possibility of instrument breakage and retrieval.

The water filled environment of the joint precludes the use of the CO_2 and the Er:YAG laser, because the synovial fluid would absorb the laser energy before contact with the target tissues of the joint itself.

Using a laser such as a Ho:YAG, enables the surgeon to perform all the techniques capable with the CO_2 laser, but because of its limited absorption by water, it transmits through fluids and can be used directly within the fluid-filled joint space.

The Ho:YAG laser vastly improves the ability to remove and sculpt diseased tissues compared with mechanical instrumentation. The small size of the tip and the easily manipulated fiberoptic hand piece reduces operating time and allows access to all recesses within the TMJ. It has been established that with a power output of 0.8 J and a pulse rate of 10 Hz (8 W), tissues are efficiently ablated without creating excessive zones of thermal damage. Using this technique, such procedures as diskectomy, diskoplasty, synovectomy, hemostasis, posterior attachment contraction, eminectomy and debridement of fibrous ankylosis can be performed on an outpatient basis through two incisions less than 2 mm each.

▮ SCAR REVISION WITH LASER

Oral and maxillofacial surgeons frequently are faced with the management of cutaneous injuries causing scar formation.

Advances in laser technology have led to increasing use of pulsed-dye lasers (PDLs), Er:YAG lasers, and CO_2 lasers. The choice of laser is influenced by the qualities of the scar, including color and texture, and the timing and types of previous treatments. PDLs have proved to be effective for treatment of hypertrophic scars and show striking improvements in scar textures. The 585 nm PDL specifically targets blood vessels within the scar tissue, leading to fibroblast proliferation and decreased collagen production. PDLs often are referred to as vascular lasers, because they have hemoglobin as their chromophore and penetrate the epidermis without de-epithelialization. By reducing scar tissue erythema and inducing collagen remodeling to flatten and soften scars, the PDL is indicated for erythematous and hypertrophic scars of the maxillofacial region. Revision usually is performed on outpatient basis without anesthesia. Most lesions show an 80 percent improvement after two PDL treatments. A period of 6 to 8 weeks between treatments is recommended to allow healing. A topical antibiotic or healing ointment is recommended for the first few postoperative days. Strict sun avoidance should be practiced to avoid stimulating pigment production in these areas.

USE OF Er: YAG LASER

Gingival hyperpigmentation is mostly caused by the physiologic deposition of melanin by melanocytes. In patients with a "gummy smile", this pigmentation causes an esthetic problem. Methods to remove this pigmentation may vary, but it seems that the most reliable and satisfactory procedure is by laser ablation. The Er:YAG laser is capable of excellent soft tissue ablation, which makes it suitable for this kind of pigmentation removal.

Applications of the laser for dental implant surgery have focused primarily on:

- Soft tissue revision
- Second stage surgery
- Decontamination of implant surfaces
- Treatment of peri-implantitis
- Implant maintenance.
- When Er:YAG and CO_2 lasers are applied (only at low power) to metal, energy reflection occurs, leaving the implant surface intact without significant alterations. The Er:YAG laser is particularly advantageous in these situations because it can eliminate soft tissue and ablate bone without damaging the implant surface.
- Nd:YAG, Ho:YAG, should not be used for implant surgery, because they harm the surface of all endosseous implants
- The 810 nm GaAlAs diode laser seems to be safe as far as possible surface alterations are concerned.
- The CO_2, Er:YAG, and diode lasers have been shown to be safe and effective for treating peri-implantitis. They can be used for the removal of peri-implant gingival overgrowths and to decontaminate implant surfaces before bony augmentations.
- The Er:YAG laser was also proposed for implant maintenance, taking advantage of its bactericidal

effect, technical simplicity and absence of postoperative pain and edema. Peri-implant infection results in inflammation of the surrounding soft tissues and can induce a breakdown of the implant supporting bone. It is associated with the presence of a subgingival microflora, which is quite similar to that in periodontal pockets and contains a large variety of Gram negative anaerobic bacteria.

LOW LEVEL LASER THERAPY

Therapeutic laser treatment, also referred to as low level, soft, cold, low level laser therapy (LLLT), offers numerous benefits. Along with the primary benefit of being nonsurgical, it promotes tissue healing and reduces edema, inflammation, and pain.

Low level laser therapy (LLLT) benefits can be performed with various wavelengths and units with different outputs. Usually, the therapeutic window for subthermal tissue interaction is 1 to 500 mW, but surgical lasers can be defocused and used as a "low level" laser.

Beneficial treatment effects have been applied in dermatologic conditions such as wounds and inflammations, neural ailments in various locations, and musculoskeletal ailments causing pain and degeneration in various sites (Figs 54.25A and B).

Laser Safety

Lasers can carry a very high risk of causing severe injury and damage.
There are three facets to laser safety:
1. The manufacturing process of the instrument
2. Proper operation of the device
3. The personal protection of the surgical team and the patient.

Primary Hazards

Primary hazards are directly caused by the laser beam. Laser radiation endangers mainly two organs; eyes and skin. In case of eyes, it can cause damage to retina, cornea and the lens. Hence, even a slight carelessness can destroy the vision permanently. Skin is much less sensitive than the eyes and the damage occurs only at higher energies.

Secondary Hazards

Secondary Hazards are related to the operation of the laser, and are independent of radiation characteristics.

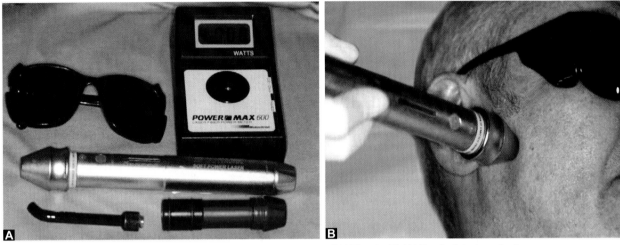

Figs 54.25A and B: (A) Low level laser therapy (LLLT) unit, (B) LLLT unit clinical application

Different tissues have different energy requirement for injury to occur. The skin may require 5 to 20 watts to create a burn injury, while retina may require 2 to 3 milliwatts to create a permanent visual field loss. The CO_2 laser does not reach the retina, because of its wavelength characteristics, whereas the Nd:YAG laser readily reaches the retina even at low levels of power. Hence, the best recommendation is to assume that injury range extends to all parts of the room. The laser can injure anyone within the room where the laser is used. Whenever the laser is in use, all persons in the room must observe all recommended specific precautions for the type of laser being used.

Duration of Exposure and Eye Protection

The longer the exposure, the higher the amount of energy delivered. The dangers vary from laser to laser. There is difference between lasers in the type of lens required to protect the eyes of the awake patient and the personnel. CO_2 lasers require clear glass or plastic of a certain density. The type of eyeshield is very specific for each type of laser. The eyeshields used with the Nd:YAG are goggles with a green tinted lens, the eyeshields used with the argon laser are an amber orange color. The optical density specifications for the eyeshields should be obtained from the laser company.

Maximum Permissible Exposure (MPE-Values)

Different body tissues have different sensitivities to light irradiation; the MPE-values are defined separately

for skin and eyes. Their physical units are W/m^2 and J/m^2. The specified MPE values always are determined by national standards.

Operating Room Safety

Patient Safety

This includes:
i. Use of noninflammable materials, wherever possible
ii. Use of eyeshields for patient (Fig. 54:28)
iii. Use of laser resistant shielding materials for surgical field and for protecting anesthesia equipment.
iv. Certain adjustments in anesthesia techniques may also decrease the potential hazards. N_2O aids burning, in the presence of significant amounts of O_2. To avoid this risk, it is recommended that O_2 supplementation be minimized during laser surgery. If G.A. is employed, attempts to keep FIO_2 at or slightly below 0.25 should be made. If I.V. sedation is used, O_2 supplementation should be kept to a minimum or avoided. The surgeon can warn the anesthesiologist to turn off the supplemental O_2 when laser is activated.

Personnel Safety

The personnel working in laser environment can be at risk for injury. Similar patterns of injury from the laser occur in the personnel as in the patients.

The rules for the absolute safety of the personnel are as follows:

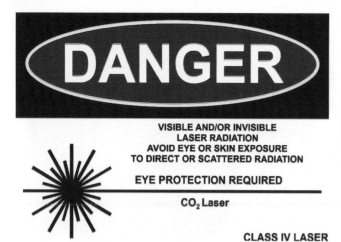

CLASS IV LASER

Fig. 54.26: Laser safety signs and labels

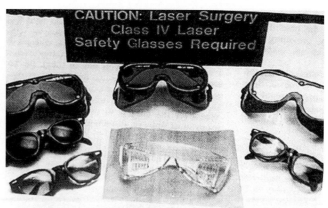

Fig. 54.27: Eye protection during laser surgery. A pair of safety glasses hung on or taped to the door to encourage entering personnel to use them. Multiple protective eyeglasses used for each laser, depending on the wavelength

i. Post signs that lasers are being used (Fig. 54.26). These signs should (a) describe the type of laser, (b) indicate the risk class of laser, (c) indicate the required safety equipment for personnel (specific eyeshields) and (d) state that if unprotected personnel enter the area, the laser is to be turned off.

ii. Eye shields to be worn at all times by all personnel including the dentist, assistant, patient, and others. Generally, protective glasses must have an optical density (OD) of at least four for the particular laser emission and device.

Laser safety glasses must protect the eye structures from the specific wavelength in use, and the information about lens protection must be imprinted on the frames of the glasses or goggles. (Figs 54.27 to 54.29).

iii. Safety shields must be used.

iv. A bucket of sterile water should be immediately available in the operating theater.

v. A laser safety officer (LSO) must be stationed at the laser unit at all times.

vi. Safety orientation for laser use should be required of all surgeon, anesthesia personnel, and operating room staff.

vii. Credentialing of surgeons for use of each type of laser and laser apparatus is needed.

Fire and explosion hazards: Lasers generate significant heat. This heat presents a fire hazard to all materials near the beam or laser knife.

Fire hazards associated with class IV lasers: Laser take many forms. Proper procedure to minimize this kind of problem should include the following:

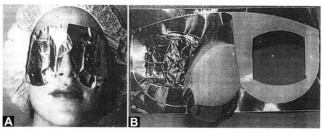

Figs 54.28A and B: (A) Use of self-adhering laser safe eyeshields, (B) Soft foam pads on the under surface of the eyeshields (laser surgical procedure being done under GA in operation theatre)

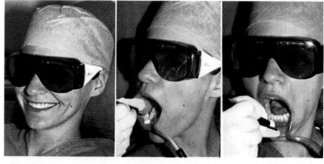

Fig. 54.29: Patient with protective eyewear in a dental clinic, during laser treatment

• Use only wet cloth or fire retardant drape materials in the operative field. No paper or plastic drapes.
• Use only non-combustible anesthetic agents.
• Avoid alcohol based topical anesthetic.
• Avoid alcohol moistened gauze while firing the laser.
• Protect tissues adjacent to the surgical site.
• Know location and operation of the nearest fire extinguisher.

- Store highly combustible or explosive materials outside the nominal hazardous zone.
- Adhere to the ANSI directive: "Nitrous oxide supports combustion and should not be used during laser surgery".

CONNECTIONS AND TRAFFIC

- All lasers require a cooling system; some use an internal fan and others use a fan and a radiator with self contained coolant. Some class IV lasers require an external source of water or air to be supplied. If so, it is imperative that the lines are connected properly and that those utilities are turned on before powering up the laser.
- Electric power cords and the footswitch cable also should be inspected each time to make sure that they are in safe condition.
- The laser and the associated hook-up components must be kept out of the mainstream of traffic.
- Fiberoptic delivery systems may need special attention, because they can be up to 3 m long and, therefore, can drape easily from the emission port to the floor. The LSO must take care to not allow

equipment casters to roll over the fiber, causing its breakage or damaging other supply lines.

STERILIZATION AND INFECTION CONTROL OF LASER UNIT

- Steam sterilization is the standard of care. The small flexible optic fibers, handpieces, or tips must be steam sterilized in separate sterilization pouches after each use. They should be kept in the sterilization pouch until ready for use. It is essential that when using fiberoptically delivered lasers, the port (connecting) end remains clean and oil free. Therefore, never run the fiber in a sterilizer cycle alongside a high speed turbine with lubricant.
- The protective housing around the laser, including the control panel and articulating arm (if applicable) should receive the spray disinfectant/wipe/spray disinfectant decontamination method, as do the dental cart and counter tops. Some delivery system components such as the large diameter erbium fiberoptic cable are not designed for steam sterilization and must be disinfected in this way.

55 Piezosurgery

▮ WHAT IS PIEZOSURGERY?

Piezosurgery is a recently developed innovative system for highly precise and safe cutting of bone, with modulated ultrasonic microvibrations/oscillations produced by piezoelectric effect.

The device used for ultrasonic cutting of bone, create microvibrations, that are caused by the Piezoelectric effect, which was first described by the French physicists, Jean and Marie Curie, in 1880. They showed that, the passage of an electric current across certain ceramics and crystals, modifies them and causes oscillations, while under mechanical pressure.

The concept of use of Piezosurgery clinically, was founded by Italian physician Tomaso Vercellotti in 1988. He developed a unit, using a modulated functional working frequency of 25 to 30 kHz.

The Piezosurgery has been developed to overcome the limits of precision and intraoperatory safety existing in traditional bone cutting instruments—rotary drills and saws. Piezosurgery allows to obtain high predictability and low morbidity in bone surgery.

Piezosurgery is a term used for a collection of ultrasonic technology devices, that apply electric vibrations, resulting from pressure to cut *bone tissue* during surgical procedures. The technique is named after piezoelectricity, which is the type of electricity these machines use.

Towards the end of the 1990s, Vercellotti teamed up with Mectron Medical Technology, a company founded by Italian engineers Fernando Bianchetti and Domenico Vercellotti dedicated to producing medical devices. The collaboration has since produced more than 30 international patents under the Piezosurgery umbrella.

Physicians use Piezosurgery by modifying the level of the ultrasonic frequency that the electric vibrations produce to cut the hard or mineralized tissue of the bone. The power can be changed to accommodate the type of *bone density* involved. During this process, the softer areas are spared, which is made possible by the narrow vibration range of the machine's tip. This manner of operation is necessary for preventing the necrosis of the bone and soft tissues.

Piezosurgery is divided into two categories, according to the branches of medicine involved. The medical devices are most commonly used for osteotomy and osteoplasty. The former term refers to a type of surgery, in which bones are lengthened, shortened or have their alignment altered. The latter term specifically refers to *plastic surgery* performed on the bones. Surgeons also use Piezosurgery for otolaryngology to treat throat or nose disorders; orthopedic surgery to repair parts of the musculoskeletal system, such as the feet and hands; and neurosurgery, which concerns ailments that affect parts of the nervous system such as the *brain* and *spine*.

As of February 2011, Piezosurgery is in its third generation of production. The third generation devices have an ultrasonic frequency range of 24,000 to 36,000 Hertz (Hz). This device has applications in various dental and medical surgical specialities.

Ideally to cut soft tissue, a frequency of 50 kHz is needed, where as Piezosurgery device uses an ultrasound frequency, in the range of 25 to 30 kHz, at which only the bone is cut. The ultrasonic vibrations, when applied to the bone with slight pressure, results in cavitation phenomenon, resulting in cutting exclusively of mineralized tissues. (Piezosurgery device, needs only a gentle pressure, as excessive pressure can be detrimental to cutting and it generates excessive heat). **The device, when used as recommended, would not cut nerves, blood vessels, brain tissues or periosteum or the schneiderian membrane** (Microvibrations 60 to 200 mm/sec). However, damage to soft tissue can occur in form of heat or mechanical damage, which can be self corrected by regeneration. (In contrast, rotary drills severely lacerate the nerve, resulting in permanent damage.) Cooling of the device is ensured by irrigation using a cooling solution,which is stored at 4 degree centigrade. **The device is optimally adjusted to target only mineralized tissue.** Piezoelectric surgery system uses ultrasonic microvibrations to create an osteotomy. These microvibrations make selective, precise and very clean bone cuts possible. It also improves the visibility of the surgical site, due to the **cavitation effect** created by coolant saline distribution and by the vibrations, the blood is essentially washed away. The Piezosurgery device does not work on soft tissues, so device causes little or no soft tissue trauma during intraoral surgery. No lacerations or burns during osteotomy are seen.In addition, surgical access is easier in the deep oral cavity in comparison to surgical burs, which use a straight handpiece. The Piezosurgery device makes a precise and tactile-controlled osteotomy. In addition, this device reduces the frequency of membrane perforation, during osteotomy in maxillary sinus bone grafting and causes minimal or no damage to nerves and blood vessels, during nerve lateralization procedures, because of its ability to cut selectively. It also makes micrometric bone cuts deep in the oral cavity, resulting in precise and easy to control osteotomies, in contrast to rotary

burs or reciprocating saws. The small handpiece and scalpel ease access to the oral cavity. The Piezosurgery system can split a very narrow ridge with minimal loss or perforation of bone. In addition, this device reduces patient fear and stress during surgery performed under local anesthesia, because it makes much less noise and vibration than conventional rotary instruments.

◼ PIEZOSURGERY DEVICE

Piezosurgery device is more powerful version of dental ultrasound scaling unit, with modulated frequency and a controlled tip vibration range. In this machine, scaling tips are replaced by saw tips and diamond points.(Fig. 55.1).

Piezosurgery Device is an Ultrasound Machine

It has a Piezoelectric handpiece and a foot switch, that are connected to a main unit, which supplies power and a peristaltic pump for irrigation. An adjustable jet of 0.60 ml/minute is delivered through the peristaltic pump. The unit is controlled by a interactive key board. There are 2 programs, Bone and Root. In Bone program, the power can be set to any of the four levels depending on the quality of the bone. In Root program, the power can be set to either Perio or Endo mode.

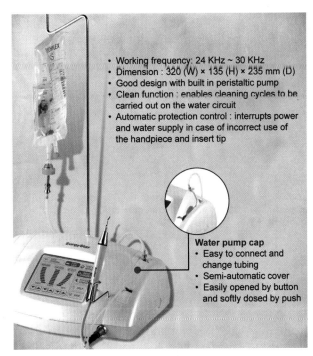

- Working frequency: 24 KHz ~ 30 KHz
- Dimension : 320 (W) × 135 (H) × 235 mm (D)
- Good design with built in peristaltic pump
- Clean function : enables cleaning cycles to be carried out on the water circuit
- Automatic protection control : interrupts power and water supply in case of incorrect use of the handpiece and insert tip

Water pump cap
- Easy to connect and change tubing
- Semi-automatic cover
- Easily opened by button and softly dosed by push

Fig. 55.1: Piezosurgery machine

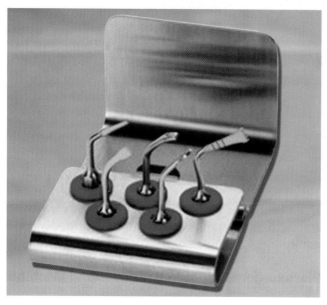

Fig. 55.2: Basic kit

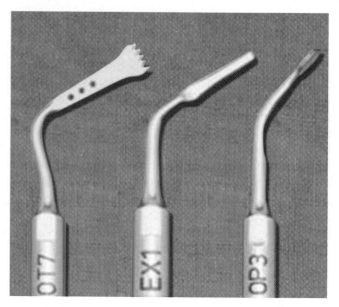

Fig. 55.4: Sharp insert tips. Tips used for osteotomy/osteoplasty

The sharp edge of insert tips enables gentle and effective treatment of the bony structures.

Sharp insert tips are used in osteotomy whenever a fine and well-defined cut in the bone structure is required.

There are for insert tips with sharp edges that are used for osteoplasty techniques and/or harvesting bone chips

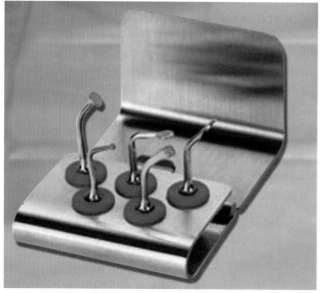

Fig. 55.3: Maxillary sinus kit is used for—Preparation of the bone windows, separation of the sinus membrane, elevation of the sinus membrane

The handpiece has several inserts or tips, some of which are shown in the Figures 55.2 to 55.7. These tips are specific for osteoplasty, osteotomy, etc. Some insert tips are gold color to treat bony tissues. This gold color is obtained by applying a coating of titanium nitride, to improve the surface hardness, which means longer working life of the tips. Steel tips are used to treat soft tissues. The micro movements are in the frequency range of 25 to 29 kHz and depending on the insert, with amplitude frequency of 60 to 210 μm. The power of the device is 5 W.

The different tips vibrate at different ultrasonic frequencies, a "selective cut" enables the clinician to cut hard tissues, while sparing fine vital anatomical structures. (Nerves, vessels and mucosa). This is the effect being used by the Piezosurgery device, in which, the electrical field is located in the handle of the saw/tip/insert. Due to the deformation caused by the electrical current, a cutting-hammering movement is produced at the tip of the instrument. Recently, specialized tips have been developed for implant site osteotomy. Diamond point tips are also available for retrograde root end filling. (Narrow tip-for osteotomy cut, Hoe like tip for collecting autogenous bone) (Figs. 55.2 to 55.7).

An oscillating tip drives the cooling irrigation fluid, making it possible to obtain effective cooling as well as good visibility (via cavitation effect), compared to conventional surgical burs and saws, even in deep spaces.

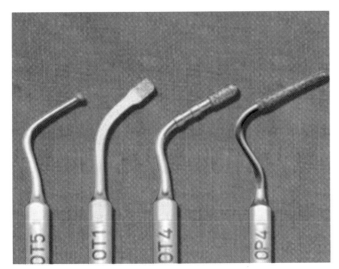

Fig. 55.5: Smoothing insert tips

The smoothing insert tips have diamond surfaces enabling precise and controlled work on the bone structures.

Smoothing insert tips are used in osteotomy when it is necessary to prepare difficult and delicate structures.

For example, those preparing for a sinus window or access to a nerve. In osteotomy, smoothing insert tips are used to obtain the final bone shape

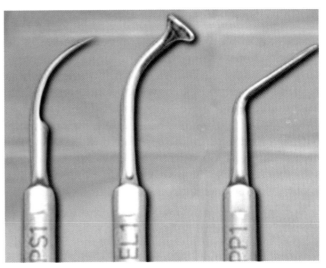

Fig. 55.6: Blunt insert tips

Blunt insert tips are used for preparing the soft tissue.

For example, for elevating Schneider's Membrane or for lateralizing nerves.

In periodontology, these tips are used for root planing

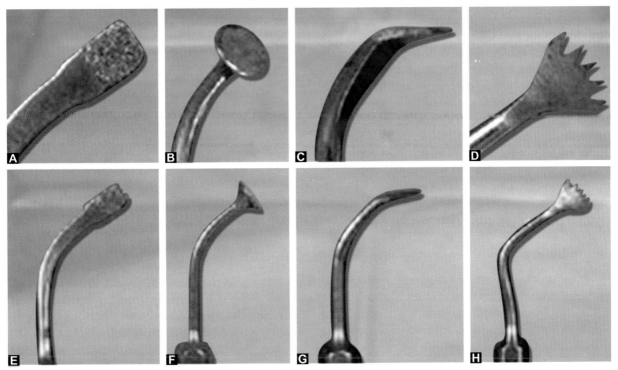

Figs 55.7A to H: A selection of available inserts, from left to right: (A) Flat scalpel, diamond tipped, titanium nitride-coated surface, (B) Cone compressor, flat, blunt, (C) Bond harvester, titanium nitride-coated surface, (D) Sharp tipped saw, titanium nitride-coated surface, (E to H) Same tips shown in different angle

▉ TECHNIQUE

Thanks to the controlled three-dimensional ultrasound microvibrations, the original Piezosurgery technology opens up a new age for osteotomy and osteoplasty in implantology, periodontology, endodontics and surgical orthodontics. The device is optimally adjusted to target only mineralized tissue. The selective and thermally harmless nature results in a low bleeding tendency. The precise nature of the instrument allows exact, clean and smooth cuts. Postoperative excellent wound healing is obtained. Its use may be extended to more complex oral, maxillofacial, craniofacial surgery cases, as well as to other interdisciplinary problems.

The machines are all similar in that they use a high-frequency back-and-forth movement of the various tips with constant irrigation to cut bone, section teeth or lift the maxillary sinus membrane. The Piezosurgery unit uses a frequency of 25 to 29 kHz, modulated with a low frequency of 10 to 60 Hz with linear vibrations of the tips between 60 and 210 μm horizontally and a 20 to 60 μm in a vertical motion. which auto adjusts according to the tip's acoustic response. The vibration amplitude is also adjustable in the range of 30 to 60 μm. This allows constant and instantaneous adaptation of the power required depending on the resistance encountered by the tip.

The handpiece makes use of 5 W of power to easily cut bone. Beside tips for preparing bone, these versatile units also come with tips to perform periodontal scaling, endodontics and other procedures.

To determine the amount of force used, the sound of the cutting can be used as a acoustic feedback. Piezosurgery needs only small amount of pressure and delivers a highly precise cut. If excessive pressure is applied, the tip dose not move and results in generation of heat.

▉ ADVANTAGES OF PIEZOSURGERY

Maximum Safety

Piezosurgical unit's physical and mechanical properties have several clinical advantages (Tables 55.1 and 55.2). Novice as well as experienced surgeons will appreciate these many advantages. Piezo ultrasonic units have over traditional surgical methods. The increased visibility afforded by the cavitation effect creates a clear, bloodless field. One can see better, when Piezosurgery device is used to cut bone in posterior areas or when trying to remove a root tip at the bottom of a blood-

Table 55.1: Advantages of the use of piezosurgery device

- Micrometric cutting action—Precise, secure to limit tissue damage, esp. to osteocyte, less damage to bone at structural and cellular level compared to other techniques. Very safe and less traumatic than conventional drills, due to the absence of macrovibrations.
- Selective cutting action: minimum soft tissue damage maximum intraoperative visibility, blood free operative site (cavitation effect)
- Minimum surgical stress-excellent tissue handling
- Excellent tissue healing
  - Ease of use and control
  - Ease of use and control
  - Safer cutting in complex anatomic areas, sparing vital structures
  - Sterile water environment for better asepsis-free from contamination
  - Less swelling, less postoperative pain
  - The unit has programs that allow you to cut, carve, or polish

Table 55.2: Indications of piezosurgical device in oral surgery

It is used for osteotomy, bone graft harvesting-chips and blocks, direct maxillary sinus lift window creation, lifting of sinus membrane, and removal of impacted teeth.

- Atraumatic dental extraction
- Extraction of impacted teeth
- Osteogenic distraction
- Endodontic surgery/apex surgery
- Cyst removal
- Osteotomy/corticotomy
- Bone harvesting-chips and blocks
- Implant site development—Maxillary sinus lift, ridge expansion (crystal splitting), alveolar nerve decompression, bone harvesting

filled socket. The cavitation effect clears the field by the bursting of water bubbles under high pressure. This causes cleansing of the osseous crest. There is also a hemostatic effect on the cut surfaces thanks to cavitation and in part to the production of nascent oxygen.

The increased safety with which delicate surgical procedures can be performed is one of the greatest benefits of Piezo ultrasonic technology; soft tissues are not harmed if touched by the tip. Hard and soft tissues are cut at different frequencies, and with the instrument's tip vibrating at ultrasonic frequencies tuned for hard tissues, it provides a "selective cut" that enables the clinician to cut hard tissues while sparing fine anatomical structures. This action is so precise that even a novice to the technology can remove the shell from a raw chicken egg while leaving the membrane intact.

Manufacturers claim less surgical trauma is produced to bone ,in implant surgery, resulting in earlier osseointegration, but these claims have not been verified by multicenter scientific studies.

One important factor in implant success is position of implant for an ideal final prosthesis and not necessarily placing implant in the area of maximum bone. To achieve such a ideal implant position, the local site need to be modified with either osteoplasty, alveolar ridge splitting, bone augmentation or sinus floor elevation. Piezoelectrical surgery can be used to perform these tasks in much simpler manner as compared to conventional surgical techniques.

Ultrasonic devices are very helpful in cutting of bone in multiple piece maxillary surgery due to high safety level. (Microscopic examination of bony fragments, showed no signs of coagulative necrosis. The vitality of pulpal tissue was maintained. Reduction in postoperative bleeding and hematoma formation was striking.

During rhinoplasty procedure, chisel and mallet technique, which is blind, unguarded method can lacerate soft nasal tissue and damage principal vessels, such as nasal angular artery and may increase the risk of bleeding and periorbital ecchymosis. Piezoelectric device used for rhinoplasty avoids these problems.

Main advantage is that Peizosurgery insert tips are very strong, resistant to fracture and last longer. Tips can easily reach difficult areas for osteotomy such as lower border of mandible and pterygoid region. These tips very useful in pterygoid disjunction in LeFort I osteotomy, and lower border cut of the mandible in sagittal split osteotomy, giving cut at the lateral surface of ramus for intraoral vertical ramus osteotomy and inferior alveolar nerve lateralization. (Figs 55.8 to 55.11).

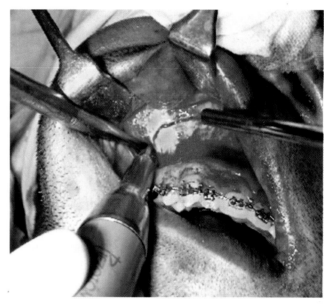

Fig. 55.9: Clinical use of the tip for LeFort I osteotomy (*Courtesy:* Dr Vidya Rattan)

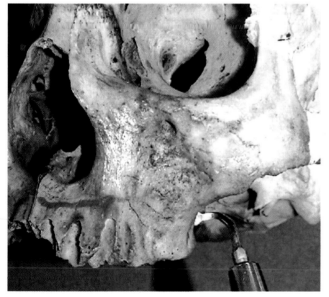

Fig. 55.8: Special design of the angulated insert tip can easily reach pterygoid region for planned cut for LeFort I osteotomy (*Courtesy:* Dr Vidya Rattan)

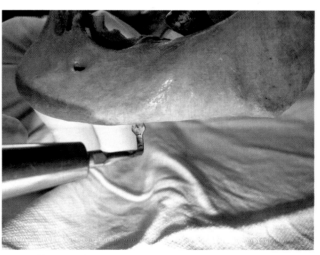

Fig. 55.10: Insert tip is very convenient for lower border cut in case of sagittal split osteotomy of mandible (*Courtesy:* Dr Vidya Rattan)

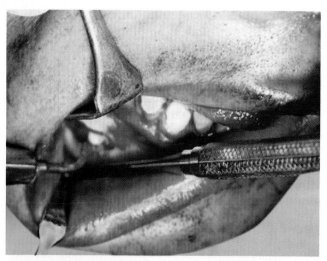

Fig. 55.11: Diamond insert for working near the nerve. Mental nerve being lateralized in a case of mandibular hyperplasia planned for lower border osteotomy (*Courtesy:* Dr Vidya Rattan)

■ BIOLOGICAL EFFECTS ON BONE CUT BY PIEZOSURGERY DEVICE

The effects of mechanical instruments on the structures of bone and the viability of cells is important in regenerative surgery.

Research has shown that there is preservation of osteocytes and favorable osseous repair and remodeling after the use of Piezosurgery device, than harvesting with carbide or diamond burs. Piezoelectric bone surgery seems to be more efficient in the first phases of bony healing. It induces an earlier increase in bone morphogenesis proteins (BMP-4 and TGF-β2 proteins), and fewer proinflammatory cytokines, neo-osteogenesis is considerably more and controls the inflammatory process better, and stimulates remodeling of bone as early as 56 days after treatment.

■ DISADVANTAGE/LIMITATION

The speed of cutting bone is slow as compared to drills and conventional saws thus increasing the operation time. The technique can be difficult to learn. It increases the working pressure which can impede the vibration of devices, that transform the vibrational energy into heat, so if not careful in adjustments, the tissues can be damaged.

Clinical Success

A recent study on human subjects showed ultrasonic surgery can cut the perforation rate by 75 percent for maxillary sinus lifting cases. The results found a total of seven sinus perforations out of 100 maxillary sinus surgeries in the study, as compared to 30 perforations out of 100, when the procedures were performed with rotary instruments. Additionally, all seven perforations occurred while a hand instrument was used during the elevation.

When using an ultrasonic surgical tool in the posterior of the mouth cutting a bone block from the ramus or sectioning bone around a third molar, there is less chance of damage to the soft tissue than when using sharp rotary instruments. Lateral nerve repositioning also is much safer using the piezosurgery. The smaller cut afforded by the piezoultrasonic tip also lends itself to making the most precise cut prior to splitting a thin ridge for expansion.

Benefits for Patients

Another aspect of piezo ultrasonic surgery that dentists and patients will appreciate is the increase in post-operative comfort and the faster healing rate. This technology allows the surgeon to cut precisely with less heat transmitted to damage the osteocytes. Less bone is removed with the cutting tips than with a surgical bur, resulting in less swelling, less pain and faster healing.

Research shows the bone adjacent to the site cut by piezosurgery does not necrose. Instead, it leaves living osteocytes directly adjacent to the surgical site, which promotes faster healing.

It also is possible to harvest autograft bone granules of the optimum size of 500 μm with living osteocytes using a specialized chisel tip. Autogenous bone is the gold standard of bone grafting materials and is cost effective compared with bottled bone. (Figs 55.12 to 55.16)

Recent Developments (Fig. 55.17)

The newest application for the piezo ultrasonic surgery unit is creating an implant osteotomy using special diamond-coated tips that also are suited for lifting the maxillary sinus membrane through the implant osteotomy. This procedure has traditionally been done by tapping osteotomes with a mallet to create a green stick fracture of the sinus floor. Then the membrane is elevated by packing bone graft material into the site.

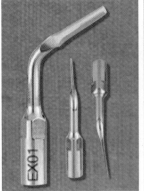
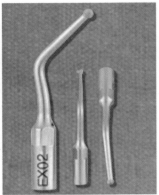
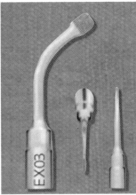

Fig. 55.12: Use of various piezo tips
- When extracting remaining root rests.
- Easy removal can be made even in case of impacted third molars as well as of other hard-to-extract teeth.
- Easy extraction of teeth without destroying the bone of the thin Labial Plate and Buccal Plate about the anterior teeth.
- Applied to Ridge expansion techniques aimed at narrow areas.
- Used for bone surgery for both orthopedic and cosmetic purpose

(Caution) Maximum efficiency: Water 100%, Power 50%, Swing 60%

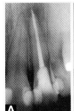
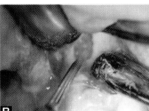
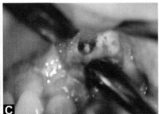
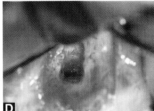
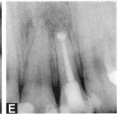

Figs 55.13A and E: Apicoectomy procedure using piezosurgery device : (A) Apicoectomy after endodontic treatments due to the periapical cyst in the lateral incisor of the left upper jaw, (B) The expansion of exit area infected with the periapical cyst and the removal of the cyst using and Ex01 piezo tip, (C) The clean elimination of the periapical cyst, (D) Conducting the retrofilling with the MTA after removing the infected root apex using the Ex01 piezo tip and cleaning its area with the Ex02 piezo tip, (E) Postoperative X-ray after six months

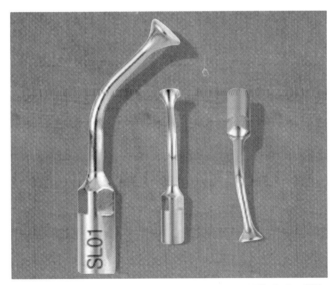

(Caution) Maximum efficiency: Water 70%, Power 30%, Swing 60%

Fig. 55.14: Sinus membrane elevator tips
- Applied to the initial separation of the maxillary sinus membrane.
- Able to separate the membrane surrounding the window without leaving perforations.
- Making the insertion of an instrument for lift and augmentation of the sinus membrane easy.

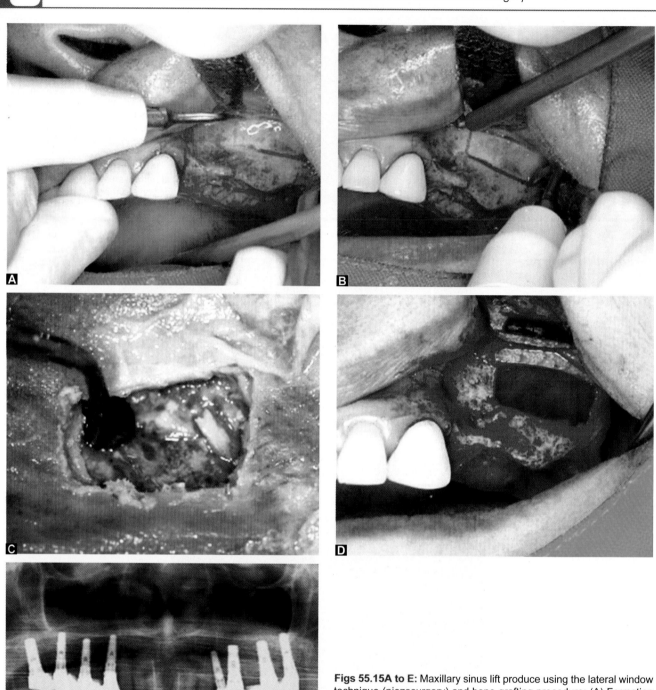

Figs 55.15A to E: Maxillary sinus lift produce using the lateral window technique (piezosurgery) and bone grafting procedure: (A) Formation of window around the maxillary left premolars and molars using a BS piezo tip, (B) Figure showing the safe formation of a window on the lateral maxillary sinus, (C) Separating the maxillary sinus membrane around the window at the initial stage using the SIO1 after taking out the window bone block and thus preventing the tearing of the membrane resulting from a subsequent use of an instrument at the time of the initial separation of the sinus membrane, (D) Figure showing the lift and augmentation of the sinus membrane without any tear, (E) Picture displaying a perfect elevation and the ensuring placement of dental prostheses (after nine months)

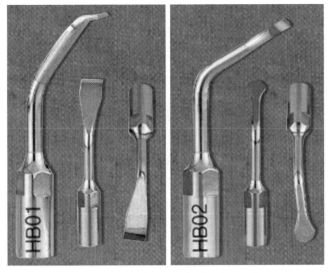

- Mess for osteoplastic operation or collecting bone clip.
- Osteoplasty for high precision.
- Osteoplasty of sinus lift without any damage to soft tissue

Figs 55.16A to F: Bone harvesting technique: (A) Exposure of the defect in buccal plate, (B) Bone harvesting, (C) Allograft, (D) Implant placement, (E) Defect covered with bone graft, (F) Final rehabilitation

However, the traditional method has two negatives. First, it is possible to tear the maxillary sinus membrane when fracturing and lifting the sinus floor. Second, patients find it to be a frightening procedure that has even been associated with creating labyrinthine concussion and positional vertigo.

Using the Piezo unit, the sinus membrane can be lifted in a less threatening and gentler manner. The osteotomy can be created with a pilot drill of the piezo to 1 to 2 mm below the floor of the sinus . Then the diamond-coated tips, of increasing diameters (from 1.35 mm to 2.80 mm), are designed to widen this access canal to the Schneiderian membrane. Finally, when performing this procedure with the Piezotome, the Intralift "trumpet tip" is used in the osteotomy. This uses irrigation in a hydrodynamic effect to lift the membrane. Patient acceptance is much greater with this method when compared with the osteotome and mallet.

Keep in mind the various tips are unit-specific because they are tuned to work only with the specific unit for which they were designed. It also is important to remember there is a learning curve as the operator gains an understanding of how much pressure and contact speed is optimum with each tip, and cutting with the piezo ultrasonic will be slower than with a rotary drill and bur. Speed will increase with experience, but will still require a bit more time. However, the advantages of the technology in terms of safety, accuracy and patient acceptance of ultrasonic procedures outweigh any disadvantages of reduced cutting speed.

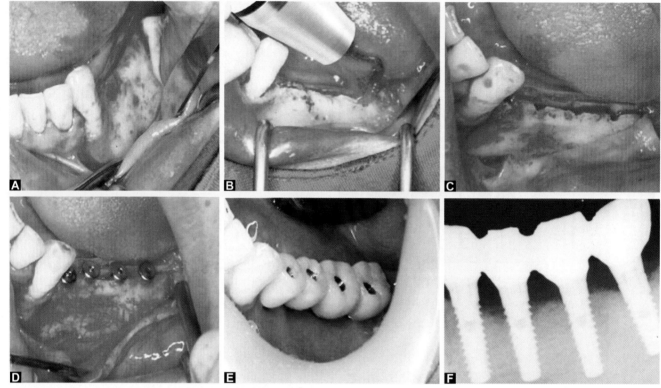

Figs 55.17A to F: Ridge split technique for implant insertion: (A) Exposure of a alveolar ridge, (B and C) Ridge spliting technique, (D) Implants insertion, (E) Final prosthesis, (F) X-ray after 8 months

■ BIBLIOGRAPHY

1. Budd JC, Gekelman D, White JM. Temperature rise of the post and on the root surface during ultrasonic post removal. Int Endod J 2005;38:705–11.

2. Chiriac G, Herten M, Schwarz F, Rothamel D, Becker J. Autogenous bone chips: influence of a new piezoelectric device (Piezosurgery) on chip morphology, cell viability and differentiation. J Clin Periodontol 2005;32:994–9.

3. Dominik J Hoigne, Stefan Stübinger, Oliver Von Kaenel, Sonia Shamdasani and Paula Hasenboehler. Piezoelectric osteotomy in hand surgery: first experiences with a new technique BMC Musculoskeletal Disorders 2006,7:36.

4. Dong-Seok Sohn, Mi-Ra Ahn, Won-Hyuk Lee, Duk-Sung Yeo So-Young Lim Piezoelectric Osteotomy for Intraoral Harvesting of Bone Blocks. Int J Periodontics Restorative Dent 2007;27(2):127–31.

5. Eggers G. et al. Piezosurgery: an ultrasound device for cutting bone and its use and limitations in maxillofacial surgery. British journal of oral and Maxillofacial Surgery 2004;42:451-453.

6. Happe A. Use of a piezoelectric surgical device to harvest bone grafts from the mandibular ramus: report of 40 cases. Int J Periodontics Restorative Dent. 2007;27(3):241-249.

7. Hema Seshan, Kranti Konuganti, and Sameer Zope Piezosurgery in periodontology and oral implantology. Indian Soc Periodontol. 2009;13(3):155–156.

8. Mectron Piezosurgery Brochuer

9. Preti G, Martinasso G, Peirone B, et al. Cytokines and growth factors involved in the osseointegration of oral titanium implants positioned using piezoelectric bone surgery versus a drill technique: a pilot study in minipigs. J Periodontol 2007; 78:716–22.

10. Robiony M, Polini F, Costa F, Vercellotti T, Politi M. Piezoelectronic bone cutting in multipiece maxillary osteotomies. J Oral Maxillofac Surg 2004;62:759–61.

11. Schlee M, Steigmann M, Bratu E, Garg AK. Piezosurgery: basics and possibilities. Implant Dent. 2006;15(4):334–40.

12. Schlee M. et al. Piezosurgery: Basic and Possibilities. Implant Dentistry 2006;15(4):334–338.

13. Vercellotti T, Nevins ML, Kim DM, et al. Osseus response following resective therapy with piezosurgey. Int Periodontics Restorative Dent 2005;25:543–9.

14. Vercellotti T, Pollack AS. A new bone surgery device: sinus grafting and periodontal surgery. Compend Contin Educ Dent. 2006;27(5):319–25.

Appendices

S. No.	Complications	Causes	Prevention	Management
A.	**Intraoperative complications**			
a.	**Soft-tissue injuries**			
1.	Mucosal tears	i. Improper surgical technique: (Inadequate size of flap) ii. Improper handling of instruments: (careless retraction) iii. Use of excessive and uncontrolled forces.	i. Proper surgical technique (Proper designing of flap) ii. Proper handling of instruments iii. Use of controlled force.	Closure of tear after completion of surgical procedure.
2.	Punctures (Elevator slipping off)	Uncontrolled force (elevator) *Common areas:* i. Upper—posterior palate ii. Lower—tongue and floor of the mouth.	i. Use of controlled force ii. Supporting the alveolus from lingual and palatal sides with fingers iii. Proper grip of instruments (Elevators should always be used with an index finger, as a guide, down to the shank of handle towards the tip, to act as a "stop", in case the instrument slips).	*Depends upon size:* i. *Small:* Closure not required; allowed to heal with 2° intention ii. *Large:* Closure indicated; and allowed to heal with 1° intention *Deep punctures:* Suturing may block drainage from depth of wound. Therefore, wound is left open for drainage; and allowed to heal with 2° intention.
3.	Inadvertent incisions	Lack of attention *Common sites:* lips and cheeks.	Surgeon should be constantly alert, while taking the blade; from tray back to tray; or from staff back to staff.	Depends upon the length of incision i. *Small:* No need for suturing ii. *Large:* Requires suturing.

4.	Thermal injuries	i. It may leave a thick ugly scar
		  Using hot instruments directly from autoclave
		  Instruments that feel warm with gloves on;
		  are sufficient to cause tissue damage
		ii. Overheating of rotary instruments (handpieces)
		iii. *Predisposition (Common sites):* Lips, cheeks and angles of the mouth.
			i. Allow instruments to cool down
			ii. *For speed-cooling:* immerse in normal saline
			iii. Regular maintenance of rotary instruments
			iv. Proper retraction to protect lips and cheeks, etc.
				It can leave ugly, thick scars.
				i. Application of vaseline
				ii. Scar-revision, if present; at a later date.

Contd...

S. No.	Complications	Causes	Prevention	Management
5.	Abrasion and avulsion injuries	Use of rotary instruments with long shanks of burs/drills; rubbing onto soft tissues *Predisposition:* (Common sites): Lips, cheeks and corners of mouth.	i. Surgeons should be alert/attentive; while using rotary instruments ii. Adequate retraction or protection of soft tissues, while using these instruments.	*Depends upon size and site:* Palliative ii. Area-covered with vaseline iii. Revision of scar, at a later stage.
6.	*Crush injuries:* Gingival tissues lacerated by blades of forceps	i. Carelessness ii. *Common occurrence:* Upper and lower lips getting entangled with forceps while extracting molars *Maxillary tooth:* Patient will inform of pain *Mandibular tooth:* Severe crush injury, as the area is anesthetized.	i. Surgeon should remain alert and attentive ii. Careful retraction of soft-tissues, especially the lips.	Palliative
7.	Ecchymosis	Secondary bleeding internally (a) mild and (b) severe.	Atraumatic surgical technique.	a. Mild: Reassurance to the patient b. Treat with cold or hot packs depending upon when the patient is seen c. Use of proteolytic enzymes (serratiopeptidase 20 mg/day).
8.	*Surgical emphysema:* Air pushed in tissue spaces	It follows the use of air-driven turbine for bone/tooth sectioning. It develops rapidly with a crackling feeling.	Avoid using air-driven instruments for oral surgical procedures.	Absorption is spontaneous, within 1–2 weeks i. Observe signs and symptoms ii. Control of infection.
b.	**Injuries to hard tissues: (teeth and bone)** **A. Teeth** **a. Injuries to tooth being extracted**			
1.	Fractures of teeth/roots	a. *Major cause:* Improper surgical technique: (i) Improper or no elevation prior to application of forceps. (ii) Inappropriate/excessive application of force applied over forceps during extraction b. *Other causes:* Presence of following factors increase the likelihood of fracture of teeth/roots: i. Tooth weakened by carious process or large restoration ii. *Hasty extraction:* Impatient at the time of extraction iii. *Abnormal root morphology:* Ankylosed roots, devitalized roots, divergent roots, dilacerated roots and slender roots iv. Dense alveolar bone.	a. Preoperative assessment of root morphology, and carious lesions b. Planning surgical removal. c. *Good surgical technique:* i. Proper selection of instruments ii. Proper use of instruments iii. Proper application of elevators iv. Proper application of forceps and v. Use of controlled force	Ideally, all roots should be removed. Some apical fragments are difficult or hazardous to remove; because of proximity to inferior alveolar nerve, or the antral floor. Such root fragments are best left *in situ.* Generally, the removal or a root fragment depends upon (i) vitality of the tooth, (ii) length of the root, (iii) whether the root was infected or not, (iv) whether the tooth was luxated or not, and (v) whether the patient is immunocompromised or not. Root fragments lesser than the apical third, or 5 mm, with a vital pulp in a healthy patient can be left alone; while those greater than 5 mm, with necrotic pulps and with periapical radiolucent areas should be removed; unless the risks of so doing outweighs potential gain. Both the retention of root apex and information given to the patient should be recorded.

Contd...

S. No.	Complications	Causes	Prevention	Management
2.	Displacement of teeth/roots			
a.	Displacement of teeth/roots in soft-tissues			
	i. Displacement under the mucoperiosteal flap	i. Thin cortical plate, ii. Uncontrolled force, and iii. Fenestration in cortical plates	Use controlled force, and support the alveolus during extraction.	Exploration and removal Sometimes radiographs may be required. i. Attempt should be made for its retrieval; Manipulation or pushing the root piece back into its socket should be tried
	ii. Displacement in the lingual pouch, and	i. Thin lingual cortical plate in region of mandibular third molar	Support of one finger over lingual cortical plate, in order to prevent tooth being pushed into submandibular fossa.	ii. Suitable medications should be prescribed (antibiotics, analgesics) iii. If unsuccessful, or beyond the capabilities of the operator, refer to oral and maxillofacial surgeon.
	iii. Displacement through the lingual cortex of bone in submandibular space	ii. Fenestrations of bone; where roots are in direct communication with submandibular space (In case of fenestration, it is unpreventable) iii. Breaking of lingual cortex due to fusion with the tooth/root.		
	iv. Teeth/roots displaced in pterygopalatine fossa	i. Highly placed, unerupted maxillary third molars with conical fused roots ii. Inadequate access, and iii. Careless technique. Predisposition:	i. Preoperative assessment (suitable radiographs) ii. Careful surgical technique iii. Sometimes unpredictable.	i. Take appropriate radiographs ii. Referral to oral and maxillofacial surgeon.
	v. Teeth/roots displaced into maxillary sinus	i. Maxillary posterior teeth are in close proximity with floor of maxillary sinus Teeth commonly involved second premolars, and molars, especially teeth having conical roots, and partially erupted maxillary third molars. *Commonly involved root:* Palatal root of maxillary first molar ii. Large antral cavity close to the apices of posterior teeth iii. *With advancing age, there is increase in pneumatization:* The teeth appear to be protruding into the antral cavity in a radiograph. In three dimensions, the bone of the antral floor may be very thin; and at times the root apices may contact with antral lining iv. Solitary molar tooth in atrophic maxillary alveolus v. Molar roots with large splayed roots close to antral floor.	i. Preoperative assessment (proximity of roots of molars with floor of maxillary sinus, especially third molar) ii. Use of controlled force iii. Support the alveolus iv. Leave the apical third of maxillary molar palatal roots; unless there is an indication for their removal *NB:* Patient should be informed of such a possibility before extraction.	*Confirmation:* 1. Inspection of extraction socket 2. *Nose-blowing test:* Patient is instructed to gently blow through the nose, against closed nostrils. There is passage of air through the socket, due to increase in the intra-antral pressure. The expelled air produces bubbling with blood in the socket; or if socket is empty, a fine wisp of cotton wool is held near the extraction socket. It will be deflected by the stream of air. It is essential to use gentle pressure to identify oro-antral communication (OAC). Overenthusiastic blowing may actually produce a breach in continuity of antral floor 3. Instruments, such as, suction tips and probes through the socket into the antrum in an attempt to confirm the defect. This maneuver could create a communication, if not

Contd...

S. No.	Complications	Causes	Prevention	Management
				existed. Treatment is delayed for (a) further radiographic evaluation and confirmation. The ideal way to manage oro-antral communication (OAC), is to close immediately before the passage of saliva through the defect which may cause sinusitis (b) Defect less than 2 mm: Blood clot gets organized. (c) Defect greater than 2 mm: Hemostatic agents are inserted in the socket and the socket is sutured.(d) If failure; then surgical closure is undertaken: (i) Raise the three-sided buccal mucoperiosteal flap, and advance it over the socket. (ii) Release the periosteum at the base of flap well beyond the reflection of sulcus. (iii) Achieve complete closure. (iv) Closure assisted by reducing the height of socket wall. (v) Refer to oral and maxillofacial surgeon for sinus exploration and retrieval of the roots. (vi) Information and assurance to the patient. (vii) Details notified in the record. (viii) *Sinus regimen:* Avoid blowing nose for 10-14 days. Broad spectrum antibiotics taken for seven days. Regular use of nasal drops and decongestants. (ix) If immediate closure of oro-antral communication (OAC) is not possible, the patient should be referred to oral and maxillofacial surgeon.
b.	Aspiration of teeth/roots in tracheobronchial tree	Careless technique	Careful technique	Refer to chest surgeon (Bronchoscopy and exploration)
c.	Swallowing of teeth/roots in gastrointestinal tract	i. Careless technique ii. Uncooperative patient iii. Mentally challenged patients	Careful technique	Refer to gastroenterologist (gastroendoscopy).

Contd...

S. No.	Complications	Causes	Prevention	Management
B.	**Injuries to adjacent teeth**			
1.	Subluxation/luxation/ fracture	i. *Improper surgical technique:* Placement of elevator, and use of inappropriate forceps, uncontrolled force, and application of force directly over the adjacent tooth, ii. Injudicious use of mouth props, laryngoscopes, oro-endotracheal tubes, airways, especially during extraction under GA.	i. Proper surgical technique (Proper placement of elevators, and use of proper forceps) ii. Use of controlled force iii. Force to be applied on the tooth to be extracted unless the adjacent tooth is also to be extracted.	a. *Subluxation:* Tooth is stabilized with wire or acrylic splint b. *Luxation:* i. Reimplanted immediately and stabilized with splints ii. Endodontic therapy—planned *NB:* During the period of stabilization, the tooth is kept free of occlusion.
2.	Fracture of cusps, incisal edges, restorations, and artificial crowns, etc.	i. Large carious lesions ii. Poorly condensed amalgam restoration iii. Poor retention of restoration iv. Application of excessive force.	i. Preoperative assessment (clinical and radiological) ii. Avoid placing instruments against fillings, (avoid putting heavy leverage against fillings) iii. Use—Proper instruments *NB:* Necessary to warn patient in advance.	i. Application of temporary filling after procedure ii. Plan – permanent restoration subsequently. *NB:* Care taken not to allow filling material to fall in the socket (foreign body reaction).
3.	Extraction of a wrong tooth	i. Carelessness ii. Improper communication (Referred patients, particularly by orthodontists).	i. Careful extraction ii. Referred cases; check the charts iii. In doubt, communicate and confirm with referring specialist iv. Mark the tooth with indelible pencil.	i. Replace tooth as soon as possible; and stabilize with wire or splint/arch bar Plan for endodontic treatment ii. Inform orthodontist (referring specialist) iii. (Revise—Treatment plan and accommodate the mistake) iv. Inform the patient.
C.	**Fractures**			
a.	Fracture of maxillary alveolus	i. Improper placement of instruments ii. Uncontrolled force (excessive force can lead to fracture of tooth or root) iii. Inadequate support to alveolus iv. Fusion of alveolar bone with the tooth, (common in maxillary second and third molar regions) v. Thinness of alveolar cortical bone.	i. Preoperative assessment (Maxillary sinus and tuberosity) ii. Use of controlled force iii. Adequate support to alveolus during extraction iv. Remove tooth surgically (Removal of buccal bone/sectioning of teeth).	a. Bone completely detached from periosteum: i. Completely detached bone cannot be replaced. Often it remains attached to the tooth and is removed with it. ii. Reposition the flap and obtain complete closure. If the fragment cannot be removed from the tooth, the mucoperiosteum should be carefully separated from the bone using an instrument such as a periosteal elevator, or Mitchell's trimmer; to avoid tearing of the gingiva/mucoperiosteum. Sometimes, the bone fragments can be detached from the tooth with a fine fissure bur or a Coupland's chisel. This is done when the bone has mucoperiosteum attached to it. Such bone can be retained.

Contd...

S. No.	Complications	Causes	Prevention	Management
	b. Fracture of maxillary tuberosity: It is a type of alveolar fracture	a. *Predisposition:* Common sites: (i) Isolated, overerupted maxillary 2nd and 3rd molars, (ii) Presence of a large antrum weakens the maxillary alveolus. b. Application of excessive/uncontrolled force c. Large splayed root mass of maxillary second and third molars d. Fusion of unerupted maxillary third molar to roots of second molar.	i. Preoperative assessment (radiographs): maxillary sinus and tuberosity) Good surgical technique ii. Support alveolar bone during extraction, use of controlled force. iii. Perform extraction surgically (remove locking buccal bone, sectioning of teeth).	b. Bone attached to soft-tissues (periosteum) i. Bone retained iii. Achieve complete closure a. *Small fragment:* Examine the fractured portion of tuberosity adherent to the tooth. Separate the periosteum from the bone, and the bone is removed along with the tooth. Section and remove the tooth leaving bone segment attached to periosteum b. *Large fragment:* (i) Stop/abandon the extraction. Equilibrate the tooth. (ii) If partially extracted: (1) Remove the tooth surgically; and leave the bone fragment attached to the periosteum; or (2) Section the crown; leave roots *in situ.* Roots can be removed later, when tuberosity is more stable (approximately 6–8 weeks) (3) Splint the tooth; if necessary (4) If sinus is involved, (Large segment involving bone forming floor of the antrum. It may result into oro-antral communication) (5) Antibiotics and analgesics (6) *Sinus regimen:* nasal drops and decongestants (7) Refer to oral and maxillofacial surgeon.
	c. Fracture of mandible	a. Predisposition: (i) Common situation: vertically impacted mandibular third molar, (ii) atrophic mandible b. *Poor surgical technique:* Carelessness, and excessive force with elevators c. Other situations are examples of pathological fractures: (i) Large cysts, (ii) Tumors, (iii) Generalized osteoporosis, (iv) Paget's disease, (v) Osteogenesis imperfecta, (vi) Hyperparathyroidism, (vii) Osteomyelitis, previous therapeutic irradiation (Osteodystrophies: osteitis deformans, fibrous dysplasia, fragilitas ossium).	*Prevention:* (i) Preoperative assessment: Surgery should be carried out only after proper preoperative assessment. Good history, clinical and radiological examination, construction of splints preoperatively; and planning to do such cases in a proper environment. ii. Careful elevation ii. Use of controlled force iii. *NB:* Difference between simple extraction and extraction of mandibular third molar.	If fracture occurs during the course of extraction; the procedure should be stopped, appropriate radiographs are taken. Explanation should be given to the patient's and relatives. Prescribe antibiotics and analgesics. Liquid diet i. Fracture: Reduction and fixation ii. Patient should be warned about the possibility of fracture, before the operation iii. Refer to oral and maxillofacial surgeon.

Contd...

S. No.	Complications	Causes	Prevention	Management
D.	**Other complications**			
1.	Breakage of instruments (Elevator tips, burs/drills)	i. *Excessive force:* Straight elevators, inadequate torque ii. Fault in manufacturing iii. Old overused instruments	i. Use controlled force ii. Use good quality instruments.	i. Debridement ii. Attempt to remove the broken piece iii. Radiographs iv. If failure, refer to oral and maxillofacial surgeon.
2. a.	TM joint injury Trauma to the capsule	Stretching of capsule of TM joint Forceps applied during extraction are transmitted during extraction to TM joint Postoperative pain and limitation of movement.	Adequate stability to TM joint during extraction i. Adequate manual support of lower jaw during extraction ii. Support alveolus iii. *Difficult extraction:* Resort to surgical extraction.	Conservative management: Rest to the joint. (Soft diet, hot water fomentation external over joint, analgesics, and restriction of mouth opening).
b.	Dislocation of condyles	i. Application of excessive force ii. Failure to support the mandible; with extracting a difficult tooth. Mandible should be adequately supported. The dental forces applied to the teeth cause larger displacing forces than the left hand can provide as a support iii. More likely to occur under GA when masticatory muscles are relaxed, particularly, injudicious the lower border of	i. History of previous dislocation ii. Use of controlled force iii. Support the jaw Additional support can be obtained by asking the patient to bite on the mouth props. These transfer part of the dis-placing forces to maxillary teeth.	Correction to be done immediately a. Standing in front of the patient b. Standing behind the patient i. Reduction is done, with the thumbs wrapped with gauze or a bandage, to avoid injury by teeth, and placed on the occlusal surfaces of mandibular posterior teeth, and fingers under use of mouth gags, to force open the jaws to force open the jaws. Mandible is then pushed down-wards, backwards, rotating the chin upwards. With this maneuver, the condyles are moved down-wards and backwards over the articular eminences of temporal bone. Subsequently, upwards to regain its position in the glenoid fossa. ii. Patient should be warned not to open his mouth too widely or to yawn for a few days postoperatively. Patient is instructed to support the jaw during yawning. iii. Extraoral bandage support for the joint is applied, and worn until tenderness in the affected joint subsides. iv. Failure to reduce dislocation—reduction can be attempted under 5–10 mg of IV/IM valium

Contd...

S. No.	Complications	Causes	Prevention	Management
				v. Failure to reduce the dislocation; or if there is resistance encountered, LA solution is injected high in the buccal sulcus, bilaterally adjacent to maxillary third molar region, similar to the technique of posterior superior alveolar nerve block. This helps in paralysing lateral pterygoid muscles and overcoming muscular spasm. Under GA it is easy to reduce dislocation. It is valuable to check the occlusion, at the end of any extraction or surgical procedure.
3.	Involvement of maxillary sinus: Oro-antral fistula (OAF)	*Predisposition:* Maxillary sinus closely related to roots of the teeth. Oroantral communication (OAC)/ oroantral fistula (OAF); frequently produced in cases of roots with close proximity to antral floor.	*Preoperative assessment:* of relationship of sinus floor to roots of teeth (radiographs).	Depends upon the size of defect a. *Small opening:* (< 2 mm) Surgical closure: Not necessary. Blood clot is organized and retained b. *Large opening:* Large (> 2 mm) Surgical closure is required. Flap is designed and the defect is closed c. *Sinus regimen:* To prevent sinusitis: Antibiotics, nasal drops and nasal decongestants (to keep nasal cavity and the ostium patent; encourage drainage from sinus) d. In case of an established oro-antral fistula (OAF), refer patient to oral and maxillofacial surgeon.
4.	*Hemorrhage:* Primary hemorrhage: a. Hemorrhage at the time of surgery Reactionary hemorrhage: b. Hemorrhage within few hours after surgery, when vasoconstriction of damaged blood vessels has ceased Secondary hemorrhage: c. Hemorrhage up to 14 days postoperatively, as a result of infection.	(A) Local and (B) General A. Local: i. Bleeding from arteriole or vessel ii. Granulation tissue iii. Crush injury B. General: (1) Natural and (2) Acquired (a) Natural: i. Hemophilia A ii. Hemophilia B (b) Acquired: 1. Anemia (Severe) 2. Hypertension (uncontrolled) 3. Vitamin K deficiency 4. Vitamin C deficiency 5. Anticoagulation therapy 6. Liver diseases 7. Idiopathic thrombocytopenia	1. *Preoperative assessment:* a. Good medical history (personal and family history of blood relatives; of bleeding tendency) b. History of previous relevant episodes; particularly following tooth extraction (with full details) c. *Appropriate investigations:* Prothrombin time (PT), Plasma thromboplastin time (PTT), Bleeding time (BT), Platelet count (PC), and International normalized ratio (INR) d. *Suspected cases:* Refer the patient to hematologist for necessary investigations e. Good surgical technique	1. Must have a good suction apparatus, and have a clear vision of operative field a. Control the hemorrhage from soft tissues: (a) Methods of controlling hemorrhage i. Mechanical pressure in the form of finger/thumb pressure ii. Electric cauterisation iii. Injection of local anesthetic containing a vasoconstrictor (adrenaline), for relief of pain as well as for vasoconstriction. iv. *Suturing;* particularly, figure-of-eight type, across the margins of the socket v. Acrylic splint; immediate denture

Contd...

S. No.	Complications	Causes	Prevention	Management
		8. Hemorrhagic disorders 9. Under GA, if oxygenation is insufficient.	i. Careful handling of tissues to avoid unnecessary trauma ii. Placing a gauze pack over the socket for at least ten minutes; with application of biting pressure; to allow blood clot to form inside the socket iii. Remove all granulation tissue iv. Avoid crushing of tissue v. Good knowledge of anatomy of surgical area vi. Instructions to patient; not to disturb clot by avoiding vigorous mouth rinsing or chewing, or putting external agents (tongue, fingers). 2. *Observation:* At the completion of procedure, observe the patient in the office for 15 minutes; then change the pack just prior to patient's departure.	vi. Clamping of bleeding vessel and ligation with 3/0 or 4/0 ligature, or coagulation with diathermy. b. Methods of controlling hemorrhage from bone: Bone bleeding is controlled in the following ways: i. Packing the socket with gauze under pressure ii. Crushing or burnishing the bone. It is done with a hemostat or any other blunt instrument. This is applicable to small areas. It crushes the bony channels iii. Application of hemostatic substances:absorbable sponges: gelatin foam (gelfoam), surgicel or fibrin foam, etc. These substances are placed in the socket in small amount. These control bleeding by providing a clotting matrix and stabilization of the clot iv. Application/smearing of bone wax into relevant spaces in bone marrow with the help of an instruments such as burnisher or Mitchell's trimmer. It is rarely used, and is effective in stopping extensive bleeding from extraction sockets, especially, if inferior alveolar artery/vein is damaged. *Drawback:* It is poorly absorbed and may contribute to postoperative infection v. A block of impression compound is moulded over the area to offer compression or special acrylic splint constructed.

Contd...

S. No.	Complications	Causes	Prevention	Management
5.	Late supine hypotensive syndrome (LSHS) of pregnancy	*Predisposition:* Usually occurs in late pregnancy; 10% as per American literature Patient complains of faints. *Mechanism:* Pressure of fetus over inferior vena cava (IVC). There is decrease in venous return (VR), hence less cardiac output (CO); hence less blood pressure (BP); and hence cerebral ischemia; that leads to feeling of faint.	i. Put the patient in upright position ii. Treatment sessions should be of short durations iii. Avoid recumbent position.	i. Turn the patient on one side ii. Treatment sessions of short durations mechanism: venous return (VR) is increased, cardiac output (CO) is restored, blood pressure (BP) is increased. Cerebral flow to brain is restored.
E.	**Postoperative complications**			
1.	Bony spicules	Improper debridement	Proper debridement—surgical procedure	i. Removal and/or filing of bone.
2.	Hemorrhage	Poor surgical technique	a. Postoperative instructions: i. Avoid violent exercises, stimulants, very hot food or drinks, for the rest of the day, ii. Avoid vigorous or repeated mouth rinsing or chewing; it disturbs the clot and promotes bleeding iii. *Observation:* At the completion of procedure, observe the patient in the office for 15 minutes; then change the pack just prior to patient's departure.	i. Examination of the mouth: in order to determine the site and amount of hemorrhage ii. Clean the area off the blood clots iii. Application of a gauze pack over the site of hemorrhage. Patient is asked to hold it under biting pressure. Application of tannic acid on the portion of the pack relation to the site of hemorrhage. It helps to arrest hemorrhage iv. In case of tear in gingiva, it is advisable to apply suture under LA. When hemorrhage is found to be in the gingiva surrounding a tooth socket, figure-of-eight type of suturing across the socket. *Advantages:* (i) Causes tension in mucoperiosteum; which helps in arresting hemorrhage, coming from soft tissues, (ii) It protects the blood clot from disintegration, (iii) Hemorrhage from bone: as described earlier, (iv) If these measures fail, refer the patient to nearest hospital, for further management.

Contd...

S. No.	Complications	Causes	Prevention	Management
3.	Fibrinolytic alveolitis: (Dry socket, alveolar osteitis, localized osteitis alveolalgia, alveolar ostecmyelitis) It involves part or whole of the walls of socket; or the lamina dura. Geoffrey Howe, defined it as well recognized, but ill understood complication of extraction of teeth. Characteristics: The condition is characterized by acute pain, bony walls of the socket are denuded of blood clot.	Etiology: Not clear/obscure. Trauma and infection; together. They cause inflammation of marrow spaces of alveolar bone. That liberates tissue activators which convert plasminogen in blood clot to plasmin. This dissolves blood clot and releases kinins from kininogen; which is present in blood clot. The final result is of dissolution of blood clot and severe pain. Predisposing factors: i. Infection of socket occurring either before, during or after the extraction—may be an exciting factor. ii. Trauma: It is true that the condition may follow the use of excessive force during extraction. However, it is not always the case; and complications may occur after very easy extractions. iii. Vasoconstrictors: Many authorities feel that vasoconstrictors used in LA solution may predispose to dry socket, by interfering with blood supply of bone, and they point out that the condition occurs more frequently under LA than GA. Thus, vasoconstrictors cannot be the basic cause of the condition, but may well be a contributing factor. iv. Mandibular teeth show higher incidence of dry sockets than maxillary teeth. Mandible has much more dense bone and is less vascular than maxilla. However, anatomical studies	Following measures should be employed i. Scaling of the teeth; any gingival inflammation should be treated prior to extraction ii. Minimum amount of local anesthetic solution necessary for producing analgesia should be administered iii. Teeth should be removed in the least traumatic manner possible iv. Prophylatic use of antibiotics especially metronidazole from the day of extraction for 3–4 days reduces the incidence of dry socket significantly. It also has been shown to provide prompt relief from pain; if given in large doses for 5 days v. Wound debridement vi. Nerve blocks—preferred to LA infiltration.	Not a progressive disease Aim: (i) Relief of pain, and (ii) Speed of resolution (a) Procedure: i. Irrigation of debris and debridement: Socket is irrigated with warm normal saline and all degenerating blood clots are removed. Sharp bony margins should be either excised with rongeur forceps or smoothened with a bone file ii. or a drill Medicated dressing/Iodoform gauze or composed of zinc oxide eugenol on cotton wool should be packed loosely and not tightly; as it may set hard and be difficult to remove. The dressing is composed of: Eugenol, Balsam of Peru, Chlorobutanol, and Benzocaine Dressing—first 24 hours; then every alternate day; then every 3–4 days for more than 2 weeks iii. Broad-spectrum antibiotics. (b) Other measures: Analgesics, and hot Saline mouthbaths

Contd...

S. No.	Complications	Causes	Prevention	Management
		revealed that the blood supply to alveolus in lower molar region is not poorer than that of the other regions of the jaw. Lower teeth usually are more difficult to extract than upper teeth. v. *Gravity:* Mandibular sockets become contaminated with food debris. vi. Existence of systemic etiological factor. There is with a insufficient evidence to support this concept. However, increased titer of fibrinolytic substances as has been demonstrated in alveolar bone of patients afflicted with dry socket. vii. *Bacteriological origin:* A number of bacteria are known to possess fibrinolytic activity. It has been recently postulated that *Treponema denticola* may have an etiological role in the genesis of dry socket. viii. Pregnant women and those taking oral contraceptives appear to be more susceptible than others.		c. Regular follow-ups. d. If pain persists; it may require chemical cauterization of exposed bare painful bone. *Procedure:* i. Isolation and drying of dry socket ii. Application of a small quantity of carbolized resin to bear bony walls pair of tweezers iii. Zinc oxide eugenol cotton wool dressing is inserted over the caustic and left *in situ* for 3 days. The dressing relieves pain but delays healing. Alternatively, Whitehead's varnish on a piece of ribbon gauze can also be used and left *in situ* for 2–3 weeks. It is not very effective in controlling pain. At the time of removal of the pack the socket will be seen granulating.
4.	*Nerve injuries:* i. Nerve injuries without significance: Naso-palatine and buccal nerves. ii. Nerves posing problems: Inferior alveolar, mental, and lingual nerves.			The anesthesia/paresthesia lasts for periods lasting from a few days to many months, depending upon the amount of damage sustained by the involved nerves. Such patients should be seen at regular intervals until sensation returns to normal. The nature and extent of sensory loss should be carefully elicited and recorded at each visit; so that the rate of recovery is determined; and necessary supportive treatment is instituted.

Contd...

S. No.	Complications	Causes	Prevention	Management
	a. Inferior alveolar nerve	i. Close proximity of mandibular third molar roots to inferior alveolar nerve ii. *Careless surgical technique:* Movements of roots likely to cause damage; especially, when the roots are curved around the canal, or grooved by it.	a. Preoperative assessment: (radiographs). Sometimes roots of third molar are grooved, notched, or perforated by the contents of inferior alveolar neurovascular bundle. b. During procedure: Careful surgical technique: (i) while cutting the teeth, and (ii) while using a bur/currette	a. Replace the severed portions of nerve; within the canal. Allow proximal end to regenerate. Regeneration usually takes 2–6 months and sometimes years. b. Decompression is required; if there is nerve impingement or entrapment. c. Microvascular surgery is required for anastomosis and grafting. d. Referral to oral and maxillofacial surgeon. e. Patient should be warned of such consequences.
	b. Lingual nerve	*Predisposition:* Lingual nerve is in close proximity to roots of mandibular third molar i. Risk of damage while taking incision, and during elevation of lingual periosteum ii. While manipulation of lingual mucoperiosteal flap iii. Risk of direct trauma from burs or chisels used for removal of bone, or sectioning of the tooth iv. Injury during injection is rare.	i. Good knowledge of anatomy ii. *Careful surgical technique:* (proper placement of incision, careful bone removal, retraction and less manipulation of lingual flap).	i. Refer to oral and maxillofacial surgeon ii. Patient should be warned preoperatively about the possible consequences and the probable outcome.
	c. Mental nerve	Surgery in the area of mental nerve i. Overextension of relieving incision in the depth of mucobuccal fold, in premolar region ii. Removal of bone encroaching on mental foramen just below and between premolar root apices iii. Careless retraction of the flap in the vicinity of mental foramen iv. Incision and drainage of abscesses situated in the region of premolars.	a. Good knowledge of anatomy b. Good surgical technique: (i) Proper planning of incision, and (ii) Careful reflection of mucoperiosteal flap, (iii) Incision and drainage of abscesses be done by Hilton's method, in order to minimize risk of damaging mental nerve, and (iv) Protection of mental nerve with a retractor.	i. Assurance to the patient ii. Refer to oral and maxillofacial surgeon.
5.	*Injury to TM joint:* Postoperative traumatic arthritis	(i) Difficult extractions, (ii) Prolonged surgical procedures on unsupported mandible.	(i) Difficult extractions may be done surgically, (ii) Support mandible during surgical procedures.	a. Rest to joint b. Analgesics and anti-inflammatory agents.

Contd...

S. No.	Complications	Causes	Prevention	Management
6.	Acute osteomyelitis (OML)	*Predisposing factors:* Traumatic extraction of lower molars under LA, in the presence of acute gingivitis, periodontitis, or pericoronitis.	*Precautions:* The following measures to be undertaken prior to undertaking any surgical intervention: (i) To do prophylactic scaling of teeth, whenever indicated. (ii) To treat acute conditions first, and control the infections	For details of management, refer to the chapter on "Osteomyelitis".
7.	Infection/suppuration at the site	Lack of aseptic technique: inadequate preparation of the site, inadequate sterilization of instruments, etc.	i. Use of aseptic technique, and ii. Use of atraumatic technique.	i. Use of antibiotics, and ii. May be incision and drainage.
8.	Failure to complete the operation	a. Inadequacy of anesthesia: It includes: (i) faulty technique, and (ii) insufficient dosage of LA agent b. Lack of cooperation from the patient c. Lack of facilities d. Lack of skills.	i. Careful preoperative assessment, and ii. Careful treatment planning.	i. Plan to do the procedure in a place with proper facilities, and with proper anesthesia ii. Dental surgeon should be calm, courteous, and confident iii. *Nervous patients:* Use premedication.

Appendix 2: Complications following the use of local anesthetic solution in dentistry

S. No	Complications	Causes	Prevention	Management
A.	**Complications arising from drugs or chemicals used**			
1.	Soft-tissue injury	Self-inflicted trauma (lips and cheeks) Common in children, and mentally and physically challenged adults.	Warn the patient's parents or guardians against biting lips or tongue	*Symptomatic:* Comprises of analgesics, antibiotics and topical anesthetic gel for relief of pain Depends upon injury
2.	Sloughing of tissues (tissue ischemia and necrosis) i. Epithelial desquamation. ii. Sterile abscess iii. Necrosis	i. *Predisposition:* Commonly seen in hard palate, as in the region of nasopalatine, and greater palatine nerves, because the mucoperiosteum is tightly attached to the bone. It occurs at the site of injection. Necrosis leads to painful ulceration. ii. Related to volume of solution injected iii. Application of topical LA agent for prolonged period iv. Use of vasoconstrictors (usually epinephrine), resulting in tissue ischemia and necrosis (Guinta 1975).	i. Use LA agent with short duration action. ii. Use less amount of LA agent (minimal effective dose) iii. Warn the patient against application of hot items.	*Symptomatic:* Consists of analgesics, topical anesthetics, and bland diet, etc. Usually resolves within 1–2 weeks. An established abscess may require incision and drainage.
B.	**Complications arising from injection techniques**			
1.	Needle stick injuries	Careless technique	Careful of sharp instruments Prophylactic vaccination of HBV infection to be taken and maintained Inform the patient of the technique and the procedure	If injury involves a patient with AIDS, then i. The concerned authority should be informed ii. Postexposure prophylaxis PEP to be considered
2.	Needle breakage	1°: Sudden unexpected movements by patient 2°: (i) Size of needle. Breakage is common in thin (smaller diameter or of larger gauge) needles. (ii)Previously bent needles. (iii) Redirection of needles inside the tissues. (iv) Defect in manufacturing. Nicking of blood vessels during injection of LA agent	Use of proper gauge of needle (for nerve blocks; 25 gauge needles). Insertion of needle, few mm away from the hub Do not redirect the needle once completely in the tissues. Always use needles of good quality	Remain calm. Do not panic If the needle is visible, and is outside the soft-tissue, catch it with a hemostat and remove it If not visible, refer the patient to oral and maxillofacial surgeon.
3.	Hematoma		Good knowledge of anatomy. Use short needle for posterior superior alveolar nerve block. Minimize the number of needle penetrations.	a. Immediate; If the area is accessible, application of pressure for 2–3 minutes. Observe the patient at least 12 hours b. Delayed: (i) Assurance to the patient (ii) External ice application (iii) Symptomatic treatment: consisting of analgesic; muscle relaxant, and (iv) Antibiotic cover symptomatic; and consists of

Contd...

S. No.	Complications	Causes	Prevention	Management
4.	Infection	i. Contamination of needles ii. Improper preparation of site iii. Needle passing through an area of infection iv. LA solution deposited under pressure; as in intraligamental injection (deposit bacteria).	i. Preparation of site prior to penetration ii. Careful handling of needles (avoid touching nonsterile surface). iii. Avoid multiple injections with same needle iv. Use disposable needles v. Proper handling of dental cartridges (a) Store cartridges with a cover or a container (b) Clean the diaphragm with antiseptic prior to its use (c) Use cartridge only once.	i. Analagesics ii. Antibiotics iii. Physiotherapy iv. Muscle relaxants v. Incision and drainage, if necessary.

5.	Failure to obtain local analgesia	a. Faulty technique:
		  i. Deposition of LA agent far away from nerve
		  ii. Accidental intravascular administration
		b. Anatomical aberrations
		  i. Abnormal innervation
		  ii. Additional innervation
		c. Abnormal reaction to effect of LA agent
		d. Injecting in an infected area.
			i. Good knowledge of anatomy
			ii. Good surgical technique
				Not required
				i. Repeat the injections
				ii. Consider anesthetising additional nerve supply
				iii. In the presence of infection select higher block techniques.

6.	Postinjection herpetic lesions	Reactivation of dormant herpes virus particles by trauma of injection. Usually, seen in patients with history of recurrent herpes labialis, particularly, in the terminal distribution of trigeminal nerve (Inferior alveolar nerve, superior labial branch of infraorbital nerve) in a previously anesthetized nerve.	i. Preanesthetic assessment: history of recurrent herpes infections ii. Delay surgical intervention in the active stage.	Symptomatic
C. Complication arising from both				
1.	Pain on injection	i. Careless injection ii. Blunt needles iii. Rapid deposition of LA solution iv. Needles with barbs (pain while withdrawal) v. High temperature of LA solution.	i. Use sharp needles ii. Proper technique iii. Use sterile LA solution iv. Use topical LA agen prior to injection v. Inject LA solution slowly vi. Temperature of the solution should be approximately the same as room temperature, i.e. avoid using refrigerated cartridges.	Not required

Contd...

S. No.	Complications	Causes	Prevention	Management
2.	Burning on injection	i. Rapidity of injection ii. Contamination of LA cartridge (alcohol, or cold–sterilizing solutions iii. High temperature of LA solution iv. Altered pH of solution.	i. Slow injection ii. Cartridges to be stored at room temperature.	Not required
3.	Trismus	i. Trauma to muscles, and blood vessels in infratemporal and pterygomandibular fossae ii. Solution containing alcohol or cold sterilizing solutions (contamination due to storage) iii. LA agents are mild myotoxic iv. Hemorrhage leads to irritation of muscles v. Low-grade infection.	i. Use sharp, sterile and disposable needles ii. Proper handling of needles iii. Avoid contamination of needles iv. Avoid multiple injections into the same area v. Use minimum effective volumes of LA agent vi. Aspiration before injection.	*Symptomatic: and consists of:* i. Physiotherapy with jaw stretcher (Heister) ii. Heat therapy iii. Warm saline rinse iv. Analgesics v. Muscle relaxants vi. Brisement force under sedation.
4.	Edema	i. Trauma during injection ii. Infection iii. Allergy (angioedema) iv. Hemorrhage v. Injection of irritating solutions such as cold-sterilizing solutions vi. Proper storage of cartridges.	i. Preoperative assessment (history) ii. Careful handling of LA armamentarium iii. Atraumatic technique.	*Find out the cause:* allergy; antihistaminic, breathing compromised; then basic life support (BLS) is instituted (Airway, breathing, and circulation; ABC). Administration of epinephrine, antihistaminics, and corticosteroids. Refer to oral and maxillofacial surgeon.
5.	Blanching of skin	i. Trauma to blood vessel by needle, ii. Intravascular administration.	Use of aspiration technique, and avoid intra-arterial administration of local anesthetic agents.	Usually, a transient phenomenon. No treatment is required.
6.	Persistent paresthesia or anesthesia	i. Injection of LA solution near a nerve with contaminated LA solution with cold sterilizing solution, ii. Trauma to nerve sheath iii. Hemorrhage in and around nerve sheath.	i. Strict adherence to injection protocol ii. Careful surgical technique iii. Proper handling of dental cartridges.	Reassurance to the patient (Tincture of time) Prescribe B_1, B_6, B_{12} vitamin tabs. Observe the patient for two months; if no improvement, refer the patient to oral and maxillofacial surgeon Most paresthesias resolve within 8 weeks.

Contd...

S. No.	Complications	Causes	Prevention	Management
7.	Facial nerve paresis/ paralysis	i. Injection of LA solution in the capsule, or the deeper lobe of parotid gland ii. Injection superficially, into muscles of facial expression.	i. Good knowledge of anatomy ii. Follow the standard protocol for LA technique.	Explanation and assurance to the patient. Unilateral loss of motor function. It is transient and lasts for few hours, depending upon agent used, and its volume injected. Inability to voluntarily close the eye. Eye-dressing is given. Contact lenses should be removed
8.	Persistent (prolonged) pain	*Poor surgical technique:* i. Subperiosteal injection of local anesthetic agent, and tearing of periosteum by tip of the needle, ii. Needle tip with barbs, iii. Ischemic necrosis (use of vasocons- trictors: excess amount, less dilution).	i. Good surgical technique; avoid subperiosteal injection, and tearing of periosteum. Infiltration anesthesia should be given paraperiosteally, and not subperiosteally ii. Avoid needles with barbs iii. Use vasoconstrictors with maximum dilution.	Symptomatic

Index

Page numbers followed by '*f*' refer to figure and '*t*' for table.